Clinical Geriatric Psychopharmacology

Fourth Edition

Clinical Geriatric Psychopharmacology

Fourth Edition

Edited by

Carl Salzman, M.D.

Professor of Psychiatry

Harvard Medical School

Massachusetts Mental Health Center

Boston, Massachusetts

LIPPINCOTT WILLIAMS & WILKINS
A **Wolters Kluwer** Company

Philadelphia • Baltimore • New York • London
Buenos Aires • Hong Kong • Sydney • Tokyo

Acquisitions Editor: Charles W. Mitchell
Developmental Editor: Michael Standen, Joyce A. Murphy
Marketing Manager: Adam Glazer
Project Editor: David Murphy
Compositor: Maryland Composition Co., Inc.
Printer and Binder: Maple Press

3rd edition 1998 Williams & Wilkins
2nd edition 1992 Williams & Wilkins
1st edition 1984 Williams & Wilkins

530 Walnut Street
Philadelphia, 19106
Pennsylvania

351 West Camden Street
Baltimore, Maryland 21201 USA

Library of Congress Cataloging-in-Publication Data

Clinical geriatric psychopharmacology / edited by Carl Salzman.—4th ed.
   p. ; cm.
   Includes bibliographical references and index.
   ISBN 0-7817-4380-X
  1. Geriatric psychopharmacology. I. Salzman, Carl.
   [DNLM: 1. Mental Disorders—Aged. 2. Mental Disorders—drug therapy—Aged. 3. Psychotropic Drugs—therapeutic use—Aged. WT 150 C64031 2004]
RC451.4.A5C523 2004
618.97'68918—dc22

                                   2004015197

10 9 8 7 6 5 4 3 2 1

Dedication

To Rachel, Joshua, Judith P.,
and to Jessie and Harry Salzman

Preface

Since the last edition of Clinical Geriatric Psychopharmacology (CGP) was published in 1998, geriatric medicine, geriatric psychiatry, neuroscience, and psychopharmacology have witnessed explosive growth of clinical and research information. It is my hope that this fourth edition will continue to serve as a guide for psychotropic drug use in the elderly as well as an archival resource for researchers and students of geriatric psychopharmacology.

What are some of the more notable scientific and clinical advances that underlie prescription of psychotropic drugs to older individuals since the last edition was published? In basic neuroscience and pharmacokinetics, there has been an ever-expanding database on age-related changes in the brain's response to psychotropic drug medication and the body's disposition of such medication. The importance of changes in pharmacokinetics as well as in neurotransmission, gene transduction, and protein formation in the central nervous system as affected by age and by medication is beginning to inform the creation of new classes of therapeutic medications and ultimately will determine how drugs will be selected for any individual elderly patient. Our improved understanding of patterns of prescribing and costs of medicine, both of which are discussed in this fourth edition, are beginning to play an increasingly important role in public policy that will provide a basis for treatment of emotional and psy-

chiatric disorders of the elderly. In the domains of schizophrenia, psychosis, and agitation, new antipsychotic drugs have become available and patterns of drug selection and prescribing have dramatically shifted away from first-generation antipsychotics to the so-called second-generation or atypical antipsychotic medications. For bipolar illness, clinicians now have a broader range of mood-stabilizing medications that can be prescribed to the elderly as well as a growing database on the use of auxiliary medications such as antipsychotics and ion channel blockers. The field of late-life depression has probably seen the largest growth in scientific and clinically relevant information. Predictors and correlates of treatment response, genetic determinants of response and side effects, imaging studies of the depressed elderly brain are but a few of the new neuroscience that is covered in this fourth edition. New antidepressants as well as new techniques for augmenting partial or incomplete response to these drugs have also become available. There is more information on the appropriate use of ECT, treatment of psychotic depression, and the neuroscience underlying all antidepressant treatment.

The neurobiological mechanisms that may cause late-life anxiety and disturbed sleep are slowly coming into focus. There has also been expansion in neuroscience and clinical prescribing information for anxiety and sleep disorders as well, although not to the extent of depression research. Anxiety is now treated with a broader spectrum of psychotropic drugs, as are the anxiety-spectrum disorders and sleep disorders.

In addition to depression, the field of dementia continues to experience tremendous growth from new discoveries regarding the genetic basis as well as the pathophysiology of Alzheimer's disease. New medications are also available for the treatment of dementia which slow the progress of the disorder.

The fourth edition of Clinical Geriatric Psychopharmacology, like the previous three, is multiauthored. Some authors have contributed to previous editions, some are new. All are leaders in their geriatric clinical or research subspecialty. In most cases, these authors have gathered and published the data upon which their clinical and pharmacological discussions are based. Returning authors have updated their prior chapters; others have written entirely new chapters.

CGP IV continues to provide a trio of appendices. The first updates the list of psychotropic drugs and their dosages for the elderly in CGP III, augmenting this information with brief clinical descriptions of the drugs effects. The second appendix highlights the interaction between psychotropic drugs and their metabolizing enzymes. Clinical research during the past five years indicates that most drug interactions occur because of the influence of one drug upon the metabolism of another. Because the elderly commonly receive multiple medications, the likelihood of these enzyme-based interactions increases as does their clinical salience. The third appendix expands on the drug interaction tables in CGP III, presenting clinical effects of interactions of seven classes of psychotropic medications, with severity ratings and references.

Producing a multiauthored volume

that preserves a coherent style from chapter to chapter, retains each author's perspective, and meets the goal of archival review and reader accessibility is a complex task, and editorial decisions are often difficult. As in previous editions, text citations have been limited for readability and edited to provide narrative consistency throughout the book.

As with the preparation of the third edition of this volume, I was assisted by the invaluable editorial companionship of Joyce Chayes Nevis. She was able to read chapters and help me edit them not only for prose style and grammar but for content and relevance. As with CGP III, the actual preparation of the chapters was again managed capably by the skills and good humor of Valerie Charles. I would also like to thank Jessica Hudson for her exceptional help with tables and bibliographies. I thank all three for their patience as well as their enormous skill and effort in helping to prepare this Fourth Edition of Clinical Geriatric Psychopharmacology.

A sad note. One of the authors, Dr. J. Chris Gillin died of a long illness during the preparation of this edition. Chris was an extraordinary scientist, scholar, and psychiatrist, as well as a wonderful husband and father. Despite his illness, he updated his chapter from the Third Edition of Clinical Geriatric Psychopharmacology. This newly revised chapter will stand as a memorial to him and a reminder to his family, colleagues, friends, and patients of his brilliance, warmth and his generosity.

Lastly, I would like to thank the authors. Each is a leader in the field; preparation of any textbook chapter is often a burden to a busy researcher and clinician. I trust that this fourth edition of Clinical Geriatric Psychopharmacology will reward their efforts, their time, and their expertise.

Contributing Authors

Darrell R. Abernethy, M.D., Ph.D.
Clinical Director
National Institute on Aging/NIH
    Gerontology Research Center
Baltimore, Maryland

George S. Alexopoulos, M.D.
Professor of Psychiatry
Cornell University Medical College
Director, Weill-Cornell Institute of
    Geriatric Psychiatry
White Plains, New York

Sonia Ancoli-Israel, Ph.D.
Professor of Psychiatry
University of California, San Diego
Director, Sleep Disorder Clinic
Veterans Administration San Diego
    Health System
San Diego, California

Jerry Avorn, M.D.
Associate Professor of Medicine
Harvard Medical School
Chief, Division of
    Pharmacoepidemiology and
    Pharmacoeconomics
Department of Medicine
Brigham and Women's Hospital
Boston, Massachusetts

Anjan Chatterjee, M.D.
The Gertrude H. Sergievsky Center
Department of Neurology
College of Physicians and Surgeons of
    Columbia University
New York, New York

Catherine J. Datto, M.D.
Instructor, Department of Psychiatry
University of Pennsylvania
Philadelphia VA Medical Center
Philadelphia, Pennsylvania

J. Christian Gillin, M.D.
Professor of Psychiatry
Codirector, Sleep and Chronobiology
    Laboratory
University of California, San Diego
San Diego, California

Gary L. Gottlieb, M.D., M.B.A.
Professor of Psychiatry
Harvard Medical School
President, Brigham and Women's
    Hospital
Chairman, Partners Psychiatry and
    Mental Health System
Boston, Massachusetts

David J. Greenblatt, M.D.
Professor and Chair
Department of Pharmacology and
    Experimental Therapeutics
Professor of Medicine, Psychiatry, and
    Anesthesia
Tufts University School of Medicine
Boston, Massachusetts

Dilip V. Jeste, M.D.
Professor of Psychiatry and
    Neurosciences
University of California, San Diego
San Diego, California

Ira R. Katz, M.D., Ph.D.
Professor of Psychiatry
University of Pennsylvania
Director, Section on Geriatric Psychiatry
Director, Mental Illness Research
  Education and Clinical Center
Veterans Administration Medical Center
Philadelphia, Pennsylvania

Helen H. Kyomen, M.D., MS
Clinical Instructor
Department of Psychiatry and Division
  on Aging
Harvard Medical School
Boston, Massachusetts
Assistant Psychiatrist
McLean Hospital
Belmont, Massachusetts

Barry D. Lebowitz, Ph.D.
Chief, Geriatric Treatment and
  Preventive Interventions Research
  Branch
National Institute of Mental Health
Rockville, Maryland

Darin M. Lerner, M.D.
Staff Psychiatrist
Granite House
Westminster, Maryland

Benjamin Liptzin, M.D.
Chair, Department of Psychiatry
Baystate Health System
Springfield, Massachusetts
Professor and Deputy Chair,
  Department of Psychiatry
Tufts University School of Medicine
Boston, Massachusetts

Thomas C. Neylan, M.D.
Medical Director
Posttraumatic Stress Disorders Program
San Francisco Veterans Affairs Medical
  Center
University of California, San Francisco
San Francisco, California

Peter D. Nowell, M.D.
Assistant Professor
Dartmouth Hitchcock Medical Center
The Cheshire Medical Center
Lebanon, New Hampshire

Jason T. Olin, Ph.D.
Associate Director, Clinical
  Development and Medical Affairs
Forest Research Institute
Jersey City, New Jersey

David W. Oslin, M.D.
Assistant Professor, Department of
  Psychiatry
University of Pennsylvania
Philadelphia VA Medical Center
Philadelphia, Pennsylvania

Quentin R. Regestein, M.D.
Associate Professor of Psychiatry
Harvard Medical School
Director, Sleep Clinic
Brigham and Women's Hospital
Boston, Massachusetts

Charles F. Reynolds III, M.D.
Professor of Psychiatry, Neorology, and
  Neuroscience
Department of Psychiatry
University of Pittsburgh, School of
  Medicine
Pittsburgh, Pennsylvania

Steven P. Roose, M.D.
Professor of Clinical Psychiatry
Department of Psychiatry
College of Physicians and Surgeons of
  Columbia University
New York State Psychiatric Institute
New York, New York

Jeremy A. Sable, M.D.
Clinical Instructor, Department of
  Psychiatry
University of California, San Diego
San Diego, California

Harold A. Sackeim, Ph.D.
Chief, Department of Biological
  Psychiatry
New York State Psychiatric Institute
Professor, Departments of Psychiatry
  and Radiology
College of Physicians and Surgeons of
  Columbia University
New York, New York

Carl Salzman, M.D.
Professor of Psychiatry
Harvard Medical School
Director of Psychopharmacology
Massachusetts Mental Health Center
Boston, Massachusetts

Andrew Satlin, M.D.
Executive Director, Clinical
    Development and Medical Affairs
Novartis Pharmaceuticals
East Hanover, New Jersey
Research Associate in Psychiatry
Harvard Medical School
Boston, Massachusetts
Research Associate
McLean Hospital
Belmont, Massachusetts

Lon S. Schneider, M.D.
Professor of Psychiatry, Neurology, and
    Gerontology
Department of Psychiatry
University of Southern California
Los Angeles, California

Javaid I. Sheikh, M.D.
Professor of Psychiatry
Department of Psychiatry and
    Behavioral Sciences
Associate Dean for Veterans Affairs
Stanford University School of Medicine
Stanford, California
Chief of Staff, VA Palo Alto Health Care
    System
Palo Alto, California

Gary W. Small, M.D.
Professor of Psychiatry and
    Biobehavioral Sciences
Director, Center on Aging
University of California Los Angeles
Los Angeles, California

Trey Sunderland, M.D.
Chief, Geriatric Psychiatry Branch
National Institute of Mental Health
Bethesda, Maryland

Pierre N. Tariot, M.D.
Professor of Psychiatry, Medicine, Neurology,
    Aging and Developmental Biology
University of Rochester School of
    Medicine
Director of Psychiatry, Monroe
    Community Hospital
Rochester, New York

Lisa L. von Moltke, M.D.
Research Assistant Professor
Department of Pharmacology and
    Experimental Therapeutics
Tufts University School of Medicine
Boston, Massachusetts

Philip S. Wang, M.D., Dr.P.H.
Assistant Professor of Medicine
Harvard Medical School
Director, Mental Health Research
Division of Pharmacoepidemiology and
    Pharmacoeconomics
Department of Medicine
Brigham and Women's Hospital
Boston, Massachusetts

Daniel Weintraub, M.D.
Assistant Professor, Department of
    Psychiatry
University of Pennsylvania
Philadelphia VA Medical Center
Philadelphia, Pennsylvania

Michelle Wiersgalla, M.D.
Staff Psychiatrist
Hennepin Faculty Associates
Hennepin County Medical Center
Minneapolis, Minnesota

Robert C. Young, M.D.
Professor, Department of Psychiatry
Weill Medical College of Cornell
    University
New York, New York

George S. Zubenko, M.D., Ph.D.
Professor, Department of Psychiatry
University of Pittsburgh School of Medicine
Adjunct Professor of Biological Sciences
Carnegie-Mellon University
Pittsburgh, Pennsylvania

Contents

Part 3: Geriatric Agitation and Behavior Disorders

Part 4: Affective Disorders

Ira R. Katz, Catherine J. Datto, Daniel Weintraub, David W. Oslin

George S. Alexopoulos, Darin M. Lerner, Carl Salzman

Part 5: Anxiety and Related Disorders (Panic, Obsessive Compulsive, Phobias)

Part 6: Sleep Disorders

Part 7: Dementia and Memory Disorders

Part I: Overview

Chapter 1

Older Americans and Mental Illness

Barry D. Lebowitz

Jason T. Olin

The global population is growing older, gaining nearly 30 years of life expectancy in this century. In the United States, the number of persons aged 65 and above has grown by a factor of 11—from 3 million (about 4% of the population) in 1900 to over 35 million (12.4% of the population) in 2000. In 2000, for example, over 2 million Americans are estimated to have reached their 65th birthdays. In that same year, 1.8 million Americans over the age of 65 died, yielding a net increase of 238,000 older persons in that year alone. This growth will continue increasing at a slow but steady pace but will accelerate as the "baby boomers" of the post–World-War-II birth cohort reach late life. By 2030, about one American in five will be age 65 or older.[1]

The older population itself is growing older. Between 2002 and 2050, the population aged 65 and above will double in the United States, whereas, in that same period, the population aged 85 and above (also referred to as the "old-old") will increase by a factor of four: By 2030, there will be 70 million older Americans.[2] The group 85 and older remains the fastest-growing cohort in the U.S. population.

This population growth itself has been enough to create serious pressure on available healthcare and social service resources. Mental health professionals in general and geriatric psychiatrists in particular have responded to this increase in population by actively stimulating and leading the development of specialized clinical settings, research centers, and training and professional certification programs.[3,4]

Characteristics of U.S. Elderly

Developing approaches to the understanding and treatment of mental disorders in late life requires attention to three characteristics of the population of older persons: (1) population heterogeneity (gender, race, age); (2) chronic illness and comorbidity (existence of concurrent mental and medical illness); and (3) senescence (the effects of normal processes of development and change).

Population Heterogeneity

The multiplicity within even one set of demographic characteristics among U.S. elderly is extremely broad, and the interaction of these characteristics has important physical and mental health implications.

Gender

The gender effect in aging is perhaps the most pervasive of all sources of heterogeneity. Women live longer than men, about 7 years on average, and outnumber men 7 to 5 in the population aged 65 and above. For those 85 and older, women outnumber men 9 to 4. Older women are at greater risk than men of living alone, of being poor, and of having a broad array of functional disabilities that lead to increased risk of long-term hospitalization and institutionalization.[5] Nearly half of all older women are widowed (45%), and 40% of older women live alone. Most older men live with a spouse; widowed men tend to remarry. Older women are about twice as likely to be living in poverty as older men (12.2% versus 7.5%).[1]

Studies of the biology of gender differences have led to some provocative suggestions about the role of hormones in aging. For example, until quite recently estrogen replacement therapy (ERT) given to older women was believed to reduce rates of coronary artery disease, hip fracture, and stroke[6]; more recent data, however, show that the risks of ERT use are possibly greater than previously thought.[7] Studies of ERT for Alzheimer's disease (AD) indicate a decreased risk,[8,9] but this theory does not appear beneficial for symptomatic relief.[10] Estrogen changes in the perimenopausal period may be related to increased depressive symptomatology,[11,12] although data are inconclusive[13,14]: some ERT preparations may increase depressive symptomatology or have mood-altering side effects[15–17] whereas others do not.[18]

Racial and Ethnic Differences

Race or ethnicity is another important source of heterogeneity in the older population. In 2000, the population of older persons was 84% white. Rapid growth suggests that minority populations are projected to represent 25.4% of older Americans in 2030—up from 16.4% in 2000. Between 1999 and 2030, the white population 65 and older is projected to increase by 81% compared with 219% for older minorities, including Hispanics (328%), African Americans (131%), Native American, Eskimos, Aleuts (147%), and Asians and Pacific Islanders (285%).[1,2] Poverty varies among different subgroups of the population and is particularly acute in the African American population, in which 22% over 65 live in poverty. The highest poverty rates (38.3%) are experienced by older Hispanic women, who live alone or with nonrelatives.[1,2]

Race and ethnicity are of particular interest in the field of psychopharmacology, in which dosing strategies and side-effect profiles based on ethnic differences have been widely reported.[19–21] Pharmacogenetic studies have also identified significant differences among racial and ethnic groups regarding metabolism of some psychotropic drugs. These differences, however, are not specific to the elderly.[22]

Chronic Illness and Comorbidity

Chronic disease as well as concomitant mental and physical illness prevails in the population over age 65. In 1998, among those 65 to 74 years old, 28.8% reported a limitation caused by a chronic condition. In contrast, over half (50.6%) of those 75 years and over reported being limited by chronic conditions.[1] Among elderly patients, arthritis, high blood pressure, and heart disease are the most prevalent chronic illnesses. Dementia of the Alzheimer's type (AD) now afflicts approximately 4 million U.S. elderly, and this number is projected to rise to 14 million by the year 2050.[23] Dementia is the most common reason for admission to a long-term care institution, accounting for 50% of admitting diagnoses.

Commonly observed physical conditions act in combination and include arthritis (49%), hypertension (36%), hearing impairments (30%), heart disease (27%), orthopedic impairment (18%), cataracts (17%), sinusitis (12%) and diabetes (10%).[1] The extent to which each of these common conditions coexists with mental disorder may have serious implications for treatment planning.[24] Many medical conditions can also present with psychiatric, cognitive, emotional, and behavioral components; these include hypertension, delirium, electrolyte imbalance, and thyroid disorders. Coexisting mental illness, particularly depression or cognitive impairment, alters the course, treatment response, and outcome of physical illness. Concomitant mental and physical illness in late life also intensifies disability from the physical illness, predicts mortality, and significantly increases resource use.[24,25]

Depression in response to illness or physical symptoms may seem a natural and inevitable reaction to a highly stressful situation, regardless of age. However, controlled studies of pharmacologic treatment of elderly depressed persons with stroke, arthritis, cancer, ischemic heart illness, chronic lung disease, and Parkinson's disease indicate that depression is not inevitable and can and should be treated.[26] Comorbidity of physical illness with depression may increase functional disability. This is of considerable importance, as eligibility for benefits or services is often determined by level of function and not by diagnosis. Almost three-fourths (73.6%) of those aged 80 years and older report at least one disability; over half (57.6%) of those over 80 have one or more severe disabilities, and 34.9% in this age group report needing assistance as a result of disability.[1]

Functional disability represents a truly "final pathway" for the various conditions and illnesses of older people. Reducing unnecessary disability and achieving optimum function therefore remain legitimate goals for treatment and rehabilitation. Concomitant physical illness and emotional disturbance in the geriatric patient suggest the need for multidisciplinary comprehensive assessment[27] even though many older adults receive their psychiatric treatment from primary care providers.[28]

Normal Age-Related Change

Persons over the age of 65, commonly called "old," "elderly," or "geriatric," comprise a heterogenous age sample with a 40-year age range. In general, expectable age-related changes in biological, psychological, cognitive, and behavioral functioning have significant impact in late life. These changes occur in nervous system structure and function, in body composition, in vision and hearing, and in function of the gastrointestinal, musculoskeletal, cardiorespiratory, genitourinary, and reproductive systems. Some of these changes affect mental function in important ways. For example, the efficacy of central nervous system (CNS) neurotransmitters, which decreases during normal aging, affects reaction time and certain aspects of memory performance.[29–31] Nonetheless, variability in these functions and in performance is very high across the spectrum of older-age individuals in our population.[32,33]

Just as differentiating changes associated with normal development from those caused by illness is important, recognizing that not all age-associated change is negative is similarly significant: old age also holds the potential for positive and creative growth.[34] The ability to develop new skills for adaptation ("resilience") and to learn new strategies in the face of loss ("reserve capacity" or "plasticity") are capabilities that can promote the potential for rehabilitation and maintain independence.[35] Wisdom may be one of the most significant benefits of growing old.[36]

Nevertheless, we recognize that degenerative dementias such as AD evolve during adulthood. Thus, age-related cognitive decline, also referred to as age-associated memory impairment or mild cognitive impairment, might not be so benign as previously thought.[37,38] Epidemiologic data suggest that individuals with mild cognitive impairment are at risk for added psychiatric symptomatology as well.[39] Creative problem-solving that involves abstraction and rapid information processing becomes more difficult, as does adaptation to new situations, which also takes longer. Appropriate care therefore requires careful assessment and evaluation of diverse aspects of the elderly person's lifestyle.

The use of psychotropic medications can be more complicated for persons over 85 or those residing in nursing homes,[40] but the potential for using them successfully as part of the treatment of mental disorders that occur at the very end of the life cycle continues to increase. This potential for success is linked to the clinician's knowledge in three critical areas: the broad range of mental health interventions; changes in central nervous system receptor-site sensitivity; and changes in how drugs are distributed throughout the body of the older patient—particularly the old-old—most of whom are frail and vulnerable.

Benefits of Treatment

The relief of suffering through clinical intervention for late-life mental disturbance is held to be no longer sufficient rationale for expenditure of increasingly scarce healthcare resources. A number of additional dimensions and outcomes determine the treatment decision. Many beneficial outcomes for treatment of late-life mental disorders have been identified[41]; they include:

1. Managing symptomatology and minimizing severity of illness
2. Reducing risk of relapse or recurrence
3. Optimizing functional ability
4. Improving overall health status
5. Reducing inappropriate use of health care resources
6. Preventing suicide
7. Improving quality of life

Moreover, the National Institutes of Health Consensus Panel[26,42] identifies the following consequences of *not* providing treatment:

1. Development of chronic illness
2. Increased risk of cognitive impairment
3. Worsened coexisting physical illnesses
4. Suicide
5. Poor compliance with medical treatments
6. Increased overall use of healthcare resources
7. Impaired social functioning
8. Reduced overall quality of life

In general, we have good reason for therapeutic optimism, especially in light of the impressive gains in research on the diagnosis and treatment of the mental disorders of late life. In particular, the quality and power of pharmacotherapeutics for mental disorders, documented by the report of the National Advisory Mental Health Council on treatment efficacy,[43] hold promise; a recent Cochrane Review also supports the general efficacy of antidepressants.[44]

Although progress is encouraging, obstacles to full recovery or to optimal response to psychoactive drugs treatment remain. These include poor compliance resulting from nontolerable side effects of treatment, limitations of the medical delivery system, inadequate social support, eccentric personality features, adverse psychosocial factors and life events, and a heavy burden of disabling illness. Hidden self-treatment, particularly with alcohol or over-the-counter drugs, may present additional problems with respect to treatment response as well as to the development or exacerbation of symptoms of mental disorder.

Rates of Mental Disorders

As diagnostic classification becomes more specific and epidemiologic methods more refined, estimates and projections become more certain. Existing prevalence estimates should therefore be regarded strictly as "order of magnitude"; lack of significant information in some areas (personality disorders and bipolar illness, for example) indicates that insufficient data preclude even rough approximation. And, like all population figures, subgroup differences may be concealed within an overall rate.

The primary source for prevalence rates of major disorders remains the National Institute of Mental Health Epidemiologic Catchment Area Study (ECA), a 5-site population study using criteria from the *Diagnostic and Statistical Manual of Mental Disorders,* third edition (DSM-III), carried out in the early and mid-1980s. Yet these values have been criticized for underestimating mental illness in older adults by misattributing psychiatric symptoms to cognitive impairment, normal aging, or medical comorbidities.[45] Rates of mental disorder are presented in Table 1.1.

Estimates of the incidence of mental disorder diagnoses among older persons range from 12 to 22%; rates of clinically significant symptoms that do not meet full criteria for a mental disorder diagnosis are likely to be higher. Given the heterogeneity of the older population, the complexities in clinical presentation and course, and the confounding impact of comorbidity and normal developmental change, determining the epidemiology of mental disorders in the elderly is a very complex task.

Dementia

The prevalence of AD in the United States in 1997 was 2.32 million, 68% of whom were female. Prevalence is projected to nearly quadruple in the next 50 years, by which time approximately 1 in 45 Americans will have AD. The annual number of new-incident cases is currently 360,000.[46] Risk for dementia, which consists primarily of AD, increases with age; for persons aged 65 and older, the prevalence rate ranges from 2%[47] to 12%.[48] For the cohort of persons aged 85 and older, the risk of dementia is approximately 1 in 4.[49] Although age is the most consistently cited risk factor for AD of the nonfamilial type,[50] recent reports examining the "oldest old" suggest that the risk for AD may level off at age 95.[51]

Incidence rates for AD increase with age, with ethnic minorities making up an increasing proportion of those afflicted.[52] AD rates rise from 2.8 per 1000 person-years in the age group 65–69 years to 56.1 per 1000 person-years in the age group 90 years and older; rates nearly triple from the 75th to 79th year and in the 80-to-84-year age groups, but the relative increase is much less thereafter.[53] Thus AD may be best conceptualized as an "aging"-related disorder rather than simply an "age"-related one.

Many healthy older persons subjectively complain of everyday *memory problems* that have significant impact on their lives. Longitudinal objective data indicate that memory performance declines as age progresses, and older people score significantly below normal younger subjects on standardized memory tests. These individuals are not (as yet) demented. However, the majority of those labeled with mild cognitive impairment (showing slight impairment in cognitive function, usually memory), are likely to develop AD.[54]

Prevalence of AD is somewhat greater among women,[55,56] but incidence is equal between genders.[57,58] Given nearly equal incidence, the gender difference in dementia prevalence may reflect several factors: (1) the condition progresses more slowly in women; (2) women with dementia survive longer than men with dementia; (3) men have higher mortality rates generally; and (4) those with dementia may die of other causes. The effects of dem-

Table 1.1. Prevalence of Mental Disorders, United States, Age 65+[a]

Disorder	Total	Men	Women
Cognitive impairment	4.9%	1.0%	4.7%
Depression	2.5%	1.4%	3.3%
Anxiety	5.5%	3.6%	6.8%
Schizophrenia	0.1%	0.1%	0.1%
Sleep[b]	40.0%		
Alcohol abuse	0.9%	1.8%	0.3%

Table based on ECA data.
[a] Gender percentages have been weighted to account for the greater number of living elderly women than men. (The combined percentages for men and women therefore are not equal to the total.)
[b] Not based on ECA.

ographic components, specifically gender and education as risk factors, therefore, remain controversial with regard to dementia.

AD pathogenic research has focused on genetic transmission and the accumulation of β amyloid in the brain as key mechanisms.[59] The presence of apolipoprotein E (ApoE), a plasma protein involved in the transport of cholesterol and encoded by a gene on chromosome 19, is considered a significant biological risk factor for AD, possibly due to its effect on clearance of β amyloid. ApoE4 is present in 24 to 31% of the adult population without AD, whereas 34 to 65% of individuals with AD have this allele,[60] which does not seem to speed up the course of AD.[61] Although testing for the ApoE genotype does not provide enough sensitivity or specificity for diagnostic use, this genotype may represent a biological risk factor that, in combination with other aging-related stressors, increases risk for dementia.

Somewhat more controversial is the evidence that higher intelligence may protect against AD.[62,63] Future research is required to verify this and other potential protective factors.

Behavioral symptoms have long been considered a defining feature of AD, but efforts to study and treat them have been challenging. Published estimates of the prevalence of behavior symptoms such as those evinced in AD patients with depression and psychosis vary widely by setting and definition but tend to cluster in the 25 to 50% range.[39,64,65] Longitudinal studies suggest that the risk of developing these symptoms is 50 to 80% over the course of the illness.[66,67] More recent efforts have led the Food and Drug Administration to conclude that treatment indications for specific aspects of AD, such as psychosis or depression, are more likely to be considered for therapeutic claims rather than broad definitions.[68] Most recently, diagnostic criteria for psychosis and depression have been generated.[69–71]

Delirium

Delirium is common in both demented and nondemented elderly patients during and after hospitalization and is a strong predictor of death (18 to 47% mortality) if not treated promptly and appropriately.[72] Because symptoms frequently resemble those of cognitive impairment, the problem is often one of recognizing the underlying cause. Treating the wrong cause can lead to iatrogenic problems as or more intense than the presenting problem(s).

Depression

Depressive symptomatology in late life is more heterogeneous than in adulthood[73–75] due to the intermittence or infrequency of symptom.[76] Individuals with depressive symptoms are more likely to develop depression, and depressive symptoms can persist for at least a year.[77] Recent specific diagnostic categories have addressed this limitation,[78] but they have yet to be adopted by the research community at large. Others have noted that depression can occur in late life without the presence of sadness.[79]

The ECA survey study[80] reported a one-year prevalence rate for major depression in men and women aged 65 and older at about 1%. This contrasts with findings in young and mid-adulthood in which rates of major depression are higher (between 2 and 3%); the disorder is much more common in women than in men.[81,82]

Different age and gender patterns appear if the threshold for a diagnosis of depression is lowered by including depressive symptoms or if criteria are broadened to include other affective disorders such as adjustment, dysthymic, and bipolar disorders.[83] The number of depressed symptoms increases with age[84] and is more common in women.[85]

When the definition of depression is broadened to include all affective disorders, rates of all depressions combined are found to increase with age.[86] For persons aged 75, women have a prevalence rate of about 9% and men a rate of 3.5%.

A large community sample[87] reports rates ranging from 4 to 26%, depending on the breadth of definition used. Minor depression is commonly found in medical patients, with prevalence rates in the 20% range for older medical outpatients.[77,88] Symptomatic depression that does not meet full diagnostic criteria may also be significantly disabling and is highly related to impaired daily functioning and reduced quality of life.[42,89]

Depression is underdiagnosed in primary care settings.[90] In contrast to the higher rates of depressive symptoms reported among older women, older white men have a suicide rate twice that of their adolescent counterparts and 10 times that of older women. Among the highest rates (when categorized by gender and race) are suicide deaths for white men over 85, with a rate of 59 out of 100,000 (http://www.nimh.nih.gov/research/suifact.htm). Older men who have committed suicide have unique clinical profile patterns: (1) relatively few belong to ethnic minorities and even fewer older minority women commit suicide; (2) suicide rates rise with age in later life, and men aged 85 and over are at more risk than those aged 65 to 75[2]; (3) evidence from psychological autopsy studies indicates that most elderly suicide victims experienced a major depression that was typically first onset and uncomplicated by other disorders such as substance abuse[91]; and (4) most elderly suicide victims visited a primary care physician within a month of their suicide, and their depression was neither recognized nor treated.[92-94] With increased age, the relative importance of the contribution of depression to suicide risk is magnified. The typical clinical profile of the older person who commits suicide is late onset, nonpsychotic, unipolar depression of moderate severity uncomplicated by substance abuse or personality disorder.

Depression in Parkinson's disease (PD) appears common. Epidemiologic studies suggest prevalence rates between 24 to 42%,[95] underscoring the need to determine etiology and validate treatments. Al-though psychiatric problems can result secondarily from difficulties in adjusting to PD or its treatment, evidence exists that neuropsychiatric changes are intrinsic to the disease process, particularly to depression.[95] Whatever the cause, depression leads to significant morbidity and suffering in individuals with PD.

A small body of research has indicated, not surprisingly, that individuals with PD have lower levels of serotonin than non-depressed individuals.[96] Others have hypothesized a role for dopaminergic function[97,98] and cortical changes,[99] but both have been little studied. Regarding treatment, no well-controlled trials have been conducted. Despite the common use of selective serotonin reuptake inhibitors (SSRIs), concern remains for the possibility of a "serotonin syndrome," which can occur when an SSRI is coadministered with selegiline.

Depression commonly occurs in AD, sometimes preceding the dementia diagnosis. Converging evidence from neuropathologists, epidemiologists, primary clinicians, and those conducting clinical trials support the existence of a specific depression that occurs in AD. Thus, an NIMH work group recently developed provisional diagnostic criteria for depression of Alzheimer's disease (dAD)[70,71] with two aims: to facilitate hypothesis-driven research that can lead to a better understanding of the depression that co-occurs in AD and to generate more homogeneous cohorts for treatment studies.

Depression of AD is similar to a major depressive episode, but the severity threshold of this disorder is lower than for a major depressive episode. Most individuals with AD do not develop major depressive episodes. Depression of AD requires the presence of a minimum of three symptoms for a period of two weeks, compared to five or more for a major depressive episode. In addition to the symptoms of major depressive episode, irritability and social isolation/withdrawal are included, and symptoms are not required to be present "nearly every day." Individuals must meet criteria for AD, and the symptoms should best be accounted for by dAD. Note that having dAD does not necessarily rule out the presence of other diagnoses, including psychosis of AD.

Anxiety

Ten to 20% of elderly persons suffer from significant symptoms of anxiety. In terms of age and gender effects, persons aged 65 and older have lower 1-year rates of generalized anxiety (omitting panic and depression) than the population as a whole; older women, however, have nearly twice the rate of older men.[100,101] Phobia is the highest anxiety-related illness among the elderly, with a reported 6-month prevalence of 16%; in contrast, panic disorder is very uncommon, with rates of 0.04% for males and 0.41% for females aged 65 and older.[101] One-year prevalence rates of generalized anxiety disorder (excluding panic and depression) among persons aged 65 and older by gender and ethnicity are as follows: white males, 1.0%; African American males, 0.3%; white females, 2.9%; African American females, 3.7%.[101–103]

In general, stressful life events are weakly related to onset of generalized anxiety. The onset of anxiety is more common among younger women than older women, but older men are more likely to report onset of anxiety than their younger counterparts.[100] As noted, anxiety and depression commonly coexist, and anxiety is a common feature of many medical conditions (e.g., gastrointestinal, cardiovascular, and pulmonary), as well as a side effect of many commonly used medications (e.g., steroids, pressor amines, and hormones).[100]

A number of demographic factors have also been related to overall one-year prevalence rates of generalized anxiety in all ages, including urban residence (vs. rural), lower occupational class, lower income, and divorce.[104] Whether social factors and life events specifically relevant to the elderly (e.g., widowhood, onset of illness, life events of children) are related

to onset of anxiety has not been carefully studied.

Schizophrenia

The study of schizophrenia in late life offers an opportunity to examine roles of family history and gender differences in terms of timing of disease. Schizophrenia is primarily a disorder of early onset. One-year prevalence rates of schizophrenia are highest among those aged 18 to 29 (1.2%) and 30 to 44 (1.5%). Recent research suggests existence of a less common form of schizophrenia with late-life onset. Persons aged 45 to 64 have about half the rate of the younger age groups (0.6%), with few gender differences reported.[105] Few epidemiologic studies of late-onset schizophrenia exist.[106–108] Incidence rates of 12.6 per 100,000 population per year have been reported for cases of DSM-III-R–defined schizophrenia with first onset after 44 years of age.[108]

In clinical studies, gender differences have been found in various aspects of schizophrenia, including symptom presentation, cognitive impairment, neuroleptic response, tardive dyskinesia, age of onset, and course of illness.[107] Gender differences in age of onset are significant: males predominate in early onset forms of the illness, and females predominate in late-onset forms.

The etiology and pathology of late-onset schizophrenia and very late-onset schizophrenia-like psychosis are discussed in more detail in Chapter 6. Compared with early-onset and age-matched controls, the late-onset group is more likely to be female, to have a better functional history (work, marriage), and to have a greater frequency of paranoid subtype symptoms. Comparable family history and premorbid adjustment during childhood, however, suggest that both early- and late-onset patients have a genetic and/or early environmental predisposition to the disease.[107]

Sleep Problems

The prevalence of self-reported sleep disturbance as well as objective assessments of sleep impairments increases with age: most older persons complain of some sort of sleep disturbance (109). Relative to younger age groups, older people report more frequent night awakening, early morning awakening, "fragile" sleep, and greater use of sedative-hypnotic medication.[110] Over time, however, sleep complaints do not increase in older people, even after a 15-year period.[111] Persons who sleep on average less than 7 hours per night have a mortality rate 1.5 times greater than those who sleep 8 hours per night.[112] About one of every 3 older women complains of sleep problems—about twice the rate of complaints by older men.[86,113,114]

Sleep problems can result from normal aging (e.g., disturbances in circadian sleep–wake rhythm and increased sleep fragmentation) and secondary to medical illness (especially pain-related disorders and respiratory and neurological diseases) as well as psychiatric disorders (depression, dementia, anxiety).[109] Like other coexisting medical conditions, sleep disorders can contribute to exacerbation of medical and psychiatric problems. For example, older persons with sleep disturbance are more likely to have clinically significant depressive symptoms 2 weeks after reporting multiple sleep disturbances.[115]

Alcohol Dependence and Abuse

Alcohol abuse and dependence as a comorbid condition of mental disorders in the elderly has received limited attention. This may in part reflect lack of a clear definition of alcoholism in later life[116] and the relatively low proportion of alcoholics among the elderly, compared with younger populations. The 1-year prevalence rates of alcoholism are 3.1% for elderly men and 0.46% for elderly women[117] and, depending on the sample, a range of 2 to 17% respectively.[118] The predominance of males over females reporting alcohol dependence among young adults is also true for their older counterparts, although there is evidence

that 12% of elderly women drink in excess of recommended guidelines.[119]

Relatively few studies of coexisting alcohol dependence and mental disorder are available for the elderly population. Among 128 persons aged 55 and older, a prevalence rate of 21% was reported for substance-use disorders (primarily alcohol)[120]; the most frequent mental disorders comorbid with alcohol dependence were affective disorders (59%), and about half of persons with this dual diagnosis also received a personality disorder diagnosis. Others found that 36% of older adults with major depression who had been discharged from a psychiatry inpatient service had a concurrent diagnosis of alcoholism.[121] These 3 related diagnoses of alcoholism, depression, and personality disorder in older persons pose significant challenges for prevention and treatment efforts.

Problems in the Use of Psychotropic Drugs

Treatment of late-life mental disorder is confounded by age-related changes in CNS sensitivity to psychotropic drugs (pharmacodynamics) as well as changes in the aging body's ability to metabolize and excrete these drugs (pharmacokinetics). Older persons are also particularly vulnerable to the side effects of many drugs commonly used to treat medical and mental illnesses. Anticholinergic and cardiovascular reactions in particular are examples of drug-induced toxicity that can create problems as grave as those for which the medication was originally intended.

Chapter 2 includes an overview of principal psychotropic side effects commonly found in older people. Subsequent chapters in this volume present detailed description of these reactions in relation to the spectrum of specific disorders and classes of psychotropic drugs as well as of the actions of these drugs on the aging metabolic, excretory, and central nervous systems.

Consideration of three descriptive categories may be helpful in formulating treatment plans for older adults with specific mental health problems: the nature of the problems in need of treatment, treatment modalities, and treatment providers. Factors within each category necessarily influence other factors.

Nature of the Problem

Regardless of age, the context in which mental or behavior symptoms occur triggers the treatment-planning process. The search for predisposing, precipitating, and aggravating factors that influence the onset and magnitude of symptoms is critical. This process enables the clinician to decide whether a psychotropic drug is indicated and, if so, what concomitant psychosocial approaches may also be appropriate.

Identifying recent situational or psychosocial environmental changes in the patient's life related to the onset and/or severity of symptoms, such as onset or exacerbation of disease or death of a loved one, points strongly to a role for behavioral or psychosocial interventions ranging from family consultation to individual psychotherapy. These types of problems or crises may also explain troubled sleep, a change in eating behavior, increased anxiety, or dysphoria.

The use of psychotropic medications is more likely to be considered in three types of circumstances: in the absence of a solid history of a psychological problem arising in reaction to situational factors; in the absence of prior history of specific or related problems that respond to behavioral or psychosocial interventions; and in the presence of symptoms that cause significant discomfort, dysfunction, or risk to the individual.

Treatment Modalities

Healthcare practice basically follows a conservative route—the pursuit of maximum efficacy with the least risk. Common sense reminds us that psychosocial interventions are physiologically less risky than somatic treatments. Hence, psychosocial approaches are typically considered first for mental health problems. However, for some serious mental disorders in later life (e.g., major depression and schizophrenia), psychosocial interventions are insufficient. In some instances, pharmacotherapy is indicated to reduce greater risks, such as suicide, which is most prevalent among older members of the population.

Because psychiatric problems are inadequately and often inaccurately described in terms that are either somatic or nonsomatic, whether the patient should be treated with drugs or with psychotherapy is not the most useful way to pose the treatment question. Whenever pharmacotherapy is indicated for psychiatric symptoms, it should be accompanied by complementary rather than competitive mental health interventions as well. This recommendation is relevant for the primary care provider and the mental health specialist alike. For example, when a sleeping disorder indicates the need for a hypnotic, counseling and follow-up reevaluation of the patient's sleeping behavior are crucial to obtain and evaluate optimum symptom relief.

The compelling need for psychotropic medication is linked to the need for complementary psychosocial intervention for reasons ranging from drug compliance difficulties to enhancing the overall ability of the older individual to cope in the specific setting where he or she resides. The safety as well as the efficacy of psychotropic drugs may depend as much on the involvement of the patient's support system and attention to psychosocial dynamics of the immediate environment as on necessary pharmacologic considerations.

Risk Versus Benefit Considerations

Balancing a range of factors in relation to psychotropic drug use is more complex with older patients than with younger patients, and once psychotropic medication is prescribed for an older patient, follow-up typically requires more diligence than with younger adults. The fact that older patients are more likely to have more than one illness and to be taking multiple medications complicates management. Age-related alterations in CNS sensitivity and altered distribution and excretion mechanisms, as well as increased likelihood of additional health problems and prescription of concomitant medications for new or ongoing conditions lower the threshold to toxicity in later life. Hence, potential adverse interactions require consideration not only when initiating drug treatment but also at regular intervals thereafter. Those in the 85 and older age group require particularly careful monitoring.

Determining how long to continue effective drug treatment involves more than long-term safety and side-effect considerations. Close attention to the course of psychiatric disorders and to interventions that can help modify mental and behavioral symptoms in later life may permit tapering or terminating psychotropic drug administration once clinical remission or stabilization occurs.

Treatment Settings

What has been called a "continuum of care" exists in most communities, at least in theory, and is available to most people. Depending on the needs and preferences of the individual patient and family, treatment in the home, in community facilities, or in long-term institutional settings may be appropriate and optimal. Each setting has a defined and necessary function within an overall system of care. The clinical challenge is to provide appropriate types of mental healthcare within each setting.

Managed Care

The traditional private practice/fee-for-service approach to the provision of medical care in the United States has been supplanted by various organized systems referred to as *managed care*. These systems are characterized by financial arrangements based on capitation; geographic coverage; emphasis on ambulatory care; vertical integration of primary care providers, community hospitals, and referral specialists; and restricted use of tertiary care and the academic health center.[122] Forms of managed care include health maintenance organizations and preferred-provider organizations. These organizations control costs by limiting physician-patient interaction, establishing formal practice guidelines, and routine application of utilization review and prior approval procedures for all nonemergency care.[123] One effective approach to controlling costs is to control the clinical case mix by restricting access of those patients or providers who are likely to require or request substantial amounts of costly care. (In Texas, a Consumer's Union report found that 70% of mental health claim denials are overturned on appeal.)

This type of control is a major concern for persons with late-life mental disorders in which complex patterns of comorbidity and disability may significantly challenge healthcare management requirements. For example, cognitive impairment may double the length of stay for geriatric patients hospitalized for physical illness.[124]

The proliferation of specialized organizations that fund mental health treatment services (behavioral health "carve-out" companies) continues, though market consolidation has occurred over the past decade. The term *behavioral health* defines a broad range of mental health, substance abuse, counseling, employee assistance, and crisis intervention services. These organizations contract directly with employers or with managed care organizations for provision of these specialized services under fixed-fee arrangements; one organization then assumes all responsibility for the covered services. Great concern has arisen that this emerging pattern will result in significant problems for patients because of the failure of a healthcare organization to recognize, diagnose, and treat mental disorders appropriately.[125] This risk is particularly great with respect to the care of geriatric patients who characteristically present with complex patterns of comorbidity and who may be seriously disadvantaged by the separation of "behavioral health" services from other health services.

Primary Care

The scope of responsibility of the primary care sector continues to expand and to be redefined in the emerging healthcare system in the United States. At the level of training, emphasis is moving from specialty and subspecialty care to primary care. The stated goal of many involved in system reform is to allocate as many as one-half of the medical residency positions to primary care disciplines. The primary care physician will therefore assume greater responsibility for diagnosis, treatment, and long-term management in all areas of healthcare, including care of older patients with mental disorders. Moreover, in most organized systems, access to specialty and subspecialty care will be through the primary care provider, who will serve as referral resource, case manager, and "gatekeeper." In this context, identification can be problematic: in approximately half the patients with depressive disorders, these conditions are not recognized by their primary care physicians.[126,127]

The population of primary care patients is characterized by a very high degree of psychiatric morbidity. A rough rule of "thirds" characterizes the present situation of care of older persons in need of mental health services: approximately one in three receives care from a mental health professional; another third is treated in primary care; and another third receives no care at all.[126,127] However, primary care settings have been used successfully to stage interventions to treat depression. The Improving Mood-Promoting Access to Collaborative Treatment (IMPACT) collaborative care management program for late-life depression found

that, at 12 months, 45% of patients experienced 50% or greater reduction in depressive symptoms from baseline compared with 19% of usual care participants.[128]

Another important concern with emphasis on primary care is the issue of appropriateness of treatments provided. For example, clinicians too often prescribe drugs with significant anticholinergic and mood-altering effects for their elderly patients (see Chapter 2), even when more appropriate treatments are available.[129,130] When specialty psychiatric units in a general hospital are compared with medical units for treatment of depressed elderly, the quality of mental healthcare and long-term outcome of depression significantly improves with mental health specialty care, but the quality of medical care is higher in the medical unit.[131] Widespread use of treatment or practice guidelines, such as those from the Agency for Health Care Policy and Research[132] or expert consensus guidelines[133] from leading geriatric psychiatrists, might result in improved appropriateness of treatment.

At the same time, guidelines for appropriate referral from primary to specialty care and back again need to be developed and validated. One approach would provide several patient parameters along which referral from primary to specialty care could be made: patients with complex or uncertain diagnoses; those who are suicidal or severely ill; those who have failed to respond to an adequate trial of a first-line, guidelines-based treatment; and patients in need of specialty services such as electroconvulsive therapy, experimental treatment, or nonorthodox ("off-label") treatment. Similarly, referral from specialty care to primary care is suggested when patients are stabilized, or after a treatment plan for a first-line therapy has been established.

Nursing Homes

In 1997, 17,000 nursing homes in the United States had a capacity for 1.6 million beds and an occupancy rate of 88%. Two-thirds of these nursing homes were proprietary (operated for profit), with over 90% of residents over the age of 65. Although only 5% of the older population is in nursing homes at any given point in time, approximately 20% of elders will spend some time in a nursing home during their lifetimes. The population of the nursing home is predominantly "old-old" and female, with moderate to high levels of disability and functional impairment. Virtually all nursing home residents have a diagnosable mental disorder; studies reporting 80 to 90% prevalence rates are not uncommon[134,135]; two of the most predominant conditions are dementia with behavior problems and dementia with depression.[136]

Psychopharmacologic treatment approaches are common in nursing homes. Antipsychotic medications are frequently used to manage some of the more difficult behavior problems of patients with dementia as well as those with severe agitation (see Chapter 7). Excessive or inappropriate use of antipsychotics has been identified as a significant problem, and federal regulations (Omnibus Budget Reconciliation Act of 1987) are now in place to manage use of neuroleptics and sedative hypnotics. Evidence indicates that application of these regulations has significantly reduced neuroleptic usage.[137,138] In contrast, depression is undertreated in the nursing home. Although only a very small portion of patients who could benefit from antidepressant treatment actually receive it,[139] the number of nursing home residents receiving antidepressants has been increasing.[140]

Clinician Misperceptions in Use of Psychotropic Medications

The growth of geriatrics as a rigorous clinical and scientific discipline in the last two decades has increased the interest, familiarity, and confidence of clinicians working with older patients. Only in the recent past, major later-life changes were dismissed as inevitable concomitants of the aging process rather than possible pathological manifestations of underlying illness. Unfortunately, even when disease is correctly diagnosed in the geriatric patient, therapeutic skepticism and many misperceptions that impeded treatment planning in the 1970s for those 65 and older may now reappear for those 85 and older. Inaccurate views of the efficacy of psychotropic drugs is one of these misperceptions, interfering with their use for elderly patients.

Personal philosophies as well as clinical factors influence the use of psychotropics in treating older patients, and misconceptions in both areas have interfered with proper treatment decisions. Popular misperceptions of psychotropic medications as "chemical restraints," "shackles," or "mind-control agents" can obscure their therapeutic impact. Before entering the clinical domain of deciding whether or not or how to use psychotropic drugs in the treatment plan for a given geriatric patient, some perspectives both inside and outside the doctor-patient relationship require consideration, particularly those of safety and the clinician's view of life expectancy.

Overzealous concern about safety in the use of drugs can compound inadequate understanding of the efficacy of psychopharmacologic treatment approaches for older patients. Caution is appropriate—and indeed necessary—in treating elderly persons with psychotropic medication. But if such caution is too great, it can do patients a serious disservice by depriving them of an important therapeutic option. A balance of *primum non nocere* (first do no harm) and state-of-the-art knowledge regarding expectable age-related physiological changes, concomitant physical illness, and sound diagnostic and follow-up practices is necessary for aging patients.

Our understanding of the needs of the geriatric patient and of the contribution of geriatric psychopharmacology to those needs has grown rapidly and substantively in the past 20 years. The need for additional knowledge upon which to develop new approaches to the clinical care of sick old people is now apparent and pressing. Research, education, and new practice models will provide the foundation for the next phase in the development of geriatric treatment. Fulfilling the promise of these developments requires the sustained and creative efforts of investigators, educators, and clinicians.

References

1. Administration on Aging. A profile of older Americans: 2001. (Available online at http://www.aoa.gov/aoa/stats/profile/default.htm)
2. U.S. Census Bureau. National Population Projections. I. Summary Files. (NP-T3) Projections of the total resident population by 5-year age groups, and sex with special age categories: middle series, 1999 to 2100. (Available online at http://www.census.gov/population/www/projections/natsum-T3.html)
3. Lebowitz BD. The future of clinical research in mental disorders of late life. *Schizophr Res* 1997; 27:261–267.
4. Halpain MC, Harris MJ, McClure FS, et al. Training in geriatric mental health: needs and strategies. *Psychiatr Serv* 1999;50:1205–1208.
5. Davis K. *The unfinished agenda: improving the well being of older people living alone.* New York: Commonwealth Fund, 1993.
6. Grady D, Rubin SM, Petitti DB, et al. Hormone therapy to prevent disease and prolong life in postmenopausal women. *Ann Intern Med* 1992; 117:1016–1037.
7. Writing Group for the Women's Health Initiative investigators. Risks and benefits of estrogen plus progestin in healthy postmenopausal women. Principal results from the Women's Health Initiative randomized controlled trial. *JAMA* 2002;288:321–333.
8. Paganini-Hill A, Henderson VW. Estrogen deficiency and risk of Alzheimer's disease in women. *Am J Epidemiol* 1994;140:256–261.
9. Zandi PP, Carlson MC, Plassman BL, et al; Cache County Memory Study Investigators. Hormone replacement therapy and incidence of Alzheimer's disease in older women: the Cache County Study. *JAMA* 2002;288: 2170–2172.
10. Hogervorst E, Yaffe K, Richards M, et al. Hormone replacement therapy to maintain cognitive function in women with dementia (Cochrane Review). In: The Cochrane Library, Issue 3, 2002. Oxford: Update Software.
11. Hallonquist JD, Seeman MV, Lang M, et al. Variation in symptom severity over the menstrual cycle of schizophrenics. *Biol Psychiatry* 1993;33:207–209.
12. Riecher-Rossler A, Hafner H, Dutsch-Strobel A, et al. Further evidence for a specific role of estradiol in schizophrenia? *Biol Psychiatry* 1994; 36:492–495.
13. Grigoriadis S, Kennedy SH. Role of estrogen in the treatment of depression. *Am J Ther* 2002; 9:503–509.
14. Blehar MC, Oren DA. Women's increased vulnerability to mood disorders: integrating psychobiology and epidemiology. *Depression* 1995; 3:3–12.
15. Goodwin FK. *The recognition and treatment of depression in medical practice.* Washington, DC: American Medical Association Council on Scientific Affairs, 1991.
16. Manolio TA, Furberg CD, Shemanski L, et al. Associations of postmenopausal estrogen use with cardiovascular disease and its risk factors in older women. *Circulation* 1993;88:2163–2171.
17. Handa VL, Landerman R, Hanlon JT, et al. Do older women use estrogen replacement? Data from the Duke Established Populations for Epidemiological Studies of the Elderly (EPESE). *J Am Geriatr Soc* 1996;44:1–446.
18. Schneider LS, Small GW, Hamilton SH, et al. Estrogen replacement and response to fluoxetine in a multicenter geriatric depression trial. Fluoxetine Collaborative Study Group. *Am J Geriatr Psychiatry* 1997;5:97–106.
19. Ballenger JC, Davidson JR, Lecrubier Y, et al. Consensus statement on transcultural issues in depression and anxiety from the International Consensus Group on Depression and Anxiety. *J Clin Psychiatry* 2001;62 (Suppl 13):47–55.
20. Lin KM. Biological differences in depression and anxiety across races and ethnic groups. *J Clin Psychiatry* 2001;62 (Suppl 13):13–19; discussion 20–21.
21. Jann MW, Cohen LJ. The influence of ethnicity and antidepressant pharmacogenetics in the treatment of depression. *Drug Metabol Drug Interact* 2000;16:39–67.
22. Pollock BG. Issues in psychotropic drug development for the elderly. In: Bergener M, Brockelhurst JC, Finkel SI, eds. *Aging, health, and healing.* New York: Springer, 1995:235–242.
23. Statistics: About Alzheimer's Disease. A fact sheet prepared by the Alzheimer's Association. Available online at http://www.alz.org/ResourceCenter/FactSheets/FSAlzheimerStats.pdf
24. Charlson M, Peterson JC. Medical comorbidity and late-life depression: what is known and what are the unmet needs? *Biol Psychiatry* 2002; 52:226–235.
25. Katz IR. On the inseparability of mental and physical health in aged persons: lessons from depression and medical comorbidity. *Am J Geriatr Psychiatry* 1996;4:1–16.
26. Lebowitz BD, Pearson JL, Schneider LS, et al. Diagnosis and treatment of depression in late life. Consensus statement update. *JAMA* 1997; 278:1186–1190.
27. Bruce ML. The association between depression and disability. *Am J Geriatr Psychiatry* 1999;7: 8–11.
28. Ünützer J. Diagnosis and treatment of older

adults with depression in primary care. *Biol Psychiatry* 2002;52:285–292.

29. Cohen GD. *The brain in human aging.* New York: Springer, 1988.

30. Schaie KW. The hazards of cognitive aging. *Gerontologist* 1989;29:484–493.

31. Tobin JD. Physiological indices of aging. In: Danon D, Shock NW, Marois M, eds. *Aging: a challenge to science and society. Vol. 1, Biology.* New York: Oxford University Press, 1981.

32. Tabbarah M, Crimmins EM, Seeman TE. The relationship between cognitive and physical performance: MacArthur studies of successful aging. *J Gerontol A Biol Sci Med Sci* 2002;57: M228–M235.

33. Seeman TE, Lusignolo TM, Albert M, et al. Social relationships, social support, and patterns of cognitive aging in healthy, high-functioning older adults: MacArthur studies of successful aging. *Health Psychol* 2001;20:243–255.

34. Cohen GD. Creativity with aging: four phases of potential in the second half of life. *Geriatrics* 2001;56:51–54, 57.

35. Freund AM, Baltes PB. Selection, optimization, and compensation as strategies of life management: correlations with subjective indicators of successful aging. *Psychol Aging* 1998;13:531–543.

36. Baltes PB, Staudinger UM. Wisdom. A meta-heuristic (pragmatic) to orchestrate mind and virtue toward excellence. *Am Psychol* 2000;55: 122–136.

37. Goldman WP, Morris JC. Evidence that age-associated memory impairment is not a normal variant of aging. *Alzheimer Dis Assoc Disord* 2001; 15:72–79.

38. Bennett DA, Wilson RS, Schneider JA, et al. Natural history of mild cognitive impairment in older persons. *Neurology* 2002;59:198–205.

39. Lyketsos CG, Lopez O, Jones B, et al. Prevalence of neuropsychiatric symptoms in dementia and mild cognitive impairment: results from the cardiovascular health study. *JAMA* 2002; 288:1475–1483.

40. Datto CJ, Oslin DW, Streim JE, et al. Pharmacologic treatment of depression in nursing home residents: a mental health services perspective. *J Geriatr Psychiatry Neurol* 2002;15:141–146.

41. Pearson JL, Reynolds CF, Kupfer DJ, et al. Outcome measures in late-life depression. *Am J Geriatr Psychiatry* 1995;3:191–197.

42. NIH Consensus Development Panel. Diagnosis and treatment of depression in late life. *JAMA* 1992;268:1018–1024.

43. National Advisory Mental Health Council. Health care reform for Americans with severe mental illnesses. *Am J Psychiatry* 1993;150: 1447–1465.

44. Wilson K, Mottram P, Sivanranthan A, et al. Antidepressants versus placebo for the depressed elderly (Cochrane Review). In: The Cochrane Library, Issue 3, 2002. Oxford: Update Software.

45. Jeste DV, Alexopolous GS, Bartels SJ, et al: Consensus statement on the upcoming crisis in geriatric mental health. *Arch Gen Psychiatry* 1999; 56:848–853.

46. Brookmeyer R, Gray S, Kawas C. Projections of Alzheimer's disease in the United States and the public health impact of delaying disease onset. *Am J Public Health* 1998;88:1337–1342.

47. Jorm AF. *The epidemiology of Alzheimer's disease and related disorders.* London: Chapman & Hall, 1990.

48. Evans DA, Funkenstein HH, Albert MS, et al. Prevalence of Alzheimer's disease in a community population of older persons: higher than previously reported. *JAMA* 1989;262:2551–2556.

49. Jorm AF, Korten AE, Henderson AS. The prevalence of dementia: a quantitative integration of the literature. *Acta Psychiatr Scand* 1987;76: 456–479.

50. Ritchie K, Kildea D, Robine JM. The relationship between age and the prevalence of senile dementia: a meta-analysis of recent data. *Int J Epidemiol* 1992;21:763–769.

51. Ritchie K, Kildea D. Is senile dementia "age-related" or "aging-related"?—evidence from meta-analysis of dementia prevalence in the oldest old. *Lancet* 1995;346:931–934.

52. Valle R, Lee B. Research priorities in the evolving demographic landscape of Alzheimer's disease and associated dementias. *Alzheimer's Dis Assoc Disord* 2002;16 (Suppl 2):S64–S76.

53. Kukull WA, Higdon R, Bowen JD, et al. Dementia and Alzheimer's disease incidence: a prospective cohort study. *Arch Neurol* 2002;59: 1737–1746.

54. Petersen RC, Doody R, Kurz A, et al. Current concepts in mild cognitive impairment. *Arch Neurol* 2001;58:1985–1992.

55. Rocca WA, Hofman A, Brayne C, et al. Frequency and distribution of Alzheimer's disease in Europe: a collaborative study of 1980–1990 prevalence findings. *Ann Neurol* 1991;30:381–390.

56. Schoenberg BS, Anderson DW, Haerer AF. Severe dementia: prevalence and clinical features in a biracial U.S. population. *Arch Neurol* 1985; 42:740–743.

57. Bachman DL, Wolf PA, Linn RT, et al. Incidence of dementia and probable Alzheimer's disease in a general population: the Framingham study. *Neurology* 1993;43:515–519.

58. Paykel ES, Brayne C, Huppert FA, et al. Incidence of dementia in a population older than 75 years in the United Kingdom. *Arch Gen Psychiatry* 1994;51:325–332.

59. Selkoe DJ. Alzheimer's disease is a synaptic failure. *Science* 2002;298:789–791.

60. American College of Medical Genetics/American Society of Human Genetics Working Group (ACMG/ASHG) on ApoE and Alzheimer's Disease. Statement on the use of apolipoprotein E testing for Alzheimer's disease. *JAMA* 1995;274:1627–1629.

61. Murphy GM Jr, Taylor J, Kraemer HC, et al. No association between apolipoprotein E epsilon 4 allele and rate of decline in Alzheimer's disease. *Am J Psychiatry* 1997;154:603–608.

62. LaRue A, Jarvik LF. Cognitive function and prediction of dementia in old age. *Int J Aging Hum Dev* 1987;25:79–89.

63. Snowdon DA, Kemper SJ, Mortimer JA, et al. Linguistic ability in early life and cognitive

function and Alzheimer's disease in late life. Findings from the Nun Study. *JAMA* 1996;275: 528–532.

64. Cummings JL, Ross W, Absher J, et al. Depressive symptoms in Alzheimer's disease: assessment and determinants. *Alzheimer Dis Related Disord* 1995;9:87–93.

65. Finkel SI, Burns A, Cohen G. Overview, in Behavioral and psychological symptoms of dementia (BPSD): a clinical and research update. *Int Psychogeriatr* 2000; 12(Suppl 1):13–18.

66. Reisberg B, Franssen E, Sclan S, et al. Stage specific incidence of potentially remediable behavioral symptoms in aging and Alzheimer's disease. *Bull Clin Neurosci* 1989;54:95–112.

67. Rosen J, Zubenko G. Emergence of psychosis and depression in the longitudinal evaluation of Alzheimer's disease. *Biol Psychiatry* 1991;29: 224–232.

68. Laughren T. A regulatory perspective on psychiatric syndromes in Alzheimer's disease. *Am J Geriatr Psychiatry* 2001;9:340–345.

69. Jeste DV, Finkel SI. Psychosis of Alzheimer's disease. *Am J Geriatr Psychiatry* 2000;8:29–32.

70. Olin JT, Schneider LS, Katz IR, et al. Provisional diagnostic criteria for depression of Alzheimer's disease. *Am J Geriatr Psychiatry* 2002; 10:125–128.

71. Olin JT, Katz IR, Meyers BS, et al. Provisional diagnostic criteria for depression of Alzheimer's disease: rationale and background. *Am J Geriatr Psychiatry* 2002;10:129–141.

72. Kelly KG, Zisselman M, Cutillo-Schmitter T, et al. Severity and course of delirium in medically hospitalized nursing facility residents. *Am J Geriatr Psychiatry* 2001;9:72–77.

73. Blazer DG. Epidemiology of late-life depression. In: Schneider LS, Reynolds CF, Lebowitz BD, et al., eds. *Diagnosis and treatment of depression in late life.* Washington, DC: American Psychiatric Press, 1994:9–19.

74. Chen L, Eaton WW, Gallo JJ. Understanding the heterogeneity of depression through the triad of symptoms, course and risk factors: a longitudinal, population-based study. *J Affect Disord* 2000;59:1–11.

75. Flint AJ. The complexity and challenge of non-major depression in late life. *Am J Geriatr Psychiatry* 2002;10: 229–232.

76. Lyness JM, King DA, Cox C, et al. The importance of subsyndromal depression in older primary care patients: prevalence and associated functional disability. *J Am Geriatr Soc* 1999;47: 647–652.

77. Lyness JM, Caine ED, King DA, et al. Depressive disorders and symptoms in older primary care patients: one-year outcomes. *Am J Geriatr Psychiatry* 2002;10:275–282.

78. Lavretsky H, Kumar A. Clinically significant non-major depression: old concepts, new insights. *Am J Geriatr Psychiatry* 2002;10:239–255.

79. Gallo JJ, Rabins PV. Depression without sadness: alternative presentations of depression in late life. *Am Fam Physician* 1999;60:820–826.

80. Weissman MM, Bruce ML, Leaf PJ, et al. Affective disorders. In: Robins LN, Regier DA, eds. *Psychiatric disorders in America.* New York: Free Press, 1991:53–80.

81. Myers JK, Weissman MM, Tischler GL, et al. Six-month prevalence of psychiatric disorders in three communities. *Arch Gen Psychiatry* 1984; 41:959–970.

82. Blazer D. Mood disorders: epidemiology. In: Kaplan HI, Sadock BJ, eds. *Comprehensive textbook of psychiatry.* 7th ed. Baltimore: Williams & Wilkins, 1995;1:1298–1308.

83. Radloff LW. The CES-D scale: a self-report depression scale for research in the general population. *Appl Psychol Meas* 1977;1:385–401.

84. Kessler RC, Foster C, Webster PS, House JS. The relationship between age and depressive symptoms in two national surveys. *Psychol Aging* 1992;7:119–126.

85. Steffens DC, Levy RM, Wagner R, et al. Sociodemographic and clinical predictors of mortality in geriatric depression. *Am J Geriatr Psychiatry* 2002;10:531–540.

86. Romanoski AJ, Folstein MF, Nestadt G, et al. The epidemiology of psychiatrist-ascertained depression and DSM-III depressive disorders. *Psychol Med* 1992;22:629–655.

87. Blazer DG, Burchett B, Service C, et al. Association of age and depression among the elderly: an epidemiological exploration. *J Gerontol (Medical Sciences)* 1991;46:M210–M215.

88. Oxman TE, Barrett JE, Barrett J, Gerber P. Symptomatology of late-life minor depression among primary care patients. *Psychosomatics* 1990;31:174–180.

89. Bruce ML. Depression and disability in late life: directions for future research. *Am J Geriatr Psychiatry* 2001;9:102–112.

90. Garrard J, Rolnick SJ, Nitz NM, et al. Clinical detection of depression among community-based elderly people with self-reported symptoms of depression. *J Gerontol A Biol Sci Med Sci* 1998;53:M92–M101.

91. Conwell Y, Brent D. Suicide and aging I: patterns of psychiatric diagnosis. *Int Psychogeriatr* 1995;7:149–164.

92. Conwell Y. Suicide in elderly patients. In: Schneider LS, Reynolds CF, Lebowitz BD, Friedhoff AJ, eds. *Diagnosis and treatment of depression in late life.* Washington, DC: American Psychiatric Press, 1994:397–418.

93. Vassilas CA, Morgan HG. Elderly suicides' contact with their general practitioner before death [Letter to the editor]. *Int J Geriatr Psychiatry* 1994;9:1008–1009.

94. Conwell Y, Duberstein PR, Caine ED. Risk factors for suicide in later life. *Biol Psychiatry* 2002; 52:193–204.

95. Slaughter JR, Slaughter KA, Nichols D, et al. Prevalence, clinical manifestations, etiology, and treatment of depression in Parkinson's disease. *J Neuropsychiatry Clin Neurosci* 2001;13: 187–196.

96. Mayeux R, Stern Y, Cote L, et al. Altered serotonin metabolism in depressed patients with Parkinson's disease. *Neurology* 1984;34:642–646.

97. Brown A, Gershon S. Dopamine and depression. *J Neural Transm* 1993; 91:75–109.

98. Mayberg H, Solomon D. Depression in Parkinson's disease: a biochemical and organic viewpoint, in behavioral neurology of movement disorders. In: Weiner WJ, Lang AE, eds. *Ad-*

vances in neurology. Vol. 65. New York: Raven, 1995:49–60.

99. Rogers D, Lees AJ, Smith E, et al. Bradyphrenia in Parkinson's disease and psychomotor retardation in depressive illness: an experimental study. *Brain* 1987;110:761–776.

100. Stanley MA, Beck JG. Anxiety disorders. *Clin Psychol Rev* 2000;20(6):731–754

101. Blazer DG, George LK, Hughes D. The epidemiology of anxiety disorders: an age comparison. In: Salzman C, Lebowitz BD, eds. *Anxiety in the elderly: treatment and research.* New York: Springer, 1991:17–30.

102. Eaton WW, Dryman A, Weissman MM. Panic and phobia. In: Robins LN, Regier DA, eds. *Psychiatric disorders in America: the epidemiologic catchment area study.* New York: Free Press, 1991: 155–179.

103. Sable JA, Jeste DV. Anxiety disorders in older adults. *Curr Psychiatry Rep* 2001;3(4):302–307.

104. Blazer DG, Hughes D, George LK, et al. Generalized anxiety disorder. In: Robins LN, Regier DA, eds. *Psychiatric disorders in America: the epidemiologic catchment area study.* New York: Free Press, 1991:180–203.

105. Keith SJ, Regier DA, Rae DS. Schizophrenic disorders. In: Robins LN, Regier DA, eds. *Psychiatric disorders in America.* New York: Free Press, 1991:33–52.

106. Palmer BW, McClure FS, Jeste DV. Schizophrenia in late life: findings challenge traditional concepts. *Harv Rev Psychiatry* 2001;9:51–58.

107. Howard R, Rabins PV, Seeman MV, et al. Late-onset schizophrenia and very-late-onset schizophrenia-like psychosis: an international consensus. The International Late-Onset Schizophrenia Group. *Am J Psychiatry* 2000;157: 172–178.

108. Copeland JRM, Dewey ME, Scott A, et al. Schizophrenia and delusional disorder in older age: community prevalence, incidence, comorbidity and outcome. *Schizophr Bull* 1998;24: 153–161.

109. Phillips B, Ancoli-Israel S. Sleep disorders in the elderly. *Sleep Med* 2001;2:99–114.

110. NIH Consensus Statement. The treatment of sleep disorders of older people. Mar 26–28, 1990;8(3):1–22.

111. Skoog I, Steen B, Persson G, et al. A 15-year longitudinal cross-sectional population study on sleep in the elderly. In: Albarede JL, Morely JE, Roth T, Vellas BJ, eds. *Sleep disorders and insomnia in the elderly.* New York: Springer, 1993: 137–146.

112. Kripke D, Simons R, Garfinkel M, Mammond C. Short and long sleep and sleep pills. *Arch Gen Psychiatry* 1979;36:103–116.

113. Bixler EO, Kales A, Soldatos CR, et al. Prevalence of sleep disorders in the Los Angeles metropolitan area. *Am J Psychiatry* 1979;136: 1257–1262.

114. Bixler EO, Vgontzas AN, Lin HM, et al. Insomnia in central Pennsylvania. *J Psychosom Res* 2002;53:589–592.

115. Roberts RE, Shema SJ, Kaplan GA, et al. Sleep complaints and depression in an aging cohort: A prospective perspective. *Am J Psychiatry* 2000; 157:81–88.

116. Liberto JG, Oslin DW, Ruskin PE. Alcoholism in older persons: a review of the literature. *Hosp Community Psychiatry* 1992;43:975–984.

117. Helzer JE, Burnam A, McEnvoy LT. Alcohol abuse and dependence. In: Robins LN, Regier DA, eds. *Psychiatric disorders in America.* New York: Free Press, 1991:81–115.

118. Johnson I. Alcohol problems in old age: a review of recent epidemiological research. *Int J Geriatr Psychiatry* 2000;15:575–581.

119. Blow FC. Treatment of older women with alcohol problems: meeting the challenge for a special population. *Alcohol Clin Exp Res* 2000;24: 1257–1266.

120. Speer DC, Bates KB. Comorbid mental and substance disorders among older psychiatric patients. *J Am Geriatr Soc* 1992;40:886–890.

121. Blixen CE, McDougall GJ, Suen LJ. Dual diagnosis in elders discharged from a psychiatric hospital. *Int J Geriatr Psychiatry* 1997;12: 307–313.

122. Lebowitz BD, Gottlieb GL. Clinical research in the managed care environment. *Am J Geriatr Psychiatry* 1995;3:21–25.

123. Gold MR, Hurley R, Lake T, et al. A national survey of the arrangements managed-care plans make with physicians. *N Engl J Med* 1995; 333:1678–1683.

124. Torian L, Davidson E, Fulop G, et al. The effects of dementia on acute care in a geriatric medical unit. *Int Psychogeriatr* 1992;4:231–239.

125. Estes CL. Mental health services for the elderly: key policy elements. In: Gatz M, ed. *Emerging issues in mental health and aging.* Washington, DC: American Psychological Association, 1995.

126. Mulrow CD, Williams JW, Gerety MB, et al. Case-finding instruments for depression in primary care settings. *Ann Intern Med* 1995;122: 913–921.

127. Sturm R, Wells KB. How can care for depression become more cost effective. *JAMA* 1995; 273:51–58.

128. Ünützer J, Katon W, Callahan CM, et al. Collaborative care management of late-life depression in the primary care setting: a randomized controlled trial. *JAMA* 2002;288:2836–2845.

129. Willcox SM, Himmelstein DU, Woolhandler S. Inappropriate drug prescribing for the community dwelling elderly. *JAMA* 1994;272: 292–296.

130. Hanlon JT, Schmader KE, Boult C, et al. Use of inappropriate prescription drugs by older people. *J Am Geriatr Soc* 2002;50:26–34.

131. Norquist G, Wells KB, Rogers WH, et al. Quality of care for depressed elderly patients hospitalized in the specialty psychiatric units or general medical wards. *Arch Gen Psychiatry* 1995;52: 695–701.

132. Depression Guidelines Panel. Depression in primary care, vol. 2: treatment of major depression. Clinical practice guideline no. 5. Rockville, MD: US Department of Health and Human Services, Public Health Service, Agency for Health Care Policy and Research. AHCPR publ. no. 93-0551, April 1993.

133. Alexopoulos GS, Katz IR, Reynolds CF, et al. The Expert Consensus Guideline Series: Pharmacotherapy of depressive disorders in older

patients. A Postgraduate Medicine Special Report. 2001. The McGraw-Hill Companies, Inc.

134. German PS, Rovner BW, Burton LC, et al. The role of mental morbidity in the nursing home experience. *Gerontologist* 1992;32:151–158.

135. Katz IR, Rovner BW. Psychiatric disorders in the nursing home: a selective review of studies related to clinical care. *Int J Geriatr Psychiatry* 1993;8:75–87.

136. Evers MM, Samuels SC, Lantz M, et al. The prevalence, diagnosis and treatment of depression in dementia patients in chronic care facilities in the last six months of life. *Int J Geriatr Psychiatry* 2002;17:464–472.

137. Rovner BW, Edelman BA, Cox MP, Schmuely Y. The impact of antipsychotic drug regulations (OBRA-87) on psychotropic prescribing practices in nursing homes. *N Engl J Med* 1992;327:168–173.

138. Snowden M, Roy-Byrne P. Mental illness and nursing home reform: OBRA-87 ten years later. Omnibus Budget Reconciliation Act. *Psychiatr Serv* 1998;49:229–233.

139. Heston LL, Garrard J, Makris L, et al. Inadequate treatment of depressed nursing home elderly. *J Am Geriatr Soc* 1992;40:1117–1122.

140. Datto CJ, Oslin DW, Streim JE, et al. Pharmacologic treatment of depression in nursing home residents: a mental health services perspective. *J Geriatr Psychiatry Neurol* 2002;15:141–146.

Supplemental Readings

General

Busse EW, Blazer DG, eds. Geriatric psychiatry. New York: Van Nostrand Reinhold, 1998.

Coffey CE, Cummings JL, Eds. *The american psychiatric press textbook of geriatric neuropsychiatry 2nd edition.* Washington, DC: American Psychological Association Press, 2000.

Gatz M, ed. *Emerging issues in mental health and aging.* Washington, DC: American Psychological Association Press, 1995.

Hocking LB, Koenig HG, Blazer DG. Epidemiology and geriatric psychiatry. In: Tsuang MT, Tohen M, Zahner GEP, eds. *Textbook in psychiatric epidemiology.* New York: John Wiley & Sons, 1995:437–448.

Murphy E, Alexopoulos G. *Geriatric psychiatry: key research topics for clinicians.* New York: John Wiley & Sons, 1995.

Nelson JC ed. *Geriatric psychopharmacology.* New York: Marcel Dekker, 1998.

Zarit SH, Zarit JM. Mental disorders in older adults. New york: Guilford, 1998.

Gender and Racial Differences

American Psychiatric Association. *Ethnic minority elderly: a task force report of the American Psychiatric Association.* Washington, DC: American Psychiatric Association Press, 1994.

Callahan CM, Wolinsky FD. The effect of gender and race on the measurement properties of the CES-D in older adults. *Med Care* 1994;32:341–356.

Canetto SS. Elderly women and suicidal behavior. In: Canetto SS, Lester D, eds. *Women and Suicidal Behavior.* New York: Springer, 1995:215–233.

Johnson RJ, Wolinsky FD. Gender, race and health: the structure of health status among older adults. *Gerontologist* 1994;34:24–35.

Primary Care

Hendrie HC, Callahan CM, Levitt EE, et al. Prevalence rates of major depressive disorders. *Am J Geriatr Psychiatry* 1995;3:119–131.

Regier DA, Narrow WE, Rae DS, et al. The de facto U.S. mental and addictive disorders system: epidemiologic catchment area prospective 1-year prevalence rates of disorders and services. *Arch Gen Psychiatry* 1993;50:85–94.

Nursing Homes

Reichman WE, Katz PR, Reichman K eds. *Psychiatric care in the nursing home.* New York, Oxford University Press, 1996.

Rubinstein RL, Lawton MP, Rubinstein RA eds. *Depression in long-term and residential care: advances in research and treatment.* New York: Springer Pub Co, 1997.

Epidemiology of Disorders in Late Life

Alcohol and Substance Abuse

Beresford TP. Alcoholism in the elderly. *Int Rev Psychiatry* 1993;5:477–483.

Solomon K, Manepalli J, Ireland GA, Mahon GM. Alcoholism and prescription drug abuse in the elderly. *J Am Geriatr Soc* 1993;41:57–69.

Anxiety

Alexopoulos GS, Meyers BS, Young RC, et al. Anxiety in geriatric depression: effects of age and cognitive impairment. *Am J Geriatr Psychiatry* 1995;3:108–118.

Casten RJ, Parmelee PA, Kleban MH, et al. The relationships among anxiety, depression and pain in a geriatric institutionalized sample. *Pain* 1995;61:271–276.

Flint AJ. Epidemiology and comorbidity of anxiety disorders in the elderly. *Am J Psychiatry* 1994;151:640–649.

Schneider LS. Overview of generalized anxiety disorder in the elderly. *J Clin Psychiatry* 1996;57(suppl 7):34–45.

Dementia

Advisory Panel on Alzheimer's Disease. *Alzheimer's disease and related dementias: acute and long-term care services, 1996.* NIH publ. no. 96-4136. Washington, DC: U.S. Government Printing Office, 1996.

Devanand DP, Sano M, Tang MX, et al. Depressed mood and incidence of Alzheimer's disease in the elderly living in the community. *Arch Gen Psychiatry* 1996;53:175–182.

Huppert FA, Brayne C, O'Connor DW, eds. *Dementia and normal aging.* Cambridge, Eng.: Cambridge University Press, 1994.

Depression

Gallo JJ, Anthony JC, Muthén BG. Age differences in the symptoms of depression: a latent trait analysis. *J Gerontol (Psychological Sciences)* 1994;49:P251–264.

Tannock C, Katona C. Minor depression in the aged: concepts, prevalence and optimal management. *Drugs Aging* 1995;6:278–292.

Schizophrenia

Castel DJ, Murray RM. The epidemiology of late-onset schizophrenia. *Schizophr Bull* 1993;19:691–700.

Lamberti JS, Tariot PN. Schizophrenia in nursing home patients. *Psychiatr Ann* 1995;25:441–448.

Sleep Problems

Ford DE, Kamerow DB. Epidemiologic study of sleep disturbance and psychiatric disorders: an opportunity for prevention? *JAMA* 1989;262:1479–1484.

Mellinger GD, Balter MB, Uhlenhuth EH. Insomnia and its treatment: prevalence and correlates. *Arch Gen Psychiatry* 1985;42:225–232.

Rodin J, McAvay G, Timko C. A longitudinal study of depressed mood and sleep disturbances in older adults. *J Gerontol* 1988;43:P45–53.

Drug Prescribing, Adverse Reactions, and Compliance in Elderly Patients

Jerry Avorn

Philip Wang

As with many aspects of drug use in the elderly, the relatively high consumption of medications by patients over age 65 is a two-edged sword. While comprising only about 13% of the U.S. population, those over 65 consume over 30% of all prescription medications.[1] Ninety percent of Americans 65 and older use one or more medications regularly, with over 40% taking 5 or more different drugs concurrently.[2] Nonprescription drug use by the elderly has also been increased over time with over two-thirds of those 65 and older using at least one over-the-counter medication.[3,4] The high level of use of both prescription and nonprescription medications, although not surprising considering the greater burden of morbidity borne by the older population, has been cited as a cause for both alarm and reassurance.[2,3,5]

Prescription-Drug Use Concerns

The answer to the question "How much is too much?" in geriatric drug use is akin to asking whether the proverbial medicine cabinet is half full or half empty. One source of concern is about the high level of medication consumption in older patients (polypharmacy) and the potential problems it can cause: aging, even normal aging, brings with it a decreased capacity to metabolize and excrete drugs, increasing the risk of adverse drug effects if doses are not appropriately adjusted for these factors—as often they are not. A second source of polypharmacy concern in older patients is based on the greater prevalence of coexisting illnesses or physiological conditions that can interact adversely with a given medication. A clear example of this is the postural hypotension commonly seen in patients taking older tertiary amine tricyclic antidepressants (TCAs) such as amitriptyline: in a younger patient, this may be unnoticed or merely bothersome; an older patient, however, is likely to have diminished ability to accelerate heart rate in response to decreased blood pressure. Similarly, if an older person with autonomic insufficiency is also taking a diuretic for congestive heart failure and a β-blocker for hypertension, the combined effect of drugs and age-related loss of cardiovascular resilience is likely to lower blood pressure even more. If a TCA is then added, the postural hypotension that may result can cause disabling symptoms, falls, or even hip fracture.

A third reason for concern about the high levels of drug use relates to compliance. Although noncompliance with prescribed regimens does not necessarily increase with advancing age, its likelihood does rise with an increase in the number of prescribed medications (discussed in more detail later). Consequently, the more drugs in a regimen, the greater the likelihood that a patient of any age will fail to take the complete regimen as directed. This is of particular concern because patients may not omit the most trivial medications in the regimen—continuing, for example, to take a stool softener faithfully but missing doses of an antihypertensive.

A final reason for concern over the high level of medication use by the elderly is its financial impact. Although not commonly appreciated by prescribers, a high proportion of persons over 65 in the United States do not have health insurance that adequately covers their pharmaceutical expenses. Conventional Medicare insurance covers virtually no outpatient drug charges; such coverage generally must be purchased separately at additional cost, unless a patient is sufficiently indigent to qualify for Medicaid, which does provide comprehensive drug benefits. As a result, for many older patients, pharmaceutical expenditures represent one of their highest out-of-pocket healthcare costs. It had been hoped that this situation would change with the enrollment of increasing numbers of U.S. elderly persons in managed care plans, many of which cover pharmaceutical expenditures. However, many plans have found the high cost of this benefit unsustainable and have actively disenrolled older patients in recent years. Other plans have resorted to imposing growing surcharges for full pharmaceutical coverage for their Medicare enrollees. In countries with more highly developed social welfare programs, drug expenditures by the elderly are generally covered more completely. While this eases the burden on the individual patient and makes noncompliance for financial reasons less common, such universal coverage transfers the fiscal onus to the healthcare system itself, for which the cost of geriatric pharmacotherapy looms increasingly large each year.[6]

The cost of drug therapy for the elderly escalated rapidly throughout the 1980s and 1990s, outstripping the rate of growth of other components of healthcare. The cost of pharmacotherapy as a fraction of the nation's entire healthcare expenditure has remained modest, at about 10%. When used astutely, medications can indeed be one of the most cost-effective interventions in healthcare if they make it possible for patients to avoid or shorten hospital care, achieve a higher functional status, or prevent acute illness altogether. Proponents of this view question whether the large numbers of medications consumed by the elderly represent a problem or a boon, and argue that the "ideal" level of medication used by older patients is more a function of the intelligence with which the prescriber constructs the regimen, whatever its size, than the length of the drug list itself. For some conditions, including depression, there is also concern that medications may in fact be underused by the elderly population.[7,8,9]

Psychotropic drugs constitute a significant portion of prescription drugs used by the elderly. After hormone replacements, cardiovascular drugs, analgesics, GI medications and hypoglycemic agents, drugs with psychotropic properties, are the most frequently prescribed drugs taken by older people.[2,10] Usage is particularly high in nursing homes.[11] In the general hospital population, over a third of older patients hospitalized for medical-surgical care receive psychotropic drugs.[12] Older people who take psychotropic medication also use more prescription drugs of other kinds and tend to consult their physicians about drug use more than those who do not.[13]

These high rates of psychotropic medication utilization by the elderly are likely to continue increasing over time. As newer antidepressant, antipsychotic, and hypnotic agents have become widely available, psychotropic medication use has grown rapidly in all strata of the population.[14]

Given this situation, care providers and policymakers increasingly face important questions about the quality of care: is drug use in the elderly too high? If so, can it be reduced? Are there other conditions, such as depression, in which drugs are underutilized? How can psychotherapeutic benefits be enhanced and adverse effects minimized? What is the impact of factors such as polypharmacy, age, type, and severity of concomitant disease, and adverse reactions on the drug use of older patients? What effect should these factors have on prescribing decisions for psychotropic drugs? How does the special situation of nursing home care influence drug use, and how should it? What prescribing pitfalls confront prescribers, and how can they optimize their prescribing practices? What barriers to compliance with drug regimens face patients? How can care providers strengthen adherence to drug regimens?

Issues surrounding these and allied questions underlie the main topics of this chapter: drug prescribing patterns, particularly psychotropic drug prescribing; use of over-the-counter (OTC) drugs; common side effects of psychotropic drugs, particularly in relation to functional and structural age-related changes; polypharmacy, drug interactions, and adverse reactions; an approach to rational prescribing; and compliance guidelines.

Over-the-Counter Medication Concerns

Medications obtained without a prescription have, for generations, been a useful way for people to control symptoms without incurring the expense or difficulty of a formal encounter with a physician. However, the diminished physiological reserve of the elderly and their greater susceptibility to drug side effects present special problems with regard to OTC medications. These concerns have intensified in recent years with decisions by the Food and Drug Administration (FDA) to make a number of medications available over the counter that previously had been available by prescription only, such as histamine receptor antagonists and nonsteroidal anti-inflammatory drugs (NSAIDs). While such liberalization has resulted in benefits for the public, this trend also

poses new problems. OTC medications have the potential for becoming important yet hidden components of a patient's drug regimen. Even if the physician takes a very careful medication history (a practice increasingly slighted in the ever-shortening office visit routine), the patient is often not prodded to include drugs taken without a prescription. Patients often fail to volunteer such information in the mistaken belief that if a drug is available over the counter, its effects cannot be serious enough to warrant mentioning it to the physician.

Yet such omissions can be troublesome. In the realm of psychoactive substances, a variety of OTC sleep remedies contain antihistamines such as diphenhydramine (e.g., Benadryl), which can exert powerful sedating and anticholinergic effects in older patients. Because of the capacity of anticholinergic drugs to reduce secretions, they are a common constituent of many cold and allergy preparations as well. The increasingly widespread sale of NSAIDs over the counter has raised concerns about the capacity of these drugs to raise blood pressure and reduce renal function, especially in elderly patients, in addition to their prodigious capacity to cause gastropathy that often results in hemorrhage. In addition, both histamine receptor antagonists and NSAIDs have been cited as rare causes of confusion in elderly individuals.[15]

Preparations containing iron have long been favored "tonics" of the elderly and are widely advertised in numerous forms. However, overall, their use probably does more harm than good. An older person consuming an adequate diet should need little or no iron supplementation, and supplementary iron (whether received over the counter or prescribed by a physician without an adequate workup) can actually be counterproductive if it masks a treatable underlying cause. One worrisome example of this is early-stage colon malignancy for which iron deficiency anemia could provide a warning in time for resection and cure; but this may be hidden if ongoing blood loss is merely treated by iron supplementation without attempt at diagnosis. Reliance on vitamin supplements or other "tonics" to treat fatigue, lethargy, loss of libido, or related symptoms should be considered a possible indication that the actual underlying cause may be depression or another medical problem that could be treated more appropriately.

Prevelance of Psychotropic Drug Use

Among therapeutic drug classes, psychotics are prescribed to a disproportionately large percentage of elderly patients,[16] which raises a number of questions. The elderly are more vulnerable to the side effects of all drugs, psychotics in particular, because of changes in pharmacodynamic processes in the central nervous system (CNS) (see Chapter 4) and in the pharmacokinetic processes of distribution, metabolism, and excretion (see Chapter 5). In addition, drug dependence is a risk with particular classes of drugs such as benzodiazepines, and in only a small number of cases is a stop date noted.[17,18] Finally, excessive and inappropriate use of antipsychotics, as well as benzodiazepines—particularly for elderly patients in nursing homes and acute care hospitals—poses the risk of specific adverse reactions, discussed later.

Because older patients are likely to take many more medications than their younger counterparts, the chance that an elderly individual will be taking more than one medication with similar side effects increases, as does the risk of adverse drug interactions. In a study comparison of a nursing home population with a comparable number of community-dwelling ambulatory patients, 60% of nursing home residents and 23% of community dwellers were prescribed drugs with anticholinergic effects, and high proportions of patients in each population (but more in the nursing home group) received three or more of these medications concomitantly.[19] These findings suggest that prescribers did not choose selectively from available psychotics in a given class, with attention to the illness/drug profile of the individual patient to minimize rather than contribute to additive anticholinergic side effects.

Potentially inappropriate use of psychotropic medications by the elderly may have improved recently, given the attention this issue has received in the last two decades. However, recent data from the second half of the 1990s suggest that use of potentially suboptimal psychotropic agents (e.g., amitriptyline and long-acting benzodiazepines) continue to be among the most prevalent inappropriate drug regimens prescribed for the elderly.[20,21]

Psychotropic Prescribing Practices in Selected Settings

The National Medical Care Surveys (NAMCS) indicate that almost half of all visits to physicians resulting in diagnosis of mental disorder were to nonpsychiatrists and that the largest users of nonspecialized "psychiatric" services were women over 65.[22] Other national data reveal that one-third of all office visits of elderly patients involve prescription of one or more drugs with psychiatric effects that were either intended or unintended.[23,24]

The rate of benzodiazepine prescribing increases significantly with age.[25] Although these drugs may be associated with serious side effects of sedation and impaired cognition in older people, their prescription is often suboptimal in outpatient settings. Dosage and choice of drug are often inappropriate (e.g., continuing usage of hypnotics with a very long half-life). U.S. data comparing drug use in over 2000 ambulatory elderly persons point to several important changes in consumption trends: use of hypnotic drugs declined from 8.5 to 6.3%; use of long-acting hypnotics decreased somewhat, and use of shorter-acting agents increased; prescribing long half-life benzo-diazepines decreased as did use of nearly all products containing barbiturates.[26]

Hospital Inpatients

National surveys of drug use in the United States focus on the ambulatory elderly, and public attention and scrutiny often highlight nursing home residents. Yet the use of psychotropic drugs by elderly people in the hospital setting also merits continuing study and clinical attention because patients over 65, who represent just 14% of the population, account for about 40% of hospital days in the United States.[27]

A review of prescribing practices for haloperidol in the general hospital found that patients receiving this antipsychotic drug were most often elderly (mean age of 66), were seriously ill, had longer lengths of stay, and were prescribed this drug primarily to manage severe agitation. Most elderly haloperidol recipients did not have a pretreatment psychiatric consultation; those who did, however, were more likely to have a positive response to the drug.[28] Over twice as many elderly patients receive antipsychotics in the hospital than receive them as outpatients (31% and 16%, respectively).[29] This is often the result of automatic orders for medications for insomnia or postoperative behavioral disturbances that are written on an "as needed" basis whenever an older patient is hospitalized—a tradition that persists despite its irrationality.[30]

Nursing Home Residents

Increasing attention has been drawn to the nursing home as a particularly important, problematic, and interesting setting for medication and the elderly. Each year the number of older persons in the United States who reside in nursing homes increases, and the utilization of acute-care hospitals declines. As a result, on any day in the United States, more elderly people are in nursing homes (currently approaching two million) than in acute-care facilities.[31] The progressive reduction in length of hospital stay for the older person has resulted in an increase in the acuteness and severity of illnesses cared for in nursing homes. However, until recently, these settings have not been included prominently in most physician training programs or in clinical research. Many physicians and other healthcare professionals are still able to complete their training with little or no systematic exposure to a long-term care facility, and research on healthcare interventions and delivery still largely ignores these complex institutions and those who reside in them.

Ironically, although nursing home residents represent the most frail elderly with the most complex medical problems, they often receive intense pharmacologic therapy with only minimal physician input and supervision. Focus on the characteristics of nursing home drug use have, in general, found very high levels of use of psychoactive medications, even in patients for whom CNS disease was not a primary indication for nursing home admission.[32–34]

In recent decades, the number of nursing home residents has risen from 2.5 to 5% of the U.S. population over 65.[35] Frequent use of psychotropic drugs in nursing homes is well documented, occurring for as many as one third to three quarters of long-term care residents.[32–34] Prescribing of antipsychotics in particular varies with the prescriber's nursing home practice: the more beds visited, the more prescriptions issued. The prevalence of antipsychotic drug use varies widely among homes, but correspondence exists between increased usage and nursing home size. Findings such as these led to the conclusion that neuroleptics were often being prescribed for institutionalized elderly patients more to induce sleep and manage confusion and nighttime disturbance than to treat a specific diagnosis.[36]

Estimating the prevalence of psychiatric disturbance in nursing homes is often difficult, and available reports vary greatly. Although assessments by investigators in one study found that 85% of nursing home residents had diagnoses of psychiatric disorders (for which psychotropic treatment might be appropriate), the records contained no mention of psychiatric diagnosis in two-thirds of these cases.[37] Before the mandated federal guidelines of 1987 (discussed later), psychotropic drug prescription for nursing home residents was generally unaccompanied by documentation of either symptoms or mental disorder[38,39]; while the proportion appears to have improved since the implementation of these guidelines, many residents on psychotropic medications still lack documented indications.[40]

Although psychotropic dosage is also high in alternative care settings such as rest homes, more critical concerns in this setting are lack of medical supervision, poor documentation of patient status, and low staff competency—all of which can lead to excessive use (for example, use of two or more neuroleptics concurrently).[41] The high PRN use of these drugs, lack of a stop-date on prescriptions, and chronic use without meaningful clinical review have all been observed in several surveys of long-term care facility drug use.[42,43]

Approaches to Improving Prescription Practices

The last 20 to 30 years have witnessed the emergence of several approaches to improving prescribing practices and providing the most effective and least burdensome pharmacologic treatment for the elderly. These approaches include nursing home regulatory and educational models, definition of drug utilization and "appropriateness" measures, and closer attention to medication withdrawal.

Prescribing Regulations in Nursing Homes

For decades, reports in both scientific publications and the lay media alleged overuse of psychoactive medications, particularly neuroleptics, as "chemical restraints."[44] Their primary goal was alleged to be sedation of nursing home residents so that they would be less difficult to manage and could consequently reduce demands on staff time. Despite emergence of the field of geriatric psychopharmacology and publication of numerous recommendations urging judicious use of such drugs, in the 1980s federal regulators perceived that excessive use had not diminished and argued that more stringent controls were necessary. The Institute of Medicine also highlighted excessive or inappropriate use of antipsychotics and tranquilizers, suggesting low quality of care.[45] In 1990, as a result of longstanding concern over misuse of these drugs, neuroleptics became the first drug class to have their appropriate and inappropriate use defined and enforced by the federal government in a given setting.

Earlier legislation—the Omnibus Budget Reconciliation Act (OBRA) of 1987—contained new regulations that for the first time defined acceptable and unacceptable indications for the use of neuroleptic medications for elderly residents of nursing homes. Based partially on Institute of Medicine recommendations, Congress also mandated a uniform resident assessment system in nursing homes. Begun in 1990, this assessment process included guidelines and criteria for using and monitoring psychotropic drugs.[46]

These federal regulations also mandated assessment and screening of nursing home patients to identify undiagnosed psychiatric illness, particularly depression and psychosis that might be amenable to pharmacotherapy or other treatment, if identified. However, even greater concern focused on the problem of overuse of sedating medications in nursing home residents, particularly those with cognitive impairment. Specifically prohibited was the use of any psychotropic drug or physical restraints "administered for purposes of discipline or convenience and not required to treat the resident's medical symptoms.'' For all patients prescribed neuroleptics, regular attempts to reduce the dose and provide behavioral interventions were required in an effort to discontinue the drugs, unless this approach was not feasible clinically. Acceptable use of neuroleptics requires the presence of specific indications, including behavior that poses a threat to the patient or to others. By contrast, unacceptable indications include merely annoying behavior that does not pose such a risk. Measures also required that reduced use of neuroleptic medications not be accompanied by a corresponding increase in the use of physical restraints to manage disruptive patients.

Calls for reduced use of sedating medications of all kinds for the elderly have often been met with concern about potential ''breakouts'' of agitated behavior among nursing home residents. These fears have generally not been borne out, at the level of institutions or of individual patients. However, implementation of these requirements on a large scale nationwide did provide an example of an ongoing problem at the interface between regulation and clinical care: the absence of a clear plan for systematic surveillance or evaluation of the effects of the new regulations, even when such follow-up would have been both feasible and useful. This massive regulatory transformation of pharmacotherapy for large numbers of geriatric nursing home patients throughout the country during this period was one of the largest uncontrolled, unsupervised clinical experiments in the nation's history. Fortunately, a number of investigators mounted their own studies of the effects of these regulations, and results proved surprisingly reassuring.[47,48] Use of neuroleptic drugs decreased substantially following implementation of the new regulations, without evidence of widespread chaos or patient harm.

Advantages of the Institutional Setting

Although nursing homes may be uniquely susceptible to regulatory control, they also offer a set of attributes that make them fertile settings for quality improvement efforts in geriatric prescribing, particularly in relation to psychoactive drugs. First, although physician involvement is often minimal, there is provision for regular periodic review of both drug regimens and their effectiveness by prescribers, which does not occur as systematically in the outpatient setting. Second, these facilities are required by law to be staffed with nurses and serviced by pharmacists who potentially can serve vital surveillance roles in monitoring drug regimens. However, some critics argue that the demands of nursing home staff drive a large proportion of psychoactive drug prescribing by physicians, through requests by nurses and aides for what has been called ''chemical crowd-control.'' Managing agitated patients in the face of limited staffing can be daunting, and staffing constraints may lie behind many such requests for pharmacologic solutions. Ironically, even though monthly review by a consultant pharmacist was mandated by the Health Care Financing Administration (HCFA) as early as 1974 for all Medicare-licensed long-term care facilities, this surveillance apparently did not adequately control the high-use levels of tranquilizing medications, resulting in the imposition of stricter federal regulations through additional federal requirements years later.[47,48]

In addition to the continuous presence of healthcare professionals who may be well situated to monitor the need for medications, the long-term care facility at its best can also provide surveillance of these effects. In the nursing home, residents can be observed around the clock, performing activities of daily living alone and in interaction with their peers. This can offer enormous advantages over the often chaotic and unsupervised outpatient setting, making it possible to define therapeutic goals and determine whether they are being met as well as to detect drug side effects. Quality improvement programs in some nursing homes have begun to take advantage of these opportunities to maximize the benefit-risk relationship in prescribing for the frail elderly, although this approach is still far from common.

Such settings also hold the opportunity to attempt cautious, safe withdrawal of medications that may no longer be needed—an important aspect of ongoing drug regimen review for the elderly. For example, whether or not a previously agitated patient still requires neuroleptic therapy is often not clear, or whether a complex and potentially troublesome regimen of antihypertensive medications can be adjusted to reduce the symptoms it may be causing. Such withdrawal can be performed much more readily and safely in an environment of round-the-clock professional supervision. In an era of managed care, as capitation increases the economic incentive to reassess all forms of therapy, such drug regimen review and withdrawal may receive a level of attention previously thought unattainable.

Educational Approaches to Prescribing in Nursing Homes

Other nonregulatory approaches to improving the use of psychoactive drugs in these settings include a model built on the concept of academic "detailing."[49,50] This model is based on the premise that an impressive amount of prescribing-practice change occurs because sales representatives of pharmaceutical companies interact one-on-one with physicians in their offices to influence their use of specific drugs, even though the interactions are geared primarily to increasing the sales of a given company's products. The academic detailing model is based on the notion that such effective behavior-change strategies can work equally well in the service of medical-school-based, scientifically driven information about optimal prescribing.

Originally developed in outpatient settings, this approach was modified for the special needs of geriatric psychopharmacology and implemented and rigorously evaluated in controlled trials in nursing homes in Massachusetts and Tennessee.[51]

In the Massachusetts study, 12 typical long-term care facilities were randomly assigned to receive an experimental educational intervention of academic detailing or to serve as controls. Psychoactive drug use for each patient in all facilities was recorded, and residents were given a detailed, functional, and cognitive assessment. In the experimental nursing homes, educational outreach sessions were conducted with nurses and aides separately, including special sessions for staff working the night shift. Physicians who prescribed psychoactive medications heavily were seen in their offices for individual educational visits. All sessions were conducted by a clinical pharmacist with experience in long-term care, based on a curriculum developed by geriatricians. A series of color "un-advertisements" were used to summarize the best available current information on rational use of neuroleptics, benzodiazepines and other hypnotics, and antidepressants. Significant reductions were achieved in the use of the "counter-detailed" medications, including long-acting benzodiazepines, neuroleptics, highly anticholinergic antidepressants, and antihistamines used as hypnotics. In the postintervention follow-up, blinded reassessment of residents in these facilities revealed several changes. The most striking was a significant improvement in memory in patients in the experimental homes who had been taking neuroleptics prior to the intervention.

Collaborative Care Models

A related approach to improving the use of psychoactive drugs by the elderly has been developed for use in primary care settings. This approach employs collaborating personnel to support the primary care physician's management of depression to increase the quality of prescribed treatments, patient compliance, and clinical outcomes. Although earlier models have been successful, they were limited by the fact that they employed psychiatrists as the collaborating personnel and required a generally high level of intensity.[52]

Subsequent refinements attempted to increase the feasibility and cost efficiency of these collaborative care models by using less highly trained personnel as care managers. One model for quality improvement in the care of elderly depressed patients was recently tested in the IMPACT trial (Improving Mood and Promoting Access to Collaborative Treatment), an intervention shown to be significantly more effective than usual care at improving both the quality and outcomes of prescribed depression treatments.[53]

Drug Use Review and "Appropriateness" Measures

A number of trends in healthcare have coalesced to increase enthusiasm for review of all drug regimens in both ambulatory and institutional settings to determine their clinical appropriateness. This needed review has been energized, in part, by the increasing proliferation of computer-based drug dispensing, and reimbursement programs that make automated surveillance of the drug regimens of thousands or even millions of individuals possible.[54] This approach has been encouraged by the concurrent development of the quality improvement movement in medicine, which strives to define optimal, evidence-based care and move clinical decisions in that direction. Such efforts have also been fueled by the proliferation of managed care and capitated payment arrangements in which all medical care for an individual is provided in exchange for a single, fixed, annual compensation. Not surprisingly, the elderly are a population of particular concern in this area for a number of reasons: they consume the largest number of medications; they are at greater risk for complications of drug therapy; and they are disproportionately represented in Medicaid and nursing home programs, both of which have been in the forefront in developing large computer-based programs to track medication use (initially for reimbursement purposes).

The maturation of clinical geriatric pharmacology as a discipline in its own right set the stage for creation of standards of "appropriate" versus "inappropriate" drug therapy for the elderly. Data from randomized clinical trials or rigorous observational studies are often not adequate to quantify the risks and benefits of specific regimens in the elderly; the consensus of experts provides a readily available, if less ideal, alternative basis for such determinations. This approach has been used to identify specific kinds of prescribing to be avoided for elderly patients. For example, one set of appropriateness measures developed for use in nursing homes defined the use of specific agents as inappropriate in older institutionalized patients. When these criteria were applied to actual drug utilization data on nursing home residents, over 40% of patients were found to be taking one or more "inappropriate" prescriptions.[55]

Advocates of such an approach argue that even in the absence of specific clinical trial data describing the effects of a given drug in the elderly, the best available alternative is the opinion of experts on what constitutes appropriate drug use. In contrast, skeptics argue that apart from a modest number of obvious examples, judging the clinical appropriateness of any given prescription on the basis of a computerized database of orders is difficult without being able to evaluate the unique clinical situation of a particular patient. Still others object that many drug utilization review algorithms are based on "potentially problematic" drug interactions or drug-disease interactions that may be of theoretical concern but often do not produce actual harm in many real-life clinical situations. Despite these concerns, computer-based drug-regimen review, particularly for older patients, represents a promising first step in quality improvement programs. The increasing automation of drug utilization data can set the stage for truly beneficial screening of prescriptions to reduce the risk of severe adverse events or of potentially lethal drug or drug-allergy interactions. A major agenda for this field in coming years will consist of the development of generalizable, evidence-based rules for such algorithms to minimize their potential for confusion and enhance their utility for patients. A major step forward in this direction is the ACOVE project (Assessing the Care Of Vulnerable Elders), which produced a comprehensive set of evidence-based recommendations for the care of a wide range of clinical conditions in the elderly.[56-58]

Medication Withdrawal

Just as the apartments of many elderly patients over the years become lined with photographs of grandchildren, souvenirs from trips, and memorabilia collected over decades, so the drug regimens of many older individuals can, over the years, become cluttered with years of accreted drug therapies, often initiated by multiple physicians. Many prescribers may have left only minimal records describing the reason for therapy, or none at all. One of the most useful acts the clinician can perform for elderly patients is a careful drug-by-drug review of each regimen. This is ideally accomplished when a new older patient is first seen, but it should be performed on an ongoing basis, at least annually. This can be difficult for a number of reasons. The most challenging is the dramatically shortened amount of time available for evaluating an elderly patient, even at the initial visit, in an increasingly cost-constrained environment. In addition, many physicians are reluctant to "rock the boat" in a stable patient taking multiple medications even if indications for some remain unclear and the dose for others seems higher than is desirable.

Despite this, compelling reasons argue against a "don't rock the boat" perspective. First, even if a patient appears stable on numerous medications of dubious purpose, knowing whether an existing level of fatigue, occasional forgetfulness, or gait instability represents a side effect of an unneeded drug is not possible. Second, between visits, patients may well develop an intercurrent illness such as influenza or gastroenteritis, causing hypovolemia that can lead to acutely reduced metabolism and excretion of some of these drugs, which can render a useless but "innocent" drug immediately problematic. Third, even the most cost-conscious managed care executive will realize that a few extra minutes spent discontinuing a long-acting benzodiazepine or lowering an excessive dose of an antihypertensive can be highly cost effective if such action prevents a fall that can result in a fractured hip or obviates the need for a costly workup for mistakenly diagnosed dementia.

Common Side Effects of Psychotropic Drug Use

As people age, they are increasingly likely to experience side effects of drugs of all kinds (Table 2.1). The elderly are more vulnerable to the adverse drug reactions of psychotropic drugs than younger adults because of several age-related factors. First, altered sensitivity to psychotropic drugs associated with age-related changes in the CNS causes some older people to experience toxicity from doses routinely prescribed for younger adults whereas others may not respond at all to therapeutic doses. Second, the body's ability to metabolize and excrete drugs tends to decrease with age, leading to higher levels of unmetabolized drug at the receptor site and a prolonged sojourn of drugs in the body. Third, older people are more likely to take a variety of drugs for treatment of age-related medical illness, and the interaction among medical, OTC, and psychotropic drugs can create important problems.[59] Each of these factors—altered sensitivity to drugs, altered drug disposition, and polypharmacy—alone or together may be responsible for the increased incidence and sensitivity to

Table 2.1.   Side Effects of Psychoactive Drugs in Older People

Drug Effect	Symptoms
Decreased CNS arousal level	Sedation, apathy, fatigue, withdrawal, depressed mood, disinhibition, confusion
Peripheral anticholinergic blockade	Dry mouth, constipation, atonic bladder, blurry vision
Central anticholinergic blockade	Confusion, disorientation, agitation, assaultiveness, visual hallucinosis
α-Adrenergic blockade and central pressor blockade	Orthostatic hypotension
Dopaminergic blockade	Extrapyramidal symptoms, tardive dyskinesia

psychotropic drug side effects associated with aging.

Sedation

In older patients, the effects of hypnotics (prescribed or OTC) may persist into the next day so that the patient is drowsy or even asleep for part of the day.[60,61] Daytime sedation commonly contributes to nighttime insomnia, thus perpetuating the need for sedating drugs at bedtime. In older patients, daytime sedation may be associated with a sense of isolation, helplessness, depression, and confusion. The problem of daytime sedation from psychotropic drugs is compounded when other drugs with sedative effects are also prescribed.

Confusion

Psychotropic drugs may produce confusion, disorientation, restlessness, and forgetfulness. Among older medical or surgical patients, severe confusional states may result from the interaction of psychotropic drugs with medical drugs. Confusion may also begin as restlessness, difficulty concentrating, and rapidly declining recall of recent information in the older person. In more severe cases, agitation, misidentification of familiar people, wandering, and combativeness may occur. This syndrome intensifies in unfamiliar surroundings: older patients who have been recently hospitalized, or have

moved, or have entered a nursing home are particularly susceptible. Confusion is also often worse at night and may be exacerbated by sedating drugs.[62]

Confusion, disorientation, and agitation associated with psychotropic drug use may be seen in their most severe forms in the hospital intensive care unit. Here the older patient may try to get out of bed or pull out tubes, catheters, and sutures; or become frightened, paranoid, and combative. Repetitive stereotyped behavior, delirium, and visual and tactile hallucinations may also occur. In severe cases of drug toxicity, symptoms of confusion, disorientation, and agitation may be life-threatening if an older person becomes unable to eat or participate in self-care activities or becomes self-destructive. In the hospital, these symptoms may interfere with medical and nursing care, and the patient may become unmanageable. In the nursing home, the resident may assault other residents, staff, and family members or become self-mutilating.

Orthostatic Hypotension

In the elderly patient, orthostatic hypotension is a frequent side effect of some neuroleptics and antidepressants. This condition may precipitate falls that result in fractures and may induce stroke or even myocardial infarction; patients with cervical osteoarthritis or low cardiac output seem especially susceptible. Orthostatic hypotensive episodes are especially common at night when the patient may awaken to urinate.

Falls and Fractures

It has long been known that psychotropic medications can increase an older person's risk of falls and fractures. Risk factors include dose-dependent increases in sedation, confusion, cognitive deficits, ataxia, diplopia, and vertigo. The relationship between benzodiazepine use and falls,[63] as well as hip fractures, has repeatedly been confirmed.[64]

However, the clinical implications of such findings have been complicated by the fact that benzodiazepines given for psychiatric indications may be quite beneficial for some patients. For this reason, subsequent research has sought to further identify particular agents, together with their half-lives, dosages, and durations of use, that may be especially dangerous and therefore avoided.[65-67] Examining the risks of hip fracture posed by other psychotropic classes is also important, because these classes may sometimes be substituted for benzodiazepines. Even psychotropic classes thought to be "safer" in the elderly, such as newer antidepressants[68] and newer, nonbenzodiazepine sedative-hypnotics,[69] can significantly increase the risks of falls and hip fractures.

Cardiac Side Effects

Alterations in the rate, rhythm, and force of myocardial contraction may occur with advanced age or with increasing plasma drug levels, which may be a consequence of old age. These effects are more hazardous in the patient with preexisting cardiac pathology, and so, because older people tend to be more likely to have cardiac disease than younger adults, the vulnerability to serious cardiac toxicity from psychotropic drugs increases. These effects occur most commonly with antidepressants but have also been reported with lithium and neuroleptics. Alterations in heart rate and rhythm are due to the effect of some psychotropic drugs on the cardiac conduc-

tion system and are often reflected in characteristic ECG changes (see Chapters 9 and 12 for more detailed discussion).

Extrapyramidal Symptoms

Extrapyramidal signs and symptoms caused by neuroleptic drugs are often indistinguishable from those caused by idiopathic Parkinson's disease.[70-72] These include tremor, rigidity, and akinesia or bradykinesia, effects characterized by decreased mobility, energy and speech, and mask-like facies. Because the older akinetic patient may appear apathetic, withdrawn, and depressed, bradykinesia is often misdiagnosed as depression. In contrast, another extrapyramidal side effect, akathisia, resembles agitation. Elderly patients with drug-induced akathisia cannot remain still; they alternately sit and stand frequently and pace. Such patients may have "restless legs" and describe their muscles as "tense" or "jittery," or they may have choreiform movements of the hands and trunk. Because akathisia may be misinterpreted as agitation, the older patient is sometimes given an increased dose of neuroleptic, which can worsen symptoms. Other parkinsonian symptoms produced by neuroleptics resemble those of the clinical illness, i.e., shuffling gait, pill-rolling tremor at rest, and cogwheel rigidity. In an older patient with preexisting Parkinson's disease, drug-induced parkinsonian side effects aggravate the movement disorder and may be disabling. Large population-based observational studies have shown increased risk of initiating a drug appropriate for the treatment of idiopathic Parkinson's disease (e.g., levodopa) for patients taking neuroleptics, particularly high-potency agents such as haloperidol. This problem is also seen in older patients prescribed metoclopramide (Reglan), a drug used for gastrointestinal symptoms that is chemically related to the neuroleptics.[73]

Of particular concern is tardive dyskinesia, an extrapyramidal syndrome resulting from chronic neuroleptic use. Symptoms include repetitive involuntary motions, usually of the facial muscles. This can be particularly distressing for elderly patients because it can intensify already compromised movement and can seriously affect the ability to engage in social and daily activities. Tardive dyskinesia can occur after only brief use of neuroleptic drugs in older patients. Once symptoms have begun, cessation of the offending drug may not eliminate the problem and may even exacerbate it.

In addition to vigilance for these specific, more readily apparent adverse effects, keeping in mind that any homeostatic system under CNS control may be weakened by age and further weakened by drugs acting on the CNS is also important. This may include control, body sway, the thermoregulatory mechanism, and bowel and bladder control, all of which may be compromised by use of psychotropic drugs. The converse of psychoactive drugs causing somatic symptoms is the precipitation of brain-related symptoms by somatic therapies (Table 2.2). These, too, are myriad and include: the agitation or somnolence that can result in overreplacement or underreplacement of thyroid hormone; the lethargy, fatigue, and depression-like symptoms that can result from β-blockers used to treat hypertension or angina pectoris; or the hallucinations, nightmares, and delirium that can result

Table 2.2.   Examples of Drug-Induced Psychiatric Symptoms

Symptom	Possible Drug Cause
Sexual dysfunction	Thiazides, β-blockers
Hallucinations, psychosis	Levodopa, procainamide, corticosteroids
Confusion	Antidepressants, benzodiazepines, digoxin, antihistamines
Agitation	Bronchodilators (xanthines, β-agonists), "activating" antidepressants

from L-dopa used to treat idiopathic Parkinson's disease.

Ageism, Polypharmacy, and Adverse Drug Reactions

In assessing the possibility of an adverse drug event in an older patient, distinguishing between drug-induced illness and illness from other causes is critically important. It is almost never appropriate to consider a symptom in an older patient merely "a result of the normal aging process."[74] The mistaken belief that clinically troublesome symptoms result from old age per se has been called "ageism," a phrase coined to highlight its similarity to other terms such as sexism, racism, or antisemitism, in which a single demographic characteristic of an individual—whether it be gender, skin color, national origin, religion, or number of years since birth—is seen as a reliable marker for other characteristics of that person. Chronological age per se is not an adequate explanation of or cause for dementia, mood disorders, fatigue, or a host of somatic symptoms such as incontinence or shortness of breath. This erroneous belief can have the dangerous result of preventing an adequate diagnostic workup for a condition (such as depression or a secondary dementia) that could respond well to therapy.

The problem of ageism is particularly important in relation to the recognition of adverse drug events, which may present with symptoms readily mistaken by the unwary for "the problems of normal aging." The detection and treatment of drug-induced illness—*preferably by eliminating the offending drug rather than by treating the side effect with yet another medication*—can be among the most effective and rewarding interventions in all of geriatric practice. When an elderly patient or family member incorrectly attributes a treatable illness to aging is unfortunate; when this is done by a physician, it is inexcusable. The following proposition is a clinically useful overstatement: *Any new symptom in an older patient should be considered a possible drug side effect until proven otherwise.* Although this expectation will often not be borne out, such a posture is a helpful reminder to the clinician to consider possibilities that might otherwise be ignored.

Openness to the possibility of drug-induced illness should be paired with particular attention to "crossover" relationships between somatic and psychiatric treatments and symptoms (Table 2.3). A drug side effect may be fairly evident when the symptom is fatigue and the offending agent is a sedative/hypnotic. However, somatic symptoms are frequently caused by psychoactive drugs, just as CNS symptoms can be caused by somatic therapies. For example, anticholinergic side effects caused by a variety of psychoactive drugs (each discussed separately in more detail in the chapters that follow) illustrate the protean ways in which the effects of these drugs on the parasympathetic nervous system can present as symptoms that have nothing to do with the brain itself.[75] Psychoactive medications with strong anticholinergic side effects include low-potency neuroleptics such as thioridazine and chlorpromazine, tertiary amine tricyclic antidepressants such as amitriptyline or imipramine, as well as all of the antihistamines, which have become popular hypnotics because

of their low cost and OTC availability (particularly diphenhydramine).

Review of the vegetative functions managed by the parasympathetic nervous system makes clear how interference with this system by anticholinergic drugs can disrupt normal physiology and produce symptoms. Normal parasympathetic function makes possible, among other things, the secretion of saliva, intestinal motility, and contraction of the detrusor muscle of the bladder. Medications that interfere with such functions, even though their target organ may be the brain, can result in myriad symptoms throughout the body. Reduced salivary function causes dry mouth, problems with denture use, difficulty swallowing, and reduced pleasure in eating. Interference with colonic motility can produce or exacerbate constipation, which in turn can result in a host of other problems, ranging from abdominal pain to fecal impaction. Impaired contraction of the detrusor muscle of the bladder can be particularly important in older men, in whom benign prostatic hypertrophy is common. In these patients, micturition is often accomplished only by strong contraction of the bladder muscle that is required to push urinary flow beyond the obstructing prostate. When an anticholinergic medication is added to the regimen and reduces the strength of such contraction, worsened prostatic symptoms can

Table 2.3.   Psychotropic Drug Use in the Elderly

- Inventory all medications, including nonpsychoactive drugs
- Screen the list to eliminate unnecessary or duplicative prescriptions
- Select drugs that are most appropriate for the elderly, affordable, and least likely to interact with other medications or comorbidity
- Define a clear indication for each prescribed medication and an assessable therapeutic goal
- Educate the patient about proper use and potential side effects of each drug
- Document each drug's effectiveness in achieving its desired therapeutic outcome; adjust regimen accordingly
- Monitor for adverse drug events, particularly those presenting as new symptoms
- Assess compliance and respond to noncompliance as needed
- Reassess regimen on an ongoing basis

Adapted from Avon J. Care Guide on Medications and the Elderly. Prepared for the American College of Physicians.

occur, including increased hesitancy and difficulty emptying the bladder and even acute urinary retention. Since Freud, psychiatrists have been trained to see intimate connections between genitourinary function and mental life, but in a given patient the pharmacologic association may remain obscure. The astute clinician must be prepared to attribute symptoms far from the brain to the use of medications for mood or sleep that had been directed primarily at the CNS.

A number of studies have reviewed hospital admissions to determine the frequency of drug-related problems that led to hospitalization. Estimates vary widely depending upon the population studied and criteria used, but most studies of admissions of patients over age 65 found medication-related admissions rates to be between 2% and 11%.[76,77] Studies of iatrogenic illness occurring in hospitalized patients have consistently identified drug side effects as the most common cause.[76] Many studies assessing the preventability of drug-related illness found that up to half of such events could have been prevented.[77] The risk of adverse reactions and interactions may increase further when drugs are prescribed PRN without adequate monitoring; older people living alone are more subject to harmful PRN-related interactions because of lack of supervision. The hospital emergency room is also a frequent site of adverse drug interactions.

In addition to the increased risk of adverse drug interactions in the elderly, drugs given to treat one disorder may exacerbate another. For example, β-blockers as a treatment for neuroleptic-resistant psychosis are contraindicated in the patient with asthma, congestive heart failure, or atrioventricular conduction defects. In older persons with multiple pathology, several conditions—cardiovascular, thyroid, or pulmonary, as well as electrolyte imbalance—may all be exacerbated by drugs taken to treat other disease.[78,79]

Nutritional Status and Drug Effects

Nutritional status can have important consequences for drug effects in some elderly patients, particularly those who are malnourished. At greatest risk of malnutrition are those severely incapacitated mentally or physically, socially isolated with chronic health problems, and those who lack good nutritional habits. Among psychogeriatric patients, 30% receive inadequate amounts of protein (indicated by low plasma albumin and serum transferring levels), a problem more prevalent among patients with dementia than those with psychosis.[80] Coingestion of specific foods may also affect the serum concentrations of psychotropic medications. For example, concomitant intake of grapefruit juice has been shown to raise concentrations of several drugs with psychotropic effects through inhibition of enzymes of the cytochrome P-450 system located in the intestinal wall.[81] In addition to altered plasma proteins, nutritional status may affect other physiological functions, which in turn may alter psychotropic drug effects. For example, urinary pH, often altered by diet or disease, can play an important role in the excretion of several psychotropics. Amitriptyline, desmethylimipramine, imipramine, and nortriptyline are excreted in greater concentration when the urine has an acidic pH than when it's alkaline.

Diet and nutritional status have direct relevance to prescribing monoamine oxidase inhibitors (MAOIs) (see Chapter 9). Although reluctance to use MAOIs for elderly patients because of fear of drug–food interactions may be somewhat exaggerated, the patient taking these drugs must avoid specific tyramine-rich foods such as aged cheese, pickled fish, yeast extracts, and broad-bean pods. Interaction of these foods with MAOIs may produce fatal hypertension or hyperthermia.

Compliance

Many perfectly conceived pharmacologic regimens do not achieve their goals because prescribers are unaware of the very high level of noncompliance that occurs with both acute and chronic drug regimens. Records of actual filled prescriptions make clear that how patients do (or do not) take their medications may bear strikingly little resemblance to what the physician intended.

Overall Compliance and Older Patients

In general, only scant evidence suggests that older age itself is a risk factor for noncompliance, although the complexity of the regimen is an important barrier to proper use. The use of three or more drugs a day places elderly people at particular risk for poor compliance.[82] Compliance with one regimen does not necessarily mean that a patient will comply with another, and physicians cannot estimate compliance behavior on the basis of past drug-use histories, particularly if "extra" drugs are found in the patient's home. Noncompliance may precipitate an increase in dose or addition of a new agent to obtain the desired therapeutic outcome in what is incorrectly thought to be a "treatment-resistant case."[83]

A particularly important insight has been the difference observed in drug use in controlled clinical trials compared with drug-taking behavior in the "real" world. For example, recent randomized controlled clinical trials among elderly populations with depression have been instrumental in showing that antidepressants alone, and especially in combination with psychotherapies, can significantly prevent or delay recurrence.[84] However, clinical trials are generally based in academically affiliated medical centers or conducted by experienced contract research organizations. By definition, they involve only physicians and patients who have volunteered to participate in these activities. Before the regimen begins, a lengthy form, signed by both patient and investigator, stipulates in detail what the new therapy is, its expected benefits, and its potential risks. Drug use is monitored frequently,

much more intensively than in normal practice, and surveillance of both desired and untoward drug effects is careful and frequent. Patients who consider dropping out of the study are often given special attention and urged to "stick it out" if no obvious harm is being experienced. Inevitably, these measures are pursued to a much lesser extent in routine clinical practice. The benefits and risks of a therapy are rarely described in the same detail as in a clinical trial, and surveillance of drug taking, therapeutic effects, and adverse outcomes is far less meticulous.

In addition to being a poor predictor of compliance behavior, the clinical trial—on which virtually all of our understanding of a drug's efficacy is based—may also be a poor predictor of a drug's outcome in routine care. The *efficacy* of a treatment is its best possible performance under ideal settings, usually as measured in a clinical trial. However, the *effectiveness* of that treatment is its performance in actual practice settings, which may be quite different. For example, TCAs and selective serotonin reuptake inhibitors (SSRIs) may be similar in efficacy in a controlled clinical-trial setting, in which doses of the former can be titrated through use of serum drug determinations to achieve ideal levels, and patients and physicians can be urged to remain in the trial despite side effects. However, in actual practice, where serum drug-level monitoring is far less complete and there is no study nurse urging the patient and physician to "treat through" side effects, patterns of compliance and therefore of drug effectiveness for the two antidepressant categories may well differ.

Compliance with antidepressants in the elderly poses another set of special problems. Medications for angina or arthritis generally produce symptomatic benefits at the time they are taken, making compliance less of a problem. Antihypertensive drugs, by contrast, virtually never produce any symptomatic benefit. While they promise prevention of catastrophic illness years in the future, they may also produce uncomfortable side effects that are very much in the present.[85] Antidepressant therapy in the elderly often represents an even more difficult compliance problem. Most of these drugs are unlikely to yield much therapeutic benefit in the early weeks of therapy but are likely to cause a variety of unpleasant side effects. All this occurs in patients who, by virtue of their underlying depression, are likely to have problems with somatization, hopelessness, and despair. Thus, in assessing apparent treatment failure in older patients prescribed antidepressants, poor compliance must be at the top of the differential diagnosis.

Types of Noncompliance

Three common forms of drug treatment noncompliance occur in the elderly: underuse, overuse, and alteration of schedules and doses. Underuse of drugs because of forgetting is common in older people and especially prevalent among those who are isolated or are cognitively impaired. Forgetting to take a dose of a drug is likelier if a patient takes several drugs, each with a different dosage schedule. Although the most common compliance problem seen in practice is the failure of the patient to take enough medication, in geriatric psychopharmacology the converse may also be seen. We ask patients to continue to take some prescribed medications (such as antidepressants or antihypertensives) that may make them feel sick because of side effects, but we expect them *not* to regularly take other basic medications (such as benzodiazepine hypnotics or tranquilizers) that may actually make them feel better, and, if discontinued, can precipitate uncomfortable symptoms. These are not intuitively obvious concepts, and the wise clinician will not expect these notions to come readily to patients. Because of this, overcompliance with some psychoactive drugs in the elderly can be a common and dangerous problem in drug-taking behavior.

Some older patients who are acutely ill may take more than the prescribed dose of a medication in the mistaken belief that more of the drug will speed their recovery. Deliberate overuse of prescription drugs, however, is relatively rare among the elderly. Older patients may also change the dose or administration time of their medications to accommodate their own daily schedule. A reduction in dose initiated by the patient to diminish side effects has been termed "intelligent noncompliance."[86] A common noncompliant behavior of the elderly is deliberate underuse of a prescribed drug. Some elderly patients may try to save money by lowering the dose or sharing medications. Others may save medications for future use by stopping a particular regimen early. Some may stop medications when symptoms abate, believing that the condition has been cured; others may discontinue medication if symptoms persist, believing it is not working. The latter may occur particularly if the onset of therapeutic action in the elderly is delayed for several weeks, as is often the case for antidepressants. This phenomenon shows the need for careful, consistent discussion with patients and/or their caregivers of drug-taking schedules and their purpose.

Techniques for Improving Compliance

Many factors may contribute to noncompliance in older patients.[87–89] These include inadequate information regarding the necessity for drug treatment, unclear prescribing directions, and an inadequate doctor–patient relationship. One common reason for noncompliance is that patients often are not clearly told the name and purpose of the medication. However, even patients who have this information may not be significantly more compliant than those who do not—a reminder that drug noncompliance is a complex phenomenon. Adherence to instructions may vary according to individual personality, site of care, health beliefs, the drug prescribed, the disease being treated, and the side effects experienced (Table 2.1).

The Patient–Doctor Relationship

Elderly patients often leave a physician's office without a clear understanding of what is expected of them. An excessively authoritarian approach by the healthcare provider can result in an encounter in which the patient feels inhibited and does not ask questions or report observations about a drug's effects. The authoritarian approach may also be ineffective in bringing about lifestyle changes and new health behaviors required by chronic illness and drug treatment. Communication with the patient is the best antidote to noncompliance. No medication should be started without a brief discussion of its purpose, expected effect, and potential side effects. In follow-up visits, appropriate compliance should not be assumed. On a regular basis, and at least once or twice each year, the patient should be asked to bring in all medications for a thorough review. On other occasions, it is often helpful to open a conversation on compliance in the following way: "I see you're taking a lot of different drugs. Sometimes patients on this many medications have trouble being sure that they take every dose. Does this ever happen to you?" This is a far more effective way to begin a discussion of compliance than the question, "You're taking all your pills, right?" or, even worse, avoiding the subject altogether.

The Health Belief Model

Much practical insight on compliance behavior has come from the health belief model developed nearly 30 years ago.[90] This formulation is based on the concept that how or even whether a patient follows the physician's instructions depends upon the patient's perception of a number of factors:

- Personal susceptibility to a given medical problem
- Severity of the consequences of that problem
- Potential benefit of a given health behavior (e.g., taking a prescription as directed)
- Barriers to engaging in that health behavior, which may be psychological, social, or economic.

Each of these areas can be touched on briefly in a concise discussion with the patient to clarify whether the patient has a problem in any of these domains.

Other Psychosocial Variables

A variety of mental disorders may themselves adversely affect the ability of elderly patients to comply with prescribed treatment regimens. Chief among these are dementia and other conditions that impair cognition. Such impairment can produce forgetfulness or confusion regarding doses and treatment schedules, which may be induced or exacerbated by drugs. Anxiety disorders and alcohol misuse in the elderly may also lead to noncompliance through similar mechanisms. Depressive symptoms are also emerging as an important cause of medication noncompliance in the elderly.[91] The mechanism by which depression could affect compliance may involve detrimental effects on adherence with preventive medications, including poor motivation, pessimism over the effectiveness of treatments, decrements in attention and memory, decreased self-care, and even intentional self-harm. In addition, depression has been associated with greater sensitivity to unpleasant side effects from medications.[92] Other psychosocial variables may affect a patient's compliance with medications. For example, poorly motivated patients comply poorly, and poor motivation may be a response to an unenthusiastic provider. Some elderly patients may not read, write, or understand enough English to understand prescribing directions. Other identifiable and potentially correctable factors are the patient's inability to schedule appointments, long waiting times, and the cost of treatment. The latter has been a source of increasing concern as more and more elderly Americans find it difficult to pay for their increasingly expensive drug regimens.[93] These mental disorders and psychosocial variables may be among the few modifiable factors that clinicians can influence and thereby increase a patient's adherence.

Decreasing Multiple Medications

An important factor contributing to drug treatment noncompliance in older people is the total number of times per day drugs must be taken. The more drugs taken and the more varied the doses and dosage schedules, the more noncompliance is likely to occur.[94] Thus, the single best way to enhance compliance is to prune the medication regimen rigorously of all but necessary medications. This has two added benefits. First, it will protect the patient from unnecessary side effects because a drug with no therapeutic value will, by definition, have a benefit-to-risk ratio of zero. Second, prudent reduction of the number of necessary medications will help contain costs, which will be of direct benefit to either the patient or the healthcare system itself. (A corollary of this statement is that a drug with no therapeutic benefit also has zero cost-effectiveness.)

Once the regimen has been stripped of all unnecessary medications, formulations should be prescribed that minimize the total number of medications taken each day and the number of times each day that medications must be taken. This can be accomplished by choosing combination products in appropriate dose ratios (as in the case of antihypertensive medications) or those that do not require numerous daily doses. The downside to the latter approach is that drugs requiring the fewest daily doses are often those with the longest half-lives, a feature that can present its own important pharmacokinetic problems in the elderly. The tradeoff between shorter-acting drugs, generally preferable in older patients, and the desire to reduce the number of daily doses must be resolved for each patient on a drug-by-drug basis.

A variety of aids are widely available to help the older patient on multiple drugs maintain good compliance.[95] These range from simple pillboxes that can be prefilled by the patient or a caregiver to more elaborate electronic devices such as electronic pill bottles that emit a loud beeping sound if the lid is not removed in a timely manner according to preprogramed instructions. The increasing versatility of computer and telecommunications hardware and software has led to experimental work on automated telephone systems for patients with memory impairment that can phone the patient at predetermined intervals with a reminder to take a particular dose. Given the decreasing cost of such interventions and the increase in resource use caused by noncompliance, such high-tech solutions to the problem of noncompliance are likely to become more common in the coming years.

Type of Dosage and Identification

A frequent source of confusion that impairs the recognition of noncompliance is the inability of the patient to identify the particular drug that he or she is taking. If asked, patients often respond that they are taking "a little white pill" or "a little yellow pill." Since many tablets and capsules have very similar appearances, it is not surprising that an older patient may misidentify a pill and take the wrong medication. Another source of confusion is the noninterchangeability of trade name and generic drugs; if different preparations of the same drug are prescribed by different physicians, the patient may not recognize the duplication, which can lead to overdose. Conversely, because pharmacies or health plans frequently change the supplier of a given product to get the best price, patients may find that their gray and red capsule is now black and green. This can result in overuse (if the patient does not recognize that the two drugs are the same and takes both) or in underuse (if the patient feels the wrong medication was dispensed, instead of the "usual pill"). It is useful, therefore, for the caregiver to check all drugs at periodic intervals.

Computerized Models

The rapidly increasing prevalence of automated prescription records could offer an ideal opportunity for detecting noncompliance. Computerized pharmacy refill records make it possible to determine with speed, accuracy, and efficiency when patients are failing to refill prescriptions at the appropriate times. Such accurate and cost-efficient means of assessing compliance may be extremely important in light of evidence that the accuracy of patients' self-reports of compliance behavior may be extremely poor.[96] Compliance assessed through automated refill data can then set the stage for targeted interventions designed to address such noncompliance before it results in adverse clinical consequences.

Directions and Specificity

The search for better compliance and therapeutic outcome should start with addressing several specific questions before prescribing a medication for an elderly patient:

- Does the patient have sensory, cognitive, or literacy problems?
- How many physicians does this patient consult?
- Can the patient manage and tolerate an additional drug?
- How should the standard adult dose be modified?
- Which side effects are likely to occur? Which interactions?
- What dosage form is best for this patient? Can the patient administer the dosage form selected?
- Does the patient live alone? Is special packaging required for this patient? Is other assistance necessary to arrange or supervise the drug regimen?
- Can the patient afford the regimen prescribed?
- What monitoring is necessary to evaluate outcomes and adjust the regimen accordingly?

Once this process is complete, information and its exchange are key to drug compliance. Good communication enables the provider to work toward achieving effective treatment in several ways: by evaluating prior and current response and expected compliance characteristics; by augmenting understanding of the patient's health status, beliefs, motivation, and socioeconomic status; and by heightening the patient's understanding of the goals, promises, and limitations of a particular regimen. Communication is also necessary to help motivate and encourage patients to participate fully in an agreed-upon regimen in an informed and intelligent manner. For these efforts, emphasis is on removing barriers and implementing enabling strategies.

Instructions should be given in language the patient is most likely to understand. Counseling, either individually or in groups, is one of the most effective strategies for achieving compliance. Adherence may be heightened by a combination of specific written and verbal instructions together with easy-to-use packaging. Imprecise instructions (e.g., "take as directed") and instructions not printed in large letters are more likely to result in poor compliance.

Conclusion

Optimal use of drugs by the elderly, particularly psychotropic medications, will be an increasingly important issue as the population over 65 (and especially over 85) continues to increase dramatically. The basic principles delineated in this chapter can aid rational drug prescription: careful evaluation before use begins and frequent monitoring thereafter; knowledge of age-related pharmacokinetic and pharmacodynamic changes to provide a foundation for understanding the increased vulnerability of older people to the side effects and adverse reactions to psychotropic drugs; surveillance for drug-induced illness; awareness of compliance behavior; and heightened attention to goals for the older person's overall functional status. Taken together, these elements can help clarify each patient's specific psychotropic drug needs and how those needs can best be met.

This overview of drug prescribing and taking makes clear that medication use in the older population can be one of the most powerful determinants of geriatric health and illness, depending upon how intelligently such therapy is prescribed. The blessing and the curse of geriatric pharmacotherapy is that older patients are far more likely than their younger counterparts to have illnesses that can be treated effectively or even prevented by the wise use of drugs; yet, at the same time, they are at a substantially greater risk for illnesses caused by such intervention. Several specific considerations will enable the astute clinician to maximize the benefit that can be achieved from drug therapy in older patients:

- Becoming familiar with the altered physiology that is seen even with healthy aging, as well as the more severe changes that come with disease in old age
- Using drug therapy—particularly psychoactive drug therapy—only after a thorough diagnostic workup clarifies that such an approach is appropriate
- Ensuring that symptoms in an older patient are never just written off as "the result of old age" without seeking a clearer and potentially treatable underlying cause, particularly one that might be easily reversed, such as a drug side effect
- Choosing the agent and the dose appropriate for the altered characteristics of the geriatric patient
- Identifying at the outset clear subjective or behavioral goals for the use of each psychoactive medication prescribed and periodically performing a system-

atic assessment of how well a given drug is meeting these goals
- Closely monitoring how the patient is using the prescribed medication, being alert to the frequent problems of poor compliance

Consideration of these issues will be well worth the modest time it requires and will enable the clinician to wield the powerful double-edged risk-benefit sword to provide the greatest benefit and least risk of harm to the older patient.

References

1. Grossberg GT, Grossberg JA. Epidemiology of psychotherapeutic drug use in older adults. *Clin Geriatr Med* 1998;14(1):1–5.
2. Kaufman DW, Kelly JP, Rosenberg L, et al. Recent patterns of medication use in the ambulatory adult population of the United States: The Slone Survey. *JAMA* 2002;287(3):337–344.
3. Stoehr GP, Ganguli M, Seaberg EC, et al. Over-the-counter medication use in an older rural community: the MoVIES Project. *J Am Geriatr Soc* 1997;45(2):158–165.
4. Hanlon JT, Fillenbaum GG, Ruby CM, et al. Epidemiology of over-the-counter drug use in community dwelling elderly: United States perspective. *Drugs & Aging* 2001;18(2):123–131.
5. Lassila HC, Stoehr GP, Ganguli M, et al. Use of prescription medications in an elderly rural population: the MoVIES Project. *Ann Pharmacother* 1996;30:589–595.
6. Schneeweiss S, Walker AM, Glynn RJ, et al. Outcomes of reference drug pricing for angiotensin-converting enzyme inhibitors. *N Engl J Med* 2002; 346:822–829.
7. Luber MP, Meyers BS, Williams-Russo PG, et al. Depression and service utilization in elderly primary care patients. *Am J Geriatr Psychiatry* 2001; 9:169–176.
8. Ünützer J, Simon G, Belin TR. Care for depression in HMO patients aged 65 and older. *J Am Geriatr Soc* 2000;48:871–878.
9. Ünützer J, Katon W, Russo J. Patterns of care for depressed older adults in a large-staff model HMO. *Am J Geriatr Psychiatry* 1999;7:235–243.
10. Schappert SM. Ambulatory care visits to physician offices, hospital outpatient departments, and emergency departments: United States, 1997. *Vital Health Stat* 1999;143(13):i–iv, 1–39.
11. Sorensen L, Foldspang A, Gulmann NC, et al. Determinants for the use of psychotics among nursing home residents. *Int J Geriatr Psychiatry* 2001;16(2):147–154.
12. Wancata J, Benda N, Meise U, et al. Use of psychotropic drugs in gynecological, surgical, and medical wards of general hospitals. *Int J Psychiatry Med* 1998;28(3):303–314.
13. Aparasu RR, Mort JR, Sitzman S. Psychotropic

prescribing for the elderly in office-based practice. *Clin Ther* 1998;20(3):603–616.

14. Olfson M, Marcus S, Druss B, et al. National trends in outpatient treatment of depression. *JAMA* 2002;287:203–209.

15. McEvoy GK, ed. *American Hospital Formulary Service drug information.* Bethesda, MD: American Society of Health System Pharmacias, 1995.

16. Mort JR, Aparasu RR. Prescribing potentially inappropriate psychotropic medications to the ambulatory elderly. *Arch Intern Med* 2000; 160(18):2825–2831.

17. Weinert CR. Epidemiology of psychiatric medication use in patients recovering from critical illness at a long-term acute-care facility. *Chest* 2001;119(2):547–553.

18. Egan M, Moride Y, Wolfson C, et al. Long-term continuous use of benzodiazepines by older adults in Quebec: prevalence, incidence and risk factors. *J Am Geriatr Soc* 2000;48(7):811–816.

19. Blazer DG II, Federspiel CF, Ray WA, et al. The risk of anticholinergic toxicity in the elderly: a study of prescribing practices in two populations. *J Gerontol* 1983;38(1):31–35.

20. Zhan C, Sangl J, Bierman AS, et al. Potentially inappropriate medication use in the community-dwelling elderly. *JAMA* 2001;286:2823–2829.

21. Pitkala KH, Strandberg TE, Tilvis RS. Inappropriate drug prescribing in home-dwelling, elderly patients. *Arch Intern Med* 2002;162: 1707–1712.

22. Schurman RA, Kramer PD, Mitchel JB. The hidden mental health network: treatment of mental illness by nonpsychiatrist physicians. *Arch Gen Psychiatry* 1985;42:89–94.

23. Knapp DA, Michocki RJ. Drug prescribing for very elderly ambulatory patients. *J Am Geriatr Soc* 1985;35:1036.

24. Ancill RJ, Embury GD, MacEwan GW, et al. The use and misuse of psychotropic prescribing for elderly psychiatric patients. *Can J Psychiatry* 1988; 33:585–589.

25. Woods JH, Katz JL, Winger G. Benzodiazepines: use, abuse, and consequences. *Phamacol Rev* 1992;44(2):151–347.

26. Stewart RB, May FE, Moore MT, et al. Changing patterns of psychotropic drug use in the elderly: a five-year update. *Drug Intell Clin Pharm* 1989; 23:610–613.

27. National Center for Health Statistics. Health, United States, 1994. Hyattsville, MD: Public Health Service, 1995.

28. Wise TN, Mann LS, Jani N, et al. Haloperidol prescribing practices in the general hospital. *Gen Hosp Psychiatry* 1989;11:368–371.

29. Antonijoan RM, Barbonoj MJ, Torrent J, et al. Evaluation of psychotropic drug consumption related to psychological distress in the elderly: hospitalized vs. nonhospitalized. *Neuropsychobiology* 1990;23:25–30.

30. Linden M, Thiels C. Epidemiology of prescriptions for neuroleptic drugs: tranquilizers rather than antipsychotics. *Pharmacopsychiatry* 2001; 34(4):150–154.

31. Spillman BC, Lubitz J. New estimates of lifetime nursing home use: have patterns of use changed? *Med Care* 2002;40(10):965–975.

32. Draper B, Brodaty H, Low LF, et al. Use of psychotics in Sydney nursing homes: associates with depression, psychosis, and behavioral disturbances. *Int Psychogeriatr* 2001;13(1):107–120.

33. Borson, S, Doane K. The impact of OBRA '87 on psychotropic drug prescribing in skilled nursing facilities. *Psychiatr Serv* 1997;48:128–996.

34. Wancata J, Benda N, Meise U, et al. Psychotropic drug intake in residents newly admitted to nursing homes. *Psychopharmacology* 1997;134(2): 115–120.

35. Healthcare Finance Administration Review; Medicare and Medicaid Supplement, 1996.

36. Gurwitz JH, Soumerai SB, Avorn J. Improving medication prescribing and utilization in the nursing home. *J Am Geriatr Soc* 1990;38(5): 542–552.

37. Garrard J, Makris L, Dunham T, et al. Evaluation of neuroleptic drug use by nursing home elderly under proposed Medicare and Medicaid regulations. *JAMA* 1994;271:358–362.

38. Burns BJ, Larson DB, Goldstrom ID, et al. Mental disorder among nursing home patients: preliminary findings from the National Nursing Home Survey Pretest. *Int J Geriatr Psychiatry* 1988; 3:27–35.

39. Cantu TG, Korek JS. Prescription of neuroleptics for geriatric nursing home patients. *Hosp Community Psychiatry* 1989;40:457–467.

40. Siegler EL, Capezuti E, Maislin G, et al. Effects of a restraint reduction intervention and OBRA '87 regulations on psychoactive drug use in nursing homes. *J Am Geriatr Soc* 1997;45(7):791–796.

41. Avorn J, Dreyer P, Connelly K, et al. Use of psychoactive medication and the quality of care in rest homes: findings and policy implications of a state-wide study. *N Engl J Med* 1989;320:227–232.

42. Beers M, Avorn J, Soumerai SB, et al. Psychoactive medication use in intermediate-care facility residents. *JAMA* 1988;260:3016–3020.

43. Buck JA. Psychotropic drug practice in nursing homes. *J Am Geriatr Soc* 1988;36:409–418.

44. Everitt DE, Fields D, Avorn J, et al. Resident behavior and staff distress in the nursing home. *J Am Geriatr Soc* 1991;39:792–798.

45. Institute of Medicine Committee on Nursing Home Regulation. *Improving the quality of care in nursing homes.* Washington, DC: National Academy Press, 1986.

46. Morris JN, Hawes C, Fries BE, et al. Designing the national resident assessment instrument for nursing homes. *Gerontologist* 1990;30(3):293–307.

47. Shorr RI, Fought RL, Ray WA. Changes in antipsychotic drug use in nursing homes during implementation of the OBRA-87 regulations. *JAMA* 1994;271:358–362.

48. Streim JE. OBRA regulations and psychiatric care in the nursing home. *Psychiatr Ann* 1995; 25:413–418.

49. Avorn J, Soumerai SB. Improving drug-therapy decisions through educational outreach: a randomized controlled trial of academically based "detailing." *N Engl J Med* 1983;308:1457–1463.

50. Avorn J, Soumerai SB, Everitt DE, et al. A randomized trial of a program to reduce the use of psychoactive drugs in nursing homes. *N Engl J Med* 1992;327:168–173.

51. Ray WA, Blazer DG, Schaffner W, et al. Reducing antipsychotic prescribing for nursing home patients: a controlled trial of effect of an educational visit. *Am J Public Health* 1987;77:1448–1450.
52. Katon W, Von Korff M, Lin E, et al. Collaborative care management to achieve treatment guidelines; impact on depression in primary care. *JAMA* 1995;273:1026–1031.
53. Unutzer J, Katon W, Callahan CM, et al. Collaborative care management of late-life depression in primary care. *JAMA* 2002;288:2836–2845.
54. Avorn J. Geriatric drug epidemiology and health services research based on large-scale computerized datasets. In: Moore SR, Teal TW, eds. *Geriatric drug use: clinical and social perspectives.* New York: Pergamon Press, 1985.
55. Zhan C, Sangl J, Bierman AS, et al. Potentially inappropriate medication use in the community-dwelling elderly: findings from the National 1996 Medical Expenditure Panel Survey. *JAMA* 2001;286:2823–2829.
56. Wenger NS, Shekelle PG, and the ACOVE Investigators. Assessing care of vulnerable elders: ACOVE project overview. *Ann Intern Med* 2001;135(8):642–646.
57. Shekelle PG, MacLean CH, Morton SC, et al. Assessing care of vulnerable elders: methods for developing quality indicators. *Ann Intern Med* 2001;135(8):647–652.
58. Knight EL, Avorn J. Quality indicators for appropriate medication use in vulnerable elders. *Ann Intern Med* 2001;135(8):703–710.
59. Avorn J, Gurwitz JH, Rochon P. *Prinicples of pharmacology. Geriatric Medicine: An evidence-based approach.* 4th edition. C.K. Cassel, et al., ed. New York: Springer, 2003.
60. Monane M, Glynn RJ, Avorn J. The impact of sedative-hypnotic use on sleep symptoms in elderly nursing home residents. *Clin Pharmacol Ther* 1996;59:83–92.
61. Everitt DE, Avorn J, Baker MW. Clinical decision making in the evaluation and treatment of insomnia. *Am J Med* 1990;89:357–362.
62. Cassel CK, Leipzig RM, Cohen HJ, et al. *Geriatric Medicine: An evidence-based approach.* 4th ed. Springer-Verlag New York, Inc. 2003
63. Leipzig RM, Cummings RG, Tinetti ME. Drugs and falls in older people: a systematic review and meta-analysis: I. Psychotropic drugs. *J Am Geriatr Soc* 1999;47:30–39.
64. Ray WA, Griffin MR, Schaffner W, et al. Psychotropic drug use and the risk of hip fracture. *N Engl J Med* 1987;316:363–369.
65. Ray WA, Griffin MR, Downey W. Benzodiazepines of long and short elimination half-life and the risk of hip fracture. *JAMA* 1989;262:3303–3307.
66. Herings RC, Stricker BH, de Boer A, et al. Benzodiazepines and the risk of hip falling leading to femur fractures. *Arch Intern Med* 1995;155:1801–1807.
67. Wang PS, Bohn RL, Glynn RJ, et al. Hazardous benzodiazepine regimens in the elderly: effects of half-life, dosage, and duration on risk of hip fracture. American Journal of Psychiatry 2001;158:892–898.
68. Thapa PB, Gideon P, Cost TW, et al. Antidepres-

sants and the risk of falls among nursing home residents. *N Engl J Med* 1998;339:875–882.
69. Wang PS, Bohn RL, Glynn RJ, et al. Zolpidem use and hip fractures in the elderly. *J Am Geriatr Soc* 2001;49:1685–1690.
70. Avorn J, Monane M, Everitt DE, et al. Clinical assessment of extrapyramidal signs in nursing home patients given antipsychotic medication. *Arch Intern Med* 1995;99:48–54.
71. Avorn J, Bohn RL, Mogun H, et al. Neuroleptic drug exposure and treatment of parkinsonism in the elderly: a case-control study. *Am J Med* 1995;99:48–54
72. Kalish SC, Bohn RL, Mogun H, et al. Antipsychotic prescribing patterns and the treatment of extrapyramidal symptoms in older people. *J Am Geriatr Soc* 1995;43:969–973.
73. Avorn J, Gurwitz JH, Bohn RL, et al. Increased incidence of L-dopa therapy following metoclopramide use. *JAMA* 1995;274:1780–1782.
74. Gurwitz JH, Avorn J. The ambiguous relationship between aging and adverse drug reaction. *Ann Intern Med* 1991;114:956–966.
75. Monane M, Avorn J, Beers MH, et al. Anticholinergic drug use and bowel function in nursing home patients. *Arch Intern Med* 1993;153:633–638.
76. Doucet K, Chassagne P, Trivalle C, et al. Drug-drug interactions related to hospital admissions in older adults: a prospective study of 1000 patients. *J Am Geriatr Soc* 1996;44:944–948.
77. Classen DC, Pestotnik SL, Evans RS, et al. Adverse drug events in hospitalized patients: excess length of stay, extra costs, and attributable mortality. *JAMA* 1997;277(4):301–306.
78. Monane M, Gurwitz JH, Bohn RL, et al. The impact of thiazide diuretics on the initiation of lipid-reducing agents in the elderly: a population-based analysis. *J Am Geriatr Soc* 1997;45:71–75.
79. Avorn J, Glynn RJ, Gurwitz JH, et al. Adverse pulmonary effects of topical B-blockers used in the treatment of glaucoma. *J Glaucoma* 1993;2:158–165.
80. Cornoni-Huntley JC, Huntley RR, Feldman JJ, eds. *Health status and well-being of the elderly: National Health and Nutrition Examination (NHANE) Survey.* New York: Oxford University Press, 1990.
81. Fuhr U. Drug interactions with grapefruit juice. Extent, probably mechanism and clinical relevance. *Drug Safety* 1998;18:251–272.
82. Col N, Fanale JE, Kronholm P. The role of medication noncompliance and adverse drug reactions in hospitalization of the elderly. *Arch Intern Med* 1990;150:841–845.
83. Benner JS, Glynn RJ, Mogun H, et al. Long-term persistence in use of statin therapy in elderly patients. *JAMA* 2002;288:455–461.
84. Reynolds CF, Frank E, Perel JM, et al. Nortriptyline and interpersonal psychotherapy as maintenance therapies for recurrent major depression. *JAMA* 1999;281:39–45.
85. Monane M, Bohn RL, Gurwitz JH, et al. Compliance with antihypertensive therapy among elderly Medicaid enrollees: the roles of age, gender, and race. *Am J Public Health* 1996;86:1805–1808.
86. Weintraub M. Compliance: is it really an issue.

In: Lamy PP, Fedder DO, eds. *The pharmacist and the elderly: do they speak the same language?* Baltimore: Center for the Study of Pharmacy and Therapeutics for the Elderly, 1980:59–74.

87. Salzman C. Medication compliance in the elderly. *J Clin Psychiatry* 1995;56:18–22.

88. Haynes RB, McKibbon KA, Kanani R. Systematic review of randomized trials of interventions to assist patients to follow prescriptions for medications. *Lancet* 1996;348:383–386.

89. Roter DL, Hall JA, Merisca R, et al. Effectiveness of interventions to improve patient compliance: a meta-analysis. *Med Care* 1998;36:1138–1161.

90. Becker MH, Maiman LA. Sociobehavioral determinants of compliance with health and medical care recommendations. *Med Care* 1975;13:10–24.

91. Wang PS, Bohn RL, Knight E, et al. Noncompliance with antihypertensive medications: the impact of depressive symptoms and psychosocial factors. *J Gen Intern Med* 2002;17:504–511.

92. Waxman H, McCreary G, Weinnt R, et al. A comparison of somatic complaints among depressed and nondepressed older patients. *Gerontologist* 1987;85:501–507.

93. Steinman MA, Sands LP, Covinsky KE. Self-restriction of medications due to cost in seniors without prescription coverage. *J Gen Intern Med* 2001;16(12):793–799.

94. Eisen SA, Miller DK, Woodward RS, et al. The effect of prescribed daily dose frequency on patient medication compliance. *Arch Intern Med* 1990;150:1881–1884.

95. Ware GJ, Holdford NGH, Davison JH, et al. Unit dose calendar packaging and elderly patient compliance. *NZ Med J* 1991;104:495–497.

96. Wang PS, Benner JS, Glynn RJ, et al. How well do patients report non-compliance with antihypertensive medications?: A comparison of self-report vs. filled prescriptions. *Pharmacoepidemiol and Drug Saf* 2004;13:4–19

Table 2.3 References

Grossberg GT, Grossberg JA. Epidemiology of psychotherapeutic drug use in older adults. *Clin Geriatr Med* 1998;14(1):1–5.

Hanlon JT, Fillenbaum GG, Ruby CM, et al. Epidemiology of over-the-counter drug use in community dwelling elderly: United States perspective. *Drugs & Aging* 2001;18(2):123–131.

Kaufman DW, Kelly JP, Rosenberg L, et al. Recent patterns of medication use in the ambulatory adult population of the United States: The Slone Survey. *JAMA* 2002;287(3):337–344.

Lassila HC, Stoehr GP, Ganguli M, et al. Use of prescription medications in an elderly rural population: The MoVIES Project. *Ann Pharmacother* 1996;30:589–595.

Luber MP, Meyers BS, Williams-Russo PG, et al. Depression and service utilization in elderly primary care patients. *Am J Geriatr Psychiatry* 2001;9:169–176.

Schappert SM. Ambulatory care visits to physician offices, hospital outpatient departments, and emergency departments: United States, 1997. *Vital Health Stat* 1999;143(13):i–iv,1–39.

Schneeweiss S, Walker AM, Glynn RJ, et al. Outcomes of reference pricing for angiotensin-converting-enzyme inhibitors *N Engl J Med* 2002;346:822–829.

Sorenson L, Foldspang A, Gulmann NC, et al. Determinants for the use of psychotics among nursing home residents. *Int J Geriatr Psychiatry* 2001;16(2):147–154.

Stoehr GP, Ganguli M, Seaberg EC, et al. Over-the-counter medications in an older rural community: the MoVIES Project. *J Am Geriatr Soc* 1997;45(2):158–165.

Unützer J, Simon G, Berlin TR. Care for depression in HMO patients aged 65 and older. *J Am Geriatr Soc* 2000;48:871–878.

Unützer J, Katon W, Russo J. Patterns of care for depressed older adults in a large-staff model HMO. *Am J Geriatr Psychiatry* 1999;7:235–243.

Wancata J, Benda N, Meise U, et al. Use of psychotropic drugs in gynecological, surgical, and medical wards of general hospitals. *Int J Psychiatry Med* 1998;28(3):303–314.

Supplemental Readings

General

Avorn J. The role of medications. In: Berg R, Cassell J, eds. *Health promotion and disability prevention in the second fifty: report of a committee of the Institute of Medicine.* Washington, DC: National Academy Press, 1990.

Avorn J, Gurwitz JH, Rochon P. Principles of pharmacology. *Geriatric medicine: an evidence-based approach.* 4th ed. C.K. Cassel, et al., eds. New York: Springer 2003.

Avorn J. Medications and the elderly: current status and opportunities. *Health Affairs* 1995;14:276–278.

Avorn J, Gurwitz JH. Principles of pharmacology. In: Cassel CK, Cohen HJ, Larsen, et al., eds. *Geriatric medicine.* 3rd ed. New York: Springer-Verlag, 1996.

Chrischilles EA, Foley DJ, Wallace RB, et al. Use of medications by persons 65 and over: data from the established populations for epidemiologic studies of the elderly. *J Gerontol* 1992;47:MI37–144.

Gurwitz JH. Suboptimal medication use in the elderly. The tip of the iceberg [Editorial]. *JAMA* 1994;272:316–317.

Hanlon JT, Fillenbaum GG, Ruby CM. Epidemiology of over-the-counter drug use in community dwelling elderly: United States perspective. *Drugs & Aging* 2001;18(2):123–131.

Kaufman DW, Kelly JP, Rosenberg L, et al. Recent patterns of medication use in the ambulatory adult population of the United States. *JAMA* 2002;287:337–344.

Shekelle PG, MacLean CH, Morton SC, et al. Assessing care of vulnerable elders: methods for developing quality indicators. *Ann Int Med* 2001;135:647–652.

Schwartz JB. Clinical pharmacology. In: Hazzard WR, Bierman EL, Blass JP, et al., eds. *Principles of geriatric medicine and gerontology.* 3rd ed. New York: McGraw-Hill, 1994.

Wilcox SM, Himmelstein DU, Woolhandler S. Inappropriate drug prescribing for the community-dwelling elderly. *JAMA* 1994;272:292–296.

Zhan C, Sangl J, Bierman AS, et al. Potentially inappropriate medication use in the community-dwelling elderly: findings from the National 1996 Medical Expenditure Panel Survey. *JAMA* 2001; 286:2823–2829.

Nursing Home Drug Use

Avorn J, Dreyer P, Connelly K, Soumerai SB. Use of psychoactive medication and the quality of care in rest homes: findings and policy implications of a state-wide study. *N Engl J Med* 1989;320: 227–232.

Avorn J, Gurwitz JH. Drug use in the nursing home. *Ann Intern Med* 1995;123:195–204.

Avorn J, Soumerai SB, Everitt DE, et al. A randomized trial of a program to reduce the use of psychoactive drugs in nursing homes. *N Engl J Med* 1992;327:168–173.

Elon R, Pawlson LG. The impact of OBRA on medical practice within nursing facilities. *J Am Geriatr Soc* 1992;40:958–963.

Forman DE, Coletta D, Kenny D, et al. Clinical issues related to discontinuing digoxin therapy in elderly nursing home patients. *Arch Intern Med* 1991;151:2194–2198.

Garrard J, Makris L, Dunham T, et al. Evaluation of neuroleptic drug use by nursing home elderly under proposed Medicare and Medicaid regulations. *JAMA* 1991;265(4):463–467.

Garrard J, Chen V, Dowd B. The impact of the 1987 federal regulations on the use of psychotropic drugs in Minnesota nursing homes. *Am J Public Health* 1995;85(6):771–776.

Gurwitz J, Soumerai SB, Avorn J. Improving medication prescribing and utilization in the nursing home. *J Am Geriat Soc* 1990; 38:542–552.

Ray WA, Taylor JA, Meador KG, et al. Reducing antipsychotic drug use in nursing homes. A controlled trial of provider education. *Arch Intern Med* 1993;153:713–721.

Rovner BW, Edelman BA, Cox MP, Shmuely Y. The impact of antipsychotic drug regulations on psychotropic prescribing practices in nursing homes. *Am J Psychiatry* 1992;149:1390–1392.

Shorr RI, Fought RL, Ray W A. Changes in antipsychotic drug use in nursing homes during implementation of the OBRA-87 regulations. *JAMA* 1994;271:358–362.

Sorenson L, Foldspang A, Gulmann NC, et al. Determinants for the use of psychotics among nursing home residents. *Int J Geriatr Psychiatry* 2001;16(2): 147–154.

Svarstad BL, Mount JK. Nursing home resources and tranquilizer use among the institutionalized elderly. *J Am Geriatr Soc* 1991;39:869–875.

Winograd CH, Pawlson LG. OBRA 87-a commentary. *J Am Geriatr Soc* 1991;39:724–726.

Adverse Drug Reactions

Bates DW, Cullen D, Laird N, et al. Incidence of adverse drug events and potential adverse drug events: implications for prevention. *JAMA* 1995; 274:29–34.

Bates DW, Spell N, Cullen DJ, et al., for the Adverse Drug Events Study Group. The costs of adverse drug events in hospitalized patients. *JAMA* 1997; 277:307–311.

Beers M, Avorn J, Soumerai SB, et al. Psychoactive medication use in intermediate-care facility residents. *JAMA* 1988;260:3016–3020.

Beers MH, Ouslander JG, Fingold SF, et al. Inappropriate medication prescribing in skilled-nursing facilities. *Ann Intern Med* 1992;117:684–689.

Beers MH, Ouslander JG, Rollingher I, et al. Explicit criteria for determining inappropriate medication use in nursing home residents. *Arch Intern Med* 1991;151:1825–1832.

Brennan TA, Leape LL, Laird N, et al. Incidence of adverse events and negligence in hospitalized patients: results from the Harvard Medical Practice Study I. *N Engl J Med* 1991;324:370–376.

Campbell AJ. Drug treatment as a cause of falls in old age: a review of the offending agents. *Drugs Aging* 1991;1:289–302.

Classen DC, Pestotnik SL, Evans RS, et al. Adverse drug events in hospitalized patients: excess length of stay, extra costs, and attributable mortality. *JAMA* 1997;277(4):301–306.

Cummings SR, Nevitt MC, Browner WS, et al. Risk factors for hip fracture in white women. Study of Osteoporotic Fractures Research Group. *N Engl J Med* 1995;332:767–773.

Gurwitz JH, Avorn J. The ambiguous relation between aging and adverse drug reactions. *Ann Intern Med* 1991;114:956–966.

Leape LL, Bates DW, Cullen Dl, et al. Systems analysis of adverse drug events. *JAMA* 1995;274:35–43.

Thapa PB, Gideon P, Fought RL, et al. Psychotropic drugs and risk of recurrent falls in ambulatory nursing home residents. *Am J Epidemiol* 1995;142: 202–211.

Compliance

Donovan JL. Patient decision making. The missing ingredient in compliance research. *Int J Technol Assess Healthcare* 1995;11:443–455.

Eisen SA, Miller DK, Woodward RS, et al. The effect of prescribed daily dose frequency on patient medication compliance. *Arch Intern Med* 1990; 150:1881–1884.

Glickman L, Bruce EA, Caro FG, Avorn J. Physicians' knowledge of drug costs for the elderly. *J Am Geriatr Soc* 1994;42:992–996.

Monane M, Bohn R, Gurwitz JH, et al. Noncompliance with congestive heart failure therapy in the elderly. *Arch Intern Med* 1994;154:433–437.

National Council on Patient Information and Education. Focusing on communication, compliance, FDA Med Guide proposal in 1996. *Formulary* 1996;31:389–398.

Salzman C. Medication compliance in the elderly. *J Clin Psychiatry* 1995;56(suppl 1):18–22.

Stephenson BJ, Rowe BH, Haynes B, et al. Is this patient taking the treatment as prescribed? *JAMA* 1993;269:2779–2781.

Urquhart J. Patient compliance as an explanatory variable in four selected cardiovascular studies. In: Crarner JA, Spilker B, eds. *Patient compliance in medical practice and clinical trials.* New York: Raven Press, 1991:301–322.

Chapter 3

The Cost of Psychotropic Drug Use for the Elderly

Helen H. Kyomen

Gary L. Gottlieb

The past decade has witnessed significant development in new psychotropic drug treatments for elderly patients. Improved tolerance and efficacy have given older adults the opportunity for improvement in symptoms, function, quality of life, and morbidity and mortality. However, the daily *costs* of these treatments can be staggering and, in the context of the socioeconomics of later life, large segments of the older population may have little or no access to these advances. Policymakers continue to wrestle with developing rational plans to provide insurance for prescription drugs for the elderly—a challenge that must be met if the potential of ongoing discovery is to be translated into true treatment effectiveness.

Until recently, only about 65% of Medicare beneficiaries have had some outpatient prescription drug coverage, largely obtained from former employer-sponsored insurance coverage, Medicaid, privately paid Medigap coverage, and Medicare components of Health Maintenance Organizations (HMOs); for relatively small population subgroups, medications have been provided by the Veterans Administration health system, state-sponsored pharmacy-assistance programs, or local community programs.[1] Inadequate prescription drug coverage has been, and will continue to be, associated with compromised compliance with drug therapy and consequent adverse health outcomes for Medicare beneficiaries.[2]

In contrast to the explosive increases in expenditures for drugs, benefits from Social Security and Supplemental Security Income have increased by only modest recent changes in the Consumer Price Index.[3] Poor elderly persons without Medicaid coverage spend approximately 50% of their total income on out-of-pocket healthcare costs. Primary expenditures are Medicare deductibles and coinsurance, premiums for private (Medigap) insurance, and prescription drugs.[4] The near-poor (within 125% of the federal poverty line) spend 30%. Almost 60% of Medicare beneficiaries with incomes below the federal poverty line did not receive Medicaid assistance in 1997.[4] Anecdotal reports abound of low-income elderly persons who have stopped using essential drugs in order to pay for food,[5] and cost of health services is the single most important reason cited in the 1991–1996 Medicare Current Beneficiary Survey by Medicare beneficiaries who did not see a physician for a medical condition in a recent year.[6] This survey did not separate out-of-pocket psychotropic prescription drug cost from other costs associated with a medical visit, but growing out-of-pocket costs for prescription drugs certainly must have been an important component of this treatment barrier.

The three primary sources of drug coverage for about 65% of Medicare beneficiaries with some current outpatient prescription coverage have been:

1. Employer-sponsored insurance policies. About 45% of Medicare beneficiaries with outpatient prescription drug coverage receive this coverage from former employers.[1]
2. Medicaid coverage. About 17% of Medicare beneficiaries with outpatient prescription drug coverage have sufficiently limited incomes and assets to qualify for coverage through Medicaid. In all states, Medicaid coverage includes prescription drugs, subject to locally developed formularies.
3. Medigap supplemental insurance. About 14% of Medicare beneficiaries with outpatient prescription drug coverage purchase supplemental (Medigap) insurance.[1] However, this type of coverage is limited; among the 10 standard Medigap policies, only 3 offer prescription drug coverage. In 2002, two modest coverage policies required a $250 deductible and 50% copayment, with coverage limited to $1250 annually. Each of these two plans costs $1900 per year (for prescription and other "gap" coverage, i.e., coverage falling between Medicare and supplemental payment). One more extensive plan has the same $250 deductible and 50% copayment, but coverage is limited to $3000 annually and the cost is $3250 per year. Because of high copayments, high deductibles, and benefit caps, few Medicare beneficiaries purchase Medigap plans with supplemental drug coverage. Only about 19% of elderly persons with privately purchased Medigap policies have coverage for drugs.[1]

Currently when additional drug coverage sources—i.e., Medicare + Choice (newly renamed Medicare Advantage), the Veterans Administration, Pharmaceutical Assistance Programs, and local or community programs—are aggregated, only about 65% of the Medicare beneficiary population have had some kind of outpatient prescription drug coverage.

Elderly persons with restricted ability to pay for prescription drugs use fewer medications, on average, and suffer adverse health outcomes as a consequence. Ominous consequences of inadequate nonpsychotropic and psychotropic prescription drug coverage result:

1. Substantially reduced use of statin medications occurs among Medicare beneficiaries with coronary heart disease or history of myocardial infarction and inadequate pharmacy benefit coverage; estimated usage rates are 4.1% for Medicare patients with no drug coverage versus 27.4% for patients with employer-sponsored drug coverage ($p < 0.001$).[7]
2. (a) Immediate and sustained 35% reductions ($p < 0.001$) occur in the use of essential medications (defined as cardiac drugs, chronic obstructive pulmonary disease and asthma medications, insulin, anticonvulsants, and anticoagulants).
   (b) Concomitantly, admissions to nursing homes increase significantly (doubling in rate) among low-income elderly persons unable to purchase needed medications when, as in New Hampshire, a short-term (11-month) cap of 3 prescriptions/month was legislatively imposed.[8] In most cases, the elderly persons admitted to nursing homes in this situation stayed there permanently.
3. Among regular users of antipsychotic medications, significant decreases in the use of antipsychotics, sedative hypnotic agents, antidepressants, and lithium occurs (21%, $p < 0.001$), as well as twice the number of mental health emergency and day hospital services (approximately a 48% increase in visits per patient per month, $p < 0.001$) during prior 3 months. These consequences were documented in New Hampshire during the 11-month period when the 3 prescriptions/month cap was in place.[9] Under these conditions, increased state costs for mental healthcare for the people affected by

this cap on psychotropic and other medications surpassed prescription drug savings by a factor of 17.

4. The New Hampshire 3 prescriptions/ month cap led to patient-level changes in standard monthly doses of essential medications (for heart disease, asthma/chronic obstructive pulmonary disease, diabetes mellitus, seizure, and coagulation disorders) of 34.4% (mean change in standard doses) for the period in which the cap was in force, compared to the baseline period. Comorbid conditions associated with the largest relative reduction in essential drug use were psychoses/bipolar disorders, anxiety/sleep problems, and chronic pain.[10]

These data suggest that the effects of inadequate psychotropic drug coverage may have especially strong adverse consequences for elderly persons with chronic health problems.

2003 Medicare Prescription Drug Legislation

The Medicare Prescription Drug, Improvement, and Modernization Act of 2003 extensively updates the Medicare program and provides for Medicare Part D, a new program for prescription drug benefits, effective January 1, 2006. Under Medicare Part D, beneficiaries will be able to obtain prescription drug coverage by enrolling in a private prescription drug plan or in an HMO or other plan that accepts Medicare capitation and extends a drug benefit. From the spring of 2004 until January 1, 2006, implementation of an Interim Drug Program will endorse privately issued drug discount cards for Medicare beneficiaries through various card sponsors, such as Pharmaceutical Benefit Managers, wholesale and retail pharmacy delivery systems, and insurers. These medication discount cards will cost about $30 per year. The 2003 law also provides for medication treatment management programs for those with multiple chronic conditions, high prescription drug use, and probable increased drug expenses.

These revisions to Medicare have limitations but they are extremely important: Outpatient prescription drugs, including psychotropics, have not yet been covered by Medicare, the basic health insurance for most Americans over 65. This Act also plans to increase Medicare payments to doctors and hospitals, hasten marketing of lower-cost generic drugs, and offer employers subsidies to encourage them to continue their drug coverage to retirees.

The Medicare Act of 2003 affects Medigap policies with a drug benefit. Medicare beneficiaries with a Medigap plan with prescription drug coverage may continue their current Medigap plan with drug benefits or they may enroll in Medicare Part D. If those with Medigap coverage with prescription drug coverage decide to enroll in Medicare Part D later, a late-enrollment charge may be levied if the Medigap policy is not equivalent to Medicare Part D. Those enrolling in Medicare Part D from the start may enroll in another Medigap plan without prescription drug coverage, or they may keep their current Medigap plan but drop its drug benefits and pay a lower premium. People who reach age 65 after January 1, 2006, will likely only be able to enroll in a Medigap policy without drug benefits. As the Act is now written, after January 1, 2006, people will not be able to purchase a supplemental policy to offset deductibles and copayments for drug policies.

This legislation provides for the most extensive changes to Medicare since the Medicare program was initiated in July 1966. In addition to the new Medicare Part D, additional changes include: expansion and renaming of the Medicare + Choice program to Medicare Advantage; medication therapy management programs for patients with multiple chronic conditions, high numbers of prescriptions, and likely high drug expenses; coverage of screening and disease management programs, such as initial physical examinations and cardiovascular disease and diabetes screening; changes in reimbursements to hospitals and physicians including ongoing development of the prospective payment system for inpatient psychiatric care; improved rural healthcare provisions; a demonstration project for recovery audits to identify underpayments or overpayments and collect overpayments; and changes in the acquisition systems for durable medical equipment and other products to provide for a competitive bidding process.

Rise in Prescription Drug Costs

The 2003 Medicare Prescription Drug legislation was enacted against a background during the 1990s when the cost of prescription drugs was the fastest-growing component of national health expenditures.[11] In 2001, the average price per prescription rose 10 percent to $49–$50.[12] This 10%-in-one-year change is typical of recent prescription drug price increases. Such price escalations, combined with steep increases in prescription drug use, especially of newer and more expensive drugs, has resulted in substantial growth in prescription drug expenditures. Consumers spent 17 percent more ($22.6 billion) for prescription drugs in 2001 than in 2000.[13] These increases derive from three main sources[12]:

1. Increased number of prescriptions—responsible for approximately 39% of additional cost
2. Price increases—accounting for approximately 37% of additional cost
3. Greater use of newer, higher-cost drugs—responsible for approximately 24% of additional cost

These concerns are especially pertinent for the elderly, as one-third of all prescription drug purchases in the United States are made by or for people age 65 years or older. More than 85% of Medicare beneficiaries take prescription drugs, with the typical Medicare subscriber filling almost 30 prescriptions per year.[14,15] Data derived from the National Health and Nutrition Examination Survey indicate that among persons 65 years or older, 49% of men and 59% of women use 2 or more prescription drugs regularly.[16]

Medicare beneficiaries without prescription drug coverage have paid higher prices at retail than the prices paid by those with drug coverage.[17] The price differential between cash customers (i.e., elderly persons without prescription drug coverage) and those with drug coverage has been, on average, approximately 15%; for one-quarter of the most commonly used drugs, the price differential is even larger—over 20%. Moreover, the price differential between cash customers and those with third-party coverage grew substantially larger between 1996 and 1999—findings on analyses of data from the Medicare Current Beneficiary Survey, the Medical Expenditure Panel Survey, and on data from pharmacy audits conducted by the consulting firm Intercontinental Marketing Services Health, covering over 90% of the most commonly prescribed drugs.

Demographics of Medication Use

Medication use among Medicare beneficiaries increases with income and age and decreases with high function and health status.[18-22] In addition, white Medicare beneficiaries are more likely to use prescription drugs than nonwhites, even when controlling for such factors as health status, income, and education.[18,23,24] Many near-poor and low-income Medicare beneficiaries may be particularly vulnerable to underuse of essential drugs because they are simultaneously more likely to be ill, less likely to have employer-sponsored coverage, and not poor enough to qualify for Medicaid.[20,25] Even beneficiaries with prescription drug coverage frequently face high copayments and other limitations that restrict the appropriate use of prescription drugs.[8,26-28]

The most important determinant of whether or not medications are purchased by Medicare beneficiaries is the out-of-pocket cost entailed in individual prescription drug purchases. Out-of-pocket payments for prescription drugs have been growing at an even faster pace than aggregate drug costs. Without prescription drug coverage within Medicare, this disturbing trend was expected to accelerate in coming years. Table 3.1 summarizes these trends for the period 1992–2000.

Based on a large sample of elderly participants in the Survey of Asset and Health Dynamics among the oldest-old, a strong link was found between lack of prescription drug coverage and underuse of prescribed medications due to costs.[29] These data provide self-report evidence from beneficiaries that the cause of reduced drug use was cost and not lesser need for medication. Additional disconcerting findings also emerged: among elderly persons without drug coverage, minorities were four times more likely to report underuse due to cost than white respondents; people with low incomes (i.e., household income < $10,000) were three times more likely to report underuse for cost reasons; and people in poor health were three times more likely to report underuse due to cost than those in very good or excellent health.[29]

Data from a longitudinal survey of some 7,000 elderly households (Elderly Health Supplement to the Panel Study of Income Dynamics)[20] revealed that among Medicare beneficiaries who use prescription drugs, a large percentage of their cost (67%) is paid out of pocket, resulting in an average of 3.1% of household income being spent on out-of-pocket payments for drugs. The distribution of these payments is considerably skewed, with 7% of elderly households spending at least 10%, and 1% spending over a quarter of household income on drugs.

Effect of Prescription Drug Coverage on Use

Among Medicare beneficiaries, lack of availability of prescription drug coverage as well as out-of-pocket costs, even when these are relatively small in magnitude, correlate negatively with medication use.[2] That is, Medicare beneficiaries with prescription drug coverage are substantially more likely to purchase prescribed medications. Those who must pay for prescription drugs out of pocket, including copayments, deductibles, and other cost-sharing mechanisms, are less likely to fill their prescriptions. Whether these factors have a differential effect with regard to psychotropic medications compared to all drugs is not known. It is possible that psychotropic drugs are even less likely to be purchased than other prescription medications: facing out-of-pocket drug costs or

Table 3.1. Prescription Drug Spending by Medicare Beneficiaries, 1992 and 2000[a]

Prescription spending per beneficiary	Prescriptions/year[b] (annual average)	Cost per prescription (annual average)	Time period (annual average)
1992	$559	19.6	$28.50
2000	$1205	28.5	$42.30
Change, 1992–2000	+ 116%	+ 45%	+ 48%

a. Source: Families USA Foundation. Cost overdose: growth in drug spending for the elderly, 1992–2010. *Families USA Publication No. 00-107*. Washington, DC: Families USA; 2000.
b. Average number of prescriptions filled, not number of drugs

even a copayment, an elderly patient may rather purchase, for example, medications for acute symptom relief (e.g., analgesics) over those needed for management of a chronic condition, like most psychiatric disorders. For elderly patients living on limited fixed incomes, out-of-pocket costs for maintenance psychotropic drug treatment may exceed available financial resources.

When prescription drug reimbursement was limited in New Hampshire to three prescriptions per month for elderly and disabled Medicaid recipients,[8,9,27] an immediate and sustained reduction (46%) occurred in the number of prescriptions used by those receiving multiple drugs—a reduction extending across all classes of prescription medications.[27] The three comorbid conditions associated with the largest relative reductions in essential drug use were psychoses/bipolar disorders, anxiety/sleep problems, and chronic pain.[10] Use of antipsychotic medications for patients with schizophrenia, as well as use of sedative hypnotic agents, antidepressants, and lithium, all dropped significantly during the period in which the New Hampshire cap was in place; for example, among regular users of antipsychotic agents, medication use decreased 21.2% ($p < 0.001$) during this period.[9] Also, a concomitant increase in outpatient and emergency mental health services (approximately 48% increase in visits per patient per month, $p < 0.001$) occurred during the period of the three prescriptions/month cap. The aggregate mental health services cost increases exceeded the prescription drug cost savings attributable to the cap by seventeen fold.

Increases in prescription drug insurance copayment need not be very large for the cost sharing to decrease drug utilization. Medicaid claims made on behalf of predominately elderly South Carolina residents[30] reveal a significant drop in prescription drug use (from 24.8 to 23 claims per eligible recipient per year, 7.3%) occurred after South Carolina im-

plemented a fifty-cent copayment per prescription.

The 2003 Medicare Prescription Drug, Improvement, and Modernization Act may provide greater access to prescription drug coverage for more elderly, but this legislation is not without limitations. Monthly premiums are estimated to be an average of $35 in 2006, increasing to a $58 average in 2013. Under a voluntary plan, starting in 2006, Medicare beneficiaries who pay the $35 average per month will have 75% of prescription drug costs covered up to $2,250 (approximately $4,000 in 2013) after paying a $250 deductible. Coverage then recommences with a sliding scale copayment after beneficiaries have paid $3,600 ($6,400 in 2013) out of pocket for prescription drugs. To encourage companies to maintain drug benefits for their retirees, the government will pay 28% of the costs that companies incur for each retiree—between $250 and $5,000. Whether these cost-sharing arrangements will be adequate to promote appropriate drug utilization remains to be seen.

Medicare Beneficiaries With and Without Prescription Drug Coverage

Medicare enrollees without prescription drug coverage have received fewer medications and spend less on drugs than those with drug coverage. On average, noncovered beneficiaries filled 17.6 prescriptions at a cost of about $550 in 1998. In contrast, beneficiaries with medication coverage filled 24.1 prescriptions and spent about $999 in that year—an 82% difference in expenditures.[31]

Based on 1998 Medicare Current Beneficiary Survey data, estimates reveal that covered Medicare beneficiaries in self-reported poor health spent $910 more in total for drugs than their noncovered counterparts; the covered versus noncovered utilization differential for persons with or without one or more chronic condition had also widened in recent years. Although female beneficiaries, on average, obtain many more prescriptions (by 46%) than males, the covered/noncovered prescription drug differential among males is wider than that for females. Noncovered males use 40% fewer prescriptions than covered males, while noncovered females use 17% fewer than covered females. Covered beneficiaries in poor health also fill almost 15 more prescriptions, on average, than noncovered enrollees in poor health. Covered beneficiaries with one or more chronic conditions receive more prescriptions than their uncovered counterparts, with large differences in use and spending between covered and noncovered beneficiaries with incomes below the federal poverty level.

For all levels of income, prescription drug utilization was higher for covered beneficiaries. The lower the beneficiary's income, the larger the difference in prescription drug utilization. The largest discrepancy occurs among Medicare beneficiaries with incomes below the federal poverty level: fourteen prescriptions annually. These data highlight the degree to which the covered/noncovered differentials in prescription drug utilization and spending patterns have widened significantly in recent years.[31]

Whether these utilization and spending differentials hold for psychotropic medications is not known: data permitting analysis specific to psychoactive medications are not available. However, there is no reason to assume that these trends are less important for Medicare beneficiaries with psychiatric disorders, either alone or in combination with other illnesses.

Demographic and health history differences between Medicare beneficiaries with and without prescription drug coverage are most pronounced with regard to earnings per household. Among beneficiaries without prescription drug coverage, the proportion of elderly beneficiaries with low household incomes is much higher than among beneficiaries with coverage. This differential is shown graphically in Figure 3.1.

Psychotropic Drug Utilization

Although empirical sales data providing detail sufficient to segregate costs of psychotropic drugs from other classes of medications are limited, psychotropic drugs comprise a large fraction of prescription drugs used by Medicare beneficiaries. Based on Medicare Current Bene-

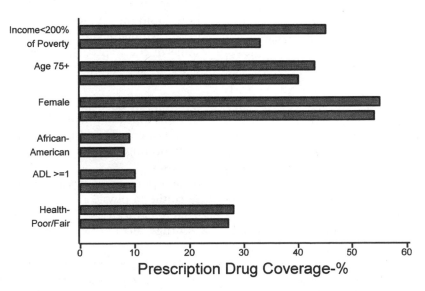

Figure 3.1. Characteristics of Medicare Beneficiaries Without [1st Bar] and With [2nd Bar] Prescription Drug Coverage, 1999.

ficiary Survey data, psychotherapeutic drugs are estimated to constitute the fourth largest category of medications reported by noninstitutionalized Medicare beneficiaries, comprising 7% of all drugs used.[32] Drug categories used more frequently were cardiac drugs (15%), cardiovascular drugs (10%), and diuretics (7%).

Antidepressants are among the most frequently prescribed medications for Medicare beneficiaries. For example, analysis of claims for payment of outpatient prescription drugs among Medicare beneficiaries enrolled in prescription benefit plans managed by a large prescription benefit management company (Merck-Medco Managed Care), purchasers were categorized according to ten separate medical conditions based on the pattern of prescription drugs purchased in 1998.[14] Depression was one of the 10 categories, and depression prevalence in this sample of 375,000 beneficiaries aged 65 years or older was estimated at 10.3%. Comparative estimated prevalence rates for arthritis, diabetes, and cancer were 16.1%, 7.6%, and 3.2%, respectively.

In 1998, average total expenditures for all drugs among persons with at least one prescription were $1343 (median $895). For depression, the average total expenditure among persons with at least one prescription was $2293 (median $1760). Among the ten established disease categories, only diabetes ($2324) and acid-peptic disease ($2305) had higher average prescription drug costs than depression. On average, the total out-of-pocket expenditure for prescription drugs in 1998 in this analysis was $164. For depression, the average out-of-pocket expenditure was $274. Among the ten disease categories, only diabetes had higher average out-of-pocket costs—$280—than depression.[14] In 2001, for all prescription drug expenditures (i.e., for *all* purchasers, not limited to Medicare beneficiaries), more money was spent on the antidepressant drug categories for which drug sales were tracked[12]; expenditures for the antipsy-

chotic medications category was ranked thirteenth. These data probably underestimate actual expenditures for all elderly Medicare beneficiaries[14] because the Merck-Medco system serves only employer-based plans, and elderly persons with employer-sponsored drug coverage are thought to be healthier, younger, and, on average, to have higher incomes than the Medicare population as a whole (see Table 3.2).[33]

Data on expenditure patterns for psychotropic medications other than antidepressants and antipsychotics prescribed for elderly persons have not been analyzed, representing a significant gap in current knowledge about psychotropic drug utilization among elderly consumers. Rational planning for adequate financing of pharmaceutical treatments for neuropsychiatric conditions in the elderly cannot be undertaken without these data.

Psychotropic Drug Costs and Compromised Patients

In clinical practice, some geropsychiatric patients who are struggling financially commonly use a number of different practical methods to reconcile their limited household income with the need to take expensive medication. The following are some of the approaches that patients in these circumstances have followed:

1. Purchasing only part of their prescriptions and then taking medications on only some days of the month
2. Rationing medications, taking smaller doses
3. Stopping a medication without consulting a physician
4. Self-medicating with over-the-counter drugs, alcohol, or other substances

Any of these actions can result in severely compromised geropsychiatric care, and clinicians treating elderly patients must be alert to signs that these treatment-

Table 3.2.   Comparative Costs of Psychotropic Medications

Antidepressant Medication

Norpramin	10 mg capsules	$0.74/capsule
Desipramine (generic)	10 mg capsules	$0.18/capsule
Pamelor	10 mg capsules	$1.53/capsule
Nortriptyline (generic)	10 mg capsules	$0.30/capsule
Celexa (citalopram)	10 mg capsules	$2.22/tablet
Lexapro (escitalopram)	10 mg capsules	$2.07/tablet
Paxil (paroxetine)	10 mg capsules	$2.50/tablet
Prozac	10 mg capsules	$3.07/capsule
Fluoxetine (generic)	10 or 20 mg capsules	$1.13/capsule
Zoloft (sertraline)	25 or 50 mg capsules	$2.33/tablet
Effexor XR (venlafaxine)	37.5 mg capsules	$2.37/capsule
Wellbutrin SR (bupropion)	100 mg tablets	$1.60/tablet

Antipsychotic Medication

Haloperidol (generic)	0.5 05 or I mg tablets	$0.09/tablet
Perphenazine (generic)	2 mg tablets	$0.34/tablet
Stelazine	2 mg tablets	$1.13/tablet
Trifluoperazine (generic)	2 mg tablets	$0.44/tablet
Abilify (aripiprazole)	10 or 15 mg tablets	$8.87/tablet
Geodon (ziprasidone)	20 mg capsules	$3.75/capsule
Risperdal (risperidone)	0.25 mg tablets	$2.73/tablet
Seroquel (quetiapine)	25 mg tablets	$1.44/tablet
Zyprexa (olanzapine)	5 mg tablets	$5.83/tablet

Sedative/Hypnotic Medication

Ativan	0.5 mg tablets	$0.97/tablet
Lorazepam (generic)	0.5 mg tablets	$0.47/tablet
Serax	10 mg tablets	$1.10/capsule
Oxazepam (generic)	10 mg tablets	$0.43/capsule
Ambien (zolpidem)	5 mg tablets	$1.93/tablet
Sonata (zaleplon)	5 mg tablets	$2.03/capsule

*These are self-pay prices offered (circa August 2003) by a U.S.-based, internationally accessible commercial pharmacy. These prices do not take into account discounts or insurance coverage. Dosage levels are the more commonly prescribed units for an elderly patient.

compromising actions may be taking place. When such behaviors are suspected, alerting family members or other caregivers is certainly indicated, and referral of the patient to community elderly-assistance programs may be necessary.

For some of the newer psychotropic drugs, pharmaceutical manufacturers have developed drug assistance programs to aid patients unable to purchase needed medication. These programs usually require a prescribing healthcare professional's involvement to provide documentation regarding the patient's need for the drug, as well as information from the patient regarding income, assets, expenses, and insurance coverage. Though often very helpful, these programs involve a time delay while applications for assistance are processed. These delays are longer for some pharmaceutical companies than for others, depending in part on the level of documentation of need that must be provided. Commonly such drug assistance programs require that the medications provided be sent to the healthcare professional's office rather than to the patient, and this procedure may result in an interruption of treatment and subsequent relapse. Dependence on the ''good-will'' provision of free medications is an inadequate basis for psychotropic drug treatment of elderly patients with limited financial resources!

Conclusions

Most low-income elderly Medicare beneficiaries lack coverage for psychotropic and
other important medications, resulting in
avoidable deterioration of health (especially among those with chronic illnesses)
and the avoidable use of expensive institutional services. Rapidly escalating drug
costs, more restrictive drug-coverage policies, and a dramatic increase in size of
the elderly population have exacerbated
these problems. To recapitulate:

- Prescription drugs are an increasingly
  important part of the healthcare needs
  of Medicare beneficiaries, and psychotropic medications are among the prescription drugs most frequently used by
  large numbers of this population.
- Out-of-pocket prescription drug costs
  impose large financial burdens on Medicare beneficiaries, particularly those
  with low income.
- Coverage for prescription drugs has varied widely among Medicare beneficiaries. Although employer-based coverage frequently is comprehensive, it is
  available for only a minority of the Medicare population. Medigap coverage
  does not provide high-value (cost-effective) coverage for psychotropic prescription drugs.
- Coverage for psychotropic prescription
  drugs may be more variable among
  Medicare beneficiaries than is coverage
  for prescription drugs generally, but
  credible data addressing this issue are
  not available.
- Elderly persons pay higher prices for
  prescription drugs, including psychotropic medications, than do persons
  with conventional health insurance coverage.
- Prescription drug expenditures vary
  dramatically across the Medicare population, with some beneficiaries paying
  substantially more for psychotropic
  medications and other drugs, both out
  of pocket and in aggregate, than other
  beneficiaries.

- Medicare beneficiaries without prescription drug coverage or with limited
  coverage use fewer prescriptions than
  otherwise comparable Medicare beneficiaries with adequate prescription drug
  coverage.
- Credible evidence shows that reduced
  prescription drug utilization among elderly people is associated with adverse
  health outcomes.
- Although research data are not available, clinical experience affirms that adverse health outcomes from reduced or
  absent prescription drug use are more
  prevalent for psychotropic medications
  than for other drugs.

Even with the new Medicare 2003 legislation, the experience of the past several
years with regard to prescription drug-cost
acceleration and the effects of inadequate
prescription drug coverage suggests that
Medicare prescription coverage should
maintain at least the following features:

1. Standardized eligibility criteria and
   standard benefits, based on need, without regard to place of residence
2. Progressive cost-sharing (i.e., a sliding-
   scale mechanism) so that the poorest
   and sickest participants do not encounter greater barriers for use
3. Comprehensive drug pharmacy so that
   coverage encompasses medications of
   all categories, including psychotropic
   agents that have been shown to be safe
   and effective
4. Vigorous monitoring mechanisms to
   encourage use of lower-cost generic
   drugs and agents that are clearly cost
   effective

The programs proposed by the 2003
Medicare legislation offer many construc-
tive changes. However, in the first months
since its passage, data reveal that these
changes will cost one-third more than initially projected. Praise and criticism for
this legislation remain to be tested.

References

1. Davis M, Poisal J, Chullis G, et al. Prescription drug coverage, utilization, and spending among Medicare beneficiaries. *Health Aff* 1999;18: 231–243.
2. Adams AS, Soumerai SB, Ross-Degnan D. The case for a Medicare drug benefit: a critical review of the empirical evidence. *Annu Rev Public Health* 2001;22:49–61.
3. Social Security Administration, U.S. Department of Health and Human Services. *Fact sheet: 1999 Social Security changes.* Baltimore, MD: Social Security Administration, 1998.
4. Gross DJ, Alecxih L, Gibson MJ, et al. Out-of-pocket health spending by poor and near-poor elderly Medicare beneficiaries. *Health Serv Res* 1999;34:241–254.
5. *Wall Street Journal.* The uncovered: drugs costs can leave elderly a grim choice: pills or other needs. New York, NY: November 17, 1998.
6. Murray LA, Poisal JA. Barriers to physician care for Medicare beneficiaries. *Health care Fin Rev* 1998;19:101–104.
7. Federman AD, Adams AS, Ross-Degnan D, et al. Supplemental insurance and use of effective cardiovascular drugs among elderly Medicare beneficiaries with coronary heart disease. *JAMA* 2001; 286:1732–1739.
8. Soumerai SB, Ross-Degnan D, Avorn J, et al. Effects of Medicaid drug-payment limits on admission to hospitals and nursing homes. *N Engl J Med* 1991;325:1072–1077.
9. Soumerai SB, McLaughlin TJ, Ross-Degnan D, et al. Effects of limiting Medicaid drug-reimbursement benefits on the use of psychotropic agents and acute mental health services by patients with schizophrenia. *N Engl J Med* 1994;331: 650–655.
10. Fortess EE, Soumerai SB, McLaughlin TJ, et al. Utilization of essential medications by vulnerable older people after a drug benefit cap: importance of mental disorders, chronic pain, and practice setting. *J Am Geriatr Soc* 2001;49: 793–797.
11. Levit K, Cowan C, Lazenby H, et al. Health spending in 1998: signals of change. *Health Aff* 2000;19:124–132.
12. National Institute for Health Care Management Research and Educational Foundation. *Prescription drug expenditures 2001: another year of escalating costs.* Washington DC: 2002.
13. *Wall Street Journal.* Prescription-drug spending jumps 17%. New York, NY: March 29, 2002.
14. Steinberg EP, Gutierrez B, Momani A, et al. Beyond survey data: a claims-based analysis of drug use and spending by the elderly. *Health Aff* 2000; 19:198–211.
15. Health Care Financing Administration, U.S. *Department of Health and Human Services. Medicare & Choice: Changes for the year 2000.* Baltimore, MD: Healthcare Financing Administration, 2001.
16. Centers for Disease Control and Prevention, National Center for Health Statistics. National health and nutrition survey (NHANES). *Patterns of prescription drug use in the United States, 1988–94.* Atlanta GA: Center for Disease Control and Prevention, 2002. Available at http://www.cdc.gov/nchs/nhanes.htm

17. U.S. Department of Health and Human Services. *Prescription drug coverage, spending, utilization, and prices.* Report to the President. Washington DC: U.S. Department of Health and Human Services, April 2000.
18. Blustein J. Drug coverage and drug purchases by Medicare beneficiaries with hypertension. *Health Aff* 2000;19:219–230.
19. Lillard LA, Rogowski J, Kington R. Insurance coverage for prescription drugs: effects on use and expenditures in the Medicare population. *Med Care* 1999;37:926–36.
20. Rogowski J, Lillard LA, Kington R. The financial burden of prescription drug use among elderly persons. *Gerontologist* 1997;37:475–482.
21. Stuart B, Coulson NE. Use of outpatient drugs as death approaches. *Healthcare Fin Rev* 1994;15: 63–82.
22. Johnson RE, Mullooly JP, Greenlick MR. Morbidity and medical care utilization of old and very old persons. *Health Serv Res* 1990;25: 639–665.
23. Khandker RK, Simoni-Wastila LJ. Differences in prescription drug utilization and expenditures between Blacks and Whites in the Georgia Medicaid populations. *Inquiry* 1998;35:78–87.
24. Fillenbaum GG, Hanlon JT, Corder EH, et al. Prescription and nonprescription drug use among black and white community-residing elderly. *Am J Public Health* 1993;83:1577–1582.
25. Soumerai SB, Ross-Degnan D. Inadequate prescription-drug coverage for Medicare enrollees—a call to action. *N Engl J Med* 1999;340: 722–728.
26. Soumerai SB, Ross-Degnan D. Experience of state drug benefit programs. *Health Aff* 1990;9: 36–54.
27. Soumerai SB, Avorn J, Ross-Degnan D, et al. Payment restrictions for prescription drugs under Medicaid: effect on therapy, cost, and equity. *N Engl J Med* 1987;317:550–556.
28. Reeder CE, Nelson AA. The differential impact of copayment on drug use in a Medicaid population. *Inquiry* 1985;22:396–403.
29. Steinman MA, Sands LP, Covinsky KE. Self-restriction of medications due to cost in seniors without prescription coverage: a national survey. *J Gen Intern Med* 2001;16:793–799.
30. Nelson AA, Reeder CE, Dickson WM. The effect of a Medicaid drug co-payment program on the utilization and cost of prescription services. *Med Care* 1984;22:724–736.
31. Poisal JA, Murray L. Growing differences between Medicare beneficiaries with and without drug coverage. *Health Aff* 2001;20:74–85.
32. Waldron CH, Poisal JA. Five most commonly used types of pharmaceuticals. *Healthcare Fin Rev* 1999;20:119–123.
33. Poisal JA, Murray LA, Chulis GS, Cooper BS. Prescription drug coverage and spending for Medicare beneficiaries. *Healthcare Fin Rev* 1999;20: 15–27.

Supplemental Readings

Centers for Medicare and Medicaid Services: Medicare Modernization Act. http://www.cms.hhs.gov/medicarereform; February, 2004.

Center for Medicare/Medicaid Services. National Healthcare Expenditures Projections: 2000–2010. http://www.hcfa.gov/stats/NHE-proj/proj2000/proj2000, March, 2001.

Healthcare Financing Administration. *A Profile of Medicaid: Chartbook 2000:* U.S. Department of Health and Human Services, September 2000.

Healthcare Financing Administration. *Medicare 2000: 35 Years of Improving Americans' Health and Security.* U.S. Department of Health and Human Services, 2000.

Katzelnick DJ, Kobak KA, Greist JH, et al. Effect of primary care treatment of depression on service use by patients with high medical expenditures. *Psychiatr Serv* 1997;48:59–64.

Larsen PD, Martin JL. Polypharmacy and elderly patients. *AORN J* 1999;69:619–628.

NIHCM. *Prescription Drug Expenditures in 2001: Another Year of Escalating Costs.* Washington, DC, National Institute for Healthcare Management, 2002.

Shea DG. Parity and prescriptions: policy developments and their implications for mental health in later life. *Generations* 2002;26:83–89.

Strain JJ, Lyons JS, Hammer JS, et al. Cost offset from a psychiatric consultation-liaison intervention with elderly hip fracture patients. *Am J Psychiatry* 1991;148:1044–1049.

Thomas CP, Ritter G, Wallack SS. Growth in prescription drug spending among insured elders. *Health Aff* 2001;20:265–277.

Ünützer J, Patrick DL, Simon G, et al. Depressive symptoms and the cost of health services in HMO patients age 65 years and older. *JAMA* 1997;277:1618–1623.

USDHHS. *Mental Health: A Report of the Surgeon General.* Rockville, MD, U.S. Department of Health and Human Services, 1999.

Part II: The Aging Process and Response to Psychotropic Drugs

Chapter 4

Neurotransmission in the Aging Central Nervous System

Trey Sunderland

Mental capacities decline as age increases, but the central nervous system (CNS) actually functions at very complex levels, usually until the last moment of life. Indeed, as the brain ages, it is perhaps impressive that most normal functions are preserved.

Traditionally, individual neurotransmitters such as norepinephrine, dopamine, serotonin, γ-aminobutyric acid (GABA), acetylcholine, and glutamic acid have been associated directly with specific groups of neuronal pathways and implicated in particular CNS functions. For instance, norepinephrine and serotonin pathways are often associated with mood regulation; dopamine is linked primarily with coordination of muscular movement, cognitive function, and symptoms of psychosis, although some dopamine pathways are also associated with mood; acetylcholine, one of the more ubiquitous neurotransmitters in the CNS, also functions in muscular coordination as well as in REM sleep. It is implicated in mood regulation, and, most importantly, plays a central role in memory function; GABA, like acetylcholine, is present in the synapses of many different neuronal pathways throughout the CNS and may serve as a link between sets of neurons (e.g., dopamine and acetylcholine, norepinephrine and serotonin) as well as being implicated in the symptoms of anxiety. However, whereas GABA is a major inhibitory neurotransmitter in the CNS, glutaminergic acid is one of the important excitatory amino acids, with actions throughout the cortex.

Less well known are the various neuromodulator and effector systems that interconnect these major neurotransmitters with biological actions. This process of signal transduction probably also undergoes subtle changes during aging, thereby altering the sensitivity, efficacy, and regulation of neurotransmission.[1,2] The most obvious effector systems that change with age are the sex hormones (e.g., estrogen, testosterone, DHEA), but many other hormones are also involved (e.g., oxytocin and vasopressin).[3–5] Further study of these hormones on the traditional neurotransmitter systems during aging is necessary.

CNS functions involving movement, perception, cognition, speech, memory, and emotion are thought to emanate from complex interconnections of neurons that cluster to form nuclei or groups of nuclei located in discrete areas of the brain. From these nuclei, neuronal pathways transmit messages from one brain location to another via the synthesis, release, and complex interactions of chemical neurotransmitters. The same neurotransmitters communicate among all the nerves of a particular neuronal pathway. Specific brain pathways have thus come to be identified with the name of the principal neurotransmitter produced by their neurons and the various effector systems known as second messengers. The precise relation among different brain functions and specific neurotransmitters remains only partially charted, even within the dedicated neuronal pathways. Moreover, some neurotransmitters are found in more than one neuronal pathway or effector system and therefore may be associated with several different functions in the brain, each with its own cascade.

The Neurotransmission Process

Neurotransmitters, once viewed simply as chemical messengers that joined the presynaptic and postsynaptic neurons like an electrical spark across a gap, are now seen as part of the neurotransmission process. The process includes neurotransmitters, neurohormones, and neuromodulators, all of which contribute to the transfer of information from one cell to another. Starting with the amino acid and enzymatic precursors, neurotransmitters are generally synthesized and stored in vesicles in the presynaptic nerve ending. As a signal is conducted down through the body of a neuron to the nerve ending, the neurotransmitter is released into the synaptic cleft, initiating a sequence of chemical events that carry a neuronal signal across the synapse to the next neuron. The released neurotransmitter also regulates further presynaptic synthesis and release, thereby maintaining a balance of neurotransmitter manufacture, storage, and release into the synapse.

In a classical sense, release of neurotransmitter is governed by several factors: entrance of extracellular calcium into the presynaptic nerve ending; the amount of neurotransmitter already present in the synapse; and the activity of a receptor located on the presynaptic nerve terminal. The presynaptic receptor (or autoreceptor) functions like a thermostat in a home heating system. If a high level of neurotransmitter is available in the synapse, the autoreceptor shuts off further presynaptic neurotransmitter release. When neurotransmitter levels fall, the autoreceptor

initiates the release of more neurotransmitter from presynaptic storage. Impaired function of the autoreceptor, manifest as either subsensitivity or hypersensitivity to synaptic neurotransmitter, contributes to dysregulated neuronal function.

On the far side of the synapse, the postsynaptic neuron contains protein molecules embedded in the membrane that surrounds an enlarged, bulbous nerve terminal. These molecules form discrete receptors, and each receptor generally binds with only one specific neurotransmitter, although binding may be influenced by other substances such as peptide molecules (known as neuromodulators), hormones (neurohormones), cyclic nucleotides (neuromediators) or growth factors (neurotrophic factors).

A single neurotransmitter may have several subtypes of receptors that differ in structure and function even though they share a common neurotransmitter. Receptor sites are located in the membrane of the presynaptic nerve terminal as well as in the postsynaptic neuronal membrane, and may thus respond distinctively to the aging process as well as to psychotropic drugs. Receptors often change in function, depending on the availability of neurotransmitters. For example, when neurotransmitter is in short supply, receptor sites can increase in number and sensitivity to available neurotransmitter in an attempt to maintain usual levels of neurotransmitter function—the process of "upregulation." When excess neurotransmitter is available in the synaptic cleft, receptors usually decrease in number and sensitivity—the process of "downregulation." Psychotropic drugs may alter the available supply of neurotransmitter, causing either "up" or "down" regulation.

In some neuronal pathways, the binding of a neurotransmitter to its receptor site continues the neuronal message directly without intervening steps. In others, neurotransmission is more complex and occurs in several steps. For example, direct neurotransmission occurs along

GABA and acetylcholine pathways as well as some dopamine and serotonin pathways. Neurotransmission along other dopamine and serotonin pathways, as well as in all norepinephrine neurotransmission, is considerably more complex.

The first step in all neurotransmission, direct or complex, involves release of neurotransmitter itself—the "first messenger"—which delivers the neuronal "message" across the synaptic cleft by binding to the receptor site. In complex neurotransmission, norepinephrine, dopamine, or serotonin molecules bind to receptor-site proteins that either stimulate or inhibit further synaptic events. When stimulated, the protein activates an enzymatic transformation of energy-containing molecules that serve as a "second messenger" and continue transmission of neuronal information. For example, in some norepinephrine, dopamine, and serotonin neurons, the enzyme adenylate cyclase catalyzes conversion of the energy-containing molecule adenosine triphosphate (ATP) to cyclic AMP (cAMP), the second messenger. In other norepinephrine and serotonin neurons, the enzyme phospholipase C catalyzes transformation of a polyphosphoinositide molecule to the second messengers inositol triphosphate (IP_3) and diacylglycerol (DAG). The neurotransmitter message is then amplified by cAMP or IP_3, activating yet another enzyme (known as protein kinase), which carries out the specific function of the neuron or continues transmission of the neuronal signal along the pathway. Whether direct or complex, transmission of the neuronal signal across the synaptic cleft to the receptor site initiates the functional response of that neuron.

After receptor-site binding, most of the neurotransmitter is taken back into the presynaptic nerve terminal (reuptake), where a small portion is metabolized by the enzyme monoamine oxidase (MAO), which has two forms, MAO_A and MAO_B. Small amounts of norepinephrine, dopamine, and serotonin are metabolized in their respective presynaptic nerve end-

ings. Remaining portions of neurotransmitter not taken back into the presynaptic nerve ending are metabolized and removed from further synaptic activity. Some neurotransmitters that bind to the postsynaptic receptor site (e.g., acetylcholine and GABA) are metabolized and removed from further synaptic activity by enzymes present either in the synapse or in the postsynaptic nerve terminal. Nonmetabolized portions of the neurotransmitter are stored for future release.

These two processes, metabolism and reuptake, maintain a balance among neurotransmitter synthesis, release, and amount in the synapse. Other substances (neuromodulators), also manufactured and released to the synaptic receptor site, may alter receptor binding, sensitivity, or second-messenger responsivity. Thus, the final common pathway of protein function can be altered in multiple ways. Within these complex synaptic events, many functional derangements are possible, leading to alterations in neuronal function and resultant protein deployment. When synaptic dysfunction occurs throughout a neuronal pathway, clinical symptoms may develop. In general, most symptoms of disturbed thinking, memory, muscular coordination, and emotion are thought to result from alteration in these events, specifically variation in amounts and activities of neurotransmitter in the synapse, number or sensitivity of receptor sites, and functional response of the second-messenger system of effector proteins within the cell. Thus, although the neurotransmission cascade has expanded well beyond the neurotransmitter itself, it still focuses on the neurotransmitter signal as the key initiating event, although it quickly moves on to include the downstream effector systems that are now becoming the targets for pharmacologic manipulation.

The concept of vertical integration within isolated neurotransmitter systems has come under intense scrutiny over the last decade. Neurotransmitters and their associated effector systems, including first and second messengers, are now viewed as integrators of information. Rather than being separate and parallel neurotransmitter highways, cooperation and coordination across multiple neurotransmitter systems occurs, with sharing of signaling molecules and biologic mechanisms involved in those cascades. Perhaps most importantly, the receptor-based neurotransmitter systems can be viewed as a biologic amplification system with the transcription of multiple copies of messenger ribonucleic acid (mRNA) and endpoint proteins as the ultimate outcome measures.

Using the glutamate system as an illustrative example, ionotropic (voltage dependent) receptors and metabotropic (G-protein-mediated) receptors must also be considered. Both of these types of receptors can be affected by aging. Focusing first on the ionotropic receptors, specifically the N-methyl-D-aspartate (NMDA) receptor that is calcium permeable, a clear-cut effect of aging occurs. Calcium ($Ca++$) has long been associated with possible explanations of brain aging,[6] but, more recently, great progress has been made in identifying important, rate-limiting steps in calcium-dependent neurotransmission that may be affected by aging. A special focus of interest has been change within voltage-dependent calcium channel receptors such as NMDA. Specifically, the amplitude and duration of calcium-dependent hyperpolarization differs over the aging process.[7-9] Changes in calcium-dependent synaptic plasticity and transmission within the hippocampus have also been identified, thereby altering synaptic transmission with brain aging.[10,11] Long-term potentiation (LTP) decays more rapidly with aging while long-term depression (LTD) increases in older animals, perhaps due to changes in stimulation thresholds,[12,13] thereby making the addition of new memories more difficult with aging.

In addition to age-related changes in synaptic neurotransmission, postsynaptic signaling pathways are also dysregulated with aging, including the activity of down stream protein phosphatases and kinases[10,14] For instance, within metabotropic receptors, an age-related increase in the protein phosphatase activity of calcineurin (CaN) can lead to the dephosphorylation of downstream proteins such as cAMP response element binding (CREB) or the bcl-2 protein BAD.[15-18] The net result of this dysregulation would indeed be increased susceptibility to neurotoxicity and cell death in different brain areas.[19] In another pathway, glycogen synthase kinase-3 (GSK-3), a serine/threonine kinase, is a major protein in the regulation of apoptosis through its effects on downstream gene transcription factors (including c-jun, β-catenin and Myc) indicating that the GSK-3 cascade is also important in normal aging.[20-22] Because it regulates β-amyloid protein,[23] GSK-3 has also been linked to the pathogenesis of Alzheimer's disease (AD), suggesting a role for GSK-3 antagonists in the therapeutics of AD.

These two age-related changes, enzyme phosphorylation and gene transmission, represent only a fraction of the age-associated postsynaptic alteration. Many more will be identified as potential targets of future drug treatments in the elderly.

Effect of Age on Neurotransmitters

Reduced transmission of neuronal messages in the aging brain, whether associated with changes in the amount and activity of neurotransmitter or with reduced sensitivity to it, is thought to be associated with some of the more prevalent emotional, behavioral, and cognitive disorders of elders. The question of receptor malleability is quite important in aging studies. The ability of a receptor to upregulate or downregulate in response to drugs may decrease with age.[24] Since the elderly may take many drugs that affect neurotransmitter supply, the reduced ability of these receptors to upregulate or downregulate may be responsible, in part, for an older patient's increased or decreased responsiveness to medications. Age-related changes regarding specific neurotransmitters in the human CNS are presented in Tables 4.1 to 4.6 and are discussed in detail in the sections that follow.

Norepinephrine

Norepinephrine has long been known to participate in regulating mood, arousal, and memory. A catecholamine neurotransmitter produced from the amino acid precursor tyrosine, norepinephrine enters the terminal end of the catecholaminergic neuron where it is converted to norepinephrine through a series of enzymatic transformations to become a biogenic amine. First, the enzyme tyrosine hydroxylase and its cofactor biopterin convert tyrosine to 3,4-dihydroxyphenylalanine (dopa). The rate of this enzymatic conversion regulates the rate of norepinephrine synthesis to the extent that reduced availability or activity of tyrosine hydroxylase, tyrosine, or biopterin decreases norepinephrine's synthesis. Because catecholamine biosynthesis uses less than 2% of the body's tyrosine, the enzyme level usually regulates the rate of synthesis. The second catalytic step in the conversion involves a decarboxylase enzyme that rapidly converts dopa to dopamine, with vitamin B_6 as a cofactor. However, a reduced vitamin B_6 level does not significantly reduce norepinephrine synthesis. In the third and final transformation, dopamine is converted to norepinephrine by the enzyme dopamine β-hydroxylase (DβH), with ascorbic acid as a cofactor. Once synthesized, norepinephrine is stored in intraneuronal vesicles, awaiting calcium-dependent release into the synaptic cleft, where, as the first messenger, it initiates the neurotransmission process by binding to both presynaptic and postsynaptic receptors.

At least three receptors—α_1-, α_2-, and the β-receptors—are important in norepinephrine neurotransmission. The α_1-receptors are postsynaptic, linked to the phospholipase C enzyme system, which in turn acts on various phosphoinositides, producing the second messengers IP_3 and DAG. IP_3 activates the release of intracellular calcium and DAG activates protein kinase C to continue the path of neurotransmission. The α_2-receptors (primarily presynaptic) as well as the β-receptors (postsynaptic) activate adenylate cyclase, which then converts ATP to cAMP. The presynaptic α_2-receptor serves as a feedback or "thermostat"-type regulator of further synthesis or presynaptic release of norepinephrine: "turning on" α_2-receptors "turns off" norepinephrine synthesis and release. The effect of norepinephrine on postsynaptic β- and presynaptic α_2-receptor cAMP is thought to mediate the primary neuronal messages of norepinephrine, in particular the regulation of mood. Altered sensitivity of either the postsynaptic β- or presynaptic α_2-receptor, or both, to norepinephrine is associated with affective illness in humans.

While tonic sympathoadrenal activity generally increases with aging,[25] decreased norepinephrine activity has been assumed in the brains of older people. However, data supporting this assumption are sparse and sometimes contradictory. The aging process is thought to change the rate and amount of central norepinephrine synthesis. Overall, the aging brain has fewer neurons in the locus ceruleus—the major center for norepinephrine-containing cells in the brainstem that projects to much of the cortex.[26,27] Also, reduced activity of tyrosine hydroxylase and dopa decarboxylase enzymes in the brains of older people suggests reduced norepinephrine synthesis.[26] In addition, MAO_B, which is partly responsible for the metabolic breakdown of norepinephrine, increases with age in humans.[28] Nonetheless, the norepinephrine content of the cerebrospinal fluid (CSF) increases, especially in older men,[29] and 3-methoxy-4-hydroxyphenylglycol (MHPG), a metabolite of norepinephrine, increases with age in selected brain areas (see Table 4.1).[26,27,30,31]

Table 4.1.   Age-Related Changes in the Noradrenergic System

Noradrenergic Markers[a]	Location	Techniques	Findings
Adrenergic neurons			
Mann (1991)	Locus ceruleus	Cell counts	Decreased
G-protein coupling			
Insel (1993)	Animal cortex	Forskolin	Decreased
α_2-receptor			
Sastre & Garcia-Sevilla (1994)	Cortex, platelets	^{3}H-Yohimbine	Decreased
Supiano & Hogikyan (1993)	Cortex, platelets	^{3}H-Yohimbine	Decreased
Pascual et al. (1992)	Cortex, platelets	Autoradiography	Decreased
Kalaria & Andorn (1991)	Hypothalamus	^{3}H-Clonidine	Decreased
β-receptors			
Mendelson & Paxinos	Cortex	B2 Autoradiography	Decreased
Arango et al. (1990)	Cortex	b1 Autoradiography	Decreased
Kalaria et al. (1989)	Cortex	b2 Autoradiography	Unchanged
Plasma NE			
Esler et al. (2002)	Subcortical areas	Norepinephrine turnover	Increased
Featherstone et al. (1987)	Plasma	Isotope dilution	Decreased Clearance
Goldstein et al. (1983)	Plasma	Norepinephrine levels	Increased
MHPG			
Hartikainen et al. (1991)	Selected brain areas	Biochemical assay	Unchanged
Gottfries (1990)	Cerebrospinal fluid	Biochemical assay	Increased

[a] Complete reference citations at end of chapter.

Although data on brain levels of adrenergic receptors in humans are sparse, growing evidence points to age-related reduction in the number of α- and β-receptors in various animal species.[32] However, brain levels of adenylate cyclase and cAMP are thought to remain unchanged during the aging process, suggesting that age-related adrenergic function is more a result of changes in receptor function than in postreceptor enzymatic (second messenger) function. Although β-receptors located on human lymphocytes have been found in similar numbers in older and in younger patients, these receptors appear less responsive when stimulated by norepinephrine.[33,34] Similarly, α_2 receptor density on platelets may be reduced in older humans.[35]

Whether age-related reduction in norepinephrine activity results from impaired function of regulatory proteins or from a dissociation between receptor located events (such as binding and protein regulation) and postreceptor events (such as enzymatic synthesis of second messengers) is not known. After release into the synaptic cleft, most of the norepinephrine is taken up into the presynaptic nerve ending; some is stored in vesicles for release back into the synapse; some is metabolized.

Presynaptic metabolism of norepinephrine results from the activity of MAO in its two forms, MAO_A and MAO_B. Because the activity of MAO in the presynaptic nerve endings (Table 4.1), particularly in form B, increases with age, central norepinephrine metabolism also increases with age, leading to decreased amounts of neurotransmitter. However, plasma and CSF norepinephrine levels increase, at least in older men.[29] Whether this increase is secondary to reduced metabolism or results from an actual increase in production is not yet known. Nonetheless, the finding of increased norepinephrine levels illustrates one of the many contradictions in available knowledge of the aging noradrenergic system and emphasizes the need for further study.

Dopamine

Perhaps the best-known CNS neurotransmitter, dopamine is associated with clinical disorders such as schizophrenia and Parkinson's disease and, to a lesser extent, Alzheimer's disease. As with norepinephrine, changes in nigrostriatal function and dopamine neurotransmission occur with age. Even the phenotypic markers of dopamine neurons decrease with age, as shown with nuclear receptor-related growth factor 1 (Nurr1) changes over time.[35]

Dopamine is another catecholamine associated with several functions in the brain, each mediated through three distinct pathways. The first, the *nigrostriatal tract,* controls complex muscular movements and posture. Reduced dopamine concentrations in this pathway cause the stiffness, tremor, and muscular dyscoordination associated with Parkinson's disease. A second pathway, the *tuberoinfundibular tract,* is associated with the production and release of prolactin, a hormone associated with sexual function and lactation. Altered dopamine levels in this tract influence breast growth and milk production in both men and women. Neurotransmission in the third pathway or set of pathways, the *mesolimbic and mesocortical,* is less well understood. Altered dopamine neurotransmission in these pathways is implicated in the development and course of psychosis in schizophrenia. In association with other neurotransmitters, dopamine may also play a role in memory function and mood regulation. In fact, a general decline in the function of prefrontal dopamine connections has led to models explaining the cognitive decline of aging.[35,36]

Dopamine synthesis follows the same process of enzymatic transformation as norepinephrine. In dopamine synthesis, however, the enzyme DβH (which converts dopamine to norepinephrine) is absent, and dopamine is the final product of the synthesis. Because the activity of the enzymes tyrosine hydroxylase and dopa decarboxylase decreases with age, reduced dopamine synthesis and neurotransmission may result (Table 4.2). In addition, the number of dopamine neurons in the nigrostriatal tract decreases with age, reducing overall dopaminergic neurotransmission in the important pathway controlling motor movement, perhaps establishing the basis for many of the motor problems of the elderly.[37]

There are at least five subtypes of dopamine receptors: D_1, D_2, D_3, D_4, and D_5. D_1-receptors alter adenylate cyclase activity and cAMP production and are found primarily on the postsynaptic neuronal membrane. D_2-receptors do not use the adenylate cyclase/cAMP second-messenger linkage, and in some cases D_2-receptors may actually inhibit adenylate cyclase. Some D_2-receptors function as autoreceptors, located on the presynaptic neurons. Although aging is associated with a significant decrease in D_2-receptors, D_1-receptors may actually increase with age. Younger adults have more D_2- than D_1-receptors; in contrast, in older persons, the ratio of D_1- to D_2-receptors may increase up to threefold, suggesting a significant change in the type of dopamine neurotransmission during the aging process. The function of D_3-receptors is not yet known.

Recent years have seen dramatic advances in the documentation of these dopaminergic changes with age. Using spectroscopic techniques and various imaging techniques with ligands to measure the D_2-receptor and the dopamine transporter, investigators have repeatedly confirmed age-related decreases in striatum and other dopaminergic areas (Table 4.2). Furthermore, molecular biology techniques have also revealed decreases in the mRNA for the transporter that correlate with increased age in animals and humans.[38] Interestingly, measures of the metabolite byproduct of dopamine, homovanillic acid (HVA), are stable in the CSF with age, despite marked reduction

Table 4.2.   Age-Related Changes in the Dopaminergic System

Dopaminergic Marker[a]	Location	Techniques	Findings
Dopaminergic neurons			
Morgan et al. (1987)	Substantia nigra	Cell count	Decreased
Nurr1 immunoreactivity			
Chu et al. (2002)	Substantia nigra	Postmortem immunoflorescence	Decreased
Dopamine transporter			
Pirker et al. (2000)	Striatum	^{123}I β-CIT SPECT	Decreased
Mozley et al. (1999)	Basal ganglia	^{99}Tc-TRODAT-1 SPECT	Decreased
Van Dyck et al. (1995)	Striatum	^{123}I β-CIT SPECT	Decreased
Volkow et al. (1994)	Basal ganglia	$[^{11}C]$ Cocaine PET	Decreased
Bannon et al. (1992)	Nigrostriatum	mRNA	Decreased
DeKeyser et al. (1990)	Nigrostriatum	Postmortem assay	Decreased
Dopamine receptor			
Wang et al. (1995)	Basal ganglia	^{18}F-NMS PET	Decreased
Roth & Joseph (1994)	Striatum (rat)	mRNA	Decreased
Rinne et al. (1993)	Striatum	^{11}G-raclopride PET	Decreased
Tyrosine hydroxylase			
McGeer (1981)	Caudate	Postmortem TH assay	Decreased
MAO enzyme			
Robinson et al. (1977)	Hypothalamus	Postmortem benzylamine assay	Normal
Homovanillic acid			
Miura et al. (2002)	Cortex, striatum (rat)	Biochemical assay	
Bareggi et al. (1985)	Cerebrospinal fluid	Biochemical assay	Increased

[a] Complete reference citations at end of chapter.

in dopamine neurons in both normal and AD patients.

The most frequent clinical result of reduced dopamine transmission in older people is impaired movement coordination, as seen in the tremor and rigidity of Parkinson's disease. However, the actual pattern of cell loss in normal persons and those with Parkinson's disease is quite different, suggesting that Parkinson's disease is not simply an extension of normal aging.[39] This difference is further supported by the recent finding of a genetic abnormality in the long arm of chromosome 4 in one large family pedigree of patients with Parkinson's disease.[40] Functional imaging studies in normal and Parkinson's disease have connected the age-associated cognitive declines with the dopamine system.[41]

Because typical neuroleptic drugs block dopamine neurotransmission in the nigrostriatal tract, they also can produce Parkinson-like effects (extrapyramidal symptoms). Age-related decline of dopamine neurotransmission in the nigrostriatal tract therefore leads to increased susceptibility of older people to acute neuroleptic-induced extrapyramidal symptoms. Alterations in the D_1:D_2-receptor ratio may also increase the susceptibility of older individuals to the chronic effects of neuroleptic usage, such as tardive dyskinesia. With use of such new atypical neuroleptics as clozapine, risperidone, and olanzapine, this side-effect profile can be reduced significantly.

Serotonin

Serotonin receptors have been associated increasingly with psychiatric conditions ranging from obsessive compulsive disorder to schizophrenia to depression and AD. Although no specific disorder unique to older individuals can be attributed to changes in serotonin, this neurotransmitter participates in the regulation of mood, appetite, sleep, and aggression, and may even play a role as a "pacemaker" of the aging process (Table 4.3). For these reasons, age-related changes in the activity of serotonin may be more important than previously recognized. Accordingly, the serotonin system has been linked to age-related behavior problems and cognitive decline, perhaps as a modifying influence rather than the primary cause.[42]

Synthesis of serotonin, like that of norepinephrine and dopamine, occurs in the presynaptic neuron, where two enzyme transformations occur. First, an amino acid, tryptophan, enters the terminal end of the neuron and is converted to 5-hydroxytryptophan (5-HTP) by tryptophan hydroxylase and a biopterin cofactor. This step in the enzymatic conversion process determines the rate of serotonin synthesis. Second, a decarboxylase enzyme rapidly converts 5-HTP into 5-hydroxytryptamine (5-HT)—serotonin. The amount of serotonin synthesized is governed by both enzyme-conversion steps.

A tremendous change has occurred in the nomenclature for the various 5-HT receptors. Currently many cloned subtypes are best organized under the classification of $5-HT_1$ and $5-HT_2$ "families" of receptors, each with its own distinctive functions. Autopsy studies show that both 5-HT itself and the $5-HT_2$ receptor numbers may decrease in the cortex with age while remaining relatively stable in the hippocampus and striatum (Table 4.3). Similarly, functional imaging studies with positron emission tomography (PET) ligands document cortical decreases in $5-HT_2$ binding.[43]

Postmortem studies of human brains show loss of $5-HT_1$ receptors with age[44] as well as reduced numbers of $5-HT_2$ receptors in the frontal cortex (but not the hippocampus). These postmortem findings

Table 4.3. Age-Related Changes in the Serotonergic System

Serotonergic Markers[a]	Location	Techniques	Findings
5-HT transporter			
Yamamoto et al. (2002)	Thalamus & midbrain	^{11}C-McN5652 PET	Decreased
Kuikka et al. (2001)	Midbrain	^{123}I nor-β-CIT SPECT	Decreased
Pirker et al. (2000)	Selected brain areas	^{123}I β-CIT SPECT	Decreased
Marcussen et al. (1987)	Neocortex	^{121}I β-CIT SPECT	Decreased
5-HT$_{1A}$-receptor			
Parsey et al. (2002)	Selected brain areas	^{11}C-WAY PET	No change
Tauscher et al. (2001)	Selected brain areas	^{11}C-WAY PET	Decreased
Burnet et al. (1994)	Hippocampus	mRNA	Increased
Marcussen et al. (1987, 1984)	Striatum	^{3}H-IMI binding	No change
Middlemiss et al. (1986)	Frontal cortex	^{3}H-8OH-DPAT	Decreased
5-HT$_{2A}$-receptor			
Wang et al. (1995); Sparks (1989)	Frontal, occipital	^{18}F-NMS PET	Decreased
Burnet et al. (1994)	Hippocampus	mRNA	Unchanged
Tryptophan hydroxylase			
Kloppel et al. (2001)	Raphe nuclei	TH immunochemistry	Unchanged
Meek (1977)	Selected brain areas		Decreased
Serotonergic levels			
Severson et al. (1995); Gottfries et al. (1979)	Selected brain areas	Cell count	Decreased
5-HIAA			
Muira et al. (2002)	Selected brain areas	Biochemical assay	Decreased
Bareggi et al. (1985)	Cerebrospinal fluid	Biochemical assay	Increased

[a] Complete reference citations at end of chapter.

are supported by in vivo human brain imaging with PET scans that visualize reduced spiroperidol binding in the caudate and putamen and the frontal cortex.[45] Although the functional significance of these receptor changes is not known, evidence suggests that normal older subjects are less sensitive than younger persons to the behavioral effects of a drug that increases serotonin function, suggesting an age-related reduction in either serotonin production or receptor activity.[46] Concentrations of serotonin and its metabolite 5-hydroxyindoleacetic acid (5-HIAA), however, remain unchanged in selected brain areas across the life span,[47] suggesting that the amount of available serotonin is unaffected by age. Because serotonin is generally metabolized by MAO_A, whether the well-characterized increase in MAO_B levels affect the metabolism of serotonin is unclear.

Despite the contradictory nature of research data currently available, most clinical evidence suggests that the function and sensitivity of serotonin receptors decreases with advanced age. If a pattern of decreased serotonergic activity or responsiveness is confirmed, the changes in sleep, appetite, and mood common in older persons may be explained by this age-related decrease in serotonin function. Furthermore, increasing evidence suggests a modulatory influence of serotonin on memory and other behaviors most closely associated with acetylcholine function.[48]

Acetylcholine

The acetylcholine system is perhaps most associated with change over time. Given the strong link between acetylcholine and memory, it is not surprising that researchers and clinicians alike look to this system when assessing age-related memory loss or the possible onset of Alzheimer's disease. In contradistinction to the serotonin data, cholinergic information regarding the CNS is relatively consistent, pointing to an overall decrease in functional capacity as

well as increased sensitivity to pharmacologic challenge.[49–51]

Acetylcholine is one of the first identified and most common CNS neurotransmitters. Synthesized in the presynaptic neuron from dietary choline, it requires only one enzymatic transformation—conversion to acetylcholine by the synthesizing enzyme choline acetyltransferase (CAT), typically found in or around nerve endings. The choline concentration in the nerve cell determines the amount of acetylcholine synthesis. As with other neurotransmitters, synthesized acetylcholine is stored in presynaptic vesicles prior to release into the synaptic cleft. Measurement of acetylcholine is technically difficult and is usually accomplished by indirect bioassays.

Acetylcholine neurotransmission occurs with its release into the synapse and to the acetylcholine postsynaptic receptor site without coupling to adenylate cyclase. Newly synthesized acetylcholine is more readily released than stored acetylcholine. As with the MOA neurotransmitters (norepinephrine, dopamine, and serotonin), a presynaptic autoreceptor regulates the release of acetylcholine. Because acetylcholine undergoes metabolism by acetylcholinesterase, its neurotransmission depends on a balance between neurotransmitter synthesis and metabolism, which is significantly altered in such illnesses as AD.

Distinct pharmacologic properties define the two classes of acetylcholine receptors—muscarinic and nicotinic. Although cholinergic receptors in the CNS have been classified almost exclusively as muscarinic, both types of cholinergic receptors are present. Furthermore, at least five subtypes of muscarinic receptor—M_1 to M_5—are postulated to exist, although the postsynaptic (M_1) and presynaptic (M_2) cholinergic receptors are the two that can be characterized by currently available pharmacologic techniques, each with a different function.[32,52] Recent brain imaging techniques have determined that aging individuals are more likely to show increased M_2 binding in vivo than younger individuals,[53] perhaps suggesting a lower concentration of synaptic acetylcholine.

Information about the effects of normal aging on the cholinergic system are limited and at times contradictory (Table 4.4). Because of the difficulty in measuring acetylcholine directly, the effect of age on total brain acetylcholine is not known. An age-related shrinking of cholinergic neurons in the basal forebrain probably occurs, with resultant decline in cholinergic innervation throughout the brain.[54] This is consistent with prior findings of reduced acetylcholine synthesis and muscarinic receptor binding in aged brains[55,56] and with findings of a general decline in sleep parameters with age.[57]

Acetylcholine plays a significant role in memory storage and retrieval.[58] Experiments with both humans and animals reveal that a reduction in acetylcholine level impairs memory and problem-solving ability. Further, drugs with anticholinergic properties can cause severe disruption of acetylcholine neurotransmission in the CNS of some persons, resulting in confusion and disorientation.[50,59] By implication, a reduced amount of the acetylcholine-synthesizing enzyme CAT is thought to be responsible for at least some of the memory decline in both normal aging and AD.[58,60] In AD, marked disturbance in cholinergic function includes decreased quantity of CAT, fewer cholinergic neurons in the basal forebrain, fewer M_2 muscarinic and nicotinic receptors, and altered responsiveness to cholinergic drugs.[49,61–64]

It is tempting to suggest that the memory losses of normal aging might also re-

Table 4.4.   Age-Related Changes in the Cholinergic System

Cholinergic Markers[a]	Location	Techniques[b,c]	Findings
Cholinergic neurons			
Mesulam et al. (1987)	Basal forebrain (rodent)	Cell count	Decreased
Choline Level			
Brooks et al. (2001)	Frontal lobe	magnetic resonance imaging	Unchanged
G-protein coupling			
Cutler et al. (1994)	Basal ganglia	Carbachol stimulation	Decreased
M_1, M_2-receptors			
Podruchny et al. (2003)	Cortex	[^{18}F]-FP-TZTP PET	Increased
Lee et al. (1996)	Cortex	[^{11}C]-TRB PET	Normal
Suhara et al. (1993)	Cortex	[^{11}C]-NMPB PET	Decreased
Nordberg et al. (1992)	Cortex and other areas	Human autopsy	Normal or mixed
Nicotinic receptor			
Nordberg et al. (1992)	Cortex and thalamus	^{3}H-Nicotine binding	Decreased
Flynn & Mash (1986)	Thalamus	Human autopsy	Decreased
Acetylcholinesterase			
Mesulam et al. (1991)	Cerebral cortex	Immunoassay	No change
Nakano et al. (1986)	Cerebrospinal fluid	Biochemical assay	Increased
Choline acetyltransferase			
Court et al. (1993);	Cortex and other	Human autopsy	Decreased or
Allen et al. (1983)	areas		normal
Scopolamine infusion			
Sunderland et al. (1995)	Cerebral perfusion	SPECT study	Increased sensitivity
Molchan (1992)	Cognitive/behavioral	Drug challenge	Increased sensitivity

[a] Complete reference citations at end of chapter.
[b] NMPB, N-methyl-4piperidylbenzilate; TRB, tropanylbenzilate. [c] FP-TZTP, 3-(3-(3-[^{18}F]Flouropropyl) thio)-1,2,5-thiadiazol-4-yl)-1,2,5,6-tetrahydro-1-methylpyridine.

sult from age-related but less massive changes in the cholinergic system than those seen with AD.[64,65] At the very least, the increased sensitivity of older persons to the anticholinergic properties of psychoactive and other medications may well result in gradual age-related changes in the cholinergic system.[50] From a pharmacologic perspective, the only modest response of AD patients to cholinergic replacement drugs suggests an inherent irreversible failure in the acetylcholine system itself. Findings of altered signal transduction with age[66] and the possibility that AD patients show evidence of differential upregulation of the acetylcholine system after chronic anticholinergic stimulation[67] are also consistent with this hypothesis. However, irreversible structural changes in all cases cannot always be assumed since evidence shows detectable serum anticholinergic activity in older community-based persons that is related to cognitive performance.[68]

Benzodiazepine-GABA Receptor Complex

Like acetylcholine, GABA is widely distributed in the CNS. Unlike acetylcholine, however, GABA is not widely distributed in other parts of the body; only trace amounts are found in peripheral nerves and other tissues. Within the CNS, GABA functions as an inhibitory neurotransmitter and therefore plays a major role in modulating neuronal transmission. GABA receptors are generally divided into two subtypes: $GABA_A$, thought to be involved in feeding behavior, anticonvulsive activity, and anxiety; and $GABA_B$, associated with cardiovascular modulation, analgesia, and depression.[69] Not surprisingly, alterations in GABA function are implicated in various neurologic or psychiatric disorders. Reduced GABA neurotransmission is a central feature of Huntington's chorea and an important factor in Parkinson's disease, tardive dyskinesia, and epilepsy.

GABA is produced from the conversion of glutamic acid by the enzyme glutamic acid decarboxylase (GAD) and a pyridoxal cofactor (vitamin B_6). Although the activity of this synthesizing enzyme decreases during normal aging, whether such activity actually reduces the levels of GABA has not been confirmed. Because GABA is unstable in postmortem tissue, increasing by up to 30 to 40% within 2 minutes of death, testing the effects of aging is difficult. However, age-related decreases in GABA occur in the CSF, markedly so in older women (Table 4.5).

Unlike other neurotransmitters, GABA is not stored in presynaptic vesicles. Rather, it is released directly into the synapse after synthesis. After this release, GABA binds to its postsynaptic receptor without coupling to adenylate cyclase, where it functions as an inhibitory neurotransmitter by decreasing the firing rate of the postsynaptic neuron. Some GABA receptors are closely linked to other receptors that appear to accept only benzodiazepine molecules. The interdependent complex formed by the interaction of these two sets of receptors is hypothesized to operate in the following ways. GABA enhances the binding of a benzodiazepine molecule to its receptor sites; the benzodiazepine in turn sensitizes the GABA receptor to its own neurotransmitter, thus enhancing GABA activity. Activation of the benzodiazepine–GABA receptor complex opens a channel in the neuronal membrane that permits negatively charged chloride ions to enter the neuron from outside the cell. An increase in intracellular chloride causes the electrical activity of the cell membrane to decrease, thereby dampening or inhibiting neurotransmission.

Owing to the paucity of human postmortem data on the effects of aging on the benzodiazepine–GABA receptor complex, most available information is derived from animal studies. Unfortunately, results from experiments in animals have been confusing and sometimes contradictory. For example, benzodiazepine-receptor binding in rats increases with age in the dentate gyrus[70] and decreases in the

Table 4.5.   Age-Related Changes in the GABAergic System

GABAergic Markers[a]	Location	Techniques	Findings
GABA neurons			
Allen et al. (1983)	Selected brain areas	Human autopsy	Decreased
GABA receptors			
Vela et al. (2003)	Hippocampus (rodent)	α_1 subunit mRNA	Increased
Suhara et al. (1993)	10 Brain regions	$[^{11}C]$ Ro 15-4513 PET	No change
Glutamic acid decarboxylase			
Giardino et al. (2002)	Cerebral cortex (rodent)	GAD mRNA	Increased
McGeer (1981)	Thalamus	Human autopsy	Decreased
GABA levels			
Grachev & Apkarian (2001)	Prefrontal cortex	$[^1H]$ magnetic resonance	Decreased
Bareggi et al. (1985);	Cerebrospinal fluid	Biochemical assay	Decreased
Hare et al. (1982)			

[a]Complete reference citations at end of chapter.

cortex, but only if measured in the morning.[71] Similar contradictions and evidence for circadian variations have also been found in rat GABA-receptor binding[71,72] and receptor message[73] perhaps suggesting differential effects in different cortical areas. In animals, aging does not alter the sensitivity of the rat benzodiazepine receptors to GABA modulation,[74] suggesting a dynamic interaction between these two receptors with age.[75] Similarly, PET studies with GABA ligands fail to show any age-related decrease in GABA receptors.[76] This finding contrasts with clinical observations of increased sensitivity of elderly humans to benzodiazepines.[77] Recent data suggest that exogenous GABA and GABA agonists may restore visual cortical discrimination in older monkeys,[78] suggesting that such reversal of age-related GABA decline might also be helpful in humans.

Glutamate

Glutamate, considered one of the major excitatory amino acids (EAAs), is associated with several receptors in the CNS (i.e., NMDA, D, L-α-amino-3-hydroxy-5-methyl-4-isoaxole-propionate [AMPA], kainite, and metabrotropic). Glutamate and other EAAs are thought to have an important role in neuronal plasticity and cell regulation. However, in excess, these neurotransmitters can be neurotoxic, leading to suggestions that the EAAs may be involved in neurodegeneration, which in turn may lead to memory loss in normal aging as well as more serious cognitive disruption in conditions such as AD and Parkinson's disease. A summary of the age-related changes in the glutamate system is found in Table 4.6.

The idea that a balanced level of gluta-minergic neurotransmission is important in the CNS comes from several sources. For instance, the NMDA receptor has been implicated in the formation of long-term potentiation and the neuronal plasticity associated with memory consolidation.[79,80] This association is further enhanced by the concentration of NMDA receptors in the hippocampus and frontal cortex, and the finding in animals that pharmacologic blockade of these receptors can lead to memory impairment.[81,82] Furthermore, excessive glutaminergic stimulation can lead to neuronal toxicity, presumably due, at least in part, to excessive entry of calcium into the cell. While human autopsy data concerning neuronal markers and receptor subtypes is relatively sparse, there is some suggestion of a slight decrease in receptor number with age in the cerebellum, basal ganglia and selected other areas of brain.[83,84]

Table 4.6. Age-Related Changes in the Glutaminergic System

Glutaminergic Markers[a,b]	Location	Techniques[c]	Findings
N-acetyl Aspartate levels			
Grachev & Apkarian (2001)	Cortex	[^{1}H] Magnetic resonance	Decreased
Brooks et al. (2001)	Frontal lobe	[^{1}H] Magnetic resonance	Decreased
Glutamate levels			
Kornhuber et al. (1993)	Putamen	[^{3}H]-Glutamate	No change
EEA transporter			
Procter et al. (1988)	Cortex	Neurochemical assay	Decreased
NMDA-receptor			
Villares and Stavale (2001)	Basal ganglia	[^{3}H]-Glutamate binding	Decreased
Court et al. (1993)	Cortex	[^{3}H]-MK-801 binding	Stable
Johnson et al. (1993)	Cerebellum	[^{3}H]-MK-801 binding	Increased
Piggott et al. (1992)	Frontal cortex	[^{3}H]-MK-801 binding	Decreased

[a] complete reference citations at end of chapter.
[b] EEA, excitatory amino acid; NMDA, N-methyl-o-aspartate.

The possibility of increased glutaminergic stimulation with age, leading to excessive excitability and neuronal toxicity, is an appealing hypothesis given the recent data suggesting that memantine (a NMDA-antagonist) is of benefit to AD subjects with moderate to severe disease.[85] However, the human data supporting an absolute increase in glutaminergic activity are lacking. Rather, a shift in glutaminergic–cholinergic, glutaminergic–serotonergic or glutaminergic–hormonal interactions may be more important in the aging process.[86] Many more specific imaging and pharmacologic studies are needed to explore these hypotheses.

Effect of Psychotropic Drugs on Neurotransmisison

The pervasive view of psychotropic drugs has revolved around the immediate pharmacologic effects of these agents as MOA reuptake blockers, as modulators of MOA metabolism, or as receptor blockers in specific neurotransmitter receptors. Although these descriptions adequately characterize the initial effects of these agents, they have never fully explained the delayed benefit derived from psychotropic agents or the ultimate mechanism of their therapeutic effects. In fact, these initial pharmacologic effects have led to many overly simplistic theories explaining complex psychiatric disorders such as depression and schizophrenia with single-neurotransmitter deficit or overactivity hypotheses. Current preclinical research focuses on the homeostatic mechanism associated with the downregulation of β-adrenergic receptors and the resultant changes in protein kinase activity in targeted neurons. Other potentially important sites of change include the α_2-adrenergic receptor, dopamine receptor (D_1), several serotonin receptors (i.e., 5-HT_{1A} and 5-HT_2), and the linked changes in downstream signal transduction and neuronal circuitry. Simply put, the current emphasis in psychotropic drug research is on the effects of medications on multiple signaling pathways.

Historically the monoaminergic hypothesis of depression was based on the theory that chronically inadequate norepinephrine levels eventually result in behavioral symptoms of depression. Heterocyclic antidepressants increase norepinephrine and, in some cases, serotonin and dopamine availability at the synapse. This neurochemical activity was thought to explain part of the therapeutic antidepressant effect of these drugs, which involves blocking the presynaptic reuptake of nor-epinephrine, serotonin, or dopamine, thereby increasing availability within the synaptic cleft. A second, more current, hypothesized mechanism involves the modulation of both presynaptic and post-synaptic receptors. The net result of altered presynaptic receptor activity reportedly increases or decreases synthesis and releases neurotransmitter into the synaptic cleft via the autoreceptor's thermostat-like feedback mechanism. Increased or decreased postsynaptic receptor function in response to varying levels of neurotransmitter thus maintains stable neurotransmission.

Another traditionally held hypothesized mechanism involves increased norepinephrine, serotonin, and dopamine availability resulting from inhibiting the metabolism of these neurotransmitters by MAO inhibitors rather than from blocking their reuptake. Because the activity of MAO_B located in the presynaptic nerve ending increases in the brains of aging humans, neurotransmitter metabolism presumably increases, resulting in decreased neurotransmitter availability. Although no data indicate that increased presynaptic metabolism of these three neurotransmitters in older people actually results in reduced levels of neurotransmitter in the synapse, increased MAO_B activity with age suggests that MAO inhibitors may be particularly useful antidepressants for older patients. Clinical research in this area is inadequate.

The longstanding explanation of pharmacologic benefits of neuroleptic drugs in schizophrenia revolves around the purported overactivity of dopaminergic neurons in this condition, particularly in the striatum. Rather than increasing neurotransmitter availability (as antidepressants do for norepinephrine, dopamine, and serotonin), neuroleptics are thought to *decrease* dopamine neurotransmission by blocking dopamine binding at dopamine receptor sites. Indeed, dopaminergic blockade in the mesolimbic pathway can diminish symptoms of psychosis as well as

other forms of disordered behavior. Concomitantly, dopamine blockade in the nigrostriatal tract can disrupt the regulation of complex muscular movement, producing the characteristic "neuroleptic" extrapyramidal symptoms of stiffness, tremor, and restlessness. These side effects are more frequent and more severe in older patients because diminished dopamine neurotransmission accompanies normal aging. However, as with the antidepressants, current neuroleptic research focuses on the downstream regulation of G proteins linked to dopamine receptors and the possibility of "uncoupling" between receptors and various second-messenger systems that lead to disrupted neuronal circuitry in schizophrenia and other psychotic disturbances.

In addition to their presumed site of therapeutic activity, neuroleptics and cyclic antidepressants, as well as many other drugs commonly taken by older patients, block postsynaptic acetylcholine receptor sites, resulting in *decreased* acetylcholine neurotransmission. By blocking acetylcholine receptor sites in the aging CNS, which already experiences reduced acetylcholine neurotransmission, these drugs may produce serious toxic effects such as confusion, disorientation, and memory loss. Blockade of peripheral CNS acetylcholine receptors produces anticholinergic effects such as dry mouth, constipation, and urinary retention. These side effects are more frequent and severe in older than in younger patients, partly because the cholinergic systems of elders have less functional reserve and partly because their pharmacologic sensitivity to anticholinergic drugs is greater.[50]

Age-Related Central Nervous System Alterations in Receptor Sensitivity and Psychotropic Drug Effects

In general, older patients seem to be more susceptible than their younger counterparts to the therapeutic and toxic effects of psychotropic drugs. This increased responsiveness can be explained by four important factors. First, age-related changes in cell number and size of specific brain centers, as well as alteration in neurotransmitter sensitivity, may heighten the pharmacologic effect of a drug. Second, certain neurotransmitter receptors may be selectively affected by age-related changes at presynaptic and postsynaptic receptors. Third, age-related changes in the receptor itself, whether located at the actual neurotransmitter binding site or within the second messenger or the effector system, may change sensitivity to the available neurotransmitter. Altered binding of the neurotransmitter to its receptor site may affect its sensitivity to blockade by some psychotropic drugs. Fourth and most simply, altered drug disposition in the aging body generally results in *higher concentration* of psychotropic drugs at CNS receptor sites (see Chapter 5).

The hypothesis of increased receptor sensitivity to psychotropic drugs in older people assumes an enhanced drug response for any concentration of drug at a receptor. This important assumption continues to guide the clinical use of psychotropic drugs: for any given drug dose, clinicians can expect older individuals to have a heightened therapeutic and toxic response. For example, older people are generally sensitive to anticholinergic side effects, often developing toxicity manifest as cognitive and behavioral disturbance at doses only half those given to younger adults.[50,59] Increased receptor sensitivity may also account for the increased effects of benzodiazepines and lithium in the elderly. Research studies suggesting increased density and sensitivity of benzodiazepine binding sites with age may explain the heightened sensitivity of the aging CNS to the sedating effects of long-acting benzodiazepines for any given drug concentration. Enhanced receptor-site sensitivity may also explain the therapeutic efficacy of lithium in elderly patients at plasma concentrations substantially lower than those necessary for younger adults.

Patients with AD who have severe acetylcholine cell loss and reduced neurotransmission are especially sensitive to the anticholinergic effects of drugs.

Similar reasoning may explain the increased sensitivity of older patients to the dopamine-blocking property of neuroleptics. Because dopamine neurotransmission in the nigrostriatal tract may decrease with age, increased dopamine receptor sensitivity to additional dopamine blockade by a neuroleptic may explain the greater incidence and severity of extrapyramidal symptoms in older patients receiving these drugs. This increased responsivity to neuroleptics may be proportional to the decreased number of D_2-receptors.[37] Because the number of serotonin receptors (i.e., 5-HT$_1$ and 5-HT$_2$) also changes significantly with age, research data show that normal elderly persons respond differently to drugs that selectively alter serotonin function.[46]

Although these clinical and research observations may support the concept of *increased* receptor-site sensitivity in older people, some research data actually support *decreased* receptor-site response to drugs. For example, although the number of postsynaptic β-noradrenergic receptor sites decreases with age, one research report notes that older patients are *less sensitive* than younger patients to the effect of drugs that alter norepinephrine receptor sites, resulting in reduced response to cyclic antidepressants.[28] This finding may, in fact, explain why some elderly patients seem resistant to these drugs and require high doses.

Evidence points to the probable association of both increased and decreased receptor-site sensitivity with aging. To date, however, data are insufficient to explain the relation between altered receptor-site sensitivity and the effects of psychotropic drugs in the elderly. To clarify these issues, important additional factors must be studied. Interaction among several factors—altered receptor sensitivity and altered pharmacokinetics (see Chapter 5), other medications, nutritional status, and medical health or disease—are not yet sufficiently understood. Any aspect of these complex factors, alone or in combination, may ultimately verify the basis of altered sensitivity to psychotropic drugs in older patients.

Nonetheless, the clinical manifestations of altered receptor sensitivity are apparent in the patterns of drug effects in elderly patients. Whether these effects result specifically from altered receptor sensitivity, altered kinetics, uncoupling of receptor and effector systems, or other factors, enhanced response to both the therapeutic and the toxic effects of psychotropic drugs is reasonably certain in the elderly. The salient fact is that older patients are more likely to develop unwanted side effects from psychotropic drugs and to require lower dosage regimens. Unfortunately, this concept often leads to the inadequate pharmacologic treatment of the elderly who are suffering from true psychiatric conditions. Increased sensitivity in the elderly is certainly a reason to be cautious and to generally use lower doses of psychotropic medications, but it is not an excuse for inadequate treatment.

References

1. Fowler CJ, Cowburn RF, O'Neill C. Brain signal transduction disturbances in neurodegenerative disorders. *Cell Signal* 1992;4:1–9.
2. Mattson MP. Activities of cellular signaling pathways: a two-edged sword? *Neurobiol Aging* 1991; 12:343–346.
3. Gandy S. Estrogen and neurodegeneration. *Neurochem Res* 2003;28:1003–1008.
4. Ishunina TA, Swaab DF. Neurohypophyseal peptides in aging and Alzheimer's disease. *Ageing Res Rev* 2002;1:537–558.
5. Norbury R, Cutter WJ, Compton J, et al. The neuroprotective effects of estrogen on the aging brain. *Exp Gerontol* 2003;38:109–117.
6. Khachaturian ZS. The role of calcium regulation in brain aging: reexamination of a hypothesis. *Aging (Milano)* 1989;1:17–34.
7. Landfield PW, Pitler TA. Prolonged Ca2+-dependent afterhyperpolarizations in hippocampal neurons of aged rats. *Science* 1984;226: 1089–1092.
8. Disterhoft JF, Thompson LT, Moyer JR Jr., et al. Calcium-dependent afterhyperpolarization and learning in young and aging hippocampus. *Life Sci* 1996;59:413–20.
9. Landfield, PW. Aging-related increase in hippocampal calcium channels. *Life Sci* 1996;59: 399–404.
10. Foster TC, Sharrow KM, Masse JR, et al. Calcineurin links Ca2+ dysregulation with brain aging. *J Neurosci* 2001;21:4066–4073.
11. Barnes C. Plasticity in the ageing central nervous system. *Int Rev Neurobiol* 2001;45:339–354.
12. Foster TC, Norris CM. Age-associated changes in Ca (2+)-dependent processes: relation to hippocampal synaptic plasticity. *Hippocampus* 1997;7:602–612.
13. Kamal A, Biessels GJ, Duis SE, et al. Learning and hippocampal synaptic plasticity in streptozotocin-diabetic rats: interaction of diabetes and ageing. *Diabetologia* 2000;43:500–506.
14. Davis S, et al. Dysfunctional regulation of alpha-CaMKII and syntaxin 1B transcription after induction of LTP in the aged rat. *Eur J Neurosci* 2000;12:3276–3282.
15. Tong G, Shepherd D, Jahr CE. Synaptic desensitization of NMDA receptors by calcineurin. *Science* 1995;267:1510–1512.
16. Genazzani AA, Carafoli E, Guerini D. Calcineurin controls inositol 1,4,5-trisphosphate type 1 receptor expression in neurons. *Proc Natl Acad Sci U S A* 1999;96:5797–5801.
17. Norris CM, Blalock EM, Chen KC, et al. Calcineurin enhances L-type Ca(2+) channel activity in hippocampal neurons: increased effect with age in culture. *Neuroscience* 2002;110: 213–225.
18. Adachi M, Imai K. The proapoptotic BH3-only protein BAD transduces cell death signals independently of its interaction with Bcl-2. *Cell Death Differ* 2002;9:1240–1247.
19. Griffith WH, Jasek MC, Bain SH, et al. Modification of ion channels and calcium homeostasis of basal forebrain neurons during aging. *Behav Brain Res* 2000;115:219–233.
20. Hetman M, Cavanaugh JE, Kimelman D, et al. Role of glycogen synthase kinase-3beta in neuronal apoptosis induced by trophic withdrawal. *J Neurosci* 2000;20:2567–2574.
21. Bijur GN, Jope RS. Proapoptotic stimuli induce nuclear accumulation of glycogen synthase kinase-3 beta. *J Biol Chem* 2001;276:37436–37442.
22. Gould TD, Zarate CA, Manji HK. Glycogen synthase kinase-3: a target for novel bipolar disorder treatments. *J Clin Psychiatry* 2004;65:10–21.
23. Phiel CJ, Wilson CA, Lee VM, et al. GSK-3alpha regulates production of Alzheimer's disease amyloid-beta peptides. *Nature* 2003;423:435–439.
24. Pedigo NW, Jr. Neurotransmitter receptor plasticity in aging. *Life Sci* 1994;55:1985–1991.
25. Seals DR, Esler MD. Human ageing and the sympathoadrenal system. *J Physiol* 2000;528:407–417.
26. Vijayashankar N, Brody H. A quantitative study of the pigmented neurons in the nuclei locus coeruleus and subcoeruleus in man as related to aging. *J Neuropathol Exp Neurol* 1979;38:490–497.
27. McGeer EG. Neurotransmitter systems in aging and senile dementia. *Prog Neuropsychopharmacol* 1981;5:435–445.
28. Scarpace PJ, Abrass LB. Alpha- and beta-adrenergic receptor function in the brain during senescence. *Neurobiol Aging* 1988;9:53–58.
29. Raskind MA, Peskind ER, Veith RC, et al. Increased plasma and cerebrospinal fluid norepi-

nephrine in older men: differential suppression by clonidine. *J Clin Endocrinol Metab* 1988;66: 438–443.

30. Oreland L, Gottfries CG. Brain and brain monoamine oxidase in aging and in dementia of Alzheimer's type. *Prog Neuropsychopharmacol Biol Psychiatry* 1986;10:533–540.

31. Gottfries CG. Neurochemical aspects on aging and diseases with cognitive impairment. *J Neurosci Res* 1990;27:541–547.

32. Vestal RE, Wood AJ, Shand DG. Reduced B-adrenoceptor sensitivity in the elderly. *Clin Pharmacol Ther* 1979;26:181–186.

33. Kalaria RN, Andorn AC. Adrenergic receptors in aging and Alzheimer's disease: decreased alpha 2-receptors demonstrated by [3H]p-aminoclonidine binding in prefrontal cortex. *Neurobiol Aging* 1991;12:131–136.

34. Mendelsohn FAO, Paxinos G. *Receptors in the human nervous system*. San Diego: Academic Press, 1991.

35. Supiano MA, Hogikyan RV. High affinity platelet alpha 2-adrenergic receptor density is decreased in older humans. *J Gerontol* 1993;48: B173–B179.

36. Braver TS, Barch DM. A theory of cognitive control, aging cognition, and neuromodulation. *Neurosci Biobehav Rev* 2002;26:809–817.

37. Rinne JO, Hietala J, Ruotsalainen U, et al. Decrease in human striatal dopamine D2 receptor density with age: a PET study with [11C]raclopride. *J Cereb Blood Flow Metab* 1993;13: 310–314.

38. Bannon MJ, Poosh MS, Xia Y, et al. Dopamine transporter mRNA content in human substantia nigra decreases precipitously with age. *Proc Natl Acad Sci U S A* 1992;89:7095–7099.

39. Palmer AM, DeKosky ST. Monoamine neurons in aging and Alzheimer's disease. *J Neural Transm Gen Sect* 1993;91:135–159.

40. Polymeropoulos MH, Higgins JJ, Golbe LI, et al. Mapping of a gene for Parkinson's disease to chromosome 4q21-q23. *Science* 1996;274:1197–1199.

41. Kaasinen V, Rinne JO. Functional imaging studies of dopamine system and cognition in normal aging and Parkinson's disease. *Neurosci Biobehav Rev* 2002;26:785–793.

42. Gareri P, De Fazio P, De Sarro G. Neuropharmacology of depression in aging and age-related diseases. *Ageing Res Rev* 2002;1:113–134.

43. Wang GJ, Volkow ND, Logan J, et al. Evaluation of age-related changes in serotonin 5-HT2 and dopamine D2 receptor availability in healthy human subjects. *Life Sci* 1995;56:PL249–PL253.

44. Middlemiss DN, Palmer AM, Edel N, et al. Binding of the novel serotonin agonist 8-hydroxy-2-(di-n-propylamino) tetralin in normal and Alzheimer brain. *J Neurochem* 1986;46:993–996.

45. Wong DF, Wagner HN Jr., Dannals RF, et al. Effects of age on dopamine and serotonin receptors measured by positron tomography in the living human brain. *Science* 1984;226:1393–1396.

46. Lawlor BA, Sunderland T, Mellow AM, et al. A preliminary study of the effects of intravenous m-chlorophenylpiperazine, a serotonin agonist, in elderly subjects. *Biol Psychiatry* 1989;25: 679–686.

47. Wester P, Hardy JA, Marcusson J, et al. Serotonin concentrations in normal aging human brains:

relation to serotonin receptors. *Neurobiol Aging* 1984;5:199–203.

48. Tottori K, Nakai M, Uwahodo Y, et al. Attenuation of scopolamine-induced and age-associated memory impairments by the sigma and 5-hydroxytryptamine(1A) receptor agonist OPC-14523 (1-[3-[4-(3-chlorophenyl)-1-piperazinyl]-propyl]-5-methoxy-3,4-dihydro-2[1H]-quinolinone monomethanesulfonate). *J Pharmacol Exp Ther* 2002;301:249–257.

49. Sunderland T, Tariot PN, Cohen RN, et al. Anticholinergic sensitivity in patients with dementia of the Alzheimer type and age-matched controls. A dose-response study. *Arch Gen Psychiatry* 1987;44:418–426.

50. Molchan SE, Martinez RA, Hill JL, et al. Increased cognitive sensitivity to scopolamine with age and a perspective on the scopolamine model. *Brain Res Brain Res Rev* 1992;17:215–226.

51. Terry AV Jr., Buccafusco JJ. The cholinergic hypothesis of age and Alzheimer's disease-related cognitive deficits: recent challenges and their implications for novel drug development. *J Pharmacol Exp Ther* 2003;306:821–827.

52. Ehlert FJ, Roeske WR, Yamamura HI. Muscarinic receptors and novel strategies for the treatment of age-related brain disorders. *Life Sci* 1994;55:2135–2145.

53. Podruchny TA, Connolly C, Bokde A, et al. In vivo muscarinic 2 receptor imaging in cognitively normal young and older volunteers. *Synapse* 2003;48:39–44.

54. Mesulam MM, Mufson EJ, Rogers J. Age-related shrinkage of cortically projecting cholinergic neurons: a selective effect. *Ann Neurol* 1987;22: 31–36.

55. Gibson GE, Peterson C. Aging decreases oxidative metabolism and the release and synthesis of acetylcholine. *J Neurochem* 1981;37:978–984.

56. Freund G. Cholinergic receptor loss in brains of aging mice. *Life Sci* 1980;26:371–375.

57. Reynolds CF III, Kupfer DJ. Sleep research in affective illness: state of the art circa 1987. *Sleep* 1987;10:199–215.

58. Bartus RT, Dean RL III, Beer B, et al. The cholinergic hypothesis of geriatric memory dysfunction. *Science* 1982;217:408–414.

59. Drachman DA. Memory and cognitive function in man: does the cholinergic system have a specific role? *Neurology* 1977;27:783–790.

60. Coyle JT, Price DL, DeLong MR. Alzheimer's disease: a disorder of cortical cholinergic innervation. *Science* 1983;219:1184–1190.

61. Sunderland T, Tariot PN, Newhouse PA. Differential responsivity of mood, behavior, and cognition to cholinergic agents in elderly neuropsychiatric populations. *Brain Res* 1988;472: 371–389.

62. Whitehouse PJ, Martino AM, Antuono PG, et al. Nicotinic acetylcholine binding sites in Alzheimer's disease. *Brain Res* 1986;371:146–151.

63. Mash DC, Flynn DD, Potter LT. Loss of M2 muscarinic receptors in the cerebral cortex in Alzheimer's disease and experimental cholinergic denervation. *Science* 1985;228:1115–1117.

64. Picciotto MR, Zoli M. Nicotinic receptors in aging and dementia. *J Neurobiol* 2002;53:641–655.

65. Casu MA, Wong TP, De Koninck Y, et al. Aging causes a preferential loss of cholinergic innerva-

tion of characterized neocortical pyramidal neurons. *Cereb Cortex* 2002;12:329–337.

66. Cutler R, Joseph JA, Yamagami K, et al. Area specific alterations in muscarinic stimulated low Km GTPase activity in aging and Alzheimer's disease: implications for altered signal transduction. *Brain Res* 1994;664:54–60.

67. Sunderland T, Esposito G, Molchan SE, et al. Differential cholinergic regulation in Alzheimer's patients compared to controls following chronic blockade with scopolamine: a SPECT study. *Psychopharmacology (Berl)* 1995;121:231–241.

68. Mulsant BH, Pollock BG, Kirshner M, et al. Serum anticholinergic activity in a community-based sample of older adults: relationship with cognitive performance. *Arch Gen Psychiatry* 2003; 60:198–203.

69. Matsumoto RR. GABA receptors: are cellular differences reflected in function? *Brain Res Brain Res Rev* 1989;14:203–225.

70. Fanelli RJ, McNamara JO. Effects of age on kindling and kindled seizure-induced increase of benzodiazepine receptor binding. *Brain Res* 1986;362:17–22.

71. Niles LP, Pulido OM, Pickering DS. Age-related changes in GABA and benzodiazepine receptor binding in rat brain are influenced by sampling time. *Prog Neuropsychopharmacol Biol Psychiatry* 1988;12:337–344.

72. Ito Y, Ho IK, Hoskins B. Cerebellar GABAA and benzodiazepine receptor characteristics in young and aged mice. *Brain Res Bull* 1988;21: 251–255.

73. Vela J, Gutierrez A, Vitorica J, et al. Rat hippocampal GABAergic molecular markers are differentially affected by ageing. *J Neurochem* 2003; 85:368–377.

74. Kochman RL, Sepulveda CK. Aging does not alter the sensitivity of benzodiazepine receptors to GABA modulation. *Neurobiol Aging* 1986;7: 363–365.

75. Giardino L, Zanni M, Fernandez M, et al. Plasticity of GABA(a) system during ageing: focus on vestibular compensation and possible pharmacological intervention. *Brain Res* 2002;929: 76–86.

76. Suhara T, Inoue O, Kobayashi K, et al. No age-related changes in human benzodiazepine receptor binding measured by PET with [11C]Ro 15-4513. *Neurosci Lett* 1993;159:207–210.

77. Pomara N, Stanley B, Block R, et al. Increased sensitivity of the elderly to the central depressant effects of diazepam. *J Clin Psychiatry* 1985;46: 185–187.

78. Leventhal AG, Wang Y, Pu M, et al. GABA and its agonists improved visual cortical function in senescent monkeys. *Science* 2003;300:812–815.

79. Bliss TV, Collingridge GL. A synaptic model of memory: long-term potentiation in the hippocampus. *Nature* 1993;361:31–39.

80. Ikonomovic MD, Sheffield R, Armstrong DM. AMPA-selective glutamate receptor subtype immunoreactivity in the aged human hippocampal formation. *J Comp Neurol* 1995;359:239–252.

81. Muller WE, Scheuer K, Stoll S. Glutamatergic treatment strategies for age-related memory disorders. *Life Sci* 1994;55:2147–2153.

82. Ingram DK, Spangler EL, Iijima S, et al. Rodent models of memory dysfunction in Alzheimer's

disease and normal aging: moving beyond the cholinergic hypothesis. *Life Sci* 1994;55:2037–2049.

83. Kornhuber ME, Kornhuber J, Retz W, et al. L-glutamate and L-aspartate concentrations in the developing and aging human putamen tissue. *J Neural Transm Gen Sect* 1993;93:145–150.

84. Villares JC, Stavale JN. Age-related changes in the N-methyl-D-aspartate receptor binding sites within the human basal ganglia. *Exp Neurol* 2001; 171:391–404.

85. Reisberg B, Doody R, Stoffler A, et al. Memantine in moderate-to-severe Alzheimer's disease. *N Engl J Med* 2003;348:1333–1341.

86. McEwen BS. Sex, stress and the hippocampus: allostasis, allostatic load and the aging process. *Neurobiol Aging* 2002;23:921–939.

Table 4.1 References

Arango V, Ernsberger P, Marzuk PM, et al. Autoradiographic demonstration of increased 5-HT2 and β-adrenergic receptor binding sites in the brains of suicide victims. *Arch Gen Psychiatry* 1990; 47:1038–1047.

Esler M, Hastings J, Lambert G, et al. The influence of aging on the human sympathetic nervous system and brain norepinephrine turnover. *Am J Physiol Regul Integr Comp Physiol* 2002;282: R909–R916.

Featherstone JA, Veith RC, Flatness D, et al. Age and alpha-2 adrenergic regulation of plasma norepinephrine kinetics in humans. *J Gerontol* 1987;42: 271–276.

Goldstein DS, Lake CR, Chernow B, et al. Age-dependence of hypertensive-normotensive differences in plasma norepinephrine. *Hypertension* 1983;5: 100–104.

Gottfries CG. Neurochemical aspects of aging and diseases with cognitive impairment. *J Neurosci Res* 1990;27:541–547.

Hartikainen R, Soininen H, Reinihainen KJ, et al. Neurotransmitter markers in the cerebrospinal fluid of normal subjects: effects of aging and other confounding factors. *J Neural Transm Gen Sect* 1991;84:103–117.

Insel PA. Adrenergic receptor, G proteins, and cell regulation: implications for aging research. *Exp Gerontol* 1993;28:341–348.

Kalaria RN, Andorn AC. Adrenergic receptors in aging and Alzheimer's disease: decreased alpha 2-receptors demonstrated by [^{3}H]p-aminoclonidine binding in prefrontal cortex. *Neurobiol Aging* 1991;12:131–136.

Kalaria RN, Andorn AC, Tabaton M, et al. Adrenergic receptors in aging and Alzheimer's disease: increased beta 2-receptors in prefrontal cortex and hippocampus. *J Neurochem* 1989;53: 1772–1781.

Mann DMA. Is the pattern of nerve cell loss in aging and Alzheimer's disease a real, or only an apparent, selectivity? *Neurobiol Aging* 1991;12:340–343.

Mendelsohn FAO, Paxinos G, eds. *Receptors in the human nervous system.* San Diego: Academic Press, 1991.

Pascual J, del Arco C, Gonzalez AM, et al. Quantitative light microscopic autoradiographic localization of a_2-adenoreceptors in the human brain. *Brain Res* 1992;585:116–127.

Sastre M, Garcia-Sevilla JA. Density of alpha-2A adrenoceptors and G_i proteins in the human brain: ratio of high-affinity agonist sites to antagonist sites and effect of age. *J Pharmacol Exp Ther* 1994; 269:1062–1072.

Supiano MA, Hogikyan RV. High affinity platelet a_2-adrenergic receptor density is decreased in older humans. *J Gerontol Biol Sci* 1993;48:B173–B179.

Table 4.2 References

Bannon MJ, Poosch MS, Xia Y, et al. Dopamine transporter mRNA content in human substantia nigra decreases precipitously with age. *Proc Natl Acad Sci USA* 1992;89:7095–7099.

Bareggi SR, Franceschi M, Smirne S. Neurochemical findings in cerebrospinal fluid in Alzheimer's disease. In: Gottfries CG, ed. *Normal aging, Alzheimer's disease, and senile dementia: aspects on etiology, pathogenesis, diagnosis, and treatment.* Brussels: Editions de l'Université de Bruxelles, 1985:203–212.

Chu Y, Komptolit K, Cochran EJ, et al. Age-related decreases in Nurr1 immunoreactivity in the human substantia nigra. *J Comp Neurol* 2002;450: 203–214.

DeKeyser J, Ebinger G, Vauquelin G. Age-related changes in the human nigrostriatal dopaminergic system. *Ann Neurol* 1990;27:157–161.

McGeer EG. Neurotransmitter systems in aging and senile dementia. *Prog Neuropsychopharmacol* 1981; 5:435–445.

Morgan DG, May PC, Finch CE. Dopamine and serotonin systems in human and rodent brain: effects of age and neurodegenerative disease. *J Am Geriatr Soc* 1987;35:334–345.

Mozley PD, Acton PD, Barraclough ED, et al. Effects of age on dopamine transporters in healthy humans. *J Nuc Med* 1999;40:1812–1817.

Pirker W, Asenbaum S, Hauk M, et al. Imaging serotonin and dopamine transporters with 123I-beta-CIT SPECT: binding kinetics and effects of normal aging. *J Nucl Med* 2000;41:36–44.

Rinne JO, Heitala J, Ruotsalainen U, et al. Decrease in human striatal dopamine D_2 receptor density with age: a PET study with [^{11}C] raclopride. *J Cereb Blood Flow Metab* 1993;13:310–314.

Robinson DS, Sourkes TL, Nies A, et al. Monoamine metabolism in human brain. *Arch Gen Psychiatry* 1977;34:89–92.

Roth GS, Joseph JA. Age-related changes in the translational and posttranscriptional regulation of the dopaminergic system. *Life Sci* 1994;55: 2031–2035.

Van Dyck CH, Seibyl JP, Malison RT, et al. Age-related decline in striatal dopamine transporter binding with Iodine-123-β-SPECT. *J Nucl Med* 1995;36:1175–1181.

Volkow ND, Fowler JS, Wand GJ, et al. Decreased dopamine transporters with age in healthy human subjects. *Ann Neurol* 1994;36:237–239.

Wang GJ, Volkow ND, Logan J, et al. Evaluation of age-related changes in serotonin 5-HT$_2$ and dopamine D$_2$ receptor availability in healthy human subjects. *Life Sci* 1995;56:249–253.

Table 4.3 References

Bareggi SR, Franceschi M, Smirne S. Neurochemical findings in cerebrospinal fluid in Alzheimer's disease. In: Gottfries CG, ed. *Normal aging, Alzheimer's disease, and senile dementia: aspects on etiology, pathogenesis, diagnosis, and treatment.* Brussels: Editions de l'Université de Bruxelles, 1985:203–212.

Burnet PWJ, Eastwood SL, Harrison PJ. Detection and quantification of 5-HT$_{1A}$ and 5-HT$_{2A}$ receptor mRNAs in human hippocampus using a reverse transcriptase-polymerase chain reaction (RT-PCR) technique and their correlation with binding site densities and age. *Neurosci Lett* 1994; 178:85–89.

Gottfries CG, Gottfries I, Johansson B, et al. Acid monoamine metabolites in human cerebrospinal fluid and their relations to age and sex. *Neuropharmacology* 1979;10:665–672.

Kuikka JT, Tammela L, Bergstrom KA, et al. Effects of ageing on serotonin transporters in healthy females. *Eur J Nucl Med* 2001;28:911–913.

Marcussen J, Oreland L, Winblad B. Effect of age on human brain serotonin (S-1) binding sites. *J Neurochem* 1984;43:1699–1705.

Marcussen JO, Alafuzoff I, Backstrom IT, et al. 5-Hydroxytryptamine-sensitive [^{3}H]imipramine binding of protein nature in the human brain: II. Effect of normal aging and dementia disorders. *Brain Res* 1987;425:137–145.

Meek JL, Bertilsson L, Cheney DL, et al. Aging-induced changes in acetylcholine and serotonin content of discrete brain nuclei. *J Gerontol* 1977; 129–131.

Middlemiss DN, Palmer AM, Edel N, et al. Binding of the novel serotonin agonist 8-hydroxy-2-(di-*n*-propylamino) tetralin in normal and Alzheimer brain. *J Neurochem* 1986;46:993–996.

Miura H, Qiao H, Ohta T. Influence of aging and social isolation on changes in brain monoamine turnover and biosynthesis of rats elicited by novelty stress. *Synapse* 2002;46:116–124.

Parsey RV, Oquendo MA, Simpson NR, et al. Effects of sex, age and aggressive traits in man on brain serotonin 5-HT1A receptor binding potential measured by PET using [C-11]WAY-100635. *Brain Res* 2002;954:173–182.

Pirker W, Asenbaum S, Hauk M, et al. Imaging serotonin and dopamine transporters with 123I-beta-CIT SPECT: binding kinetics and effects of normal aging. *J Nucl Med* 2000;41:36–44.

Severson JA, Marcusson JO, Osterburg HH, et al. Elevated density of [^{3}H] binding in aged human brain. *J Neurochem* 1985;45:1382–1389.

Sparks DL. Aging and Alzheimer's disease: altered cortical serotonergic binding. *Arch Neurol* 1989; 46:138–140.

Tauscher J, Verhoeff NP, Christensen BK, et al. Serotonin 5-HT1A receptor binding potential declines with age as measured by [11C]WAY-100635 and PET. *NeuroPsychopharmacology* 2001;24: 522–530.

Wang GJ, Volkow ND, Fowler JS, et al. Evaluation of age-related changes in serotonin 5-HT2 and dopamine D2 receptor availability in healthy human subjects. *Life Sci* 1995;56:249–253.

Yamamoto M, Suhara T, Okubo Y, et al. Age-related decline of serotonin transporters in living human brain of healthy males. *Life Sci* 2002;71:751–757.

Table 4.4 References

Allen SJ, Benton JS, Goodhardt MJ, et al. Biochemical evidence of selective nerve cell changes in the normal aging human and rat brain. *J Neurochem* 1983;41:256–265.

Brooks JC, Roberts N, Kemp GJ, et al. A proton magnetic resonance spectroscopy study of age-related changes in frontal lobe metabolite concentrations. *Cereb Cortex* 2001;11:598–605.

Court JA, Perry EK, Johnson M, et al. Regional patterns of cholinergic and glutamate activity in the developing and aging human brain. *Dev Brain Res* 1993;74:73–82.

Cutler R, Joseph JA, Yamagami K, et al. Area specific alterations in muscarinic stimulated low K_m GTPase activity in aging and Alzheimer's disease: implications for altered signal transduction. *Brain Res* 1994;664:54–60.

Flynn DD, Mash DC. Characterization of L-[^{3}H] nicotine binding in human cerebral cortex: comparison between Alzheimer's disease and the normal. *J Neurochem* 1986;47:1948–1954.

Lee KS, Frey KA, Koeppe RA, et al. In vivo quantification of cerebral muscarinic receptors in normal human aging using positron emission tomography and [^{11}C]-tropanyl benzilate. *J Cereb Blood Flow Metab* 1996;16:303–310.

Mesulam MM, Mufson EJ, Rogers J. Age-related shrinkage of cortically projecting cholinergic neurons: a selective effect. *Ann Neurol* 1987;22:31–36.

Mesulam MM, Geula C. Acetylcholinesterase-rich neurons of the human cerebral cortex: cytoarchitectonic and ontogenetic patterns of distribution. *J Comp Neurol* 1991;306:193–220.

Molchan SE, Martinez RA, Hill JL, et al. Increased cognitive sensitivity to scopolamine with age and a perspective on the scopolamine model. *Brain Res Rev* 1992;17:215–226.

Muller WE, Stoll L, Schubert T, et al. Central cholinergic functioning and aging. *Acto Psychiatr Scand* 1991;366(suppl):34–43.

Nakano S, Kato T, Nakamura S, et al. Acetylcholinesterase activity in cerebrospinal fluid of patients with Alzheimer's disease and senile dementia. *J Neurol Sci* 1986;75:213–223.

Nordberg A, Alafuzoff I, Winblad B. Nicotinic and muscarinic subtypes in the human brain: changes with aging and dementia. *J Neurosci Res* 1992;31:103–111.

Podruchny T, Connolly C, Bodke A, et al. In vivo muscarinic 2 receptor imaging in cognitively normal young and older volunteers. *Synapse* 2003; 48:39–44.

Suhara T, Inoue O, Kobayashi K, et al. No age-related changes in human benzodiazepine receptor binding measured by PET with [^{11}C]R513. *Neurosci Lett* 1993;159:207–210.

Sunderland T, Esposito G, Molchan SE. Differential cholinergic regulation in Alzheimer's patients compared to controls following chronic block-

ade with scopolamine: a SPECT study. *Psychopharmacology* 1995;121:231–241.

Table 4.5 References

Allen SJ, Benton JS, Goodhardt MJ, et al. Biochemical evidence of selective nerve cell changes in the normal aging human and rat brain. *J Neurochem* 1983;41:256–265.

Bareggi SR, Franceschi M, Smirne S. Neurochemical findings in cerebrospinal fluid in Alzheimer's disease. In: Gottfries CG, ed. *Normal aging, Alzheimer's disease, and senile dementia: aspects on etiology, pathogenesis, diagnosis, and treatment.* Brussels: Editions de l'Université de Bruxelles, 1985:203–212.

Giardino L, Zanni M, Fernandez M, et al. Plasticity of GABA(a) system during ageing: focus on vestibular compensation and possible pharmacological intervention. *Brain Res* 2002;929:76–86.

Hare TA, Wood JH, Manyam BV, et al. Central nervous system gamma-aminobutyric acid activity in man; relationship to age and sex as reflected in CSF. *Arch Neurol* 1982;39:247–249.

McGeer EG. Neurotransmitter systems in aging and senile dementia. *Prog Neuropsychopharmacol* 1981; 5:435–445.

Suhara T, Inoue O, Kobayashi K, et al. No age-related changes in human benzodiazepine receptor binding measured by PET with [^{11}C]Ro 15-4513. *Neurosci Lett* 1993;159:207–210.

Vela J, Gutierrez A, Vitorica J, et al. Rat hippocampal GABAergic molecular markers are differentially affected by ageing. *J Neurochem* 2003;85:368–377.

Table 4.6 References

Brooks JC, Roberts N, Kemp GJ, et al. A proton magnetic resonance spectroscopy study of age-related changes in frontal lobe metabolite concentrations. *Cereb Cortex* 2001;11:598–605.

Court JA, Perry EK, Johnson M, et al. Regional patterns of cholinergic and glutamate activity in the developing and aging human brain. *Dev Brain Res* 1993;74:73–82.

Grachev ID, Apkarian AV. Aging alters regional multichemical profile of the human brain: an *in vivo* 1H-MRS study of young versus middle-aged subjects. *J Neurochem* 2001;76:582–593.

Johnson M, Perry EK, Ince PG, et al. Autoradiographic comparison of the distribution of [^{3}H]-MK801 and [^{3}H]-CNQX in the human cerebellum during development and aging. *Brain Res* 1993;615:259–266.

Kornhuber ME, Kornhuber J, Retz W, et al. L-glutamate and L-aspartate concentrations in the developing and aging human putamen tissue. *J Neural Trans [GenSect]* 1993;93:145–150.

Piggott MA, Perry EK, Perry RH, et al. [^{3}H]-MK-801 binding to the NMDA receptor complex, and its modulation in human frontal cortex during development and aging. *Brain Res* 1992;588:277–286.

Procter AW, Lowe SL, Palmer AM, et al. Topographical distribution of neurochemical changes in Alzheimer's disease. *J Neurol Sci* 1988;84:125–140.

Villares JC, Stavale JN. Age-related changes in the N-methyl-D-aspartate receptor binding sites within the human basal ganglia. *Exp Neurol* 2001;171:391–404.

Supplemental Readings

General

Allen SJ, Benton JS, Goodhardt MJ, et al. Biochemical evidence of selective nerve cell changes in the normal aging human and rat brain. *J Neurochem* 1983;41:256–265.

American Psychiatric Association. *Task force report: tardive dyskinesia.* Washington, DC: American Psychiatric Association, 1980.

Bjorntorp P. Neuroendocrine ageing. *J Intern Med* 1995;238:401–404.

Calderini G, Toffano G. Phospholipid methylation, ³H-diazepam, and ³H-GABA bonding in the cerebellum of aged rats. In: Giacobini E, Filogamo G, et al., eds. *The aging brain: cellular and molecular mechanisms of aging in the nervous system.* New York: Raven, 1982:87–92.

Creasey H, Rapoport SI. The aging human brain. *Ann Neurol* 1985;17:2–10.

Davies P. Neurotransmitter-related enzymes in senile dementia of the Alzheimer type. *Brain Res* 1989;171:319–327.

Dekosky ST, Palmer AM. Neurochemistry of aging. In: Albert ML, Knoefel JE, eds. *Clinical neurology of aging.* New York: Oxford University Press, 1994:79–101.

Desbordes P, Cohadon F. Brain water and aging. *J Gerontol* 1987;42:655–659.

Desjardins GC, Beaudet A, Meaney MJ, et al. Estrogen-induced hypothalamic beta-endorphin neuron loss: a possible model of hypothalamic aging. *Exp Gerontol* 1995;30:253–267.

Ershler WB, Sun WH, Binkley N. The role of interleukin-6 in certain age-related diseases. *Drugs Aging* 1994;5:358–365.

Fairbairn A, Blessed G. Nicotinic receptor abnormalities in Alzheimer's and Parkinson's disease. *J Neurol Neurosurg Psychiatry* 1987;50:806–809.

Feldman RD, Limbird LE, Nadeau J, et al. Alterations in leukocyte β-receptor affinity with aging. *N Engl J Med* 1984;310:815–819.

Fliers E, Swaab DF. Neuropeptide changes in aging and Alzheimer's disease. In: Swaab DF, Fliers E, Mirmiran M, et al., eds. *Progress in brain research.* Vol. 70. Amsterdam: Elsevier Science Publishers, 1986:141–152.

Flynn DD, Mash DC. Characterization of L-[³H] nicotine binding in human cerebral cortex: comparison between Alzheimer's disease and the normal. *J Neurochem* 1986;47:1948–1954.

Fulop T, Seres I. Age-related changes in signal transduction. *Drugs Aging* 1994;5:366–390.

Henry JM, Roth GS. Solubilization of striatal D-2 dopamine receptors: evidence that apparent loss during aging is not due to membrane sequestration. *J Gerontol* 1986;41:129–135.

Houston HG, McClelland RJ. Age and gender contributions to intersubject variability of the auditory brainstem potentials. *Biol Psychiatry* 1985;20:419–430.

Katzman R, Terry R. Normal aging of the nervous system. In: Katzman R, Rowe JW, eds. *Principles of geriatric neurology.* Philadelphia: FA Davis, 1994;18–47.

Komiskey HL, Raemont LM, Mundinger KL. Aging: modulation of GABA_A binding sites by ethanol and diazepam. *Brain Res* 1988;458:37–44.

Leake A, Ferrier IN. Alterations in neuropeptides in aging and disease. *Drugs Aging* 1993;3:408–427.

Mann JJ, Petito C, Stanley M, et al. Amine receptor binding and monoamine oxidase activity in postmortem human brain tissue: effect of age, gender, and postmortem delay. In: Burrows GD, Norman TR, Dennerstein L, eds. *Clinical and pharmacological studies in psychiatric disorders.* London: John Wiley & Sons, 1985:37.

Marcusson J, Oreland L, Winblad B. Effect of age on human brain serotonin (S-1) binding sites. *J Neurochem* 1984;43:1699–1705.

McGeer PL, McGeer EG, Suzuki J, et al. Aging, Alzheimer's disease, and the cholinergic system of the basal forebrain. *Neurology* 1984;34:741–745.

Memo M, Spano PF, Kobayashi H, et al. Brain catecholamine receptor function during aging. In: Barbagallo-Santgiorgi G, Exton-Smith AN, eds. *The aging brain: neurological and mental disturbances.* New York: Plenum, 1980:15–24.

Missale C, Govoni S, Pasinetti G, et al. Age-dependent changes in the mechanisms regulating dopamine uptake in the central nervous system. *J Gerontol* 1986;41:136–139.

Mooradian A. Effect of aging on the blood-brain barrier. *Neurobiol Aging* 1988;9:31–39.

Morgan DG, May PC, Finch CE. Dopamine and serotonin systems in human and rodent brain: effects of age and neurodegenerative disease. *J Am Geriatr Soc* 1987;35:334–345.

Palmer AM, DeKosky ST. Monoamine neurons in aging and Alzheimer's disease. *J Neural Trans [GenSect]* 1993;91:135–159.

Perry EK, Perry RH, Smith CJ, et al. Acetylcholinesterase activity in cerebrospinal fluid of patients with Alzheimer's disease and senile dementia. *J Neurol Sci* 1986;75:213–223.

Perry EK, Piggott MA, Court JA, et al. Transmitters in the developing and senescent human brain. *Ann NY Acad Sci* 1993;695:69–72.

Powers RE. Neurobiology of aging. In: Busse EW, Coffey CE, eds. *Textbook of geriatric psychiatry.* Washington, DC: American Psychiatric Press, 1996:35–69.

Raskind MA, Peskind ER, Lampe TH, et al. Cerebrospinal fluid vasopressin, oxytocin, somatostatin, and β-endorphin in Alzheimer's disease. *Arch Gen Psychiatry* 1986;43:382–388.

Reichlmeier K, Iwangoff P, Enz A. Enzymatic changes in the aging brain and some aspects of its pharmacological intervention with ergot compounds. In: Eisdorfer C, Fann WE, eds. *Psychopharmacology and aging.* New York: Spectrum, 1980:13–46.

Rossor MN, Iversen LL, Reynolds GP, et al. Neurochemical characteristics of early and late onset types of Alzheimer's disease. *Br Med J* 1984;288:961–964.

Roth GS. Changes in tissue responsiveness to hormones and neurotransmitters during aging. *Exp Gerontol* 1995;30:361–368.

Rowe JW, Minaker KL, Sparrow D, et al. Age-related failure of volume-pressure-mediated vasopressin release. *J Clin Endocrinol Metab* 1982;54:661–664.

Schmidt AW, Peroutka SJ. 5-Hydroxytryptamine receptor "families." *FASEB J* 1989;3:2242–2249.

Schmucker DL. Aging and drug disposition: an update. *Pharmacol Rev* 1985;37:133–148.

Spokes EG. An analysis of factors influencing measurements of dopamine, noradrenaline, glutamate decarboxylase and choline acetylase in human post-mortem brain tissue. *Brain* 1979;102:333–346.

Swaab DF, Fliers E, Partiman TS. The suprachiasmatic nucleus of the human brain in relation to sex, age and senile dementia. *Brain Res* 1985;342:37–44.

Wurtman RJ, Zeizel SH. Brain choline: its sources and effects on the synthesis and release of acetylcholine. In: Corkin S, Davis KL, Growdon JH, et al., eds. *Alzheimer's disease: a report of progress in research.* New York: Raven, 1983:303–314.

Yamamura HI. Neurotransmitter receptor alterations in age-related disorders. In: Enna SJ, Samorajski T, Beer B, eds. *Brain neurotransmitters and receptors in aging and age-related disorders.* Vol. 17. New York: Raven, 1981:143–147.

Chapter 5

Kinetics and Dynamics of Psychotropic Drugs in the Elderly

Lisa L. von Moltke

Darrell R. Abernethy

David J. Greenblatt

The time course and intensity of the effect of any drug depends on its affinity for a receptor/effector site and on its concentration at that site. In general, drug concentration at the receptor site is dependent at least in part on the concentration in blood, which in turn is determined by three pharmacokinetic factors: absorption, distribution, and clearance. Receptors in the central nervous system (CNS) are within a sanctuary created by the blood–brain barrier (BBB). Here and in other protected sites, drug concentrations can also be influenced by the function of active transporters. Rational selection of any drug, as well as establishment of correct dosage and dosing schedules, is based not only on an understanding of the drug's pharmacological effects but also on these pharmacokinetic characteristics, which may be altered by natural changes in the structure and function of the human body during the aging process. Age and age-related illness are associated with decreased cardiac output, decreased renal and hepatic blood flow, increased body fat, decreases and alterations in some plasma proteins, and decreased activity of a number of hepatic enzymes responsible for drug metabolism. Nutritional deficiency or excess may also influence psychotropic drug pharmacokinetics. Additionally, the presence of polypharmacy, which increases with age, increases the possibility of both pharmacokinetic and pharmacodynamic interactions in a population that is uniquely susceptible to both the occurrence and the serious sequelae of such events.

The effect of aging on the pharmacokinetics of psychotropic drugs has received considerable research attention in recent years. Numerous studies suggest that old age is associated with pharmacokinetic alterations that, in general, decrease the body's efficiency and ability to clear a number of psychotropic drugs. Together with altered central nervous system (CNS) sensitivity to such drugs, these pharmacokinetic changes may explain the increased sensitivity of older patients to both the therapeutic and the toxic effects of psychoactive medications.

Understanding the impact of aging on drug disposition as well as on CNS function is key to effective geriatric therapeutics, especially because the "therapeutic index" (the ratio of the amount of drug that causes toxicity to the amount required for therapeutic effect) for psychotropic drugs may be lower for older patients than for younger ones. The resulting decreased margin of safety requires that the clinician understand both the predictable changes in psychotropic drug disposition (pharmacokinetics) and CNS effects (pharmacodynamics) in the geriatric patient.

Basic Pharmacokinetic Principles and the Aging Process

Pharmacokinetics is the discipline that describes and predicts the time course of absorption, distribution, biotransformation, and elimination of a drug. Pharmacodynamics describes the time course of the biochemical, physiological, and neurobehavioral effects of drugs. More simply stated, pharmacokinetics describes what the human body does to the drug, whereas pharmacodynamics describes what the drug does to the body. A third approach that has acquired increasing importance over the last decade is kinetic-dynamic modeling, in which time as a variable is removed, and drug effect is evaluated in direct relation to its concentration either in blood or at a hypothetical site of pharmacodynamic action.

In the absence of coexisting disease, the physiological changes associated with aging result in a number of well-studied and predictable alterations in psychotropic drug pharmacokinetics. Separately and together, these changes influence the circulating concentration of a drug and its concentration at the receptor site.

Absorption

The rate of drug absorption from the gastrointestinal (GI) tract after oral administration influences the time course and intensity of initial drug action. The completeness of absorption (absolute bioavailability) influences all phases of the plasma concentration curve. A variety of factors, including drug efflux transport protein activity and interactions with other medications, can influence absorption. It must be emphasized that incomplete bioavailability after oral dosage may result from presystemic extraction as well as incomplete absorption.[1,2] The presence of cytochrome P450 (CYP3A) isoforms in the intestine, as well as multiple cytochrome and glucuronidation enzymes in the liver, can result in extensive metabolism of an orally administered drug before the dose arrives in the systemic circulation from the GI tract and portal circulation. Oral bioavailability of drugs that undergo extensive first-pass metabolism can be increased if the function of these first-pass enzymes is inhibited.[3] Although not a result of actual changes in absorption, the net effect is for less drug to be metabolized (extracted) before reaching the systemic circulation. The higher amount of intact drug reaching the systemic circulation can lead to both higher peak levels and greater overall drug exposure. The clinical picture appears similar to what would be seen if more drug had been absorbed or administered initially.

The transport protein P-glycoprotein (P-gp) is now known to have an important role in pharmacokinetic processes including absorption.[4–7] Acting as an efflux transport protein in the small intestine, this member of the ABC transporter superfamily acts to limit transport of recognized substrates across the intestinal mucosa by inhibiting the movement across the epithelial cell and returning the substrate to the intestinal lumen. Hence, it helps determine oral bioavailability for these substrates. In addition, substances that result in an increase or decrease in the function of P-gp can lead to a decrease or increase (respectively) in oral bioavailability of substrates.

Effect of Aging

In theory, absorption of orally ingested drugs from the GI tract may be altered because of age-related reductions in gastric acid and mesenteric blood flow, as well as reduced size of the absorbing surface and changes in transport of drugs across the intestinal epithelial membrane. Although the rate of absorption of drugs may in some cases decrease as a result of delayed gastric emptying or abnormal gastric motility associated with aging, the extent of absorption of psychotropic drugs is not significantly altered by the aging process unless overt GI pathology exists.[8]

Evidence exists that CYP3A activity decreases with age.[8,9] It is not currently known whether or how aging affects P-gp in the intestine or other sites. Since the elderly use more medications than younger people, the possibilities for changes in absorption due to chelation, or pH, and motility changes from these concomitant medications also increase. Multiple medications also increase the risk of exposure to drug interactions with metabolizing enzymes and P-gp that can affect presystemic extraction and absorption, respectively.

Clinical Implications

Drugs with anticholinergic properties used by elderly patients decrease intestinal motility and therefore may delay the rate of absorption, resulting potentially in a delayed clinical effect. Examples of such drugs include atropine, scopolamine, meperidine, neuroleptics, and cyclic antidepressants. Antacids containing aluminum, magnesium, and calcium, in addition to milk of magnesia, can also delay absorption of psychotropic drugs by altering their ionization as well as by delaying gastric emptying time.

Drugs with a large component of presystemic extraction due to CYP3A, such as triazolam and nefazodone, may require dosing adjustments in elderly individuals to prevent higher than expected peak levels. The presence of multiple medications may cause interactions involving transporters and/or metabolizing enzymes at the level of absorption and bioavailability. Clinicians need to remain alert for both toxicity (usually due to inhibition) and loss of efficacy (usually due to induction), which may result.

Distribution

After a drug is absorbed, it is distributed throughout the body. "Volume of distribution" (V_d) is a hypothetical quantity having units of volume that indicates how extensively a particular drug is distributed throughout the body. Because all psychotropic drugs except lithium are lipid soluble, the V_d of these agents denotes the theoretical size of the peripheral space—presumably consisting mainly of lipoidal or adipose tissues—in which lipid-soluble drugs will be sequestered. The V_d for lithium (a relatively water-solu-ble compound) is related to the total body water in which lithium could be distributed.

The ability to distribute into the central nervous system (CNS) is an obvious requirement for psychoactive drugs. Those medications in clinical use have the physiochemical characteristics necessary to allow them to cross the blood–brain endothelium in spite of its barrier function. Some studies in animals that completely lack P-gp show higher brain uptake of some psychotropic drugs in these "knock out" models than in genetically intact animals,[10] suggesting that P-gp has some role in determining the final CNS distribution of these medications. To date, there are no reports on humans totally lacking in P-gp. Consequently, the spectrum of variability in P-gp activity in the blood–brain barrier of humans is likely to be much smaller than that represented in the comparative paradigm of "knockout" versus intact animals. Similarly, the variations in CNS distribution of currently available psychotropic medications that are attributable to P-gp in humans are likely to be smaller than those reported in these animal studies.

Effect of Aging

As people age, lean muscle mass and total body water decrease, while total body fat tends to increase relative to total body weight.[11] Neuroleptics, antidepressants, anticonvulsants, anxiolytics, and sedative-hypnotics are lipid-soluble compounds. Therefore, a given dosage of a drug from one of these classes will be distributed or diluted more extensively in the peripheral body tissues of an older patient than of a younger patient. Gender may influence drug distribution in a similar way because women have a greater proportion of adipose tissue than men do, regardless of age (Fig. 5.1). In contrast, lithium is relatively water soluble. Peripheral distribution of lithium therefore decreases in elderly patients, and the drug remains more concentrated in the central compartment.[12]

Little is known about how normal aging affects the blood–brain barrier,

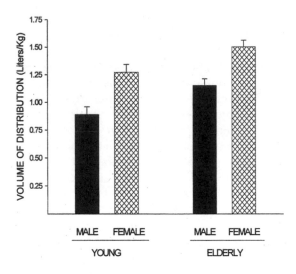

Figure 5.1. Mean ($\pm$ SE) pharmacokinetic volume of distribution (V_d) of the lipophilic psychotropic drug trazodone in relation to age and gender in a study of intravenous trazodone administered to a series of healthy volunteers. Note that V_d is greater in women than in men and in elderly than in young subjects.

either wholly or only specific elements of it, such as P-gp. Medications that alter the effect of P-gp function in the blood–brain barrier could change the distribution profile for medications which are substrates for this transporter.[13–16] Since the elderly use more medications concurrently, these interactions may be more probable in aging individuals. Interactions would be expected to be most pronounced for drugs that are normally excluded from the CNS by P-gp. As an example, under experimental conditions, investigators have shown that it is possible to decrease the apparent function of P-gp in humans with the administration of an inhibitor (quinidine). Subsequent administration of very high doses of the P-gp substrate loperamide, which is effectively excluded from the CNS under normal circumstances, resulted in central opioid effects with respiratory depression.[17]

Clinical Implications

Alterations in V_d may have several potential clinical implications. The elimination half-life ($t_{1/2}$) of a drug is directly proportional to V_d (if clearance is unchanged) according to the following relationship:

$$t_{1/2} = (0.693 \times V_d)/\text{Clearance} \quad \text{(Eq. 5.1)}$$

Thus an increase in V_d in elderly individuals prolongs the elimination half-life, even if clearance is unchanged. This by itself will have no effect on the steady-state concentration (C_{ss}) during multiple dosage, as C_{ss} depends on dosing rate and clearance; however, the time necessary to attain C_{ss} may be prolonged, and the fluctuation in drug concentration between doses will decrease if the dose interval remains constant. The implications of increased V_d after single doses are not yet clear. Although elimination half-life and therefore duration of action may, in principle, be prolonged, in actual fact the duration of action could be shortened in the elderly. This occurs because the duration of action of single doses of lipophilic psychotropic drugs usually depends, at least in part, on distribution rather than on elimination or clearance.

Investigations are necessary to determine whether changes in BBB P-gp function can result in clinically relevant increases or decreases in drug penetration for medications that are able to penetrate the BBB in spite of being found to be P-gp substrates in vitro or in animal models. Such changes in CNS distribution could be one possible mechanism for the subtle interindividual differences in drug efficacy or toxicity that clinicians observe.

Protein Binding

When drugs enter the systemic circulation, they may bind to plasma albumin and, to a lesser extent, to red blood cells and α_1-acid glycoprotein. All psychotropic drugs except lithium are moderately to extensively protein bound.

Protein-bound drugs exist in reversible equilibrium with the unbound fraction. The extent of protein binding may fluctuate in any given individual or may vary widely among individuals, even those of the same age and sex. The free *fraction* of drug is the proportion of the total drug concentration that is not bound to protein. In contrast, the free *concentration* is the absolute concentration of unbound drug. Under circumstances in which only the unbound drug can be cleared by the liver ("restrictive clearance"), free *fraction* and free *concentration* are determined by independent and unrelated physiological and biological factors[18] (Fig. 5.2).

Protein-binding characteristics vary among drugs. Cyclic antidepressants bind to both albumin and α_1-acid glycoprotein, but the free fraction depends more on levels of α_1-acid glycoprotein. For benzodiazepines and neuroleptics, the free fraction depends mainly on albumin levels. Lithium does not bind to plasma proteins.

In principle, only the free drug concentration is available for diffusion out of the vascular system to sites of activity in brain tissue. However, protein binding may or may not restrict the capacity of the liver to biotransform or clear a drug. For some psychotropic drugs (e.g., chlordiazepox-

ide, diazepam, alprazolam, lorazepam), clearance is largely restricted by plasma binding; for many others (the benzodiazepine midazolam, most tricyclic antidepressants, selective serotonin reuptake inhibitors [SSRIs], and neuroleptics), binding does not restrict clearance. For restrictively cleared drugs, alterations in protein binding alone have no effect either on steady-state plasma concentrations of unbound drug or on clinical effect[18] (Fig. 5.3).

Effect of Aging

Plasma albumin levels tend to decrease with age, although levels do not necessarily fall below the "normal" range. Decreased albumin concentration is generally associated with decreased capacity for drug binding, although the mechanism is not well understood. Free fractions of some psychotropic drugs may increase in older people, especially in the 8th or 9th decades of life, and α_1-acid glycoprotein levels increase moderately with increasing age.[19] Again, such changes by themselves do not imply a change in either free drug concentration or clinical effect.

Clinical Implications

Decreases in plasma albumin levels may in part be *associated with* (but not necessarily be the *cause of*) the clinically observed increases in prevalence of toxicity of some

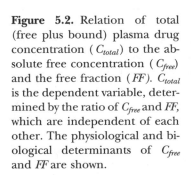

Figure 5.2. Relation of total (free plus bound) plasma drug concentration (C_{total}) to the absolute free concentration (C_{free}) and the free fraction (*FF*). C_{total} is the dependent variable, determined by the ratio of C_{free} and *FF*, which are independent of each other. The physiological and biological determinants of C_{free} and *FF* are shown.

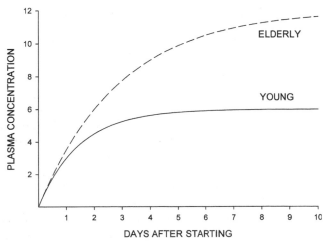

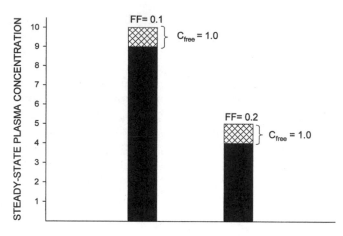

Figure 5.3. *Left:* A drug whose hepatic clearance is restricted by protein binding is administered continuously at a constant dosing rate. If free fraction (*FF*) is 0.1, free concentration (C_{free}) is 1.0 units, bound concentration is 9.0 units, and total concentration (C_{total}) is 10.0 units. *Right:* An intervening factor causes a decrease in plasma protein binding, and FF increases to 0.2; nothing else changes—the dosing rate and the clearance of free drug remain constant. Therefore, C_{free} is unchanged at steady-state, and the pharmacological effect of the drug is also unchanged at steady-state. However, C_{total} falls to 5.0.

psychotropic drugs in older people. For example, increased CNS sedation from benzodiazepines has been associated with age-related decreases in plasma albumin levels and increased fraction of unbound drug. It is more likely that such associations are caused by reduced hepatic clearance and/or increased drug sensitivity than by altered free fraction as such. Malnutrition may also decrease the concentration of albumin and thus increase the free fraction of neuroleptics and benzodiazepines. Physical illness may be associated with increased α_1-acid glycoprotein, causing wide differences among older people in the binding of cyclic antidepressants. In elderly patients without other factors predisposing to toxicity (such as impaired hepatic clearance), decreased plasma binding alone probably plays only a minor role in psychotropic drug toxicity.

Psychotropic drugs may be displaced from binding sites by other drugs that compete for the same sites. This may result in transiently higher levels of unbound drug, which may in turn produce a transient increase in pharmacodynamic effect. The consensus among investigators in this field is that clinically important in-

teractions attributable to protein-binding displacement are very rare.[20]

Hepatic Metabolism and Clearance

Lithium is cleared by renal excretion, but essentially all other psychotropic drugs are cleared by hepatic biotransformation. After oral dosage, substrates of cytochrome P-450-3A isoforms (Table 5.1) may also undergo substantial metabolism in the GI tract because this cytochrome is present in the intestinal mucosa as well as the liver.[3]

When a drug is taken orally, it passes through the liver via the portal and hepatic veins before entering the systemic circulation. Drug biotransformation in the GI tract mucosa and/or by the liver during the "first pass" from the portal circulation is collectively termed "presystemic extraction." This may account for the poor bioavailability of many psychotropic drugs after oral dosage.[1,2] "High-extraction" drugs that undergo high presystemic extraction include all neuroleptics, all tricyclic, SSRI, and "mixed mechanism" antidepressants (with the exception of trazodone), buspirone, and two benzodiazepines (triazolam and mi-

Table 5.1. Representative Psychotropic Drugs Metabolized Entirely or in Part by Human Cytochrome P-450-3A Isoforms

Sedatives, hypnotics, and anxiolytics
  Alprazolam
  Bromazepam
  Diazepam
  Midazolam
  Triazolam
  Zolpidem

Antidepressants
  Amitriptyline
  Citalopram
  Clomipramine
  Imipramine
  Mianserin
  Nefazodone

Neuroleptics
  Clozapine
  Haloperidol
  Quetiapine

dazolam). CYP3A activity appears to decrease with age.[9] Therefore, after an older patient is given an oral dose of one of these CYP3A-dependent high-extraction drugs, a relatively larger fraction of drug reaches the systemic circulation than in a younger patient. In the case of very short half-life drugs, such as triazolam and midazolam, the clinical result could be a more intense drug-induced sedative effect for the geriatric patient.[21,22] Decreases in hepatic blood flow with age have been mentioned by some investigators to explain decreases in hepatic clearance of some medications. However, hepatic blood flow will only influence the clearance of high-extraction drugs given intravenously. Further, the phenomenon of decreased clearance in the elderly is observed for a number of drugs that have clearance values that are not flow-dependent, such as diazepam and alprazolam. Additional in vitro evidence suggests that CYP3A and possibly some CYP2C activity and expression may decrease with age.

Hepatic clearance of drugs with *low* presystemic extraction (such as benzodiazepines other than midazolam and tria-

zolam) also depends upon hepatic enzyme activity. The activity of these enzymes controls a series of metabolic transformations that ultimately inactivate the drug and prepare it for elimination. For many psychotropic drugs, intermediate metabolic steps produce metabolites that are pharmacologically active.

The initial enzymatic transformation for many psychotropic drugs is demethylation, which yields an "active metabolite." For example, chlordiazepoxide and diazepam are demethylated to desmethylchlordiazepoxide and desmethyldiazepam, respectively. The cyclic antidepressant amitriptyline is demethylated to nortriptyline, imipramine to desipramine, and doxepin to desmethyldoxepin (Table 5.2). Demethylated active metabolites undergo further enzymatic transformations, which in turn may produce additional active metabolites. The initial metabolic steps generally are oxidative processes mediated by the hepatic cytochrome P-450 drug-metabolizing system.

A second category of drug biotransformation involves synthetic reactions such as glucuronide, sulfate, or acetyl conjugation. These synthetic processes are relatively uninfluenced by aging. In the case of acetylation, the acetylator polymorphism ("slow" vs. "rapid") is more important than any age-related change. Some psychotropic drugs that are first oxidized to pharmacologically active metabolites are ultimately inactivated by synthetic biotransformation, resulting in inactivation of the administered drug. However, three benzodiazepines (oxazepam, lorazepam, and temazepam) are directly biotransformed via glucuronide conjugation.

Clinical Implications

During multiple dosage with a psychotropic drug, C_{ss} depends directly on dosage rate and inversely on clearance as follows:

$$C_{ss} = \text{Dosing rate/Clearance} \qquad \text{(Eq. 5.2)}$$

Thus impairment of clearance associated with old age implies an increase in C_{ss}

Table 5.2.   Representative Psychotropic Drugs Metabolized by Demethylation

Drug	Metabolite	Pharmacologic Activity
Diazepam	Desmethyldiazepam	Yes
Chlordiazepoxide	Desmethylchlordiazepoxide	Yes
Adinazolam	Desmethyladinazolam	Yes
Imipramine	Desipramine	Yes
Amitriptyline	Nortriptyline	Yes
Doxepin	Desmethyldoxepin	Yes
Fluoxetine	Norfluoxetine	Yes
Sertraline	Desmethylsertraline	No[a]
Venlafaxine	O-Desmethylvenlafaxine	Yes
Citalopram	Desmethylcitalopram	Not established
Clozapine	Norclozapine	Not established

[a] Desmethylsertraline has weak SSRI activity but produces cytochrome inhibition similar to that of parent drug.

at any given dosing rate (Fig. 5.4). Therefore, a need for reduced daily dosage of many psychotropic drugs should be anticipated for elderly persons. Additionally, coadministration of any medication that is an inhibitor of any enzyme that determines the clearance of a given drug can also lead to increases in C_{ss}. In general, medications that are completely dependent on one enzyme for clearance are more vulnerable to these kinds of potentially significant kinetic interactions.

Renal Clearance

As hepatic clearance refers to the capacity of the liver to eliminate drugs via biotransformation, renal clearance refers to the capacity of the kidney to excrete the drug unchanged in the urine. Lithium and the hydroxylated metabolites of tricyclic anti-

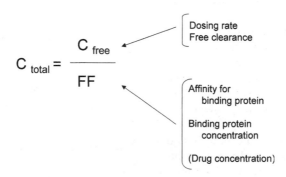

Figure 5.4. A hypothetical drug is administered at the same constant rate to a young patient and an elderly one, with the assumption that the drug's V_d is the same in both patients. Clearance of the drug, however, is 50% lower in the elderly person than in the young individual. Equation 4.2 indicates that steady-state plasma concentration is twice as high in the elderly patient as in the younger (12 vs. 6 units). Equation 4.1 indicates that elimination half-life will be twice as long in the elderly patient (2.0 vs. 1.0 days), thereby prolonging the time necessary to attain steady-state after dosage initiation.

depressants undergo significant renal clearance.

Effect of Aging

Renal blood flow and glomerular filtration rate decrease as a function of increasing age.[23] For drugs such as lithium, which is cleared by the kidney without prior hepatic or intestinal metabolism, clearance is proportional to the glomerular filtration rate. Since this usually decreases during the aging process, renal excretion of lithium is often impaired. Congestive heart failure, diabetes, or hypertension—common medical problems in the elderly—further reduce renal function.

Clinical Implications

Decreased lithium clearance illustrates the primary effect of reduced renal function associated with aging on psychotropic drugs. Although V_d may slightly decrease with age (because of reduced relative amounts of total body water), the consequence of reduced renal clearance is much more important than the change in V_d: the elimination half-life is prolonged from an average of 24 hours in the young adult to 36 hours in the older patient. The result is higher values of lithium C_{ss}, with increased likelihood of higher plasma levels and toxicity.

Other medications may alter psychotropic drug excretion through the kidneys. For example, sodium-depleting diuretics, which older people often take for hypertension, and nonsteroidal antiinflammatory drugs may cause further lithium retention, leading to higher plasma and intracellular lithium levels and an increased likelihood of toxicity. Reduced renal blood flow resulting from impaired cardiac function in the elderly also impairs renal clearance.

Impaired renal function also reduces clearance of active and potentially toxic substances such as the water-soluble hydroxy metabolites of cyclic antidepressants or risperidone. If renal clearance of cyclic metabolites decreases with age, older patients may be exposed to potential cardiac toxicity.[24,25]

Steady-State Plasma Levels and Drug Accumulation

Psychotropic drugs generally are not given only once but, rather, are administered repeatedly for long periods of time. When the interval between doses is less than the elimination half-life—as is often the case with psychotropic drugs—the drug begins to accumulate in the plasma. Accumulation continues until the rate of drug entry into the body equals the rate of elimination. This point is known as the steady-state condition, with the associated C_{ss}. Since the *rate* of accumulation of any drug depends on its elimination half-life, roughly four to five half-lives are required before a drug reaches steady state if the dose and the dosing interval remain constant.

In contrast, the *extent* of accumulation depends only on the dosing rate and clearance, as indicated by equation 5.2. If the dosing rate is constant, C_{ss} will increase inversely with clearance. Reduced hepatic or renal clearance in the elderly, therefore, not only prolongs a drug's elimination half-life (assuming V_d is unchanged) but also raises its C_{ss} during multiple dosage[26] (Fig. 5.4).

Effect of Aging

Pharmacokinetic changes after single doses predict the consequences of multiple-dose administration for many drugs with linear kinetics. Pharmacokinetics for drugs which eventually inhibit or induce their own clearance are more complex, and single doses are not as useful in predicting the kinetic profile which will occur with multiple doses. Impaired drug clearance after a single dose in aged individuals should predict an increased steady-state plasma drug concentration with multiple dosing (Fig. 5.4). Drugs with nonlinear kinetics (such as paroxetine, phenytoin or nefazodone) pose an additional hazard because C_{ss} may increase disproportionately as the dosing rate is increased. C_{ss} of psychotropic drugs may also be influenced by other drugs that alter hepatic metabolism. Drugs that impair hepatic metabolism increase the plasma concentration of most psychotropic drugs for any given dosage. Conversely, drugs that stimulate or induce hepatic metabolism decrease steady-state plasma levels.

Clinical Implications

Higher steady-state plasma levels for any given dose are expected in older patients and are likely to increase the concentration of drug at the CNS receptor site. For the older patient, increased concentration often means an increased likelihood of toxicity—one of the reasons that lower dosages are necessary. Because time to reach steady-state is increased, rapid changing of dosing schedules for psychotropic drugs in older patients therefore may be unwise; little therapeutic benefit may result, and the risk of toxicity may increase.

Since older patients are likely to take a variety of drugs (in addition to psychotropics) that potentially alter hepatic metabolism, the likelihood of variations in steady-state plasma levels of psychotropic drugs increases. For this reason, caution is necessary when prescribing additional drugs in conjunction with psychotropic drugs.

Pharmacodynamics and Aging

Clinical observations indicate that elderly patients are more susceptible than younger adults to a number of drug effects, particularly sedation, anticholinergic toxicity, extrapyramidal effects, and orthostatic hypotension. Based on early knowledge of the age-related changes in drug pharmacokinetics, increased sensitivity to a given dosage of drug in older individuals was simply attributed to decreased drug clearance and increased drug accumulation. However, it is now apparent that for many of these side effects, aged patients also experience increased responses, even when drug is present at the same concentration as in younger patients. To better describe these phenomena, techniques to link drug disposition (pharmacokinetics) to drug effect (pharmacodynamics) are used, allowing examination of drug effect at any given plasma-drug concentration.[27] Currently available information indicates that elderly patients may have greater sensitivity to psychotropic drug-induced sedation, anticholinergic activity, and orthostatic hypotension, even at modest plasma drug levels.[28-30]

Pharmacokinetics of Specific Drug Groups

As a general principle, the pharmacokinetic profile of psychotropic drugs is altered in aging, leading to prolonged elimination half-life, and, for many drugs, reduced clearance and elevated plasma levels. Studies of these pharmacokinetic parameters in relation to specific drug groups are summarized in Table 5.3. As a rule, studies in elderly populations are still insufficient. Because the elderly are an increasingly diverse group, studies done on small numbers of healthy volunteers within a narrow age range (e.g., 65–75) may not be wholly predictive of the elderly patients clinicians will see in their practices. Claims that statistically significant decrements in clearance or increases in AUC in the 20–30% range are "clinically insignificant" for the elderly population should be viewed critically and with skepticism given the difference in the kinetic-dynamic relationship that may exist for many elderly patients.

Sedatives, Hypnotics, and Anxiolytics

All benzodiazepines metabolized by the cytochrome P-450 family of enzymes have impaired clearance in elderly humans,[9,31-33] as does zolpidem, an imidazo-

Table 5.3.   Studies of Psychotropic Drug Pharmacokinetics

Pharmacokinetic Parameter	Age-Related Changes
	NEUROLEPTICS
	HALOPERIDOL
Steady-state plasma level	
Dysken et al. (1994)	No differences in plasma levels between elderly and younger patients
Aoba et al. (1985)	No differences in plasma levels between elderly and younger patients
	THIORIDAZINE
Acute plasma level	
Cohen & Sommer (1988)	Parent compound and active metabolite higher in elderly
Elimination half-life	
Musze & Vanderheeren (1977)	Doubles from age 27 to 64
Martensson & Roos (1973)	
	ZIPRASIDONE
Clearance	
Wilner et al. (2000)	Clearance reduced in the elderly
Snoeck et al. (1995)	Clearance reduced in the elderly
	QUETIAPINE
Clearance	
deVane and Nemeroff (2001)	Clearance reduced in the elderly
	MOOD STABILIZERS
	LITHIUM
Steady-state plasma level	
Hewick et al. (1977)	Decreased dose needed to produce therapeutic levels
Elimination half-life	
Hardy et al. (1987)	Wide variability (20.4–35 hr); twice as long in elderly as in young (40 vs. 20 hr)
Davis et al. (1973)	
Schou (1968)	
Clearance	
Hardy et al. (1987)	Wide variability (1.2–23.6 mg/min); lower in elderly than younger individuals
Chapron et al. (1982)	
	VALPROIC ACID
Elimination half-life	
Bauer et al. (1985)	Doubled or tripled in elderly compared with young patients
	TRICYCLIC ANTIDEPRESSANTS
	AMITRIPTYLINE
Steady-state plasma level	
Nies et al. (1977)	Higher in elderly than in young (138 vs. 82 μg/L); correlated with age

(continued)

Table 5.3.   *(continued)*

Pharmacokinetic Parameter	Age-Related Changes

Elimination half-life
Ogura et al. (1983)   Significantly increased in elderly compared with young (27 vs. 15 hr)
Schultz et al. (1983)   Prolonged in elderly compared with young (21.7 vs.16.2 hr)
Henry et al. (1981)   Mean = 37.3 hr; not compared with young

Clearance
Schultz et al. (1983)   Mean = 0.29 L/hr/kg; not compared with young
Ogura et al. (1983)
Henry et al. (1981)   No difference by age; significantly reduced in elderly compared with young

CLOMIPRAMINE

Steady-state plasma level
Kunik et al. (1994)   Therapeutic levels reached at lower does than in midlife patients

DESIPRAMINE

Steady-state plasma level
Nelson et al. (1985)   Young and elderly had levels > 115 µg/L and increased 2-hydroxy-desipramine

Kitanaka et al. (1982)   Elderly had increased 2-hydroxydesipramine: desipramine ratios (0.86) compared with young (0.55)

Elimination half-life
Abernethy et al. (1985)   31 hr in elderly men vs. 21 hr in young men
Nelson et al. (1985)   Slightly prolonged in elderly men but not in elderly women
Cutler et al. (1984)   26 hr mean; wide variation (11–46 hr)
Antal (1982)   21 hr
Nies et al. (1977)   75–92 hr (from imipramine)

Clearance
Antal (1982)   1.78 L/hr/kg; not compared with younger sample

DOXEPIN

Steady-state plasma level
Leinonen & Ylitalo (1991)   No relation between concentrations of doxepin, demethyldoxepin, or combination on efficacy

Clearance
Ereshefsky et al. (1988)   Weak but significant reduction in oral clearance with age

IMIPRAMINE

Steady-state plasma level
Bjerre et al. (1981)   Higher in elderly but wide variability; increased dosage resulted in
Nies et al. (1977)   increased plasma levels; disproportionate rise in desipramine metabolite

Elimination half-life
Abernethy et al. (1985)   Significantly prolonged in elderly (27 hr) compared with young subjects (17 hr)
Nies et al. (1977)   23.8 hr for elderly compared with 19.0 hr for younger subjects
Hrdina et al. (1980)   23–26 hr

Clearance
Benetello et al. (1990)   Reduced clearance in elderly males (0.396 L/hr/kg) compared with younger subjects (0.851 L/hr/kg)

(continued)

Table 5.3. *(continued)*

Pharmacokinetic Parameter	Age-Related Changes
	MAPROTILINE
Elimination half-life	
Hrdina et al. (1980)	32 hr
	NORTRIPTYLINE
Steady-state plasma level	
Bupp & Preskorn (1991)	Positive but weak correlation with age; large variation
Kumar et al. (1987)	No difference between young and elderly when concentrations were adjusted for dosage
Young et al. (1985)	Concentrations of E10-hydroxynortriptyline significantly elevated in elderly (173 vs. 92 µg/L/hr)
Kragh-Sorensen et al. (1980) Dawling et al. (1980)	Proportional to dose, increased with age
Elimination half-life	
Turbots (1980)	No significant correlation between $t_{1/2}$ and age
Dawling et al. (1980)	Half-life twice as high in elderly (45 vs. 26 hr)
Clearance	
Schneider et al. (1990)	Reduced in elderly (20 vs. 54 L/hr); correlated with age; inversely correlated with creatinine clearance
Dawling et al. (1980)	

ATYPICAL ANTIDEPRESSANTS

NEFAZODONE

Steady-state plasma level	
Barbhaiya et al. (1996)	Slightly higher in elderly than in young (972.3 vs 489.6 mg/ mL); higher in women
Elimination half-life	
Barbhaiya et al. (1996)	No difference in elderly (7.1 hr) compared with young

BUPROPION

Clearance	
Sweet et al (1995)	Clearance reduced compared to young subjects

TRAZODONE

Steady-state plasma level	
Montelone et al. (1989)	No correlation with age
Elimination half-life	
Bayer et al. (1983)	30% higher in older subjects (11.6 vs. 6.4 hr)
Volume of distribution	
Greenblatt et al. (1987)	Higher in elderly men than women (1.15 vs. 0.89 L/kg)
Clearance	
Greenblatt et al. (1987)	Clearance significantly lower in elderly
Bayer et al. (1983)	Lower in elderly (6.3 vs. 10.8 L/hr)

VENLAFAXINE

Steady-state plasma level	
Klamerus et al. (1996)	No difference in plasma levels in elderly; higher in women

(continued)

Table 5.3.   *(continued)*

Pharmacokinetic Parameter	Age-Related Changes
Elimination half-life	
Klamerus et al. (1996)	4.7 hr
Clearance	
Kalmerus et al. (1996)	No difference in elderly, 1.16 L/hr/kg
Steady-state plasma level of O-desmethyl venlafaxine	
(active metabolite ODMV)	No difference in elderly; higher in women
Klamerus et al. (1996)	11.9 hr
Elimination half-life (ODMV)	
Klamerus et al. (1996)	
Clearance	
Klamerus et al. (1996)	0.34 L/hr/kg

REBOXETINE

Clearance	
Bergmann et al. (2000)	Clearance reduced in the elderly
Poggesi et al. (1999)	Clearance reduced in the elderly

SEROTONIN REUPTAKE INHIBITOR ANTIDEPRESSANTS

FLUOXETINE

Steady-state plasma level	
Benfield et al. (1986)	No age effect on plasma fluoxetine or desmethylfluoxetine concentrations
Elimination half-life	
Ayd (1988)	No difference
Lemberger (1985)	72 hr
Volume of distribution	
Bergstrom et al. (1988)	No difference (26 L/kg)
Clearance	
Harvey & Preskorn (2001)	No difference between young and elderly
Bergstrom et al. (1988)	No difference
Lemberger et al. (1985)	30 L/hr

FLUVOXAMINE

Steady-state plasma level	
Wilde et al. (1993)	Higher in elderly (873 vs. 592 mg/L); difference not considered clinically significant
Elimination half-life	
Wilde et al. (1993)	Slightly longer in elderly than in young volunteers (25.9 vs. 17.4 hr)

PAROXETINE

Steady-state plasma levels	
Lundmark et al. (1988)	Higher in elderly patients (46 vs. 36.3 mg/mL)
Hebenstreit (1988)	Wide variability

(continued)

Table 5.3.   *(continued)*

Pharmacokinetic Parameter	Age-Related Changes
Elimination half-life Bayer et al. (1988) Lundmark (1988)	Increases with dose 20 mg/day: 30 hr 30 mg/day: 38 hr Higher in elderly than in young volunteers (21 hr)

CITALOPRAM

Clearance Gutierrez and Abramowitz (2000) Overø et al. (1985)	No difference between young and elderly Lower clearance in the elderly

SERTRALINE

Steady-state plasma level Warrington (1991)	No difference between elderly and young
Elimination half-life Warrington (1991)	32 hr; no significant difference between young and elderly but slightly higher in both elderly men and women
Clearance Ronfeld et al. (1997)	Clearance reduced in elderly men compared to young men

BENZODIAZEPINES

ALPRAZOLAM

Gastrointestinal absorption Greenblatt et al. (1983)	Faster in elderly women than elderly men and young subjects; peak plasma concentration higher in elderly women than in elderly men or young subjects
Protein binding Greenblatt et al. (1983)	No change
Volume of distribution Greenblatt et al. (1983)	Slightly decreased
Elimination half-life Kroboth et al. (1990) Greenblatt et al. (1983)	Slight increase in women Slightly prolonged in elderly females, significantly prolonged in elderly males
Clearance Kroboth et al. (1990) Greenblatt et al. (1990)	Slight decrease Decreased compared with young; significantly lower in older men than older women

CHLORDIAZEPOXIDE

Gastrointestinal absorption Shader et al. (1977)	Peak plasma levels delayed (lower peak plasma levels)
Protein binding Roberts et al. (1978)	No change
Volume of distribution Roberts et al. (1978) Shader et al. (1977)	Increased Increased

(continued)

Table 5.3.   *(continued)*

Pharmacokinetic Parameter	Age-Related Changes
Clearance	
Roberts et al. (1978)	Decreased
Shader et al. (1977)	Decreased
Elimination half-life	
Greenblatt et al. (1989)	Prolonged
Roberts et al. (1978)	Prolonged
Shader et al. (1977)	Prolonged

DESMETHYLDIAZEPAM

Gastrointestinal absorption	
Shader et al. (1981)	No change
Ochs et al. (1979)	Delayed in elderly women but not in elderly men; peak plasma levels lower in elderly
Protein binding	
Shader et al. (1981)	Slightly decreased; trend toward increased free fraction
Volume of distribution	
Shader et al. (1981)	Increased with age
Divoll et al. (1980)	Higher in elderly women than in men
Klotz & Müller-Seydlitz (1979)	Increased
Elimination half-life	
Salzman et al. (1983)	Prolonged
Shader et al. (1981)	Very prolonged in older men (128 vs. 62 hr) but unchanged in older women
Klotz et al. (1975)	Prolonged
Clearance	
Shader et al. (1981)	Decreased slightly in older men; increased slightly in older women
Klotz & Müller-Seydlitz (1979)	Decreased

DESALKYLFLURAZEPAM

Steady-state plasma level	
Greenblatt et al. (1981)	Significantly higher in elderly vs. young men (81 vs. 53 Mg/L); not significantly higher in elderly vs. young women
Elimination half-life	
Hilbert et al. (1984)	Less significantly prolonged in elderly women (120 vs. 90 hr)
Greenblatt et al. (1981)	Active metabolite of flurazepam and quazepam: significantly prolonged in elderly men (160 vs. 74 hr)

DIAZEPAM

Gastrointestinal absorption	
Salzman et al. (1983)	Slightly delayed
Protein binding	
Ochs et al. (1981)	Decreased
Greenblatt et al. (1980)	Decreased
Macklon et al. (1980)	Decreased
Volume of distribution	
Greenblatt et al. (1980)	Increased with age, more in older women than in older men
Ochs et al. (1981)	Age effect minimal in unbound diazepam
Macklon et al. (1980)	Increased
MacLeod et al. (1979)	No change (possible increase)

(continued)

Table 5.3.   *(continued)*

Pharmacokinetic Parameter	Age-Related Changes
Elimination half-life	
Salzman et al. (1983)	Prolonged
Greenblatt et al. (1980)	Prolonged; longer in elderly men than women
MacLeod et al. (1979)	No change
Klotz et al. (1975)	Prolonged
Kanto et al. (1979)	Prolonged
Clearance	
Ochs et al. (1981)	Decreased
Greenblatt et al. (1980)	Decreased
Macklon et al. (1980)	Decreased
MacLeod et al. (1979)	No change
Kanto et al. (1979)	Decreased

LORAZEPAM

Gastrointestinal absorption	
Greenblatt et al. (1979a)	Slightly decreased absorption 80–100% complete
Protein binding	
Divoll et al. (1982)	Larger free fraction
Kraus et al. (1978)	Trend toward decreased protein binding
Volume of distribution	
Kraus et al. (1978)	No change
Elimination half-life	
Greenblatt et al. (1979a)	No change
Greenblatt et al. (1979b)	No change
Kraus et al. (1978)	No change
Swift et al. (1985)	Significantly longer in elderly than in young volunteers (19.8 hr vs. 11.2 hr)

OXAZEPAM

Gastrointestinal absorption	
Salzman et al. (1983)	Slightly delayed
Greenblatt et al. (1980b)	Relatively slow and erratic; peak plasma concentration reached sooner in men and lower in men than in women
Protein binding	
Greenblatt et al. (1980b)	High correlation between reduced albumin and increased free fraction
Shull et al. (1976)	No change
Volume of distribution	
Greenblatt et al. (1980)	No relation to age or gender
Shull et al. (1976)	Slightly increased
Elimination half-life	
Salzman et al. (1983)	No change
Ochs et al. (1981)	
Shull et al. (1976)	
Greenblatt et al. (1980)	Shorter in men than in women; slightly prolonged in older women; not significantly affected by age

(continued)

Table 5.3. *(continued)*

Pharmacokinetic Parameter	Age-Related Changes
Clearance	
Salzman et al. (1983)	No change
Ochs et al. (1981)	
Shull et al. (1976)	
Greenblatt et al. (1980)	No significant changes in elderly
	TRIAZOLAM
Elimination half-life	
Greenblatt et al. (1991)	Longer in elderly but not significantly
Greenblatt et al. (1983)	
Clearance	
Greenblatt et al. (1991)	Highly significant decrement compared with young subjects
Greenblatt et al. (1983)	
Smith et al. (1983)	No age-related changes
	ZOLPIDEM (nonbenzodiazepine hypnotic)
Clearance	
Olubodun et al. (2003)	Clearance significantly reduced in the elderly

Table prepared by Carl Salzman.

pyridine hypnotic metabolized mainly by CYP3A isoforms.[34] Benzodiazepines metabolized by glucuronide conjugation (oxazepam, lorazepam, temazepam) undergo minimal age-related change in clearance. For all drugs in this category, reduced dosage in geriatric patients is strongly recommended, because many studies indicate both increased intrinsic-sensitivity and the possibility of impaired clearance. Clearance of the nonbenzodiazepine buspirone is not altered in the elderly, but it is not known whether there are any pharmacodynamic differences.

Antidepressants

Cyclic antidepressants are high-clearance drugs that have been extensively studied in elderly patients, in whom bioavailability may increase and drug clearance decrease.[35–37] Each of these changes results in a higher C_{ss} at any given dosage.

Tertiary amine tricyclic antidepressants such as imipramine, amitriptyline, doxepin, trimipramine, and clomipramine may be demethylated to active desmethyl metabolites. The ratio of parent compound to desmethyl metabolite at steady state depends in part on demethylation, a metabolic step that may become less efficient with advanced age. As a result, when older patients are treated with one of these tertiary antidepressant compounds, the amount of parent drug can be higher than the amount of metabolite, especially when compared with younger patients. Because the parent tertiary amine tends to be more sedating than the secondary amine metabolite, older patients who receive tertiary amines may experience more frequent and more severe sedative side effects.

Both the tertiary amine and the secondary amine metabolites are further metabolized to active hydroxy metabolites (e.g., 10-hydroxyamitriptyline and 10-hydroxynortriptyline, 2-hydroxyimipramine and 2-hydroxydespiramine). Commercially available secondary amines such as desipramine and nortriptyline also produce hydroxy metabolites, which are water soluble and are excreted through the kidneys, with clearance depending on renal function. Because renal clearance declines with age, the hydroxy metabolites may accumulate to a greater extent in older patients. Each of the pharmacokinetic changes noted for cyclic antidepressants indicates that doses of these drugs to achieve similar plasma concentrations of pharmacologically active drug and metabolite may decrease by 50 to 75%.

Among SSRI and mixed-mechanism antidepressants, clearance of trazodone, sertraline, citalopram, escitalopram, nefazodone, and fluoxetine may be impaired in the elderly. A need for reduced dosage should be anticipated.

Lithium

Age-related changes in lithium pharmacokinetics occur in tandem with the age-related decline in renal function. Considerable reduction in renal clearance may occur, although variation among elderly individuals is wide. Elevated plasma lithium levels commonly result from decreased clearance in older patients, even following low doses. No data are available regarding age-related pharmacodynamics of lithium, but older patients appear to be more likely to develop neurotoxicity, even at low-therapeutic plasma levels.

Neuroleptics

Age-specific studies of the pharmacodynamics of phenothiazines and haloperidol are scant, owing to difficulties with an analytical method sensitivity as well as with initiating studies in healthy volunteers. As noted, however, elderly people are reportedly more sensitive to neuroleptic side effects, particularly sedation, orthostatic hypotension, and anticholinergic symptoms.

Most of the newer atypical antipsychotics show some differences in elderly patients. Quetiapine shows a large decrease in oral clearance in older patients, with recommendations to lower starting doses. Olanzapine clearance is reduced

in older women who are nonsmokers. Risperidone itself does not appear to have altered kinetics, but the renal clearance of the active metabolite 9-OH risperidone is reduced with increasing age. Both ziprasidone and aripiprazole are reported to have some decrease in clearance, but full data in a nonsupplement peer-reviewed publication are not available. Data that are available on ziprasidone suggest that elderly women in particular may be at risk for increased drug exposure and accumulation as compared with young women, though half-lives are extended in both elderly men and women.

Using Pharmacokinetic Information in Prescribing Psychotropic Drugs

For the research scientist, pharmacokinetic data on psychotropic drugs enhance knowledge of basic age-related changes in physiology and how these changes affect drug disposition. For the clinician, however, information concerning the alterations caused by psychotropic drug pharmacokinetics can directly assist in the prescription of these drugs to elderly patients by providing a rational basis for clinical prescribing practices.

Absorption

Although the aging process does not importantly alter the absorption of orally prescribed psychotropic drugs, absorption may be delayed by the presence of antacids, food, or anticholinergic drugs. In most cases, when the patient receives regular repeated doses after steady state has been reached, this delay is not of major clinical importance. However, if a psychotropic drug is given for a specific immediate clinical effect, such as calming anxiety or inducing sleep, a reduced rate of absorption may delay the onset of the drug effect. For example, if an older patient plans to take a hypnotic drug and then go to sleep at a given hour, absorption of this hypnotic could be delayed if the patient also receives other medications with antacid or anticholinergic effects. In these circumstances, the hypnotic should be taken before the anticipated bedtime on a relatively empty stomach or with small amounts of liquid. Bioavailability, which is affected by factors including absorption, may be unexpectedly higher in the elderly in some of the situations detailed above. Initiating treatment with smaller doses can prevent toxicity.

Clearance

As a general principle, drug clearance decreases with age. This alteration produces higher values of C_{ss} at any given dosing rate. Further, because a longer time is required before effective C_{ss} is reached, therapeutic benefits and/or toxicity may be delayed. Since the metabolism of psychotropic drugs can be altered not only by aging but also by many other factors, such as medical disease and concurrent medications, the clinician must consider all of these factors when prescribing these drugs.

Protein Binding

Although reduced protein binding (increased free fraction) of a number of drugs occurs in old age, there is little evidence that this change by itself alters the pharmacodynamic effects of psychotropic drugs in the elderly. Nonetheless, increased free fraction, particularly when attributed to substantially reduced plasma albumin concentrations, may be an important clinical marker for other factors that can predispose to psychotropic drug toxicity. These include impaired renal function or reduced hepatic metabolizing capacity, leading to reduced drug clearance or increased drug sensitivity due to debility. Reduced protein binding may also influence the interpretation of total (free plus bound) serum or plasma concentrations obtained during therapeutic monitoring. Assuming that clearance is restricted by protein binding, an increased free fraction by itself will cause a reciprocal reduction in the total plasma concentration. Thus reduced protein binding of certain drugs in the elderly may have the effect of reducing the therapeutic and toxic plasma concentration ranges when the assay procedure measures the total (free plus bound) plasma drug concentration.

Comment

Age-related pharmacokinetic alterations may play an important role in the tendency of older people to have exaggerated responses to psychotropic drugs. Most experienced clinicians treating elderly patients with psychotropic drugs intuitively incorporate pharmacokinetic information in their prescribing practice. They take the frail or sick nature of their older patients into account and prescribe lower doses, provide small dose increments in a more gradual manner, and monitor drug effects closely. They have adopted the adage "Start low, go slow," a useful guideline reflecting current knowledge of age-related alterations in psychotropic drug pharmacokinetics and pharmacodynamics. In the absence of contradictory kinetic data, it remains good advice. However, because of the prolonged time that may be necessary before a psychotropic drug reaches effective steady-state concentration, one further suggestion may be offered to the clinician: "Don't quit." In other words, rather than discontinuing treatment prematurely, the clinician should allow sufficient time—waiting until adequate plasma concentrations and the presumed necessary receptor-site drug concentrations occur—before assessing therapeutic efficacy.

Although not an intrinsic part of the aging process, polypharmacy appears to be such a predictable part of aging that it cannot be ignored or separated as a consideration in anticipating pharmacokinetic changes in the elderly. Polypharmacy increases the possibilities for drug interactions and interactions with potent inhibitors or inducers of metabolism or those involving drugs with narrow therapeutic indices, which have the potential to produce profound kinetic changes that are far more drastic than those commonly seen as a result of the aging process alone. Continuing attention to careful use of those medications which are most likely to be involved in clinically significant interactions continues to be an important part of care for this group of individuals which include some of those most vulnerable to any adverse outcomes.

Acknowledgments. Supported in part by grants MH-58435, AG-17780, DK-58435, DA-05258, DA-13209, DA-58496, AT-01381 and RR-00054 from the U.S. Department of Health and Human Services. The authors are grateful for the assistance of Richard I. Shader and Jerold S. Harmatz.

References

1. Greenblatt DJ. Presystemic extraction: mechanisms and consequences. *J of Clin Pharm* 1993; 33:650–656.
2. Greenblatt DJ, von Moltke LL, Shader RI. The importance of presystemic extraction in clinical psychopharmacology. *Journal of Clinical Psychopharmacology* 1996;16:417–419.
3. Thummel KE, Wilkinson GR. In vitro and in vivo drug interactions involving human CYP3A. *Ann Rev of Pharm and Tox* 1998;38:389–430.
4. Ayrton A, Morgan P. Role of transport proteins in drug absorption, distribution and excretion. *Xenobiotica* 2001;31:469–497.
5. Kim RB. Transporters and drug disposition. *Current Opinion in Drug Discovery & Development* 2000; 3:94–101.
6. Wacher VJ, Salphati L, Benet LZ. Active secretion and enterocytic drug metabolism barriers to drug absorption. *Adv Drug Delivery Rev* 2001; 46:89–102.
7. Matheny CJ, Lamb MW, Brouwer KL, Pollack GM. Pharmacokinetic and pharmacodynamic implications of P-glycoprotein modulation. *Pharmacotherapy* 2001;21:778–796.
8. Greenblatt DJ, Sellers EM, Shader RI. Drug disposition in old age. *N Engl J Med* 1982;306: 1081–1088.
9. Cotreau MM, von Moltke LL, Greenblatt DJ. The influence of age and sex on the clearance of cytochrome P450 (CYP) 3A substrates. *Clinical Pharmacokinetics* (in press).
10. Uhr M, Steckler T, Yassouridis A, Holsboer F. Penetration of amitriptyline, but not of fluoxetine, into brain is enhanced in mice with blood-brain barrier deficiency due to Mdr1a P-glycoprotein gene disruption. *Neuro Psychopharmacology* 2000;22:380–387.
11. Borkan GA, Hults DE, Gerzof SG, et al. Age changes in body composition revealed by computed tomography. *J Gerontol* 1983;38:673–677.
12. Chaperon DJ, Cameron IR, White LB, et al. Observations on lithium distribution in the elderly. *J Am Geriatr Soc* 1982;30:651–655.
13. Fromm MF. P-glycoprotein: a defense mechanism limiting oral bioavailability and CNS accumulation of drugs. *Int J Clin Pharmacol Ther* 2000; 38:69–74.
14. Kim RB, Fromm MF, Wandel C, et al. The drug transporter P-glycoprotein limits oral absorption and brain entry of HIV-1 protease inhibitors. *J of Clin Inv* 1998;101:289–294.
15. von Moltke LL, Greenblatt DJ. Drug transporters in psychopharmacology—are they important? *J of Clin Psychopharmacology* 2000;20: 291–294.
16. von Moltke LL, Greenblatt DJ. Drug transporters revisited. *J of Clin Psychopharmacology* 2001;21: 1–3.
17. Sadeque AJ, Wandel C, He H, et al. Increased drug delivery to the brain by P-glycoprotein inhibition. *Clin Pharm & Ther* 2000;68:231–237.
18. Greenblatt DJ, Sellers EM, Koch-Weser J. Importance of protein binding for the interpretation of serum or plasma drug concentrations. *J of Clin Pharma* 1982;22:259–263.
19. Abernethy DR, Kerzner L. Age effects on alpha-1-acid glycoprotein concentration and imipramine plasma protein binding. *J Am Geriatr Soc* 1984;32:705–708.
20. Sellers EM. Plasma protein displacement interactions are rarely of clinical significance. *Pharmacology* 1979;18:225–227.
21. Abernethy DR, Greenblatt DJ, Shader RI. Benzodiazepine hypnotic metabolism: drug interaction and clinical implications. *Acta Psychiatr Scand* 1986;74(suppl 332):32–38.
22. Greenblatt DJ, Harmatz JS, Shapiro L, et al. Sensitivity to triazolam in the elderly. *N Eng J of Med* 1991;324:1691–1698.
23. Davies DF, Shock NW. Age changes in glomerular filtration rates, effective renal plasma flow, and tubular excretory capacity in adult males. *J Clin Invest* 1950;29:496–506.
24. Kitanka I, Ross RJ, Cutler NR, et al. Altered hydroxydesipramine concentrations in elderly depressed patients. *Clin Pharmacol Ther* 1982;31: 51–55.
25. Young RC, Alexopoulos GS, Shamoian CA, et al. Plasma 10-hydroxynortriptyline in elderly depressed patients. *Clin Pharmacol Ther* 1984;35: 540–544.
26. Nies A, Robinson DS, Friedman MJ, et al. Relationship between age and tricyclic antidepressant plasma levels. *Am J Psychiatry* 1977;134: 790–793.
27. Abernethy DR. Problematic factors in pharmacodynamic studies. In: Kroboth PD, Smith RB, Juhl RP, eds. *Pharmacokinetics and pharmacodynamics. Vol 2: Current Problems and Potential. Solu-*

tions. Cincinnati: Harvey Whitney Books, 1988: 60–74.

28. Thompson TL, Moran MG, Nies AS. Psychotropic drug use in the elderly. *N Engl J Med* 1983; 308:134–138, 193–199.

29. Greenblatt DJ, Allen MD, Shader RI. Toxicity of high-dose flurazepam in the elderly. *Clin Pharmacol Ther* 1978;215:86–91.

30. Cutler NR, Narang PK. Implications of dosing tricyclic antidepressants and benzodiazepines in geriatrics. *Psychiatr Clin North Am* 1984;7: 845–861.

31. von Moltke LL, Greenblatt DJ, Harmatz JS, et al. Psychotropic drug metabolism in old age: principles and problems of assessment. In: Bloom FE, Kupfer DJ, eds. *Psychopharmacology: the fourth generation of progress.* New York: Raven, 1995:1461–1477.

32. Greenblatt DJ, Shader RI, Harmatz JS. Implications of altered drug disposition in the elderly: studies of benzodiazepines. *Journal of Clinical Pharmacology* 1989;29:866–872.

33. Greenblatt DJ, Harmatz JS, Shader RI. Clinical pharmacokinetics of anxiolytics and hypnotics in the elderly: therapeutic considerations. *Clinical Pharmacokinetics* 1991;21:165–177, 262–273.

34. Olubodun JO, Ochs HR, von Moltke LL, et al. Pharmacokinetic properties of zolpidem in elderly and young adults: possible modulation by testosterone in men. *Br J of Clin Pharm* 2003;56: 297–304.

35. Schultz P, Turner-Tamiyasu K, Smith G, et al. Amitriptyline disposition in young and elderly normal men. *Clin Pharmacol Ther* 1983;33: 360–366.

36. Abernethy DR, Greenblatt DJ, Shader RI. Imipramine and desipramine disposition in the elderly. *J Pharmacol Exp Ther* 1985;232:183–188.

37. von Moltke LL, Greenblatt DJ, Shader RI. Clinical pharmacokinetics of antidepressants in the elderly: therapeutic implications. *Clinical Pharmacokinetics* 1993;24:141–160.

Table 5.3 References

Abernethy DR, Greenblatt DJ, Shader RI. Imipramine and desipramine disposition in the elderly. *J Pharmacol Exp Ther* 1985;232:183–188.

Antal EJ, Lawson IR, Alderson LM, et al. Estimating steady state desipramine levels in noninstitutionalized elderly patients using single dose disposition parameters. *J Clin Psychopharmacol* 1982;2: 193–198.

Aoba A, Kakita Y, Yamaguchi N, et al. Absence of age effect on plasma haloperidol neuroleptic levels in psychiatric patients. *J Gerontol* 1985;40: 303–308.

Ayd FJ Jr. Fluoxetine: an antidepressant with specific serotonin uptake inhibition. *Int Drug Ther Newslett* 1988;2:5–11.

Barbhaiya RH, Buch AB, Greene DS. A study of the effect of age and gender on the pharmacokinetics of nefazodone after single and multiple doses. *J Clin Psychopharmacol* 1996;16:19–25.

Bayer AJ, Pathy MSJ, Ankier SI. Pharmacokinetic and pharmacodynamic characteristics of trazodone in the elderly. *Br J Clin Pharmacol* 1983;16: 371–376.

Bayer AJ, Roberts NA, Allen EA, et al. The pharmacokinetics of paroxetine in the elderly. *Acta Psychiatr Scand* 1988;80(suppl 350):85–86.

Benfield P, Heel RC, Lewis SP. Fluoxetine. A review of its pharmacodynamic and pharmacokinetic properties and therapeutic efficacy in depressive illness. *Drugs* 1986;32:481–508.

Bergmann JF, Laneury JP, Duchene P, et al. Pharmacokinetics of reboxetine in healthy, elderly volunteers. *Eur J Drug Metab Pharmacokinet* 2000;25: 195–198.

Bergstrom RF, Lemberger L, Farid NA, et al. Clinical pharmacology and pharmacokinetics of fluoxetine: a review. *Br J Psychiatr* 1988;153(suppl 3): 47–50.

Bupp SJ, Preskorn SH. The effect of age on plasma levels of nortriptyline. *Ann Clin Psychiatry* 1991; 3:61–65.

Chapron DJ, Cameron IR, White LB, et al. Observations on lithium disposition in the elderly. *J Am Geriatr Soc* 1982;30:651–655.

Cohen BM, Sommer BR. Metabolism of thioridazine in the elderly. *J Clin Psychopharmacol* 1988;8: 336–339.

Cutler NR, Narang PK. Implications of dosing tricyclic antidepressants and benzodiazepines in geriatrics. *Psychiatr Clin North Am* 1984;7: 845–861.

Dawling S, Crome P, Braithwaite R. Pharmacokinetics of single oral doses of nortriptyline in depressed elderly hospital patients and young healthy volunteers. *Clin Pharmacokinet* 1980;5: 394–401.

DeVane CL, Nemeroff CB. Clinical pharmacokinetics of quetiapine: an atypical antipsychotic. *Clin Pharmacokinet* 2001;40:509–522.

Divoll M, Greenblatt DJ. Effect of age and sex on lorazepam protein binding. *J Pharm Pharmacol* 1982;34:122–123.

Dysken MW, Johnson SB, Holden L, et al. Haloperidol concentrations in patients with Alzheimer's dementia. *Am J Geriatr Psychiatry* 1994;2:124–133.

Ereshefsky L, Tran-Johnson T, Davis CM, et al. Pharmacokinetic factors affecting antidepressant drug clearance and clinical effect: evaluation of doxepin and imipramine—new data and review. *Clin Chem* 1988;34:863–880.

Greenblatt DJ, Allen MD, Harmatz JS, et al. Diazepam disposition determinants. *Clin Pharmacol Ther* 1980a;27:301–312.

Greenblatt DJ, Allen MD, Locniskar A, et al. Lorazepam kinetics in the elderly. *Clin Pharmacol Ther* 1979a;26:103–113.

Greenblatt DJ, Divoll M, Abernethy DR, et al. Alprazolam kinetics in the elderly. *Arch Gen Psychiatry* 1983;40:287–290.

Greenblatt DJ, Divoll M, Harmatz JS, et al. Kinetics and clinical effects of flurazepam in young and elderly noninsomniacs. *Clin Pharmacol Ther* 1981; 30;475–486.

Greenblatt DJ, Divoll M, Harmatz JS, et al. Oxazepam kinetics: effects of age and sex. *J Pharmacol Exp Ther* 1980b;215:86–91.

Greenblatt DJ, Divoll MK, Abernethy DR, et al. Reduced clearance of triazolam in old age: relation to antipyrine capacity. *Br J Clin Pharm* 1983d;15: 303–309.

Greenblatt DJ, Divoll MK, Soong MH, et al. Age and gender effects on chlordiazepoxide kinetics: relation to antipyrine disposition. *Pharmacology* 1989b;38:327–334.

Greenblatt DJ, Harmatz JS, Shapiro L, et al. Sensitivity to triazolam in the elderly. *N Engl J Med* 1991; 324:1991–1998.

Gutierrez M, Abramowitz W. Steady-state pharmacokinetics of citalopram in young and elderly subjects. *Pharmacotherapy* 2000;20:1441–1447.

Hardy BG, Shulman KI, Mackenzie SE, et al. Pharmacokinetics of lithium in the elderly. *J Clin Psychopharmacol* 1987;7:153–158.

Harvey AT, Preskorn SH. Fluoxetine pharmacokinetics and effect on CYP2C19 in young and elderly volunteers. *J Clin Psychopharmacol* 2001;21: 161–166.

Hewick DS, Newbury P, Hopwood S, et al. Age as a factor affecting lithium therapy. *Br J Clin Pharmacol* 1977;4:201–205.

Hilbert JM, Chung M, Radwanski E, et al. Quazepam kinetics in the elderly. *Clin Pharmacol Ther* 1984; 36:566–569.

Hrdina PD, Rovei P, Henry JF, et al. Comparison of single-dose pharmacokinetics of imipramine and maprotiline in the elderly. *Psychopharmacology* 1980;70:29–34.

Kanto J, Maenpaa M, Mantyla R, et al. Effect of age on the pharmacokinetics of diazepam given in conjunction with spinal anesthesia. *Anesthesiology* 1979;51:154–159.

Kitanaka I, Ross RJ, Cutler NR, et al. Altered hydroxydesipramine concentrations in elderly depressed patients. *Clin Pharmacol Ther* 1982;31: 51–55.

Klamerus KJ, Parker VD, Rudolph RL, et al. Effects of age and gender on venlafaxine and O-desmethylvenlafaxine pharmacokinetics. *Pharmacotherapy* 1996;16:915–923.

Klotz U, Avant GR, Hoyumpa A, et al. Effects of age and liver disease on disposition and elimination of diazepam in adult man. *J Clin Invest* 1975;55: 347–359.

Klotz U, Müller-Seydlitz P. Altered elimination of desmethyldiazepam in the elderly. *Br J Clin Pharmacol* 1979;7:119–120.

Kragh-Sørensen P, Larsen NE. Factors influencing nortriptyline steady-state kinetics; plasma and saliva levels. *Clin Pharmacol Ther* 1980;28:796–803.

Kraus JW, Desmond PV, Marshall JP, et al. Effects of aging and liver disease on disposition of lorazepam. *Clin Pharmacol Ther* 1978;24:411–419.

Kroboth PD, McAuley JW, Smith RB. Alprazolam in the elderly: pharmacokinetics and pharmacodynamics during multiple dosing. *Psychopharmacology* 1990;100:477–484.

Kumar V, Smith RC, Reed K, et al. Plasma levels and effects of nortriptyline in geriatric depressed patients. *Acta Psychiatr Scand* 1987;75:20–28.

Kunik ME, Pollock BG, Perel JM, et al. Clomipramine in the elderly: tolerance and plasma levels. *J Geriatr Psychiatry Neurol* 1994;7:139–143.

Leinonen E, Ylitalo P. The influence of ageing on serum levels of tertiary tricyclic antidepressants. *Hum Psychopharmacol* 1991;6:139–146.

Lemberger L, Bergstrom RF, Wolen RL, et al. Fluox-

etine: clinical pharmacology and physiologic disposition. *J Clin Psychiatry* 1985;46:14–19.

Lundmark J, et al. Paroxetine: pharmacokinetic and antidepressant effect in the elderly. *Psychopharmacology* 1988;96:211.

Macklon AF, Barton M, James O, et al. The effect of age on the pharmacokinetics of diazepam. *Clin Sci* 1980;59:479–483.

Martensson E, Roos BE. Serum levels of thioridazine in psychiatric patients and volunteers. *Eur J Clin Pharmacol* 1973;6:181–186.

Musze RG, Vanderheeren FAJ. Plasma levels and half lives of thioridazine and some of its metabolites. *Eur J Clin Pharmacol* 1977;11:141–147.

Nelson JC, Jatlow PI, Mazure C. Desipramine plasma levels and response in elderly melancholic patients. *J Clin Psychopharmacol* 1985;5:217–220.

Nies A, Robinson DS, Friedman MJ, et al. Relationship between age and tricyclic antidepressant plasma levels. *Am J Psychiatry* 1977;134:790–793.

Ochs H, Greenblatt DJ, Divoll M, et al. Diazepam kinetics in relation to age and sex. *Pharmacology* 1981;23:24–30.

Ochs HR, Greenblatt DJ, Allen MD, et al. Effect of age and Billroth gastrectomy on absorption of desmethyldiazepam from clorazepate. *Clin Pharmacol Ther* 1979;26:449–456.

Olubodun JO, Ochs HR, von Moltke LL, et al. Pharmacokinetic properties of zolpidem in elderly and young adults: possible modulation by testosterone in men. *Br J of Clin Pharm* 2003;56: 297–304.

Overø KF, Toft B, Christophersen B, et al. Kinetics of citalopram in elderly patients. *Psychopharmacology* 1985;86:253–257.

Poggesi I, Pellizzoni C, Fleishaker JC. Pharmacokinetics of reboxetine in elderly patients with depressive disorders. *Int J Clin Pharmacol Ther* 2000; 38:254–259.

Roberts RK, Wilkinson GR, Branch RA, et al. Effect of age and parenchymal liver disease on the disposition and elimination of chlordiazepoxide (Librium). *Gastroenterology* 1978;75:479–485.

Ronfeld RA, Tremaine LM, Wilner KD. Pharmacokinetics of sertraline and its N-demethyl metabolite in elderly and young male and female volunteers. *Clinical Pharmacokinetics* 1997;32(Supp 1):22–30.

Salzman C, Shader RI, Greenblatt DJ, et al. Long versus short half-life benzodiazepines in the elderly: kinetics and clinical effects of diazepam and oxazepam. *Arch Gen Psychiatry* 1983;40: 293–297.

Schneider LS, Cooper TB, Suckow RF, et al. Relationship of hydroxynortriptyline to nortriptyline concentration and creatinine clearance in depressed elderly outpatients. *J Clin Psychopharmacol* 1990;10:333–337.

Schou M. Lithium in psychiatric therapy and prophylaxis. *J Psychiatr Res* 1968;6:69–95.

Schulz P, Turner-Tamiyasu K, Smith G, et al. Amitriptyline disposition in young and elderly normal men. *Clin Pharmacol Ther* 1983;7:360–366.

Shader RI, Greenblatt DJ, Ciraulo DA, et al. Effect of age and sex on disposition of desmethyldiazepam formed from its precursor clorazepate. *Psychopharmacology* 1981;75:193–197.

Shader RI, Greenblatt DJ, Harmatz JS, et al. Absorption and disposition of chlordiazepoxide in young and elderly male volunteers. *J Clin Pharmacol* 1977;17:709–718.

Shull HJ, Wilkinson GR, Johnson R, et al. Normal disposition of oxazepam in acute viral hepatitis and cirrhosis. *Ann Intern Med* 1976;84:420–425.

Smith RB, Divoll M, Gillespie WR, et al. Effect of subject age and gender on the pharmacokinetics of oral triazolam and temazepam. *J Clin Psychopharmacol* 1983;3:172–176.

Snoeck E, Van Peer A, Sack M, et al. Influence of age, renal and liver impairment on the pharmacokinetics of risperidone in man. *Psychopharmacology (Berl)* 1995;122:223–229.

Sweet RA, Pollock BG, Kirshner M, et al. Pharmacokinetics of single- and multiple-dose bupropion in elderly patients with depression. *J Clin Pharmacol* 1995;35:876–884.

Turbott J, Norman TR, Burrows GD, et al. Pharmacokinetics of nortriptyline in elderly volunteers. *Commun Psychopharmacol* 1980;4:225–231.

Warrington SJ. Clinical implications of the pharmacology of sertraline. *Int Clin Psychopharmacol* 1991; 2(suppl):11–21.

Wilde MI, Plosker GL, Benfield P. Fluvoxamine. An updated review of its pharmacology, and therapeutic use in depressive illness. *Drugs* 1993;46: 895–924.

Wilner KD, Tensfeldt TG, Baris B, et al. Single- and multiple-dose pharmacokinetics of ziprasidone in healthy young and elderly volunteers. *Br J Clin Pharmacol* 2000;49(Suppl 1):15S–20S.

Supplemental Readings

General References and Review Articles

Baumann P. Care and depression in the elderly: comparative pharmacokinetics of SSRIs. *International Clinical Psychopharmacology* 1998;13(suppl. 5):S35–S43.

Benetello P, Furlanut M, Zara G, et al. Imipramine pharmacokinetics in depressed geriatric patients. *Int J Clin Pharmacol Res* 1990;10:191–195.

Bjerre M, Gram LF, Kragh-Sorensen P, et al. Dose-dependent kinetics of imipramine in elderly patients. *Psychopharmacology* 1981;75:354–357.

Byerly MJ, DeVane CL. Pharmacokinetics of clozapine and risperidone: a review of recent literature. *J of Clin Psychopharmacology* 1996;16: 177–187.

Crooks J, O'Malley K, Stevenson IH. Pharmacokinetics in the elderly. *Clin Pharmacokinet* 1976;1: 280–296.

Dawling S, Crome P, Braithwaite R. Pharmacokinetics of single oral doses of nortriptyline in depressed elderly hospital patients and young healthy volunteers. *Clin Pharmacokinet* 1980;5: 394–401.

Dehlin O, Killingsjo H, Linden A, et al. Pharmacokinetics of alprazolam in geriatric patients with neurotic depression. *Pharmacol Toxicol* 1991;68: 121–124.

DeVane CL, Nemeroff CB. Clinical pharmacokinetics of quetiapine: an atypical antipsychotic. *Clin Pharmacokinet* 2001;40:509–522.

DeVane CL, Liston HL, Markowitz JS. Clinical phar-

macokinetics of sertraline. *Clin Pharmacokinet* 2002;41:1247–1266.

Durnas C, Loi CM, Cusack BJ. Hepatic drug metabolism and aging. *Clin Pharmacokinet* 1990;19: 359–389.

Felix S, Sproule BA, Hardy BG, et al. Dose-related pharmacokinetics and pharmacodynamics of valproate in the elderly. *J Clin Psychopharmacol* 2003; 23:471–478.

Fleishaker JC, Hulst LK, Ekernäs S, Grahnén A. Pharmacokinetics and pharmacodynamics of adinazolam and N-desmethyladinazolam after oral and intravenous dosing in healthy young and elderly volunteers. *J Clin Psychopharmacol* 1992;12: 403–414.

Fleishaker JC, Phillips JP, Smith TC, Smith RB. Multiple-dose pharmacokinetics and pharmacodynamics of adinazolam in elderly subjects. *Pharm Res* 1989;6:379–386.

Friedel RO. Pharmacokinetics in the geropsychiatric patient. In: Lipton MA, DiMascio A, Killam KF, eds. *Psychopharmacology: a generation of progress.* New York: Raven, 1978:1499–1505.

Furlant M, Benetello P. The pharmacokinetics of tricyclic antidepressant drugs in the elderly. *Pharmacol Res* 1990;22:15–25.

Gammans RE, Westrick ML, Shea JP, et al. Pharmacokinetics of buspirone in elderly subjects. *J Clin Pharmacol* 1989;29:72–78.

Gareri P, Stilo G, Bevacqua I, et al. Antidepressant drugs in the elderly. *General Pharmacology* 1998; 30:465–475.

Greenblatt DJ. Benzodiazepine hypnotics: sorting the pharmacokinetic facts. *J Clin Psychiatry* 1991; 52(suppl):4–10.

Greenblatt DJ. Presystemic extraction: mechanisms and consequences. *J Clin Pharmacol* 1993;33: 650–656.

Greenblatt DJ. Principles of pharmacokinetics and pharmacodynamics. In: Nemeroff CB, Schatzberg AF, eds. *American Psychiatric Press Textbook of Psychopharmacology.* Washington, DC: American Psychiatric Press, 1995:125–136.

Greenblatt DJ. The importance of presystemic extraction in clinical psychopharmacology. *J Clin Psychopharmacol* 1996;16:417–419.

Greenblatt DJ, Abernethy DR, Shader RI. Pharmacokinetic aspects of drug therapy in the elderly. *Ther Drug Monit* 1986;8:249–255.

Greenblatt DJ, Allen MD, Locniskar A, et al. Lorazepam kinetics in the elderly. *Clin Pharmacol Ther* 1979;26:103–113.

Greenblatt DJ, Divoll M, Abernethy DR, et al. Alprazolam kinetics in the elderly. *Arch Gen Psychiatry* 1983;40:287–290.

Greenblatt DJ, Harmatz JS. Kinetic-dynamic modeling in clinical psychopharmacology. *J Clin Psychopharmacol* 1993;13:231–234.

Greenblatt DJ, Harmatz JS, Shader RI. Clinical pharmacokinetics of anxiolytics and hypnotics in the elderly: therapeutic considerations. *Clin Pharmacokinet* 1991;21:165–177, 262–273.

Greenblatt DJ, Sellers EM, Shader RI. Drug disposition in old age. *N Engl J Med* 1982;306:1081–1088.

Greenblatt DJ, Shader RI, Abernethy DR. Current status of benzodiazepines. *N Engl J Med* 1983;309: 354–358.

Greenblatt DJ, Shader RI, Harmatz JS. Implications

of altered drug disposition in the elderly: studies of benzodiazepines. *J Clin Pharmacol* 1989;29: 866–872.

Greenblatt DJ, von Moltke LL, Harmatz JS, et al. Pharmacokinetics, pharmacodynamics, and drug disposition. In: Davis KL, Charney D, Coyle JT, et al., eds. *Neuropsychopharmacology: the fifth generation of progress.* Philadelphia: Lippincott Williams and Wilkins, 2002:507–524.

Greenblatt DJ, von Moltke LL. Sedative-hypnotic and anxiolytic agents. In: Levy RH, Thummel KE, Trager WF, Hanster PD, et al., eds. *Metabolic Drug Interactions.* Philadelphia: Lippincott, Williams and Wilkins, 2002:259–270.

Greenblatt DJ, von Moltke LL, Shader RI. Pharmacokinetics of psychotropic drugs. In: Nelson JC, ed. *Geriatric Psychopharmacology.* New York: Marcel Dekker, 1998:27–41.

Greenblatt DJ, von Moltke LL, Schmider J, et al. Inhibition of human cytochrome P450-3A isoforms by fluoxetine and norfluoxetine: in vitro and in vivo studies. *J Clin Pharmacol* 1996;36:792–798.

Hämmerlein A, Derendorf H, Lowenthal DT. Pharmacokinetic and pharmacodynamic changes in the elderly: clinical implications. *Clinical Pharmacokinetics* 1998;35:49–64.

Harris RZ, Benet LZ, Schwartz JB. Gender effects in pharmacokinetics and pharmacodynamics. *Drugs* 1995;50:222–239.

Hebenstreit GF, Fellerer K, Zochling R, et al. A pharmacokinetic dose titrated study in adult and elderly depressed patients. *Acta Psychiatr Scand* 1988;80(suppl 350):81–84.

Henry JF, Altamura C, Gomeni R, et al. Pharmacokinetics of amitriptyline in the elderly. *Int J Clin Pharm Ther Toxicol* 1981;19:1–5.

Hrdina PD, Rovei P, Henry JF, et al. Comparison of single-dose pharmacokinetics of imipramine and maprotiline in the elderly. *Psychopharmacology* 1980;70:29–34.

Kinirons MT, Crome P. Clinical pharmacokinetic considerations in the elderly. An update. *Clin Pharmacokinet* 1997;33:302–312.

Laurijssens BE, Greenblatt DJ. Pharmacokinetic-pharmacodynamic relationships for benzodiazepines. *Clin Pharmacokinet* 1996;30:52–76.

Le Couteur DG, McLean AJ. The aging liver: drug clearance and oxygen diffusion barrier hypothesis. *Clinical Pharmacokinetics* 1998;34: 359–373.

Lundmark K, Thomsen IS, Fjord-Larsen T, et al. Paroxetine: pharmacokinetic and antidepressant effects in the elderly. *Acta Psychiatr Scand* 1988; 80(suppl 350):76–80.

Montamat SC, Cusack BJ, Vestal RE. Management of drug therapy in the elderly. *N Engl J Med* 1989; 321:303–309.

Nies A, Robinson DS, Friedman MJ, et al. Relationship between age and tricyclic antidepressant plasma levels. *Am J Psychiatry* 1977;134:790–793.

Parikh C. Antidepressants in the elderly: challenges for study design and their interpretation. *Br J Clin Pharmacol* 2000;49:539–547.

Pollock BG, Perel JM, Reynolds CF III. Pharmacodynamic issues relevant to geriatric psychopharmacology. *J Geriatr Psychiatry Neurol* 1990;3:221–228.

Robinson DS. Age-related factors affecting antidepressant drug metabolism and clinical response.

In: Nandy K, ed. *Geriatric Psychopharmacology.* New York: Elsevier/North Holland, 1979:17–31.

Salzman C. Recent advances in geriatric psychopharmacology. In: American Psychiatric Association. *Annual Update in Psychiatry.* Washington, DC: American Psychiatric Press, 1990.

Salzman C, Shader RI, Greenblatt DJ, Harmatz JS. Long vs. short half-life benzodiazepines in the elderly. *Arch Gen Psychiatry* 1983;40:293–297.

Schmider J, Greenblatt DJ, von Moltke LL, Shader RI. Relationship of in vitro data on drug metabolism to in vivo pharmacokinetics and drug interactions: implications for diazepam disposition in humans. *J Clin Psychopharmacol* 1996;16:267–272.

Schmucker DL. Drug disposition in the elderly: a review of the crucial factors. *J Am Geriatr Soc* 1984; 32:144–149.

Schmucker DL. Aging and drug disposition: an update. *Pharmacol Rev* 1985;37:133–148.

Shader RI, von Moltke LL, Schmider J, et al. The clinician and drug interactions—an update. *J Clin Psychopharmacol* 1996;16:197–201.

Spina E and Scordo MG. Clinically significant drug interactions with antidepressants in the elderly. *Drugs Aging* 2002;19:299–320.

Thompson TL, Moran MG, Nies AS. Psychotropic drug use in the elderly. *N Engl J Med* 1983;308: 134–138, 193–199.

Triggs EJ, Nation RL, Ashley JJ. Pharmacokinetics in the elderly. *Eur J Clin Pharmacol* 1975;8:55–62.

Tumer N, Scarpace PJ, Lowenthal DT. Geriatric pharmacology: basic and clinical considerations. *Annu Rev Pharmacol Toxicol* 1992;32:271–302.

Vestal RE. Aging and pharmacology. *Cancer* 1997;80: 1302–1310.

von Moltke LL, Greenblatt DJ, Harmatz JS, Shader RI. Cytochromes in psychopharmacology. *J Clin Psychopharmacol* 1994;14:1–4.

von Moltke LL, Greenblatt DJ, Harmatz JS, Shader RI. Psychotropic drug metabolism in old age: principles and problems of assessment. In: Bloom FE, Kupfer DJ, eds. *Psychopharmacology: the fourth generation of progress.* New York: Raven, 1995:1461–1469.

von Moltke LL, Greenblatt DJ, Schmider J, et al. Metabolism of drugs by cytochrome P450-3A isoforms: implications for drug interactions in psychopharmacology. *Clin Pharmacokinet* 1995; 29(suppl 1):33–43.

von Moltke LL, Greenblatt DJ, Shader RI. Clinical pharmacokinetics of antidepressants in the elderly. Therapeutics implications. *Clin Pharmacokinet* 1993;24:141–160.

Willmore LJ. The effect of age on pharmacokinetics of antiepileptic drugs. *Epilepsia* 1995;36(suppl 5): S14–S21.

Willmore LJ. Antiepileptic drug therapy in the elderly. *Pharmacology and Therapeutics* 1998;78: 9–16.

Young RC, Alexopoulos GS, Shamoian CA, et al. Plasma 10-hydroxynortriptyline and ECG changed in elderly depressed patients. *Am J Psychiatry* 1985;142:866–868.

Absorption

Evans MA, Triggs EJ, Cheung M, et al. Gastric emptying rate in the elderly: implications for drug therapy. *J Am Geriatr Soc* 1981;29:201–205.

Gorrod JW. Absorption, metabolism, and excretion of drug in geriatric subjects. *Gerontol Clin* 1974; 16:30–42.

Greenblatt DJ, Divoll MK, Abernethy DR, et al. Age and gender effects on chlordiazepoxide kinetics: relation to antipyrine disposition. *Pharmacology* 1989;38:327–334.

Greenblatt DJ, Divoll MK, Harmatz JS, Shader RI. Antipyrine absorption and disposition in the elderly. *Pharmacology* 1988;36:125–133.

Holt PR, Balint JA. Effects of aging on intestinal lipid absorption. *Am J Physiol* 1993;264:G1–G6.

Iber FL, Murphy PA, Connor ES. Age-related changes in the gastrointestinal system: effects on drug therapy. *Drugs Aging* 1994;5:34–48.

Moore JG, Tweedy C, Christian PE, Datz FL. Effect of age on gastric emptying of liquid-solid meals in man. *Dig Dis Sci* 1983;28:340–344.

Richey DP. Effects of human aging on drug absorption and metabolism. In: Goldman R, Rochstein M, Sussman ML, eds. *The physiology and pathology of aging*. New York: Academic Press, 1975:59–63.

Shader RI, Greenblatt DJ, Harmatz JS, et al. Absorption and disposition of chlordiazepoxide in young and elderly male volunteers. *J Clin Pharmacol* 1977;17:709–712.

Body Habitus and Drug Distribution

Barlett HL, Puhl SM, Hodgson JL, Buskirk ER. Fat-free mass in relation to stature: ratios of fat-free mass to height in children, adults, and elderly subjects. *Am J Clin Nutr* 1991;53:1112–1116.

Bemben MG, Massey BH, Bemben DA, et al. Age-related patterns in body composition for men aged 20–79 yr. *Med Sci Sports Exerc* 1995;27: 264–269.

Borkan GA, Hults DE, Gerzof SG, et al. Age changes in body composition revealed by computed tomography. *J Gerontol* 1983;38:673–677.

Chapron DJ, Cameron IR, White LB, et al. Observations on lithium distribution on the elderly. *J Am Geriatr Soc* 1982;30:651–655.

Greenblatt DJ, Divoll M, Abernethy DR, Shader RI. Physiologic changes in old age: relation to altered drug disposition. *J Am Geriatr Soc* 1982; 30(Nov suppl):S6–S10.

Scavone JM, Friedman H, Greenblatt DJ, Shader RI. Effect of age, body composition, and lipid solubility on benzodiazepine tissue distribution in rats. *Arzneimittelforschung* 1987;37:2–6.

Schwartz RS, Shuman WP, Bradbury VL, et al. Body fat distribution in healthy young and older men. *J Gerontol* 1990;45:M181–185.

Drug Metabolism and Clearance

Abernethy DR, Greenblatt DJ, Shader RI. Imipramine and desipramine disposition in the elderly. *J Pharmacol Exp Ther* 1985;232:183–188.

Albrecht S, Ihmsen H, Hering W, et al. The effect of age on the pharmacokinetics and pharmacodynamics of midazolam. *Clin Pharmacol Ther* 1999;65:630–639.

Amsterdam JD, Fawcett J, Quitkin FM, et al. Fluoxetine and norfluoxetine plasma concentrations in major depression: a multicenter study. *Am J Psychiatry* 1997;154:963–969.

Axelsson R. On the pharmacokinetics of thioridazine in psychiatric patients. In: Sedvall G, Uvnas B, Zotterman Y, eds. *Antipsychotic drugs: pharmacodynamics and pharmacokinetics*. New York: Pergamon, 1976:353–358.

Barbhaiya RH, Buch AB, Greene DS. A study of the effect of age and gender on the pharmacokinetics of nefazodone after single and multiple doses. *J Clin Psychopharmacol* 1996;16:19–25.

Barbhaiya RH, Shukla UA, Greene DS. Single-dose pharmacokinetics of nefazodone in healthy young and elderly subjects and in subjects with renal or hepatic impairment. *Eur J Clin Pharmacol* 1995;49:221–228.

Barnhill JG, Greenblatt DJ, Miller LG, et al. Kinetics and dynamic components of increased benzodiazepine sensitivity in aging animals. *J Pharmacol Exp Ther* 1990;253:1153–1161.

Bergmann JF, Laneury JP, Duchene P, et al. Pharmacokinetics of reboxetine in healthy, elderly volunteers. *Eur J Drug Metab Pharmacokinet* 2000;25: 195–198.

Bertz RJ, Kroboth PD, Kroboth FJ, et al. Alprazolam in young and elderly men: sensitivity and tolerance to psychomotor, sedative and memory effects. *Journal of Pharmacology and Experimental Therapeutics* 1997;281:1317–1329.

Cohen BM, Sommer BR. Metabolism of thioridazine in the elderly. *J Clin Psychopharmacol* 1988;8: 336–339.

Curry SH. Metabolism and kinetics of chlorpromazine in relation to effect. In: Sedvall G, Uvnas B, Zotterman Y, eds. *Antipsychotic drugs: pharmacodynanics and pharmacokinetics*. New York: Pergamon, 1976:343–352.

de Vries MH, Raghoebar M, Mathlener IS, et al. Single and multiple oral dose fluvoxamine kinetics in young and elderly subjects. *Ther Drug Monit* 1992;14:493–498.

Divoll M, Greenblatt DJ, Harmatz JS, Shader RI. Effect of age and gender on disposition of temazepam. *J Pharm Sci* 1981;70:1104–1107.

Fleishaker JC, Phillips JP, Smith TC, et al. Multiple-dose pharmacokinetics and pharmacodynamics of adinazolam in elderly subjects. *Pharm Res* 1989;6:379–386.

George J, Byth K, Farrell GC. Age but not gender selectively affects expression of individual cytochrome P450 proteins in human liver. *Biochem Pharmacol* 1995;50:727–730.

Gex-Fabry M, Balant-Gorgia AE, Balant LP. Therapeutic drug monitoring of olanzapine: the combined effect of age, gender, smoking, and comedication. *Ther Drug Monit* 2003;25:46–53.

Gram LF, Christiansen J. First pass metabolism of imipramine in man. *Clin Pharmacol Ther* 1975;17: 555–563.

Greenblatt DJ, Abernethy DR, Locniskar A, et al. Effect of age, gender, and obesity on midazolam kinetics. *Anesthesiology* 1984;61:27–35.

Greenblatt DJ, Abernethy DR, Locniskar A, et al. Age, sex and nitrazepam kinetics: relation to antipyrine disposition. *Clin Pharmacol Ther* 1986;38: 697–703.

Greenblatt DJ, Divoll M, Abernethy DR, et al. Antipyrine kinetics in the elderly: prediction of age-related changes in benzodiazepine oxidizing capacity. *J Pharmacol Exp Ther* 1982;220:120–126.

Greenblatt DJ, Divoll MK, Harmatz JS, Shader RI. Antipyrine absorption and disposition in the elderly. *Pharmacology* 1988;36:125–133.

Greenblatt DJ, Divoll M, Harmatz JS, et al. Oxazepam kinetics: effects of age and sex. *J Pharmacol Exp Ther* 1980;215:86–91.

Greenblatt DJ, Friedman H, Burstein ES, et al. Trazodone kinetics: effect of age, gender, and obesity. *Clin Pharmacol Ther* 1987;42:193–200.

Greenblatt DJ, Harmatz JS, Shader RI. Factors influencing diazepam pharmacokinetics: age, sex, and liver disease. *Int J Clin Pharmacol* 1978;16:177–179.

Greenblatt DJ, Harmatz JS, Shapiro L, et al. Sensitivity to triazolam in the elderly. *N Engl J Med* 1991;324:1691–1698.

Guthrie S, Cooper RL, Thurman R, Linnoila M. Pharmacodynamics and pharmacokinetics of ethanol, diazepam and phenobarbital in young and aged rats. *Pharmacol Toxicol* 1987;61:308–312.

Gutierrez M, Abramowitz W. Steady-state pharmacokinetics of citalopram in young and elderly subjects. *Pharmacotherapy* 2000;20:1441–1447.

Harvey AT, Preskorn SH. Fluoxetine pharmacokinetics and effect on CYP2C19 in young and elderly volunteers. *J Clin Psychopharmacol* 2001;21:161–166.

Herman RJ, Wilkinson GR. Disposition of diazepam in young and elderly subjects after acute and chronic dosing. *Br J Clin Pharmacol* 1996;42:147–155.

Holazo AA, Winkler MB, Patel IH. Effects of age, gender and oral contraceptives on intramuscular midazolam pharmacokinetics. *J Clin Pharmacol* 1988;28:1040–1045.

Israili ZH. Age-related changes in the pharmacokinetics of some psychotropic drugs and its clinical implications. In: Nandy K, ed. *Geriatric Psychopharmacology.* New York: Elsevier/North Holland, 1979:31–62.

Jannuzzi G, Gatti G, Magni P, et al. Plasma concentrations of the enantiomers of fluoxetine and norfluoxetine: sources of variability and preliminary observations on relations with clinical response. *Ther Drug Monit* 2002;24:616–627.

Klamerus KJ, Parker VD, Rudolph RL, et al. Effects of age and gender on venlafaxine and *O*-desmethylvenlafaxine pharmacokinetics. *Pharmacotherapy* 1996;16:915–923.

Komiskey HL, Buck MA, Mundinger KL, et al. Effect of aging on anticonflict and CNS depressant activity of diazepam in rats. *Psychopharmacology* 1987;93:443–448.

Kraus JW, Desmond PV, Marshall JP, et al. Effects of aging and liver disease on disposition of lorazepam. *Clin Pharmacol Ther* 1978;24:411–419.

Lane HY, Chang YC, Chang WH, et al. Effects of gender and age on plasma levels of clozapine and its metabolites: analyzed by critical statistics. *J Clin Psychiatry* 1999;60:36–40.

Le Couteur DG, McLean AJ. The aging liver: drug clearance and oxygen diffusion barrier hypothesis. *Clin Pharmacokinet* 1998;34:359–373.

Leinonen E, Ylitalo P. The influence of ageing on

serum levels of tertiary tricyclic antidepressants. *Hum Psychopharmacol* 1991;6:139–146.

Lindeman RD. Changes in renal function with aging: implications for treatment. *Drugs Aging* 1992;2:423–431.

Loi CM, Vestal RE. Drug metabolism in the elderly. *Pharmacol Ther* 1988;36:131–149.

Ochs HR, Greenblatt DJ, Friedman H, et al. Bromazepam pharmacokinetics: influence of age, gender, oral contraceptives, cimetidine, and propranolol. *Clin Pharmacol Ther* 1987;41:562–570.

Olubodun JO, Ochs HR, von Moltke LL, et al. Pharmacokinetic properties of zolpidem in elderly and young adults: possible modulation by testosterone in men. *Br J Clin Pharmacol* 2003;56:297–304.

O'Malley K, Crooks J, Duke E, et al. Effect of age and sex on human drug metabolism. *Br Med J* 1971;3:607–609.

Overø KF, Toft B, Christopersen L, Gylding-Sabroe JP. Kinetics of citalopram in elderly patients. *Psychopharmacology* 1985;86:253–257.

Paine MF, Shen DD, Kunze KL, et al. First-pass metabolism of midazolam by the human intestine. *Clin Pharmacol Ther* 1996;60:14–24.

Platten H-P, Schweizer E, Dilger K, et al. Pharmacokinetics and the pharmacodynamic action of midazolam in young and elderly patients undergoing tooth extraction. *Clin Pharmacol Therapeut* 1998;63:552–560.

Poggesi I, Pellizzoni C, Fleishaker JC. Pharmacokinetics of reboxetine in elderly patients with depressive disorders. *Int J Clin Pharmacol Ther* 2000;38:254–259.

Richey DP. Effects of human aging on drug absorption and metabolism. In: Goldman R, Rochstein M, Sussman ML, eds. *The physiology and pathology of aging.* New York: Academic Press, 1975:59–63.

Robin DW, Hasan SS, Edeki T, et al. Increased baseline sway contributes to increased losses of balance in older people following triazolam. *J Am Geriatr Soc* 1996;44:300–304.

Ronfeld RA, Tremaine LM, Wilner KD. Pharmacokinetics of sertraline and its *N*-demethyl metabolite in elderly and young male and female volunteers. *Clin Pharmacokinet* 1997;32(suppl 1):22–30.

Salzman C, Shader RI, Greenblatt DJ, Harmatz JS. Long vs. short half-life benzodiazepines in the elderly. *Arch Gen Psychiatry* 1983;40:293–297.

Schultz P, Turner-Tamiyasu K, Smith G, et al. Amitriptyline disposition in young and elderly normal men. *Clin Pharmacol Ther* 1983;33:360–366.

Smith MT, Heazlewood V, Eadie MJ, et al. Pharmacokinetics of midazolam in the aged. *Eur J Clin Pharmacol* 1984;26:381–388.

Snoeck E, Van Peer A, Sack M, et al. Influence of age, renal and liver impairment on the pharmacokinetics of risperidone in man. *Psychopharmacology* (Berl) 1995;122:223–229.

Stijnen AM, Danhof M, van Bezooijen CFA. Increased sensitivity to the anesthetic effect of phenobarbital in aging BN/BiRij rats. *J Pharmacol Exp Ther* 1992;261:81–87.

Sweet RA, Pollock BG, Kirshner M, et al. Pharmacokinetics of single- and multiple-dose bupropion in elderly patients with depression. *J Clin Pharmacol* 1995;35:876–884.

Timmer CJ, Paanakker JE, VanHal HJM. Pharmacokinetics of mirtazapine from orally administered tablets: Influence of gender, age and treatment regimen. *Human Psychopharmacology* 1996;11: 497–509.

Transon C, Lecour S, Leeman T, et al. Interindividual variability in catalytic activity and immunoreactivity of three major human liver cytochrome P450 isozymes. *Eur J Clin Pharmacol* 1996;51: 79–85.

Trounce JR. Drug metabolism in the elderly. *Br J Clin Pharmacol* 1975;2:289–291.

Vestal RE, Norris AG, Tobin JD, et al. Antipyrine metabolism in man: influence of age, alcohol, caffeine and smoking. *Clin Pharmacol Ther* 1975; 18:425–432.

Wilner KD, Tensfeldt TG, Baris B, et al. Single- and multiple-dose pharmacokinetics of ziprasidone in healthy young and elderly volunteers. *Br J Clin Pharmacol* 2000;49 (Suppl 1):15S–20S.

Woodhouse KW, Mutch E, Williams FM, et al. Effect of age on pathways of drug metabolism in human liver. *Age Ageing* 1984;13:328–334.

Protein Binding

Abernethy DR, Kerzner L. Age effects on alpha-1-acid glycoprotein concentration and imipramine plasma protein binding. *J Am Geriatr Soc* 1984;32: 705–708.

Bauer LA, Davis R, Wilensky A, et al. Valproic acid clearance: unbound fraction and diurnal variation in young and elderly adults. *Clin Pharmacol Ther* 1985;37:679–700.

Bender AD, Post A, Meier JP, et al. Plasma protein binding of drugs as a function of age in adult human subjects. *J Pharm Sci* 1975;64:1711–1713.

Divoll M, Greenblatt DJ. Effect of age and sex on lorazepam protein binding. *J Pharm Pharmacol* 1982;34:122–123.

du Souich P, Verges J, Erill S. Plasma protein binding and pharmacologic response. *Clin Pharmacokinet* 1993;24:435–440.

Greenblatt DJ, Sellers EM, Koch-Weser J. Importance of protein binding for the interpretation of serum or plasma drug concentrations. *J Clin Pharmacol* 1982;22:259–263.

Hayes MJ, Langman MJS, Short AH. Changes in drug metabolism with increasing age. II. Phenytoin clearance and protein binding. *Br J Clin Pharmacol* 1975;2:73–79.

Javaid JI, Kendricks K, Pandey GN. High-affinity binding of tricyclic antidepressants to human plasma involves alpha-1-acid glycoprotein. Presented at the annual meeting of the American College of Neuropsychopharmacology. San Juan, Puerto Rico, December 1982.

MacKichan JJ. Protein binding drug displacement interactions: fact or fiction? *Clin Pharmacokinet* 1989;16:65–73.

MacLennan WJ, Martin P, Mason BJ. Protein intake and serum albumin in the elderly. *Gerontology* 1975;23:360–367.

McElnay JC, D'Arcy PF. Protein binding displacement interactions and their clinical importance. *Drugs* 1983;25:495–513.

Oravcová J, Böhs B, Lindner W. Drug-protein binding studies: new trends in analytical and experimental methodology. *J Chromatography* 1996;677: 1–28.

Sansom LN, Evans AM. What is the true clinical significance of plasma protein binding displacement interactions? *Drug Safety* 1995;12:227–233.

Sellers EM. Plasma protein displacement interactions are rarely of clinical significance. *Pharmacology* 1979;18:225–227.

Wallace S, Whiting B, Runcie J. Factors affecting drug binding in plasma of elderly patients. *Br J Clin Pharmacol* 1976;3:327–330.

Wood M. Plasma drug binding: implications for anesthesiologists. *Anesth Analg* 1996;65:786–804.

Wright JD, Boudinot FD, Ujhelyi MR. Measurement and analysis of unbound drug concentrations. *Clin Pharmacokinet* 1996;6:445–462.

Part III: Geriatric Agitation and Behavior Disorders

Chapter 6

Diagnosis of Disordered Behavior, Agitation, and Psychosis

Dilip V. Jeste

Jeremy A. Sable

Carl Salzman

One of the more distressing problems associated with severe physical, neurologic, or psychiatric illness in late life is a progressive loss of voluntary control of behavior. Older people with dementia, psychosis, or severe physical illness often exhibit disturbed, disruptive, and even potentially dangerous behaviors that include agitation, screaming, wandering, irritability, and assaultiveness. Because these behaviors can be quite distressing and unsafe for the older patient as well as to the patient's family and caregivers, psychopharmacologic treatment is frequently necessary.

Characteristics of Disordered Behavior

Disordered behavior—commonly referred to as agitation and defined as "inappropriate verbal, vocal, or motor activity"[1,2]—is not uncommon in late life, particularly in patients with dementia and in older residents of nursing homes. Agitation is understood as resulting from an interaction among personality, physical and mental conditions, and environmental factors, both physical and psychological.[3] From 50 to 80% of patients with primary degenerative dementia show sig-

nificant disruptive behavior at some point during their illness.[4,5] Paranoia is present in about one-third of these patients, and violence, hallucinations, and delusions are present in more than 20% of these patients.[6,7] Together, psychosis and agitation comprise important predictors of caregiver distress and early institutionalization of patients, thereby imposing a substantial burden on both the caregivers and the health care system as a whole.[8,9] Three categories of agitated behavior have been carefully described[2]; they are listed in Table 6.1.

Causes of Behavioral Symptoms

The complex of symptoms known as agitation, the most frequent form of disordered behavior, unlike other symptoms in older people, does not arise from a single diagnostic entity but commonly emerges from many conditions including (1) chronic organic mental disorders, particularly dementia; (2) delirium and acute confusional states; (3) delusional disorder; (4) early-onset schizophrenia; (5) late-onset schizophrenia; and (6) major mood disorders. Although considerable overlap occurs among these categories of agitation, a careful clinical evaluation of the behavioral signs and symptoms of each is necessary to determine if an underlying reversible cause exists as well as to plan for appropriate treatment.

Dementia

As people age, the risk of developing primary degenerative dementia such as Alz-

Table 6.1.   Types of Agitated Behavior

Aggressive behavior	Inappropriate physical nonaggressive behavior	Inappropriate verbal agitated behavior
Hitting	Pacing	Complaining
Kicking	Robing or disrobing	Constant requests for attention
Pushing	Repetitious mannerism	Negativism
Scratching	Escape behavior	Screaming
Tearing		
Cursing		
Grabbing		
Biting		
Spitting		

From Cohen-Mansfield, J. Agitated behaviors in the elderly, II: preliminary results in the cognitively deteriorated. *J Am Geriatr Soc* 1986;34:722–727. Reprinted with permission.

heimer's disease (AD) increases. The loss of intellectual and cognitive skills that occurs in AD and related dementias leads to disorientation, confusion, severe memory impairment, and misinterpretation of reality. These impairments frequently cause older people with dementia to feel that they are not in control of themselves and their lives, which in turn can exacerbate their behavioral disturbances. Patients may also have difficulty integrating visual, auditory, olfactory, and tactile stimuli, which may further complicate cognitive impairment as the disease progresses. Visual hallucinations, the most common type of hallucinations in AD,[10] tend to be associated with impaired cognition and rapid cognitive decline, each of which contributes to increased agitation.

Behavioral symptoms associated with the degenerative changes of dementia include anxiety, wandering (particularly at night), restlessness, and, in later stages, severe agitation. Paranoid thinking and fearfulness, belligerence, and unprovoked outbursts of rage may also occur, particularly when orientation, memory, and logical thinking deteriorate. In the early stages of dementia, agitation typically occurs when the older person feels frustrated by his or her forgetfulness or loss of functional capacities. In the later

stages, more extreme agitation develops when an older individual cannot follow directions and becomes oppositional or even psychotic.

Disordered behavior (or agitation) associated with dementia may fluctuate during the course of a day. Some patients with dementia are quite calm in a familiar, nonthreatening environment. However, these patients frequently become quite upset and agitated in an unfamiliar environment (such as a doctor's office) or when asked to perform a cognitively challenging task that may require concentration or memory. At such times, the patient may become irascible, argumentative, and difficult to manage. Reasoning is often impossible with patients in this state as they may become more agitated and even psychotic if not removed from the threatening situation.

In nursing homes, agitation is commonly seen and represents one of the more difficult problems for caregivers. Agitated, as well as yelling, crying-out, or physically or verbally assaulting demented patients can be observed in almost any nursing home, often strapped in a Geri chair and seated by the nursing station or in a room alone. In some cases, a visit from a family member may reduce agitation; at other times, a family visit may exacerbate agitation.

Agitation in a hospital setting frequently interferes with the treatment being administered. The older patient with dementia may yell all night, try to get out of bed, or pull out intravenous or nasogastric tubes or catheters. The unfamiliar hospital environment may cause disorientation, thereby worsening agitation. For elderly patients with dementia, the experience of hospitalization appears to induce a state of terror, and the response of attempting to escape leads to increased agitation. These behaviors have been subject to considerable investigation and can be quantified on a rating scale. Table 6.2 lists and describes a number of instruments that have been used to measure behavioral disturbances.

Mild or occasional disordered behavior in patients with dementia can be treated without medication. Every effort should be made to provide a quiet and consistent environment that includes sufficient orientation cues. In addition to environmental adaptation, behavior therapy, structured activities, social contact, and education of caregivers have been found to reduce the need for psychotropic medication in some individuals.[11] It is impor-

tant to address other factors that may be influencing behavior, particularly medical illness, medication effects, pain, and the possibility of recent loss. During advanced stages of dementia, severe behavior problems may develop that require medication as part of overall management (see Chapter 20).

Psychosis of AD has recently been recognized as a distinct syndrome,[12] which may provide a more specific target for antipsychotic medications in the future. Cumulative 3-year incidence of psychosis in patients with AD is approximately 50%.[13] Risk factors for the development of psychosis of AD include parkinsonian gait, bradyphrenia, and accelerated cognitive decline. Typical symptoms of psychosis of AD include paranoid delusions of theft (by spouse or caregiver) and infidelity (by spouse). Psychosis of AD tends to be characterized by delusions that are neither bizarre nor complex; they include frequent misidentification phenomena, hallucinations, more commonly visual than auditory, and absence of previous history or family history of psychosis.

Diagnostic criteria for psychosis of AD are:

1. Delusions and/or visual or auditory hallucinations present.

Table 6.2.   Instruments Used to Measure Behavioral Disturbance[a]

Scale	Symptoms Measured
CERAD (Consortium to Establish a Registry for Alzheimer's Disease) Tariot et al. (1995)	Multidimensional; includes anger as well as global and specific dimensions of agitation
Neuropsychiatric Inventory Cummings et al. (1994)	Anxiety, depression, agitation, disinhibition, behavioral retardation, psychosis, cognition
Overt Aggression Scale Kunik et al. (1994)	Verbal and physical aggression
Functional Rating Scale Crockett et al. (1989)	Depression, anxiety, apathy, aggression, psychosis
BEHAVE-AD Reisberg et al. (1987)	Aggression, affective disturbance, psychosis, anxiety, inappropriate activity
Cohen-Mansfield Agitation Inventory Cohen-Mansfield (1986)	Inappropriate activity, aggression, vocalization, complaining, negativism, wandering

[a] Complete reference citations at end of chapter.

2. Criteria for dementia of the Alzheimer type.
3. Hallucinations and/or delusions not present continuously prior to onset of symptoms of dementia.
4. Hallucinations and/or delusions have been present, at least intermittently, for 1 month or longer and are severe enough to disrupt functioning.
5. Criteria for schizophrenia, schizoaffective disorder, delusional disorder, or mood disorder with psychotic features have never been met.
6. Psychotic symptoms do not occur exclusively during course of a delirium.
7. Symptoms are not caused by another general medical condition, drug abuse, or medication.

Delirium

Behavior problems and disordered thinking in the elderly may signify delirium as well as dementia. Because delirium in older people is a potentially life-threatening condition, careful differential diagnosis is essential; *one is often mistaken for the other.* In contrast to the gradual onset of dementia, the onset of delirium is often more sudden and manifests as fluctuating consciousness as well as marked confusion, disorientation, and reduced memory. Paranoid delusions may occur, as well as visual, tactile, and sometimes auditory hallucinations. It is not unusual to observe a delirious elderly patient trying to pick insects from skin or clothes. Delirious behavior may include extreme restlessness or motor agitation, irritability, and assaultiveness, and tends to respond poorly to reason or reassurance.

Delirium can arise from acute onset of a new medical illness or exacerbation of a preexisting chronic illness, from drug reactions or interactions, and from fever or trauma. Chronic illness and acute illness (acute confusional state), drug toxicity (toxic confusional state), as well as infections and fevers must therefore be borne in mind when any elderly patient suddenly becomes acutely confused, agitated, or psychotic.

Illnesses common in elderly individuals increase vulnerability to development of delirium. For example, an older patient who develops congestive heart failure or pneumonia may become delirious. Nursing home residents with urinary tract or upper respiratory infections who become dehydrated also frequently manifest symptoms of delirium. Differentiating the behavioral features of delirium from those of dementia is therefore extremely important so that an underlying medical condition can be appropriately treated.

Delirium may also result from age-related heightened sensitivity to drugs, from drug overdose, or from drug interactions. Elderly patients often take multiple medications, sometimes without their physicians' knowledge, and often do not follow instructions consistently. They are thus at high risk for harmful drug interactions, which can lead to toxic delirium, sometimes referred to as acute confusional state. One of the most prevalent causes of drug-induced delirium in older persons arises from the anticholinergic properties of a variety of drugs, including antipsychotic and antiparkinsonian agents as well as tricyclic antidepressants. This toxic confusional state (also known as CNS anticholinergic syndrome) is characterized by a marked disturbance of short-term memory, impaired attention, disorientation, anxiety, visual and auditory hallucinations, and disordered thinking. Diagnosis in the older patient may be difficult because peripheral anticholinergic signs (e.g., dry mouth, constipation, paralytic ileus, vertigo, urinary retention, increased intraocular pressure, and cardiac arrhythmias) are not always present.

Drug-induced delirium is difficult to recognize in elderly patients who may have been confused, agitated, or psychotic before the onset of the drug-related state. Because anticholinergic toxicity in these patients is often signaled by exacerbation of preexisting disordered behavior, the toxicity may be attributed erroneously to the previous behavior. Delirious states produced by drugs or illness may also occur in older patients hospitalized for treatment of a medical or surgical illness. For example, the older patient in an intensive care unit recovering from surgery and receiving a variety of medications for severe pain may become delirious. Because psychotropic medications may contribute to delirium in some instances, they are often discontinued along with the other medications.

Delusional Disorder

The term *delusional disorder* applies to elderly patients who present with nonbizarre delusions and do not have prominent hallucinations. Subgroups of these disorders are categorized according to the predominant delusional theme: erotomanic, grandiose, jealous, persecutory, and somatic. Delusions are especially common in patients in nursing homes, where they are often misdiagnosed and undertreated.[14,15] The presence of delusions is associated with behavioral disruption and may actually be a cause of agitation and disruptive behavior.[14]

In some older patients, the delusional idea may not seriously compromise functioning or require treatment. Other older patients, however, may engage in disputes with community figures or family members who are objects of their paranoid delusions and accusations, and their actions can create situations requiring psychiatric intervention. A frequent delusional theme is that the patient's spouse is having an affair. Paranoid delusions usually cannot be altered by reasoning with the patient, and such attempts may produce agitation and rage. If the situation becomes potentially unsafe, psychotropic medication treatment may be warranted. When both members of a couple share a common delusion, it is known as a paranoid *folie à deux*.

Other important syndromes in the differential diagnosis of delusional disorder include organic mental syndromes and mood disorders. The paranoid symptoms of late-life delusional disorder usually differ in form and content from those associated with organic mental disorders, bipolar illness, and chronic paranoid schizophrenia. In organic mental disorders, paranoid symptoms accompany cognitive dysfunction and a history of progressive intellectual decline; in contrast, patients with delusional disorder have an intact sensorium. In elderly patients with either primary bipolar or unipolar mood disorders, delusions are a secondary development, and paranoid ideas may be present only during extreme mood states. In contrast, the patient with primary paranoid delusions usually remains relatively free of a major mood disturbance. Finally, elderly patients with chronic paranoid schizophrenia, in contrast to those with paranoid delusions associated with affective disorder, typically have past histories of severe social and functional disability, often with pronounced hallucinations and formal thought disorder.

Early-Onset Schizophrenia

Many patients with schizophrenia survive into old age, but data on the long-term course of their illness are sparse. Although outcomes are overall heterogeneous,[16] existing data suggest that a large majority of older patients with early-onset schizophrenia (EOS) continue to be symptomatic and impaired, but often with modest improvement in psychopathology.[17] Approximately 20% of patients experience either a remission or a significant improvement in symptoms over time[18] whereas approximately 20% of patients experience a gradual worsening with age.[19] Elderly patients with EOS generally exhibit fewer and less severe positive symptoms than do their younger counterparts[20]; negative symptoms, however, tend to persist into late life. Typical cognitive deficits observed in community-dwelling outpatients with EOS do not worsen over time and usually do not represent progressive dementia.[21–23] Although prevalence of dementia is high among chronically institutionalized patients with schizophrenia,[24,25] less than 10% of all the elderly schizophrenia patients are in long-term institutions today. The cognitive status of older patients with EOS is a more important determinant of their ability to function independently and perform activities of daily living than noncognitive symptoms.[24,26] Of course, like other older individuals, elderly patients with EOS may develop comorbid dementia with age. Managing such patients can be challenging because of their frequent episodes of agitation and increased sensitivity to psychotropic medications.

Late-Onset Schizophrenia

Schizophrenia appearing for the first time in the fifth, sixth, or seventh decade also requires consideration in the differential diagnosis of elderly patients who manifest agitated or psychotic symptoms. Although the condition is relatively uncommon, approximately 15% of all patients with schizophrenia may have onset of symptoms after the age of 45.[27–29] The syndrome is characterized by persecutory delusions and auditory (rarely visual) hallucinations, but no significant cognitive impairment or major affective disturbance. Characteristics of late-onset schizophrenia (LOS) are shown in Table 6.3.

The term "paraphrenia" has been used in the past to describe patients who develop symptoms of schizophrenia after age 45. However, little consensus exists on the meaning of the term, and this patient population reveals no difference in symptom profile between "paraphrenia" and "schizophrenia." According to criteria in *Diagnostic and Statistical Manual of Mental Disorders III, Revised* (DSM-III-R), schizophrenic patients with onset after 45 years of age were considered to have LOS.[30] The DSM-IV, however, does not make this specification, and all patients fulfilling symptom criteria are diagnosed with schizophrenia without regard to age of onset. Although formal diagnostic criteria are not currently specified for LOS, it is recognized as a distinct clinical entity that can be differentiated from EOS.

LOS is similar to EOS in terms of clinical presentation of "positive" symptoms and the chronic nature of the disorder. LOS differs from EOS in its preponderance among women compared to men, less prominent "negative" symptoms, such as social withdrawal or emotional blunting, and better premorbid level of function.[28,29] Many patients have bizarre, idiosyncratic delusions that differ from

Table 6.3.   Characteristics of Late-Onset Schizophrenia (onset after age 44)

Clinical symptoms	• Bizarre delusions, usually of persecutory type • Auditory hallucinations • Inappropriate affect and looseness of association uncommon
Risk factors	• More common in women than in men • A positive family history of schizophrenia more likely than in general population • Increased prevalence of hearing and visual deficits
Neuropsychological deficits	• Prefrontal/temporal function impairment • No evidence of progressive dementia
Brain imaging results	• Ventricles somewhat larger than those in normal subjects but smaller than those in AD patients • Areas of signal hyperintensity larger and more numerous than in normal individuals
Treatment response	• Symptomatic improvement with relatively low doses of antipsychotics • Increased risk of persistent tardive dyskinesia with typical antipsychotics

the persecutory or grandiose delusions seen in patients with AD or delusional disorder. Looseness of association and inappropriate affect are uncommon in LOS.

Neuropsychologic studies reveal a corresponding overall pattern of cognitive functioning between patients with LOS and EOS[31] except that those with LOS demonstrate significantly less impairment on measures of learning, cognitive flexibility, and organization of semantic memory compared to those with EOS.[32] Unlike patients with AD, patients with LOS (and EOS) show no significant deficit in delayed recall and no evidence of progressive cognitive deterioration.[33] Several brain imaging studies identify larger cerebral ventricles, and a preliminary study reports a larger thalamus in patients with LOS compared with similarly aged patients with EOS.[34] Functional imaging studies are needed to corroborate these findings.

For most patients with LOS, onset of illness occurs during middle age. Onset after age 65 usually represents *very-late-onset schizophrenia-like psychosis* typically secondary to general medical conditions or may be a precursor of dementia.[35] Compared to LOS, this group of disorders tends to be much more heterogeneous and is characterized by lower prevalence of negative symptoms, higher prevalence of visual hallucinations and sensory deficits, lack of family history of schizophrenia, and progressive cognitive deterioration. Differences between very-late-onset schizophrenia-like psychosis and LOS are shown in Table 6.4.

Mood Disorder

Many elderly patients with depressive disorders experience slowed thinking and behavior as well as impaired memory (sometimes referred to as dementia of depression or pseudodementia). Some depressed older persons may also become agitated, particularly if they have somatic delusions or dementia. These patients may be seen pacing, wringing their hands, pulling at their hair and clothes, crying, and complaining endlessly.

Late-life agitated psychotic depression in its most severe form can lead to physical exhaustion. The agitated state associated with depressive disorders in elderly individuals is sometimes mistaken for anxiety, especially in the well-functioning older patient. An apprehensive facial expression associated with repetitive concerns

Table 6.4. Comparison of Late-Onset Schizophrenia (LOS) versus Very-Late-Onset Schizophrenia-Like Psychosis (VLOSLP)

	LOS	VLOSLP
Age of Onset (yrs)	40–60	>65
Prevalence of Negative Symptoms	somewhat lower compared to EOS	significantly lower compared to EOS
Prevalence of Visual Hallucinations	similar to EOS	higher
Family History of Schizophrenia	similar to EOS	rare
Prevalence of Sensory Deficits	similar to normal subjects	significantly higher compared to EOS
Course	nonprogressive	progressive cognitive deterioration
Optimal Doses of Antipsychotics	25%–50% of doses used in EOS	10%–20% of doses used in younger adults

Table 6.5.   Characteristics of Agitation and Anxiety

Agitation	Anxiety
A state primarily of physical and behavioral activation	A state primarily of inner apprehension, fear, dread
Usually worse at night	May be worse at night; often worse in the early morning hours
Commonly associated with rage and irritability	Commonly associated with depression
Worse in early evening (sundowning)	No sundowning
Often correlates with cognitive decline	Independent of cognitive decline
Independent of past history of anxiety	Past history of anxiety or anxiety disorders not unusual; past history of depressive disorders not unusual

about money, health, and family tends to suggest a state of high anxiety together with the depressed mood. In such patients, agitation must be carefully distinguished from anxiety; guidelines for differentiating these two disorders appear in Table 6.5.

Conclusion

Although the manifestations of disordered behavior and psychotic thinking are obvious in elderly patients, their causes may be unclear. Accurate diagnostic evaluation, particularly in differentiating between dementia and delirium, is necessary before appropriate treatment is begun, as discussed in the next chapter.

Acknowledgement. This work was supported, in part, by National Institute of Mental Health grants MH49671, MH43693, MH59101, and by the Department of Veterans Affairs

References

1. Cohen-Mansfield J. Agitated behaviors in the elderly II. Preliminary results in the cognitively deteriorated. *J Am Geriatr Soc* 1986;34:722–727.
2. Cohen-Mansfield L, Marx M, Werner P. Agitation in elderly persons: an integrative report of findings in a nursing home. *Int Psychogeriatr* 1992;4:221–240.
3. Cohen-Mansfield J, Deutsch LH. Agitation: subtypes and their mechanisms. *Semin Clin Neuropsychiatry* 1996;1:325–339.
4. Houlihan DJ, Mulsant BH, Sweet RA, et al. A naturalistic study of trazodone in the treatment of behavioral complications of dementia. *Am J Geriatr Psychiatry* 1994;2:78–85.
5. Rosen J, Mulsant BH, Wright B. Agitation in severely demented patients. *Ann Clin Psychiatry* 1992;4:207–215.
6. Lake JT, Grossberg GT. Management of psychosis, agitation, and other behavioral problems in Alzheimer's disease. *Psychiatr Ann* 1996;26:274–279.
7. Swearer JM, Drachman DA, O'Donnell BF, Mitchell AL. Troublesome and disruptive behaviors in dementia. *J Am Geriatr Soc* 1988;36:784–790.
8. Coen RF, Swanwick GRJ, O'Boyle CA, Coakley D. Behavior disturbance and other predictors of carer burden in Alzheimer's disease. *Int J Geriatr Psychiatry* 1997;12:331–336.
9. Stern Y, Tang M, Albert MS, et al. Predicting time to nursing home care and death in individuals with Alzheimer's disease. *JAMA* 1997;277:806–812.
10. Holroyd S. Visual hallucinations in a geriatric psychiatry clinic: Prevalence and associated diagnoses. *J Geriatr Psychiatry* 1996;9:171–175.
11. Cohen-Mansfield J. Nonpharmacologic interventions for inappropriate behaviors in dementia: a review and critique. *Am J Geriatr Psychiatry* 2001;9:361–381.
12. Jeste DV, Finkel SI. Psychosis of Alzheimer's Disease and related dementias: diagnostic criteria for a distinct syndrome. *Am J Geriatr Psychiatry* 2000;8:29–34.
13. Paulsen JS, Salmon DP, Thal LJ, et al. Incidence of and risk factors for hallucinations and delusions in patients with probable AD. *Neurology* 2000;54:1965–1971.
14. Morriss RK, Rovner BW, Folstein MF, German PS. Delusions in newly admitted residents of nursing homes. *Am J Psychiatry* 1990;147:299–302.
15. Chandler JD, Chandler JE. The prevalence of neuroopsychiatric disorders in a nursing home population. *J Geriatr Psychiatry Neurol* 1988;1:71–76.
16. Carpenter WT, Kirkpatrick B. The heterogene-

ity of the long-term course of schizophrenia. *Schizophr Bull* 1988;14:645–652.

17. Jeste DV, Twamley EW, Eyler Zorrilla LT, et al. Aging and outcome in schizophrenia: a cross-sectional study of 290 community-dwelling older patients with schizophrenia and 144 normal comparison subjects. *Acta Psychiatr Scand* 2002; 107:1–8.

18. McGlashan TH. A selective review of recent North American long-term followup studies of schizophrenia. *Schizophr Bull* 1988;14:515–542.

19. Belitsky R, McGlashan TH. The manifestations of schizophrenia in late life: a dearth of data. *Schizophr Bull* 1993;19:683–685.

20. Ciompi L. Catamnestic long-term study on the course of life and aging of schizophrenics. *Schizophr Bull* 1980;6:606–618.

21. Heaton RK, Gladsjo JA, Palmer BW, et al. Stability and course of neuropsychological deficits in schizophrenia. *Arch Gen Psychiatry* 2001;58: 24–32.

22. Eyler Zorrilla LT, Heaton RK, McAdams LA, et al. Cross-sectional study of older outpatients with schizophrenia and healthy comparison subjects: no differences in age-related cognitive decline. *Am J Psychiatry* 2000;157:1324–1326.

23. Evans JD, Negron AE, Palmer BW, et al. Cognitive deficits and psychopathology in hospitalized versus community-dwelling elderly schizophrenia patients. *J Geriatr Psychiatry Neurol* 1999;12: 11–15.

24. Twamley EW, Doshi RR, Nayak GV, et al. Generalized cognitive impairments, everyday functioning ability, and living independence in patients with psychosis. *Am J Psychiatry* 2002; 159(12): 2013–2020.

25. Davidson M, Harvey P, Welsh KA, et al. Cognitive functioning in late-life schizophrenia: a comparison of elderly schizophrenic patients with Alzheimer's disease. *Am J Psychiatry* 1996;153: 1274–1279.

26. Evans JD, Heaton RK, Paulsen JS, et al. The relationship of neuropsychological abilities to specific domains of functional capacity in older schizophrenia patients. *Biol Psychiatry* 2003; 53(5):422–430.

27. Jeste DV, Eastham JH, Lacro JP, et al. Management of late-life psychosis. *J Clin Psychiatry* 1996; 57(suppl 3):39–45.

28. Harris MJ, Jeste DV. Late-onset schizophrenia: an overview. *Schizophr Bull* 1988;14:39–55.

29. Jeste DV, Harris MJ, Krull A, et al. Clinical and neuropsychological characteristics of patients with late-onset schizophrenia. *Am J Psychiatry* 1995;152:722–730.

30. American Psychiatric Association. *Diagnostic and statistical manual of mental disorders, third edition-revised.* Washington, DC: American Psychiatric Press, 1987.

31. Heaton R, Paulsen J, McAdams LA, et al. Neuropsychological deficits in schizophrenia: Relationship to age, chronicity and dementia. *Arch Gen Psychiatry* 1994;51:469–476.

32. Paulsen JS, Romero R, Chan A, et al. Impairment of the semantic network in schizophrenia. *Psychiatry Res* 1996;63:109–121.

33. Palmer BW, Bondi MW, Twamley EW, et al. Are late-onset schizophrenia-spectrum disorders neurodegenerative conditions?: Annual rates of change on two dementia measures. *J Neuropsychiat Clin Neurosci* 2003;15:45–92.

34. Corey-Bloom J, Jernigan T, Archibald S, et al. Quantitative magnetic resonance imaging of the brain in late-life schizophrenia. *Am J Psychiatry* 1995;152:447–449.

35. Howard R, Rabins PV, Seeman MV, Jeste DV, and the International Late-Onset Schizophrenia Group. Late-onset schizophrenia and very-late-onset schizophrenia-like psychois: an international consensus. *Am J Psychiatry* 2000;157: 172–178.

Table 6.2 References

Crockett D, Tuokko H, Koch W, et al. The assessment of everyday functioning using the Present Functional Questionnaire and the Functional Rating Scale in the elderly samples. *Clin Gerontol* 198;8:3–5.

Cummings JL, Mega M, Gray K, et al. The neuropsychiatric inventory: comprehensive assessment of psychopathology in dementia. *Neurology* 1994;44: 2308–2314.

Kunik ME, Yudofsky SC, Silver JM, Hales RE. Pharmacologic approach to management of agitation associated with dementia. *J Clin Psychiatry* 1994; 55:13–17.

Reisberg B, Borenstein J, Salob SP, et al. Behavioral symptoms in Alzheimer's disease: phenomenology and treatment. *J Clin Psychiatry* 1987;48:9–15.

Tariot PN, Mack JL, Patterson MB, et al, and the Behavioral Pathology Committee of the Consortium to Establish a Registry for Alzheimer's Disease. The Behavior Rating Scale for Dementia of the Consortium to establish a registry for Alzheimer's disease. *Am J Psychiatry* 1995;152: 1349–1357.

Supplemental Readings

Arnold SE, Trojanowski JQ, Gur RE, et al. Absence of neurodegeneration and neural injury in the cerebral cortex in a sample of elderly patients with schizophrenia. *Arch Gen Psychiatry* 1998;55: 225-232.

Berezin MA, Liptzin B, Salzman C. The elderly person. In: Nicholi A, ed. *Harvard guide to modern psychiatry.* 2nd ed. Cambridge, MA: Harvard University Press, 1988:665–680.

Bland RC. Demographic aspects of functional psychoses in Canada. *Acta Psychiatr Scand* 1977;55: 369–380.

Blessed G, Wilson ID. The contemporary natural history of mental disorder in old age. *Br J Psychiatry* 1982;141:59–67.

Bleuler M. *The schizophrenic disorders: long-term patient and family studies.* Trans. Clemens SM. New Haven: Yale University Press, 1978.

Bridge TP, Wyatt RJ. Paraphrenia: paranoid states of late life; European research. *J Am Geriatr Soc* 1980; 28:193–200.

Busse EW. Problems affecting psychiatric care of the aging. *Geriatrics* 1960;15:673–680.

Castle DJ, Wessely S, Howard R, Murray RM. Schizophrenia with onset at the extremes of adult life. *Int J Geriatr Psychiatry* 1997;12:712–717.

Charatan FB. Acute confusion in the elderly. *Hosp Physician* 1976;12:8–10.

Cohen CI, Cohen GD, Blank K, et al. Schizophrenia and older adults. An overview: directions for research and policy. *Am J Geriatr Psychiatry* 2000;8: 19–828.

Cohen-Mansfield J, Marx MS, Rosenthal AS. Dementia and agitation in nursing home residents: how are they related? *Psychol Aging* 1990;5(1):3–8.

Copeland JR, Dewey ME, Scott A, et al. Schizophrenia and delusional disorder in older age: community prevalence, incidence, comorbidity, and outcome. *Schizophr Bull* 1998;24:153-61.

Cooper AF, Porter R. Visual acuity and ocular pathology in the paranoid and affective psychoses of later life. *J Psychosom Res* 1976;20:97–105.

Craig TJ, Bregman Z. Late onset schizophrenia-like illness. *J Am Geriatr Soc* 1988;36:104–107.

Cullum CM, Heaton RK, Harris MJ, Jeste DV. Neurobehavioral and neurodiagnostic aspects of late-onset psychosis. *Arch Clin Neuropsychol* 1994;9(5): 371–382.

Eastham JH, Jeste DV. Differentiating behavioral disturbances of dementia from drug side effects. *Int Psychogeriatr* 1996;8(Suppl 3):429–434.

Fick DM, Agostini JV, Inouye SK. Delirium superimposed on dementia: a systematic review. *JAGS* 2002;50(10):1723–1732.

Fish F. Senile schizophrenia. *J Ment Sci* 1960;106: 938–946.

Flint AJ, Rifat SL, Eastwood MR. Late-onset paranoia: distinct from paraphrenia? *Int J Geriatr Psychiatry* 1991;6:103–109.

Funding T. Genetics of paranoid psychoses of later life. *Acta Psychiatr Scand* 1961;37:267–282.

Gierz M, Jeste DV. Physical comorbidity in elderly schizophrenic and depressed groups. *Am J Geriatr Psychiatry* 1993;1:165–170.

Gold DD. Late age of onset schizophrenia: present but unaccounted for. *Compr Psychiatry* 1984;25: 225–237.

Green MF, Kern RS, Braff DL, Mintz J. Neurocognitive deficits and functional outcome in schizophrenia: are we measuring the "right stuff"? *Schizophr Bull* 2000;26:119–136.

Halpain M, Heaton SC, Warren KA, et al. Health care utilization patterns in late-life schizophrenia: case histories. In: Bergener M, Brocklehurst J, Kanowski S, eds. *Aging, Health, and Healing.* New York: Springer Publishing Company, Inc., 1995:585–592.

Harris MJ, Jeste DV. Psychiatric disorders of late life: schizophrenia and delusional disorder. In: Kaplan HI, Sadock BJ, eds. *Comprehensive textbook of psychiatry.* 6th ed. Baltimore: Williams & Wilkins, 1995:2569–2571.

Harris MJ, Cullum CM, Jeste DV. Clinical presentation of late-onset schizophrenia. *J Clin Psychiatry* 1988; 49:356–360.

Harris MJ, Jeste DV. Late-onset schizophrenia: an overview. *Schizophr Bull* 1988;14:39–55.

Harvey PD, Howanitz E, Parrella M, et al. Symptoms, cognitive functioning, and adaptive skills in geriatric patients with lifelong schizophrenia: a comparison across treatment sites. *Am J Psychiatry* 1998;155:1080–1086.

Herbert ME, Jacobson S. Late paraphrenia. *Br J Psychiatry* 1967;113:461–469.

Howard R, Castle D, Wessely S, Murray RM. A comparative study of 470 cases of early- and late-onset schizophrenia. *Br J Psychiatry* 1993;163:352–357.

Howard R, Graham C, Sham P, et al. A controlled family study of late-onset non-affective psychosis (late paraphrenia). *Br J Psychiatry* 1997;170: 511–514.

Jeste DV, Harris MJ, Pearlson GD, et al. Late-onset schizophrenia: studying clinical validity. *Psychiatr Clin North Am* 1988;11:1–14.

Jeste DV, Paulsen J, Harris MJ. Late-onset schizophrenia and other related psychoses. In: Bloom FL, Kupfer DJ, eds. *Psychopharmacology: the fourth generation of progress.* New York: Raven Press, 1995: 1437–1446.

Jeste DV, Gladsjo JA, Lindamer LA, Lacro JP. Medical comorbidity in schizophrenia. *Schizophr Bull* 1996;22:413–430.

Jeste DV, Harris MJ, Grant I, Thal L. Psychopathology in dementia. *Bull Clin Neurosci* 1989;54: 51–58.

Jeste DV, Gierz M, Harris MJ. Pseudodementia: myths and reality. *Psychiatry Ann* 1990;20:71–79.

Jeste DV, Symonds LL, Harris MJ, et al. Non-dementia non-praecox dementia praecox? Late-onset schizophrenia. *Am J Geriatr Psychiatry* 1997;5: 302–317.

Katz MM, Itil TM. Video methodology for research in psychopathology and psychopharmacology. *Arch Gen Psychiatry* 1974;31:204–210.

Kay DA, Roth M. Environmental and hereditary factors in the schizophrenias of old age. *J Ment Sci* 1961;107:649.

Kay DWK. Late paraphrenia and its bearing on the aetiology of schizophrenia. *Acta Psychiatr Scand* 1963;39:159–169.

Lacro JP, Jeste DV. Physical comorbidity and polypharmacy in older psychiatric patients. *Biol Psychiatry* 1994;36:146–152.

Larson CA, Nyman GE. Age of onset in schizophrenia. *Hum Hered* 1970;20:241–247.

Liptzin B, Salzman C. Psychiatric aspects of aging. In: Rowe JR, Besdene R, eds. *Geriatric medicine.* 2nd ed. Boston: Little, Brown, & Co, 1988: 355–374.

McGlashan TH. Predictors of shorter-, medium-, and longer-term outcome in schizophrenia. *Am J Psychiatry* 1986;143:50–55.

Miller BL, Benson F, Cummings JL, et al. Late-life paraphrenia: an organic delusional syndrome. *J Clin Psychiatry* 1986;47:204–207.

Mintzer JE. Underlying mechanisms of psychosis and aggression in patients with Alzheimer's disease. *J Clin Psychiatry* 2001;62:23–25.

Naimark D, Jackson E, Rockwell E, Jeste DV. Psychotic symptoms in Parkinson's disease patients with dementia. *J Am Geriatr Soc* 1996;44(3): 296–299.

Oberlander M. Managing problem behaviors of elderly patients. *Hosp Community Psychiatry* 1976; 27(5):325–330.

Palmer BW, Heaton RK, Gladsjo JA, et al. Heterogeneity in functional status among older outpatients with schizophrenia: employment history, living situation, and driving. *Schizophr Res* 2002; 55:205-215.

Palmer BW, Heaton RK, Jeste DV. Extrapyramidal symptoms and neuropsychological deficits in schizophrenia. *Biol Psychiatry* 1999;45:791-794.

Patterson TL, Klapow JC, Eastham JH, et al. Correlates of functional status in older patients with schizophrenia. *Psychiatric Res* 1998;80:41-52.

Prager S, Jeste DV. Sensory impairment in late-life schizophrenia. *Schizophr Bull* 1993;19(4): 755–772.

Rabins P, Pauker S, Thomas J. Can schizophrenia begin after age 44? *Compr Psychiatry* 1984;25: 290–293.

Robertson EE, Mason-Browne NL. Review of mental illness in the older age group. *Br Med J* 1985;2: 1076–1079.

Rockwell E, Krull AJ, Dimsdale J, Jeste DV. Late-onset psychosis with somatic delusions. *Psychosomatics* 1994;35:66–72.

Roth M. The natural history of mental disorder in old age. *J Ment Sci* 1955;101:281–301.

Roth M, Morrissey JD. Problems in the diagnosis and classification of mental disorder in old age, with a study of case material. *J Ment Sci* 1952;98:66–80.

Seeman MV. Psychopathology in women and men: focus on female hormones. *Am J Psychiatry* 1997; 154:1641–1647.

Spencer T. The management of behavior disorders in the geriatric patient. *Md State Med J* 1969;18: 73–76.

Steinhart MJ. Psychiatric aspects and management of aging patients. *NY State J Med* 1974;74: 976–978.

Symmonds LL, Olichney JM, Jernigan TL, et al. Lack of clinically significant gross structural abnormalities in MRIs of older patients with schizophrenia and related psychoses. *J Neuropsychiatry Clin Neurosci* 1997;9:251-258.

Vital and Health Statistics. Chronic conditions and impairments of nursing home residents. *US Dept of Health, Education and Welfare publ. no. (HRA) 74-1707*. Data from the National Survey (series K, no. 22). Washington, DC: US Government Printing Office, 1973.

Vital and Health Statistics. Measures of chronic illness among residents of nursing and personal care homes, June-August 1969. *US Dept of Health, Education, publ. no. (HRA) 74-1709*. Data from the National Survey (series 12, no. 24). Washington, DC: US Government Printing Office, 1974.

Volavka J. Late-onset schizophrenia: a review. *Compr Psychiatry* 1985;26:148–156.

Wilson JD, Mathis E. Nursing home management of behavior problems in the geriatric patient. *J Arkansas Med Soc* 1968;65:210–213.

Wragg R, Jeste DV. Overview of depression and psychosis in Alzheimer's disease. *Am J Psychiatry* 1989;146(5):577–587.

Chapter 7

Treatment of Late-Life Disordered Behavior, Agitation, and Psychosis

Dilip V. Jeste

Jeremy A. Sable

Carl Salzman

Agitation and psychosis arising in the context of late-life psychiatric disorders, dementia, and delirium can be both disruptive and potentially harmful to elderly patients and caregivers. Although a variety of nonpharmacologic techniques can be successful for milder states of agitation and disruptive behavior, pharmacologic therapy is invariably necessary for more severe states. A number of different classes of psychotropic medications are currently used to treat severe agitation and psychotic behavior.

The United States Food and Drug Administration (FDA) does not specify agitation in dementia as an indication for treatment with psychotropic medication[1]; the use of psychotropic agents for this purpose therefore has been off-label. However, agitation as a symptom across disorders (dementia, bipolar disorder, and schizophrenia) has been approved as an indication for use of intramuscular olanzapine.

Antipsychotics are still the first-choice treatments because of their reliable therapeutic effects, although their use is limited by side effects. A variety of nonantipsychotic agents have been used to reduce agitation including antidepressants, anticonvulsants, β-blockers, benzodiazepines, cholinesterase inhibitors, and hormones.

General Principles for Antipsychotic Treatment

Antipsychotics are the most widely prescribed psychotropic drugs for institutionalized elderly patients.[2] Studies of antipsychotic use in older people suggest that these drugs have modest efficacy in treating disruptive behavior, and their use is accompanied by a high frequency of side effects.[3] The Nursing Home Reform Amendments of the Omnibus Reconciliation Act of 1987[2,4] resulted in both substantially reduced use of antipsychotics[5,6] and establishment of dosing guidelines appropriate for elderly patients.[2]

Antipsychotic drugs, given to patients of all ages, are used to improve logical thinking and to decrease loose associations, social withdrawal, ideas of reference, hallucinations, and delusions. In elderly patients, antipsychotics are also used to alleviate agitation, belligerence, and assaultiveness, as well as to aid nighttime sleep. Individuals with dementia complicated by disordered behavior, particularly nursing home residents, are commonly treated with antipsychotics. Patients with schizophrenia and mood disorders with psychotic features may also benefit from antipsychotics.[2,7–10]

Although antidepressants and electroconvulsive therapy are the primary treatments for the severe depression that can accompany agitated psychotic states (agitated psychotic depression) in older people (see Chapters 9 and 13), antipsychotic drugs are frequently required to treat the delusions and/or hallucinations and may also be useful for the insomnia or agitation that may accompany the depressive syndrome. Antipsychotics are also used as part of the treatment of agitated bipolar patients (see Chapter 12).

Since their arrival, the newer atypical antipsychotic medications have rapidly become the first-line treatment for older patients with psychosis and agitation. Existing data suggest that the atypical antipsychotics are at least as efficacious for the treatment of schizophrenia and better tolerated than the conventional antipsychotics.[11] Because of their distinct pharmacology (i.e., 5-HT$_2$ and D$_2$ antagonism), risk of movement disorders with these agents is significantly reduced compared to the corresponding risk with conventional antipsychotics at comparable dosages. The reduced risk for movement disorder side effects suggests a prescribing advantage for the elderly.

Clinical Pharmacology

Several age-related physiological changes may influence the activity and side effects of antipsychotic medications. These changes include reduced cardiac output (and concomitant reduction in renal and hepatic blood flow, relative to younger persons), reduced glomerular filtration rate, possible reduction in hepatic metabolism, and increased fat content.[12] These changes may alter the absorption, distribution, metabolism, and excretion of medications and may result in prolonged drug effects (see Chapter 5). Age-related changes in receptor-site activity may further influence drug response in elderly patients, although not all of these receptor-site mechanisms are currently well understood.

Absorption

Antipsychotic drugs are usually given to elderly patients in oral form, except in emergencies. They are absorbed well, and no significant delay in absorption occurs in older patients compared with younger ones. However, gastric emptying time and passage of antipsychotics through the intestine may be slowed by age-related decreases in gut motility, by the anticholinergic effects of antipsychotics themselves, by antacids, and by the antiparkinsonian drugs often coadministered with antipsychotics.

Protein Binding

Antipsychotic drugs are highly protein bound, with affinity for α-1-acid glycoprotein (AGP) and albumin. AGP is an acute-phase reactant protein that increases markedly in patients with schizophrenia, depression, inflammation, cancer, and other disorders. Albumin concentrations are depressed by the aging process, physical disease, or malnutrition. Decreased levels of these proteins will lead to decreased protein binding and a resultant increase in the percentage of free (unbound) drug, which provides the potential for increased toxicity.

Volume of Distribution

The aging process is associated with decreases in total body water and muscle mass and an increase in adipose tissue. Because most antipsychotic drugs are lipid soluble, they have an increased volume of distribution in the older person's body (see Chapter 5). Antipsychotic drugs that are stored in the lipid compartments of cells are released very slowly from these storage sites after use is discontinued. Clinical or toxic effects may therefore persist for weeks.

Metabolism

Antipsychotic drugs are metabolized primarily by the liver. Age-related changes in hepatic metabolism and blood flow have long been thought to result in reduced drug metabolism in elderly patients. Conclusive evidence of diminished metabolic capacity in this age group, however, is unavailable.

Receptor-Site Alterations

Elderly patients may be more sensitive to the therapeutic and toxic effects of antipsychotics because of age-related decreases in dopamine and acetylcholine neurotransmission in the central nervous system (CNS) (see Chapter 4). This sensitivity increases markedly in older patients who have structural pathological changes in the brain such as those found in dementia.

Pretreatment Evaluation

Before prescribing an antipsychotic drug for an elderly patient with severely disordered behavior or psychosis, a comprehensive medical, psychiatric, and psychosocial evaluation is essential. Past and current drug and alcohol use, as well as a list of prescribed and over-the-counter (OTC) medications and nutritional and herbal supplements are important. The presence of concomitant medical illness or polypharmacy frequently complicates the treatment of older patients with agitation or psychosis; evaluation may reveal reversible medical factors that might contribute to the behavioral disturbance. In addition, age-related sensory deficits and cognitive impairment may interfere with patient adherence to prescribed medication regimens resulting in unintentional incorrect medication doses or erroneous dosing schedules. Psychosocial evaluation may reveal precipitating stress, such as a death in the family or a move to unfamiliar surroundings, which may explain a sudden change in the elderly person's behavior.

Dosage and Administration

Starting dosages of antipsychotics for older patients should be one-fifth to one-quarter those prescribed for younger adults, and dosage should be increased gradually or decreased according to clinical response or development of side effects. (The relative severity of side effects from oral dosages of antipsychotic drugs for elderly patients is presented in Table 7.1.) Initially, antipsychotic drugs should be given to elderly patients in divided doses (two or three times a day) because patients may not be able to tolerate the side effects associated with large, single daily doses. Once a patient is clinically stable on a maintenance dose without any bothersome side effects, a trial of once-daily dosing may be attempted. Individual patient circumstances should determine the use of single or divided doses.

Antipsychotic drugs that require relatively few milligrams to produce a clinical effect are termed high-potency compounds, in contrast to low-potency agents, which require more milligrams for efficacy. The use of the term "potency" in this context, however, refers to *relative* potency on a milligram-for-milligram basis rather than to differential efficacy. In general, *low-potency* antipsychotics tend to be strongly sedating, hypotensive, and anticholinergic but produce only mild or moderate extrapyramidal symptoms. In contrast, *high-potency* antipsychotics produce frequent and severe extrapyramidal symptoms but are less sedative, less hypotensive, and less anticholinergic. Only one antipsychotic should be prescribed at a time to minimize side effects and to evaluate the individual drug's effectiveness.

For the elderly patient with schizophrenia who requires maintenance medication but whose intake of oral preparations is unreliable, the long-acting depot form of either fluphenazine or haloperidol can be administered intramuscularly every 1 to 4 weeks. (Currently, no atypical antipsychotic is available as a long-acting preparation, although a depot form of risperidone is being developed.) Antipsychotic medication administered in this way is much more potent than comparable doses administered orally. However, intramuscular injections for the thin, frail older patient with small muscle mass may be painful, and absorption may be erratic and unpredictable. Intramuscular admin-

Table 7.1. Relative Severity of Antipsychotic Drug Side Effects[a]

| Side Effect | Conventional | | Atypical (Second Generation) | | | | | |
	Low Potency e.g. thioridazine	High Potency e.g. haloperidol	Clozapine	Risperidone	Olanzapine	Quetiapine	Ziprasidone	Aripiprazole
Anticholinergic	2–3	0–1	3	0	1–2	1–2	0	0
Decreased BP	2–3	0	3	0–1	0–1	1–2	0	0
Sedation	2–3	0–1	3	1	2	2	1	1
Weight Gain	2–3	0–1	3	1–2	3	2	1	1
EPS	1–2	3	0–1	1–2	0–1	0–1	0–1	0–1
Tardive Dyskinesia	1–2	2–3	0–1	0–1	0–1	0	0	0
Increased Prolactin	1–2	2–3	0	2	0	0	0	0
Seizures	1–2	0–1	3	0	0	0	0	0
Agranulocytosis	0	0	2	0	0	0	0	0

[a] Severity Range:
0 = absent
1 = mild
2 = moderate
3 = marked

istration should therefore be avoided in such a patient whenever possible. For elderly patients who are unable to swallow tablets or capsules, either liquid or rapidly dissolving tablets are possible alternatives. Although antipsychotics are occasionally given intramuscularly to elderly patients without apparent adverse effects, systematic safety studies are lacking.

Although a majority of elderly patients require lower doses of antipsychotics than those doses given to younger patients, some older patients may require doses comparable to those given to their younger counterparts. Intensely disturbed elderly patients, for example, may require higher doses, and intramuscular injections may be necessary in emergency situations. Traditionally, the high-potency agent haloperidol has been used for emergency purposes. Because of its potential for inducing motoric side effects, haloperidol is generally administered in combination with an anticholinergic agent such as benztropine, which may not be well tolerated by older patients. An intramuscular preparation of the atypical antipsychotic ziprasidone has recently become available for emergency use, and intramuscular olanzapine is expected to be approved by the FDA in the near future. Although no data are currently available regarding their use in elderly patients, intramuscular preparations of atypical agents are expected to provide a valuable alternative for patients who may be sensitive to motoric side effects of antipsychotics or who cannot tolerate anticholinergic medication.

Once the dosage of an antipsychotic becomes stable and clinical response has been achieved with minimal side effects, the total daily dose may be given at one time. For the elderly patient with nighttime agitation, the daily dose should be given 1 to 2 hours before the disturbance usually occurs, to take advantage of the drug's sedating effects. Among those taking antipsychotics are patients with chronic schizophrenia who have been taking antipsychotics for many years. As these patients age, however, their dosage requirements may change. Oral or intramuscular doses must therefore be monitored and adjusted to the lowest effective dose.

Side Effects of Antipsychotics

Older patients are more sensitive to the side effects of antipsychotics, probably because of increased receptor-site sensitivity in the aging brain. Side effects of antipsychotic drugs that affect older people are sedation, orthostatic hypotension and arrhythmia, anticholinergic reactions, and movement disorders, particularly extrapyramidal symptoms (EPS) and tardive dyskinesia (TD). In the current era of atypical antipsychotics, the incidence of movement disorders has decreased somewhat; however, awareness about the potential for weight gain, as well as for changes in glucose and lipid metabolism with antipsychotics, is increasing.

Sedation

Sedation is one of the most common side effects of antipsychotic drugs in older patients mediated primarily via histaminic receptor blockade. Although sedation is traditionally associated with conventional, low-potency antipsychotics (e.g., chlorpromazine), it is also frequently caused by the atypical agents clozapine, olanzapine, and quetiapine. Antipsychotics with sedating qualities can be helpful for the elderly patient who has insomnia or is severely agitated during the day.

In elderly patients, sedative side effects may persist long after the drug has been administered and may ultimately interfere with the older patient's level of arousal throughout the day. Sedation may therefore impair the mental functioning of elderly people and may exacerbate disorientation and confusion in those with cognitive impairment. Most importantly, sedation associated with antipsychotics may increase risk of falls and fractures in elderly patients, thereby contributing significantly to their morbidity and mortality.[13–15] Although the sedative effects of antipsychotics may be therapeutic, oversedation in older individuals is very common and may even occur with agents believed to possess minimal sedating effects (Table 7.1). Sedation due to antipsychotics usually disappears after 1 to 3 weeks of treatment, although in older persons this period may be prolonged. Oversedation may also occur due to drug–drug interactions when antipsychotics are administered in combination with other CNS depressants such as narcotic analgesics.

Cardiovascular Effects

Important antipsychotic-induced cardiovascular effects in elderly patients include orthostatic hypotension and cardiac arrhythmia. Orthostatic hypotension is more common in older than in younger people and may be exacerbated by blockade of peripheral α-adrenergic receptors. Conventional low-potency antipsychotics, as well as clozapine, risperidone, and quetiapine have a particular tendency to cause hypotension via this mechanism. Elderly patients with low cardiac output, as well as those receiving additional medications that block α-adrenergic receptors, are especially vulnerable to this adverse effect.

Orthostatic hypotension also results from the effects of the antipsychotic on CNS vasoregulatory centers. Most hypotensive episodes occur early in the course of treatment, especially after intramuscular administration. A sudden decrease in blood pressure may cause the older patient to fall or to sustain a stroke or even a myocardial infarct. The combination of drug-induced orthostatic changes and age-related loss of postural reflexes leads to a dramatic increase in risk of falls in older people. Therefore, orthostatic hypotensive episodes are particularly dangerous at night, when the older patient awakens to urinate and gets out of bed quickly. If a patient experiences antipsychotic-induced hypotension, treatment with drugs such as ephedrine, amphetamines, or epinephrine should be avoided. Ephedrine or amphetamines may aggravate or activate agitation and may exacerbate psychotic symptoms. Epinephrine is likely to lower blood pressure due to its β-adrenergic agonist activity. No specific treatments for antipsychotic-induced hypotension are currently available. General treatment measures include reducing the dose or changing antipsychotics, maintaining fluid and electrolyte balance, temporarily avoiding antihypertensive medications, and asking the patient to rise slowly from supine or seated positions.

With particular regard to cardiac effects, tachycardia seems to occur primarily as a result of the anticholinergic properties of antipsychotics. Heart rates of more than 90 beats per minute are not uncommon in older patients who take these drugs. Epidemiologic studies provide evidence that several conventional antipsychotics increase the risk of sudden cardiac death.[16] Specifically, certain antipsychotics can induce prolongation of the QTc interval (heart-rate corrected QT interval, which is normally less than 440 milliseconds [msec]). QTc prolongation is of concern because it can potentiate a lethal ventricular arrhythmia, *torsade de pointes*. The high-potency agent pimozide and the low-potency agent thioridazine are associated with maximal QTc prolongation.[17] Among the atypical antipsychotics, ziprasidone is associated with the greatest QTc prolongation (i.e., 6–10 msec).[18] However, the low observed rate of QTc interval prolongation beyond 500 msec (the cutoff value for significantly increased risk of arrhythmia) and the absence of dose-dependent QTc interval increases or significant drug–drug interactions suggest that the risk of serious cardiac arrhythmia with ziprasidone may not increase significantly compared to the risk with the other atypical antipsychotics. Data on elderly patients with preexisting cardiovascular disease who would be at highest risk are not currently available. Such patients should be carefully evaluated before they begin any antipsychotic medication. In particular, extreme caution is required in prescribing drugs with anticholinergic properties or those that produce orthostatic hypotension.

Anticholinergic Reactions

The anticholinergic side effects of antipsychotic drugs in the presence of the age-related decrease in cholinergic function can lead to serious problems for the elderly patient. Low-potency conventional agents (e.g., chlorpromazine) and clozapine are the most anticholinergic antipsychotics. The likelihood of anticholinergic toxicity increases when anticholinergic drugs (e.g., benztropine, trihexyphenedyl) are used to treat extrapyramidal symptoms produced by antipsychotics. Concomitant use of other medications with anticholinergic side effects (such as antiparkinsonian medications, meperidine, and tricyclic antidepressants) increases the risk of severe toxicity. For example, in a general hospital setting, low-potency antipsychotics may be prescribed together with narcotics for the treatment of severe pain and/or restlessness.

Peripheral Symptoms

Peripheral anticholinergic manifestations of antipsychotics include dry mouth, blurred vision, constipation, urinary retention, and exacerbation of glaucoma. Dry mouth may lead to the loss of porcelain dental fillings or a change in the fit of denture plates and may contribute to loss of food taste. To counteract this condition, the older patient may ingest large amounts of water, which may adversely affect electrolyte balance and kidney function. Constipation, which is often a problem in older patients, can be aggravated by antipsychotics, with potentially serious consequences such as paralytic ileus.

Blurred vision may exacerbate preexisting visual acuity problems. Urinary retention secondary to prostatic hypertrophy, a particularly common problem in older men, may lead to the development of bladder or ascending renal infection.

CNS Anticholinergic Manifestations

CNS anticholinergic toxicity occurs more frequently and with greater severity in older patients, probably because of already diminished cholinergic function in the CNS. Symptoms include disorientation, impaired recent memory, and confusion; in more severe cases, visual hallucinations, assaultiveness, irritability, and belligerence can occur. The agitation and confusion of CNS anticholinergic toxicity is often mistaken for worsening psychiatric or medical illness, which can lead to increased antipsychotic dosage and consequent worsening of symptoms.

Antipsychotic-Induced Movement Disorders I: Extrapyramidal Reactions

Elderly patients are especially susceptible to the movement disorders produced by antipsychotic drugs. These movement disorders may be subdivided into two broad categories. The first, movement disorders that develop acutely (or within a few weeks) following drug administration, are commonly termed EPS. In elderly patients, these effects are predominantly akathisia and parkinsonian symptoms, both of which are usually reversible upon drug discontinuation. The second category consists of movement disorders that appear with considerable passage of time after the drug was first prescribed and may persist long after discontinuing the medication. By far the most common late-appearing ("tardive") disorder in the elderly, as in younger patients, is TD, although other tardive movement disorders may occur as well.

As a group, atypical antipsychotics are associated with a significantly reduced frequency of EPS compared to conventional antipsychotics. Among the atypical agents, risperidone carries the greatest risk for EPS. Regarding conventional antipsychotics, the incidence and severity of EPS in the elderly, as in younger patients, correlates with the potency of the antipsychotic drug (see Choice of Antipsychotics section). Less severe forms of EPS (e.g., dystonic reactions and drug-induced parkinsonism) occur with reduced frequency and intensity with lower-potency agents (e.g., chlorpromazine) compared to higher-potency agents (e.g., haloperidol). The issue of whether or not some high-potency drugs, especially when given in depot preparation, may intensify tardive dyskinesia remains unresolved.

Akathisia

The most common drug-induced EPS in elderly patients, akathisia, is characterized by motor restlessness and muscular tension, particularly in the legs, and is experienced as a desire to move. The incidence of akathisia increases until it peaks in the seventh decade. Patients complain of a need or desire to move around continuously, as well as of nervousness, anxiety, or fidgetiness. They may repeatedly cross and uncross their legs, stamp their feet, change posture frequently, rock, sway, or even run about the room. A hallmark of the condition is that it primarily involves the lower extremities. Akathisia is sometimes difficult to distinguish from the more generalized restlessness of agitation or anxiety. Asking the older person who experiences these symptoms whether or not leg muscles feel tense, stiff, or jittery—muscular feelings usually reported when akathisia is present—can be helpful for differentiation. Akathisia can last for weeks or months.

When akathisia is mistaken for agitation and the clinician raises the antipsychotic dosage, the condition usually worsens. The preferred treatment for older persons with akathisia is antipsychotic dose reduction and using either atypical or relatively low-potency conventional antipsychotics. If these treatments prove ineffective, an anticholinergic agent should be tried. Other drugs found useful for this condition include propranolol and benzodiazepines such as lorazepam. Some patients with severe akathisia require a combination of medications for maximum relief.

Antipsychotic-Induced Parkinsonism

Antipsychotic-induced parkinsonism (AIP) is significantly more common in elderly patients than in younger persons, with peak incidence occurring in the eighth decade.[2] Among patients over age 60, the prevalence of AIP exceeds 50%,[19] and according to some studies, 75% of elderly patients treated chronically with antipsychotics may develop the syndrome,[20] compared to between 15% and 40% of younger people. Symptoms of AIP including bradykinesia, rigidity, tremor, and loss of postural reflexes, closely resemble those of idiopathic Parkinson's disease (PD). In AIP, tremor tends to be less prominent, however, and the characteristic festinating gait of idiopathic PD may not be present. The incidence of postural reflex abnormalities in AIP is unknown, but it may contribute to falls in elderly patients. In a study of 56 elderly psychotic patients receiving very low doses of one of three antipsychotic medications (haloperidol, thioridazine, and risperidone), AIP was most frequently associated with haloperidol.[21]

After developing, AIP can last for weeks, months, or even longer, especially if antipsychotic treatment continues. The treatment of AIP in elderly patients can be difficult. Reduction of antipsychotic dosage should be considered first, along with switching to an atypical antipsychotic. Treatment with anticholinergic drugs commonly used in younger patients may be associated with anticholinergic toxicity in older patients. Because some patients do *not* experience remission in AIP over time, they may require antiparkinsonian drugs continuously for as long as they receive the antipsychotic. In elderly patients who develop anticholinergic toxicity, amantadine can be used.

Acute Dystonic Reaction

Dystonic reactions consist of spasms of the face, neck, back, or extraocular muscles. Of all the antipsychotic-induced EPS, acute dystonic reactions are the only ones that are *less common* in older than in younger patients. Unlike dystonic reactions in younger adults, these reactions do not appear to be related to dosage in the elderly. The Pisa syndrome, a drug-induced dystonic reaction seen predominantly in elderly patients, is a condition in which the trunk is flexed to one side.

Dystonic reactions in elderly patients can almost invariably be treated with one or two doses of an appropriate anticholinergic drug, such as 0.5 to 1 mg of benztropine (Cogentin) or 25 mg of diphenhydramine (Benadryl). However, because of the risk of anticholinergic toxicity as well as memory impairment in the elderly, anticholinergic drugs should not be given any longer than necessary. Lowering the antipsychotic dose may also help to reduce dystonic symptoms.

Antipsychotic-Induced Movement Disorders II: Tardive Dyskinesia

The first cases of TD were described only 5 years after discovery of the usefulness of antipsychotics in treating psychosis and associated behavior disorders. The tardive disorders (in contrast to acute extrapyramidal reactions) occur, by definition, late in the course of treatment and sometimes persist after the drug is discontinued. Interestingly, increased antipsychotic dosage may suppress the movements, at least temporarily. There may also be a period of time following decreased dosage or discontinuation of the offending antipsychotic when the movements may actually *increase* in severity. Although the term "dyskinesia" is often used to refer to any hyperkinetic movement disorder, conditions such as tardive dystonia and tardive tics are also forms

of tardive dyskinesia. Generally, however, *tardive dyskinesia* refers to a relatively specific, and still the most common, form of movement disorder.

Although dyskinetic movements may arise spontaneously in older people in the absence of drugs or medical illnesses, this occurs uncommonly. Spontaneous orofacial dyskinesias may be associated with known neurological disorders that include Huntington's chorea, encephalitis, and Wilson's disease, but these dyskinesias probably account for a small number of orofacial dyskinesias in old age.

Clinical Appearance

Appearing late in the course of treatment with antipsychotics, the precise time of onset of TD varies from person to person. Although the disorder does not usually appear until after at least three months of treatment, in older persons it can appear earlier—in some cases after as little as one month of treatment. According to the DSM-IV definition, TD may occur after at least three months of antipsychotic exposure in patients under 60 years of age and after a minimum of one month of exposure in older patients. Prevalence estimates of TD among outpatients over the age of 65 being treated with antipsychotic drugs are as high as 35%.[22]

Although the movements of TD are usually described as choreoathetoid (random writhing or jerking), they may be rhythmic and may be confused with tremor. The oscillating rhythmic movements of TD are much lower in frequency than those of parkinsonian tremor (3 cycles per second or less compared with the tremor of parkinsonism, which ranges from 4 to 7 cycles per second). Clinically, if the movements are obviously repetitive, they can be counted in a 5- to 10-second period to determine if there are more or less than three movements per second.

TD involves the orofacial region more commonly in older than in younger patients. Occasionally, repetitive blinking or eyebrow movements occur, but they are less common than movements of the lower face. Orofacial movements impair talking and eating; excoriation of the tongue and lips is frequent, as are numerous dental problems.

Pursing or puckering of the lips and anteroposterior, lateral, or rotary chewing movements of the jaw also occur. With considerable tongue movement, it is sometimes difficult to separate lip and jaw movements. Other movements include lip smacking, blowing, and snouting. The chewing movements may be difficult to distinguish from the chewing movements of an edentulous older person and therefore require close observation.

With more severe TD, not only do movements of the face, hands, and feet become more apparent, but other body parts are affected as well. The neck is often involved, and rhythmic rolling, rocking choreiform movements of the shoulders and trunk may be seen. Abnormal hip movements can occur and are easiest to see when the patient walks. The arms and legs may also be affected, and, in very severe cases, abnormal movements in the diaphragmatic, pharyngeal, and intercostal musculature may develop. Severe TD, which may occur in as many as 10% of patients with the disorder, can impair writing and interfere with performing other tasks requiring manual dexterity. When pharyngeal and diaphragmatic musculature is involved, respiration may be compromised; however, only rarely is dyskinesia life threatening. Curiously, regardless of the severity of the movements, they generally disappear during sleep.

For the elderly patient experiencing TD, the gross irregular movements that characterize the disorder are especially burdensome because they occur at the same time of life that motor coordination decreases and tremor increases. Both physical *and* psychological problems are consequently compounded. Orofacial movements cause great embarrassment and tend to foster social isolation, which may already be a problem for some older patients.

Course

The course of TD can be quite variable. In some older patients, it progresses rapidly over a period of several months, after which it stabilizes and then is only slowly progressive. In others, it does not appear to progress at all and may actually improve gradually over time, even in patients who remain on antipsychotics. Approximately one-third of elderly patients who discontinue use of conventional antipsychotics improve significantly within the following 2 years. After a patient has had TD for a year or more, symptoms do not worsen significantly, even if treatment with conventional antipsychotics continues. Unfortunately, predicting the severity of TD is impossible, even when the condition is recognized early in its development. The likelihood of reversal of TD after antipsychotic withdrawal decreases with age.

Risk Factors

Several factors have been implicated as increasing the risk of developing TD. These include advanced age, cumulative exposure to conventional antipsychotics, alcohol abuse/dependence, early extrapyramidal symptoms, medical comorbidity, female gender, mood disorder, and ethnicity.

Age. Elderly patients are at greater risk of developing TD than younger patients.[23] Several age-related CNS changes, particularly alterations in dopaminergic and other neurochemical receptors may influence the development of this condition, although the mechanisms underlying these changes are not clear.[24] The cumulative annual incidence of TD in older patients treated with conventional antipsychotics is between 25% and 30%,[23,25] which is five to six times greater than the annual incidence of 4% to 5% reported in younger patients. The condition is also more persistent in older than in younger patients.[26] Increased risk of TD in older patients occurs even with relatively low doses of antipsychotics at early stages of treatment.[27]

Cumulative Exposure to Conventional Anti-psychotics. As indicated earlier, length of exposure (i.e., cumulative antipsychotic dose) is a risk factor for the development of TD. For example, in 435 older patients (mean age 65.5 years), the cumulative incidence of TD was 29%, 52%, and 60% after 1,2, and 3 years of antipsychotictreatment, respectively.[23,27] This is an important risk factor for many elderly patients, particularly for those living in long-term psychiatric institutions or nursing homes who may have been treated for extended periods of time.

Alcohol Abuse/Dependence. Both young adult and older patients with schizophrenia and a history of alcohol abuse or dependence are at increased risk for developing TD. The mechanisms underlying possible alcohol-mediated susceptibility to TD are not known, but they may be both peripheral and central.

Early-Onset Extrapyramidal Symptoms. The presence of EPS before or early in the course of treatment is a risk factor for TD, especially in elderly patients.[23,28,29] Patients who develop acute parkinsonism develop TD at a significantly faster rate than patients who do not.[30] Antipsychotic doses should be monitored carefully in patients who have baseline movement disorders or develop EPS such as AIP soon after beginning treatment.

Medical Comorbidity. Elderly patients with concomitant medical illnesses are more likely to have orofacial dyskinesias than those who are not medically ill. Orofacial dyskinesias in the edentulous older patient may also increase the severity of TD.

Gender. Female gender has been held an important risk factor for TD.[31] Several elements point to increased risk for women developing TD; these include longer hospitalizations, exposure to larger doses of antipsychotics, and longer durations of antipsychotic treatment. However, recent large-scale studies of older patients have not found gender an independent risk factor for developing TD.[23,25,27]

Mood Disorders. TD may be more prevalent in patients with schizophrenia and coexisting mood disorders (both unipolar and bipolar) than in those with only schizophrenia.[32] Further studies are necessary to more precisely determine to what extent the presence of a mood disorder in an older patient who is receiving antipsychotics increases the risk for developing TD.

Other Risk Factors. The risk of TD may be influenced by ethnicity; for example, African-Americans appear to have a higher risk than Caucasians of developing TD. Other suggested risk factors include use of depot antipsychotics, history of drug interruptions or holidays, diabetes and smoking. Patients with dementia, brain damage, and mental retardation may also be at increased risk for developing TD.

Treatment of Tardive Dyskinesia

Before elderly patients are treated for TD, they require a comprehensive physical and neurological evaluation (Table 7.2); treatment of elderly patients is similar to that of younger patients.[33,34] Current recommendations are to reduce the antipsychotic to the lowest possible dose or to change to an atypical antipsychotic. Atypical antipsychotics have a lower risk of TD compared to conventional agents.[35–38] In particular, the risk of TD measured over a 9-month period in older patients receiving low doses (i.e., median dose 1 mg/day) of risperidone was found to be 5 to 6 times lower than the corresponding risk with haloperidol.[39]

Another necessary step is to taper and to withdraw any anticholinergic medications, as these drugs have been shown to exacerbate the movement disorder. Any stimulating medications such as diet pills, OTC allergy preparations, and decongestants, should also be discontinued. Benzodiazepines and β-blockers are sometimes helpful in reducing the severity of dyski-

Table 7.2.   Workup of Geriatric Patients with Suspected Tardive Dyskinesia

1. Complete physical examination, including detailed neurological and mental status examinations
2. Complete history, with special inquiries regarding
   - History of exposure to antipsychotics, L-dopa, lithium, estrogens, stimulants, toxins (including carbon monoxide, manganese, other transition metals)
   - History of rheumatic fever or Sydenham's chorea in early life
   - Family history of movement disorder
   - History of thyroid disease, polycythemia, systemic lupus erythematosus
3. Routine blood work, including electrolytes, glucose, complete blood count
4. Thyroid function tests
5. Urine drug screen for stimulants and transition metals
6. EEG
7. CT scan

netic movements but should be used with caution in elderly patients because of their potential adverse effects.

No medication has proven to be consistently effective for the treatment of TD, but some interest has emerged in using antioxidant compounds such as vitamin E (alpha-tocopherol). Although data conflict somewhat,[40] a metaanalysis reports that 12 of 18 trials produced positive results for the treatment of TD.[41] Patients with mild TD or more recent onset (less than 5 years) have a better response. Studies of vitamin E for treating TD have generally used 400 to 1600 IU/day. Few studies have focused on antioxidant treatment in older patients.

To help prevent TD, antipsychotics (even atypical agents) should be used only when absolutely necessary and low doses of medication should be prescribed. Anticholinergic agents should not be used routinely for treatment of extrapyramidal symptoms as they may worsen the condition.

Other Tardive Syndromes

Apart from the typical choreoathetoid movements of TD, other tardive syndromes have been described, although less often in older patients than in younger ones. Current case reports indicate that tardive akathisia and tardive Tourette's may be more common than

tardive dystonia in the elderly, but further research is needed to confirm these observations.[42]

Neurologic Side Effects

Neurological side effects are common in elderly patients. They include neuroleptic malignant syndrome and grand mal seizures.

Neuroleptic Malignant Syndrome

Neuroleptic malignant syndrome (NMS) is a rare but potentially lethal disorder that usually evolves over a period of 1 to 3 days. Although this syndrome is primarily seen in patients aged 20 to 40, it has been reported in patients over age 60. The clinical picture often includes extrapyramidal and autonomic dysfunction, including severe rigidity and dystonia, coarse tremor, and fever. Tachycardia, diaphoresis, tachypnea, hypertension or hypotension, urinary incontinence, elevated creatine phosphokinase levels, leukocytosis, and myoglobinuria are also evident. Although NMS has been thought to be related to the dopamine D_2-receptor blockade by conventional antipsychotics, occasional cases of NMS have been reported with atypical agents.[43,44] However, overall, atypical antipsychotics carry a significantly lower risk of NMS compared to that of conventional antipsychotics.

If NMS is at all suspected, antipsychotics should be discontinued immediately. Although many patients respond to drug discontinuation with rapid improvement, severe cases may require admission to an intensive care unit for intravenous hydration and supportive medical management. Although young adult patients respond well to dantrolene or bromocriptine, the therapeutic and toxic effects of these drugs in elderly patients have not been studied specifically, and dosage guidelines have therefore not been specified. As with most other drugs given to older patients, low doses are advised.

Grand Mal Seizures

Antipsychotics can lower the seizure threshold and thereby induce seizures in previously seizure-free patients. Elderly patients are more susceptible to seizures, particularly if they have a history of prior seizures, electroconvulsive therapy, or preexisting CNS pathology. Obtaining a careful history is therefore necessary. Since seizures are frequently also associated with increasing dosages of antipsychotic drugs rapidly, dosage increases in older patients for whom antipsychotic drugs are relatively new should be gradual.

Miscellaneous Side Effects

Additional antipsychotic side effects seen less frequently in older patients than in younger ones include hypothermia and hyperthermia, jaundice, agranulocytosis, weight gain, and dermatoses.

Hypothermia and Hyperthermia

Because of their effect on the thermoregulatory functions of the hypothalamus, antipsychotics are occasionally associated with decreased body temperature. This side effect is more common with phenothiazines than with other neuroleptic subclasses and is more likely to occur in older patients with hypothyroidism.

Antipsychotic drugs have also been associated with a dramatic *increase* in body temperature (hyperthermia). Although elderly patients are not necessarily more susceptible to this side effect, those with structural or functional disorders of the hypothalamus or hypothalamic-pituitary axis may be particularly vulnerable.

Jaundice

In rare cases, antipsychotics of the phenothiazine class, particularly chlorpromazine, produce obstructive jaundice. In contrast, other chemical classes of antipsychotics, such as the butyrophenones, thioxanthines, indoles (molindone), and dibenzoxazepines (loxapine), have not been associated with the disorder. Although jaundice is not more likely to occur in older people and is reversible upon discontinuation of the phenothiazine antipsychotic, older patients with a history of obstructive jaundice or liver disease should not be treated with drugs of this class.

Agranulocytosis

A side effect marked by reduced white blood cell count, agranulocytosis is a rare syndrome that develops within the first 8 weeks of antipsychotic treatment and resolves with dicontinuation of the offending medication. Agranulocytosis has been reported with various antipsychotics, both conventional low-potency agents such as chlorpromazine as well as atypical agents, particularly clozapine. In a review of 11,555 patients treated with clozapine, older age was found to be associated with a significantly increased risk of agranulocytosis.[45] Moreover, elderly patients experience greater mortality compared to younger patients from antipsychotic-induced agranulocytosis.

Weight Gain and Diabetes

Many antipsychotic medications can induce weight gain in younger patients.[46] Elderly patients who are frail or poorly nourished may benefit from this effect; however, weight gain may also aggravate preexisting cardiovascular disease or osteoarthritis in this population. Although the conventional antipsychotics (with the exception of molindone) frequently contribute to weight gain, this side effect has increasingly become associated with the atypical antipsychotics.

In young and middle-aged patients, growing evidence shows that weight gain associated with the atypical antipsychotics may exacerbate or perhaps induce diabetes mellitus.[47,48] In an analysis of 45 published cases of new-onset diabetes mellitus (DM) and diabetic ketoacidosis (DKA) associated with atypical antipsychotics in patients under age 60, 44% of the cases were related to clozapine, 42% to olanzapine, and only 7% to each of risperidone and quetiapine respectively.[49] Although this analysis did not establish causation or incidence of diabetes with specific antipsychotics, it supports the notion that clozapine and olanzapine are associated with diabetes to a greater extent than the other atypical agents. In a separate study, 805 cases of DM were identified in patients taking atypical antipsychotic medications. Of these, 384 were treated with clozapine, 289 with olanzapine, and 132 with risperidone.[50–52] Among the patients with new-onset DM, DKA was reported in 100 of the patients treated with olanzapine, 80 of those treated with clozapine, and 36 of those treated with risperidone.

Among patients who developed hyperglycemia or DM while taking clozapine or olanzapine, more than 60% were identified within 6 months of starting treatment. In addition, 25 deaths were reported among patients being treated with clozapine and olanzapine, and five deaths were reported among patients being treated with risperidone. This analysis suggests that clozapine and olanzapine are more likely than is risperidone to either precipitate or unmask diabetes in susceptible individuals. At the other end of the spectrum, the two most recently FDA approved atypical antipsychotics, ziprasidone and aripiprazole, are believed to be even less likely to induce weight gain than any of the other atypical antipsychotics.

Additional studies, particularly those involving older adults, are needed to substantiate this claim.

Hyperprolactinemia

Hyperprolactinemia is a by-product of the D_2 dopamine-blocking activity, the classic mechanism of action of conventional antipsychotics as well as risperidone. Evidence suggests that clozapine and olanzapine cause some prolactin elevation.[53] Hyperprolactinemia can inhibit the production of gonadal hormones, and thus, has been associated with various side effects including amenorrhea, galactorrhea, gynecomastia, and sexual dysfunction.[54] Over the long term, elevated prolactin levels may compromise bone-mineral density and lead to osteoporosis.[55] More data are needed, however, in order to determine whether antipsychotics can increase the risk of osteoporosis.[56]

Dermatoses

Antipsychotic drugs are associated with occasional rashes that subside after drug discontinuation. The rash tends to be an intensely itchy maculopapular eruption that appears all over the body. Because this condition is likely to result from an individual drug allergy, use of a drug from a different compound class usually does not produce another rash. Rashes as side effects of antipsychotics are not more common in older persons than in younger ones.

Antipsychotic drugs are also associated with increased photosensitivity to sunburn but not to suntanning. Older patients living in sunny southern climates who are being treated with antipsychotics should be warned about this effect. Topical sunscreens should be used to prevent sunburn, and sunglasses that effectively screen out ultraviolet light should be worn to protect the eyes.

An extremely rare dermatological side effect of antipsychotics is a purple-gray pigmentation of the skin. This condition is most likely to occur in patients who have been on high antipsychotic doses for long periods of time, but it is not more common in older people. In addition to being unsightly and disfiguring, it may also mask skin changes associated with the development of other diseases and may thus interfere with diagnosis. This pigmentation is reversible, but many months elapse before normal skin color returns.

Ophthalmologic Side Effects

Thioridazine can cause an irreversible pigmentary retinopathy that appears to be dose related (i.e., > 800 mg/day). Mesoridazine may also be associated with this problem, but to a smaller degree. Older patients taking these medications should have routine ophthalmologic examinations.

Syndrome of Inappropriate Antidiuretic Hormone Secretion

Antipsychotics have been associated with the syndrome of inappropriate antidiuretic hormone secretion (SIADH), which results in lower serum sodium levels. Although the majority of cases have involved conventional antipsychotics, SIADH has been reported in association with atypical agents, including clozapine and risperidone.[57,58] Risk factors for SIADH include older age and use of antipsychotics in combination with other agents such as antidepressants, thiazide-like diuretics, and nonsteroidal anti-inflammatory drugs (NSAIDs).[59] Moreover, elderly patients who may be physically debilitated prior to antipsychotic treatment may be particularly susceptible to SIADH. Sodium values that might be well tolerated in younger persons (e.g., 125–130 mmol/L) may cause considerable confusion, disorientation, and memory impairment in elderly patients. SIADH must be differentiated from excessive water intake that can occur with psychosis, and the diagnosis can usually be made by measuring urine osmolality: In the case of SIADH, it is still relatively high; when water intoxication occurs, it is extremely low.

Choice of Antipsychotics

Several types of antipsychotic drugs are available, each with a distinct chemical structure. With the advent of the more recent generation of antipsychotics, drugs are now categorized as either "conventional" or "atypical." Conventional antipsychotics include phenothiazines (e.g., chlorpromazine), butyrophenones (e.g., haloperidol), thioxanthenes (e.g., thiothixene), dibenzoxazepines (e.g., loxapine), and indolones (e.g., molindone).

Conventional Antipsychotics

Conventional antipsychotic drugs are therapeutically equivalent for the management of symptoms of severe late-life behavior disorders and psychosis. They differ only in milligram potency and side-effect profile. Selection of any one conventional antipsychotic in preference to another, therefore, is based on the pharmacokinetic and side-effect profile of each drug (Table 7.1) and the patient's history of prior drug response, or lack thereof. If an older patient does not respond to an antipsychotic, another should be tried, preferably of a different chemical class. Studies of antipsychotic treatment in the elderly are presented in Table 7.3.

Phenothiazines

The chemical structure of the three subtypes of phenothiazine agents, in order of progressively increasing potency, are (1) aliphatic side-chain (e.g., chlorpromazine), (2) piperidine side-chain (e.g., thioridazine), and (3) piperazine side-chain (e.g., acetophenazine, perphenazine, trifluoperazine, and fluphenazine).

Chlorpromazine. The oldest and traditionally one of the most widely used antipsychotics, chlorpromazine is a low-potency phenothiazine of the aliphatic side-chain group. Its metabolism is complex, resulting in pharmacologically active metabolites that include those produced in the

Table 7.3. Antipsychotic Treatment of Agitation in the Elderly: Controlled Studies

Drug(s)	Study[a]	Mean Age	Dose[b] (mg)	Results[c]
ACETOPHENAZINE				
Acetophenazine (A), Imipramine (IMI)s Trifluoperazine (TFP)	Honigfeld & Newall (1965)	66	A: 20–126 IMI: 25–150 TPF: 2–12	Acetophenazine and trifluoperazine equally effective in reducing motor disturbance, psychosis, thinking disorder; acetophenazine better than trifluoperazine in decreasing irritability and improving social competence
Acetophenazine (A), Chlorpromazine (CPZ)	Sheppard et al. (1964)	73	A: 41–80 CPZ: 52–100	Both drugs effective in reducing paranoia; acetophenazine better for delusions and bizarre posture
Acetophenazine	Chesrow & Kaplitz (1963)	—	20	Excellent or good results in 85% of subjects by clinical observation and 93% by psychological tests
Acetophenazine	Hamilton & Bennett (1962a)	61	60	Acetophenazine much superior to placebo for improved behavior and reduced assaultiveness
Acetophenazine, phenobarbital	Welborn (1961)	—	80	Drugs equally effective but only one-third of patients responded
CHLORPROMAZINE				
Chlorpromazine, pentylene, tetrazol, reserpine, placebo	Robinson (1969)	80	—	Chlorpromazine patients deteriorated faster than placebo patients
Chlorpromazine (CPZ), placebo	Barton & Hurst (1966)	76.5	CPZ: 137.5	Chlorpromazine superior for agitation
Chlorpromazine (CPZ), reserpine-pipradol, placebo	Abse & Dahlstrom (1960)	79	CPZ: 75	No difference between drug and placebo
Chlorpromazine, placebo	Seager (1955)	72.5	150–225	Chlorpromazine superior to placebo in reducing psychotic symptoms
FLUPHENAZINE				
Fluphenazine enanthate, doctor's choice	Raskind et al. (1979)	71.5	5 mg q. 2 weeks	Fluphenazine enanthate better than doctor's choice for paranoid hostility; caused depression and retardation

HALOPERIDOL

Drugs	Reference	Age	Dose	Findings
Haloperidol (H), trazodone (TR), placebo	Teri et al. (2000)	75.3 (H) 73.2 (TR)	H:1.8 TR: 200	Comparable, modest reduction in agitation in haloperidol and trazodone groups, but not greater than placebo or behavioral techniques significantly better
Standard-dose haloperidol (H_s), low-dose haloperidol (H_l), placebo	Devanand et al. (1998)	72.1	H_s: 2–3 H_l: 0.50–0.75	Standard-dose haloperidol superior to low dose and placebo for treatment of psychosis and agitation in AD; standard dose produced more severe EPS
Haloperidol (H), trazodone (TR)	Sultzer et al. (1997)	72	H: 1–5 TR: 50–250	Drugs equal in efficacy; more side effects with haloperidol
Haloperidol (H), oxazepam (OX), diphenhydramine (DPH)	Coccaro (1990)	59	H: 1.5 OX: 30 DPH: 49	All three drugs equal in modest efficacy
Haloperidol (H), clopenthixol (CL)	Gotestam et al. (1981)	80.6	H: 0.5 CL: 5	More behavioral deterioration with haloperidol
Haloperidol (H), chlormethiazole (C)	Ter Haar (1977)	65+	H: 2.5 C: 576	Haloperidol better in reducing aggression, confusion, and depression; less sedating than chlormethiazole
Haloperidol (H), thioridazine (T)	Smith et al. (1974)	76.5	H: 2 T: 106.7	Drugs equal in efficacy
Haloperidol (H), placebo	Sugerman et al. (1964)	71.6	1–4.5	Haloperidol much better than placebo in reducing overactivity, restlessness, and tension; EPS common with this drug

LOXAPINE

Drugs	Reference	Age	Dose	Findings
Loxapine (L)s Haloperidol (H)	Petrie et al. (1982)	72.5	L: 21.9 H: 4.6	Equal improvement on all scales for both drugs; both better than placebo; more sedation, retardation, and orthostatic hypotension with haloperidol; drugs equal in producing EPS

(continued)

Table 7.3. *(continued)*

Drug(s)	Study[a]	Mean Age	Dose[b] (mg)	Results[c]
THIORIDAZINE				
Thioridazine (T), behavioral diazepam (D), placebo	Stotsky (1984)	76.4	T: 10–200 D: 20–40	Thioridazine better than diazepam on all ratings; both equally sedating
Thioridazine (T), placebo; loxapine (L) Loxapine thioridazine	Barnes et al. (1982)	65+	T: 62.5 L: 10.5	Drugs equal on all scales; both drugs better than only modest improvement in most patients. more sedating and produced more EPS; caused hypotension.
Thioridazine (T), haloperidol (H)	Cowley & Glen (1979)	65+	T: 153 H: 2.1	Both equal in efficacy
Thioridazine (T), adjustment haloperidol (H)	Rosen (1979)	69	T: 58 H: 1.3	Drugs equal in therapeutic efficacy and social
Thioridazine (T), fluphenazine (F) gain, and	Branchey et al. (1978)	67	T: 84–285 F: 1.5–5	Drugs equal in therapeutic efficacy. Fluphenazine produced rigidity; strong hypotension, weight prolonged the QT interval with thioridazine
Thioridazine (T), diazepam (DZ)	Covington (1975)	80	T: 33 DZ: 7.2	Thioridazine superior to diazepam on all ratings
Thioridazine (T), diazepam (D) behavioral	Cervera (1974)	—	T: 79 DZ: 12	Drugs equal for anxiety, agitation, and tension; thioridazine better than diazepam for improvement
Thioridazine, stimulating thiothixene	Katz & Itil (1974)	—	—	Thioridazine more calming; thiothixene more
Thioridazine (T), fluoxymesterone, alone nicotinic acid, placebo	Lehmann & Ban (1974)	—	T: 75–100	BPRS total score improved only on combination of thioridazine and fluoxymesterone; thioridazine best only for blunted affect

Drugs	Reference	Age	Dose	Comments
Thioridazine (T), diazepam (DZ)	Kirven & Montero (1973)	72.5	T: 38.9 DZ: 9	Thioridazine better than diazepam for anxiety, diazepam better than thioridazine for agitation, insomnia, and depression
Thioridazine, haloperidol (H), chlorpromazine (CPZ)	Birkett & Boltuck (1972)	80.5	T: 25–100 H: 0.5–2 CPZ: 25–100	Statistically equal effect on Blood Pressure (BP) from all 3 drugs; chlorpromazine and thioridazine cause large decrease in BP
Thioridazine (T), haloperidol (H)	Tsuang et al. (1971)	72.6	T: 113 H:	Drugs equal for treatment of excitement, irritability, hostility, and suspiciousness
Thioridazine (T), haloperidol (H), chlorpromazine (CPZ), oxazepam (OX), tybamate (TYB)	Tewfik et al. (1970)	73	T: 50–150 H: 4.5 CPZ: 50–150 OX: 20–30 TYB: 700–950	None helpful; oxazepam has fewest side effects, haloperidol most; thioridazine and chlorpromazine produce least deterioration
Thioridazine (T), amitriptyline, fluoxymesterone, meprobamate, tybamate	Lehmann & Ban (1967)	72	T: 75–150	Thioridazine better than all other drugs for irritability and excitement
Thioridazine (T)	Judah et al. (1959)	63	75–500	Thioridazine caused marked decrease in agitation, improved socialization, mild EPS
THIOTHIXENE				
Thiothixene/placebo	Finkel et al. (1995)	85	0.25–18	Thiothixene more effective than placebo in reducing agitation
Thiothixene/placebo	Rada & Kellner (1976)	75.5	15	Thiothixene and placebo equal on all ratings
Thiothixene/doctor's choice	Mohler (1970)	69.9	75–90	No improvement with thiothixene
TRIFLUOPERAZINE				
Trifluoperazine	Hamilton & Bennett (1962b)	71	71	Drug not effective; cause EPS

[a] Complete citations for references at end of chapter.
[b] Dose expressed in mean daily dose, when given.
[c] EPS, extrapyramidal symptoms; BPRS, Brief Psychiatric Rating Scale; BP, blood pressure.

liver as well as by prehepatic gut metabolism. Chlorpromazine is potentially more toxic and less therapeutically predictable in older patients because of age-related changes in liver and prehepatic gut metabolism. In addition, the drug produces marked sedation, orthostatic hypotension, and anticholinergic symptoms, and has been associated with the development of cholestatic jaundice, dermatological side effects, agranulocytosis, thermoregulatory disorders, and seizures.

For these reasons, the routine use of chlorpromazine is not recommended for older patients. Should a clinician wish to use this drug, however, 10 to 25 mg orally is the recommended initial dose; the therapeutic dosage range for older patients is between 50 and 200 mg per day. Intramuscular doses are approximately four times more potent than comparable oral doses.

Thioridazine. The most commonly used antipsychotic of the piperidine phenothiazine class, was used frequently in the past for older patients with behavioral disturbances, particularly behaviors with agitation components. The advantage of this medication for the geriatric patient lies in the relatively low incidence of EPS associated with its use. However, like chlorpromazine, thioridazine produces orthostatic hypotension and marked sedation. Thioridazine is also one of the most anticholinergic of all antipsychotic drugs and therefore, should not be used in conjunction with other anticholinergic medications.

More recent evidence regarding the cardiovascular risks associated with thioridazine has further limited its use in older patients. It significantly prolongs the QT interval, has been associated with numerous cases of *torsade de pointes*, and has been implicated in an excessive number of sudden deaths compared with other antipsychotics.[60–62] Consequently, in July 2000, the FDA issued a "black box" warning regarding risk of conduction abnormalities with thioridazine in order to discourage

its use unless other agents are not effective.[63] Any elderly patient should receive a baseline electrocardiogram (EKG) prior to starting treatment with thioridazine, and cardiac status should be monitored at regular intervals during dosage titration.

Dosages of thioridazine above 800 mg per day have been associated with pigmented retinopathy and loss of vision; daily doses must not exceed 800 mg per day. Although this ceiling limits the usefulness of thioridazine for the general population of severely psychotic patients, considerably lower doses are usually effective for agitated older people. Nevertheless, any older patient with impaired retinal function should have a pretreatment eye examination before thioridazine is used, as well as routine eye examinations thereafter.

Piperazines. Four piperazine derivatives are in common use. In order of increasing milligram potency, they are: acetophenazine, perphenazine, trifluoperazine, and fluphenazine. These drugs share class characteristics: They are all relatively nonsedating and produce a relatively low incidence of orthostatic hypotension, compared with aliphatic (chlorpromazine) and piperidine (thioridazine) derivatives. Piperazine phenothiazines, however, all produce a high incidence of EPS.

Acetophenazine, the piperazine derivative with the lowest milligram potency of the four mentioned, is associated with the least severe EPS. Since it also produces relatively mild sedation and orthostatic hypotension, it is particularly useful in treating both cognitive and behavioral disturbances of older persons associated with dementia or psychosis. The initial recommended dose is 10 mg; the therapeutic dosage range is 10 to 100 mg per day.

Perphenazine, a piperazine phenothiazine particularly helpful for hyperexcited, aggressive, or very agitated older patients, is relatively nonsedating and nonhypotensive; it is associated, however, with slightly more severe EPS than acetophenazine. The initial dose is 2 to 4 mg; the therapeutic dosage range is 4 to 32 mg per day.

Trifluoperazine shares many characteristics with perphenazine but produces slightly more intense EPS. The initial dose is 1 to 2 mg; the therapeutic dosage range is 2 to 15 mg per day.

Fluphenazine is the most potent of the piperazine phenothiazines. Like haloperidol, it has almost no sedating or hypotensive effects but produces marked EPS. The initial recommended dose is 0.25 to 0.5 mg; the therapeutic dosage range is 0.5 to 4.0 mg per day.

In addition to oral forms, fluphenazine is also available in long-acting forms given by injection. The effect of fluphenazine decanoate lasts approximately 14 days; fluphenazine enanthate lasts approximately 21 days. Intramuscular fluphenazine in elderly patients is four to five times more potent than fluphenazine taken orally. The intramuscular route of administration is accompanied by the assumption that approximately equal amounts of drug are released each day. However, this assumption may not hold for any given elderly patient, since decreased muscle mass may alter the rate and regularity of release of these drugs into systemic circulation. As a general guideline, elderly patients should not receive more than 0.25 to 0.5 mL of depot intramuscular fluphenazine every 14 to 21 days.

Because fluphenazine use is associated with a high incidence of EPS, older patients receiving depot fluphenazine may be vulnerable to prolonged severe toxicity. Long-acting forms of fluphenazine should thus be administered to elderly patients with extreme caution.

Butyrophenones

HALOPERIDOL, the only antipsychotic of the butyrophenone chemical class in current use, is extensively prescribed for elderly patients for relief of agitation, psychosis, and "sundowning." Like fluphenazine, with which it shares most characteristics, haloperidol is a highly potent antipsychotic. Because it possesses almost no sedating or orthostatic hypotensive properties, it is a particularly safe drug in this regard for older patients.

However, haloperidol is associated with marked EPS and can produce severe akinesia that may be confused with the psychomotor retardation of depression or dementia in older patients. EPS may be mitigated by lower starting doses, followed by lower therapeutic doses. Initial doses should be 0.25 to 0.5 mg; the daily dosage range for the elderly patient should be 0.5 to 4.0 mg per day.

Haloperidol decanoate is available for treatment of psychosis and agitation in patients who may have difficulty complying with oral medications. The use of haloperidol decanoate is associated with the same problems as fluphenazine decanoate. Haloperidol decanoate can usually be given on a less frequent basis than fluphenazine decanoate, and monthly injections are usually sufficient.

Thioxanthenes

THIOTHIXENE, the most widely prescribed antipsychotic drug in this chemical class, has been used extensively by elderly patients. Like other antipsychotics, it is clinically effective for several types of symptoms including agitation, psychosis, and restlessness. In its effect, potency, and side effects, thiothixene resembles trifluoperazine. Because it is a high-potency antipsychotic, it produces relatively modest sedation and orthostatic hypotension but is associated with severe EPS, which may be mitigated by the use of low doses. The initial recommended dose is 1 mg; the therapeutic dosage range is between 1 and 15 mg per day.

Dibenzoxazepines

LOXAPINE, the most frequently used antipsychotic of this chemical class, is comparable in therapeutic effect and side-effect profile to perphenazine. It may produce some initial transient drowsiness in older patients and is also associated with EPS. Because one of the metabolites of loxapine is amoxapine, a tricyclic antidepressant drug, loxapine has been suggested for patients with schizophrenia who develop depression, as well as for patients with psychotic depressions. However, the safety and efficacy of loxapine in older patients have not yet been studied. Initial doses of loxapine are 10 mg; the daily dosage range is 10 to 100 mg per day.

Indolones

MOLINDONE, the only indolone currently available for clinical use, is a potent antipsychotic drug with clinical and adverse effects resembling those of perphenazine. It has relatively few sedating properties and is the only antipsychotic not associated with weight gain. Initial recommended doses are 5 to 10 mg; the therapeutic dosage range is 10 to 100 mg per day.

Atypical Antipsychotics

Although several definitions for "atypical" antipsychotics are in use, they are generally considered to be agents with both dopamine and serotonin-blocking activity. Atypical agents have a lower risk of movement disorders (i.e., EPS, TD) than conventional agents. Atypical antipsychotics also are more effective than conventional antipsychotics for controlling negative as well as positive symptoms of schizophrenia. Data on the use of these medications in the elderly are limited (Table 7.4). Currently six atypical antipsychotics are FDA approved: clozapine, risperidone, olanzapine, quetiapine, ziprasidone, and aripiprazole.

Clozapine

An atypical antipsychotic chemically related to the conventional antipsychotic agent loxapine, clozapine has the advantage of being effective in cases of treat-

ment-resistant schizophrenia, with a very low propensity for causing acute EPS and TD.[35,64] Unfortunately, the side-effect profile of clozapine is similar to that of conventional, low-potency antipsychotics; it can cause considerable hypotension, sedation, and anticholinergic side effects. In addition, it has the potential for causing seizures and agranulocytosis. Respiratory problems, including respiratory arrest, have been reported in elderly patients receiving doses of clozapine above 100 mg per day.[65] At lower doses of 25 to 50 mg per day, these side effects do not occur more frequently than in younger patients.[66]

Clozapine can be effective in treating psychosis and agitation in geriatric patients. Its potential for serious side effects, however, may limit its use to treatment of the most unresponsive elderly patients and those with severe TD. Based on its low propensity for inducing motoric toxicity, clozapine has been used successfully for the treatment of psychosis in elderly patients with Parkinson's disease. Because of its tendency to cause orthostatic hypotension and sedation, clozapine should be started at a very low dose (6.25 to 12.5 mg/day) and adjusted, with careful monitoring of mental status and blood pressure changes. Weekly monitoring of white blood cell counts is necessary and may further limit the use of this drug in more impaired elderly patients. Clozapine serum levels may be increased by drugs that inhibit cytochrome p450 isoenzyme 1A2 (CYP 1A2) such as ciprofloxacin, isoniazid, and fluvoxamine.[12]

Risperidone

Risperidone became available for use in the United States in December 1993. Although the incidence of EPS with risperidone is somewhat more compared to that with clozapine, it is much better tolerated by elderly patients overall. The risk of TD in older patients treated with low doses of risperidone is significantly lower compared to the corresponding risk with con-

Table 7.4.   Atypical Antipsychotic Treatment of Psychosis and Agitation in Late Life

Study[a]	Study Population [N]	Age (mean; range)	Dose (mg) (mean; range)	Results
			CLOZAPINE	
Howanitz et al. (1999)	US Veteran inpatients with schizophrenia or SAD [42]	CL: 65 CPZ: 68.5	CL: 300 CPZ: 600	Two drugs approximately equal in efficacy & tolerability. One patient in each group had a life-threatening side effect; more tachycardia and weight gain in CL group; more sedation in CPZ group
The Parkinson Study Group (1999)	Parkinson disease and drug-induced psychosis [60]	72	24.7; 6.25–60	Improvement in psychosis in clozapine group significantly greater than in placebo group; improvement in tremor without worsening of parkinsonism; one patient discontinued due to leukopenia
Sajatovic et al. (1998)	U.S. Veterans with schizophrenia [267] & other psychotic disorders [45]	63.4; 55–86	310; 12.5–900	Overall significant improvement in psychosis; less improvement & higher discontinuation rate in patients > age 65 than in younger patients
Chengappa et al. (1995)	Female patients with psychosis [12]	69; 61–82	150; 25–300	Psychotic symptoms improved markedly in 2 patients and moderately in 5; 7 of 12 patients experienced postural hypotension
Pitner et al. (1995)	Treatment-resistant or refractory psychotic patients [4]	74; 68–83	26.6; 12.5–43.75	Psychotic symptoms relieved in 2 patients after titration; clozapine-related side effects experienced by all patients, including falls (2 patients), bradycardia (2 patients), and delirium (1 patient)
Salzman et al. (1995)	Hospitalized psychotic patients [20]	72; 65–84	210; 75–350	All patients improved after clozapine; 12 reported sedation and lethargy; 4 developed serious respiratory complications (pneumonia, respiratory arrest)

(continued)

Table 7.4. *(continued)*

Study[a]	Study Population [N]	Age (mean; range)	Dose (mg) (mean; range)	Results
Frankenburg et al. (1994)	Treatment-resistant psychoses; several with parkinsonism or TD [8]	72; 68–80	135; 12.5–400	At least moderate improvement of psychosis in 6 patients after clozapine initiated; diminished symptoms in all patients with parkinsonism or TD; ataxia, falls, sialorrhea, and confusion required cessation of clozapine in 1 patient; another experienced urinary incontinence, confusion, and sedation; marked orthostasis in 2 patients
Oberholzer et al. (1992)	Alzheimer-type dementia [14] and other disorders [4]	81; 59–95	52; 12.5–200	3 patients discontinued clozapine due to adverse effects, 1 discontinued due to lack of clinical response; motor restlessness, somnolence, and acute confusional states developed in patients receiving 25–75 mg/day; clozapine well tolerated and safe in remaining 7 patients; in a second phase, 7 AD patients' psychopathology worsened after clozapine was discontinued and improved after drug was resumed
	OLANZAPINE			
Hwang et al. (2003)	Inpatients with schizophrenia [15], AD [15], delusional disorder [12], organic psychosis [12], affective psychosis [16], VD [6], brief psychosis [2], delirium [2]	74.2; 65–87	10.1; 2.5–20	80 of 94 patients (85%) completed study; majority had significant symptom improvement; 46 of 94 patients experienced 1 or more side effects, most frequently sedation, dizziness, & leg weakness; total body weight, fasting triglyceride, & fasting blood glucose levels significantly elevated from baseline

Study	Population	Age	Dose	Comments
Barak et al. (2002)	Inpatients with schizophrenia [20]	72.7	O 13.1; 5–25 H 7.2	Olanzapine produced significantly greater improvement in psychotic symptoms overall as well as in negative symptoms, particularly compared to those treated with haloperidol; weight gain in both groups not significantly different between groups
Breier et al. (2002)	PD patients with drug-induced psychosis [160]	U.S. Study: 72.6 European Study: 70.7	U.S. 4.2 Eur. 4.1	Olanzapine produced improvement in psychosis not superior to placebo, as well as some worsening of motor performance
Cummings et al. (2002) Post hoc analysis of a subgroup of DLB patients included in a larger study by Street et al. (2000)	Patients with DLB [29] living in nursing homes	83.3; 69–95	5–15	Doses of 5 & 10 mg/day of olanzapine associated with reduced psychosis without worsening of parkinsonism or cognition; 15 mg/day no different than placebo
Madhusoodanan et al. (2000)	Schizophrenia [3], SAD [8]	74.8; 60–85	10.8; 5–20	20% or greater improvement in psychotic (esp. positive) symptoms in 7 of 11 patients; improved MMSE in 9 patients; EPS decreased significantly; side effects included dizziness, sedation, diarrhea, rash, & mean weight gain of 3.5 lbs.
Street et al. (2000a); Clark et al. (2001)	Patients with AD [206] living in nursing homes	82.7	5–15	5 & 10 mg/day produced significant improvement in psychosis & agitation/aggression compared with placebo whereas improvement with 15 mg/day not significantly better than with placebo; for patients without baseline psychosis, olanzapine significantly reduced percentage of new emergence of psychosis compared to placebo; most common side effects: sedation, gait disturbance; no significant EPS or anticholinergic effects

(continued)

Table 7.4. *(continued)*

Study[a]	Study Population [N]	Age (mean; range)	Dose (mg) (mean; range)	Results
Street et al. (2000b) Subset analysis of patients 65 yrs & older from Tollefson et al. (1997), a larger study	Schizophrenia, SAD, & schizophreniform disorder [59], predominantly female	69; 65–86	O: 12.4 H: 8.7	Numeric superiority, compared with haloperidol, for reduction of psychosis, including both negative & depressive symptoms, but difference not statistically significant; EPS improved with olanzapine and worsened with haloperidol; patients in olanzapine group gained weight whereas those in haloperidol group lost weight
Sajatovic et al. (1998)	Patients with schizophrenia [27] & history of antipsychotic responsiveness	70.6; 65–80	8.4	No significant reduction in psychiatric symptoms but significant reduction in EPS; no significant effect on comorbid medical conditionsor cognition
Tollefson et al. (1997) Subset analysis from larger trial	Acute mania [8]	61–67	16	Olanzapine produced improvements in mania and psychosis compared to placebo and did not worsen depression; EPS improved; no adverse effects
Satterlee et al. (1995)	Outpatients with AD & psychosis [238]	78.6; 64–94	2.4	No statistically significant difference in either efficacy or adverse effects (EPS, weight gain, EKG changes) between olanzapine and placebo; only 69 patients received 5 mg or more of olanzapine

OLANZAPINE IM AND LORAZEPAM IM

Study	Population	Age (mean; range)	Dose	Results
Meehan et al. (2002)	Agitated patients with AD, VD, mixed dementia [272]	77.6; 54–97	L: 1.0–2.5 O: 2.5–12.5	2 hours postinjection, both drugs significantly better than placebo; 24 hours postinjection, olanzapine superior compared to lorazepam & placebo for reducing excitation; side effects of both drugs similar to placebo

QUETIAPINE

Study	Population	Age (mean; range)	Dose	Results
Tariot et al. (2000)	AD [80], PD [41], schizophrenia [32], psychosis due to vascular disease [11], delusional disorder [8], SAD [6], bipolar disorder [5], major depression with psychosis [1]	76.1; 54–94	137.5	48% of patients completed study; significant reduction in psychosis in 49%; most common side effects: somnolence, dizziness, postural hypotension
Fernandez et al. (1999)	PD [35] with drug-induced psychosis	75; 58–89	40.6	Significant improvement in psychosis in 20/24 patients; no decline in motor function; 3/24 withdrew due to side effects (orthostatic hypotension, nausea, headache)

QUETIAPINE AND RISPERIDONE

Study	Population	Age (mean; range)	Dose	Results
Mintzer et al. (2001) Subset analysis of elderly patients from a larger study by Mullen et al. (2001)	Schizophrenia and related psychotic disorders including SAD, affective psychosis, delusional disorder, dementia [92]	65–87	Q 200 R 3	Both drugs significantly improved psychotic symptoms, with no significant differences in efficacy between groups; EPS, akathisia significantly less frequent in quetiapine group compared to risperidone group.

(continued)

Table 7.4. *(continued)*

Study[a]	Study Population [N]	Age (mean; range)	Dose (mg) (mean; range)	Results
		RISPERIDONE		
Brodaty et al. (2003)	AD [180], VD [88], mixed dementia [41] in nursing homes	83	0.95	Study completed by 73% of patients in risperidone group versus 67% of patients in placebo group; significant improvement in aggression, agitation, & psychosis; at least 1 adverse event (esp. sedation, UTI) reported by 94% of patients in risperidone group (versus 92% in placebo group); EPS rate with risperidone not significantly different than with placebo
Chan et al. (2001)	AD [46], VD [12]	H: 80.8 R: 80.2	H: 0.90 R: 0.85	Only 3 patients did not complete study; both haloperidol & risperidone significantly reduced frequency & severity of behavioral symptoms; haloperidol associated with increased frequency of EPS compared to risperidone
Davidson et al. (2000)	Schizophrenia [170], schizophreniform disorder [10]	73; 54–89	3.7	Only 54% of patients completed study; however, of these, 54% had 20% or greater reduction in PANSS total score; 10% had adverse effects, including EPS, sedation, and dizziness; significant reduction in severity of preexisting EPS, low incidence of TD
De Deyn et al. (1999)	AD [229], VD [90], mixed dementia [25]	81; 56–97	R: 1.1; 0.5–4 H: 1.2; 0.5–4	Compared to placebo, both drugs associated with significantly reduced aggression; at doses of 0.75–1.5 mg/day of risperidone, EPS not significantly different from placebo, and less than with haloperidol

Study	Diagnosis [n]	Age	Dose	Results
Katz et al. (1999)	AD [456], VD [97], mixed dementia [72]	82.7	1.2; 0.5–2	Significant reductions in behavioral symptoms in patients treated with either 1 or 2 mg/day of risperidone compared to those treated with placebo; 2 mg/day of risperidone associated with increased EPS, but at 0.5 or 1mg/day, EPS comparable to placebo
Madhusoodanan et al. (1999)	Schizophrenia or SAD [103]	71	2.4	Significant improvement in psychosis for 50% of patients; well tolerated overall
Berman et al. (1996)	Schizophrenia [10]	71; 66–81	4–6	Patients titrated to 6 mg/day; 1 patient required dosage reduction to 4 mg/day after developing restlessness; overall, psychopathology and cognitive ratings improved; no serious side effects or EPS
Jeste et al. (1996)	Nursing home patients with severe behavior problems or dementia [10]	67; 47–79	3.9; 0.5–8	7 patients improved markedly from baseline; 2 others improved moderately; 1 patient worsened following initiation of risperidone and improved after drug was withdrawn; risperidone well tolerated in remaining patients
Jeste et al. (1996)	Severely agitated or psychotic nursing home patients with multiple medical problems [14]	71; 54–100	1.7; 0.25–6	2 patients developed disruptive behavior or refused medication (considered treatment failures); remaining 12 showed marked or moderate improvement in psychotic symptoms; risperidone well tolerated in all patients
Allen et al. (1995)	Lewy body dementia [3]	72; 66–78	0.66; 0.5–1.0	Marked reductions in all patients in psychotic and other behavioral symptoms; risperidone well tolerated except for worsening mild EPS in 1 patient

(continued)

Table 7.4. *(continued)*

Study[a]	Study Population [N]	Age (mean; range)	Dose (mg) (mean; range)	Results
Jeanblanc & Davis (1995)	Severely agitated or violent nursing home patients [5]	82; 77–91	1.5–2.5	Maximum benefit observed in 7–10 days in dose range of 1.5–2.5 mg/day; 2 patients developed EPS that resolved after treatment with amantadine; greater participation in social activity and ability to follow directions
Madhusoodanan et al. (1995)	Acute exacerbation of Schizophrenia [6] Schizoaffective disorder [3] Bipolar disorder [2] Senile dementia [2]	69; 61–79	4.9; 1.5–6	8 patients responded; 4 experienced reduced EPS or TD symptoms; hypotension necessitated discontinuation in 2 patients, but risperidone was otherwise well tolerated
Raheja et al. (1995)	Agitated and withdrawn patients [2]	79; 76–82	3	1 patient developed orthostatic hypotension and tremors on 4 mg/day; behavior symptoms returned when risperidone was withdrawn
Meco et al. (1994)	L-dopa-induced hallucinations [6]	71; 67–79	0.67; 0.25–1.25	Hallucinations decreased in 3 patients, disappeared completely in the other 3; severity of Parkinson's disease unchanged

[a] Complete reference citations at end of chapter.

ventional agents such as haloperidol. Treatment of patients with schizophrenia or dementia with risperidone can lead to improved global cognition after initiating treatment. Risperidone has been shown to be a useful antipsychotic in elderly patients, for whom the starting doses may be as low as 0.25 mg per day, which is considerably lower than those required for their younger counterparts.[67] Serum levels of risperidone may be increased by inhibitors of CYP 2D6, such as fluoxetine, cimetidine, and quinidine.[12]

Risperidone has been associated with a small increased risk of stoke in nursing home residents over 80. Since this population is already at very high risk for medical complications of pharmacologic therapies, the impact of these observations on prescribing atypical antipsychotic drugs for agitation in this population is unknown.

Olanzapine

Olanzapine became available in the United States in 1996. Although it is associated with a low frequency of EPS, it is quite sedating and has some potential for inducing anticholinergic effects and orthostasis in elderly patients. As with younger patients, olanzapine is associated with significant weight gain in older patients. This effect may be beneficial for elderly patients such as nursing home residents, who may have lost weight due to dementia, depression, or medical illness. However, for patients who are overweight, olanzapine may lead to undesirable weight gain as well as associated metabolic disturbances such as type 2 diabetes and dyslipidemia. Therefore, baseline body weight, blood glucose, hemoglobin A_{1c}, cholesterol and trigliceride levels are recommended for patients beginning treatment with olanzapine.

Based on the limited studies available, olanzapine is considered a safe and effective treatment for psychosis in older patients. The starting dose is 1.25 to 2.5 mg per day, and the target maintenance dose is between 5 and 15 mg/day (lower doses for patients with dementia), usually administered at bedtime. A unique feature of olanzapine for elderly patients is its availability in a rapidly dissolving oral tablet form. It can be used by patients who are unable to swallow pills because of medical illness (e.g., stroke) as wellas for rapid control of agitation and/or psychosis. Studies in younger adults identify olanzapine's mood-stabilizing properties. Thus, although studies in older patients are currently lacking, the potential exists for use of olanzapine for treatment of mania in this population. Like clozapine, olanzapine levels may be increased by CYP 1A2 inhibitors.

Olanzapine has been associated with a small increased risk of stoke in nursing home residents over 80. Since this population is already at very high risk for medical complications of pharmacologic therapies, the impact of these observations on prescribing atypical antipsychotic drugs for agitation in this population is unknown.

Quetiapine

Quetiapine was marketed in the United States in 1997. The high $5\text{-}HT_2$ to D_2-receptor blockade ratio accounts for the low potential for EPS with quetiapine. In terms of its receptor-binding profile, the most potent action of quetiapine is as an inhibitor of histamine H_1-receptors, which contributes to significant sedation. In addition, α-1-adrenergic receptor antagonism occurs, causing orthostatic hypotension, which tends to manifest as dizziness or lightheadedness in older patients. Quetiapine has very little, if any, anticholinergic potential.

Overall, quetiapine is a safe and effective agent for treating psychosis and disruptive behavior in elderly patients, with a starting dose of 12.5 to 25 mg per day. Although its shorter half-life calls for 2 or 3 doses per day, quetiapine can be effective when administered as a single bedtime dose. Because of its sedating effect, it is particularly useful for elderly patients with insomnia associated with nightime agitation or psychosis. The low frequency of EPS observed with this drug has led to its increasing role for patients with psychosis associated with Parkinson's disease. In terms of drug interactions, quetiapine levels may be increased by ketoconazole (CYP 3A4 inhibitors e.g., alprazolam, erythromycin) and decreased by CYP inducers (e.g., phenytoin, carbamazepine, barbiturates).

Ziprasidone

Ziprasidone was approved by the FDA in 2001. Although no published data on its use for elderly patients are available, clinical experience indicates that ziprasidone is becoming a useful medication for this population. In terms of its side effects, it has been associated with negligible weight gain and metabolic disturbances in younger adult patients. In addition, it has low potential for EPS, anticholinergic effects, or hyperprolactinemia. Although ziprasidone causes some prolongation of the QTc interval, this effect has not been found to have any clinical significance.

Because it can produce some physical activation, ziprasidone may be useful for elderly patients with apathy associated with dementia or negative symptoms of schizophrenia. Although anecdotal reports suggest that 20 mg per day may be an appropriate starting dose for older patients, data are not yet available to confirm whether this is a safe and effective dose. Although ziprasidone appears to interact minimally with other medications in vitro, CYP 3A4 inhibitor may increase serum levels, and carbamazepine (CYP 3A4 inducer) may reduce serum levels of ziprasidone.[68] An intramuscular formulation of ziprasidone is better tolerated than intramuscular haloperidol for younger and middle-aged adult patients with acute agitation associated with a psychotic disorder.[69]

Aripiprazole

The newest atypical antipsychotic to be approved by the FDA, aripiprazole, arrived on the U.S. market in 2002. Aripiprazole may act either as an antagonist or as a partial agonist at dopamine receptors, depending on existing levels of dopamine in the brain. Because it is also a partial agonist at the $5HT_{1A}$ receptor, aripiprazole may be the first of a new generation of antipsychotics known as *dopamine-serotonin system stabilizers*.[70] The potential for aripiprazole to autoregulate dopamine levels is expected to minimize EPS and hyperprolactinemia.[54,71] In addition, aripiprazole may possess the least α-1-adrenergic, anticholinergic, and antihistaminic potential of all the atypical antipsychotics.[72] The long half-life (i.e., 72 hours) of aripiprazole could benefit elderly patients who may not adhere to medication schedules. Controlled studies of aripiprazole in older patients are needed in order to determine safety, efficacy, and optimal dosing.

Treatment of Agitation with Non-Antipsychotic Drugs

Increasingly, nonantipsychotics have been used to treat severely agitated elderly patients. These medications have been used, particularly for patients with dementia, as alternatives to antipsychotics either for patients who may either not respond to them or tolerate their side effects or in situations where psychosis has not been established. Important to remember is that the use of a psychotropic medication for nonpsychotic agitation is considered an off-label use, as the FDA does not currently specify agitation as an indication for treatment.

Various classes of nonantipsychotic medications have been used, including drugs that affect the serotonin neurotransmission system (trazodone, buspirone, selective serotonin reuptake inhibitor [SSRI] antidepressants), anticonvulsants, β-blockers, benzodiazepines, cholinesterase inhibitors, and hormones. Although controlled data supporting the efficacy and tolerability of these agents are limited, clinical experience suggests that they can be useful for some patients. Further research is necessary to better understand the types of patients for whom these compounds may be particularly appropriate. The use of nonantipsychotic drugs to control agitation is summarized in Table 7.5.

Drugs Affecting Serotonin Neurotransmission

Trazodone, buspirone, as well as some SSRIs may be effective in treating geriatric agitation.

Trazodone

Trazodone has been widely used for the treatment of agitation and is effective both for the management of acute agitation as well as for prevention of further episodes of severe disordered behavior. In patients who respond, disruptive behaviors usually decrease significantly within 2 to 4 weeks following initiation of trazodone treatment. Doses of trazodone for treatment of agitation in elderly patients usually range from 50 to 300 mg per day. Although sedation is common, other side effects are mild and usually do not affect the older patient's physical health. Priapism, a rare side effect of trazodone in young and middle-age males, has not been reported in elderly males. Nevertheless, if penile swelling is observed, trazodone should be discontinued immediately and emergency urological consultation should be obtained.

Buspirone

The published evidence for use of buspirone in agitated elderly patients is scant relative to that of other nonantipsychotic treatments. From available studies and case reports, the dose of buspirone necessary for clinical efficacy may range from 5 mg to as much as 80 mg per day. Clinical experience suggests that doses above 40

mg per day are usually necessary in order to be effective. Therapeutic effect may not be apparent for 1 to 2 weeks at full therapeutic doses. Occasionally, buspirone may increase agitation in an elderly patient with dementia; significant sedation is unusual but can occur.

SSRI Antidepressants

Studies of SSRIs for treating agitated behavior have reported conflicting results. Anecdotal reports of SSRIs have suggested favorable results whereas double-blind studies have generally reported mixed results. Whether or not SSRI antidepressants can adequately control severely disruptive behavior seen in nursing homes and hospitals has not yet been determined. However, in milder forms of agitation, commonly seen in the early and middle stages of dementia when the patient is still living at home or in the community, clinical experience suggests that these antidepressants may significantly reduce disruptive behavior. It is important to monitor the older patient frequently, however, since SSRIs may lose their therapeutic effect as the dementia progresses and may actually worsen agitation in more severe forms of the illness. Moreover, in a large study of elderly nursing home residents, rates of falls among patients treated with SSRIs were reported to be approximately equivalent to those treated with tertiary amine tricyclic antidepressants (TCAs).[73]

Anticonvulsants

Conventional anticonvulsants, such as carbamazepine and valproate, as well as newer agents, such as gabapentin and topiramate, may also provide treatment for geriatric agitation.

Carbamazepine

An effective treatment for patients whose dementia has components of agitation, rage, combativeness, and mood lability, carbamazepine may bring about behavioral improvement within 2 to 4 weeks or

Table 7.5. Studies of Nonantipsychotic Treatment of Agitation in the Elderly

Study[a]	Study Population[b] [N]	Age[c] (mean; range)	Dose[c,d] (mg) (mean; range)	Results
ALPRAZOLAM and HALOPERIDOL				
Christensen et al. (1997)	"Organic mental syndromes" (delirium, dementia, & other cognitive disorders) [48]	83; 65–98	H: 0.64; 0.1–1.0 A: 1.0	Alprazolam as effective as haloperidol and produced less EPS
BUSPIRONE				
Levy et al. (1994)	Probable AD [20]	73[e]	60	Global ratings same with drug and placebo; buspirone improved anxiety, delusions, and aggressive symptoms over placebo
Herrmann & Eryavec (1993)	SDAT [7], MID [6], alcoholic dementia [3]	78; 65–89	15–45	Reduced agitation and aggression in 7 patients
Sakauye et al. (1993)	AD [10]	83; 75–92	60	With 60 mg/day, 22% reduction of agitation scores; maximum benefit at 30–40 mg/day
CARBAMAZEPINE				
Olin et al. (2001)	AD [21; 16 completers]	75;	388	Modest overall benefit, esp. for hostility, in patients who had previously not responded to antipsychotics
Tariot et al. (1998)	AD [33], MID [13], mixed dementia [5]	63–86 86	(serum level 4.9; 3.7–6.8)	Moderate improvement in agitation; significantly better than placebo
Tariot et al. (1994)	AD [17], MID [8]	85	304 (serum level 5.3) 288	Marked global improvements in agitation symptoms
Gleason & Schneider (1990)	Probable AD [91]	72; 60–85	200–1000	Improvements in tension, hostility, uncooperativeness and agitation

Study	Diagnosis [N]	Age	Dose	Results
Marin & Greenwald (1989)	AD [2], MID [1]	71; 70–72	100–300	Marked reduction in irritability and combativeness
Leibovici & Tariot (1988)	Dementia [2]	81,85	300,500	Agitated behavior diminished following addition of carbamazepine
Patterson (1988)	Dementia [13]	48–69	N/A	Incidents of assaultive behavior decreased ~50% following carbamazepine
Patterson (1987)	Organic brain disease [8]	52; 37–66	~400	Decreased assaultive incidents
McAllister (1985)	Mixed frontal lobe and psychiatric disorders [5]	60; 52–69	820; 400–1900	Remarkable improvement in affective lability in 5 patients
Chambers et al. (1982)	Senile dementia [19]	80	100–300	No difference between drug and placebo
CITALOPRAM				
Pollock et al. (1997)	AD [13], MID [1], dementia NOS [2]	77.6	20	Significant reduction in behavioral symptoms in majority of patients; well tolerated by most patients
CITALOPRAM and PERPHENAZINE				
Pollock et al. (2002)	AD [61], dementia NOS [16], VD [6], mixed dementia [2]	C: 80.9 P: 80.4	C: 20 P: 6.5	Significant improvement in agitation and aggression with both drugs compared to baseline; however, only citalopram was more efficacious than placebo; side effects comparable to placebo in both groups
DONEPEZIL				
Gauthier et al. (2002)	AD [207]	74.3; 48–92	?	Improvement in behavioral symptoms significantly greater than with placebo; well tolerated overall
Paleacu et al. (2002)	AD [28]	79; 54–96	9.1	Significant improvement in behavior; well tolerated
Feldman et al. (2001)	AD [290]	73.6; 48–92	?	Improvement in behavior significantly better than with placebo; well tolerated overall

(continued)

Table 7.5.   *(continued)*

Study[a]	Study Population[b] [N]	Age[c] (mean; range)	Dose[c,d] (mg) (mean; range)	Results
Tariot et al. (2001)	AD [208]	85.7; 64–102	9.5	Improvement in behavior NOT significantly different compared to placebo, but well tolerated overall
Cummings et al. (2000)	AD [332]	?	?	Significantly reduced behavior disturbance in patients taking donepezil
		ESTROGENS		
Kyomen et al. (2002); Kyomen et al. (1999)	Dementia [14]	84	CE: 0.625–2.5	Significant reduction in aggression, even at lowest dose, without adverse effects
Kyomen et al. (1991)	Probable AD [2]	71,92	CE: 1.25 DES: 2	Marked reduction in sexual and physical aggression following addition of estrogen compounds
		FLUOXETINE		
Geldmacher (1994)	Probable AD [5]	77	40	No improvement on several psychometric tests
	FLUOXETINE (F) and HALOPERIDOL (H)			
Auchus et al. (1997)	AD [15]	75.6	F: 20 H: 3.0	Neither drug more effective than placebo; both produced more side effects than placebo
		FLUVOXAMINE		
Olafsson et al. (1992)	Degenerative or MID [46]	65–93	150	Minimal improvement in irritability, anxiety, and confusion; behavior and cognition unchanged
		GABAPENTIN		
Herrmann et al. (2000)	AD [7], VD [3], FTD [1], Alcoholic dementia [1], who did not respond to antipsychotics	79.3	900	No significant change in behavior (NPI, CMAI), but improvement on CGI; high frequency of side effects such as sedation, gait instability

LORAZEPAM AND ALPRAZOLAM

Study	Diagnosis [N]	Age	Dose	Outcome
Ancill et al. (1991)	Agitated patients with dementing disorder [40]	L 78 A 80	L: 1–6 A: 0.5–3	Global ratings improved 29% in lorazepam-treated patients, 42% in those treated with alprazolam

METRIFONATE

Study	Diagnosis [N]	Age	Dose	Outcome
Cummings et al. (2001)	Probable AD [648]	74	Study A 43 Study B 50	Reduced psychiatric and behavioral symptoms including agitation; well tolerated overall

PROPRANOLOL

Study	Diagnosis [N]	Age	Dose	Outcome
Weiler et al. (1988)	Senile dementia [6]	73; 66–83	80–560	Diminished agitated behavior in all 6 patients
Greendyke et al. (1986)	Organic brain disease [10]	52; 27–75	520	Improvements in assaultive behavior
Greendyke et al. (1984)	Organic brain disease [8]	56; 43–79	465; 200–520	Marked decrease in assaultive behavior and outbursts
Jenike (1983)	Senile and presenile dementia, behavior disorder [3]	54–86	60–160	Diminished aggressive and destructive behavior
Petrie & Ban (1981)	Senile [2] and presenile dementia [1]	54–86	60–160	Agitation and wandering behavior improved

RIVASTIGMINE

Study	Diagnosis [N]	Age	Dose	Outcome
McKeith et al. (2000)	LBD [120]	73.9; 57–87	9.4	Significantly reduced anxiety, delusions, & hallucinations compared to placebo; GI side effects more frequent compared to placebo but well tolerated overall

TRAZODONE

Study	Diagnosis [N]	Age	Dose	Outcome
Houlihan et al. (1994)	Dementia patients requiring psychiatric hospitalization [22]	81; 64–91	172; 25–500	Moderate to marked improvement in 82% of patients after addition of trazodone
Lebert et al. (1994)	AD [13]	70	75	Improvement in irritability, restlessness, and anxiety for 10 patients

(continued)

Table 7.5. *(continued)*

Study[a]	Study Population[b] [N]	Age[c] (mean; range)	Dose[c,d] (mg) (mean; range)	Results
Aisen et al. (1993)	AD [16]	77	180; 100–300	Trazodone addition resulted in at least a mild benefit in 13, 10 of whom tolerated the drug
Pinner & Rich (1988)	Organic mental disorders and physically aggressive behavior [7]	63; 52–71	279; 150–400	Marked improvement in 3 patients; no improvement in 3
Simpson & Foster (1986)	Organic brain syndrome [4]	67; 62–72	375; 200–500	Improved patient cooperation and behavior
		TRAZODONE and BUSPIRONE		
Lawlor et al. (1994)	AD [10]	67 T B 30	150	Small decreases in agitation, psychosis, hostility, and disruption; no difference between buspirone and placebo
		VALPROATE		
Porsteinsson et al. (2001)	AD [40], VD [10], mixed dementia [6]	85	826; 375–1375 Serum level 45; 22–85	Mild reduction in agitation in valproate group compared to placebo but higher frequency of adverse effects
Kunik et al. (1998)	Dementia [13]	71.3; 65–82	846 Serum level 48	Significant reduction in general psychiatric symptoms, overall agitation, physical aggression, and nonaggressive physical agitation; well tolerated
Porsteinsson et al. (1997)	Dementia (including 1 with comorbid schizophrenia and 1 with comorbid SAD) [12], mental retardation (MR) [1]	81.6; 65–97	250–1500 Serum level 33–107	Reduced agitation in some patients; well tolerated

Study	Diagnosis [n]	Age	Dose	Results/Comments
Puryear et al. (1995)	Bipolar disorder [7], organic mental disorder [3], SAD [2], schizophrenia [1]	63–81	1000; 250–750 Serum level 56.5 34–82	Significant improvement in general psychiatric symptoms; well tolerated overall
Lott et al. (1995)	AD [5], MID [2], senile dementia NOS [3]	71–94	525; 375–750	Frequency of agitated behavior diminished by 50% or more in 8 patients following valproate
Sival et al. (1994)	AD [13], dementia NOS [7], MID [2], other [1]	M, 79 F, 82	481; 240–1200	Complete cessation of disturbed behavior in 26% of patients; long-term reduction of disturbed behavior in 52%
Wilcox et al. (1994)	Schizophrenia [12], bipolar [10], border-line personality [10], schizoaffective [2]	31; 19–62	1000; 750–1500	Reduced agitation and marked decrease in time spent in seclusion
Mellow et al. (1993)	Dementia [4]	70; 65–83	1750; 1000–2500	Improved behavior in 2 patients, transient improvement in 1, 1 experienced no behavior improvement
Mazure et al. (1992)	Schizoaffective disorder [1], schizophrenia [1]	63,68	1000, 2000	Dramatic decreases in agitated, assaultive, and disruptive behavior
ZOLPIDEM				
Jackson et al. (1996)	AD [2]	64,86	2.5–5	Markedly decreased agitation

[a] Complete references at end of chapter.
[b] AD, Alzheimer's disease; MID, multi-infarct dementia; NOS, not otherwise specified; SDAT, senile dementia of Alzheimer's type; VD, vascular dementia; FTD, fronto-temporal dementia; SAD, schizo-affective disorder.
[c] Age and Dose expressed in mean and range, when given.
[d] CE, conjugated estrogens; DES, diethylstibesterol; N/A, not stated.
[e] L, lorazepam; A, alprazolam.

even sooner. Relatively low doses of carbamazepine (200 to 300 mg/day) can be used, and patients are likely to respond at plasma levels below the therapeutic range used for treatment of seizures (4 to 12 g/mL). In elderly patients, sedation is the most common side effect of carbamazepine, and mild transient leukopenia develops in approximately 10% of patients. A review of the patient's medications is prudent before administering carbamazepine, as the drug is a potent metabolism-inducer. Guidelines for use of carbamazepine are described in Chapter 12.

Because carbamazepine can cause agranulocytosis, a baseline white blood cell count should be obtained before drug treatment is initiated. There is no evidence, however, to suggest that elderly patients are more susceptible to carbamazepine-induced agranulocytosis than their younger counterparts.

Valproate

Valproate is used increasingly to treat behavioral agitation in elderly patients, and a growing number of studies suggest that valproate may substantially reduce behavioral agitation without significant sedation or other cognitive side effects. Doses of valproate that have been used for treatment of agitation range from 240 to 2500 mg per day, with corresponding plasma levels of 45 to 90 mg/L. Although some patients have experienced some drowsiness and sedation, these side effects appear to be relatively mild. Before administering valproate, a review of patient medications is warranted, as this drug is known for several adverse drug interactions.

Newer Anticonvulsants

In comparison to valproate and carbamazepine, the newer anticonvulsants (e.g., gabapentin, topiramate, oxcarbazepine) may be better tolerated by older patients. However, their efficacy has not been established in controlled studies involving older adults.

Additional Nonantipsychotics

Beta-blockers

A nonantipsychotic drug that blocks postsynaptic β-adrenergic receptor sites, propranolol has been used successfully to treat agitation, assaultiveness, and explosive outbursts of rage in older psychotic or demented patients.[74] Propranolol may be preferable to antipsychotics for some older patients because it carries no risk of extrapyramidal symptoms, anticholinergic reactions, or TD.

Dosages of propranolol vary considerably for older patients, depending on the individual's psychiatric and medical condition. Starting dosages should be 10 mg two or three times a day, with increases of 10 mg each day thereafter. When no toxic effects occur, or in cases of severe agitation, more rapid dosage increments may be necessary. The therapeutic range of propranolol in most cases is between 80 and 100 mg per day. Appearance of clinical effects usually correlates with slowed pulse rate, indicating effective β-receptor blockade.

Propranolol should be used with extreme caution in patients with asthma or heart disease. It is contraindicated in patients with cardiogenic shock, sinus bradycardia, heart block (greater than first degree), and most cases of congestive heart failure. Propranolol causes bradycardia and hypotension and should be used with caution in hypotensive patients.

Because depression has also been associated with the use of propanolol, evaluation of the mood as well as the cardiovascular status of the patient is essential prior to starting propranolol therapy. Once therapy begins, vital signs must be taken regularly, and cardiovascular functioning must be monitored. To date, the reported use of propranolol for extended periods to control behavior of older patients has been scant.

Benzodiazepines

Benzodiazepines have been used widely for treating acute outbursts of agitation and other behavioral problems, although few studies in elderly patients with dementia or schizophrenia are available. Reduced agitation has been demonstrated in some patients with short-term treatment, and benzodiazepines appear to be as effective as antipsychotics in treating target symptoms. Sedation is much more likely to occur with benzodiazepine treatment than with antipsychotics. The short-acting benzodiazepines (e.g., lorazepam, alprazolam, oxazepam) are preferred over the long-acting agents (e.g., diazepam, clonazepam), and relatively small doses (lorazepam 0.5 to 4 mg/day or oxazepam 10 to 60 mg/day) are recommended. Some caution must be exercised in using benzodiazepines to treat agitation, however; use of these agents in elderly patients is associated with cognitive impairment as well as falls. In fact, for nursing home residents, although the risk of falls with short-acting benzodiazepines decreases compared to that with with long-acting agents, the risk still increases significantly above baseline.[75]

Controversy continues regarding the appropriate use of benzodiazepines for the treatment of late-life disruptive behavior. Allegations that benzodiazepines have been overused in nursing homes for behavior control have led to the establishment of regulations governing the use of benzodiazepines in nursing homes (see Chapter 16). There are concerns regarding possible behavior disinhibition, as well as memory and concentration impairment with this class of medication. Despite these concerns, occasional use of benzodiazepines to control behavior may be practical, effective, and safe for the disruptive elderly patient if appropriate guidelines for their use are followed. Although benzodiazepines have been shown to be as effective as antipsychotics for treatment of agitation in nursing home residents,[76] these data are from older studies and should not be used as current treatment recommendations. As outlined in Chapter 16, low doses and

brief use of short half-life compounds are advised.

A nonbenzodiazepine with benzodiazepine-like properties, zolpidem, has also been reported useful for the control of agitation in elderly patients with dementia.[77] Since other psychotropic drugs are available for the control of disruptive behavior, benzodiazepine-like agents should not be used as a first-line treatment. Rather, they should be reserved for those elderly patients who do not respond to other treatment approaches or who cannot tolerate other psychotropic drugs.

Cholinesterase Inhibitors

Agents known as cholinesterase (ChE) inhibitors have been developed to increase cholinergic activity in the brains of patients with AD (see Chapter 20). Three medications belonging to this class are currently approved: donepezil, rivastigmine, and galantamine. By preventing the breakdown of acetylcholine by acetylcholinesterase, these agents increase the concentration of acetylcholine. This process is believed to account for the beneficial effects of ChE inhibitors on cognition and function in patients with AD. Cholinergic dysfunction may also contribute to neuropsychiatric symptoms in patients with AD: ChE inhibitors may benefit specific symptoms such as delusions, hallucinations, agitation, anxiety, and apathy in patients with dementia.

The most common side effects of these medications are gastrointestinal, including nausea, vomiting, decreased appetite, weight loss, and diarrhea. Dizziness, headache, increased physical activity, and insomnia have also limited the use of ChE inhibitors in older patients. They are contraindicated in patients with active peptic ulcer disease and sick sinus syndrome.

These agents may offer a valuable treatment alternative for elderly patients with dementia and behavioral disturbances who cannot tolerate antipsychotic medications (e.g., those with Lewy body dementia). However, additional safety and efficacy data are needed before ChE inhibitors can be considered for approval for this purpose.

Hormones

Clinical experience suggests that female hormones may decrease aggressive behavior and inappropriate sexual behavior in elderly men. Both medroxyprogesterone as well as conjugated estrogens have been used to suppress aggressive sexual behavior in older male patients with dementia. Additional controlled studies are necessary to demonstrate the safety and efficacy of hormone treatment.

Use of Antipsychotics in Difficult Clinical Situations

Comorbid conditions of TD and parkinsonism, agitation and EPS, Parkinson disease and L-dopa–induced psychosis occur more frequently than has been recognized. Treatment of these coexisting conditions in elderly patients may be extremely difficult.

Tardive Dyskinesia, Parkinsonism, and the Elderly Patient

The coexistence of TD and parkinsonian symptoms, previously thought to be unusual, is not infrequently observed in the elderly patient. In fact, AIP may develop in over half of patients with TD. Treatment of TD often makes parkinsonism worse, and vice versa: For example, using anticholinergic medications to treat AIP frequently exacerbates TD, and decreasing these anticholinergic medications in an attempt to improve TD leads to inadequate control of the parkinsonism. Discontinuing antipsychotic treatment will reduce parkinsonian symptoms and may decrease TD, but increased agitation or psychosis will result. If discontinuing an antipsychotic is not clinically feasible, it is important to discuss with the elderly patient, when possible, which side effects are most distressing. For many elderly patients, parkinsonian symptoms are much more incapacitating than TD.

For some older psychotic or agitated patients, substituting an alternative drug or adding a medication that will facilitate reduced antipsychotic dosage may be feasible. For example, antipsychotic dosage may be reduced when a benzodiazepine or other antiagitation drug is added. Electroconvulsive therapy (ECT) may be administered for the most severe cases in which psychotic depression, TD, and AIP coexist. In some instances, electroconvulsive therapy (ECT) is effective for all three of these conditions.

Agitation and Extrapyramidal Side Effects

Akathisia and AIP may be easily confused with agitation in elderly patients. A simple and usually effective way to distinguish AIP from agitation is to determine if anticholinergic medication (such as benztropine or its equivalent) is effective. AIP is rapidly relieved by 1 to 2 mg of such a drug, whereas agitation generally either remains unaffected or may become somewhat worse.

L-Dopa–Induced Psychosis in Parkinson's Disease

Some elderly patients who are psychotic may develop PD, and some patients with PD may become psychotic (see Chapter 11). It can be quite challenging to treat a patient with psychosis *and* PD. Conventional antipsychotic drugs tend to worsen the movement disorder, whereas L-Dopa frequently induces or exacerbates psychosis. Treatment for PD is associated with the development of psychosis in as many as 60% of patients treated over long periods of time. Initially, psychosis induced by L-Dopa is usually mild, characterized by hallucinations and illusions, but it may progress to a more severe paranoid psychosis that warrants treatment.

Recent experience suggests that certain atypical antipsychotics may be effective in the management of psychosis that either coexists with PD or is a result of L-Dopa treatment. In two double-blind studies involving patients with PD with drug-induced psychosis, clozapine was reported to be safe and efficacious without worsening motor function.[78,79]

Considerable progress has been made in the pharmacologic treatment of the common and difficult clinical problem of late-life agitation and psychosis. Although one or more medication trials may be necessary, most behavior disorders can now be safely and effectively managed with appropriate pharmacotherapy.

Clinical Vignettes

Case 7.1

Mr. A., a 78-year-old retired insurance salesman with moderately advanced AD lived at home with his wife, his full-time caregiver. Mrs. A. had been assisting her husband with dressing, feeding, toileting, and bathing for several years, but admitted recent deterioration of her own health. Nonetheless, she insisted on keeping Mr. A. at home and caring for him herself. When her husband's physician suggested that she consider hiring some help at home to reduce the burden on herself, Mrs. A. claimed that she simply could not afford to hire extra help. ''Besides,'' she added, ''taking care of my husband isn't a burden.'' However, she noted that Mr. A. had declined significantly in his overall level of function over the week prior to her reporting increased apathy, reduced level of conversation, increased daytime napping, and decreased nocturnal sleep. At night, he had been getting up and wandering around the house, appearing confused and disoriented. He was eating poorly. Episodes of bladder incontinence were occurring more frequently than usual, and a few episodes of bowel incontinence, which had never occurred in the past, were present. He had refused to take a shower for several days and when Mrs. A. attempted to change his diaper, he became agitated, even combative, and very tearful. Mrs. A. became concerned and called Mr. A.'s psychiatrist to ask for a medication that would return Mr. A. to his usual self. She indicated that she had already tried increasing the dose of risperidone from 1.5 mg per day to 3 mg per day but that it had not improved his behavior at all. The psychiatrist recommended that Mrs. A. bring her husband into the urgent care center for a medical evaluation.

Upon arrival at the urgent care, Mr. A. was talking loudly and incoherently. He was extremely restless, and displayed a frightened affect. He pointed toward the floor and tugged at his wife's arm. On physical examination, Mr. A. was tachycardic with a heart rate of 115 per min. His blood pressure was $^{98}/_{55}$ in the supine position and dropped to 80/50 when he sat up. Oral temperature was 100.8°F; his skin was warm and flushed and his mucous membranes were dry; pupils were dilated. Bowel sounds were absent and bladder was distended. Mr. A. was immediately connected to a cardiac monitor and given intravenous fluids. The attending physician asked Mrs. A. what medications her husband had been receiving. Mrs. A. explained that Mr. A. was taking Elavil (amitriptyline) 75 mg at night for insomnia, hydrochlorothiazide 25 mg daily for hypertension, and risperidone 1.5 mg (3 mg for the last several days) for agitation.

The physician inquired about any recent surgeries and Mrs. A. stated that Mr. A. had undergone dental surgery a little over a week before. She explained that he had recently completed the antibiotics prescribed by the oral surgeon and that she had not seen any need to fill the prescription for painkillers that were given to her after his procedure. The physician asked Mrs. A. if she had all of Mr. A.'s medications with her and she produced the medication bottles from her purse. After examining the bottles, the physician discovered that the bottle that Mrs. A. believed to contain risperidone was actually labeled Cogentin (benztropine mesylate) 1 mg tablets. The physician explained to Mrs. A. that the medication that she had been giving her husband was making him sick.

Mr. A. was subsequently admitted to the medical intensive care unit with anticholinergic delirium and urinary retention. All of his medications were held and he was treated with intravenous physostigmine. Mr. A. also had a dental abscess and he was started on a different antibiotic and treated with intravenous morphine for the pain. His condition gradually improved with adequate hydration. Over the next several days, Mr. A.'s mental status returned to its previous baseline and he was discharged from the hospital with a referral to social services.

This case presents the not uncommon scenario of AD complicated by delirium. In this particular instance, the acute change in mental status had two precipitating sources. The first was untreated postsurgical pain, which frequently manifests with agitation in elderly individuals with dementia. The second was overuse of an anticholinergic medication (benztropine), which added to the anticholinergic effects of yet another medication (amitriptyline) being taken by the patient. The three drugs produced an intoxication syndrome. The inadvertent substitution of risperidone for benztropine (a medication commonly prescribed for treatment of extrapyramidal side effects produced by risperidone) by Mrs. A. may have been partially due to her growing caregiver burden under the stress of her husband's deterioration—illustrating one of the ways that caregiver burden can compromise the health of an elderly person with dementia. A social intervention such as in-home caregiving services, day treatment, respite care, or placement in an appropriate caregiving facility may reduce caregiver burden-related morbidity.

Case 7.2

Mrs. B., a 71-year-old retired nurse with two grown children had lived alone for 6 months after her husband had died from colon cancer. She had cared for him during the last year of his life as his illness progressed. Since her retirement several years before, Mrs. B. and her husband had moved to a rural farmhouse far away from the city. After their father's death, Mrs. B.'s children encouraged her to move back so that she could be closer to them. She seemed to spend almost all of her time alone inside the house and they became concerned about her social isolation. She had not been sleeping well ever since her husband's death and had given up her morning walk because she claimed that it was a painful reminder of her husband's absence. Still, Mrs. B. insisted that if she could take care of her husband during his illness, she could certainly take care of herself. "After all, (she was) a nurse."

During a visit to the farmhouse, however, Mrs. B.'s children noticed that she looked thin and fatigued. The food that they had brought for her a few weeks before was still unopened. When asked about her eating habits, she stated that there was "no point in eating," claiming that her body was decaying from cancer. She was certain of this fact, because she had been experiencing abdominal pain. She also remarked about a foul odor in the house that she attributed to her rotting flesh. She was preoccupied with a waxy substance on her skin that she believed was a sign of her tissues decaying. She stated that her husband's voice told her that as long as she didn't eat, they would be together soon.

Mrs. B.'s children were very concerned about her weight loss and irrational thinking. They suggested that she be evaluated by her physician, but she adamantly refused. Despite her protests, her son and daughter took her to the nearest hospital for evaluation. Her daughter petitioned for her involuntary admission to the psychiatric unit, based on the testimony of two psychiatrists who certified to the court that she was indeed gravely disabled as well as a danger to herself. Once admitted, Mrs. B. was started on 15 mg of the antidepressant mirtazepine at night to target her depression, insomnia, and decreased appetite, as well as 2.5 mg of olanzapine to reduce psychotic symptoms and to help her to regain the weight she had lost; olanzapine was titrated up to a dose of 10 mg and mirtazepine was titrated up to 30 mg at bedtime.

Unfortunately, Mrs. B. continued to eat poorly and to lose additional weight in the hospital; thus far she had lost 25 pounds, and insisted that her bowels had fallen out of her body. The attending psychiatrist on the unit decided that because of her poor insight into her delusional thinking and significant weight loss, the most appropriate intervention for Mrs. B. was ECT. She responded well to ECT within a few weeks: her affect brightened, her agitation diminished, and her appetite improved. Upon discharge from the hospital, she agreed to move into a seniors' apartment complex closer to her children. Mrs. B. was maintained on antidepressant treatment and did not experience any recurrence of psychotic symptoms.

This case illustrates the severe neurovegetative symptoms that can accompany a psychotic depression in an elderly patient. In some instances, antipsychotic medication may not be a practical treatment for such a patient if nutritional status has become precarious. ECT offers a potentially quicker treatment option for psychotic depression when a patient's physical health is at imminent risk.

Case 7.3

Mrs. C., an 80-year-old divorced woman who lived alone, had an extensive psychiatric history dating back to her mid-thirties, at which time she was hospitalized after a suicide attempt and treated with chlorpromazine. She was later diagnosed with bipolar disorder and maintained on lithium over the years. Mrs. C. had a history of alcohol abuse and had also abused various sleeping pills over the years to treat her "chronic insomnia." She had been married to a physician for many years who had prescribed her medications for her, but her drinking and chaotic lifestyle eventually led to a divorce. Since then, Mrs. C. went from doctor to doctor requesting prescriptions for alprazolam. She continued in this fashion for many years until she developed such a tolerance for the alprazolam that she required 10 mg/day in order to achieve the effect she desired.

Her primary care physician was concerned about her high dosage of alprazolam and convinced Mrs. C. to agree to switch to diazepam because of its longer elimination half-life. He explained to her that because diazepam would stay in her system longer, she would not have to take it as frequently and could avoid the withdrawal between doses. After a few days on diazepam, Mrs. C. called her physician's office to report that the medication wasn't strong enough. She complained that it did not put her to sleep the way alprazolam did. Her physician asked if she had ever taken anything else that had helped her to sleep. Mrs. C. recalled that the chlorpromazine she had received during her first hospitalization had been very sedating. Her physician wrote a prescription for 100 mg of chlorpromazine at bedtime. Mrs. C. found the medication effective, and over the following weeks, she used it up to 3 times during the daytime so that she could take naps. She then began to experience dizzy spells, especially when she got out of bed to walk to the bathroom. She also experienced cognitive clouding and urinary incontinence, particularly when she awaked from sleep.

At her next appointment, Mrs. C.'s physician observed her gait to be quite unsteady; she also seemed confused and tremulous, her speech was mildly dysarthric, and she could not provide a clear description of her activities in recent days. The physician referred Mrs. C. to the emergency department for some bloodwork and a CT head scan. Her lithium level was elevated at 1.8 and her CT scan revealed a subdural hematoma estimated to be approximately one week old. Evidently, Mrs. C. had fallen and hit her head, although she could not recall doing so. Lithium was discontinued, and she was treated with intravenous fluids and referred to neurosurgery for evacuation of the subdural hematoma.

This case illustrates the problem of polypharmacy in elderly patients. Conventional low-potency antipsychotics can produce excessive sedation, orthostatic hypotension, and anticholinergic effects. All of these effects can predispose elderly patients to falls and fractures, which lead to excessive morbidity and mortality. In this case, side effects were worsened by coadministration of diazepam, a long-acting benzodiazepine that tends to accumulate in the blood of many elderly patients. Several factors made this patient a poor candidate for such medications: her history of alcohol abuse, unreliable adherence with medication, and living alone. Because of its narrow therapeutic window and potential for toxicity, lithium also may not be an optimal choice for patients with this profile. Benzodiazepines should always be used cautiously in older patients. Shorter-acting agents, such as lorazepam, are preferred over

longer-acting agents, and benzodiazepines should not be used in combination with other sedating medications such as low-potency antipsychotics.

Case 7.4

Mr. D. was a 66-year-old divorced, retired carpenter who lived alone. About 9 months before hospital admission for leg pain, he had been diagnosed with glioblastoma multiforme, a malignant tumor in the frontal lobe of his brain for which he received radiation therapy and was treated with steroids to reduce the edema in his brain. Previously, Mr. D. had been healthy, without any other relevant medical or psychiatric history.

After uneventful surgery for repair of an inguinal hernia, Mr. D. was discharged home with a prescription for acetaminophen with codeine. One week later, he returned to the hospital emergency department complaining of pain in his left calf. After being examined by the attending physician, he was admitted to the general medical service for treatment of a deep vein thrombophlebitis (DVT). Mr. D. was anticoagulated with heparin and received meperidine and hydroxazine for his leg pain, after which he slept for several hours. That night, he awoke feeling disoriented and confused. He dialed the telephone operator and asked for the police department. Hearing the commotion, the ward nurse came over to ask if anything was wrong. Mr. D. was standing in front of the window holding a chair above his head, preparing to throw it against the window. The nurse grabbed the chair and attempted to take it away from him, but he struck out at her and called out loudly, "Help! Police!"

Shortly after, the hospital security staff arrived and the psychiatrist on call was paged. When the psychiatrist arrived, Mr. D. was sitting on his bed, surrounded by hospital security staff and several nurses. He was agitated, shouting at the staff in a belligerent tone and threatening to sue them if they did not allow him to leave the hospital. When the psychiatrist asked Mr. D. if he knew why he was in the hospital, Mr. D. looked confused, hesitated for a few moments, and then responded suspiciously, "You're not going to trick me into telling you what you want to know!" The psychiatrist attempted to reassure Mr. D., explaining to him that he was in the hospital receiving treatment for his swollen leg after his recent hernia surgery. The explanation increased Mr. D.'s paranoia, and he became more agitated and began to shout incoherently. Then he struggled to get out of his bed, lost his grip of the side bed rail and fell over, accidentally injuring the side of his head against the nightstand. The psychiatrist offered Mr. D. some medication orally, but he refused and assumed a threatening posture, gesturing violently with his hands. Based on Mr. D.'s continued danger to himself and others, the psychiatrist ordered 2 mg of haloperidol to be given intramuscularly. Mr. D. responded to the medication without adverse effects and he became less agitated over the next 10 minutes. The psychiatrist recommended discontinuing the demerol and vistaril and that a nonsteroidal antiinflammatory agent be used instead. After consulting with Mr. D.'s neurosurgeon, the decision was made to continue Mr. D.'s steroids for the time being. Bloodwork, urine and chest X-ray did not show any evidence of new infection.

The following day, Mr. D.'s daughter came to the hospital. The psychiatrist explained to her that her father's episode was not uncommon among patients with brain tumors, especially with the added effects of thrombophlebitis and medications. In addition, although Mr. D.'s condition had improved significantly overnight, he might experience recurrent episodes of confusion and agitation. Mr. D.'s daughter agreed to stay with her father to help reassure him, and over the next week, he did experience episodic agitation and paranoia. With the help of his daughter, the nursing staff was able to manage his symptoms with verbal redirection and occasional 0.5 mg oral doses of haloperidol. By the end of the week, Mr. D.'s behavior had normalized, his thrombophlebitis had resolved, and he was discharged on a lower dose of steroids.

This case illustrates the problem of postoperative delirium frequently experienced by older patients admitted to hospitals. The etiology of delirium is often multifactorial and might include infection, medication effects, untreated pain, and change in environment. This particular patient's delirium resulted from his readmission to the hospital with a DVT and receiving meperidine and hydroxazine, which are known to impair cognition and to induce delirium in elderly patients. Because of the severity of his psychosis and agitation, the patient's maintenance steroids were temporarily discontinued, based on their potential for inducing psychosis. Atypical or high-potency conventional antipsychotics (e.g., haloperidol) are preferred over low-potency agents for emergency treatment of psychosis and agitation in older patients with delirium. Low doses of these medications are recommended on a short-term basis in order to control symptoms that interfere with safety and care in the hospital setting.

Case 7.5

Mr. E., a 74-year-old married man, retired from the U.S. Navy, had been healthy until approximately 2 years previously when he stopped playing golf. He claimed that he couldn't swing the club the way he used to and became frustrated with his performance. Around the same time, Mrs. E. had begun to notice other changes in Mr. E.: he was becoming more forgetful and frequently misplaced his belongings. Although at times Mr. E. behaved quite normally, on other occasions he would become quite confused and agitated, accusing his wife of having an affair with a neighbor who lived across the street. When Mrs. E. tried to reassure him that she was not involved with another man, Mr. E. stated that he had seen the neighbor coming in and out of their bedroom and that he knew "what (they) were up to." Mrs. E. also reported that her husband was "seeing things," as he would frequently comment on people who were not present as if they were sitting in the room.

Mrs. E. arranged for her husband to be assessed by a neurologist. On examination, Mr. E. was alert and oriented to time but not to place; he thought he was at the naval base. His gait was bradykinetic, with reduced arm swing; his facial expression was masked; and there was increased tone in his extremities. He spoke very candidly of his wife's affair. Mini-Mental State Examination score was $^{24}/_{30}$, with rapid forgetting of two of three objects. The neurologist requested a CBC, chemistry, TSH, folate and Vitamin B12 levels, RPR and a brain MRI, all of which were within normal limits. He diagnosed Mr. E. with Lewy body dementia and prescribed donepezil 5 mg/day and quetiapine 100 mg at bedtime. On the way home from the neurologist's office, Mr. E. threatened to kill his wife if she did not identify the man with whom she was having an affair. Mrs. E. called 911, and the police subsequently brought Mr. E. to the emergency department for evaluation.

Mr. E. was admitted to the geriatric psychiatry unit and started on the medications prescribed by the neurologist. However, shortly after his arrival on the unit, he became belligerent with another patient, whom he accused of stealing his wallet. He struck out at the patient and then at the staff who attempted to subdue him. He was then treated with lorazepam as well as an additional 100 mg of quetiapine for his acute agitation and psychosis. The following day, he continued to exhibit agitated behavior, and his quetiapine dose was increased to 300 mg/day. He became increasingly confused, disoriented, unsteady in his gait, and eventually he fell. The psychiatrist discontinued quetiapine and lorazepam, prescribing instead valproate for Mr. E.'s impulsive, aggressive outbursts, which he tolerated without adverse effects.

During her husband's hospitalization, Mrs. E. realized that she could no longer care for him at home. She arranged for nursing home placement where he was maintained on valproate 750 mg/day and quetiapine 50 mg at bedtime. He stabilized within one month, and his episodes of hostility toward other patients were behaviorally controlled by the facility caregivers.

This case illustrates the difficulties in treating psychosis and agitation associated with Lewy body dementia. Patients frequently develop psychotic symptoms relatively early, including visual hallucinations. Although psychotic behavior and agitation often warrant use of antipsychotic medication, patients with Lewy body dementia tend to be exquisitely sensitive to these agents. Parkinsonian symptoms and gait disturbance may predispose such patients to falls, which can contribute to excessive mortality. In some cases, nonantipsychotic medications may be use adjunctively with very low doses of atypical antipsychotics to control behavioral symptoms.

Case 7.6

Mrs. F. was a 69-year-old African-American woman who lived alone with a 38-year history of schizophrenia. For many years, she had received treatment with trifluoperazine, which controlled her hallucinations and paranoia but produced parkinsonism and TD. As Mrs. F. lived an isolated existence and experienced severe negative symptoms, she was not particularly bothered by these side effects.

When she was 65 years of age, her psychiatrist changed her antipsychotic medication to olanzapine, reducing her parkinsonian symptoms and TD considerably. Over the following year, however, Mrs. F. gained approximately 25 pounds. Since starting on olanzapine, she had become less apathetic and socially withdrawn and had begun to attend a neighborhood drop-in facility. Developing some interest in socializing with other people, she was quite concerned about her weight gain. In fact, she told her psychiatrist that she preferred her old medication, because ``at least it didn't make (her) fat.''

Mrs. F.'s psychiatrist referred her to an internist to evaluate her weight gain. After examining her and ordering some laboratory tests, the internist found that she had developed type-2 diabetes (hemoglobin A_1C = 9.8), hyperten-

sion (blood pressure $^{170}/_{105}$), and mild hypercholesterolemia (total cholesterol = 226 mg/dL). She was given prescriptions for glipizide, felodipine, and simvastatin, advised to quit smoking, exercise, and modify her diet, and told that if she didn't follow the instructions she would be at high risk for a heart attack.

Several weeks later, Mrs. F. returned to her psychiatrist for a routine appointment. She appeared more disheveled and wore dark sunglasses. Her affect was flat and her speech was impoverished. She admitted that she had stopped taking olanzapine almost 2 weeks earlier, claiming that because she couldn't understand or remember all of the internist's instructions, she decided to discontinue olanzapine, as she believed that it had caused her medical problems. The psychiatrist reassured her and reminded her of the importance of staying on her antipsychotic medication. Mrs. F. was then referred to a geriatrician and visiting nurse who made regular home visits. The nurse educated Mrs. F. about her condition and monitored her diet and medications. Over time, Mrs. F. was able to lose some weight, and her blood pressure, blood glucose, and cholesterol levels normalized.

This case illustrates the challenges inherent in managing patients with early-onset schizophrenia presenting later in life. The arrival of atypical antipsychotics has reduced the incidence of movement disorders, more frequently associated with the conventional agents. However, metabolic changes such as weight gain, glucose intolerance, and dyslipidemia appear to complicate the use of some atypical antipsychotics. In addition, the improved efficacy of these medications for treating negative symptoms of schizophrenia may potentiate improved insight and awareness of symptoms as well as side effects. It is important to involve a multidisciplinary team of health providers because of the difficulties that older patients with schizophrenia may encounter in accessing and utilizing health care.

Case 7.7

Mr. G., a 68-year-old, never-married, retired aircraft engineer, lived alone. He was brought to the emergency department by the local police after firing a handgun in his apartment and calling 911. According to Mr. G., drug dealers lived in the apartment above his and had been plotting to kill him for several months. He was certain of this because he frequently heard the crack cocaine making a cracking sound through the ceiling. He believed that they were monitoring his apartment and telephone calls and that they had sent him a death threat in the mail. When the local police narcotics unit failed to respond to his demand for his neighbors' arrest, he purchased a gun and hired a security guard for protection. Mr. G. claimed that he heard the drug dealers talking outside his apartment door just as they were about to break in and kill him. He therefore fired the gun to protect himself. In the process, he sustained superficial gunshot wounds to both knees.

Mr. G.'s medical history was significant for past alcohol dependence. Approximately 4 years earlier, he suffered an ischemic L3-L4 paraplegia during surgical repair of an aortic aneurysm. The operation left him permanently wheelchair-confined, with numerous complications that included neurogenic bowel and bladder, chronic pain and nausea, and recurrent urinary tract infections. Several months prior to his emergency visit, he was admitted with urosepsis and delirium. His condition improved on intravenous antibiotics and he was transferred to a nursing home for convalescence. He was found to be withdrawn, hopeless, and unmotivated for rehabilitation. A psychiatric consultation resulted in a diagnosis of major depression. He was treated with sertraline, to which he responded at a dose of 50 mg/day. He was eventually discharged to his own apartment, where he lived for only a few weeks before becoming convinced that his neighbors were conspiring to kill him, which ultimately precipitated another visit to the emergency department.

On mental status examination, Mr. G. presented with a mask-like facial expression and bilateral resting pill-rolling tremor. He displayed worried affect, constricted in range. His thought process was logical, but his thought content revealed paranoid delusions. He denied suicidal or homicidal ideation but insight and judgment were clearly impaired. Cognitive evaluation was unremarkable; Mini Mental State Examination score was $^{29}/_{30}$. Physical examination confirmed L3-L4 paraplegia. Laboratory studies, including CBC, serum chemistry, urinalysis, TSH, Vitamin B12 and folate, RPR, and chest Xray were all within normal limits; MRI brain scan was normal for his age.

Mr. G. was admitted to the psychiatric unit for more thorough evaluation and treatment. Medical causes of psychosis, including dementia, medications and substances, and other medical conditions were ruled out. With particular regard to medications, Mr. G had been taking diazepam 15 mg TID and oxycodone 10 mg QID for chronic leg pains, and metoclopramide 15 mg QID as well as cimetidine 400 mg BID for nausea. During his hospitalization, diazepam and oxycodone doses were ta-

pered and gabapentin was substituted for treatment of neuropathic pain. A neurologic consultation suggested that Mr. G.'s parkinsonism was medication-induced; indeed, it resolved with discontinuation of metoclopramide. Cimetidine was also discontinued because of its potential for contributing to mental status changes. Mr. G. was treated with quetiapine, which was titrated up to a dose of 150 mg/day without adverse effects.

His preoccupation with drug dealers diminished somewhat; however, his insight and judgment remained impaired. He insisted on moving to a new apartment where he believed the drug dealers would be less likely to harass him. Mr. G. was followed for the next 14 months by the geropsychiatry community outreach program because of a concern regarding his adherence with medication. He continued to employ a private security guard for protection. Unfortunately, Mr. G. ultimately committed suicide. He was discovered by a visiting nurse in his apartment after taking a lethal overdose of medications.

This case illustrates the potential severity of psychosis in late-life delusional disorder. Despite appropriate treatment, psychotic symptoms frequently persist and can have disastrous consequences.

Case 7.8

Mrs. H., a 53-year-old married homemaker, was referred for psychiatric consultation by her general surgeon after she had recently been assessed for a breast lump, and was subsequently diagnosed with cancer. During the process of reviewing her treatment options, the surgeon observed Mrs. H. to be poorly focused, preoccupied, highly anxious, and at times bizarre in her behavior. Concerned about how her psychological state might affect her ability to choose and participate in an appropriate treatment, he referred her for a psychiatric evaluation. According to Mrs. H.'s husband, she had been well prior to 2 years previously, before her cancer diagnosis, without any past psychiatric history. Her husband reported that she had gradually become increasingly withdrawn, spending more time alone inside the house, and not attending social functions that she had previously enjoyed. He had observed her talking and laughing in her bedroom over the past few months when nobody was there. Mrs. H. was convinced that she was being sexually assaulted and harassed by an unidentified person. She claimed that she would go to sleep fully clothed and wake up in the morning wearing nothing but underwear. She complained of unexplained scratches on her skin and pains in her body. She described feeling terrified to leave her house, as she was certain that ''they'' would ''get (her)'' if she did. She did not believe that she had cancer, stating instead that this was ''just their way of controlling (her),'' and that she planned to seek out a second opinion from a different surgeon.

Mrs. H. had no history of previous physical illness, mood disorder, or substance abuse; she referred to a history of molestatation by an uncle during her childhood. She had a college education and a happy marriage with two children. On mental status examination, Mrs. H. was quite guarded, with anxious affect. Her thought process was tangential, and her thought content revealed persecutory delusions. She was preoccupied with a small piece of paper that had been torn out of a magazine that she found in the waiting room. She repeatedly made facial and hand gestures in disbelief, indicating her certainty that this piece of paper had special meaning for her. She was well oriented but was distracted; insight and judgment were poor. Laboratory workup results and physical examination were within normal limits, and an MRI brain scan was unremarkable.

Mrs. H. consented to treatment with loxapine, which resulted in modest improvement in her symptoms after a period of several weeks at a dose of 50 mg BID. Although she continued to show evidence of a delusional belief system, at times, she became well enough to receive treatment for her cancer and to return to her homemaking duties.

This case illustrates how delusions can compromise the insight and judgment of an older person with late-onset schizophrenia, and consequently interfere with medically necessary treatment. In such cases the use of antipsychotic medication can be life saving.

Case 7.9

Mr. J., a 76-year-old retired cattle breeder with moderately advanced Alzheimer's disease and a history of hypotensive episodes associated with cardiovascular disease, became unmanageable in a nursing home where he had functioned marginally during the prior 3 years. When staff tried to assist him in showering, he became combative, shouted racial insults, and accused them of torturing him. The nursing home administrator considered hospitalization. After the problems were discussed with the attending physician, a psychiatric consultation was requested.

At the time of consultation, Mr. J.'s medication consisted of digoxin and hydrochlorothiazide, but no supplemental potassium or neuroleptic medication was being given. According to the nursing staff, the patient's behavior had escalated when both his daughters and their families left town on vacation. The patient had not remembered being informed of their departure, and he felt abandoned and fearful that some harm had come to them. He accused nurses at the home of being responsible for his daughters' disappearance.

Physical examination and review of Mr. J.'s medical record revealed some muscle weakness, lethargy, and depressed mood in addition to recent episodes of orthostatic hypotension. After discussing these findings with the attending physician, the psychiatrist ordered a battery of studies including plasma digoxin level, plasma potassium level, and EKG. The digoxin level and EKG were normal, but the plasma potassium level was significantly lowered. Although the patient's weakness, lethargy, and depression abated dramatically after prescription of supplemental potassium, his psychotic, threatening accusations to the staff continued. Because of the patient's cardiovascular instability, the psychiatrist recommended haloperidol, slowly increased to 2 mg orally two times daily, because it produces comparatively less hypotension and sedation than a low-potency phenothiazine. Twice-daily checks for orthostatic hypotension and extrapyramidal side effects were also ordered.

The psychiatrist explained to Mr. J. that his attending physician, whom he had known and trusted for many years, wanted him to take this new medication. He readily agreed, and his psychotic behavior improved within 3 days. The psychiatrist gradually lowered and then discontinued haloperidol after the daughters' return, without a recrudescence of psychotic symptoms. The daughters were advised to take vacations at different times and to telephone their father during these vacations to reduce the likelihood of another psychotic episode.

This case illustrates the need to perform a comprehensive evaluation of an elderly patient before prescribing a neuroleptic. Electrolyte disturbance, drug toxicity, infections, and various other medical or psychosocial stresses can precipitate a psychosis. Orders for a neuroleptic in a hospital, and especially in a nursing home, should include specific orders for monitoring blood pressure and anticholinergic and extrapyramidal side effects. Antiparkinsonian agents need only be considered if extrapyramidal side effects develop; they should not be used prophylactically.

Case 7.10

Mrs. K., a 69-year-old widow with multi-infarct dementia and depression, was admitted to the hospital for diagnostic assessment and physical rehabilitation. Her family reported that she had become more difficult to manage at home because of nighttime wandering, agitation, auditory hallucinations, and paranoid accusations toward family members.

When she was admitted to the hospital, her symptoms worsened. After laboratory and other tests revealed no visible cause for her dementia and agitation, thioridazine, 50 mg twice daily, was ordered. Her symptoms improved after 3 days. However, a week later she developed parkinsonian tremor and rigidity. Benzotropine mesylate, 1 mg twice daily, was ordered, whereupon she became more confused and agitated and began having visual hallucinations. Physical examination revealed diminished bowel sounds and bladder distention. The attending physician, believing the psychosis had worsened, prescribed higher doses of thioridazine, which further aggravated the confusion, agitation, and hallucinations. Psychiatric consultation was requested.

A toxic delirium (CNS anticholinergic syndrome) was suspected, resulting from the combined anticholinergic properties of the neuroleptic and the antiparkinsonian drug. Cogentin was discontinued, and thioridazine was reduced. Within 2 days the confusion decreased, and visual hallucinations and peripheral anticholinergic signs subsided. The reduced dosage of thioridazine produced minimal extrapyramidal side effects, making the use of an antiparkinsonian drug unnecessary.

This case illustrates the sensitivity of elderly patients, especially those with organic brain dysfunction, to the anticholinergic side effects of psychotropic and other drugs. These reactions often resemble a worsening of the psychosis, sometimes leading to use of still higher doses of the offending drug. Maintaining a high index of suspicion for toxic delirium in elderly patients is important for diagnosing this common problem. The experience of Mrs. K. also illustrates the necessity of using very low starting doses of neuroleptics (50 mg of thioridazine twice daily was too high for this patient). Furthermore, because of the strong anticholinergic properties of thioridazine, an anticholinergic medication to control extrapyramidal symptoms should not be required.

Case 7.11

Mrs. L., an 82-year-old cachectic woman with hypertensive cardiovascular disease, was ad-mitted to a general hospital from a nursing home because of agitation, depression, and malnourishment. Medications upon admission to the hospital included digoxin, hydrochlorothiazide, propranolol, supplemental potassium, amitriptyline, chlorpromazine, quinidine, and diazepam (for insomnia).

An ECG revealed second-degree heart block and multifocal premature ventricular contractions; blood digoxin level was 2.4 ng/mL. Because the patient's lethargy had apparently interfered with adequate oral intake, intravenous fluids were administered. A trial discontinuation of amitriptyline, digoxin, propranolol, diazepam, and chlorpromazine resulted within a few days in increased alertness, cooperation with eating, and subsequent discontinuation of intravenous fluids. A week later Mrs. L.'s depression and apathy had decreased.

This case illustrates the common problem of polypharmacy in elderly patients. Combining a neuroleptic with other psychotropic drugs can lead to oversedation, anticholinergic effects, and cardiotoxicity. Elderly patients with CNS dysfunction are especially sensitive to the sedating effects of CNS-acting drugs, such as benzodiazepines, antidepressants, narcotics, analgesics, and antihypertensives. The effect of a combination of such drugs may lead to agitation, confusion, and combativeness; increasing the dosage of such drugs only aggravates these signs and symptoms. To avoid the toxic effects of polypharmacy, psychotropic drugs should be used only when necessary and for brief periods of time.

Case 7.12

During the postoperative recovery period, following surgery for carcinoma of the stomach, Mr. M., a 76-year-old patient with no prior history of psychiatric illness, was placed on meperidine (Demerol) and chlorpromazine for pain. Because he had trouble sleeping in the intensive care unit, which was brightly lit 24 hours a day, the dose of chlorpromazine was increased to 100 mg at bedtime, in addition to 25 mg given every 4 hours in conjunction with meperidine. One week later, when the patient was no longer in the intensive care unit, he commented to a family member that small bugs seemed to be crawling on the wall opposite his bed. He seemed amused by seeing these bugs, particularly when told they did not really exist. In the evening, however, after the family left, he grew restless and agitated and attempted to climb out of bed. He was confused and disoriented and mistook the night nursing staff for family members. He did not seem to know that he was in a hospital room or that he had undergone surgery, and he attempted to pull intravenous and drainage tubes from his body. The surgical opinion was that this man was suffering from brain metastases from his stomach carcinoma, and the family was told to prepare for imminent death.

The patient's son, a psychiatrist, was surprised by the vivid nature of the visual hallucination in the presence of an otherwise clear sensorium. He also noted that during the daytime his father did not remember the confusion and disorientation experienced the previous evening; during the day, disorientation and general memory loss were not apparent. The psychiatrist suggested to the surgeon that these symptoms might be the result of anticholinergic toxicity, and chlorpromazine dosage was reduced. Two days later, the bugs had vanished, and nighttime agitation, confusion, disorientation, and memory loss were virtually absent.

This case illustrates several common problems in the administration of neuroleptics to patients with physical disease in general hospitals. Although neuroleptics may be used to augment analgesia or to reduce agitation in the acutely ill patient, neuroleptic side effects may sometimes be diagnostically confusing. In this patient, brain metastases was an inaccurate diagnosis.

The clinical experience of Mr. M. also demonstrates the common problems of disorientation that older patients face in intensive care units in general hospitals. The use of disorienting medications may actually worsen symptoms of confusion produced by intensive care units. This patient's clinical course also illustrates development of sundowning syndrome: heightened agitation, confusion, and memory loss in the evening when perceptual stimuli decrease. Although neuroleptics are commonly used to treat sundowning syndrome, the symptoms may actually be worsened by the anticholinergic effects of drugs. In the general hospital, therefore, it is important to be aware of potential drug interactions and their toxic effects in older patients.

Case 7.13

Mr. N., a 77-year-old resident in a nursing home for 6 years following a stroke and residual left hemiparesis, complained that he could not sleep. He consistently awakened after approximately 4 hours of sleep, insisting that it was time to get up, even though it was 2:00 or 3:00 in the morning. When told by the nursing staff that it was still the middle of the night, he would insist that this was not so and become severely agi-

tated and aggressive. These symptoms progressed to the point that the nursing staff considered transferring the patient to a different nursing home unit. When interviewed, Mr. N. discussed at length his belief that one of his roommates (a man as rigid and aggressive as he) was rummaging through his belongings and planning to do him harm; on one occasion they came to blows.

Physical examination revealed the presence of a bladder infection in addition to Mr. N.'s neurologic deficits. Treatment of the bladder infection, however, failed to improve his sleep or behavior. Haloperidol was then prescribed in doses that gradually increased to 2 mg at bedtime. Mr. N.'s behavior during the night as well as during the day improved on this dosage.

Four months later, however, Mr. N was noted to have less energy, and to be mildly depressed and drooling. A diagnosis of akinesia was made, and haloperidol was discontinued, with the gradual resolution of these side effects. Unfortunately, his nocturnal agitation returned. At this point, thioridazine treatment was begun, starting at 10 mg and increasing to 10 mg three times daily. On this dosage, Mr. E. became much calmer, and when he awakened during the night, he was able to go back to sleep. His relationship with the nursing staff improved, and his paranoid delusions disappeared.

This vignette indicates both the dangers and the potential value of treatment with neuroleptics for sleep disturbance associated with psychotic levels of agitation. Whereas 30 mg of thioridazine daily helped stabilize Mr. N.'s sleep pattern and behavior, small doses of haloperidol induced unacceptable extrapyramidal side effects. This case also illustrates use of a sedating neuroleptic to help sleep, to reduce psychosis and agitation, as well as providing an example of how very small doses of a neuroleptic drug may be effective as well as toxic in elderly patients who suffer from neurologic damage.

Case 7.14

Mr. P., a 67-year-old married, retired civil service worker with a master's degree in education, presented to the emergency room with his wife. He reported a 3-month history of federal agents pursuing him because they thought he was a covert agent trying to obtain military secrets. He was also concerned that they were bugging his phone and following his car. He said that automobile license plates on the freeway would instruct him where to get off the road or to stop his car; the radio was also referring directly to him. His wife confirmed his story and said that he was becoming increasingly diffi-cult to manage at home owing to several concerns, such as his constant locking of the house and not allowing the curtains to be drawn or the phone to be used. Mr. P. also reported hearing a male voice that talked to him occasionally.

Neither Mr. P. nor his wife had a history of alcohol or other substance abuse. He denied symptoms of mania such as grandiosity, reduced need for sleep, pressure of speech, flight of ideas, or activities such as spending sprees. He also denied depressive symptoms such as almost daily depressed mood, anhedonia, significant weight change, sleep disturbances, psychomotor retardation, loss of energy, guilt, or suicidal ideation.

Mr. P.'s psychiatric history was unremarkable; family history revealed a nephew with a diagnosis of schizophrenia. Medical history was significant for gout, which had been stabilized on allopurinol for 10 years. Mental status examination showed constricted affect, delusional thought content, and poor insight; Mini-Mental State Examination Score was $^{28}/_{30}$; physical examination was unremarkable. Laboratory evaluation (including routine chemistries, complete blood count, and thyroid function tests) was significant for a serum uric acid of 7.2 mg/L. A CT scan of the head was within normal limits.

Mr. P. was admitted to the psychiatry service where he was evaluated and started on Perphenazine, 4 mg at bedtime, which was gradually increased to 16 mg per day. The patient reported feeling "safe" in the hospital, and his symptoms gradually resolved, with improved insight over a 3-week period. He was discharged after 3 weeks.

On his first follow-up evaluation (6 weeks after neuroleptic medication was begun) Mr. P. had lingual dyskinesia. Perphenazine was gradually tapered over a 6-week period with no recurrence of psychotic symptoms but also without improvement of the TD. The patient had a recurrence of his psychosis 10 months later that gradually resolved on Perphenazine at 16 mg per day, but he required maintenance neuroleptic treatment for 6 months before it could be discontinued. A third recurrence of symptoms required 4 to 8 mg of Perphenazine continuously to control paranoid ideation and ideas of reference. Mr. P.'s mild TD continued.

This case presents an example of late-onset schizophrenia with symptomatic response to neuroleptics, recurrences of psychosis, and development of TD.

Case 7.15

Mr. Q., a 59-year-old divorced, retired appliance repairman who lived in his car, presented to the emergency department requesting to have some metal splinters removed from the base of his skull. According to Mr. Q., the splinters were implanted in his skull by two women "operators" who were controlling his thoughts and occasionally physical functions via transmitted electronic signals. He continually heard the voices of the "operators" who commented on his behavior and threatened him. The patient denied any alcohol or street drug use as well as any symptoms of mood disorder (according to DSM-IV criteria).

Mr. Q.'s medical history revealed 3 prior psychiatric admissions at ages 50, 51, and 53. Neurologic workups (including CT scan and EEG) during these admissions were unremarkable. Prior to his first hospitalization, Mr. Q. had had no psychiatric contact and functioned well as an appliance repairman and as a husband and father. According to his wife and daughter, at age 47 he gradually became withdrawn and neglected personal hygiene. Mr. Q.'s business deteriorated, and he stopped working at age 49. His psychiatric history included occasional abuse of Percodan and Tylox. Medical history was significant for insulin-dependent diabetes mellitus and type IV dyslipidemia. A mental status examination revealed constricted affect, delusional content, and mild looseness of associations; his Mini-Mental State Examination Score was $^{27}/_{30}$. Physical examination was unremarkable except for mild obesity. Laboratory evaluation was notable for a glucose level of 288 mg/L, cholesterol level of 351 mg/L, and triglyceride level of 445 mg/L.

Mr. Q. was followed for several years but continued to refuse neuroleptic medication. He was hospitalized several times after becoming especially anxious and agitated because of delusions and hallucinations. His anxiety and agitation usually occurred when the "operators" were controlling his driving and he expected them to force him off the road. Milieu therapy and private access to the clinic staff worked well to help the patient feel more control over his persecutors. Unfortunately, Mr. G.'s psychosis gradually worsened and he eventually committed suicide.

This case illustrates the severity of late-life psychotic illness. Despite aggressive treatment, late-life psychotic symptoms do not always diminish.

Case 7.16

Mrs. R., a 63-year-old married homemaker with 10 years of education, was well until the age of 54 when she was hospitalized after several months of "not being herself." She and her husband both reported that she had difficulty sleeping and heard voices that interfered with her ability to concentrate. Mrs. R. had a delusion that she was "put in the computer." She became increasingly concerned about hearing "bad words" from her neighbors that emanated from within her house. The voices commented on her private life and called her names such as "wicked woman." She often yelled back in response to the voices. According to her husband, she was able to clean her house and prepare meals reasonably well. Mrs. R. had no history of either mood disorder or alcohol or other substance abuse. On mental status examination, she was pleasant and cooperative but somewhat guarded and with constricted affect. Her thought processes were tangential and her thought content was notable for a belief of being placed in a computer; she was observed to whisper frequently. Mrs. R. was well oriented but had poor concentration; insight and judgment were fair. Medical and psychiatric histories were not significant. Laboratory workup results and physical examination were within normal limits, and a MRI of the brain was unremarkable. Mrs. R. was treated with haloperidol 10 mg daily, which resulted in moderate symptomatic improvement.

This case illustrates the treatment of late-onset schizophrenia with a neuroleptic because of the patient's delusions and hallucinations.

Acknowledgments. This work was supported, in part, by the National Institute of Mental Health grants MH 43693, MH 49671, MH 45131, and by the Department of Veterans Affairs.

References

1. Laughren T. A regulatory perspective on psychiatric syndromes in Alzheimer Disease. *Am J Geriatr Psychiatry* 2001;9:340–345.
2. Sweet RA, Pollock BG. Neuroleptics in the elderly: guidelines for monitoring. *Harv Rev Psychiatry* 1995;2:327–335.
3. Salzman C. Treatment of agitation in the elderly. Meltzer HY, ed. In: *Psychopharmacology: third generation of progress.* New York: Raven Press, 1987.
4. Elon R, Pawlson LG. The impact of OBRA on medical practice within nursing facilities. *J Am Geriatr Soc* 1992;40:958–963.
5. Rovner BW, Edelman BA, Cox MP, et al. The impact of antipsychotic drug regulations on psychotropic prescribing practices in nursing homes. *Am J Psychiatry* 1992;149:1390–1392.
6. Shorr RI, Fought RL, Ray WA. Changes in antipsychotic drug use in nursing homes during implementation of the OBRA-87 regulations. *JAMA* 1994;271:358–362.
7. Morris RK, Rovner BW, Folstein MF, et al. Delusions in newly admitted residents of nursing homes. *Am J Psychiatry* 1990;147:299–302.
8. Tariot PN, Podgorski CA, Blazina L, et al. Mental disorders in the nursing home: another perspective. *Am J Psychiatry* 1993;150:1063–1069.
9. Mulsant BH, Gershon S. Neuroleptics in the treatment of psychosis in late life: a rational approach. *Int J Geriatr Psychiatry* 1993;8:979–992.
10. Jeste DV, Harris MJ, Pearlson GD, et al. Late-onset schizophrenia: studying clinical validity. *Psychiatr Clin North Am* 1988;11:1–14.
11. Davis JM, Chen N, Glick ID. A meta-analysis of the efficacy of second-generation antipsychotics. *Arch Gen Psychiatry* 2003;60:553–564.
12. Sweet RA, Pollock BG. New atypical antipsychotics. Experience and utility in the elderly. *Drugs Aging* 1998;12:115–127.
13. Gurwitz JH, Field TS, Avorn J, et al. Incidence and preventability of adverse drug events in nursing homes. *Am J Med* 2000;109:166–168.
14. Thapa PB, Gideon P, Fought RL, et al. Psychotropic drugs and risk of recurrent falls in ambulatory nursing home residents. *Am J Epidemiol* 1995;142:202–211.
15. Cumming RG. Epidemiology of medication-related falls and fractures in the elderly. *Drugs Aging* 1998;12:43–53.
16. Ray WA, Meredith S, Thapa PB, et al. Antipsychotics and the risk of sudden cardiac death. *Arch Gen Psychiatry* 2001;58:1161–1167.
17. Maixner SM, Mellow AM, Tandon R. The efficacy, safety, and tolerability of antispychotics in the elderly. *J Clin Psychiatry* 1999;60:29–41.
18. Glassman AH, Bigger JT. Antipsychotic drugs: prolonged QTc interval, *torsade de pointes,* and sudden death. *Am J Psychiatry* 2001;158:1774–1782.
19. Rajput AH. Drug-induced parkinsonism in the elderly. *Geriatric Medicine Today* 1984;3:99.
20. Hoffman WF, Labs SM, Casey DE. Neuroleptic-induced parkinsonism in older schizophrenics. *Biol Psychiatry* 1987;22:427–439.
21. Caligiuri MP, Lacro JP, Jeste DV. Incidence and predictors of drug-induced parkinsonism in older psychiatric patients treated with very low doses of neuroleptics. *J Clin Psychopharmacol* 1999;19:322–328.
22. Yassa R, Nastase C, Dupont D, et al. Tardive dyskinesia in elderly psychiatric patients: a 5-year study. *Am J Psychiatry* 1992;149:1206–1211.
23. Jeste DV, Caligiuri MP, Paulsen JS, et al. Risk of tardive dyskinesia in older patients: a prospective longitudinal study of 266 patients. *Arch Gen Psychiatry* 1995;52:756–765.
24. Mukherjee S, Wisniewski A, Bilder R, et al. Possible association between tardive dyskinesia and altered carbohydrate metabolism. *Arch Gen Psychiatry* 1985;42:205.
25. Woerner MG, Alvir JM, Saltz BL, et al. Prospective study of tardive dyskinesia in the elderly:

rates and risk factors. *Am J Psychiatry* 1998;155: 1521–1528.

26. Kane JM, Woerner M, Lieberman J. Tardive dyskinesia: prevalence, incidence, and risk factors. *J Clin Psychopharmacol* 1988;8:52S–56S.

27. Jeste DV, Lacro JP, Palmer BW, et al. Incidence of tardive dyskinesia in early stages of low-dose treatment with typical neuroleptics in older patients. *Am J Psychiatry* 1999;156:309–311.

28. Chatterjee A, Chakos M, Koreen A, et al. Prevalence and clinical correlates of extrapyramidal signs and spontaneous dyskinesia in never-medicated schizophrenic patients. *Am J Psychiatry* 1995;152:1724–1729.

29. Saltz BL, Woerner MG, Kane JM, et al. Prospective study of tardive dyskinesia incidence in the elderly. *JAMA* 1991;266:2402–2406.

30. Kane JM, Jeste DV, Barnes TRE, et al. *Tardive dyskinesia: a Task force report of the American Psychiatric Association.* Washington, DC: American Psychiatric Association, 1992.

31. Yassa R, Jeste DV. Gender differences in tardive dyskinesia: a critical review of the literature. *Schizophr Bull* 1992;18:701–715.

32. Kane JM. Tardive dyskinesia in affective disorders. *J Clin Psychiatry* 1999;60:43–47.

33. Jeste DV, Lohr JB, Clark K, et al. Pharmacological treatment of tardive dyskinesia in the 1980s. *J Clin Psychopharmacol* 1988;8:38S–48S.

34. Levinson DF, Simpson GM. Neuroleptic-induced extrapyramidal symptoms with fever. *Arch Gen Psychiatry* 1986;43:839–848.

35. Casey DE. Effects of clozapine therapy in schizophrenic individuals at risk for tardive dyskinesia. *J Clin Psychiatry* 1998;59:31–37.

36. Street JS, Tollefson GD, Tohen M, et al. Olanzapine for psychotic conditions in the elderly. *Psychiatric Annals* 2000;30:191–196.

37. Jeste DV, Rockwell E, Harris MJ, et al. Conventional vs. newer antipsychotics in elderly patients. *Am J Geriatr Psychiatry* 1999;7:70–76.

38. Jeste DV, Glazer WM, Morgenstern H. Low incidence of persistent tardive dyskinesia with quetiapine treatment of psychotic disorders in the elderly (Abstract). *Am J Geriatr Psychiatry* 2000;8: 25–26.

39. Jeste DV, Lacro JP, Bailey A, et al. Lower incidence of tardive dyskinesia with risperidone compared with haloperidol in older patients. *J Am Geriatr Soc* 1999;47:716–719.

40. Adler LA, Rotrosen J, Edson R, et al. Vitamin E treatment for tardive dyskinesia. *Arch Gen Psychiatry* 1999;56:836–841.

41. Boomershine KH, Shelton PS, Boomershine JE. Vitamin E in the treatment of tardive dyskinesia. *Ann Pharmacother* 1999;33:1195–1202.

42. Lohr JB, Jeste DV. *Neuroleptic-induced movement disorders: tardive dyskinesia and other tardive syndromes in psychiatry, revised edition.* Michels R, Cavenar JO, Jr., Brodie NKH, et al., eds. Philadelphia: J.B. Lippincott, 1988.

43. Webster P, Wijeratne C. Risperidone-induced neuroleptic malignant syndrome. *Lancet* 1994; 344:1228–1229.

44. Buckhard PR, Vingerhoets FJG, Alberque C, et al. Olanzapine-induced neuroleptic malignant synrome. *Arch Gen Psychiatry* 1999;56:101–102.

45. Alvir JMaJ, Lieberman JA, Safferman AZ, et al. Clozapine-induced agranulocytosis: incidence and risk factors in the United States. *N Engl J Med* 1993;329:162–167.

46. Allison DB, Casey DE. Antipsychotic-induced weight gain: a review of the literature. *J Clin Psychiatry* 2001;62:22–31.

47. Newcomer JW, Haupt DW, Fucetola R. Abnormalities in glucose regulation during antipsychotic treatment of schizophrenia. *Arch Gen Psychiatry* 2002;59:337–345.

48. Sernyak MJ, Leslie DL, Alarcon RD. Association of diabetes mellitus with use of atypical neuroleptics in the treatment of schizophrenia. *Am J Psychiatry* 2002;159:561–566.

49. Jin H, Meyer JM, Jeste DV. Phenomenology of and risk factors for new-onset diabetes mellitus and diabetic ketoacidosis associated with atypical antipsychotics: an analysis of 45 published cases. *Ann Clin Psychiatry* 2002;14:59–64.

50. Koller E, Schneider B, Bennett K, et al. Clozapine-associated diabetes. *Am J Med* 2001;111: 716–723.

51. Koller EA, Doraiswamy PM. Olanzapine-associated diabetes mellitus. *Pharmacotherapy* 2002;22: 841–852.

52. Koller E, Doraiswamy PM, Cross JT. Risperidone-associated diabetes. Presented at the 85th Annual Meeting of the Endocrine Society, Philadelphia, PA: June 19–22, 2002.

53. Turrone P, Kapur S, Seeman MV, et al. Elevation of prolactin levels by atypical antipsychotics. *Am J Psychiatry* 2002;159:133–135.

54. Goodnick PJ, Rodriguez L, Santana O. Aripiprizole: impact on prolactin levels. *Expert Opinion Pharmacother* 2002;3:1381–1391.

55. Halbreich U, Palter S. Accelerated osteoporosis in psychiatric patients: possible pathophysiological processes. *Schizophr Bull* 1996;22:447–454.

56. Zhang-Wong JH, Seeman MV. Antipsychotic drugs, menstrual regularity, and osteoporosis risk. *Arch Women Ment Health* 2002;5:93–98.

57. Collins A, Anderson J. SIADH induced by two atypical antipsychotics. *Int J Geriatr Psychiatry* 2000;15:282–283.

58. Ogilvie AD, Croy MF. Clozapine and hyponatraemia (letter). *Lancet* 1992;340:672.

59. Chan TY. Drug-induced syndrome of inappropriate antidiuretic hormone secretion: causes, diagnosis, and management. *Drugs Aging* 1997; 11:27–44.

60. Buckley NA, Sander P. Cardiovascular adverse effects of antipsychotic drugs. *Drug Saf* 2000;23: 215–228.

61. Mehtonen OP, Aranko K, Malkonen L, et al. A survey of sudden death associated with the use of antipsychotic or antidepressant drugs: 49 cases in Finland. *Acta Psychiatr Scand* 1991;84: 58–64.

62. Reilly JG, Ayis SA, Ferrier IN, et al. Thioridazine and sudden unexplained death in psychiatric inpatients. *Br J Psychiatry* 2002;180:515–522.

63. Zarate CA. Sudden cardiac death and antipsychotic drugs. *Arch Gen Psychiatry* 2001;58:1168–1171.

64. Kane JM, Honigfeld G, Singer J, et al. Clozapine for the treatment resistant schizophrenic: a dou-

ble-blind comparison with chlorpromazine. *Arch Gen Psychiatry* 1988;45:789–796.

65. Salzman C, Vacarro B, Lieff J, et al. Clozapine in older patients with psychosis and behavioral disruption. *Am J Geriatr Psychiatry* 1995;3:26–33.

66. Pitner JK, Mintzer JE, Pennypacker LC, et al. Efficacy and adverse effects of clozapine in four elderly psyschotic patients. *J Clin Psychiatry* 1995; 56:180–185.

67. Jeste DV, Eastham JH, Lacro JP, et al. Management of late-life psychosis. *J Clin Psychiatry* 1996; 57(suppl 3):39–45.

68. Gunasekara NS, Spencer CM, Keating GM. A review of its use in schizophrenia and schizoaffective disorder. *Drugs* 2003;62:1217–1251.

69. Brook S, Lucey JV, Gunn KP, et al. Intramuscular ziprasidone compared with intramuscular haloperidol in the treatment of acute psychosis. *J Clin Psychiatry* 2000;61:933–941.

70. Jordon S, Koprivika V, Chen R, et al. The antipsychotic aripiprazole is a potent partial agonist at the human 5-HT(1A) receptor. *Eur J Pharmacol* 2002;441:137–140.

71. Saha AR, Petrie JL, Ali MW. Safety and efficacy profile of aripiprazole, a novel antipsychotic. *Schizophr Res* 1999;36:295–296.

72. Goodnick PJ, Jerry JM. Aripiprazole profile on efficacy and safety. *Exp Opin Pharmacother* 2002; 3:1773–1781.

73. Thapa PB, Gideon P, Cost TW, et al. Antidepressants and the risk of falls among nursing home residents. *N Engl J Med* 1998;339:875–882.

74. Weiler PG, Mungas D, Bernick C. Propranolol for the control of disruptive behavior in senile dementia. *J Geriatr Psychiatry Neurol* 1988;145: 226–230.

75. Ray WA, Thapa PB, Gideon P. Benzodiazepines and the risk of falls in nursing home residents. *J Am Geriatr Soc* 2000;48:682–685.

76. Stotsky B. Psychosis in the elderly in Psychopharmacology and Aging. *Vol 6: Advances in behavioral biology.* Eisdorfer C, Faun WE, eds. New York: Plenum, 1973.

77. Jackson CW, Pitner JK, Mintzer JE. Zolpidem for the treatment of agitation in elderly demented patients. *J Clin Psychiatry* 1996;57:372–373.

78. The French Clozapine Parkinson Study Group. Clozapine in drug-induced psychosis in Parkinson's disease. *Lancet* 1999;353:2041–2042.

79. The Parkinson Study Group. Low-dose clozapine for the treatment of drug-induced psychosis in Parkinson's disease. *N Engl J Med* 1999; 340:757–776.

Table 7.3 References

Abse W, Dahlstrom WG. The value of chemotherapy in senile mental disturbances. *JAMA* 1960;174: 2036–2042.

Altman H, Mehta D, Evenson RC. Behavioral effects of drug therapy on psychogeriatric inpatients. I: Chlorpromazine and thioridazine. *J Am Geriatr Soc* 1973;21:241–248.

Barnes R, Veith R, Okimoto J, et al. Efficacy of antipsychotic medications in behaviorally disturbed dementia patients. *Am J Psychiatry* 1982;139: 1170–1174.

Barton R, Hurst L. Unnecessary use of tranquilizers in elderly patients. *Br J Psychiatry* 1966;112: 989–990.

Birkett DP, Boltuch B. Chlorpromazine in geriatric psychiatry. *J Am Geriatr Soc* 1972;20:403–406.

Branchey MH, Lee JH, Arun R, Simpson FM. High- and low-potency neuroleptics in elderly psychiatric patients. *JAMA* 1978;239:1860–1862.

Cervera AA. Psychoactive drug therapy in the senile patient: controlled comparison of thioridazine and diazepam. *Psychiatr Digest* 1974;35:15–21.

Chesrow EJ, Kaplitz SE. Acetophenazine (Tindal) in the treatment of chronically ill patients with anxiety and tension: a double-blind study. *J Am Geriatr Soc* 1963;11:445–448.

Coccaro EF, Kramer E, Zemishlany Z, et al. Pharmacologic treatment of noncognitive behavioral disturbances in elderly demented patients. *Am J Psychiatry* 1990;147:1640–1645.

Covington JS. Alleviating agitation, apprehension, and related symptoms in geriatric patients: a double-blind comparison of a phenothiazine and benzodiazepine. *South Med J* 1975;68:719–724.

Cowley LM, Glen RS. Double-blind study of thioridazine and haloperidol in geriatric patients with a psychosis associated with organic brain syndrome. *J Clin Psychiatry* 1979;40:411–419.

Devanand DP, Marder K, Michaels KS, et al. A randomized, placebo-controlled dose comparison trial of haloperidol for psychosis and disruptive behaviors in Alzheimer's disease. *Am J Psychiatry* 1998;155:1512–1520.

Finkel SI, Lyons JS, Anderson RL, et al. A randomized, placebo-controlled trial of thiothixene in agitated demented nursing home patients. *Int J Geriatr Psychiatry* 1995;10:129–136.

Gotestam KG, Ljunghall S, Olsson B. A double-blind comparison of the effects of haloperidol and *cis*-(z)–clopenthixol in senile dementia. *Acta Psychiatr Scand Suppl* 1981;294:46–53.

Hamilton LD, Bennett JL. Acetophenazine for hyperactive geriatric patients. *Geriatrics* 1962a;17: 596–601.

Hamilton LD, Bennett JL. The use of trifluoperazine in geriatric patients with chronic brain syndrome. *J Am Geriatr Soc* 1962;10:140–147.

Honigfeld G, Newall PN. Hemodynamic effects of imipramine, acetophenazine or trifluperazine in geriatric psychiatry. *Dis Nerv Syst* 1965;26: 427–429.

Judah L, Murphee D, Seager L. Psychiatric response of geriatric-psychiatric patients to Mellaril. *Am J Psychiatry* 1959;115:1118–1119.

Katz MM, Itil TM. Video methodology for research in psychopathology and psychopharmacology. *Arch Gen Psychiatry* 1974;31:204–210.

Kirven LE, Montero EF. Comparison of thioridazine and diazepam in the control of nonpsychotic symptoms associated with senility: double-blind study. *J Am Geriatr Soc* 1973;21:546–551.

Lehmann HE, Ban TA. Comparative pharmacotherapy of the aging psychotic patient. *Laval Med* 1967;38:588–595.

Lehmann HE, Ban TA. Thioridazine-geriatrics. *Psychopharmacol Bull* 1974;1:75–76.

Mohler G. Clinical trial of thiothixene (Navane) in

elderly chronic schizophrenics. *Curr Ther Res* 1970;12:377–386.

Petrie WM, Ban TA, Baney S, et al. Loxapine in psychogeriatrics: a placebo- and standard-controlled clinical investigation. *J Clin Psychopharmacol* 1982; 2:122–126.

Rada RT, Kellner R. Thiothixene in the treatment of geriatric patients with chronic organic brain syndrome. *J Am Geriatr Soc* 1976;24:105–107.

Raskind M, Alvarez C, Herlin RN. Fluphenazine enanthate in the outpatient treatment of late paraphrenia. *J Am Geriatr Soc* 1979;27:459–463.

Robinson, DB. Evaluation of certain drugs in geriatric patients. *Arch Gen Psychiatry* 1969;25:41–46.

Rosen HJ. Double-blind comparison of haloperidol and thioridazine in geriatric outpatients. *J Clin Psychiatry* 1979;40:24–31.

Seager CP. Chlorpromazine in the treatment of elderly patients. *Br Med J* 1985;1:882–884.

Sheppard C, Bhattacharyya A, DiGiacomo M, Merlis S. Effects of acetophenazine dimaleate on paranoid symptomatology in female geriatric patients. *J Am Geriatr Soc* 1964;12:884–888.

Smith GR, Taylor CW, Linkous P. Haloperidol versus thioridazine for the treatment of psychogeriatric patients. *Psychosomatics* 1974;15:134–138.

Stotsky BA. Double-blind study of thioridazine and haloperidol in geriatric patients and a psychosis associated with organic brain syndrome. *Clin Ther* 1984;6:546–549.

Sugerman AA, Williams H, Adlerstein AM. Haloperidol in the psychiatric disorders of old age. *Am J Psychiatry* 1964;120:1190–1192.

Sultzer DL, Gray KF, Gunay I, et al. A double-blind comparison of trazodone and haloperidol for treatment of agitation in patients with dementia. *Am J Geriatr Psychiatry* 1997;5(1):60–69.

Ter Haar HW. The relief of restlessness in the elderly. *Age Aging* 1977;(suppl):73–82.

Teri L, Logsdon RG, Peskind E, et al. Treatment of agitation in AD: a randomized, placebo-controlled clinical trial. *Neurology* 2000;55:1271–1278.

Tewfik GI, Jain VK, Harcup M, Magowan S. Effectiveness of various tranquilizers in the management of senile restlessness. *Gerontol Clin* 1970;12:351–359.

Tsuang MM, Min LL, Stotsky BA, Cole JO. Haloperidol versus thioridazine for hospitalized psychogeriatric patients. *J Am Geriatr Soc* 1971;19:593–600.

Welborn WS. A trial of a new tranquilizing agent in geriatric patients. *Psychosomatics* 1961;2:450–455.

Table 7.4 References

Allen RL, Walker Z, D'Ath PJ, et al. Risperidone for psychotic and behavioral symptoms in Lewy body dementia. *Lancet* 1995;346:185.

Barak Y, Shamir E, Zemishlani H, et al. Olanzapine vs. haloperidol in the treatment of elderly chronic schizophrenia patients. *Prog Neuropsychopharmacol Bio Psychiatry* 2002;26:1199–1202.

Berman I, Merson A, Rachov-Pavlov J, et al. Risperidone in elderly schizophrenic patients. *Am J Geriatr Psychiatry* 1996;4:173–179.

Breier A, Sutton VK, Feldman PD, et al. Olanzapine in the treatment of dopamimetic-induced psychosis in patients with Parkinson's disease. *Biol Psychiatry* 2002;52:438–445.

Brodaty H, Ames D, Snowdon J, et al. A randomized placebo-controlled trial of risperidone for the treatment of aggression, agitation, and psychosis of dementia. *J Clin Psychiatry* 2003;64:134–143.

Chan WC, Lam LC, Choy CN, et al. A double-blind randomized comparison of risperidone and haloperidol in the treatment of behavioural and psychological symptoms in Chinese dementia patients. *Int J Geriatr Psychiatry* 2001;16:1156–1162.

Chengappa KNR, Baker RW, Kreinbrook SB, et al. Clozapine use in female geriatric patients with psychosis. *J Geriatr Psychiatry Neurol* 1995;8:12–15.

Clark WS, Street JS, Feldman PD, et al. The effects of olanzapine in reducing the emergence of psychosis among nursing home patients with Alzheimer's disease. *J Clin Psychiatry* 2001;62:34–40.

Cummings JL, Street J, Masterman D, et al. Efficacy of olanzapine in the treatment of psychosis in dementia with Lewy bodies. *Dement Geriatr Cogn Disord* 2002;13:67–73.

Davidson M, Harvey PD, Vervarcke J, et al. A long-term, multicenter, open-label study of risperidone in elderly patients with psychosis. *Int J Geriatr Psychiatry* 2000;15:506–514.

De Deyn PP, Rabheru K, Rasmussen A, et al. A randomized trial of risperidone, placebo, and haloperidol for behavioral symptoms of dementia. *Neurology* 1999;53:946–955.

Fernandez HH, Friedman JH, Jacques C, et al. Quetiapine for the treatment of drug-induced psychosis in Parkinson's disease. *Mov Disorders* 1999; 14:484–487.

Frankenburg FR, Kalunian D. Clozapine in the elderly. *J Geriatr Psychiatry Neurol* 1994;7:129–132.

Howanitz E, Pardo M, Smelson DA. The efficacy and safety of clozapine versus chlorpromazine in geriatric schizophrenia. *J Clin Psychiatry* 1999;60:41–44.

Hwang JP, Yang CH, Lee TW, et al. The efficacy and safety of olanzapine for the treatment of geriatric psychosis. *J Clin Psychopharmacol* 2003;23:113–118.

Jeanblanc W, Davis YB. Risperidone for treating dementia-associated aggression. *Am J Psychiatry* 1995;152(8):1239.

Jeste DV, Eastham JH, Lacro JP, et al. Management of late-life psychosis. *J Clin Psychiatry* 1996; 57(suppl 3):39–45.

Katz IR, Jeste DV, Mintzer JE, et al. Comparison of risperidone and placebo for psychosis and behavioral disturbances associated with dementia: a randomized, double-blind trial. *J Clin Psychiatry* 1999;60:107–115.

Madhusoodanan S, Brecher M, Brenner R, et al. Risperidone in the treatment of elderly patients with psychotic disorders. *Am J Geriatr Psychiatry* 1999;7:132–38.

Madhusoodanan S, Brenner R, Araujo L, et al. Efficacy of risperidone treatment for psychoses associated wtih schizophrenia, schizoaffective disorder, bipolar disorder, or senile dementia in 11 geriatric patients: a case series. *J Clin Psychiatry* 1995;56:514–518.

Madhusoodanan S, Brenner R, Suresh P, et al. Efficacy and tolerability of olanzapine in elderly patients with psychotic disorders: a prospective study. *Ann Clin Psychiatry* 2000;12:11–18.

Meco G, Alessandria A, Bonifati V, et al. Risperidone for hallucinations in levodopa-treated Parkinson's disease patients. *Lancet* 1994;343: 1370–1371.

Meehan KM, Wang H, David SR, et al. Comparison of rapidly acting intramuscular olanzapine, lorazepam, and placebo: a double-blind, randomized study in acutely agitated patients with dementia. *Neuropsychopharmacology* 2002;26(4):494–504.

Mintzer J, Mullen J, Sweitzer D. Extrapyramidal symptoms in elderly patients treated with quetiapine or or risperidone. Presented at the 9th International Congress of the International Psychogeriatric Association; Sept 9–14, 2001;Nice, France.

Mullen J, Jibson MD, Sweitzer D. A comparison of the relative safety, efficacy, and tolerability of quetiapine and risperidone in outpatients with schizophrenia and other psychotic disorders: the Quetiapine Experience with Safety and Tolerability (QUEST) study. *Clin Ther* 2001;23: 1839–1854.

Oberholzer AF, Hendriksen C, Monsch AU, et al. Safety and effectiveness of low-dose clozapine in psychogeriatric patients: a preliminary study. *Int Psychogeriatr* 1992;4(2):187–195.

Parkinson Study Group. Low-dose clozapine for the treatment of drug-induced psychosis in Parkinson's disease. *N Engl J Med* 1999;340:757–763.

Pitner JK, Mintzer JE, Pennypacker LC, et al. Efficacy and adverse effects of clozapine in four elderly psychotic patients. *J Clin Psychiatry* 1995;56: 180–185.

Raheja RK, Bharwani I, Penetrante AE. Efficacy of risperidone for behavioral disorders in the elderly: a clinical observation. *J Geriatr Psychiatry Neurol* 1995;8:159–161.

Sajatovic M, Perez D, Brescan D, Ramirez LF. Olanzapine therapy in elderly patients with schizophrenia. *Psychopharmacol Bull* 1998;34:819–823.

Sajatovic M, Ramirez LF, Garver D, et al. Clozapine therapy for older veterans. *Psychiatr Serv* 1998;49: 340–344.

Salzman C, Vaccaro B, Lieff J, Weiner A. Clozapine in older patients with psychosis and behavioral disruption. *Am J Geriatr Psychiatry* 1995;3:26–33.

Satterlee WG, Reams SG, Burns PR, et al. A clinical update on olanzapine treatment in schizophrenia and in elderly Alzheimer's disease patients. *Psychopharmacol Bull* 1995;31:534.

Street JS, Clark WS, Gannon KS, et al. Olanzapine treatment of psychotic and behavioral symptoms in patients with Alzheimer disease in nursing care facilities: a double-blind, randomized, placebo-controlled trial. *Arch Gen Psychiatry* 2000;57: 968–976.

Street JS, Tollefson GD, Tohen M, et al. Olanzapine for psychotic conditions in the elderly. *Psychiatr Ann* 2000;30:191–196.

Tariot PN, Salzman C, Yeung PP, et al. Long-term use of quetiapine in elderly patients with psychotic disorders. *Clin Ther* 2000;22:1068–1084.

Tollefson GD, Beasley CM, Tran PV, et al. Olanzapine versus haloperidol in the treatment of schizophrenia and schizoaffective and schizophreniform disorders: Results of an international collaborative trial. *Am J Psychiatry* 1997;154:457–465.

Table 7.5 References

Aisen PS, Johannessen DJ, Marin DB. Trazodone for behavioral disturbance in Alzheimer's disease. *Am J Geriatr Psychiatry* 1993;1(4):349–350.

Ancill RJ, Carlye WW, Liang RA, et al. Agitation in the demented elderly: a role for benzodiazepines? *Int Clin Psychopharmacol* 1991;6:141–146.

Auchus AP, Bissey-Black C. Pilot study of haloperidol, fluoxetine, and placebo for agitation in Alzheimer's disease. *J Neuropsychiatry Clin Neurosciences* 1997;9:591–593.

Chambers CA, Bain J, Rusbottom R, et al. Carbamazepine treatment of agitation in senile dementia and overactivity-placebo-controlled double-blind trial. *IRCS Med Sci* 1982;10:505–506.

Christensen DB, Benfield WR. Alprazolam as an alternative to low-dose haloperidol in older, cognitively impaired nursing facility patients. *J Am Geriatr Soc* 1997;46:620–625.

Cummings JL, Donohue JA, Brooks RL. The relationship between donepezil and behavioral disturbances in patients with Alzheimer's disease. *Am J Geriatr Psychiatry* 2000;8:134–140.

Cummings JL, Nadel A, Masterman D, et al. Efficacy of metrifonate in improving the psychiatric and behavioral disturbances of patients with Alzheimer's disease. *J Geriatr Psychiatry Neurol* 2001;14: 101–108.

Feldman H, Gauthier S, Hecker J, et al. A 24-week randomized, double-blind study of donepezil in moderate to severe Alzheimer's disease. *Neurology* 2001;57:613–620.

Gauthier S, Feldman H, Hecker J, et al. Functional, cognitive, and behavioral effects of donepezil in patients with moderate Alzheimer's disease. *Curr Med Res Opinion* 2002;18:347–354.

Geldmacher DS, Waldman AJ, Doty L, et al. Fluoxetine in dementia of the Alzheimer's type: prominent adverse effects and failure to improve cognition. *J Clin Psychiatry* 1994;55:161.

Gleason RP, Schneider LS. Carbamazepine treatment of agitation in Alzheimer's outpatients refractory to neuroleptics. *J Clin Psychiatry* 1990; 51(3):115–118.

Greendyke RM, Kanter DR, Schuster DB, et al. Propranolol treatment in assaultive patients with organic brain disease. *J Nerv Ment Dis* 1986;174(5): 290–294.

Greendyke RM, Schuster DB, Wooton JA. Propranolol in the treatment of assaultive patients with organic brain disease. *J Clin Psychopharmacol* 1984; 4(5):282–285.

Herrmann N, Eryavec G. Buspirone in the management of agitation and aggression associated with dementia. *Am J Geriatr Psychiatry* 1993;1:249–253.

Herrmann N, Lanctot K, Myszak M. Effectiveness of gabapentin for the treatment of behavioral disorders in dementia. *J Clin Psychopharmacol* 2000;20: 90–93.

Houlihan DJ, Mulsant BH, Sweet RA, et al. A naturalistic study of trazodone in the treatment of behavioral complications of dementia. *Am J Geriatr Psychiatry* 1994;2(1):78–85.

Jackson CW, Pitner JK, Mintzer JE. Zolpidem for the treatment of agitation in elderly demented patients. *J Clin Psychiatry* 1996;57(8):372–373.

Jenike MA. Treating the violent elderly patient with propranolol. *Geriatrics* 1983;38(3):29–30, 34.

Kunik ME, Puryear L, Orengo CA, et al. The efficacy and tolerability of divalproex sodium in elderly demented patients with behavioral disturbances. *Int J Geriatr Psychiatry* 1998;13:29–34.

Kyomen HH, Hennen J, Gottlieb GL, et al. Estrogen therapy and noncognitive psychiatric signs and symptoms in elderly patients with dementia. *Am J Psychiatry* 2002;159:1225–1227.

Kyomen HH, Nobel KW, Wei JY. The use of estrogen to decrease aggressive physical behavior in elderly men with dementia. *J Am Geriatr Soc* 1991; 39(10):1110–1112.

Kyomen HH, Satlin A, Hennen J, et al. Estrogen therapy and aggressive behavior in elderly patients with moderate-to-severe dementia; results from a short-term, randomized, double-blind trial. *Am J Geriatr Psychiatry* 1999;7:339–348.

Lawlor BA, Radcliffe J, Molchan SE, et al. A pilot placebo-controlled study of trazodone and buspirone in Alzheimer's disease. *Int J Geriatr Psychiatry* 1994;9:55–59.

Lebert F, Pasquier F, Petit H. Behavioral effects of trazodone in Alzheimer's disease. *J Clin Psychiatry* 1994;55(12):526–538.

Leibovici A, Tariot PN. Carbamazepine treatment of agitation associated with dementia. *J Geriatr Psychiatry Neurol* 1988;1(2):110–112.

Levy MA, Burgio LD, Sweet R, et al. A trial of buspirone for the control of disruptive behaviors in community-dwelling patients with dementia. *Int J Geriatr Psychiatry* 1994;9:841–848.

Lott AD, McElroy SL, Keys MA. Valproate in the treatment of behavioral agitation in elderly patients with dementia. *J Neuropsychiatry Clin Neurosci* 1995;7(3):314–319.

McAllister JW. Carbamazepine in mixed frontal lobe and psychiatric disorders. *J Clin Psychiatry* 1985; 46:393–394.

McKeith I, Del Ser T, Spano P, et al. Efficacy of rivastigmine in dementia with lewy bodies: a randomized, double-blind, placebo-controlled international study. *Lancet* 2000;356:2031–2036.

Marin DB, Greenwald BS. Carbamazepine for aggressive agitation in demented patients during nursing care. *Am J Psychiatry* 1989;146(6):805.

Mazure CM, Druss BG, Cellar JS. Valproate treatment of older psychotic patients with organic mental syndromes and behavioral dyscontrol. *J Am Geriatr Soc* 1992;40(9):914–916.

Mellow AM, Solano-Lopez C, Davis S. Sodium valproate in the treatment of behavioral disturbance in dementia. *J Geriatr Psychiatry Neurol* 1993;6(4):205–209.

Olafsson K, Jørgensen S, Jensen HV, et al. Fluvoxamine in the treatment of demented elderly patients: a double-blind, placebo-controlled study. *Acta Psychiatr Scand* 1992;85:453–456.

Olin JT, Fox LS, Pawluczyk S, et al. A pilot randomized trial of carbamazepine for behavioral symptoms in treatment-resistant outpatients with Alzheimer disease. *Am J Geriatr Psychiatry* 2001;9: 400–405.

Paleacu D, Mazeh D, Mirecki I, et al. Donepezil for the treatment of behavioral symptoms in patients with Alzheimer's disease. *Clinical Neuropharmacology* 2002;25:313–317.

Patterson JF. Carbamazepine for assaultive patients with organic brain disease. *Psychosomatics* 1987; 28(11):579–581.

Patterson JF. A preliminary study of carbamazepine in the treatment of assaultive patients with dementia. *J Geriatr Psychiatry Neurol* 1988;1(1): 21–23.

Petrie WM, Ban TA. Propranolol in organic agitation. *Lancet* 1981;2:324.

Pinner E, Rich CL. Effects of trazodone on aggressive behavior in seven patients with organic mental disorders. *Am J Psychiatry* 1988;145(10): 1295–1296.

Pollock BG, Mulsant BH, Rosen J, et al. Comparison of citalopram, perphenazine, and placebo for the acute treatment of psychosis and behavioral disturbances in hospitalized, demented patients. *Am J Psychiatry* 2002;159:460–465.

Pollock BG, Mulsant BH, Sweet R, et al. An open pilot study of citalopram for behavioral disturbances of dementia: plasma levels and real-time observations. *Am J Geriatr Psychiatry* 1997;5:70–78.

Porsteinsson AP, Tariot PN, Erb R, et al. Placebocontrolled study of divalproex sodium for agitation in dementia. *Am J Geriatr Psychiatry* 2001;9: 58–66.

Porsteinsson AP, Tariot PN, Erb R, et al. An open trial of valproate for agitation in geriatric neuropsychiatric disorders. *Am J Geriatr Psychiatry* 1997; 5:344–351.

Puryear LJ, Kunik ME, Workman Jr R. Tolerability of divalproex sodium in elderly psychiatric patients with mixed diagnoses. *J Geriatr Psychiatry Neurol* 1995;8:234–237.

Sakauye KM, Camp CJ, Ford PA. Effects of buspirone on agitation associated with dementia. *Am J Geriatr Psychiatry* 1993;1(1):82–84.

Simpson DM, Foster. Improvement in organically disturbed behavior with trazodone treatment. *J Clin Psychiatry* 1986;47(4):191–193.

Sival RC, Haffmans PMJ, Van Gent PP, et al. The effects of sodium valproate in the treatment of behavioral disturbances in dementia. *J Am Geriatr Soc* 1994;42:906–909.

Tariot PN, Cummings JL, Katz IR, et al. A randomized, double-blind, placebo-controlled study of the efficacy and safety of donepezil in patients with Alzheimer's disease in the nursing home setting. *J Am Geriatr Soc* 2001;49:1590–1599.

Tariot PN, Erb R, Leibovici A, et al. Carbamazepine treatment of agitation in nursing home patients: a preliminary study. *J Am Geriatr Soc* 1994;42: 1160–1166.

Tariot PN, Erb R, Podgorski CA, et al. Efficacy and tolerability of carbamazepine for agitation and aggression in dementia. *Am J Psychiatry* 1998;155: 54–61.

Weiler PG, Mungas D, Bernick C. Propranolol for the control of disruptive behavior in senile dementia. *J Geriatr Psychiatry Neurol* 1988;1(4): 226–230.

Wilcox J. Divalproex sodium in the treatment of aggressive behavior. *Ann Clin Psychiatry* 1994;6(1): 17–20.

Supplemental Readings

General

Abse W, Dahlstrom WG. The value of chemotherapy in senile mental disturbances. *JAMA* 1960;174: 2036–2042.

Aisen PS, Deluca T, Lawlor BA. Falls among geropsychiatry inpatients are associated with prn medications for agitation. *Int J Geriatr Psychiatry* 1992;7: 709–712.

Alexopoulos GS, Silver JM, Kahn DA, et al. The Expert Consensus Guideline Series: treatment of agitation in older persons with dementia. *Postgrad Med Special report* 1998;April:1–88.

Ancill RJ, Carlyne WW, Liang RA, et al. Agitation in the demented elderly: a role for benzodiazepines? *Int Clin Psychopharmacol* 1991;6:141–146.

Arunpongpaisal S, Ahmed I, Aqeel N, et al. Antipsychotic drug treatment for elderly people with late-onset schizophrenia. *Cochrane Database Syst Rev* 2003;2:CD004162.

Barnes R, Veith R, Okimoto J, et al. Efficacy of antipsychotic medications in behaviorally disturbed dementia patients. *Am J Psychiatry* 1982;199: 1170–1174.

Barton R, Hurst L. Unnecessary use of tranquilizers in elderly patients. *Br J Psychiatry* 1966;112: 989–990.

Billig N, Cohen-Mansfield J, Lipson S. Pharmacological treatment of agitation in a nursing home. *J Am Geriatr Soc* 1991;39(10):1002–1005.

Burnside IM. Symptomatic behaviors in the elderly. In: Birren JB, Sloane RB, eds. *Handbook of mental health and aging.* Englewood Cliffs, NJ: Prentice-Hall, 1980:719–744.

Busse EW. Problems affecting psychiatric care of the aging. *Geriatrics* 1960;15:673–680.

Branchey MH, Lee H, Arun R, et al. High- and low-potency neuroleptics in elderly psychiatric patients. *JAMA* 1978;239:1860–1862.

Christensen K, Haroun A, Schneiderman LJ, et al. Decision-making capacity for informed consent in the older population. *Bull Am Acad Psychiatry Law* 1995;23:353–365.

Coccano EF, Kramer E, Zemishlany Z, et al. Pharmacologic treatment of noncognitive behavioral disturbances in elderly demented patients. *Am J Psychiatry* 1990;147:1640–1645.

Colenda CC, Mickus MA, Marcus SC, et al. Comparison of adult and geriatric psychiatric practice patterns: findings from the American Psychiatric Association's Practice Research Network. *Am J Geriatr Psychiatry* 2002;10:609–617.

Cooper TB, Robinson DS. Pharmacokinetics of neuroleptic drugs in the aged. In: Raskin A, Robinson DS, Levine J, eds. *Age and the pharmacology of psychoactive drugs.* New York: Elsevier, 1981: 181–192.

Cooper AJ. Medroxyprogesterone acetate (MPA) treatment of sexual acting out in men suffering from dementia. *J Clin Psychiatry* 1987;48(9): 368–370.

Davis JM, Dysken MW, Haberman SJ, et al. The use of survival curves in analysis of antipsychotic relapse studies. *Adv Biochem Pharmacol* 1980;24:471–481.

Davis JM, Fann WE, El-Yousef MK, et al. Clinical problems in treating the aged with psychotropic drugs. In: Eisdorfer C, Fann WE, eds. *Psychopharmacology and aging. Vol 6: Advances in behavioral biology.* New York: Plenum, 1973:111–125.

Dawson-Butterworth K. The chemopsychotherapeutics of geriatric sedation. *J Am Geriatr Soc* 1970; 18:97–114.

Devanand DP, Levy SR. Neuroleptic treatment of agitation and psychosis in dementia. *J Geriatr Psychiatry Neurol* 1995;8(suppl 1):S18–S27.

Eisdorfer C. Issues in the Psychopharmacology of the aged. In: Eisdorfer C, Fann WE, eds. *Psychopharmacology and aging. Vol 6: Advances in behavioral biology.* New York: Plenum, 1973:3–7.

Eisdorfer C. Observations on the Psychopharmacology of the aged. *J Am Geriatr Soc* 1975;23:53.

Epstein LJ. Anxiolytics, antidepressants, and neuroleptics in the treatment of geriatric patients. In: Lipton MA, DiMascio A, Killman KF, eds. *Psychopharmacology: a generation of progress.* New York: Raven, 1978:1517–1524.

Exton-Smith AN. Tranquilizers and sedatives in the elderly. *Practitioner* 1962;188:732–738.

Exton-Smith AN, Hodkinson HM, Cromie BW. Controlled comparison of four sedative drugs in elderly patients. *Br Med J* 1963;2:1037–1040.

Field TS, Gurwitz JH, Avorn J, et al. Risk factors for adverse drug events among nursing home residents. *Arch Intern Med* 2001;161:1629–1634.

Ganzini L, Heintz R, Hoffman WF, et al. Acute extrapyramidal syndromes in neuroleptic-treated elders: a pilot study. *J Geriatr Psychiatry Neurol* 1991; 4:222–225.

Gilbert PL, Harris MJ, McAdams LA, et al. Neuroleptic withdrawal in schizophrenic patients: a review of the literature. *Arch Gen Psychiatry* 1995;52: 173–188.

Glassman AH, Bigger JT, Jr. Antipsychotic drugs: prolonged QTc interval, torsade de pointes, and sudden death. *Am J Psychiatry* 2001;158: 1774–1782.

Gottlieb GL, McAllister TW, Gur RC. Depot neuroleptics in the treatment of behavioral disorders in patients with Alzheimer's disease. *J Am Geriatr Soc* 1988;36:619–621.

Gurian BS, Baker EH, Jacobson S, et al. Informed consent for neuroleptics with elderly patients in two settings. *J Am Geriatr Soc* 1990;38:37–44.

Guze BH, Baxter LR Jr. Neuroleptic malignant syndrome. *N Engl J Med* 1985;313:163–166.

Hamilton LD. Aged brain and the phenothiazines. *Geriatrics* 1966;21:131.

Helms PM. Efficacy of antipsychotics in the treatment of the behavioral complications of dementia: a review of the literature. *J Am Geriatr Soc* 1985; 33:206–209.

Houlihan DJ, Mulsant BH, Sweet RA, et al. A naturalistic study of trazodone in the treatment of behavioral complications of dementia. *Am J Geriatr Psychiatry* 1994;2:78–85.

Howard R, Ballard C, O'Brien J, et al. UK and Ireland Group for Optimization of Management in Dementia. Guidelines for the management of agitation in dementia. *Int J Geriatr Psychiatry* 2001;16: 714–717.

Howell TH, Harth JAD, Dutuch M. Sedation and analgesia in old age. *Practitioner* 1954;173: 172–173.

Jenike MA. *Handbook of geriatric psychopharmacology.* Littletown, MA: PSG, 1985.

Jeste DV. Late-onset schizophrenia: an overview. *Schizophr Bull* 1988;14:39–55.

Jeste DV, Gilbert P, McAdams LA, et al. Considering neuroleptic maintenance and taper on a continuum: need for individual, rather than dogmatic, approach. *Arch Gen Psychiatry* 1995;52:209–212.

Jeste DV, Lacro JP, Gilbert PL, et al. Treatment of late-life schizophrenia with neuroleptics. *Schizophr Bull* 1993;19(4):817–830.

Kinon BJ, Stauffer VL, McGuire HC, et al. The effects of antipsychotic drug treatment on prolactin concentrations in elderly patients. *J Am Med Dir Assoc* 2003;4:189–194.

Koller WC. Edentulous orodyskinesia. *Ann Neurol* 1983;13:97–99.

Lazarus LW. Psychotropic drug management of the organic psychoses in the elderly. In: Davis JM, Greenblatt DJ, eds. *Psychopharmacology update: new and neglected areas.* New York: Grune & Stratton, 1979:15–27.

Learoyd BM. Psychotropic drugs in the aging patient. *Med J Aust* 1972;1:1131–1133.

Lehmann HE, Ban TA. Comparative pharmacotherapy of the aging psychotic patient. *Laval Med* 1967;38:588–595.

Lehmann HE, Ban TA. Chemotherapy in aged psychiatric patients. *Can Psychiatr Assoc J* 1969;14: 361–369.

Lifshitz K, Kline NS. Psychopharmacology of the aged. In: Freeman JT, ed. *Clinical principles and drugs in the aging.* Springfield, IL: Charles C. Thomas, 1963:421–457.

Maurer AS. Management of emotional disturbances in geriatric patients. *J Am Geriatr Soc* 1973;21: 226–228.

Meyers BS, Klimstra SA, Gabriele M, et al. Continuation treatment of delusional depression in older adults. *Am J Geriatr Psychiatry* 2001;9:415–422.

Post F. The impact of modern drug treatment on old age schizophrenia. *Gerontol Clin* 1962;4:137–146.

Prien RF, Haber PA, Caffey EM. The use of psychoactive drugs in elderly patients with psychiatric disorders: survey conducted in twelve Veterans Administration hospitals. *J Am Geriatr Soc* 1975;23: 104–112.

Raskind MA, Risse SC. Antipsychotic drugs and the elderly. *J Clin Psychiatry* 1986:5(suppl):17–22.

Risse SC, Barnes R. Pharmacologic treatment of agitation associated with dementia. *J Am Geriatr Soc* 1986;34:368–376.

Ritschel WA. In: Pagliano LA, Pagliano AM, eds. *Pharmacologic aspects of aging.* St. Louis: CV Mosby, 1983:219–256.

Robinson DB. Evaluation of certain drugs in geriatric patients. *Arch Gen Psychiatry* 1969;25:41–46.

Ruths S, Straand J, Nygaard HA. Multidisciplinary medication review in nursing home residents: what are the most significant drug-related problems? The Bergen District Nursing Home (BEDNURS) study. *Qual Saf Health Care* 2003;12: 176–180.

Salzman C. Update on geriatric psychopharmacology. *Geriatrics* 1979;34:87–90.

Salzman C. Geriatric psychopharmacology. In: Gelenberg A, Bassuk E, Schoonover S, eds. *The practi-*

tioner's guide to psychiatric drugs. 3rd ed. New York: Plenum, 1981.

Salzman C. Key concepts in geriatric psychopharmacology: altered pharmacokinetics and polypharmacy. *Psychiatr Clin North Am* 1982;5:181–190.

Salzman C. Management of psychiatric problems. In: Rowe JW, Besdine RW, eds. *Health and disease in old age.* Boston: Little, Brown, 1982:115–136.

Salzman C. A primer on geriatric psychopharmacology. *Am J Psychiatry* 1982;139:67–74.

Salzman C. Basic principles of psychotropic drug prescription for the elderly. *Hosp Community Psychiatry* 1982;33:133–136.

Salzman C. Geriatric psychopharmacology. *Annu Rev Med* 1985;36:217–228.

Salzman C. Treatment of the elderly agitated patient. *J Clin Psychiatry* 1987;48(suppl):19–22.

Salzman C. Treatment of agitation, anxiety, and depression in dementia. *Psychopharmacol Bull* 1988;24:39–42.

Salzman C. Treatment of the agitated demented patient. *Hosp Community Psychiatry* 1988;39:1143–1144.

Salzman C. Recent advances in geriatric psychopharmacology. *APA Update* 1989;9:279–292.

Salzman C. Principles of psychopharmacology. In: Bienenfeld DR, ed. *Verwoert's clinical geropsychiatry.* Baltimore: Williams & Wilkins, 1990:234–249.

Salzman C, Hoffman SA, Schoonover SC. In: Bassuk LL, Schoonover SC, Gelenberg A, eds. *Practitioner's guide to psychoactive drugs.* New York: Plenum, 1983.

Salzman C, Nevis-Olesen J. Psychopharmacological and somatic treatments. In: Birren JE, ed. *Handbook of mental health and aging.* New York: Academic Press, 1992.

Salzman C, Shader RI, Pearlman M. Psychopharmacology and the elderly. In: Shader RI, DiMascio A, eds. *Psychotropic drug side effects.* Baltimore: Williams & Wilkins, 1970:261–279.

Salzman C, Shader RI, van der Kolk BA. Psychopharmacology and the geriatric patient. In: Shader RI, ed. *A manual of psychiatric therapeutics.* Boston: Little, Brown, 1975:171–184.

Salzman C, Shader RI, van der Kolk BA. Clinical psychopathology and the elderly patients. *NY State J Med* 1976;76:71–77.

Schneider LS, Pollock VE, Lyness SA. A metaanalysis of controlled trials of neuroleptic treatment in dementia. *J Am Geriatr Soc* 1990;38:553–563.

Schneider LS, Sobin PB. Neuroleptic medications in the management of psychogeriatric patients: a double-blind clinical trial. *Psychosomatics* 1990;15: 134–138.

Schneider LS, Tariot PN, Lyketsos CG, et al. National Institute of Mental Health Clinical Antipsychotic Trials of Intervention Effectiveness (CATIE): Alzheimer disease trial methodology. *Am J Geriatr Psychiatry* 2001;9:346–360.

Sewell DD, Jeste DV. Distinguishing neuroleptic malignant syndrome (NMS) from NMS-like acute medical illnesses: a study of 34 cases. *J Neuropsychiatry Clin Neurosci* 1992;4:265–269.

Siede H, Muller HF. Choreiform movements as side effects of phenothiazine medication in geriatric patients. *J Am Geriatr Soc* 1967;15:517–522.

Silverman M, Parker JB, Busse EW. A review of drugs

in the elderly psychiatric patient. *NC Med J* 1959; 20:432–482.

Sloane RB. Psychiatric problems of the aged. *Cont Educ* 1978;11:42–47.

Small GW. Psychopharmacological treatment of elderly demented patients. *J Clin Psychiatry* 1988; 49(suppl):8–13.

Spencer T. The management of behavior disorders in the geriatric patient. *Md State Med J* 1969;18: 73–76.

Spira N, Dysken MW, Lazarus LW, et al. Treatment of agitation and psychosis. In: Salzman C, ed. *Clinical geriatric psychopharmacology.* New York: McGraw-Hill, 1984:49–76.

Steinhart MJ. Psychiatric aspects and management of aging patients. *NY State Med J* 1974;74: 976–978.

Stotsky BA. Haloperidol in the treatment of geriatric patients. In: DiMascio A, Shader RI, eds. *Butyrophenones in psychiatry.* New York: Raven, 1972: 71–86.

Stotsky BA. Psychosis in the elderly. In: Eisdorfer C, Faren WE, eds. *Psychopharmacology and aging.* New York: Plenum, 1973:193–202.

Stotsky BA. Psychoactive drugs for geriatric patients with psychiatric disorders. In: Gershon S, Raskin A, eds. *Aging. Vol 2: Genesis and treatment of psychological disorders in the elderly.* New York: Raven, 1975:239–258.

Sweet RA, Pollock BG. Neuroleptics in the elderly: guidelines for monitoring. *Harv Rev Psychiatry* 1995;2:327–335.

Tariot PN, Schneider LS, Katz IR. Anticonvulsant and other non-neuroleptic treatment of agitation in dementia. *Geriatr Psychiatr Neurol* 1995;8(suppl 1):S28–S39.

Teri L, Larson EB, Reifler BV. Behavioral disturbance in dementia of the Alzheimer type. *J Am Geriatr Soc* 1988;36:1–6.

Tewfik GI, Jain VK, Harcup M, Magowan S. Effectiveness of various tranquilizers in the management of senile restlessness. *Gerontol Clin* 1970;12: 351–359.

Thompson TLH, Morgan MG, Nies AS. Psychotropic drug use in the elderly. *N Engl J Med* 1983;308: 194–199.

Tune LE, Strauss ME, Lew MF, et al. Serum levels of anticholinergic drugs and impaired recent memory in chronic schizophrenic patients. *Am J Psychiatry* 1982;139:1460–1462.

U.S. Senate Special Committee on Aging. Drugs and nursing homes. Washington, DC: Government Printing Office, 1975.

van Reekum R, Clarke D, Conn D, et al. A randomized, placebo-controlled trial of the discontinuation of long-term antipsychotics in dementia. *Int Psychogeriatr* 2002;14:197–210.

Wolff K. *Geriatric psychiatry.* Springfield, IL: Charles C Thomas, 1963;78–86.

patients with anxiety and tension: a double-blind study. *J Am Geriatr Soc* 1963;11:445–448.

Hamilton LD, Bennett JL. Acetophenazine for hyperactive geriatric patients. *Geriatrics* 1962;17: 596–601.

Honigfeld G, Newhall PN. Hemodynamic effects of imipramine, acetophenazine or trifluoperazine in geriatric psychiatry. *Dis Nerv Syst* 1965;26: 427–429.

Sheppard C, Bhattacharya A, DiGiacomo M, et al. Effects of acetophenazine dimaleate on paranoid symptomatology in female geriatric patients. *J Am Geriatr Soc* 1964;12:884–888.

Welborn WS. A trial of a new tranquilizing agent in geriatric patients. *Psychosomatics* 1961;2:1–3.

Buspirone

Cantillon M, Brunswick R, Molina D, Bahro M. Busiprone vs. haloperidol. A double-blind trial for agitation in a nursing home population with Alzheimer's disease. *Am J Geriatr Psychiatry* 1996;4: 263–267.

Colenda CC. Buspirone in treatment of agitated demented patients. *Lancet* 1988;1:1169.

Sakauye KM, Camp CJ, Ford PA. Effects of buspirone on agitation associated with dementia. *Am J Geriatr Psychiatry* 1993;1:82–84.

Tiller JWG, Dakis JA, Shaw JM. Short-term buspirone treatment in disinhibition with dementia. *Lancet* 1988;2:510.

Valproate

Lott AD, McElroy SL, Keys MA. Valproate in the treatment of behavioral agitation in elderly patients with dementia. *J Neuropsychiatry Clin Neurosci* 1995;7(3):314–319.

Mellow AM, Solano-Lopez C, Davis S. Sodium valproate in the treatment of behavioral disturbance in dementia. *J Geriatr Psychiatry Neurol* 1993;6:205–209.

Carbamazepine

Chambers CA, Bain J, Rosbottom R, et al. Carbamazepine in senile dementia and overactivity—placebo controlled double blind trial. *IRCS Med Sci* 1982;10:505–506.

Gleason RP, Schneider LS. Carbamazepine treatment of agitation in Alzheimer's outpatients refractory to neuroleptics. *J Clin Psychiatry* 1990;51: 115–118.

Leibovici A, Tariot P. Carbamazepine treatment of agitation associated with dementia. *J Geriatr Psychiatry Neurol* 1988;1:110–112.

Lemke MR. Effect of carbamazepine on agitation in Alzheimer's inpatients refractory to neuroleptics. *J Clin Psychiatry* 1995;56:354–357.

McAllister TW. Carbamazepine in mixed frontal lobe and psychiatric disorders. *J Clin Psychiatry* 1985;46(9):393–394.

Tariot PN, Mack JL, Patterson MB, et al. The Behavior Rating Scale for Dementia of the Consortium

Acetophenazine

Ayd FJ. Tranquilizers and the ambulatory geriatric patient. *J Am Geriatr Soc* 1961;8:909–914.

Chesrow EJ, Kaplitz SE, Breme JT, et al. Acetophenazine (Tindal) in the treatment of chronically ill to Establish a Registry for Alzheimer's Disease. *Am J Psychiatr* 1995;152:1349–1357.

Chlorpromazine

Abse W, Dahlstrom WG. The value of chemotherapy in senile mental disturbances. *JAMA* 1960;174: 2036–2042.

Altman H, Mehta D, Evenson RC, et al. Behavioral effects of drug therapy on psychogeriatric inpatients. I: Chlorpromazine and thioridazine. *J Am Geriatr Soc* 1973;21:241–248.

Barton R, Hurst L. Unnecessary use of tranquilizers in elderly patients. *Br J Psychiatry* 1966;112: 989–990.

Birkett DP, Boltuch B. Chlorpromazine in geriatric psychiatry. *J Am Geriatr Soc* 1972;20:403–406.

Kurland AA. Chlorpromazine in the management of the institutionalized aged psychiatric patient with chronic brain syndrome. *Dis Nerv Syst* 1955;16: 336–369.

Pollack B. The addition of chlorpromazine to the treatment program of emotional behavioral disorder in the aged. *Geriatrics* 1956;11:253–259.

Prien RF, Levine J, Cole JO. Indications for high dose chlorpromazine therapy in chronic schizophrenia. *Dis Nerv Syst* 1979;31:739–745.

Robinson DS. Elevation of certain drugs in geriatric patients. *Arch Gen Psychiatry* 1969;25:41–46.

Seager CP. Chlorpromazine in the treatment of elderly psychotic women. *Br Med J* 1955;1:882–884.

Settel E. Chlorpromazine in the treatment of senile agitation. *Gen Pract* 1956;12:74–76.

Silverman M, Parker JB, Busse EW. A review of drugs in the elderly psychiatric patient. *NC Med J* 1959; 20:428–432.

Terman LA. Treatment of senile agitation with chlorpromazine. *Geriatrics* 1955;10:520–522.

Young RC. Plasma nor 1-chlorpromazine concentrations: effects of age, race, and sex. *Ther Drug Monit* 1986;8:23–26.

Diazepam

deLemos GP, Clement WR, Nickels E. Effects of diazepam suspension in geriatric patients hospitalized for psychiatric illness. *J Am Geriatr Soc* 1965; 13:355–359.

Fluphenazine

Kane JM, Smith JM. Fluphenazine vs. placebo in patients with remitted, acute first-episode schizophrenia. *Arch Gen Psychiatry* 1982;39:473–481.

Raskind M, Alvarez C, Herlin RN. Fluphenazine enanthate in the outpatient treatment of late paraphrenia. *J Am Geriatr Soc* 1979;27:459–463.

Settel E. Treatment of anxiety and agitation with prochlorperazine in geriatric patients. *J Am Geriatr Soc* 1957;5:827–831.

Silverman M, Parker JB, Busse EW. A review of drugs in the elderly psychiatric patient. NC Med J 1959; 20:428–432.

Haloperidol

Aoba A, Kakita Y, Yamaguchi N, et al. Absence of age effect on plasma haloperidol neuroleptic levels in psychiatric patients. *J Gerontol* 1985;40: 303–308.

Ban TA, Pecknold JE. Haloperidol and the butyrophenones. In: Simpson LL, ed. *Drug treatment of mental disorder.* New York: Raven, 1975:45–60.

Devanand DP, Cooper T, Sackeim HA, et al. Low dose haloperidol and blood levels in Alzheimer's disease: a preliminary study. *Psychopharmacol Bull* 1992;28(2):169–173.

Forsman A, Ohman R. Pharmokinetic studies on haloperidol in man. *Curr Ther Res* 1976;20: 319–336.

Gerle B, Petersson B, Widmark M. Clinical experiences with haloperidol. *Svenska Lak Tidn* 1961; 58:415–418.

Gotestam KG, Ljunghell S, Olsson B. A double-blind comparison of the effects of haloperidol and Cig(2)-clopenthixol in senile dementia. *Acta Psychiatr Scand* 1981;294(suppl):46–53.

Lacro JP, Kuczenski R, Roznoski M, et al. Serum haloperidol levels in older psychotic patients. *Am J Geriatr Psychiatry* 1996;4:229–236.

Lapolla A, Nash LR. A butyrophenone (haloperidol) for the treatment of institutionalized patients. *Int J Neuropsychiatry* 1966;2:129–134.

Lovett WC, Stokes DK, Taylor LB, et al. Management of behavioral symptoms in disturbed elderly patients: comparison of trifluoperazine and haloperidol. *J Clin Psychiatry* 1987;48:234–236.

Rosen HJ. Double-blind comparison of haloperidol and thioridazine in geriatric outpatients. *J Clin Psychiatry* 1979;40:24–31.

Smith GR, Taylor CW, Linkous P. Haloperidol versus thioridazine for the treatment of psychogeriatric patients. A double-blind trial. *Psychosomatics* 1974; 15:134–138.

Solomon K. Haloperidol and the geriatric patient: practical considerations. In: FJ Ayd Jr, ed. *Haloperidol update 1958–1980.* Baltimore: Ayd Medical Communications, 1980:115–173.

Steinhart MJ. Psychotropic drugs. *Am Fam Physician* 1975;12:92–101.

Stotsky BA. Haloperidol in the treatment of geriatric patients. In: DiMascio A, Shader RI, eds. *Butyrophenones in psychiatry.* New York: Raven, 1972: 71–86.

Stotsky BA. Psychoactive drugs for geriatric patients with psychiatric disorders. In: Gershon S, Raskin A, eds. *Aging. Vol 2: Genesis and treatment of psychological disorders in the elderly.* New York: Raven, 1975:239–258.

Sugarman AA, Williams H, Adlerstein AM. Haloperidol in the psychiatric disorders of old age. *Am J Psychiatry* 1964;120:1190–1192.

Tesar GE, Murray BG, Cassem NH. Use of high-dose intravenous haloperidol in the treatment of agitated cardiac patients. *J Clin Psychopharmacol* 1985;5(6):344–347.

Tewfik GE, Jain VK, Harcup M, et al. Effectiveness of various tranquilizers in the management of senile restlessness. *Gerontol Clin* 1970;12: 351–359.

Tobin JM, Brosseau ER, Lorenz AA. Clinical evaluation of haloperidol in geriatric patients. *Geriatrics* 1970;25:119–122.

Tsuang MM, Min LL, Stotsky BA, Cole JO. Haloperidol versus thioridazine for hospitalized psychogeriatric patients. *J Am Geriatr Soc* 1971;19:593–600.

Viukari M, Salo H, Lamminsiva U, Gordin A. Tolerance and serum levels of haloperidol during parenteral and oral haloperidol treatment in geriatric patients. *Acta Psychiatr Scand* 1982;65:301–308.

Perphenazine

Ayd FJ Jr. The treatment of anxiety, agitation and excitement in the aged. *J Am Geriatr Soc* 1957;5:1–4.

Mulsant BH, Sweet RA, Rosen J, et al. A double-blind randomized comparison of nortriptyline plus perphenazine versus nortriptyline plus placebo in the treatment of psychotic depression in late life. *J Clin Psychiatry* 2001;62:597–604.

Singh AN, Saxena BM. A comparative study of prolonged action (depot) neuroleptics: pipothiazine palmitate versus fluphenazine ananthate in chronic schizophrenic patients. *Curr Ther Res* 1975;25:121–132.

Pimozide

Kushnir SL. Pimozide in the management of psychotically agitated demented patients. *J Am Geriatr Soc* 1987;35:1–3.

Propranolol

Elliot FA. The neurology of explosive rage. *Practitioner* 1976;217:51–59.

Elliot FA. Propranolol for the control of belligerent behavior following acute brain damage. *Ann Neurol* 1977;1:489–491.

Ratey JJ, Morrill R, Oxenkrug G. Use of propranolol for provoked and unprovoked episodes of rage. *Am J Psychiatry* 1983;140:1356–1357.

Schreier HA. Use of propranolol in the treatment of postencephalitic psychosis. *Am J Psychiatry* 1979;136:840–841.

Sheppard GP. High-dose propranolol in schizophrenia. *Br J Psychiatry* 1979;134:470–476.

Yorkston NJ, Zaki SA, Pitcher OR, et al. Propranolol as an adjunct to the treatment of schizophrenia. *Lancet* 1977;2:575–578.

Yudofsky S, Williams D, Gorman J. Propranolol in the treatment of rage and violent behavior in patients with chronic brain syndromes. *Am J Psychiatry* 1981;138:218–220.

Thioridazine

Ahmed A. Thioridazine in the management of geriatric patients. *J Am Geriatr Soc* 1968;16:945–947.

Altman H, Mehta D, Evenson RC. Behavioral effects of drug therapy on psychogeriatric inpatients. I:

Chlorpromazine and thioridazine. *J Am Geriatr Soc* 1973;21:241–248.

Ayd FJ. Tranquilizers and the ambulatory geriatric patient. Thioridazine side-chain sulfoxide and thioridazine side chain sulfone, in chronic psychotic patients. *J Am Geriatr Soc* 1961;8:909–914.

Ban TA. Psychopathology, Psychopharmacology and the organic brain syndromes, part II. *Psychosomatics* 1976;17:131–137.

Barksdale B. Behavior problems in nursing home patients. Treatment with thioridazine. *Curr Ther Res* 1971;13:359–363.

Beber CR. Management of behavior in the institutionalized aged. *Dis Nerv Syst* 1965;26:591–595.

Bercel NA. Clinical trial of thioridazine in private practice. *Am Pract Digest Treat* 1961;12:44–48.

Birkett DP, Boltuch B. Psychotropic drugs in old age. *J Med Soc NJ* 1973;70:647–648.

Brovins WG, Wierzbicki J. Use of thioridazine. *Mich Med* 1967;66:583–584.

Cavero CV. Evaluation of thioridazine in the aged. *J Am Geriatr Soc* 1966;14:617–622.

Cervera AA. Psychoactive drug therapy in the senile patients: controlled comparison of thioridazine and diazepam. *Psychiatr Digest* 1974;35:15–21.

Chien CP. Psychiatric treatment for geriatric patients. "Pub" or drug? *Am J Psychiatry* 1971;127:1070–1075.

Cobb AB, Wilson DP, Abide JM. Use of drugs under the Mississippi Medicaid program. *J Miss Med Assoc* 1972;13:81–85.

Cohen S. Thioridazine (Mellaril): a review. *Mind* 1964;2:134–145.

Cole JO, Stotsky BA. Improving psychiatric drug therapy: a matter of dosage and choice. *Geriatrics* 1974;39:74–78.

Covington JS. Alleviating agitation, apprehension, and related symptoms in geriatric patients: a double-blind comparison of a phenothiazine and a benzodiazepine. *South Med J* 1975;68:719–724.

Dawson-Butterwork K. The chemopsychotherapeutics of geriatric sedations. *J Am Geriatr Soc* 1970;18:719–724.

DiMascio A, Goldberg HL. Managing disturbed geriatric patients with chemotherapy. *Hosp Physician* 1975;11:35–39.

Felger HL. Thioridazine (Mellaril) in the geriatric patient. *Dis Nerv Syst* 1972;33:178–182.

Fleischl H. Effects of thioridazine on chronically regressed patients. *J Am Geriatr Soc* 1967;15:29–33.

Fraiberg PL. Control of behavioral symptoms in patients with long-term illness. *Dis Nerv Syst* 1972;33:178–182.

Hader M. The use of selected phenothiazines in elderly patients: a review. *J Mt Sinai Hosp* 1972;33:178–182.

Hamilton LD. Aged brain and the phenothiazines. *Geriatrics* 1966;21:131–138.

Hoogerbeets JD, Lawall J. Changing concepts of psychiatric problems in the aged. *Geriatrics* 1975;40:83–87.

Jackson EB. Mellaril in the treatment of the geriatric patient. *Am J Psychiatry* 1961;118:543–544.

Judah L, Murphee D, Seager L. Psychiatric response of geriatric-psychiatric patients to Mellaril (TP-21 Sandoz). *Am J Psychiatry* 1959;115:1118–1119.

Kastenbaum R, Aisenberg R. Toward a conceptual model of geriatric psychopharmacology; an experiment with thioridazine and dextroamphetamine. *Gerontologist* 1964;4:68–71.

Katz MM, Itil TM. Video methodology for research in psychopathology and psychopharmacology. *Arch Gen Psychiatry* 1974;31:204–210.

Kirven LE, Montero EF. Comparison of thioridazine and diazepam in the control of nonpsychotic symptoms associated with senility: double-blind study. *J Am Geriatr Soc* 1973;21:546–551.

Kral VA. The use of thioridazine (Mellaril) in aged people. *Can Med Assoc J* 1961;84:152–154.

Lehmann HE, Ban TA. Comparative pharmacotherapy of the aging psychotic patients. *Laval Med* 1967;38:588–595.

Lehmann HE, Ban TA. Thioridazine—geriatrics. *Psychopharmacol Bull* 1974;7:75–76.

Lehmann HE, Ban TA, Kral VA. Drugs and patients: evaluating chemicals that change human behavior. *Psychopharmacol Bull* 1970;6:48–63.

Maurer AS. Management of emotional disturbances in geriatric patients. *J Am Geriatr Soc* 1973;21:226–228.

Meyer LD. *Side effects of drugs.* New York: Excerpta Medica, 1963.

McDonald C. Problems of aging: psychoneurosis in the elderly. *Postgrad Med* 1965;38:432–437.

Musze RG, Vanderheeren FAJ. Plasma levels and half lives of thioridazine and some of its metabolites. II: Low doses in older psychiatric patients. *Eur J Clin Pharmacol* 1977;11:141–147.

Prien RF. Chemotherapy in chronic organic brain syndrome—a review of the literature. *Psychopharmacol Bull* 1973;9:5–20.

Prien RF. A survey of psychoactive drug use in the aged in Veterans Administration hospitals. *Psychopharmacol Bull* 1975;11:50–51.

Reedy WJ. An internist's observations on thioridazine in the very elderly. *J Am Geriatr Soc* 1967;15:587–592.

Ricitelli ML. Modern concepts in the management of anxiety and depression in the aged and infirm. *J Am Geriatr Soc* 1964;12:652–657.

Smith GR, Taylor CW, Linkons P. Haloperidol versus thioridazine for the treatment of psychogeriatric patients: a double-blind trial. *Psychosomatics* 1974;15:134–138.

Tonken H. Indications for phenothiazines in general practice and clinical trial with thioridazine. *Manit Med Rev* 1966;46:630–634.

Tsuang MM, Min Lu L, Stotsky BA, et al. Haloperidol versus thioridazine for hospitalized psychogeriatric patients. *J Am Geriatr Soc* 1971;19:593–600.

Thiothixene

Ban TA. Drug interactions with psychoactive drugs. *Dis Nerv Syst* 1975;36:164–166.

Ban TA. *Pharmacotherapy of thiothixene.* New York: Raven, 1978:156.

Ban TA. Some recent biochemical findings with possible therapeutic implications for schizophrenia. *J Clin Psychiatry* 1978;38:535–541.

Birkett DP, Hirschifield W, Simpson GM. Thiothixene in the treatment of diseases of the senium. *Curr Ther Res* 1972;14:775–779.

Charatan FB. Depression in old age. *NY State J Med* 1975;1:2505–2509.

Cohen BM, Sommer BR. Metabolism of thioridazine in the elderly. *J Clin Psychopharmacol* 1988;8:336–339.

Covington JS. Alleviating agitation, apprehension, and related symptoms in geriatric patients: a double-blind comparison of a phenothiazine and a benzodiazepine. *South Med J* 1975;68:719–724.

Itil TM, Unvrdi C, Wohlrabe J, et al. Drug therapy of psychosis associated with organic brain syndrome. Scientific exhibit at the American Public Health Association centennial, Atlantic City, NJ, 1972.

Katz MM, Itil TM. Video methodology for research in psychopathology and psychopharmacology. *Arch Gen Psychiatry* 1974;31:204–210.

Lehmann HE, Ban TA. Thiothixene in geriatrics. *Psychopharmacol Bull* 1970;6:123–124.

Mohler G. Clinical trial of thiothixene (Navane) in elderly chronic schizophrenics. *Curr Ther Res* 1970;12(5):377–386.

Olivros RT, Ban TA, Lehmann HE, et al. Thiothixene—its range of therapeutic activity. *Int J Clin Pharmacol* 1970;3:26–29.

Rada RT, Kellner R. Thiothixene in the treatment of geriatric patients with chronic organic brain syndrome. *J Am Geriatr Soc* 1976;24:105–107.

Sloane RB. Psychiatric problems of the aged. *Cont Educ* 1978;11:42–47.

Steinhart MJ. Drugs for the elderly psychiatric patient. *Consultant* 1978;18:137–139.

Trazodone

Greenwald BS, Marin DB, Silverman SM. Serotonergic treatment of screaming and banging in dementia. *Lancet* 1986;2:1464–1465.

Lawlor BA, Radcliffe J, Molchan SE, et al. A pilot placebo-controlled study of trazodone and buspirone in Alzheimer's disease. *Int J Geriatr Psychiatry* 1994;9:55–59.

Nair NPV, Ban TA, Hontela S, Clarke R. Trazodone in the treatment of organic brain syndromes with special reference to psychogeriatrics. *Curr Ther Res* 1973;15:769–775.

O'Neil M, Page N, Adkins WN. Tryptophan-trazodone treatment of aggressive behavior. *Lancet* 1986;2:859–860.

Pinner E, Rich CL. Effects of trazodone on aggressive behavior in seven patients with organic mental disorders. *Am J Psychiatry* 1988;145(10):1295–1296.

Simpson DM, Foster D. Improvement in organically disturbed behavior with trazodone treatment. *J Clin Psychiatry* 1986;47:191–193.

Tingle D. Trazodone in dementia. *J Clin Psychiatry* 1986;47:482.

Trifluoperazine

Brooks GW, MacDonald MG. Effects of trifluoperazine in aged depressed female patients. *Am J Psychiatry* 1961;117:932–933.

Hamilton LD, Bennett JL. The use of trifluoperazine in geriatric patients with chronic brain syndrome. *J Am Geriatr Soc* 1962;10:140–147.

Kropach K. The treatment of acutely agitated senile

patients with trifluoperazine (Stelazine). *Br J Clin Pract* 1959;13:859–862.

Lovett WC, Stokes DK, Taylor LB, et al. Management of behavioral symptoms in disturbed elderly patients: comparison of trifluoperazine and haloperidol. *J Clin Psychiatry* 1987;48:234–236.

Prien RF, Levine J, Cole JO. High-dose trifluoperazine therapy in chronic schizophrenia. *Am J Psychiatry* 1969;126:305–313.

Mesoridazine

Goldstein BJ, Dippy WE. A clinical evaluation of mesoridazine (Serentil) in geriatric patients. *Curr Ther Res* 1967;9:256–260.

Prochlorperazine

Settel E. Treatment of anxiety and agitation with prochlorperazine in geriatric patients. *J Am Geriatr Soc* 1957;5:827–831.

Shubin H, Sherson J. Prochlorperazine in the management of restive aged patients. *J Am Geriatr Soc* 1959;7(5):405–407.

Melperone

DeCuyper H, van Plaag HM, Verstraeten D. The effect of milenperone on the aggressive behavior of psychogeriatric patients. *Neuropsychobiology* 1985; 13:1–6.

Fisher R, Blair M, Shedletsky R, et al. An open dose finding study of melperone in treatment of agitation and irritability associated with dementia. *Can J Psychiatry* 1983;28(3):193–196.

Molindone

Pepper M. Clinical experience with molindone hydrochloride in geriatric patients. *J Clin Psychiatry* 1985;46(8):26–29.

Risperidone

Allain H, Tessier C, Bentue-Ferrer D, et al. Effects of risperidone on psychometric and cognitive functions in healthy elderly volunteers. *Psychopharmacology* (Berl) 2003;165:419–429.

Barak Y, Shamir E, Weizman R. Would a switch from typical antipsychotics to risperidone be beneficial for elderly schizophrenic patients? A naturalistic, long-term, retrospective, comparative study. *J Clin Psychopharmacol* 2002;22:115–120.

Barak Y. No weight gain among elderly schizophrenia patients after 1 year of risperidone treatment. *J Clin Psychiatry* 2002;63:117–119.

Ellis T, Cudkowicz ME, Sexton PM, et al. Clozapine and risperidone treatment of psychosis in Parkinson's disease. *J Neuropsychiatry Clin Neurosci* 2000; 12:364–369.

Gallucci G, Beard G. Risperidone and the treatment of delusions of parasitosis in an elderly patient. *Psychosomatics* 1995;36(6):578–580.

Jeste DV, Eastham JH, Lacro JP, et al. Management of late-life psychosis. *J Clin Psychiatry* 1996; 57(suppl 3):39–45.

Jeste DV, Klausner M, Brecher M, et al. A clinical evaluation of risperidone in the treatment of schizophrenia: a 10-week, open-label, multicenter trial ARCS Study Group. Assessment of Risperdal in a Clinical Setting. *Psychopharmacology (Berl)* 1997;131:239–247.

Koro CE, Fedder DO, L'Italien GJ, et al. Assessment of independent effect of olanzapine and risperidone on risk of diabetes among patients with schizophrenia: population based nested case-control study. *BMJ* 2002;325:243.

Koro CE, Fedder DO, L'Italien GJ, et al. An assessment of the independent effects of olanzapine and risperidone exposure on the risk of hyperlipidemia in schizophrenic patients. *Arch Gen Psychiatry* 2002;59:1021–1026.

Madhusoodanan S, Brenner R, Araujo L, et al. Efficacy of risperidone treatment for psychoses associated with schizophrenia, schizoaffective disorder, bipolar disorder, or senile dementia in 11 geriatric patients: a case series. *J Clin Psychiatry* 1995;56(11):514–518.

Marder SR, Meibach RC. Risperidone in the treatment of schizophrenia. *Am J Psychiatry* 1994;151: 825–835.

Meco G, Bedini L, Bonifati V, et al. Risperidone in the treatment of chronic schizophrenia with tardive dyskinesia. *Curr Ther Res* 1989;46(5): 876–883.

Meyer JM. A retrospective comparison of weight, lipid, and glucose changes between risperidone- and olanzapine-treated inpatients: metabolic outcomes after 1 year. *J Clin Psychiatry* 2002;63: 425–433.

Weiser M, Rotmensch HH, Korczyn AD, et al. Rivastigmine-Risperidone Study Group. A pilot, randomized, open-label trial assessing safety and pharmacokinetic parameters of co-administration of rivastigmine with risperidone in dementia patients with behavioral disturbances. *Int J Geriatr Psychiatry* 2002;17:343–346.

Yerrabolu M, Prabhudesai S, Tawam M, et al. Effect of risperidone on QT interval and QT dispersion in the elderly. *Heart Dis* 2000;2:10–12.

Zhao Q, Xie C, Pesco-Koplowitz L, et al. Pharmacokinetic and safety assessments of concurrent administration of risperidone and donepezil. *J Clin Pharmacol* 2003;43:180–186.

Atypical Antipsychotics

Ames D, Wirshing WC, Marder SR. Advances in antipsychotic pharmacotherapy: clozapine, risperidone, and beyond. *Essent Psychopharmacol* 1996; 1(1):5–26.

Barak Y, Shamir E, Zemishlani H, et al. Olanzapine vs. haloperidol in the treatment of elderly chronic schizophrenia patients. *Prog Neuropsychopharmacol Biol Psychiatry* 2002;26:1199–1202.

Breitbart W, Tremblay A, Gibson C. An open trial of olanzapine for the treatment of delirium in hospitalized cancer patients. *Psychosomatics* 2002; 43:175–182.

Clark WS, Street JS, Feldman PD, et al. The effects of olanzapine in reducing the emergence of psychosis among nursing home patients with Alzheimer's disease. *J Clin Psychiatry* 2001;62:34–40.

Fernandez HH, Trieschmann ME, Burke MA, et al. Long-term outcome of quetiapine use for psychosis among Parkinsonian patients. *Mov Disord* 2003;18:510–514.

Fernandez HH, Trieschmann ME, Burke MA, et al. Quetiapine for psychosis in Parkinson's disease versus dementia with Lewy bodies. *J Clin Psychiatry* 2002;63:513–515.

Fontaine CS, Hynan LS, Koch K, et al. A double-blind comparison of olanzapine versus risperidone in the acute treatment of dementia-related behavioral disturbances in extended care facilities. *J Clin Psychiatry* 2003;64:726–730.

Friedman JH, Fernandez HH. Atypical antipsychotics in Parkinson-sensitive populations. *J Geriatr Psychiatry Neurol* 2002;15:156–170.

Harvey PD, Napolitano JA, Mao L, et al. Comparative effects of risperidone and olanzapine on cognition in elderly patients with schizophrenia or schizoaffective disorder. *Int J Geriatr Psychiatry* 2003;18:820–829.

Hwang JP, Yang CH, Lee TW, et al. The efficacy and safety of olanzapine for the treatment of geriatric psychosis. *J Clin Psychopharmacol* 2003;23:113–118.

Jibson MD, Tandon R. A summary of research findings on the new antipsychotic drugs. *Essent Psychopharmacol* 1996;1(1):26–37.

Kane JM, Honigfeld G, Singer J, et al. Clozapine for the treatment resistant schizophrenic: a double-blind comparison with chlorpromazine. *Arch Gen Psychiatry* 1988;45:789–796.

Klein C, Gordon J, Pollak L, et al. Clozapine in Parkinson's disease psychosis: 5-year follow-up review. *Clin Neuropharmacol* 2003;26:8–11.

Madhusoodanan S, Brenner R, Alcantra A. Clinical experience with quetiapine in elderly patients with psychotic disorders. *J Geriatr Psychiatry Neurol* 2000;13:28–32.

Martin H, Slyk MP, Deymann S, et al. Safety profile assessment of risperidone and olanzapine in long-term care patients with dementia. *J Am Med Dir Assoc* 2003;4:183–188.

McManus DQ, Arvanitis LA, Kowalcyk BB. Quetiapine, a novel antipsychotic: experience in elderly patients with psychotic disorders. Seroquel Trial 48 Study Group. *J Clin Psychiatry* 1999;60:292–298.

Meehan KM, Wang H, David SR, et al. Comparison of rapidly acting intramuscular olanzapine, lorazepam, and placebo: a double-blind, randomized study in acutely agitated patients with dementia. *Neuropsychopharmacolgy* 2002;26:494–504.

Meltzer HY, Fibiger HC. Olanzapine: a new atypical antipsychotic drug. *NeuroPsychopharmacology* 1996;14:83–85.

Morgante L, Epifanio A, Spina E, et al. Quetiapine versus clozapine: a preliminary report of comparative effects of dopaminergic psychosis in patients with Parkinson's disease. *Neurol Sci* 2002;23(Suppl 2):S89–90.

Reddy S, Factor SA, Molho ES, et al. The effect of quetiapine on psychosis and motor function in parkinsonian patients with and without dementia. *Mov Disord* 2002;63:513–515.

Ritchie CW, Chiu E, Harrigan S, et al. The impact

upon extra-pyramidal side effects, clinical symptoms and quality of life of a switch from a conventional to atypical antipsychotic (risperidone or olanzapine) in elderly patients with schizophrenia. *Int J Geriatr Psychiatry* 2003;18:432–440.

Schwartz TL, Masand PS. The role of atypical antipsychotics in the treatment of delirium. *Psychosomatics* 2002;43:171–174.

Verma S, Orengo CA, Kunik ME, et al. Tolerability and effectiveness of atypical antipsychotics in male geriatric inpatients. *Int J Geriatr Psychiatry* 2001;16:223–227.

Fluoxetine

Lebert F, Pasquier F, Petit H. Behavioral effects of fluoxetine in dementia of Alzheimer type. *Int J Geriatr Psychiatry* 1994;9:590–591.

Tardive Dyskinesia

Alpert M, Diamond F, Friedhoff AJ. Receptor sensitivity modification in the treatment of tardive dyskinesia. *Psychopharmacol Bull* 1982;18:90–92.

American Psychiatric Association. *Tardive Dyskinesia Task Force report.* Washington, DC: American Psychiatric Association, 1980:25–27.

Baldessarini RJ, Cole JO, Davis JM, et al. *Tardive dyskinesia: a task force report of the American Psychiatric Association.* Washington, DC: American Psychiatric Association, 1980.

Barnes TRE, Wiles DH. Variation in oro-facial tardive dyskinesia during depot antipsychotic drug treatment. *Psychopharmacology* 1983;81:359–362.

Bourgeois M, Bouilh P, Tignot S, et al. Spontaneous dyskinesias versus neuroleptic-induced dyskinesias in 270 elderly subjects. *J Nerv Ment Dis* 1980;168:177–178.

Casey D, Gardos G, eds. *Tardive dyskinesia: from dogma to reason.* Washington, DC: American Psychiatric Press, 1986:15–32.

Casey DE. Tardive dyskinesia: epidemiologic factors as a guide for prevention and management. In: Kemali D, Racagui G, eds. *Chronic treatments in neuropsychiatry.* New York: Raven, 1985:15–24.

Cavero CV. Evaluation of thioridazine in the aged. *J Am Geriatr Soc* 1966;14:617–622.

Chacko RC, Root L, Marmion J, et al. The prevalence of tardive dyskinesia in geropsychiatric outpatients. *J Clin Psychiatry* 1985;46:55–57.

Chouinard G, Annable L, Ross-Chouinard A, et al. Factors related to tardive dyskinesia. *Am J Psychiatry* 1979;136:79–83.

Crane GE. Tardive dyskinesia in patients treated with major neuroleptics: a review of the literature. *Am J Psychiatry* 1968;124:40–48.

Crane GE, Smeets RA. Tardive dyskinesia and drug therapy in geriatric patients. *Arch Gen Psychiatry* 1974;30:341–343.

Dolder CR, Jeste DV. Incidence of tardive dyskinesia with typical versus atypical antipsychotics in very high risk patients. *Biol Psychiatry* 2003;53:1142–1145.

Doongaji DR, Jeste DV, Jape NM, et al. Effects of intravenous metoclopramide in 81 patients with tardive dyskinesia. *J Clin Psychopharmacol* 1982; 2(6):376–379.

Eastham JH, Lacro JP, Jeste DV. Ethnicity and movement disorders. *Mt Sinai J Med* 1996;63(5&6): 314–319.

Fann WE, Smith R, Davis JM, et al. *Tardive dyskinesia: research and treatment.* New York: SP Medical, 1980.

Freedman R, Kirch D, Bell J, et al. Clonidine treatment of schizophrenia. Double-blind comparison to placebo and neuroleptic drugs. *Acta Psychiatr Scand* 1982;65:35–45.

Granacher RP. Differential diagnosis of tardive dyskinesia: an overview. *Am J Psychiatry* 1981;138: 1288–1297.

Gunne LM, Haggstrom JE, Sjoquist B. Association with persistent neuroleptic-induced dyskinesia of regional changes in brain GABA synthesis. *Nature* 1984;309:347–349.

Hunter R, Earl CJ, Thornicroft S. An apparently irreversible syndrome of abnormal movements following phenothiazine medication. *Proc R Soc Med* 1964;57:758–762.

Jenike MA. Tardive dyskinesia: special risk in the elderly. *J Am Geriatr Soc* 1983;31:71–73.

Jeste DV, Caligiuri MP. Tardive dyskinesia. *Schizophr Bull* 1993;19:303–315.

Jeste DV, Caligiuri MP, Paulsen JS, et al. Risk of tardive dyskinesia in older patients: a prospective longitudinal study of 266 patients. *Arch Gen Psychiatry* 1995;52:756–765.

Jeste DV, Krull AJ, Kilbourn K. Tardive dyskinesia: managing a common neuroleptic side effect. *Geriatrics* 1990;45(12):49–54.

Jeste DV, Wyatt RJ. Changing epidemiology of tardive dyskinesia: an overview. *Am J Psychiatry* 1981; 138:297–309.

Jeste DV, Wyatt RJ. Therapeutic strategies against tardive dyskinesia: two decades of experience. *Arch Gen Psychiatry* 1982;39:803–816.

Jeste DV, Wyatt RJ. *Understanding and treating dyskinesia.* New York: Guilford Press, 1982:96.

Johnson GFS, Hunt EG, Rey JM. Incidence and severity of tardive dyskinesia increase with age. *Arch Gen Psychiatry* 1982;39:486.

Kaufmann CA, Jeste DV, Shelton RC, et al. Noradrenergic and neurological abnormalities in tardive dyskinesia. *Biol Psychiatry* 1986;21:799–812.

Klawans HL, Tanner CM, Barr A. The reversibility of "permanent" tardive dyskinesia. *Clin Neuropharmacol* 1984;7(2):153–159.

Kobayashi RM. Drug therapy of tardive dyskinesia. *N Engl J Med* 1977;296:257–260.

Lacro JP, Gilbert PL, Paulsen JS, et al. Early course of new-onset tardive dyskinesia in older patients. *Psychopharmacol Bull* 1994;30(2):187–191.

Lieberman J, Kane JM, Woerner M, et al. Prevalence of tardive dyskinesia in elderly samples. *Psychopharmacol Bull* 1984;20:382.

Mukherjee S, Rosen AM, Cardenas C, et al. Tardive dyskinesia in psychiatric outpatients: a study of prevalence and association with demographic clinical and drug history variables. *Arch Gen Psychiatry* 1982;39:466–469.

Nasrallah HA, Dunner FJ, McCalley-Whitters M, et al. Pharmacologic probes of neurotransmitter systems in tardive dyskinesia: implications for clinical management. *J Clin Psychiatry* 1986;47: 56–59.

Owens DGC, Johnstone EC, Frith CD. Spontaneous involuntary disorders of movement. *Arch Gen Psychiatry* 1982;39:452–461.

Paulsen JS, Caligiuri MP, Palmer B, et al. Risk factors for orofacial and limbtruncal tardive dyskinesia in older patients: a prospective longitudinal study. *Psychopharmacology* 1996;123:307–314.

Paulsen JS, Heaton R, Jeste DV. Neuropsychological impairment in tardive dyskinesia. *Neuropsychology* 1994;8(2):227–241.

Smith JM, Baldessarini RJ. Changes in prevalence, severity, and recovery in tardive dyskinesia with age. *Arch Gen Psychiatry* 1980;37:1368–1373.

Smith JM, Oswald OL, Kucharsky T, Waterman LJ. Tardive dyskinesia: age and sex difference in hospitalized schizophrenics. *Psychopharmacology* 1978;58:207–211.

Sutcher HD, Underwood RB, Beatty RA, Sugar O. Orofacial dyskinesia: a dental dimension. *JAMA* 1971;216:1459–1563.

Sweet RA, Mulsant BH, Rifai AH, et al. Dyskinesia and neuroleptic exposure in elderly psychiatric patients. *J Geriatr Psychiatry Neurol* 1992;5: 156–161.

Thaker GK, Tamminga CA, Alphs LD, et al. Brain gamma-aminobutyric acid abnormality in tardive dyskinesia. *Arch Gen Psychiatry* 1987;44:522–529.

Toennissen LM, Casey DE, McFarland BH. Tardive dyskinesia in the aged. *Arch Gen Psychiatry* 1985; 42:278–284.

Varga E, Sugerman AA, Varga V, et al. Prevalence of spontaneous oral dyskinesia in the elderly. *Am J Psychiatry* 1982;139:329–331.

Yassa R. Antiparkinsonian medication withdrawal in the treatment of tardive dyskinesia: a report of three cases. *Can J Psychiatry* 1985;30:440–442.

Yassa R. The course of tardive dyskinesia in newly treated psychogeriatric patients. *Acta Psychiatr Scand* 1991;83:347–349.

Yassa R, Jeste DV. Gender differences in tardive dyskinesia: a critical review of the literature. *Schizophr Bull* 1992;18(4):701–715.

Yassa R, Uhr S, Jeste DV. Gender differences in chronic schizophrenia: need for further research. In: Light E, Lebowitz B, eds. *The elderly with chronic mental illness.* New York: Springer, 1991:16–31.

Part IV: Affective Disorders

Chapter 8

Diagnosis of Late-Life Depression

Ira R. Katz

Catherine J. Datto

Daniel Weintraub

David W. Oslin

Historically the primary impetus for advances in psychiatric diagnosis has been the availability of new treatments, which in turn has led to increased specificity of diagnosis and treatment. Recent therapeutic developments in the treatment of depressive disorders include an increasing number of well-tolerated pharmacologic treatments as well as increasing evidence that certain psychotherapies are effective for older depressed adults. Availability of these treatments has led to concerns that targets for treatment should extend beyond major depressive disorder and that overly narrow definitions of depressive disorders might impede delivering of safe and effective interventions to potential treatment beneficiaries.

Two recent lines of progress have developed in the diagnosis of late-life depression. One, related to rising public health awareness of the suffering and disability that affects depressed older adults in the community, has led to advances in the recognition and diagnosis of minor, or subsyndromal depressions that do not meet criteria for major depressive disorder. The other is the rapidly evolving knowledge in neuropsychiatry and neurobiology of the aging brain in older pa-

tients with depression. Data from investigations in this area suggest diagnostic subtypes of late-life depression based on the interrelation of depression, cerebrovascular disease, and neurodegenerative disorders.

Epidemiology

The epidemiology of depression may be characterized approximately as a pyramid in which states of increasing severity occur with decreasing frequency. Studies consistently demonstrate that the number of elderly community residents who suffer from a major depression is rather low (in the range of 1 to 5%), whereas the prevalence of significant depressive symptoms is higher (at least 15 to 18%).[1] Moreover, in the community, the prevalence of major depression apparently decreases with age (at least until age 75 or 85), whereas prevalence of depressive symptoms appears to stay the same or even increase.[2] Thus, although major depression is the best understood of the depressive disorders, it must be viewed as only the "tip of the iceberg," especially in the geriatric population; other more prevalent types of depression may also cause suffering, morbidity, and disability. Major depressive disorder is also less common for elderly individuals, but those with significant depressive symptoms do not function as well as those with chronic medical conditions who are not depressed[3] and incur higher health costs than their nondepressed counterparts.[4]

If the goal of psychiatric diagnosis is the identification of elderly patients who could benefit from treatment, a key question concerns how the lower threshold should be defined. In addition to major depression, what types of depressions of lesser severity should be identified and diagnosed? Although this must be viewed as a question to be answered by empirical research, some guidance is provided in the Introduction to the *Diagnostic and Statistical Manual for Mental Disorders, IV, Text Revision* (DSM-IV-TR):

> Each of the mental disorders is conceptualized as a clinically significant behavioral or psychological syndrome or pattern that occurs in an individual and that is associated with present distress (e.g., a painful symptom) or disability (e.g., impairment in one or more important areas of functioning) or with a significantly increased risk of suffering death, pain, disability, or an important loss of freedom. In addition, this syndrome or pattern must not be merely an expectable and culturally sanctioned response to a particular event, for example, the death of a loved one (xxxvi).

Comorbidity

Other issues of current concern are related to the diagnosis of depression in the face of significant comorbidity from medical or neurologic disorders (see Chapter 11). Among the elderly, the prevalence of major depression differs by setting. Although estimates of depression range from 1 to 5% in the community, they rise to 12% among older patients hospitalized for medical or surgical conditions[5,6] and, historically, up to 20 or 25% among chronically ill but cognitively intact patients in nursing homes.[7]

Major depression is relatively uncommon among healthy elderly individuals who live independently in the community, but its prevalence increases significantly in those settings where patients have the most severe chronic diseases and disabilities. This epidemiologic pattern indicates that major depression in late life occurs in most cases as a component, complication, or consequence of comorbid medical or neurologic disease.

Life Course

A comprehensive diagnosis of depression requires knowledge of the course of symptoms over the elderly patient's lifetime. Increasing evidence shows that a cross-sectional "snapshot" of symptoms is necessary but not sufficient to provide the diagnostic information necessary to guide treatment planning especially since it is now clear that maintenance treatment can prevent recurrences of major depression in vulnerable patients.[8-14] A comprehensive understanding of a patient's depressive symptoms, remissions, relapses, and recurrences requires a lifetime diagnosis based on knowledge of the individual's psychiatric history as well as current symptoms.

Diagnosis as Process

Psychiatric diagnosis must be viewed as both a science and a process. A number of methods for classifying the depressive disorders of late life have been proposed, based on either epidemiologic findings or clinical experience.[15-18] The guidelines presented in this chapter are based on the current edition of the DSM-IV-TR because it is the most widely used typology.

Establishing presence of depressive symptoms in older individuals requires knowledge of normal aging and normative changes in role performance and social interactions as well as appreciation of the extent to which older individuals can successfully adapt to loss, disease, disability, and dependence. In fact, underlying the interest of those who treat elderly depressed patients tend to have an optimistic view of the aging process and of the impressive abilities of older people to adapt to disease and disability if they are not depressed.

Case Recognition

Evaluation of the older patient's mood and related symptoms should be an important component of any contact with a physician or nonmedical health care provider. Evidence supporting the need for a proactive approach to case identification for depression in medical care settings is compelling: Approximately 40% of older patients who commit suicide have seen a physician within 1 week of their deaths, 70% within 1 month.[19,20] Obvious opportunities therefore exist for prevention if patients with depression are identified and treated. These possibilities are not just theoretical. The lay public and many primary care providers still have basic misconceptions about what separates late-life depression as an illness from normal sadness or a normal reaction to loss, stressful life events, or disability. An unpublished survey conducted in the mid-1990s found that 93% of adults surveyed felt that depression in older people was normal when it occurred in response to a significant medical illness such as a heart attack or hip fracture. Accordingly, ongoing educational efforts are needed to emphasize that depression can be an illness, even when it occurs in a context in which it is understandable, intuitively or empathically. Training primary care physicians to recognize, diagnose, and treat depression has been shown to decrease suicide rates.[21,22] Several approaches have been proposed for case recognition. The most time-honored is the medical interview. Its effective use requires that clinicians have a high index of suspicion for depression in all cases, but especially in cases in which patients present with complaints such as excess disability, increased use of health care services, fatigue, and nonspecific aches. Following this model, clinicians should address emotional issues in some way at each visit, and should follow up with open-ended inquiries about symptoms related to depression whenever positive indications of distress, demoralization, or suffering appear. More conventional approaches to screening include the use of standardized, psychometrically validated instruments such as the Geriatric Depression Scale[23] or the Cen-

ter for Epidemiological Studies Depression (CESD) Scale.[24] Alternatively, screening may be accomplished through brief, structured inquiries.

The cardinal symptoms of depression in late life, as in other life phases, are dysphoric mood and diminished interest or pleasure in activities. Irritability may also signal an emerging depression. Because depression may manifest either as negative affects or by absence of positive affects, clinical screening should include inquiries about pleasurable activities and events in addition to inquiries about dysphoric mood and related symptoms. Findings suggest that a brief two-question screener—e.g., during the past month, have you often been bothered by little interest or pleasure in doing things? feeling down, depressed or hopeless?—may be as useful as more traditional rating scales.[25] However, in applying these methods, it is important to recall that apathy can occur in the absence of depression in disorders such as stroke or Alzheimer's disease (AD).[26,27] Nevertheless, particularly in the absence of these conditions, anhedonia and a decrease in pleasurable activities should be considered symptoms of depression. With appropriate follow-up of those who screen positive, brief screeners can be useful in facilitating case identification.

Elderly patients may come to clinical attention because they are themselves seeking help for depression, because they are seeking help for something else, or because someone else (e.g., a physician, other professional, family member, or friend) suspects depression (Table 8.1). When patients seek help specifically for depressive symptoms, the clinician should, in most cases, assume that the intensity of these symptoms warrants treatment. In some cases, to determine whether treatment is indicated, the clinician's task is to evaluate the symptoms along dimensions of severity, persistence, suffering, disability, and risk. An easily stated formula can be used to educate both the lay public and primary care pro-

Table 8.1. Reasons Older Patients Seek Help or Referral for Depression

Persistent pain (e.g., headache, backache, gastrointestinal pain)
Agitation
Apathy and withdrawal
Multiple nonspecific somatic complaints
Weight loss or appetite disturbance
Excess disability
Anxiety
Decreased memory or concentration
Easy fatigability
Lethargy
Increased use of health care services
Sleep disturbances—either insomnia or excess daytime somnolence
Interpersonal difficulties
Sexual difficulties
Unresolved grief
Alcohol abuse
Benzodiazepine abuse
Noncompliance with medical treatments

viders: It may be normal to get sad or depressed, but if someone cannot cast off a depressed state or if this state leads to disability in self-care, social activities, or role performance, or to risks related to self-destructive behavior, self-neglect, or decreased adherence to needed care, it is an illness that should be treated.

The current population of older people is from a generation that generally has stigmatized mental disorders and, at times, some individuals (perhaps most often those with stoic characters) have difficulty discussing feelings of depression, helplessness, hopelessness, or worthlessness with clinicians they do not know well. Although a diagnosis of depression can often be made after a brief clinical evaluation, at times excluding depression in a single visit can be difficult. Information from collateral sources, family, friends, or caregivers is often helpful and necessary to rule in or rule out the diagnosis of depression. However, even after all available information is reviewed, in some cases uncertainty may remain as to whether depression (either any depres-

sion or a specific depressive disorder) is present or absent. In management of these cases, the potential risks of overdiagnosis must be weighed against those of underdiagnosis (and, similarly, overtreatment and undertreatment) for each particular case. At times, a provisional diagnosis of a depressive disorder and a trial treatment may be appropriate to ensure that suffering or disability due to a possible depression has been addressed.

Strategies to ensure that late-life depression is recognized and that treatment is initiated appropriately is still needed, but recognition of marked increases in availability of treatment, largely as a result of primary care prescribing of new antidepressants, is equally important. Prevalence of antidepressant use in several geriatric primary care populations is above 10%[28,29]; other findings estimate that approximately 8% of one pharmacy-benefit population received at least one prescription for an antidepressant in 1999 and that state-to-state variation in prescribing rates was considerable.[30] Another industry source reports that sales of antidepressants are growing rapidly, with a 19% increase in 2000 alone.[31] Current rates of prescribing thus may well even be considerably higher. These figures are significant because they are comparable to or greater than estimates for the prevalence of major depression and other clinically significant depressive disorders. These rates suggest that psychiatrists and other providers will increasingly be seeing patients for evaluations and treatment planning, not at the onset of their illnesses but after one or more preliminary attempts at primary care treatment. This raises numerous questions about the limits of history-taking under such circumstances and about appropriate strategies for evaluation and treatment planning.

Pathways to Diagnosis and Diagnostic Distinctions

The diagnosis of depression is hierarchical. The first question is whether any clinically significant depression is present; the second question concerns the specific type of depression.

Psychiatric-Medical Comorbidity

An early step in the evaluation of elderly patients with any depression (not just those with symptoms of major depression) should be a review of their medical status, with particular attention to the presence and severity of medical illnesses (Table 8.2) and medications that may be associated with or the cause of the affective symptoms (Table 8.3). DSM-IV and DSM-IV-TR replaced the ill-defined diagnostic entity "organic affective disorder" with "mood disorder due to a general medical condition," allowing specification of several subtypes, including "with major depressive-like episode" (if symptoms are similar to those of major depression) and "with depressive features" (if the predominant mood is depressed but criteria for major depression are not met). This change emphasizes the clinical principle that depressions of any type may result either directly from medical or neurologic illness or from the adverse effects of medications.

To distinguish among depressions arising from the physiological effects of disease, those due to disease as a form of stress, and those that result from psychological mechanisms, a few pragmatic guidelines are available for clinicians. For example, if a medical intervention leads to alleviation of depressive symptoms without significant risk within a brief time—e.g., correction of electrolyte imbalance or a medically supervised trial dis-

Table 8.2.   Medical Illnesses Associated with Depression

CNS disease	**Nutritional deficiencies**
Alzheimer's disease	B_{12} deficiency
Stroke	Folic acid deficiency
Vascular dementia	Thiamine deficiency
Neoplasms	Iron deficiency
Parkinson's disease	Protein-calorie malnutrition
Multiple sclerosis	
Amyotrophic lateral sclerosis	**Electrolyte imbalances**
Huntington's disease	Hyponatremia
Myasthenia gravis	Hypokalemia
Paraneoplastic syndromes	Hyperkalemia
Migraine	Hypercalcemia
Endocrine disorders	**Neoplastic and systemic disease**
Hypothyroidism	Uremia
Hyperthyroidism	Liver failure
Autoimmune thyroiditis	Carcinoma of the pancreas
Hyperparathyroidism	Temporal arteritis
Diabetes mellitus	Systemic lupus erythematosus
Addison's disease	Rheumatoid arthritis
Cushing's disease	Disseminated carcinomatosis
Infectious disease	**Cardiovascular disease**
Tertiary syphilis	Myocardial infarction
Viral encephalitis	Angina pectoris
Infectious mononucleosis	Coronary bypass surgery
Influenza	
Lyme disease	
HIV infection	
Hepatitis	

Modified from Kalayam B, Shamoian CA. Treatment of depression: diagnostic considerations. In: Salzman C, ed. *Clinical Geriatric Psychopharmacology*. 2nd ed. Baltimore: Williams & Wilkins, 1992:115–135.

Table 8.3. Some Medications Associated with Toxicity in Mood Disorders

α-methyl dopa
Reserpine
Propranolol and other β-blockers
Clonidine
Thiazide diuretics
Guanethidine
Digitalis
Progesterone
L-Dopa
Glucocorticoids
Anabolic steroids
Benzodiazepines
Barbiturates
Cimetidine, ranitidine, and other H_2 blockers
Cyclosporine
Cycloserine
Metoclopramide
Neuroleptics
Disulfiram
Ethambutol
Nonsteroidal antiinflammatory agents
Opiate analgesics
Sulfonamides
Baclofen
HMGCoA inhibitors
Calcium channel blockers

Modified from DSM-IV Source Book.

continuation of medications with the potential for toxicity—the initial medical disorders should be the target of intervention. In these cases, if affective or behavioral symptoms persist after correcting physiological abnormalities or discontinuing medications, then treatment of the affective disorder should be instituted. In other cases, if the depression is thought to be related to an irreversible disorder (e.g., stroke) or to absolutely necessary medications, then initial interventions should target the depression. In still other cases, where waiting to see if the depression will respond to medical treatment may significantly extend suffering or disability (e.g., severe depression in the context of mild vitamin B_{12} deficiency), interventions that address both the depression and the medical problem should be instituted concurrently.

For managing depressions attributed to adverse effects of medications, determining whether or not the agent in question is actually necessary and whether alternative approaches for treatment are available is important. In most cases, the initial step in managing depressions thought to be related to adverse drug effects is withdrawal of the agent held to be the culprit. However, exceptions occur. For example, although treatment with interferon can lead to depression and related symptoms, treating these depressions can help patients continue with treatment and benefit from it.[32–34] Thus, even when depression is the result of an adverse drug effect, the therapeutic benefit of continuing treatment may override the judgment to alter the dose or discontinue the medication.

In applying standard criteria for the diagnosis of depressive disorders in elderly patients with significant physical illness, determining whether symptoms such as anorexia and easy fatigability are due to depression or physical illness can be difficult. DSM-IV-TR states:

> The evaluation of the symptoms of a Major Depressive Episode is especially difficult when they occur in an individual who also has a general medical condition (e.g., cancer, stroke, myocardial infarction, diabetes.) Some of the criterion items of a Major Depressive Episode are identical to the characteristic signs and symptoms of a general medical condition (e.g., weight loss with untreated diabetes, fatigue with cancer). Such symptoms should count toward a Major Depressive Episode except when they are clearly and fully accounted for by a general medical condition. For example, weight loss in a person with ulcerative colitis who has many bowel movements and little food intake should not be counted.

This is a variant of an "etiologic" strategy in which clinicians are required to determine whether symptoms should be attributed to depression as opposed to other conditions. Alternative approaches include an "inclusive" method that counts all symptoms toward the diagnosis, regardless of possible ambiguity in their etiology, and an "exclusive" one, in which all potentially ambiguous symptoms are discounted.[35-37] Of these, the inclusive approach is, in principle, more sensitive and the exclusive method more specific.

A final approach, a "substitutive" method, replaces ambiguous vegetative or somatic symptoms with unambiguous affective or ideational ones; for example, fatigue, anorexia or weight loss, psychomotor retardation, and impaired concentration could be replaced by irritability, tearfulness, social withdrawal, or feelings of being punished.[38,39] The fact that substitutive approaches to the diagnosis of major depression show reasonable agreement with other diagnostic strategies has interesting implications. From one perspective, a count of symptoms may occur along a scale that measures disease severity for which the exact nature of symptoms counted may not be of critical importance. From another perspective, however, vegetative symptoms may be specific indicators of hypothalamic dysfunction. Whether the overall severity of depression or the presence of specific indicators of neurobiological dysfunction best predicts responses to biological treatments is still not clear.

Each diagnostic approach can be used by experienced clinicians with acceptable reliability.[37] Some studies reveal significant differences in the apparent prevalence of depression in geriatric study samples; others do not. The best recommendation to the clinician working with an older patient with symptoms of depression and medical illness is to evaluate the diagnosis according to each of these methods. If the evaluations arrive at the same conclusion, then a good deal of confidence in the diagnosis is warranted. However, if the evaluations do not agree, treatment planning should depend on whether the clinical situation is best served by a diagnosis that increases sensitivity or one that enhances specificity. That is, does the context call for doing everything possible to ensure that potentially treatable sources of distress, disabil-

ity, and morbidity are addressed, or does it call for ensuring that a compelling rationale exists for any proposed interventions? The decision will, in general, be based upon severity of symptoms, levels of disability and suffering, and the values expressed by both patient and family.

Psychiatric Comorbidity

Evaluation of elderly patients for depression includes probes to determine whether they also suffer from sleep disorders or substance abuse. Without specifically considering sleep disorders, distinguishing between fatigue and decreased interests or concentration due to depression and the daytime effects of a primary insomnia (such as breathing-related sleep disorder or primary hypersomnia) may be difficult. When fatigue and daytime sleepiness are prominent symptoms, the patient's family should be asked about loud snoring, gasping for breath at night, and interrupted breathing that might indicate the presence of sleep apnea. Similarly, both the patient and family should be asked about restlessness, especially at night, and about jerky movements of the legs when patients are asleep that might indicate the presence of restless leg syndrome. When these additional symptoms are present, patients should be referred for a sleep evaluation.

Late-life depression frequently coexists with substance abuse, most commonly alcohol or sedative-hypnotic drugs. Although classic teaching suggests that late-life onset of alcohol abuse is frequently a symptom of depression, this formulation has recently been questioned.[40] When depression and alcohol abuse coexist, treatment should target both conditions; addressing only one aspect of the patient's condition is likely to result in unsatisfactory treatment outcomes.

Benzodiazepines are still frequently prescribed by primary care physicians and may be used over extended periods of time by those with subjective complaints of insomnia. Encountering older patients with significant levels of depression complicated by longstanding benzodiazepine use is not unusual. Although the first approach to treating these patients optimally should be benzodiazepine withdrawal, many patients are reluctant to try to decrease their medications. Drug withdrawal in younger adult patients who abuse benzodiazepines demonstrate that depressive features are strong predictors of difficulties in tolerating drug discontinuation.[41] Accordingly, in many cases, treating depressive symptoms to facilitate benzodiazepine withdrawal may be necessary.

Onset of Depression

Determining whether an episode of depression is the first occurrence of a major mood disorder or whether prior episodes of major depression, mania, or hypomania have occurred is important. If it is a first episode, the "lifetime diagnosis" is major depressive disorder, single episode; if one or more prior episodes have occurred, the "lifetime diagnosis" is major depressive disorder, recurrent. With a prior history of mania, the diagnosis is bipolar I disorder, most recent episode depressed. In contrast, prior history of hypomania leads to a diagnosis of bipolar II disorder, depressed.

Less severe, but significant although low, levels of depressive symptomatology (e.g., depressed mood, easy fatigability, and decreased concentration) may characterize a range of disorders: minor depression, an adjustment disorder with depressed mood, dysthymic disorder, major depression in partial remission, or some variant of bipolar disorder, depending upon prior history. For elderly patients whose current symptom pattern suggests a diagnosis of minor depression, the most important differential diagnostic distinction is whether they have ever experienced a full major depressive episode. If so, the current symptoms could represent either residua of a previous episode or the prodromal phase of an imminent recur-

rence. In these cases, the appropriate diagnosis is major depression in partial remission rather than minor depression. To prevent relapse, treatment for such patients should be directed toward the underlying major depressive disorder. If manic or hypomanic episodes have occurred previously, the correct diagnosis is bipolar disorder.

For elderly patients with major depressive disorder, distinguishing between those with initial onset in late life and those whose illness began in young adulthood or middle age is important.[42] Although not formally recognized in DSM-IV, increasing evidence suggests that *late-onset depressive* and *early onset depressive* are meaningful subtypes. Elderly patients with early onset depression have more first-degree relatives with depression than late-onset patients, suggesting a familial or genetic component to pathogenesis.[43] Late-onset depressives, in contrast, have much more chronic illness, suggesting that medical factors play a significant role.

Major Depressive Episode

DSM-IV-TR criteria for a major depressive episode (Table 8.4) are similar to those of DSM-IV and DSM-IIIR and, to a lesser extent, DSM-III. The validity of the pattern of symptoms constituting these criteria for defining a treatment-responsive syndrome of increased morbidity in older individuals is well established. However, difficulties continue to arise in applying these criteria in elderly populations for two main reasons: (1) overlap between symptoms of depression and those associated with age-related physical illnesses, and (2) concern that the diagnosis of major depression may not capture adequately many clinically significant depressions in this population. The frequency and distribution of symptoms of major depression may differ in older compared with younger patients, with fewer symptoms of guilt and self-reproach and more somatic symptoms in the older popula-

Table 8.4. Major Depression and Major Depressive Disorder

I. DSM-IV-TR Criteria for Major Depression
   A. 5 or more of the following symptoms have been present during the same 2-week period and represent a change from previous functioning; symptoms must include either (1) depressed mood or (2) loss of interest or pleasure:
     1. Depressed mood
     2. Markedly diminished interest or pleasure in all of almost all activities
     3. Significant weight loss or loss of appetite
     4. Insomnia or hypersomnia
     5. Psychomotor agitation or retardation
     6. Fatigue or loss of energy
     7. Feelings of worthlessness or excessive or inappropriate guilt
     8. Diminished ability to think or concentrate or indecisiveness
     9. Recurrent thoughts of death, recurrent suicidal ideation, or a suicide attempt or specific plan
   B. Symptoms do not meet criteria for a Mixed (depressive and manic) Episode
   C. Symptoms cause clinically significant distress or impairment in functioning
   D. Symptoms are not due to direct physiological effects of a substance (abuse of drug or medication) or a general medical condition
   E. Symptoms are not better accounted for by Bereavement
II. DSM-IV–TR Criteria for Major Depressive Disorder
   A. Presence of one (for Major Depressive Disorder, Single Episode) or more (for Major Depressive Disorder, Recurrent) Major Depressive Episode(s)
   B. The Major Depressive Episode is not better accounted for by a primary psychotic disorder
   C. A Manic Episode has never occurred

Specify: Mild, Moderate, Severe without Psychotic Features/Severe with Psychotic features
        With Catatonic, Melancholic, or Atypical Features
        In Partial Remission, In Full remission, or Chronic

---

tion.[44–46] These findings have not been universally replicated, however.

The diagnosis of major depression is usually straightforward in the physically healthy elderly, but in those with coexisting illnesses the disorder may make it difficult to evaluate expressions of affect—e.g., distinguishing between depression and states of apathy due to neurologic disorders.[26,27] For example, verbal expression of depressive symptoms may be compromised in elderly patients who experience language disturbances due to dominant hemisphere stroke so that clinicians need to rely more on behavioral observations than on verbal reports. In contrast, disturbances of emotional expression, such as aprosody due to a nondominant hemisphere stroke or mask-like facies and hypophonia due to Parkinson's disease, requires careful listening by clinicians to what is said rather than the affective tone.[47]

Little is known concerning the extent of symptomatology of major depression in the oldest old (those over 85). Comparison of daily variability in the affect of depressed elderly patients with that of normal controls from a residential care facility reveals that individuals with major depression report considerable day-to-day variability in dysphoric mood and negative affects in addition to persistently low levels of positive affect. In contrast, euthymic individuals report significant day-to-day variability in positive affect and consistently low levels of negative affect.[48] Thus the cardinal sign of depression among the "old-old" may not be presence of dysphoria but, instead, absence of positive affect. Withdrawal from usual activities and irritability also characterize depression in this age group.

Vegetative symptoms of depression listed in DSM-IV-TR are reliable indicators of depression in younger adults, and despite age-related changes in sleep and sexual functioning, they remain useful for healthy older adults,[49] at least until the ninth decade of life. However, for those elderly individuals with significant medical illnesses and disability who are most likely to experience depression, these indicators can be ambiguous. Even though somatic or vegetative symptoms may at times be nonspecific, they are often important both as indicators of depression and as sources of morbidity.

Appetite disturbances, usually decreased appetite often with significant weight loss, are common in late-life major depression. Depression is, in fact, a common cause of malnutrition among the frail elderly.[50-52] Sleep disturbances due to depression can be severe and can lead to exhaustion; physical energy may, at times, decrease to the point that the patient becomes bedridden. Psychomotor retardation may also be so severe that it resembles Parkinson's disease or leads to withdrawal, mutism, and immobility. Agitation may be severe enough to exhaust the older patient, particularly when it occurs in combination with loss of sleep and weight. Loss of sexual interest is a common symptom of major depression in both older and younger patients. Since healthy older individuals usually retain an interest in sex (although often diminished), clinicians must not overlook decreased sexual desire as a symptom of depression in a previously sexually active older person.

The idea that older patients may experience "masked depressions" or "depression without sadness" has been a recurring theme in geriatric psychiatry.[53,54] Although the term has never been well defined, it suggests a depressive syndrome even in the absence of prominent dysphoria or ideational symptoms such as guilt or self-reproach, helplessness, hopelessness, or worthlessness. Similarly, the usefulness of the term "depressive equivalents" (manifest primarily by symptoms such as chronic pain, fatigue, hypochondriasis, or excessive concern with other somatic symptoms without other significant depressive symptoms) should be reevalu-

ated. Because DSM-IV-TR allows diagnosis of a major depressive episode in the presence of either a depressed mood or markedly diminished interest or pleasure in activities, such depressions fit into the standardized diagnostic typology and use of these terms may no longer be necessary. If older patients (as well as others) have minimal dysphoria and have fully retained their ability to experience pleasure during usual activities, a diagnosable depressive disorder is unlikely.

Comorbidity of major depression and symptoms of personality disorder are common, occurring in almost one-quarter of older people with serious depressions—mostly among those with initial onset of depression in early life. These symptoms can be amplified and exaggerated by the presence of depression and may respond, at least in part, to its treatment. Controversy exists about the extent to which coexisting personality disorders affect the course of depression and the response to treatment.[55-60]

An extensive body of research has examined the validity of the diagnosis of depression across patient populations, confirming treatment in the presence of comorbid disorders as diverse as stroke, AD, Parkinson's disease, cancer, cardiac disease, chronic obstructive pulmonary disease, diabetes, and arthritis (see Chapter 11), as well as in clinical settings as disparate as primary care, inpatient rehabilitation, and long-term care.[61] The most conservative interpretation of these studies is that symptoms of major depression, and possibly of other depressive disorders, predict a therapeutic response to antidepressant medication regardless of medical or neurologic comorbidities or treatment setting.

Subtypes of Major Depression

Diagnostic guidelines for depression in younger healthy patients apply to older frail individuals. Until recently, clinicians and researchers have assumed that "depression is depression" and that current diagnostic methods remain valid across comorbid conditions and clinical settings. However, the presence of variations or subtypes of depression, in younger as well as older patients, including depression emerging in later life, can complicate the diagnosis.

Several subtypes of major depression occur in older individuals with varying degrees of frequency. These include melancholia, delusional depression, and seasonal affective disorder.

Melancholia

In the elderly, as in the young, the term "melancholic features" is used to define a severe subtype of depression that requires and is most likely to respond to somatic treatment. The diagnosis "major depression with melancholic features" may be made when the episode includes either loss of pleasure in all (or almost all) activities or a loss of mood reactivity to pleasurable stimuli and three or more of the following features: a distinct quality of the depressed mood (more like numbness than sadness), significant diurnal variation (with symptoms at their worst in the morning), early morning awakening, marked psychomotor agitation or retardation, significant anorexia or weight loss, and excessive or inappropriate guilt.

Delusional Depression

Depressions complicated by the presence of delusions may be more frequent in elderly patients than in younger adults,[62] and they may be most common in the presence of dementia or neurologic disorders. Mood disturbances and vegetative symptoms tend to be more severe in delusional depressions, and these patients are more likely to experience relapses or recurrences of their depressions. Mood-congruent delusions in late life are characterized by themes of personal inadequacy, disease, impending death, poverty, punishment, guilt, and an exaggerated sense of worthlessness. Patients may reproach themselves for exaggerated minor failures and may search for clues to confirm their negative self-evaluations.

When guilt predominates in delusional depression, the delusion is often expressed in the form of an excessive reaction to a current or past failing. The triggering episode may be remote, such as an affair forgiven by the spouse in the past but relived intensely by the patient. Nihilistic delusions may be extensions of unrealistic ideas of hopelessness and worthlessness or a wish for death and can be experienced as a conviction of being untreatable. Somatic delusions are characterized by unshakable beliefs in impaired functioning of some part of the body; for example, older patients may insist that they have cancer or that they are rotting away. Other delusions that may occur with late-life depression include paranoid or persecutory delusions and delusional jealousy. Transient auditory hallucinations can accompany delusional depression in late life. Congruent with the underlying mood disorder, hallucinated voices often berate the patient for past or present shortcomings or transgressions. Other psychotic symptoms (such as visual hallucinations, thought insertion, and thought broadcasting) do not, in general, occur in late-life depression.

Seasonal Affective Disorder

Recurring major depressive episodes may have a seasonal pattern, with a regular temporal relation between the onset of depressive episodes at a particular time of year, usually with relapses in the fall or winter. Remissions also occur at a characteristic time of year, usually spring. Seasonal affective disorder is rare in late life; when it does occur, it may be related to seasonal changes in exposure to bright light and may respond to light therapy.

Contexts of Major Depression

Elderly individuals who experience the main contextual subtypes of major depression are those who fail to thrive, nursing home residents, and persons who are bereaved.

Failure to Thrive

Depression may also occur in elderly persons in the context of inanition or failure to thrive[49]—a state marked by disability, weight loss, and biochemical evidence of subnutrition that includes anemia, hypoalbuminemia, and decreased levels of cholesterol.[63] Although failure to thrive is a common condition with a multifaceted origin, considerable clinical evidence suggests that depression is a common cause of weight loss, malnutrition, and depression in frail elderly patients. It is often a terminal state, although recognition and vigorous treatment can be lifesaving. In some patients, it may be the consequence of gradual weight loss caused by impaired appetite or diminished food intake related to self-care disability. In others, it results from the catabolic effects of acute medical illness. Thus, this diagnosis should be carefully considered in patients who experience weight loss, malnutrition, or cachexia without other apparent cause.

Depression in the Nursing Home

Major depression occurs in approximately 20 to 25% of cognitively intact nursing home residents,[7] a rate higher in order of magnitude than that for older individuals living in the community. It also occurs in a considerable number of patients with cognitive impairment. Because nursing home residents have high levels of chronic illness and consequent low levels of self-care, high rates of depression may be expected. In addition, features of the nursing home environment, including lack of a sense of control, have been suggested as factors that may worsen depression. Evidence also suggests that depression contributes to behavioral symptoms,[64] decreased participation in social activities,[65] and increased care needs.[66] Moreover, even among those frail elderly patients who require residential care, depression responds to treatment with standard antidepressants (but not to placebo).[67]

The diagnostic criteria for depression in nursing home residents is similar to those for other patients with significant disabling medical illnesses. Direct care staff, who have the most contact with patients in nursing homes, frequently have difficulty recognizing depressive symptoms.[68] Because case identification is often a barrier to care, standard rating scales (e.g., the Geriatric Depression Scale) may be used to improve case identification as well as train nursing home staff to recognize depression.[69]

In recent years, major changes in the epidemiology of depression and its treatment in nursing homes have occurred. Whereas in the 1980s approximately 10% of patients with known diagnoses of depression ever received treatment, now substantially over one-third of all nursing home residents receive an antidepressant medication.[70] Although this may have led to a significant decrease in the prevalence of depression, it also raises questions about how to ensure that depressions are adequately treated and when to discontinue medications.

Depression and Bereavement

Distinguishing between depression and bereavement is a common problem in psychiatric diagnosis, primarily because of extensive overlap in symptoms of major depression and those of normal bereavement. Almost one-quarter of widows and widowers evaluated 2 months after loss of their spouses exhibit symptoms consistent with a diagnosis of a major depressive episode.[71] Although spousal bereavement is more common among the elderly, its symptoms are less severe and its course more benign in older adults than in younger ones, perhaps because loss of a spouse is a more expectable, "on time" event for the geriatric population. Unlike other contexts in which depression occurs, depressive symptoms after spousal bereavement are more common and more severe in men than in women.

DSM-IV-TR provides guidelines that may be useful for distinguishing major depression from normal bereavement even though they have not been validated specifically in the aged. These guidelines state that the diagnosis of major depressive disorder is generally not made unless symptoms are still present 2 months after the loss. Particular symptoms not characteristic of a normal grief reaction may help distinguish normal bereavement from a major depressive episode; these include guilt about things other than actions at the time of the death, thoughts of suicide, preoccupation with worthlessness, intense psychomotor retardation, significant functional impairment, and hallucinations other than transitory experiences of the deceased person. Patients with symptoms of major depression after spousal bereavement benefit from treatment with antidepressant medications and alleviation of depressive symptoms does not complicate the process of grief.[72,73]

Nonmajor Depressive Disorders

Although major depression is the best-understood depressive disorder, it is not the only one that is clinically significant. Many clinicians and researchers who repeatedly found high levels of significant depressive symptoms in clinical populations were surprised when the NIMH Epidemiological Catchment Area studies found a low prevalence of major depression among the elderly. Although major depression is less common among older community-residing individuals than in younger adults,[74] depressive disorders whose symptoms do not meet criteria for major depression can cause significant morbidity, excess disability, and increased use of health care services. These nonmajor depressive disorders include dysthymic disorder, adjustment disorder with depressed mood, and depressive disorder not otherwise specified. The latter may include several conditions discussed as candidates for further study, including minor depression, mixed anxiety depression, and episodic recurrent depression.

These depressive disorders vary in symptomatology, severity, and duration but the severity of dysphoria associated with them can overlap with that of major depression. Clinical experience suggests that in late life, people have fewer severe personality and substance abuse disorders that could lead to high levels of dysphoria in the absence of major depression. Late-life depressions may therefore exist on more of a continuum than those seen earlier in life. Even after controlling for the severity of dysphoria, major depression differs from other depressive conditions in the extent of associated disability and mortality.[75] Thus the distinction between major depression and other depressive disorders remains valid in late life.

Dysthymic Disorder

A dysthymic disorder is characterized by depressed mood (for most of the day for most days) and two or more depression-associated symptoms that have persisted for 2 years or more (without a respite lasting more than 2 months). Patients who can be so categorized have not experienced a major depression (for the first 2 years of the disorder) and have never experienced a manic or hypomanic episode.

Adjustment Disorder

An adjustment disorder with depressed mood, characterized by development of emotional symptoms in response to an identifiable stressor (within 3 months of the onset of the stress), may be seen in late life. To meet DSM-IV criteria for adjustment disorder, symptoms must cause marked distress exceeding what could be expected from the stressor or from significant impairment in social or occupational functioning. They must also represent new pathology rather than an exacerbation of a preexisting condition, and they must resolve within 6 months of the termination of the stress (unless the stress itself becomes chronic). This diagnosis cannot be made when symptoms meet diagnostic criteria for major depression or dysthymic disorder. However, because adjustment disorders are characterized by severe distress or disability, the diagnosis implies a need for treatment. These disorders call attention to the need for psychotherapy targeted to adjustment of the provocative stressor. However, when such treatment does not lead to symptom remission, it should be supplemented with other approaches.

Depression (Not Otherwise Specified)

Depression not otherwise specified (NOS) refers to clinically significant states of depression that do not meet diagnostic criteria for major depression, dysthymic disorder, or adjustment disorder. Among elderly patients, this category may include a number of distinct conditions. *Minor depression* is manifested by depressed mood or markedly diminished interest or pleasure in activities and at least one (but fewer than four) other depression-associated features for a period of at least 2 weeks. *Recurrent brief depressive disorder* describes a condition in which the symptoms of major depression are present for at least 2 days but less than 2 weeks at least once a month for a year. *Mixed anxiety-depressive disorder* is characterized by dysphoric mood lasting at least 1 month that is accompanied by at least four of the depression-associated symptoms or those of generalized anxiety. Each of these conditions can be diagnosed only in a patient who has never had major depressive, manic or hypomanic episodes and is not dysthymic. In addition, DSM-IV includes criteria for depressive personality among those conditions that require further study. Among all of the states of depression considered, this may be the least well defined and the least applicable to study or clinical work with the elderly.

Most clinically significant depressions in primary care and other medical settings meet diagnostic criteria for minor depression.[76] Further evidence for its importance comes from findings that symptoms of minor depression may coexist with those of mild cognitive impairment,[77] and

they may be risk factors for later development of major depression,[78] which, in turn, may be a risk factor for later development of AD.[79]

Minor depression may also respond to antidepressant treatment.[80] However, results of the controlled trial stated: "Because treatment effects were less consistent for minor depression, our data suggest that clinicians should consider antidepressant treatment only for those with more severe functional impairment and a 4- to 6-week trial of watchful waiting for all others."

Neuropsychiatry of Late-Life Depression

Recent progress in the neuropsychiatry of late-life depression has developed from three foci: (1) longstanding interest in the relation between depression and Alzheimer's disease (AD)[81,82]; (2) empirical findings from neuroimaging suggesting that subclinical cerebrovascular disease may be the pathophysiologic link between general medical conditions common in the elderly and the mood disorders associated with these conditions[83–87]; and (3) converging evidence that damage to striato-pallido-thalamo-cortical pathways, whether from cerebrovascular disease or age-related neurodegeneration, can lead to additional diagnostic subtypes of late-life depression.[88–91] For example, depression in AD, vascular depression, as well as depression associated with frontal lobe impairment (the syndrome of depression with executive dysfunction), may represent treatment-relevant subtypes of major depression.[92–98] With the current state of knowledge, the practical value of these developments for diagnosis may be in helping providers recognize individuals who may be less likely to benefit from standard first-line interventions for depression and may therefore need more intensive follow up and monitoring during treatment.

Depression and Alzheimer's Disease

Knowledge of the relation between major depression and AD and related disorders has advanced steadily in geriatric psychiatry.[99] Early pioneering research[100] demonstrated that the psychopathology of late life was not amorphous; senile dementia and depression were distinct disorders. Subsequently, use of the term "pseudodementia"[101] emphasized that major depression and other psychiatric disorders can, at times, cause reversible cognitive impairment that mimics the deficits due to irreversible dementing disorders. The concept *pseudodementia* was refined, noting that patients with major depression often have real cognitive impairment[102,103]; the term "dementia syndrome of depression" was used to describe the intellectual deficits caused by depression, to indicate that there was nothing "pseudo" about observed impairments.

Whether or not the term pseudodementia was used, it became clear that patients with cognitive impairment can have either an irreversible dementia such as AD or reversible deficits due to depression.[104,105] The diagnostic issue thus became not one of either/or thinking ("is it depression or dementia?") but, rather, whether or not a treatable source of disability is present: whether or not the patient has an irreversible dementia, and does he or she also have a treatable depression that could account for at least a component of the observed disability?

More recent scientific advances include the following findings: patients with AD complicated by major depression are likely to have neuropathological lesions of brainstem aminergic nuclei[106,107] and a family history of major depression[108]; patients with major depression accompanied by reversible cognitive impairment are at increased risk for the onset of irreversible dementia over a period of several years[109,110]; and, more speculatively, a history of major depression may be a risk factor for later development of AD.[111–113] Although knowledge of the interrelation of AD and major depression is evolving, compelling evidence now proposes that depression, when present, can increase

disability[114] as well as caregiver burden and the risk of nursing home placement in patients with dementia.[115]

Thus the clinician must look for major depression occurring as a possible component, complication, or comorbidity of AD. If present, it should be treated; affective symptoms in cognitively impaired patients improve with antidepressant treatment[116] (see Chapters 9–13). If the patient has the single disorder of major depression with pseudodementia, treatment may lead to resolution of cognitive deficits. If the patient has major depression and an independent dementing disorder, treatment may lead to diminished disability. In each case, both patient and caregiver may benefit.

Reports from caregivers are necessary to evaluate depressive symptoms in patients with dementia. However, increasing evidence suggests that patients with mild-to-moderate cognitive impairment can report reliably on their current affect or mood, especially if structured cues are available to them.[117] Consequently, a rating scale such as the Cornell scale[118,119] or a diagnostic system such as the Cambridge examination for mental disorders of the elderly (CAMDEX)[120]—both of which make it possible to incorporate information from patient report, direct clinical observation, and caregiver report in estimating the severity of depressive symptoms—may be useful in assessing symptoms of major depression as a syndrome. Self-ratings such as those obtained with the Geriatric Depression Scale are also valid in the assessment of mood for patients with mild-to-moderate cognitive impairment.

In patients with AD, as well as in other older individuals, clinically significant depressive symptoms occur more often than the full syndrome of major depression. Clinical and epidemiologic studies demonstrate frequencies ranging from 0 to 87% (median, 41%) for depressed mood in patients with AD and from 0 to 86% (median, 19%) for specific depressive disorders.[121] Patients with dementia can have a spectrum of affective symptoms and disorders: they may have prolonged and uncontrolled emotional liability (perhaps more commonly in vascular dementia than in AD); they may have brief, recurrent but self-limited depressive episodes; finally, they may have persistent mild-to-moderate severe depressive symptoms.[122] Their recognition is important because they too can contribute to disability, suffering, and caregiver burden and because individuals with these symptoms can respond to treatment.

Recent provisional diagnostic criteria for depression of AD are now available (Table 8.5).[81,82] Although these provisional criteria were derived from those for major depressive episode, they contain several significant differences: (1) the proposed criteria for depression of AD requires the presence of three or more symptoms (vs. five or more for major depressive episode); (2) the presence of symptoms nearly every day is not required,

as is the case for major depressive episode; (3) criteria for the presence of irritability, social isolation, or withdrawal were added; (4) the criteria for loss of interest or pleasure were revised to reflect decreased positive affect or pleasure in response to social contact and usual activities.

Neuroimaging Findings

Structural brain imaging suggests two separable correlates of late life depression: (1) cerebral atrophy and (2) subcortical/deep white matter lesions visualized as hyperintensities on MRI ("leukoariosis"). The findings on atrophy include reports of increased ventricular–brain ratios as well as decreased volumes of specific brain regions.[85,86,123–126] They may be related to two distinct processes: neurodegeneration as a cause of depression and depression as a cause of neurodegeneration. The findings on subcortical and

Table 8.5. Provisional Diagnostic Criteria for Depression of Alzheimer's Disease

A. 3 or more of the following symptoms have been present during the same 2-week period and represent a change from a previous level of functioning. Symptoms must include depressed mood and/or decreased positive affect or pleasure.
    1. Clinically significant depressed mood
    2. Decreased positive affect or pleasure in response to social contacts and usual activities
    3. Social isolation or withdrawal
    4. Disruption in appetite
    5. Disruption in sleep
    6. Psychomotor agitation or retardation
    7. Irritability
    8. Fatigue or loss of energy
    9. Feelings of worthlessness, hopelessness, or excessive or inappropriate guilt
    10. Recurrent thoughts of death or suicidal ideation, plan, or attempt
B. Meets diagnostic criteria for Dementia of the Alzheimer's Type
C. Depressive symptoms cause clinically significant distress or disruption in functioning
D. Symptoms do not occur exclusively during a delirium
E. Symptoms are not due to direct physiological effects of a substance (abuse of drug or medication)
F. |Symptoms are not better accounted for by other conditions, such as major depressive disorder, bipolar disorder, bereavement, primary psychosis, psychosis of Alzheimer's Disease, anxiety disorders, or substance-related disorder.

Specify if :   Co-occurring onset: If onset antedates or co-occurs with the AD symptoms
                 Post-AD onset: If onset occurs after AD symptoms

Specify if: With Psychosis of AD
             With other significant behavioral signs or symptoms
             With past history of mood disorder

From JT Olin, LS Schneider, IR Katz, et al. *American Journal of Geriatric Psychiatry* 2002;10:125–128.

deep white matter hyperintensities provide evidence for associations between depression and "subclinical" cerebrovascular disease.[83–87,127–138]

Both neuropsychological and electrophysiological measures suggest that these hyperintensities, which have come to be attributed to subclinical cerebrovascular disease, can affect cerebral activity in the overlying cortex. They reveal independent associations with both age and health status and may occur in patients with AD as well as those with depression. Because subcortical and deep white-matter hyperintensities are not observed in those (relatively uncommon) patients with late-life depression who do *not* have cardiovascular (or cerebrovascular) risk factors,[139] they may reflect structural damage that mediates the increased risk of depression in those with cardiovascular disease. Repeated episodes of depression may lead to "scarring" in the form of atrophy and degeneration of specific brain structures.

Functional neuroimaging with positron emission tomography (PET) scanning shows decreased cerebral glucose metabolism either throughout the brain or, most prominently, in specific brain regions.[140–142] This contrasts with the results of PET scans of AD patients, in which the decrements in glucose metabolism are most prominent in the parietal lobe. Imaging studies of late-life depression are summarized in Table 8.6.

Earlier hopes that biological markers, including those related to neuroendocrine activity and peripheral neurochemical measures, could facilitate the diagnosis of depression or the distinction between cases of depression and dementia have not been borne out. Despite evidence that major depression has structural and physiological correlates, diagnosis remains based primarily upon behavior and reports of subjective experience. However, neuroimaging may hold promise for guiding the diagnosis of subtypes of depression. In addition, promising findings from genetic studies suggesting that genetic markers (e.g., poly-

morphisms related to the serotonin transporter promoter) may be relevant to the pathogenesis of depression or to moderating treatment responses[143–145] are all encouraging.

Results of neuroimaging studies support the validity of the diagnosis of major depression as a biomedical disorder. The hypothesis that structural changes in the brain seen as subcortical and deep white matter hyperintensities on MRI scans may be involved in the pathogenesis of a sizable subset of patients with late-onset depression has been supported through a large and growing body of research.[83–87] Other findings support the concept that late-life depression can be associated with cerebral atrophy, generalized or focal.[123–126,134–138] There is also evidence that repeated episodes of depression can lead to "scarring" in the form of atrophy and degeneration of specific brain structures.[146,147] This raises critical questions about the extent to which adequate treatment for depression throughout life can prevent neuronal loss.

Vascular Depression

Mounting evidence now supports the contention that "subclinical" cerebrovascular disease, manifest primarily by subcortical and deep white-matter lesions seen on MRI scans, may mediate the effects of a number of general medical conditions leading to late-life depression. A classic study[84] evaluated the clinical features of depression in older patients with and without the presence of these lesions and found that individuals with positive MRI findings were more likely to be older, to have underlying vascular disease, and to have depressions characterized by older age of onset, anhedonia, functional disability, and absence of psychotic features. These results suggested that older patients with depression in the context of vascular lesions exhibit vascular depressions, reflecting damage to striato-pallido-thalamo-cortical pathways.

A complementary seminal work[83] found that patients with vascular depres-

Table 8.6. Imaging Studies of Late-Life Depression

Scan	Study	Reference[a]
CT	Enlarged lateral ventricles in depressed geriatric patients	Krishnan et al. (1996) Dolan et al. (1985) Jacoby & Levy (1980)
	Greater ventricular enlargement in late-onset than in early onset geriatric depression	Alexopoulos (1992) Shima (1984) Jacoby & Levy (1980) Rossi et al. (1980)
	Enlarged ventricles associated with poor response to nortriptyline	Young (1988)
MRI	Deep white matter hyperintensities more frequently due to cerebral ischemia and located at dorsolateral prefrontal cortex in depressed subjects; these lesions appear to lateralize to the left in depressed patients	Thomas (2002) Nebes (2001) Tupler (2002)
	Older adults with MDD have smaller frontal lobe volumes and smaller orbital frontal cortex volumes	Kumar (2002) Kumar (2000) Lai (2000)
	Significant white and gray matter hyperintensity ("leukoariosis") in elderly depressed patients; associated with late onset of first episode, suicidal ideation, delusions, DST nonsuppression, poor response to antidepressant treatment	Greenwald (1996) Krishnan(1996) Salloway (1996) Wurthmann (1995) Miller (1994) Coffey (1993) Boone (1992) Kumar (1992) Leuchter (1992) Figiel (1991) Coffey et al. (1988) Fazekas et al. (1988)
	Widening of cortical sulci, temporal lobe sulci, temporal horns, sylvian fissures, lateral and third ventricles	Lidaka (1996) Krishnan(1991) Zubenko (1990)
	Widespread cortical and subcortical atrophy and basal ganglia lacunae inversely correlated with IMI binding	Husain (1991) Rabins (1991)
PET	In depressed patients, decreased cerebral glucose metabolism most prominent in frontal lobe and right hemisphere; contrasts with AD patients in whom glucose	Lesser (1994) Kumar (1993) Sackeim (1990)
	Metabolism decrements are most prominent in parietal lobe	Navarro (2002) Vasile (1996)
SPECT	In depressed patients, significantly lower uptake in left anterior frontal region; in remission the left frontal perfusion abnormality normalizes	Ito (1996)

[a] Complete reference citations at end of chapter.

sion defined in clinical terms as late-onset depression occurring in the context of significant cerebrovascular risk factors, differed from others with late-life depression in several ways: greater overall cognitive impairment and disability, specific cognitive deficits (including fluency and naming), more retardation, less agitation, less guilt feelings, and greater lack of insight.[83]

This line of investigation is important for what it may reveal about the pathogenesis of late-onset depression, opportunities for prevention, and guidelines for clinical care. Data further suggest that patients with vascular depression may exhibit slower or less complete responses to standard treatments.[96-98] If these data are confirmed, clinical trials and systematic studies to evaluate responses to both standard and novel treatments would be indicated.

Syndrome of Depression with Executive Dysfunction

Control of functions that include planning, sequencing, organizing, and abstracting—i.e., executive function—is located in the prefrontal cortex, a site of increasing importance for investigation of late-life depression. Recurring findings from neuroimaging studies in patients with primary depression (as well as those with stroke, Parkinson's disease, and other CNS disorders), together with findings from animal models, suggest that disorders of the prefrontal cortex and its projections to the amygdala and basal ganglia may underlie both depression and specific impairments in executive function.[88,89]

Disturbances to frontal subcortical systems due to stroke, subclinical cerebrovascular disease, or age-related neurodegeneration may thus lead to a syndrome of depression with impairments including decreased verbal fluency, impaired visual naming, psychomotor retardation, loss of interest in activities, and mild vegetative symptoms. Such "depression-executive-dysfunction syndrome" of late life[148] may

constitute a treatment-relevant subtype of major depression characterized by poor or slow response to antidepressant treatment with early relapse or recurrence (see Chapter 14).[90-92,94,95,148,149] This syndrome may also be associated with suspiciousness or paranoid ideation. These concepts and the data subsequent research yields will be validated in two ways: first, by the extent to which clinical features predict decreased response to standard treatment (Chapter 14) and second, by the extent to which they serve to define a patient population that may benefit from alternative interventions.

Consequences of Depression

The importance of the recognition and diagnosis of depression is best demonstrated by the consequences of depression. Depression in late life is a persistent or recurrent disorder that can result from psychosocial stress or physiological effects of disease and can lead to increased disability, cognitive impairment, exacerbation of symptoms from medical illness, physiological deterioration, increased use of health care services, and higher rates of suicide and nonsuicide mortality.[150,151]

Despite significant advances in the treatments for depression available for older patients, findings on longer-term outcomes have not changed significantly over the past generation.[152] Now, as in the past, the "rule of thirds" seems to apply: approximately one-third of patients have good outcomes with full recovery; another third recover with subsequent episodes of relapse; and the final third have some degree of chronic or persistent symptoms. Although clear differences in outcomes between younger adults and older patients are not seen, the effects of social factors on both onset of and recovery from depression tend to be weaker in older adults than in younger ones.[153]

Mounting evidence[10-14,154,155] suggests that maintenance treatment with antidepressant medications remains effective in preventing relapses and recurrences in older patients (See Chapter 14). Significant improvement of longer-term outcomes with the wider use of maintenance treatment is therefore likely. This optimistic view, however, may require some tempering by growing evidence that certain depressions may be risk factors or prodromes for dementia. Further research is needed to determine whether vigorous treatment for depression can decrease the incidence of dementia.

Suicide

The psychiatric morbidity associated with depression includes (preventable) recurrences, substance abuse, and cognitive impairment. Suicide, however, makes the most compelling case for the importance of recognizing depression in general medical care settings. Although suicide in younger populations may be attributed to a number of disorders (including substance abuse, psychoses, and personality disorders as well as depression), psychological autopsy studies of completed suicides and psychiatric evaluations of attempted-suicide survivors demonstrate that suicide among older persons is more specifically related to depression. Moreover, compelling evidence indicates that enhancing the recognition and treatment of depression in primary care can prevent suicide.[156,157]

Suicide is the tenth most common cause of death in the elderly. Although one of every five suicides in the United States is committed by a person over the age of 65 years, it is likely that underreported suicide among older persons may occur even more frequently. Because of advanced age, an older person's death from suicide may appear to result from illness or material factors.

Expression of thoughts of death and suicide occurs along a broad spectrum. At one end may be the passive wish for death from natural causes, such as during sleep; older persons may say that they would not kill themselves but would be happy not to waken. Such thoughts are not unusual

among very old people, especially those whose friends and spouses have already died. These patients do not represent a suicidal risk.

More worrisome are older people in the middle of the suicide spectrum who are chronically ill with disturbing or incapacitating disorders—individuals who have lost significant function or are aware of progressive loss of function. Examples include patients with cardiovascular disorders that limit a previously active life or older persons aware of having a progressive dementia. Although not recurrently depressed, these older patients may consider suicide by active efforts or may passively contribute to their death by not complying with their medical regimens.

At the far end of the spectrum are very old patients, usually depressed, who are actively suicidal and who may be at extreme risk of suicide. The chance of successfully completing a suicide attempt is highest among the elderly, particularly those who live alone or are experiencing recent bereavement. For these reasons, clinicians are strongly encouraged to ask an older patient who is depressed, chronically ill, or widowed about suicidal ideation. It is also important to ask about the availability of firearms as a means for committing suicide. Regardless of how clinicians may view gun ownership as a general issue, the availability of firearms for those who are depressed is a medical issue.

At the present time, white males 65 and over comprise the group at highest risk for suicide in the United States.[158] Among all age groups, a history of living alone without friends or social support, a history of alcoholism, and a history of prior psychiatric illness with prior suicide attempts all increase suicidal risk. Delusional depressed patients and depressed patients with a history of panic disorder appear to be at greatest risk. The risk is particularly high if patients hear voices commanding them to kill themselves.

The physician must evaluate the possibility that a depressed older patient will attempt suicide. Some practitioners may worry that asking a depressed person about suicide will initiate suicidal thoughts not previously present and thus contribute to a suicide attempt. Elderly patients, however, are often relieved when the topic of suicide is raised and may be eager to discuss their thoughts.

Exacerbation of Medical Morbidity

Interactions between depression and medical illnesses are complex and bidirectional (see Ch 11). Depression can lead to the onset of medical and neurological illnesses that include breast cancer,[159] myocardial infarction,[160] diabetes,[161] AD,[162–164] and osteoporosis.[165,166] In turn, these and other disorders can lead to depression. Finally, depression can interact with established medical conditions, worsening their course; this principle has been established across conditions, and, in greater detail, in disorders such as diabetes.[167–169]

One of the most evocative demonstrations that depression and related symptoms can be precursors of subsequent physical illnesses comes from long-term longitudinal studies of health and mental health in subjects initially assessed in college and followed for several decades. This research demonstrates the expected associations between depression, chronic medical illnesses, and disability when the subjects reached older ages. However, these associations could be attributed largely to a greater risk of medical illnesses in those with early depression and related symptoms, not just to an increased risk of depression in those with disabling medical conditions.[170]

For those with established medical disorders, the general medical consequences of depression in older adults can be summarized by the unifying hypothesis that depression interacts with medical or neurologic illness to modify the course of the disease by increasing the associated morbidity and disability as well as the use of health care services.[171,172] The association among depression, morbidity, and disability is a highly replicable finding from measures of disability in heterogeneous samples as well as from disease-specific measures in more homogeneous populations. For example, findings from a community sample demonstrate that the progression from depression to disability is as frequent and severe as that leading from disability to depression.[173] In contrast, evaluation of the magnitude of the disability attributable to depression in young and middle-aged adults in medical care settings shows that depression is associated with poor physical, social, and role functioning that could not be attributed to medical comorbidity[117]; the extent of disability related to depression is comparable to or worse than that of eight major chronic medical conditions.

Studies of relationships among health status, depression, and functional impairment demonstrate that depression can lead to increased disability or a negative outcome from rehabilitation in patients with stroke,[174–176] myocardial infarction,[177,178] chronic obstructive pulmonary disease,[179,180] hip fracture,[181,182] parkinsonism,[183] and arthritis[184]—all conditions affecting large numbers of elderly individuals. One pioneering study conducted with patients with chronic obstructive pulmonary disease demonstrates that treatment of depression can both reduce depressive symptoms and improve day-to-day functioning.[185]

Important questions about the mechanisms by which depression can lead to adverse health effects—either the onset of new disorders or worsening of established conditions—persist. Some specific mechanisms have been proposed. For example, some investigators suggest that decreased bone density in patients with depression may be related to hypercortisolemia.[166] Others propose that cardiac effects may be related to autonomic dysregulation in depression, perhaps as manifest by decreased heart rate variability, or to changes in platelet functioning[186–194] (see Chapter 11).

Several recent studies demonstrate associations between pain and depression among elderly patients with chronic medical illness.[195-197] The relation is apparently bidirectional; that is, high levels of pain can be both a cause and a consequence of depression. Increased pain complaints attributable to depression occur primarily in patients who also have medical illnesses that can elicit pain. In these cases, depression appears to increase the intensity of pain due to diagnosable somatic disease.

Morbidity and Costs

Increased use of general medical health services, both inpatient and outpatient, by patients with depression is readily demonstrated in both younger and older adult populations.[198] The major question in this area, however, is whether this effect remains after controlling for medical comorbidity. For both younger and older adults, substantial evidence supports the significance of this effect after controlling for medical illness.[199-201]

Investigations of older persons suggest that increased rates of hospitalization associated with nonspecific measures of poor mental health remain significant after controlling for general medical status[202] and that more outpatient visits and associated costs for inpatients with elevated scores on self-rated depression scales are significant after controlling for the number of comorbid medical conditions.[203] Additional research shows that depressed patients have longer lengths of stay as well as more hospital days subsequent to an initial hospitalization (and greater in-hospital mortality) than controls from the same population matched with respect to age, type and severity of illness, and functional status,[204] and that nursing home residents with depression use more resources,[205] even after controlling for levels of disability.

In addition to increasing the morbidity and costs associated with other medical illnesses, depression may also increase nonsuicide mortality. A generation ago, elderly depressed patients who received "adequate treatment" survived longer

than those who did not,[206] suggesting that treatment of depression in the aged could extend life. Further, depression after a myocardial infarction is associated with increased mortality, even after controlling for the severity of the patient's cardiac disease.[207,208] Research to evaluate the extent to which treatment of depression leads to decreased mortality is in progress.

Data from long-term care settings uniformly demonstrate an association between depression and decreased survival,[209-214] but some controversy remains regarding the underlying mechanism: are patients dying because they are depressed, or are they depressed because they are dying? From the researcher's perspective, the difference between these alternatives hinges on a number of technical matters related to how one quantifies medical illness and how one uses these measures in statistical analyses. From the clinician's perspective, these findings mean that although it is clear that the appropriate diagnosis and treatment of depression can improve the quality of life of many older individuals, we do not yet know how frequently it will also extend life. Regardless, the consequences of depression as well as the suffering it entails make clear that its recognition and treatment are of major importance.

Acknowledgment.. Supported by a Clinical Research Center grant from the National Institute of Mental Health, grant number MH 52129.

References

1. Gurland BJ, Cross PS, Katz S. Epidemiological perspectives on opportunities for treatment of depression. *Am J Geriatr Psychiatry* 1992;4: S7–S13.
2. Romanoski AJ, Folstein MF, Nesdadt G, et al. The epidemiology of psychiatrist-ascertained depression and DSM-III depressive disorders. Results from the Eastern Baltimore mental health survey clinical reappraisal. *Psychol Med* 1992;22:629–655.
3. Wells KB, Burman MA. Caring for depression in America: lessons learned from early findings of the Medical Outcomes Study. *Psychiatr Med* 1991;9:503–519.
4. Cole MG, Dendukuri N. Risk factors for depres-

sion among elderly community subjects: a systematic review and meta-analysis. *Am J Psychiatry* 2003;160:1147–1156.

5. Koenig HG, Meador KG, Cohen HJ, et al. Depression in elderly hospitalized patients with medical illness. *JAMA* 1988;148:1929–1936.

6. Koenig HG, O'Connor CM, Guarisco SA, et al. Depressive disorder in older medical inpatients on general medicine and cardiology services at a university teaching hospital. *Am J Geriatr Psychiatry.* 1993;1:197–210.

7. Rovner BW, Katz IR. Psychiatric disorders in the nursing home: a selective review of studies related to clinical care. *Int J Geriatr Psychiatry* 1993;8:75–87.

8. Frank E, Kupfer DJ, Perel JM, et al. Three-year outcomes for maintenance therapies in recurrent depression. *Arch Gen Psychiatry.* 1990;47:1093–1099.

9. Frank E. Long term prevention of recurrences in elderly patients. In: Schneider LS, Reynolds CF III, Lebowitz BD, et al., eds. *Diagnosis and treatment of depression in late life.* Washington, DC: American Psychiatric Press, 1994:317–329.

10. Klysner R, Bent-Hansen J, Hansen HL, et al. Efficacy of citalopram in the prevention of recurrent depression in elderly patients: placebo-controlled study of maintenance therapy. *Brit J Psychiatry* 2002;181:29–35.

11. Flint AJ, Rifat SL. Maintenance treatment for recurrent depression in late life. A four-year outcome study. *Am J Geriatr Psychiatry* 2000;8:112–116.

12. Reynolds CF III, Perel JM, Frank E, et al. Three-year outcomes of maintenance nortriptyline treatment in late-life depression: a study of two fixed plasma levels. *Am J Psychiatry* 1999;156:1177–1181.

13. Flint AJ, Rifat SL. Recurrence of first-episode geriatric depression after discontinuation of maintenance antidepressants. *Am J Psychiatry* 2000;157:1183–1184.

14. Reynolds CF III, Frank E, Perel JM, et al. Nortriptyline and interpersonal psychotherapy as maintenance therapies for recurrent major depression: a randomized controlled trial in patients older than 59 years. *JAMA* 1999;281:39–45.

15. Blazer D, Hughes DC, George LK. The epidemiology of depression in an elderly community population. *Gerontologist* 1987;27:281–287.

16. Spitzer RL, Endicott J, Robins E. Research diagnostic criteria: rationale and reliability. *Arch Gen Psychiatry* 1978;35:773–782.

17. Snaith RP. The concepts of mild depression. *Br J Psychiatry* 1987;150:387–393.

18. Clinical descriptions and diagnostic guidelines. In: World Health Organization. *International classification of diseases.* 10th ed. (ICD-10). Geneva, Switzerland: World Health Organization, Division of Mental Health, 1991.

19. Conwell Y. Suicide in elderly patients. In: Schneider LS, Reynolds CF III, Lebowitz BD, et al., eds. *Diagnosis and treatment of depression in late life.* Washington, DC: American Psychiatric Press, 1994:397–418.

20. Conwell Y. Outcomes of depression. *Am J Geriatr Psychiatry* 1996;4:S34–S44.

21. Rutz W, von Knorring L, Walinder J. Frequency of suicide on Gotland after systematic postgraduate education of general practitioners. *Acta Psychiatr Scand* 1989;80:151–154.

22. Rutz W, Carlsson P, von Knorring L, et al. Cost-benefit analysis of an educational program for general practitioners given by the Swedish Committee for the Prevention and Treatment of Depression. *Acta Psychiatr Scand* 1992;85;457–464.

23. Yesavage JA, Brink RL, Rose TL, et al. Development and validation of a geriatric depression scale. *J Psychiatr Res* 1983;17:31–49.

24. Radloff LS. The CES-D scale: a self-report depression scale for research in the general population. *Appl Psychol Meas* 1977;1:385–401.

25. Whooley MA, Avins AL, et al. Case finding instruments for depression. Two questions are as good as many. *J Gen Int Med* 1997;12:439–445.

26. Marin RS, Firinciogullari S, Biedrzycki RC. The sources of convergence between measures of apathy and depression. *J Affective Disord* 1993;28:117–124.

27. Marin RS, Firinciogullari S, Biedrzycki RC. Group differences in the relationship between apathy and depression. *J Nerv Ment Dis* 1994;182:235–239.

28. Blazer DG, Hybels CF, Simonsick EM, et al. Marked differences in antidepressant use by race in an elderly community sample: 1986–1996. *Am J Psychiatry* 2000;157:1089–1094.

29. Mamdani MM, Parikh SV, Austin PC, et al. Use of antidepressants among elderly subjects: trends and contributing factors. *Am J Psychiatry* 2000;157:360–367.

30. Mamdani MM, Herrmann N, Austin P. Prevalence of antidepressant use among older people: population-based observations. *J Am Geriatr Soc* 1999;47:1350–1353.

31. Popkin MK, Tucker GJ. Mental disorders due to a general medical condition and substance-induced disorders: mood, anxiety, psychotic, catatonic, and personality disorders. In: Widger TA, Frances AJ, Pincus HA, et al., eds. *DSM-IV sourcebook.* Washington, DC: American Psychiatric Association, 1994: 243–276.

32. Musselman DL, Lawson DH, Gumnick JF, et al. Paroxetine for the prevention of depression induced by high-dose interferon alfa. *New Engl J Med* 2001;344:961–966.

33. Mohr DC, Goodkin DE, Likosky W, et al. Treatment of depression improves adherence to interferon beta-1b therapy for multiple sclerosis. *Arch Neurol* 1997;54:531–533.

34. Capuron L, Gumnick JF, Musselman DL, et al. Neurobehavioral effects of interferon-alpha in cancer patients: phenomenology and paroxetine responsiveness of symptom dimensions. *Neuropsychopharmacol* 2002;26:643–652.

35. Cohen-Cole S, Stoudemire A. Major depression and physical illness: special considerations in diagnosis and biological treatment. *Psychiatr Clin North Am* 1987;10:1–17.

36. Hendrie HC, Callahan CM, Levitt EE, et al. Prevalence rates of major depressive disorders. *Am J Geriatr Psychiatry* 1995;3:119–131.

37. Koenig HG, Pappas P, Holsinger T. Assessing

diagnostic approaches to depression in medically ill older adults: how reliably can mental health professionals make judgments about the cause of symptoms? *J Am Geriatr Soc* 1995; 43:472–478.

38. Endicott J. Measurement of depression in patients with cancer. *Cancer* 1984;53:2243–2247.

39. Rapp SR, Vrana S. Substituting nonsomatic for somatic symptoms in the diagnosis of depression in elderly male medical patients. *Am J Psychiatry* 1989;146:1197–1200.

40. Atkinson RM. Aging and alcohol use disorders: diagnostic issues in the elderly. *Int Psychogeriatr* 1990;2:55–72.

41. Rickels K, Schweizer E, Case WG. Long term therapeutic use of benzodiazepines. I. Effects of abrupt discontinuation. *Arch Gen Psychiatry* 1990;47:899–907.

42. Alexopoulos GS, Young RC, Meyers BS, et al. Late-onset depression. *Psychiatr Clin North Am* 1988;11:101–115.

43. Krishnan KR. Biological risk factors in late life depression. *Biol Psychiatry* 2002;52:185–192.

44. Gurland BJ. The comparative frequency of depression in various adult age groups. *J Gerontol* 1976;31:283.

45. Gallo JJ, Anthony JC, Muthen BO. Age differences in the symptoms of depression: a latent trait analysis. *J Gerontol* 1994;49:251–264.

46. Rabins PV. Barriers to diagnosis and treatment of depression in elderly patients. *Am J Geriatr Psychiatry* 1996;4:79–83.

47. Ross ED, Rush AJ. Diagnosis and neuroanatomical correlates of depression in brain damaged patients. Implications for a neurology of depression. *Arch Gen Psychiatry* 1981;38: 1344–1354.

48. Lawton MP, Parmelee PA, Katz IR, Nesselroade J. Affective states in normal and depressed older people. *J Gerontol Psychol Sci* 1996;51: 309–316.

49. Gurland BJ, Dean LL, Cross PS. The effects of depression on individual social functioning in the elderly. In: Breslau LD, Haug MR, eds. *Depression and aging.* New York: Springer, 1983; 256.

50. Morley JE, Kraenzle D. Causes of weight loss in a community nursing home. *J Am Geriatr Soc* 1994;42:583–585.

51. Katz IR, Beason-Wimmer P, Parmelee PA, et al. Failure to thrive in the elderly: exploration of the concept and delineation of psychiatric components. *J Geriatr Psychiatry Neurol* 1993;6: 161–169.

52. Blaum CS, Fries BE, Fiatarone MA. Factors associated with low body mass index and weight loss among nursing home residents. *J Gerontol* 1995;50:162–168.

53. Gallo JJ, Rabins PV. Depression without sadness: alternative presentations of depression in late life. *Am Fam Physician* 1999;60:820–826.

54. Gallo JJ, Rabins PV, Lyketsos CG, et al. Depression without sadness: functional outcomes of nondysphoric depression in later life. *J Am Geriatr Soc* 1997;45:570–578.

55. Kunik ME, Mulsant BH, Rifai AH, et al. Personality disorders in elderly inpatients with major

depression. *Am J Geriatr Psychiatry* 1993;1: 38–45.

56. Abrams RC, Rosendahl E, Card C, Alexopoulos GS. Personality disorder correlates of late and early onset depression. *J Am Geriatr Soc* 1994; 42:727–734.

57. Thompson LW, Gallagher D, Czirr R. Personality disorder and outcome in the treatment of late-life depression. *J Geriatr Psychiatry* 1988;21: 133–146.

58. Abrams RC, Alexopoulos GS, Spielman LA, et al. Personality disorder symptoms predict declines in global functioning and quality of life in elderly depressed patients. *Am J Geriatr Psychiatry* 2001;9:67–71.

59. Abrams RC, Spielman LA, Alexopoulos GS, et al. Personality disorder symptoms and functioning in elderly depressed patients. *Am J Geriatr Psychiatry* 1998;6:24–30.

60. Abrams RC, Rosendahl E, Card C, Alexopoulos GS. Personality disorder correlates of late and early onset depression. *J Am Geriatr Soc* 1994; 42:727–731.

61. Katz IR. Drug treatment of depression in the frail elderly: discussion of the NIH consensus development conference on the diagnosis and treatment of depression in late life. *Psychopharmacol Bull* 1993;29:101–108.

62. Martinez RA, Mulsant BH, Meyers BS, Lebowitz BD. Delusional and psychotic depression in late life: clinical and research needs. *Am J Geriatr Psychiatry* 1996;4:77–84.

63. Institute of Medicine. *Enhancing lives, extending lives. Report of the Committee for a National Research Agenda on Aging.* Washington, DC: National Academy Press, 1991.

64. Cohen-Mansfield J, Marx MS. Relationship between depression and agitation in nursing home residents. *Compr Gerontol (B)* 1988;2: 141–146.

65. Voelkl JE, Fries BE, Galecki AT. Predictors of nursing home residents' participation in activities programs. *Gerontologist* 1995;35:44–51.

66. Fries BE, Mehr DR, Schneider D, et al. Mental dysfunction and resource use in nursing homes. *Med Care* 1993;31:898–920.

67. Katz IR, Simpson GM, Curlik SM, et al. Pharmacologic treatment of major depression for elderly patients in residential care settings. *J Clin Psychiatry* 1990;51:41.

68. Burrows AB, Satlin A, Salzman C, et al. Depression in a long-term care facility: clinical features and discordance between nursing assessment and patient interviews. *J Am Geriatr Soc* 1995;43:1118–1122.

69. McGivney SA, Mulvihill M, Taylor B. Validating the GDS Depression Screen in the nursing home. *J Am Geriatr Soc* 1994;42:490–492.

70. Datto C, Oslin D, Streim J, et al. Pharmacological treatment of depression in nursing home residents: a mental health services perspective. *J Geriatr Psychiatry and Neurology* 2002;15: 141–146.

71. Zisook S, Schuchter SR, Sledge P. Diagnostic and treatment considerations in depression associated with late-life bereavement. In: Schneider LS, Reynolds CF III, Lebowitz BD, et al., eds. *Diagnosis and treatment of depression in late*

life. Washington, DC: American Psychiatric Press, 1994:419–436.

72. Pasternak RE, Reynolds CF III, Schlernitzauer M. Acute open trial nortriptyline therapy of bereavement-related depression in late life. *J Clin Psychiatry* 1991;52:307–310.

73. Prigerson HG, Frank E, Kasl SV, et al. Complicated grief and bereavement-related depression as distinct disorders: preliminary empirical validation in elderly bereaved spouses. *Am J Psychiatry* 1995;52:22–30.

74. Blazer DG. Epidemiology of late life depression. In: Schneider LS, Reynolds CF III, Lebowitz BD, et al., eds. *Diagnosis and treatment of depression in late life.* Washington, DC: American Psychiatric Press, 1994:9–19.

75. Katz IR, Parmelee PA, Streim JE. Depression in older patients in residential care. *Am J Geriatr Psychiatry* 1995;3:161–169.

76. Koenig HG, Blazer DG III. Minor depression in late life. *Am J Geriatr Psychiatry* 1996;4:14–21.

77. Forsell Y, Jorm AF, von Strauss E, et al. Prevalence and correlates of depression in a population of nonagenarians. *Br J Psychiatry* 1995;167: 61–64.

78. Parmelee PA, Katz IR, Lawton MP. Incidence of depression in long term care settings. *J Gerontol Med Sci* 1992;47:189–196.

79. Green RC, Cupples LA, Kurz A, et al. Depression as a risk factor for Alzheimer's Disease. *Arch Neurol* 2003;60:753–759.

80. Williams JW Jr., Barrett J, Oxman T, et al. Treatment of dysthymia and minor depression in primary care: A randomized controlled trial in older adults. Clinical Trial. Multicenter Study. Randomized Controlled Trial. *JAMA.* 2000; 284:1519–1526.

81. Olin JT, Katz IR, Meyers BS, et al. Provisional diagnostic criteria for depression of Alzheimer disease: rationale and background. *Am J Geriatr Psychiatry* 2002;10:129–141.

82. Olin JT, Schneider LS, Katz IR, et al. Provisional diagnostic criteria for depression of Alzheimer disease. *Am J Geriatr Psychiatry* 2002;10: 125–128.

83. Alexopoulos GS, Meyers BS, Young RC, et al. Clinically defined vascular depression. *Am J Psychiatry.* 1997;154:562–565.

84. Krishnan KR, Hays JC, Blazer DG. MRI-defined vascular depression. *Am J Psychiatry* 1997; 154(4):497–501.

85. Kumar A, Mintz J, Bilker W, et al. Autonomous neurobiological pathways to late-life major depressive disorder: clinical and pathophysiological implications. *Neuropsychopharmacology* 2002; 26(2):229–236.

86. Kumar A, Bilker W, Jin Z, et al. Atrophy and high intensity lesions: complementary neurobiological mechanisms in late-life major depression. *Neuropsychopharmacology* 2000; 22(3):264–274.

87. Thomas AJ, O'Brien JT, Davis S, et al. Ischemic basis for deep white matter hyperintensities in major depression: a neuropathological study. *Arch Gen Psychiatry* 2002;59:785–792.

88. Liotti M, Mayberg HS. The role of functional neuroimaging in the neuropsychology of

depression. *J Clinic & Experim Neuropsychology* 2001;23:121–136.

89. Mayberg HS. Limbic-cortical dysregulation: a proposed model of depression. *J Neuropsychiatry & Clin Neurosci* 1997;9:471–481.

90. Lockwood KA, Alexopoulos GS, van Gorp WG. Executive dysfunction in geriatric depression. *Am J Psychiatry* 2002;159:1119–1126.

91. Alexopoulos GS, Kiosses DN, Klimstra S, et al. Clinical presentation of the "depression-executive dysfunction syndrome" of late life. *Am J Geriatr Psychiatry* 2002;10:98–106.

92. Alexopoulos GS, Meyers BS, Young RC, et al. Executive dysfunction and long-term outcomes of geriatric depression. *Arch Gen Psychiatry* 2000;57:285–290.

93. Alexopoulos GS, Kiosses DN, Choi SJ, et al. Frontal white matter microstructure and treatment response of late-life depression: a preliminary study. *Am J Psychiatry* 2002;159:1929–1932.

94. Kalayam B. Alexopoulos GS. Prefrontal dysfunction and treatment response in geriatric depression. *Arch Gen Psychiatry* 1999;56: 713–718.

95. Miller MD, Lenze EJ, Dew MA, et al. Effect of cerebrovascular risk factors on depression treatment outcome in later life. *Am J of Geriatr Psychiatry* 2002;10:592–598.

96. Krishnan KR, Hays JC, George LK, et al. Six-month outcomes for MRI-related vascular depression. *Depress & Anxiety* 1998;8:142–146.

97. Salloway S, Boyle PA, Correia S, et al. The relationship of MRI subcortical hyperintensities to treatment response in a trial of sertraline in geriatric depressed outpatients. *Am J Geriatr Psychiatry* 2002;10:107–111.

98. O'Brien J, Ames D, Chiu E, et al. Severe deep white matter lesions and outcome in elderly patients with major depressive disorder: follow up study. *BMJ* 1998;317:982–984.

99. Forstl H, Burns A, Luthert P, et al. Clinical and neuropathological correlates of depression in Alzheimer's disease. *Psychol Med* 1992;22: 877–884.

100. Roth M. The natural history of mental disorders in old age. *J Ment Sci* 1955;101:281–301.

101. Kiloh L. Pseudodementia. *Acta Psychiatr Scand* 1961;37:336–351.

102. Caine E. Pseudodementia. Current concepts and future directions. *Arch Gen Psychiatry* 1981; 38:1359–1364.

103. Starkstein SE, Rabins PV, Berthier ML, et al. Dementia of depression among patients with neurological disorders and functional depression. *J Neuropsychiatry Clin Neurosci* 1989;1: 263–268.

104. Reifler BV, Larson E, Hanley R. Coexistence of cognitive impairment and depression in geriatric outpatients. *Am J Psychiatry* 1982;139: 623–626.

105. Reifler BV, Larson E, Teri L, et al. Dementia of the Alzheimer's type and depression. *J Am Geriatr Soc* 1986;34:855–859.

106. Zweig RM, Ross CA, Hedreen JC, et al. The neuropathology of aminergic nuclei in Alzheimer's disease. *Ann Neurol* 1988;24:233–242.

107. Zubenko GS, Moossy J. Major depression in pri-

mary dementia. *Arch Neurol* 1988;45:1182–1186.

108. Pearlson GD, Ross CA, Lohr WD, et al. Association between family history of affective disorder and the depressive syndrome of Alzheimer's disease. *Am J Psychiatry* 1990;147:452–456.

109. Alexopoulos GS, Meyers BS, Young RC, et al. The course of geriatric depression with "reversible dementia": a controlled study. *Am J Psychiatry* 1993;150:1693–1699.

110. Kral VA. Long-term follow-up of depressive pseudodementia of the aged. *Can J Psychiatry* 1989;34:445–446.

111. Agbayewa MO. Earlier psychiatric morbidity in patients with Alzheimer's disease. *J Am Geriatr Soc* 1986;34:561–564.

112. Jorm AF, van Duijn CM, Chandra V, et al., for the EURODEM Risk Factors Research Group. Psychiatric history and related exposures as risk factors for Alzheimer's disease: a collaborative re-analysis of case-control studies. EURODEM Risk Factors Research Group. *Int J Epidemiol* 1991;20:43–47.

113. Speck CE, Kukull WA, Brenner DE, et al. History of depression as a risk factor for Alzheimer's disease. *Epidemiology* 1995;6:366–369.

114. Pearson JL, Teri L, Reifler BV, et al. Functional status and cognitive impairment in Alzheimer's patients with and without depression. *J Am Geriatr Soc* 1989;34:1117–1121.

115. Steele C, Rovner B, Chase GA, et al. Psychiatric symptoms and nursing home placement of patients with Alzheimer's disease. *Am J Psychiatry* 1990;147:1049–1051.

116. Reifler BV, Teri L, Raskind M, et al. Double-blind trial of imipramine in Alzheimer's disease patients with and without depression. *Am J Psychiatry* 1989;146:45–49.

117. Katz IR, Parmelee P. Assessment of depression in patients with dementia. *J Ment Health Aging* 1996;2:227–242.

118. Alexopoulos GS, Abrams RC, Young RC, et al. Cornell scale for depression in dementia. *Biol Psychiatry* 1988;23:271–284.

119. Alexopoulos GS, Abrams RC, Young RC, et al. Use of the Cornell scale in nondemented patients. *J Am Geriatr Soc* 1988;36:230–236.

120. Roth M, Tym E, Mountjoy CQ, et al. CAMDEX: a standardized instrument for the diagnosis of mental disorder in the elderly with special reference to the early detection of dementia. *Br J Psychiatry* 1986;149:698–709.

121. Wragg RE, Jeste D. Overview of depression and psychosis in Alzheimer's disease. *Am J Psychiatry* 1989;146:577–587.

122. Lazarus LW, Newton N, Cohler B, et al. Frequency and presentation of depressive symptoms in patients with primary degenerative dementia. *Am J Psychiatry* 1987;144:41–45.

123. Bell-McGinty S, Butters MA, Meltzer CC, et al. Brain morphometric abnormalities in geriatric depression: long-term neurobiological effects of illness duration. *Am J Psychiatry.* 2002;159:1424–1427.

124. Lai T, Payne ME, Byrum CE, et al. Reduction of orbital frontal cortex volume in geriatric depression. *Biol Psychiatry* 2000;48:971–975.

125. Sheline YI, Sanghavi M, Mintun MA, Gado MH. Depression duration but not age predicts hippocampal volume loss in medically healthy women with recurrent major depression. *J of Neurosci* 1999;19:5034–5043.

126. Sheline YI, Gado MH, Price JL. Amygdala core nuclei volumes are decreased in recurrent major depression. *Neuroreport* 1998;9:2436.

127. Krishnan KR, Gadde KM. The pathophysiological basis of late-life depression: imaging studies of the aging brain. *Am J Geriatr Psychiatry* 1996;4:22–33.

128. Coffey CE, Wilkinson WE, Weiner RD, et al. Quantitative cerebral anatomy in depression: a controlled magnetic resonance imaging study. *Arch Gen Psychiatry* 1993;50:7–16.

129. Figiel GS, Krishnan KR, Doraiswamy PM, et al. Subcortical hyperintensities on brain magnetic resonance imaging: a comparison between late-age onset and early onset elderly depressed subjects. *Neurobiol Aging* 1991;12:245–247.

130. Kumar A, Yousem D, Souder E, et al. High-intensity signals in Alzheimer's disease without cerebrovascular risk factors: a magnetic resonance imaging evaluation. *Am J Psychiatry* 1992;149:248–250.

131. Boone KB, Miller BL, Lesser IM, et al. Neuropsychological correlates of white-matter lesions in healthy elderly subjects: a threshold effect. *Arch Neurol* 1992;49:549–554.

132. Fazekas F, Niederkorn K, Schmidt R, et al. White-matter signal abnormalities in normal individuals: correlation with carotid ultrasonography, cerebral blood flow measurements, and cerebrovascular risk factors. *Stroke* 1988;9:1285–1288.

133. Leuchter AF, Newton TF, Cook IA, et al. Changes in brain functional connectivity in Alzheimer's-type and multi-infarct dementia. *Brain* 1992;115:1543–1561.

134. Baldwin RC, O'Brien J. Vascular basis of late-onset depressive disorder. *Br J Psychiatry* 2002;180:157–160.

135. Van den Berg MD, Oldehinkel AJ, Bouhuys AL, et al. Depression in later life: three etiologically different subgroups. *J Affective Disord* 2001;65:19–26.

136. Thomas AJ, Ferrier IN, Kalaria RN, et al. A neuropathological study of vascular factors in late-life depression. *J Neurol, Neurosurg & Psychiatry* 2001;70:83–87.

137. Simpson S, Baldwin RC, Jackson A, et al. Is the clinical expression of late-life depression influenced by brain changes? MRI subcortical neuroanatomical correlates of depressive symptoms. *Internat Psychogeriatrics* 2000;12:425–434.

138. Lyness JM, Caine ED, Cox C, et al. Cerebrovascular risk factors and later-life major depression. Testing a small-vessel brain disease model. *Am J Geriatr Psychiatry* 1998;6:5–13.

139. Miller DS, Kumar A, Yousem DM, et al. MRI high-intensity signals in late-life depression and Alzheimer's disease: a comparison of subjects without major vascular risk factors. *Am J Geriatr Psychiatry* 1994;49:549–554.

140. Kumar A, Newberg A, Alavi A, et al. Regional cerebral glucose metabolism in late-life depression and Alzheimer's disease: a preliminary

positron emission tomography study. *Proc Natl Acad Sci* 1993;90:7019–7023.

141. Lesser IM, Mena I, Boone KB, et al. Reduction of cerebral blood flow in older depressed patients. *Arch Gen Psychiatry* 1994;51:677–686.

142. Sackeim HA, Prohovnik I, Moeller JR, et al. Regional cerebral blood flow in mood disorders. I. Comparison of major depressives and normal controls at rest. *Arch Gen Psychiatry* 1990;47:60–70.

143. Pollock BG, Ferrell RE, Mulsant BH, et al. Allelic variation in the serotonin transporter promoter affects onset of paroxetine treatment response in late-life depression. *Neuropsychopharmacology* 2000;23:587–590.

144. Steffens DC, Svenson I, Marchuk DA, et al. Allelic differences in the serotonin transporter-linked polymorphic region in geriatric depression. *Am J Geriatr Psychiatry* 2002;10:185–191.

145. Brummett BH, Siegler IC, McQuoid DR, et al. Associations among the NEO Personality Inventory, Revised and the serotonin transporter gene-linked polymorphic region in elders: effects of depression and gender. *Psychiatr Genet* 2000;13:13–18.

146. Sheline YI, Gado MH, Kraemer HC. Untreated depression and hippocampal volume loss. *American Journal of Psychiatry* 2000;160:1516–1518.

147. Sheline YI, Wang PW, Gado MH, et al. Hippocampal atrophy in recurrent major depression. Proceedings of the National Academy of Sciences of the United States of America. 1999;93:3908–3913.

148. Alexopoulos GS. "The depression-executive dysfunction syndrome of late life": a specific target for D3 agonists? *Am J Geriatr Psychiatry* 2001;9:22–29.

149. Lockwood KA, Alexopoulos GS, van Gorp WG. Executive dysfunction in geriatric depression. *Am J Psychiatry* 2002;159:1119–1126.

150. Schneider LS, Reynolds CF III, Lebowitz BD, et al. *Diagnosis and treatment of depression in late life.* Washington, DC: American Psychiatric Press, 1994.

151. Katz IR, Alexopoulos GS. Consensus update: diagnosis and treatment of late life depression. *Am J Geriatr Psychiatry.* 1996;4:1–95.

152. Murphy E. The course and outcome of depression in late life. In: Schneider LS, Reynolds CF, Lebowitz BD, eds. *Diagnosis and treatment of depression in late life: results of the NIH Consensus Development Conference.* Washington, DC: American Psychiatric Press, 1994:81–98.

153. George L. Social factors and depression in late life. In: Schneider LS, Reynolds CF, Lebowitz BD, eds. *Diagnosis and treatment of depression in late life: results of the NIH Consensus Development Conference.* Washington, DC: American Psychiatric Press, 1994:131–154.

154. Reynolds CF III, Perel FE, Perel JM, et al. Maintenance therapies for late-life recurrent major depression: research and review circa 1995. *Int Psychogeriatr* 1995;7:27–39.

155. Reynolds CF III, Alexopoulos GS, Katz IR, et al. Chronic depression in the elderly: approaches for prevention. *Drugs & Aging* 2001;18:507–514.

156. Szanto K, Gildengers A, Mulsant BH, et al. Identification of suicidal ideation and prevention of suicidal behaviour in the elderly. *Drugs & Aging* 2002;19:11–24.

157. Alexopoulos GS, Bruce ML, Hull J, et al. Clinical determinants of suicidal ideation and behavior in geriatric depression. *Arch Gen Psychiatry* 1999;56:1048–1053.

158. Kessler RC, Berglund P, Demler O, et al. The epidemiology of major depressive disorder: results from the National Comorbidity Survey Replication (NCS-R). *JAMA* 2003;289(23):3095–3105.

159. Gallo JJ, Armenian HK, Ford DE, et al. Major depression and cancer: the 13-year follow-up of the Baltimore epidemiologic catchment area sample. *Cancer Causes & Control* 2000;11:751–758.

160. Pratt LA, Ford DE, Crum RM, et al. Depression, psychotropic medication, and risk of myocardial infarction. Prospective data from the Baltimore ECA follow-up. *Circulation* 1996;94:3123–3129.

161. Eaton WW, Armenian H, Gallo J, et al. Depression and risk for onset of type II diabetes. A prospective population-based study. *Diabetes Care* 1996;19:1097–1102.

162. Speck CE, Kukull WA, Brenner DE, et al. History of depression as a risk factor for Alzheimer's disease. *Epidemiology* 1995;6:366–369.

163. Jorm AF, van Duijn CM, Chandra V, et al. Psychiatric history and related exposures as risk factors for Alzheimer's disease: a collaborative re-analysis of case-control studies. EURODEM Risk Factors Research Group. *Int J Epidemiol* 1991;2:S43–S47.

164. Alexopoulos GS, Meyers BS, Young RC, et al. The course of geriatric depression with "reversible dementia": a controlled study. *Am J Psychiatry* 1993;150:1693–1699.

165. Schweiger U, Weber B, Deuschle M, Heuser I. Lumbar bone mineral density in patients with major depression: evidence of increased bone loss at follow-up. *Am J Psychiatry* 2000;157:118–120.

166. Michelson D, Stratakis C, Hill L. Bone mineral density in women with depression. *New Engl J Med* 1996;335:1176–1181.

167. de Groot M, Anderson R, Freedland KE, et al. Association of depression and diabetes complications: a meta-analysis. *Psychosom Med* 2001;63:619–630.

168. Anderson RJ, Freedland KE, Clouse RE, et al. The prevalence of comorbid depression in adults with diabetes: a meta-analysis. *Diabetes Care* 2001;24:1069–1078.

169. Lustman PJ, Anderson RJ, Freedland KE, et al. Depression and poor glycemic control: a meta-analytic review of the literature. *Diabetes Care* 2000;23:934–942.

170. Vaillant GE. Natural history of male psychological health, XIV: Relationship of mood disorder vulnerability to physical health. *Am J Psychiatry* 1998;155:184–191.

171. Katz IR. On the inseparability of mental and

physical health in aged persons. *Am J Geriatr Psychiatry* 1996;4:1–16.

172. Katz IR, Streim J, Parmelee P. Prevention of depression, recurrences, and complications in late life. *Prev Med* 1994;23:743–750.

173. Gurland BJ, Wilder DE, Berkman C. Depression and disability in the elderly: reciprocal relations and changes with age. *Int J Geriatr Psychiatry* 1988;3:163–179.

174. Feibel JH, Springer CJ. Depression and failure to resume social activities after stroke. *Arch Phys Med Rehabil* 1982;63:276–278.

175. Parikh RM, Robinson RG, Lipsey JR, et al. The impact of poststroke depression on recovery in activities of daily living over a 2-year follow-up. *Arch Neurol* 1990;47:786–789.

176. Mayo NE, Korner-Bitensky NA, Becker R. Recovery time of independent function poststroke. *Am J Phys Med Rehabil* 1991;70:5–12.

177. Stern MJ, Pascale L, McLoone JB. Psychosocial adaptation following myocardial infarction. *J Chron Dis* 1975;29:513–525.

178. Schleifer SJ, Macari-Hinson MM, Coyle DA, et al. The nature and course of depression following myocardial infarction. *Arch Intern Med* 1989; 149:1785–1789.

179. Schenkman B. Factors contributing to attrition rates in a pulmonary rehabilitation program. *Heart Lung* 1985;14:53–58.

180. Weaver TE, Narsavage GL. Physiological and psychological variables related to functional status in chronic obstructive pulmonary disease. *Nurs Res* 1992;41:286–291.

181. Mossey JM, Mutran E, Knott K, et al. Determinants of recovery 12 months after hip fracture: the importance of psychosocial factors. *Am J Public Health* 1989;79:279–286.

182. Mossey JM, Knott K, Craik R. The effects of persistent depressive symptoms of hip fracture recovery. *J Gerontol* 1990;45:M163–M168.

183. Starkstein SE, Mayberg HS, Leiguarda R, et al. A prospective longitudinal study of depression, cognitive decline, and physical impairments in patients with Parkinson's disease. *J Neurol Neurosurg Psychiatry* 1992;55:377–382.

184. Beckham JC, D'Amico CJ, Rice R, et al. Depression and level of functioning in patients with rheumatoid arthritis. *Can J Psychiatry* 1992;37: 539–543.

185. Borson S, McDonald GJ, Gayle T, et al. Improvement in mood, physical symptoms, and function with nortriptyline for depression in patients with chronic obstructive pulmonary disease. *Psychosom Bull* 1993;29:101–108.

186. Agelink MW, Majewski T, Wurthmann C, et al. Autonomic neurocardiac function in patients with major depression and effects of antidepressive treatment with nefazodone. *J Affective Disorders* 2001;62:187–198.

187. Carney RM, Freedland KE, Stein PK, et al. Change in heart rate and heart rate variability during treatment for depression in patients with coronary heart disease. *Psychosomatic Med* 2000;62:639–647.

188. Stein PK, Carney RM, Freedland KE, et al. Severe depression is associated with markedly reduced heart rate variability in patients with sta-

ble coronary heart disease. *J Psychosom Res* 2000; 48:493–500.

189. Krittayaphong R, Cascio WE, Light KC, et al. Heart rate variability in patients with coronary artery disease: differences in patients with higher and lower depression scores. *Psychosom Med* 1997;59:231–235.

190. Maes M, Van der Planken M, Van Gastel A, et al. Blood coagulation and platelet aggregation in major depression. *J Affective Disord* 1996;40: 35–40.

191. Carney RM, Blumenthal JA, Stein PK, et al. Depression, heart rate variability, and acute myocardial infarction. *Circulation* 2001;104: 2024–2028.

192. Lederbogen F, Gilles M, Maras A, et al. Increased platelet aggregability in major depression? *Psychiatry Res* 2001;102:255–261.

193. Musselman DL, Tomer A, Manatunga AK, et al. Exaggerated platelet reactivity in major depression. *Am J Psychiatry* 1996;153:1313–1317.

194. Yeragani VK, Balon R, Pohl R, Ramesh C. Depression and heart rate variability. *Biol Psychiatry* 1995;38:768–770.

195. Williamson GM, Schultz R. Pain, activity restriction, and symptoms of depression among community-residing elderly adults. *J Gerontol* 1992; 47:367–372.

196. Parmelee PA, Katz IR, Lawton MP. The relation of pain to depression among institutionalized aged. *J Gerontol* 1991;46:15–21.

197. Cohen-Mansfield J, Marx MS. Pain and depression in the nursing home: corroborating results. *J Gerontol* 1993;48:96–97.

198. Waxman HM, Carner EA, Blum A. Depressive symptoms and health service utilization among the community elderly. *J Am Geriatr Soc* 1983; 31:417–420.

199. Unutzer J, Patrick DL, Simon G, et al. Depressive symptoms and the cost of health services in HMO patients aged 65 years and older. A 4-year prospective study. *JAMA* 1997;277: 1618–1623.

200. Luber MP, Meyers BS, Williams-Russo PG, et al. Depression and service utilization in elderly primary care patients. *Am J Geriatr Psychiatry* 2001;9:169–176.

201. Luber MP, Hollenberg JP, Williams-Russo P, et al. Diagnosis, treatment, comorbidity, and resource utilization of depressed patients in a general medical practice. *Int J Psychiatry in Med* 2000;30:1–13.

202. Manning WG, Wells KB. The effects of psychological distress and psychological well-being on use of medical services. *Med Care* 1992;30: 541–553.

203. Callahan CM, Hui SL, Nienaber NA, et al. Longitudinal study of depression and health services use among elderly primary care patients. *J Am Geriatr Soc* 1994;42:833–838.

204. Koenig HG, Shelp F, Goli V, et al. Survival and health care utilization in elderly medical inpatients with major depression. *J Am Geriatr Soc* 1989;37:399–406.

205. Fries BE, Mehr DR, Schneider D, et al. Mental dysfunction and resource use in nursing homes. *Med Care* 1993;31:898–920.

206. Avery D, Winokur G. Mortality in depressed patients treated with electroconvulsive therapy and antidepressants. *Arch Gen Psychiatry* 1976; 33:1029–1037.

207. Frasure-Smith N, Lésperance F, Talajic M. Depression following myocardial infarction: impact on 6-month survival. *JAMA* 1993;270: 1819–1825.

208. Frasure-Smith N, Lésperance F, Talajic M. Depression and 18-month prognosis after myocardial infarction. *Circulation* 1995;91:999–1005.

209. Katz IR, Lesher E, Kleban M, et al. Clinical features of depression in the nursing home. *Int Psychogeriatr* 1989;1:5–15.

210. Rovner BW, German PS, Brant LF, et al. Depression and mortality in nursing homes. *JAMA* 1991;265:993–996.

211. Parmelee PA, Katz IR, Lawton MP. Depression and mortality among institutionalized aged. *J Gerontol* 1992;47:3–10.

212. Ashby D, Ames D, West CR, et al. Psychiatric morbidity as prediction of mortality for residents of local authority homes for the elderly. *Int J Geriatr Psychiatry* 1991;6:567–575.

213. Shah A, Phongsathorn V, George C, et al. Does psychiatric morbidity predict mortality in continuing care geriatric inpatients? *Int J Geriatr Psychiatry* 1993;8:255–259.

214. Samuels SC, Katz IR, Parmelee PA, et al. Use of the Hamilton and Montgomery-Asberg Depression Scales in the institutional elderly: relationship to measures of cognitive impairment, disability, physical illness, and mortality. *Am J Geriatr Psychiatry* 1996;4:237–246.

Table 8.6 References

Boone KB, Miller BL, Lesser IM, et al. Neuropsychological correlates of white-matter lesions in healthy elderly subjects: a threshold effect. *Arch Neurol* 1992;49:549–554.

Coffey CE, Figiel GS, Djang WT, et al. Leukoencephalopathy in elderly depressed patients referred for ECT. *Biol Psychiatry* 1988;24:143–161.

Coffey CE, Wilkinson WE, Weiner RD, et al. Quantitative cerebral anatomy in depression: a controlled magnetic resonance imaging study. *Arch Gen Psychiatry* 1993;50:7–16.

Fazekas F, Niederkorn K, Schmidt R, et al. White-matter signal abnormalities in normal individuals: correlation with carotid ultrasonography, cerebral blood flow measurements, and cerebrovascular risk factors. *Stroke* 1988;19:1285–1288.

Figiel GS, Krishnan KR, Doraiswamy PM, et al. Subcortical hyperintensities on brain magnetic resonance imaging: a comparison between late-age onset and early onset elderly depressed subjects. *Neurobiol Aging* 1991;12:245–247.

Greenwald BS, Kramer-Ginsberg E, Krishnan RR, et al. MRI signal hyperintensities in geriatric depression. *Am J Psychiatry* 1996;153:1212–1215.

Ito H, Kawashima R, Awata S, et al. Hypoperfusion in the limbic system and prefrontal cortex in depression: SPECT with anatomic standardization technique. *J Nucl Med* 1996;37(3):410–414.

Kumar A, Bilker W, Jin Z, Udupa J. Atrophy and high intensity lesions: complementary neurobiological mechanisms in late-life major depression. *Neuropsychopharmacology* 2000:22(3);264–274.

Kumar A, Mintz J, Bilker W, et al. Autonomous neurobiological pathways to late-life major depressive disorder: clinical and pathophysiological implications. *Neuropsychopharmacology* 2002:26(2); 229–236.

Kumar A, Newberg A, Alavi A, et al. Regional cerebral glucose metabolism in late-life depression and Alzheimer's disease: a preliminary positron emission tomography study. *Proc Natl Acad Sci USA* 1993;90:7019–7023.

Kumar A, Yousem D, Souder E, et al. High-intensity signals in Alzheimer's disease without cerebrovascular risk factors: a magnetic resonance imaging evaluation. *Am J Psychiatry* 1992;149:248–250.

Lai T, Payne ME, Byrum CE, et al. Reduction of orbital frontal cortex volume in geriatric depression. *Biological Psychiatry* 2000:48(10);971–975.

Lesser IM, Mena I, Boone KB, et al. Reduction of cerebral blood flow in older depressed patients. *Arch Gen Psychiatry* 1994;51:677–686.

Leuchter AF, Newton TF, Cook IA, et al. Changes in brain functional connectivity in Alzheimer's-type and multi-infarct dementia. *Brain* 1992;115: 1543–1561.

Miller DS, Kumar A, Yousem DM, et al. MRI high-intensity signals in late-life depression and Alzheimer's disease: a comparison of subjects without major vascular risk factors. *Am J Geriatr Psychiatry* 1994;49:549–554.

Navarro V, Gasto C, Lomena F, et al. Normalization of frontal cerebral perfusion in remitted elderly major depression. *Neuroimage* 2002;16:781–787.

Nebes RD, Vora IJ, Meltzer CC, et al. Relationship of deep white matter hyperintensities and apolipoprotein E genotype to depressive symptoms in older adults without clinical depression. *Am J of Psychiatry* 2001:158(6);878–884.

Sackeim HA, Prohovnik I, Moeller JR, et al. Regional cerebral blood flow in mood disorders. I. Comparison of major depressives and normal controls at rest. *Arch Gen Psychiatry* 1990;47:60–70.

Salloway S, Malloy P, Kohn R, et al. MRI and neuropsychological differences in early- and late-onset geriatric depression. *Neurology* 1996;46:1567–1574.

Thomas AJ, O'Brien JT, Davis S, et al. Ischemic basis for deep white matter hyperintensities in major depression: a neuropathological study. *Arch Gen Psychiatry* 2002;59(9):785–792.

Tupler LA, Krishnan KR, McDonald WM, et al. Anatomic location and laterality of MRI signal hyperintensities in late-life depression. *Journal of Psychosomatic Research* 2002;53(2):665–676.

Vasile RG, Schwartz RB, Garada B, et al. Focal cerebral perfusion defects demonstrated by 99mTc-hexamethylpropyleneamine oxime SPECT in elderly depressed patients. *Psychiatry Research* 1996; 67(1):59–70.

Wurthman C, Bogerts B, Falkai P. Brain morphology assessed by computed tomography in patients with geriatric depression, patients with degenerative dementia, and normal control subjects. *Psychiatry Res* 1995;61:103–111.

Supplemental Readings

General

Baldessarini RJ. *Biomedical aspects of depression and its treatment.* Washington, DC: American Psychiatric Press, 1983.

Ballenger JC. Biological aspects of depression—implications for clinical practice. In: Frances AJ, Hales RE, eds. *Review of psychiatry, vol. 7.* Washington, DC: American Psychiatric Press, 1988.

Blazer D. The diagnosis of depression in the elderly. *J Am Geriatr Soc* 1980;28:52–58.

Burkhart KS. Diagnosis of depression in the elderly patient. *Lippincotts Prim Care Pract* 2000;4: 149–162.

Butler RN, Cohen G, Lewis MI, et al. Late-life depression: how to make a difficult diagnosis. *Geriatrics* 1997;52:37, 41–42, 47–50.

Charney DS, Reynolds CF, Lewis L, et al. Depression and Bipolar Support Alliance consensus statement on the unmet needs in diagnosis and treatment of mood disorders in late life. *Arch Gen Psychiatry* 2003;60:664–672.

Cohen GD. Depression in late life. An historic account demonstrates the importance of making the diagnosis. *Geriatrics* 2002;57:38–39.

Cole MG, Bellavance F. The progress of depression in old age. *Am J Geriatr Psychiatry* 1997;5:4–14.

Conn DK, Steingart AB. Diagnosis and management of late life depression: a guide for the primary care physician. *Int J Psychiatry Med* 1997;27: 269–281.

Dalton JR, Busch KD. Depression. The missing diagnosis in the elderly. *Home Healthc Nurse* 1995;13: 31–35.

Depression and treatment of depression in late life. NIH Consensus Development Conference. November 4–6, 1991.

Devanand DP, Nelson JC. Concurrent depression and dementia: implications for diagnosis and treatment. *J Clin Psychiatry* 1985;46:389–392.

Diagnosis and treatment of depression in late life: the NIH Consensus Development Conference Statement. *Psychopharmacol Bull* 1993;29:87–100.

Glickman L, Friedman SA. Changes in behavior, mood, or thinking in the elderly. Diagnosis and management. *Med Clin North Am* 1976;60: 1297–1313.

Goldin LR, Gershon ES. The genetic epidemiology of major depressive illness. In: Frances AJ, Hales RE, eds. *Review of psychiatry, vol. 7.* Washington, DC: American Psychiatric Press, 1988.

Hall CW, ed. *Psychiatric presentations of medical illnesses: somatopsychic disorders.* New York: SP Publications, 1980.

Kales HC, Valenstein M. Complexity in late-life depression: impact of confounding factors on diagnosis, treatment, and outcomes. *J Geriatr Psychiatry Neurol* 2002;15:147–155.

Kanowski S. Depression in the elderly: clinical considerations and therapeutic approaches. *J Clin Psychiatry* 1994;55:166–173.

Katz IR. Drug treatment of depression in the frail elderly: discussion of the NIH Consensus Development Conference on the Diagnosis and Treatment of Depression in Late Life. *Psychopharmacol Bull* 1993;29:101–108.

Kim KY, Hershey LA. Diagnosis and treatment of depression in the elderly. *Int J Psychiatry Med* 1988;18:211–221.

Lebowitz BD, Pearson JL, Schneider LS, et al. Diagnosis and treatment of depression in late life. Consensus statement update. *JAMA* 1997;278: 1186–1190.

Lesseig DZ. Primary care diagnosis and pharmacologic treatment of depression in adults. *Nurse Pract* 1996;21:72, 75–76.

Lyness JM, Cox C, Curry J, et al. Older age and the underreporting of depressive symptoms. *J Am Geriatr Soc* 1995;43:216–221.

McCahill ME, Brunton SA. The elderly patient with multiple complaints. *Hosp Pract (Off Ed)* 1995;30: 49–54.

Miller MD, Schulz R, Paradis C, et al. Changes in perceived health status of depressed elderly patients treated until remission. *Am J Psychiatry* 1996;153:1350–1352.

NIH Consensus Development Panel on Depression in Late Life. Diagnosis and treatment of depression in late life. *JAMA* 1992;268:1018–1023.

Pond CD, Mant A, Kehoe L, et al. General practitioner diagnosis of depression and dementia in the elderly: can academic detailing make a difference? *Fam Pract* 1994;11:141–147.

Rapp SR, Vrana S. Substituting nonsomatic for somatic symptoms in the diagnosis of depression in elderly male medical patients. *Am J Psychiatry* 1989;146:1197–1200.

Raskin DE. Psychiatry and the elderly: diagnosis, treatment, and medical/ethical dilemmas. *Del Med J* 1988;60:371–373.

Reynolds CF III, Lebowitz BD, Schneider LS. The NIH Consensus Development Conference on the Diagnosis and Treatment of Depression in Late Life: an overview. *Psychopharmacol Bull* 1993;29: 83–85.

Reynolds CF. Depression: making the diagnosis and using SSRIs in the older patient. *Geriatrics* 1996; 51:28–34.

Rothera I, Jones R, Gordon C. An examination of the attitudes and practice of general practitioners in the diagnosis and treatment of depression in older people. *Int J Geriatr Psychiatry* 2002;17: 354–358.

Rothschild AJ. The diagnosis and treatment of late-life depression. *J Clin Psychiatry* 1996;57(suppl 5): 5–11.

Sahr N. Assessment and diagnosis of elderly depression. *Clin Excell Nurse Pract* 1999;3:158–164.

Schwenk TL. Diagnosis of late life depression: the view from primary care. *Biol Psychiatry* 2002;52: 157–163.

Unutzer J. Diagnosis and treatment of older adults with depression in primary care. *Biol Psychiatry* 2002;52:285–292.

Wilson K, Mottram P, Sivananthan A, Nightingale A. Antidepressants versus placebo for the depressed elderly (Cochrane Review). In: *The Cochrane Library*, Issue 3, 2002. Oxford: Update Software.

Winstead DK, Mielke DH, O'Neill PT. Diagnosis and treatment of depression in the elderly: a review. *Psychiatr Med* 1990;8:85–98.

Winstead DK, Mielke DH. Differential diagnosis between dementia and depression in the elderly. *Neurol Clin* 1984;2:23–35.

Zisook S, Downs NS. Diagnosis and treatment of depression in late life. *J Clin Psychiatry* 1998; 59(suppl 4):80–91.

Biological Markers in Depression

Asarch KB, Shih JC, Kulscar A. Decreased ^{3}H-imipramine binding in depressed males and females. *Community Psychopharmacol* 1981;4:425–432.

Briley MS, Raisman R, Sechter D, et al. ^{3}H-imipramine binding in human platelets—a new biochemical parameter in depression. *Neuropharmacology* 1980;19:1209–1210.

Carroll BJ. Dexamethasone suppression test. In: Hall RCW, Beresdorf TP, eds. *Handbook of psychiatric diagnostic procedures, vol. 1.* New York: SP Publications, 1984:3–28.

Dement WC, Miles LE, Carskadon MA. "White paper" on sleep and aging. *J Am Geriatr Soc* 1982; 30:25–30.

Georgotas A, Stokes PE, Hapworth WE, et al. The relationship of dexamethasone suppression test to subtypes of depression and to symptomatic severity in the elderly. *J Affective Disord* 1986;10: 51–57.

Kupfer DJ. Neuropsychological markers—EEG sleep measures. *J Psychiatr Res* 1984;18:467–495.

Kupfer DJ, Foster FG, Coble P, et al. The application of EEG sleep for the differential diagnosis of affective disorders. *Am J Psychiatry* 1978;135:69–74.

Loosen PT, Prange AJ. Serum thyrotropin response to thyrotropin-releasing hormone in psychiatric patients—a review. *Am J Psychiatry* 1982;139: 405–416.

Magni G, Schifano F, De Leo D. The dexamethasone suppression test in depressed and non-depressed geriatric medical inpatients. *Acta Psychiatr Scand* 1986;73:511–514.

Robinson DS, Davies JM, Nies A, et al. Relation of sex and aging to monoamine oxidase activity of human plasma and platelets. *Arch Gen Psychiatry* 1971;24:536–541.

Schneider LS, Severson JA, Pollock V, et al. Platelet monoamine oxidase activity in elderly depressed outpatients. *Biol Psychiatry* 1986;21:1360–1364.

Schneider LS, Severson JA, Sloane RB. Platelet ^{3}H-imipramine binding in depressed elderly patients. *Biol Psychiatry* 1985;20:1234–1237.

Teicher MH, Lawrence JM, Barber NI, et al. Increased activity and phase delay in circadian motility rhythms in geriatric depression. *Arch Gen Psychiatry* 1988;45:913–917.

Brain Imaging and Depression

Coffey CE, Figiel GS, Djang WT, et al. White matter hyperintensity on MRI: clinical and neuroanatomical correlates in the depressed elderly. *Neuropsychiatry* 1988;1:135–144.

Drevets WC. Geriatric depression: brain imaging correlates and pharmacologic considerations. *J Clin Psychiatry* 1994;55(suppl):71–81.

Hauser P, Altshuler LL, Berrettini W, et al. Temporal lobe measurement in primary affective disorder by MRI. *J Neuropsychiatry* 1988;1:128–134.

Jacoby RJ, Dolan RJ, Levy R, et al. Quantitative computerized tomography in elderly depressed patients. *Br J Psychiatry* 1983;143:124–127.

Jacoby RJ, Levy R, Bird JM. Computerized tomography and the outcome of affective disorder—a follow up study of elderly patients. *Br J Psychiatry* 1983;39:288–292.

Kalayam B, Alexopoulos GS. Prefrontal dysfunction and treatment response in geriatric depression. *Arch Gen Psychiatry* 1999;56:713–718.

Swanwick GR, Rowan M, Coen RF, et al. Clinical application of electrophysiological markers in the differential diagnosis of depression and very mild Alzheimer's disease. *J Neurol Neurosurg Psychiatry* 1996;60:82–86.

Delusional Depression

Baldwin RC. Delusional and non-delusional depression in late life—evidence for distinct subtypes. *Br J Psychiatry* 1988;152:39–44.

Coryell W, Tsuang MT. Major depression with mood-congruent or mood-incongruent psychotic features—outcome after 40 years. *Am J Psychiatry* 1985;142:479–482.

Glassman AH, Roose SP. Delusional depression—a distinct clinical entity? *Arch Gen Psychiatry* 1981; 38:424–427.

Meyers BS, Greenberg R. Late-life delusional depression. *J Affective Disord* 1986;11:133–137.

Dementia and Depression

Bulbena A, Berrios G. Pseudodementia: facts and figures. *Br J Psychiatry* 1986;148:87–94.

Caine ED. Pseudodementia. *Arch Gen Psychiatry* 1981; 38:1359–1364.

Kiloh LG. Pseudodementia. *Acta Psychiatr Scand* 1960;37:336–351.

McAllister TW. Overview of pseudodementia. *Am J Psychiatry* 1983;140:528–533.

Pearlson GD, Rabins PV, Kim WS, et al. Structural brain CT changes and cognitive deficits in elderly depressives with and without reversible dementia (pseudodementia). *Psychol Med* 1989;19: 573–584.

Snow SS, Wells CE. Case studies in neuropsychiatry: diagnosis and treatment of coexistent dementia and depression. *J Clin Psychiatry* 1981;42: 439–441.

Depression and Dementia

Alexopoulos GS, Meyers BS, Young RC, et al. The course of geriatric depression with "reversible dementia": a controlled study. *Am J Psychiatry* 1993;150:1693–1699.

Brook C, Simpson WM. Dementia, depression, or grief? The differential diagnosis. *Geriatrics* 1990; 45:37–43.

Butler RN, Finkel SI, Lewis MI, et al. Aging and mental health: diagnosis of dementia and depression. *Geriatrics* 1992;47:49–52, 55–57.

Copeland JR, Gurland BJ, Dewey ME, et al. Is there more dementia, depression and neurosis in New York? A comparative study of the elderly in New York and London using computer diagnosis AGECAT. *Br J Psychiatry* 1987;151:466–473.

Devanand DP, Nelson JC. Concurrent depression and dementia: "implications for diagnosis and treatment. *J Clin Psychiatry* 1985;46:389–392.

Gray JW, Rattan AI, Dean RS. Differential diagnosis of dementia and depression in the elderly using neuropsychological methods. *Arch Clin Neuropsychol* 1986;1:341–349.

Greenwald BS, Kramer-Ginsberg E, Marin DB, et al. Dementia with coexistent major depression. *Am J Psychiatry* 1989;146:1472–1478.

Kral VA. The relationship between senile dementia (Alzheimer's type) and depression. *Can J Psychiatry* 1983;28:304–306.

Liston EH, Jarvik LF, Gerson S. Depression in Alzheimer's disease—an overview of adrenergic and cholinergic mechanisms. *Compr Psychiatry* 1987; 28:444–457.

Merriam AE, Aronson MK, Gaston P, et al. The psychiatric symptoms of Alzheimer's disease. *J Am Geriatr Soc* 1988;36:7–12.

Reifler BV, Larson E, Hanley R. Coexistence of cognitive impairment and depression in geriatric outpatients. *Am J Psychiatry* 1982;139:623–626.

Reifler BV, Larson E, Teri L, et al. Dementia of the Alzheimer's type and depression. *J Am Geriatr Soc* 1986;34:855–859.

Zubenko GS, Mossey J. Major depression in primary dementia: clinical and neuropathological correlates. *Arch Neurol* 1988;45:1182–1186.

Depression and Institutionalized Aged

Heston LL, Garrard J, Makris L, et al. Inadequate treatment of depressed nursing home elderly. *J Am Geriatr Soc* 1992;40:1117–1122.

Katz IR, Parmelee PA, Streim JE. Depression in older patients in residential care. *Am J Geriatr Psychiatry* 1995;3:161–169.

Parmelee PA, Katz IR, Lawton MP. Depression among institutionalized aged: assessment and prevalence estimation. *J Gerontol* 1989;44: M22–M29.

Parmelee PA, Katz IR, Lawton MP. Depression and mortality among institutionalized aged. *J Gerontol* 1992;47:P3–P10.

Parmelee PA, Katz IR, Lawton MP. Incidence of depression in long-term care settings. *J Gerontol* 1992;47:M189–M196.

Phillips CJ, Henderson AS. The prevalence of depression among Australian nursing home residents: results using draft ICD-10 and DSM-III-R criteria. *Psychol Med* 1991;21:739–748.

Rovner BW, German PS, Brant LJ, et al. Depression and mortality in nursing homes. *JAMA* 1991;265: 993–996.

Drug-Induced Depression

Billings R, Stein M. Depression associated with ranitidine. *Am J Psychiatry* 1986;143:915–916.

Billings R, Tang SW, Ratkoff VM. Depression associated with cimetidine. *Can J Psychiatry* 1981;26: 260–261.

DeMuth G, Ackerman S. Alpha-methyl dopa and depression—a clinical study and review of the literature. *Am J Psychiatry* 1983;140:534–538.

Griffin S, Friedman M. Depressive symptoms in propranolol users. *J Clin Psychiatry* 1986;47:453–457.

Okada F. Depression after treatment with thiazide diuretics for hypertension. *Am J Psychiatry* 1985; 142:1101–1102.

Paykel ES, Fleminger R, Watson JP. Psychiatric side effects of antihypertensive drugs other than reserpine. *J Clin Psychopharmacol* 1982;2:14–39.

Pollack MH, Rosenbaum JF, Cassem NH. Propranolol and depression revisited: three cases and a review. *J Nerv Ment Dis* 1985;173:118–119.

Epidemiology

Blazer DG. Is depression more frequent in late life? *Am J Geriatr Psychiatry* 1994;2:193–199.

Girling DM, Barkley C, Paykel ES. The prevalence of depression in a cohort of very elderly. *J Affective Disord* 1995;34:319–329.

Gurland BJ, Cross PS, Katz S. Epidemiological perspectives on opportunities for treatment of depression. *Am J Geriatr Psychiatry* 1996;4(suppl 1):S7–S13.

Krishnan PA, Katz IR, Lawton MP. Incidence of depression in long term care settings. *J Gerontol Med Sci* 1992;47:M189–196.

Meyers BS. Epidemiology and clinical meaning of "significant" depressive symptoms in later life. *Am J Geriatr Psychiatry* 1994;2:188–191.

Late-Onset Depression

Alexopoulos GS, Meyers BS, Young RC, et al. Brain changes in geriatric depression. *Int J Geriatr Psychiatry* 1988;3:157–161.

McCullough JP, Braith JA, Chapman RC, et al. Comparison of early and late onset dysthymia. *J Nerv Ment Dis* 1990;78:577–581.

Meyers BS, Alexopoulos GS. Age of onset and studies of late-life depression. *Int J Geriatr Psychiatry* 1988; 3:219–228.

Ranga K, Krishnan R, Hays JC, et al. Clinical and phenomenological comparisons of late-onset and early onset depression. *Am J Psychiatry* 1995; 152:785–788.

Masked Depression

Keilholz P. Masked depressions and depressive equivalents. In: Keilholz P, ed. *Masked depression—an international symposium.* Berne: Hans Huber, 1973.

Lesse S. The masked depression syndrome. Results of a seventeen-year clinical study. *Am J Psychiatry* 1983;37:456–475.

Salzman C, Shader RI. Depression in the elderly. I: Relationship between depression, psychologic defense mechanisms and physical illness. *J Am Geriatr Soc* 1978;27:253–260.

Medical Illnesses and Depression

Abram HS, Moore GL, Westervelt FB Jr. Suicidal behavior in chronic dialysis patients. *Am J Psychiatry* 1971;127:1199–1204.

Blumer D, Heilbronn M. Chronic pain as a variant of depressive disease—the pain prone disorder. *J Nerv Ment Dis* 1982;170:381–394.

Cassem NH, Hackett TP. Psychological aspects of myocardial infarction. *Med Clin North Am* 1977; 61:711–721.

Cavanaugh S. Diagnosing depression in the hospitalized patient with chronic medical illness. *J Clin Psychiatry* 1984;45:13–16.

Derogatis LR, Morrow GR, Fetting J, et al. The prevalence of psychiatric disorders among cancer patients. *JAMA* 1983;249:751–757.

Dupont RM, Cullum CM, Jeste DV. Poststroke depression and psychoses. *Psychiatr Clin North Am* 1988;11:133–149.

Gold MS, Kronig MH. Comprehensive thyroid evaluation in psychiatric patients. In: Hall RCW, Beresdorf TP, eds. *Handbook of psychiatric diagnostic procedures, vol. 1.* New York: SP Publications, 1984:29–45.

Gold MS, Pottash ALC, Extein I. Hypothyroidism and depression: evidence from complete thyroid function evaluation. *JAMA* 1981;245:1919–1922.

Hoch CC, Reynolds CF, Kupfer DJ, et al. Sleep-disordered breathing in normal and pathologic aging. *J Clin Psychiatry* 1986;47:499–503.

Kathol RG, Perry F. Relationship of medical illnesses to depression—a critical review. *J Affective Disord* 1981;3:111–121.

Kelly WE, Checkley SS, Bender DA, et al. Cushing's syndrome and depression—a prospective study of 26 patients. *Br J Psychiatry* 1983;142:16–19.

Kukull WA, Koepsell TD, Inui TS, et al. Depression and physical illness among elderly general medical clinic patients. *J Affective Disord* 1986;10: 153–162.

Lowry MR, Atcherson E. Characteristics of patients with depressive disorders on entry into home hemodialysis. *J Nerv Ment Dis* 1979;167:748–751.

McCahill ME, Brunton SA. The elderly patient with multiple complaints. *Hosp Pract (Off Ed)* 1995;30: 49–54.

Robinson RG, Kubos KG, Starr LB, et al. Mood changes in stroke patients: relationship to lesion location. *Compr Psychiatry* 1983;24:555–566.

Robinson RG, Rabins PV, eds. *Aging and clinical practice—depression and coexisting physical disease.* New York: Igaku-Shoin, 1989.

Robinson RG, Starr LB, Kubos KL, et al. A two year longitudinal study of post-stroke mood disorders: findings during the initial evaluation. *Stroke* 1983; 14:736–741.

Rodin GM. Renal dialysis and the liaison psychiatrist. *Can J Psychiatry* 1980;25:473–477.

Rodin GM, Voshart K. Depression in the medically ill: an overview. *Am J Psychiatry* 1986;143:696–705.

Schiffer RB, Babigian HM. Behavioral disorders in multiple sclerosis, temporal lobe epilepsy and amyotrophic lateral sclerosis: an epidemiological study. *Arch Neurol* 1984;41:1067–1069.

Stern MJ, Pascale L, Ackerman A. Life adjustment post-myocardial infarction: determining predictive variables. *Arch Intern Med* 1977;137:1680–1685.

Morbidity and Depression

Abrams RC, Alexopoulos GS, Young RC. Geriatric depression and DSM-III-R personality disorder criteria. *J Am Geriatr Soc* 1987;35:383–386.

Baldwin RC, Jolley DJ. The prognosis of depression in old age. *Br J Psychiatry* 1986;149:574–583.

Cole MG. Age, age of onset and course of primary depressive illness in the elderly. *Can J Psychiatry* 1983;28:102–104.

Eastwood MR, Corbin SL. The relationship between physical illness and depression in old age. In: Murphy E, ed. *Affective disorders in the elderly.* New York: Churchill Livingstone, 1986.

Havens L. Clinical interview with a suicidal patient (with commentary). In: Douglas J, Brown HN, eds. *Suicide—understanding and responding.* Madison, CT: International Universities Press, 1989.

Katz IR. On the inseparability of mental and physical health in aged persons. *Am J Geriatr Psychiatry* 1996;4:1–16.

Keller MB. Chronic and recurrent affective disorders: incidence, course and influencing factors. In: Racagnio G, ed. *Chronic treatment in neuropsychiatry.* New York: Raven, 1985.

Keller MB, Lavori PW, Rice J, et al. The persistent risk of chronicity in recurrent episodes of nonbipolar major depressive disorder: a follow-up study. *Am J Psychiatry* 1986;143:24–28.

Keller MB, Shapiro RW. "Double depression." Superimposition of acute depressive episodes on chronic depressive disorders. *Am J Psychiatry* 1982;139:438–442.

Miller MD, Paradis CF, Houck PR, et al. Chronic medical illness in patients with recurrent major depression. *Am J Geriatr Psychiatry* 1996;4: 281–290.

Morgan AC. Special issues in the assessment and treatment of suicide risk in the elderly. In: Douglas J, Brown HN, eds. *Suicide—understanding and responding.* Madison, CT: International Universities Press, 1989.

Murphy E. The prognosis of depression in old age. *Br J Psychiatry* 1983;142:111–119.

Robins LN, West PA, Murphy GE. The high rate of suicide in older white men: a study testing ten hypotheses. *Soc Psychiatry* 1977;12:1–20.

Rating Scales

Beck AT, Ward CH, Mendelson M, et al. An inventory for measuring depression. *Arch Gen Psychiatry* 1961;4:561–571.

Blessed G, Tomlinson BE, Roth M. The association between quantitative measures of dementia and of senile change in the cerebral grey matter of elderly subjects. *Br J Psychiatry* 1968;114:797–811.

Copeland JR, Kelleher MJ, Kellett JM, et al. A semi-structured clinical interview for the assessment of diagnosis and mental state in the elderly: the Geriatric Mental State Schedule. I. Development and reliability. *Psychol Med* 1976;6:439–449.

Folstein MF, Folstein SE, McHugh PR. "Mini-Mental

State": a practical method for grading the cognitive state of patients for the clinician. *J Psychiatr Res* 1975;12:189–198.

Gray JW, Rattan AI, Dean RS. Differential diagnosis of dementia and depression in the elderly using neuropsychological methods. *Arch Clin Neuropsychol* 1986;1:341–349.

Gurland BJ, Fleiss JL, Goldberg K, et al. A semi-structured clinical interview for the assessment of diagnosis and mental state in the elderly: the Geriatric Mental State Schedule. II. A factor analysis. *Psychol Med* 1976;6:451–459.

Hamilton M. A rating scale for depression. *J Neurol Neurosurg Psychiatry* 1960;23:56–62.

Kahn RL, Goldfarb AI, Pollack M, et al. Brief objective measures for the determination of mental status in the aged. *Am J Psychiatry* 1960;117:326–328.

Mackinnon A, Christensen H, Cullen JS, et al. The Canberra Interview for the Elderly: assessment of its validity in the diagnosis of dementia and depression. *Acta Psychiatr Scand* 1993;87:146–151.

Mackinnon A, Christensen H, Cullen JS, et al. The Canberra Interview for the Elderly: a new field instrument for the diagnosis of dementia and depression by ICD-10 and DSM-III-R. *Acta Psychiatr Scand* 1992;85:105–113.

Chapter 9

Treatment of Depression with Tricyclic Antidepressants, Monoamine Oxidase Inhibitors, and Psychostimulants

George S. Alexopoulos

Darin M. Lerner

Carl Salzman

All antidepressants are efficacious in treating late-life depression. However, individual patients may respond to some antidepressants and not others. Clinical and research literature suggests a continuing therapeutic role for tricyclic antidepressants (TCAs) and monoamine oxidase inhibitors (MAOIs) in the eldely, especially when the illness is severe.[1] However, these agents have become less commonly used in the psychotropic treatment of late-life depression since the introduction of selective serotonin reuptake inhibitors (SSRIs) in the last decade (see Ch 10). Potentially dangerous side effects including cardiac conduction problems, orthostatic hypotension, and urinary retention, as well as annoying side effects such as dry mouth and constipation, have limited the use of TCAs. Concerns about drug–drug and drug–food interactions, in addition to side effects, may be responsible for the limited use of MAOIs. Knowledge and clinical experience in the use of these agents, however, is particularly important for psychiatrists treating inpatients, depressed elders with psychotic depression, and treatment-resistant late-life depression. Psychostimulants are not effective when taken as the only antidepressant; they are used primarily to increase energy and alertness as well as to augment the therapeutic effect of other antidepressant medications.

Tricyclic Antidepressants

TCAs are the most extensively investigated class of drugs used to treat geriatric depression. Nortriptyline, in particular, is considered the "gold-standard" against which other antidepressants are compared. Although indications for use in older persons are the same as for young adults, older patients are more likely to experience side effects because of age-related pharmacokinetic alterations in drug absorption, binding, distribution, metabolism, and excretion (discussed later and in Chapter 5). Elderly patients may also be more sensitive to the toxic effects of these drugs because of age-related altered central nervous system (CNS) neurotransmission (see Chapter 4). Older patients may develop higher plasma levels of drugs and their metabolites than younger adults while taking similar dosages because of age-related changes in hepatic clearance (see Chapter 5). Depressed elders require TCA plasma levels similar to those of younger adults, but those can usually be obtained with lower dosages than the dosages commonly prescribed for younger adults.

Despite the introduction and wide use of newer antidepressants in the last decade, TCAs have several advantages: blood levels can be measured and ECG can be used to monitor the effect of dosage increments on cardiac conductions, and a wealth of research data on treatment of depression in the elderly focuses on TCAs, especially nortriptyline.

Medical Assessment

A comprehensive medical evaluation is essential before TCA treatment begins. The medical examination of a depressed geriatric patient has two principal goals: to diagnose medical illnesses frequently associated with depression and to identify conditions that increase the risk of treatment. Patients who require TCA treatment should be evaluated for presence of cardiac disease (particularly conduction defects), endocrinopathies, vitamin deficiencies, cerebrovascular or degenerative brain diseases, glaucoma, and prostatic hypertrophy. Extensive medical history, complete physical examination (including rectal examination), and blood pressure measurement (supine, sitting, and standing) are recommended, and an ECG should always be obtained. Consultation with a cardiologist, urologist, or ophthalmologist is necessary when cardiac disease, prostatic hypertrophy, or glaucoma is suspected.

Depressed patients with thyroid disease have at best a partial response to antidepressants until the thyroid dysfunction is effectively treated. For this reason, testing thyroid functions in depressed elders is critical. Fatigue, malaise, constipation, or functional decline often are the first manifestations of thyroid disease. Physical findings suggestive of thyroid disorders may include goiter, exopthalamos, weight loss or weight gain, and heat and cold intolerance. Laboratory screening for thyroid dysfunction is essential when a patient presents with psychiatric symptoms and should include serum TSH determination; further thyroid function assessment may include serum thyroxine (T_4), serum triiodothyronine (T_3), T_3 resin uptake (T_3RU), free T_4, and free thyroxine index (FTI). Patients with hypothyroidism may develop depressive syndromes whether or not they are cognitively impaired. Hypothyroidism is a common side effect of lithium that may also lead to anxious depression, generalized anxiety, and even psychosis.

Vitamin B_{12} and folate deficiencies should be ruled out in depressed el-derly patients. Depression, apathy, and cognitive impairment may be either the first manifestations of B_{12} deficiency or part of the classical presentation of these deficiencies. Symptoms are anemia, fatigue, and pallor, together with neurologic signs such as peripheral neuropathy, spinal cord syndrome, and dementia. All depressed elderly patients should be screened for folate and B_{12} deficiency by obtaining folate and serum B_{12} levels; folate concentration is measured more accurately by RBC folate measurement than by serum folate levels. The laboratory workup for anemia should include CBC with differential, platelet count, reticulocyte count, and a peripheral smear.

Classes of TCAs

Although some older patients may respond better to one TCA than another, no predictable differences in therapeutic efficacy have yet been identified among them. However, among experts in geriatric psychiatry, 94% prefer nortriptyline as the TCA of choice.[2] Selection of a particular antidepressant for an elderly patient, therefore, is usually based primarily on differences in side effects among the drugs.

Clinical Pharmacology

TCAs are divided into two subgroups. The first—the tertiary amines—consists of amitriptyline, clomipramine, doxepin, imipramine, and trimipramine. Tertiary amine TCAs produce the most frequent and severe side effects of all antidepressants. Recent expert guidelines do not recommend the use of tertiary amine TCAs in the treatment of late-life depression.[2] The second subgroup—the secondary amines—includes nortriptyline, desipramine, maprotiline, amoxapine, and protriptyline. Nortriptyline and desipramine, although chemically related to tertiary amines, have fewer and less severe side effects. Distinguishing characteristics of TCAs are shown in Table 9.1.

Absorption

TCAs are slowly but completely absorbed. However, their anticholinergic action may

Table 9.1.   Relative Side Effects of Tricyclic Antidepressants in the Elderly Patient

Drug	Sedation	Hypotension	Anticholinergic Side Effects	Altered Cardiac Rate and Rhythm
TERTIARY AMINES				
Amitriptyline	Strong	Moderate	Very strong	Strong
Clomipramine	Strong	Strong	Strong	Strong
Doxepin	Moderate–strong	Moderate	Strong	Moderate
Imipramine	Mild	Moderate	Moderate–strong	Moderate
Trimipramine	Strong	Moderate	Strong	Strong
SECONDARY AMINES				
Amoxapine	Mild	Moderate	Moderate	Moderate
Desipramine	Mild	Mild–moderate	Mild	Mild
Maprotiline	Moderate–strong	Moderate	Moderate	Mild
Nortriptyline	Mild	Mild	Moderate	Mild
Protriptyline	Mild	Moderate	Strong	Moderate

slow gastric and intestinal motility, thus delaying absorption, which leads to high peak blood levels. In most instances, this delay in absorption has limited clinical significance.

Protein Binding

TCAs bind weakly to plasma albumin and strongly to alpha$_1$-acid-glycoprotein. Although approximately 95% of the circulating TCA is protein-bound, only the unbound fraction is biologically active and thus responsible for therapeutic effects and adverse reactions. Serum albumin levels decrease with advanced age, but alpha$_1$-acid-glycoprotein levels remain unchanged or increase.[3] The clinical significance of changes in these plasma proteins is unclear.

Hepatic Metabolism

The hepatic metabolism of TCAs proceeds through two major stages, demethylation and hydroxylation. A varying proportion of the tertiary amines is first demethylated to secondary amines. Because the rate and efficiency of demethylation decreases with advanced age, the amount of demethylated tertiary amines decreases. This process in turn leads to high plasma levels of nondemethylated tertiary amines that are more toxic than their demethylated metabolites. The decreased efficiency of demethylation may explain in part why levels of tertiary amines are higher in geriatric patients and result in greater toxicity than in their younger counterparts.

Both tertiary and secondary amines undergo aromatic hydroxylation, the primary metabolic pathway for TCAs mediated by the hepatic cytochrome P-450 IID6 (CYP IID6) enzyme system. With aging, metabolism becomes less efficient, with three important clinical consequences. First, plasma levels of imipramine, amitriptyline, desipramine, and nortriptyline for any given dose are higher than those of young people.[3] Second, age-related changes in hepatic cytochrome P-450 activity differ widely among old people, resulting in great variability in TCA plasma levels from patient to patient. Third, renal clearance decreases, prolonging the elimination of TCA metabolites. Drugs that interact with metabolic enzymes may alter blood levels of TCAs. For example, perphenazine inhibits CYP-III D6, raising blood levels of nortriptyline (and other TCAs) to potentially toxic levels (see Appendix C).

Hydroxylated Metabolites

The extensive hepatic metabolism of TCAs results in the formation of biologically active hydroxylated metabolites. Although their therapeutic efficacy is relatively weak, these metabolites may contribute to the development of cardiac toxicity. Because they are water soluble, their clearance depends on the efficiency of the kidneys. Age-associated reduction in the renal clearance of water-soluble compounds such as hydroxymetabolites may result in higher plasma levels.[4-6] Thus when TCAs are prescribed, geriatric patients tend to develop higher plasma levels of the hydroxylated metabolites than younger adults receiving comparable doses.[7,8]

The most thoroughly studied hydroxylation pathway is found in the metabolism of nortriptyline. The hydroxylated metabolite of nortriptyline (10-hydroxynortriptyline 10-OH-NT) penetrates the blood–brain barrier more freely than its parent compound. Pharmacologic characteristics of this hydroxylated metabolite that may be relevant to the treatment of depressed geriatric patients include[8-11]:

- Less than half as potent as nortriptyline in inhibiting the uptake of norepinephrine in animal studies
- Lower volume of distribution (8 L/kg)
- Shorter elimination half-life (8 hours)
- Larger free fraction than nortriptyline
- Weak anticholinergic properties: muscarinic binding is $\frac{1}{18}$ that of nortriptyline
- The Z isomer of 10-OH-NT (Z-10-OH-NT) causes bradycardia, decrements in blood pressure, and reduced cardiac output in animals
- The E isomer of 10-OH-NT (E-10-OH-NT) causes arrhythmias less frequently than nortriptyline[11]

Despite the low potential of E-10-OH-NT to cause arrhythmias, clinical evidence in geriatric depressive patients reveals that plasma levels of E-10-OH-NT[12] and combined E-10-OH-NT and ortriptyline[13] are associated with prolonged cardiac conduction. Thus the cardiotoxicity of E-10-OH-NT in elderly patients may be explained by the high E-10-OH-NT plasma concentrations (1.5 to 4 times higher than those of nortriptyline) and the large free-drug fraction of E-10-OH-NT.[11,12]

More research is needed to examine the cardiac effects of hydroxylated metabolites, but it is reasonable to regard at high cardiac risk elderly patients with plasma levels of 10-OH-NT higher than 200–250 ng/mL. Because most clinical laboratories do not measure the hydroxylated metabolites of TCAs, a pretreatment ECG should be obtained and subsequent ECGs be carefully monitored.[13] Evidence for potential cardiotoxicity is widening of the QRS or QT_c interval.

Plasma levels of the hydroxylated metabolite of desipramine 2-hydroxydesipramine (2-OH-DMI) are reported to be associated with prolonged PR and QT_c intervals.[14] However, 2-OH-DMI levels may have limited value in predicting cardiotoxicity for two reasons: the ratio of 2-OH-DMI to desipramine is 1:2,[15] and elderly patients have only 23% higher 2-OH-DMI plasma concentrations than younger patients.[15]

Volume of Distribution

Complex age-related effects on volume of distribution and metabolism prolong the elimination half-life of TCAs in elderly patients. These age-induced pharmacokinetic changes raise two clinically important questions: do older persons need the same plasma levels as younger persons for an antidepressant response? If so, do they achieve these levels at lower doses than younger adults, or do they need the same dosage?

Elderly patients may achieve higher plasma levels of TCAs, especially imipramine and amitriptyline, than younger patients while receiving equivalent doses. However, tricyclic plasma levels may have a 20-fold variation among elderly patients receiving the same dose. Measuring plasma levels is a useful clinical practice because high plasma levels are poorly tolerated in older patients.

Antidepressant response in elderly people usually requires plasma levels in the same therapeutic range as younger adults, although some patients may respond when blood levels are at a lower therapeutic range.[16] For geriatric patients, low therapeutic plasma levels of TCAs should be tried for at least 2 to 6 weeks unless urgency requires more aggressive treatment. If no response occurs at low plasma levels, levels similar to those of younger adults should be used.

Pharmacodynamics

Pharmacodynamic studies of TCAs in the elderly have recently focused on genetic contributions to drug response as well as on the sensitivity of the aging CNS to drug effects. Although genetic contributions have not yet become part of clinical practice, receptor sensitivity does directly influence prescribing practices.

Pharmacogenetics

Drug-metabolizing enzymes are under genetic control. For example, the hepatic enzyme debrisoquine hydroxylase, encoded by the CYP IID6 gene, is principally responsible for the hydroxylation of nortriptyline via the interaction between a gene's control over an enzyme and the dose of drug that will be metabolized by that enyme. This gene/dosage effect may be altered by the alleles that modify the expression of the gene. Alleles have been identified for genetic control of nortriptyline plasma concentration, as well as for the relation betwen plasma concentration and nortriptyline dose.[17] CYP IID6 allelles that result in decreased debrisoquine hydroxylase activity are associated with increased nortriptyline concentration and need for a low nortriptyline dose in elderly patients taking multiple medications.[17]

In the near future, genotyping may allow clinicians to identify elderly patients particularly vulnerable to the development of adverse effects from TCAs. Genotyping may also prove useful in predicting the dose that will be both efficacious and safe for a given individual.

Receptor Sensitivity

Elderly patients tend to be more responsive to both the therapeutic and the toxic effects of TCAs. The high sensitivity to these effects may be a consequence of age-related alteration in monoamine (norepinephrine, serotonin) as well as acetylcholine neurotransmission in the CNS[18] (see Chapter 4). Older patients with structural pathological brain changes also exhibit increased sensitivity to drugs.

The effect of age on monoamine brain neurotransmission and receptor function in humans requires further investigation. Most studies indicate that aging leads to a decline in the brain concentrations of norepinephrine, serotonin, and dopamine.[19,20] Although a compensatory increase in postsynaptic monoamine receptors should be expected, such increase may not occur in aged persons. Brain autopsy studies report a decline in the number of binding sites of postsynaptic serotonin 5-HT2 and the alpha-adrenergic brain receptors, with no change noted in presynaptic serotonin 5-HT1 and the dopamine D2 postsynaptic brain receptors[19,20] (see Chapter 4). These findings suggest that in addition to a decline in neurotransmitter concentrations, aging affects the function of postsynaptic receptors. Whether or not these changes are the cause of increased antidepressant drug sensitivity in the elderly is not known. Furthermore, not all older patients are more sensitive than their younger counterparts to antidepressant drugs.

Choice of Tricyclics

To date, studies comparing the efficacy of TCAs have failed to identify any single therapeutically superior compound. The selection of a specific TCA therefore depends on concern about side-effect profile (Table 9.1) in the individual patient and the clinician's experience with specific antidepressants. Many published reports indicate the efficacy of TCAs for treating geriatric depression; these studies are summarized in Table 9.2.

Table 9.2. Studies of Depressed Geriatric Populations Using Tricyclic Antidepressants (TCAs)

Drugs	Studies	N	(Age range; mean)	Outcome Scales	Results
			AMITRIPTYLINE		
Amitriptyline	Kyle et al. (1998)	365	73	MADRS, HAM-D, CGI	Equal efficacy, but more side effects with amitriptyline
Amitriptyline, mirtazapine	Høyberg et al. (1996)	115	60–85	HAM-D MADRS CGI	Equal efficacy on depression ratings; amitriptyline superior to mirtazapine on Global Rating
Amitriptyline, paroxetine	Geretsegger et al. (1995)	91	Mean 71	HAM-D	Equal efficacy
Amitriptyline, fluoxetine	Fairweather et al. (1993)	33	Mean 70	HAM-D	Equal efficacy; less cognitive impairment with fluoxetine
Amitriptyline, paroxetine	Hutchinson et al. (1992)	101	65+	HAM-D	Both drugs effective; fewer anticholinergic side effects with paroxetine
Amitriptyline, sertraline	Cohn et al. (1990)	241	65–82	HAM-D CGI	Equal efficacy; more side effects with amitriptyline
Amitriptyline, trazodone, mianserin	Altamura et al. (1989a)	106	60–83	HAM-D, GDS	Trazadone associated with lower prevalence of side effects (especially anticholinergic adverse effects) than amitriptyline or mianserin
Amitriptyline, fluoxetine	Altamura et al. (1989b)	28	?65	HAM-D	Significant amelioration for both groups at end point of HAM-D scores compared with baseline value; anticholinergic side effects significantly more severe, and weight gain detected only in patients receiving amitriptyline

Drug(s)	Reference	N	Age	Instruments	Comments
Amitriptyline, maprotiline	Koncevoj et al. (1989)	38	Geriatric	HAM-D, BPRS, CGI, EEG, ECG, gerontopsychiatric interview	No severe adverse reactions; side effects can be minimized with careful monitoring for cardiovascular effects and adequate activity regimen
Amitriptyline, desipramine	Wilkins et al. (1989)	15	62–95	Self-observation rating of anxiety and depression	Trend for cortisol, PRL, and GH concentrations to decline during study period; trend reversed for all three hormones in those receiving DMI
Amitriptyline, trazodone	Sauvage et al. (1987)	53	60–85	NA	Subjects responded well, indicating efficacy of *Psychopharmacology* and psychotherapy for apathetic syndrome in geriatric patients
Amitriptyline, mianserin, dothiepin	Waite et al. (1986)	23	Mean 76	?	Poor response to all treatments
Amitriptyline, diazepam, trazodone	Ather et al. (1985)	149	59–?85	HAM-D, VAS, therapeutic effect, global improvement	More favorable response with amitriptyline or trazodone than diazepam; fewer side effects with trazodone than amitriptyline; possibly more anticholinergic effects with amitriptyline
Amitriptyline, desipramine, imipramine, nortriptyline, ECT	Meyers & Mei-Tal (1985)	70	60–91 Mean 72.6	NA	Significant improvement in 15 of 24 subjects receiving HCAs: 16 of 17 receiving ECT responded; 11 of 15 receiving an antidepressant followed by ECT responded; conclusion: ECT is highly beneficial treatment
Amitriptyline, desipramine, methylphenidate	Spar & LaRue (1985)	71	47–95 Mean 71.8	POMS	"Blind" to POMS, physicians prescribed according to their own judgment; acute response to methylphenidate predicted outcome treatment with desipramine but not

(continued)

Table 9.2. *(continued)*

Drugs	Studies	N	(Age range; mean)	Outcome Scales	Results
Amitriptyline, mianserin	Branconnier et al. (1982)	75	>60–85	HAM-D, SDS, POMS, CGI, EEG	Amitriptyline and mianserin equally effective in relieving depressive symptoms; EEG results revealed significant benzodiazepine like action of mianserin; no significant impairment of cognitive functioning from mianserin; compared with heterocyclics, mianserin offers improved in the therapeutic index
Amitriptyline, nomifensine	Goldstein et al. (1982)	31	64–89	Not given	Amitriptyline more effective but caused more side effects
Amitriptyline, mianserin, trazodone	Altamura et al. (1988)	75	60–83	HAM-D	Decreased geriatric depression scores at 3 weeks; subjects receiving trazodone had fewer side effects
Amitriptyline, trazodone, mianserin. Dothiepin	Blacker et al. (1988)	176	18–80	HAM-D, global severity	Assessed efficacy of trazodone vs. mianserin, dothiepin, or AMI; trazodone associated with lower incidence of dry mouth, visual dizziness, and drowsiness
Amitriptyline	Burch et al. (1988)	74	25–80	MADRS, depression items on LEEDS, SAS	In 50 subjects 25–65 years old, antidepressant response at low plasma drug levels poorer than at medium or high levels, at which responses were equally effective

CLOMIPRAMINE (CMI)

Drug	Study	n	Dose	Measure	Results
Clomipramine	Petracca et al (1996)	58	70.6	HAM-D, MMSE, UKU	Clomipramine superior to placebo
Clomipramine	Kunik et al. (1994)	5	67–80	HAM-D	Low dose well tolerated; 42% decrease in depression ratings in previously treatment-resistant patients
Clomipramine, paroxetine	Pelicier & Schaefer (1993)	83	Mean 71	HAM-D	Equal efficacy
Clomipramine, paroxetine	Rouillon (1991)	87	60+	?	Equal efficacy
Clomipramine, paroxetine	Samuelian (1991)	59	>60	MADRS CGI	Equal efficacy
Clomipramine, paroxetine	Guillibert et al. (1989)	79	60+	HAM-D	Equal efficacy; more side effects with clomipramine

DESIPRAMINE (DMI)

Drug	Study	n	Dose	Measure	Results
Desipramine	Nelson et al. (1995)	34	>75	HAM-D plasma concentrations	Blood levels not elevated; no effect of age on clearance; elevated hydroxy blood levels; response to blood levels equivalent to younger adult responders
Desipramine	Dinan & Barry (1990)	29	20–73	Estimates of GH in blood	Used desipramine to stimulate growth hormone: 18 subjects showed blunted response; growth hormone time test unable to distinguish between patients with endogenous and nonendogenous depression; significant neuroendocrine abnormality in subset of patients with nonendogenous depression.

(continued)

Table 9.2. *(continued)*

Drugs	Studies	N	(Age range; mean)	Outcome Scales	Results
Desipramine, amitriptyline	Wilkins et al. (1989)	15	62–95	Self–observation rating of anxiety and depression	Results show trend for the cortisol, PRL, and GH concentrations to decline during study period; trend for all three hormones reversed in those receiving DMI
Desipramine, maprotiline, doxepin	Kushnir (1988)	1	102	Clinical observation	No adverse effects; maprotiline most effective of the three drugs; doxepin caused sedation; desipramine caused hallucinations
Desipramine	Nelson et al. (1988)	43	>60	OH-DMI/DMI ratio, plasma concentrations, Mann-Whitney U test	Steady-state OH-DMI and desipramine concentrations and ratios examined to determine if OH-DMI levels were elevated in subjects over age 60; higher OH-DMI concentration associated with older age
Desipramine	Kutcher et al. (1986)	19	60–85	HAM-D, DST	Therapeutic response related to plasma drug levels: plasma concentrations of 2-OH-DMI not related to therapeutic response.
Desipramine, perphenazine	Nelson et al. (1986)	31	23–78	CGI, global response	Examined relation of response to neuroleptic and DMI concentration: responders had higher DM concentrations and received higher neuroleptic doses

Drug/Treatment	Study	N	Age	Measures	Results/Conclusions
Desipramine, amitriptyline, imipramine, nortriptyline, ECT	Meyers & Mei-Tal (1985)	70	60–91 Mean 72.6	NA	Significant improvement in 15 of 24 subjects receiving HCAs; 16 of 17 receiving ECT responded; 11 of 15 receiving an antidepressant followed by ECT responded; conclusion: ECT highly beneficial treatment
Desipramine, amitriptyline, methylphenidate	Spar & LaRue (1985)	71	47–95 Mean 71.8	POMS	"Blind" to POMS, physicians prescribed according to their own judgment; acute response to methylphenidate predicted outcome treatment with desipramine but not amitriptyline
Desipramine	Cutler et al. (1984)	5	70–85	Heart rate, BP, NE concentrations in plasma	Findings suggest desipramine and nortriptyline particularly suitable for elderly patients
DOXEPIN					
Doxepin, paroxetine	Dunner et al. (1992)	271	Mean 69	HAM-D	Paroxetine superior to doxepin, with fewer side effects
Doxepin, paroxetine	Halikas (1991)	272	>60	HAM-D, Covi, Raskin, clinical observation	Equal efficacy; fewer side effects with paroxetine
Doxepin, desipramine, maprotiline	Kushnir (1988)	1	102		Maprotiline most effective—no adverse effects; doxepin caused sedation; desipramine caused hallucinations
Doxepin	Lakshmanan et al. (1986)	24	70–83	HAM-D, GDS	Significantly reduced depressive symptoms of 11 subjects treated with doxepin compared with 13 receiving placebo; no side effects recorded
Doxepin, fluoxetine	Feighner & Cohn (1985)	78	Mean 68	HAM-D	Equal efficacy
Doxepin, imipramine	Neshkes et al. (1985)	36	55–81	HAM-D BP	Equal efficacy; greater orthostatic decrease in BP with imipramine
Doxepin, maprotiline	Gwirtsman et al. (1983)	38	>65	?	Maprotiline superior to doxepin

(continued)

Table 9.2. *(continued)*

Drugs	Studies	N	(Age range; mean)	Outcome Scales	Results
			IMIPRAMINE		
Imipramine, sertraline	Forlenza et al. (2000)	55	>60	MADRS, CGI, MMSE	Equal efficacy; imipramine associated with more side effects
Imipramine, reboxetine	Katona et al. (1999)	347	74.5	HAM-D.MADRS, CGI	Equal efficacy; imipramine better for dysthymia
Imipramine, paroxetine	Katona et al. (1998)	198	74	MADRS, CGI, Cornell	Equal efficacy; paroxetine fewer anticholinergic side effects
Imipramine, buspirone	Schweizer et al. (1998)	177	72	HAM-D, CGI, HAM-A	Imipramine superior to buspirone and placebo; buspirone superior to placebo
Imipramine, milnacipran	Tignol et al. (1998)	147	74.1	HAM-D, MADRS, CGI, COVI anxiety, MMSE, WAIS	Equal therapeutic efficacy; more anticholinergic side effects with imipramine
Imipramine, nefazodone	van Laar et al. (1995)	12	60–70	Driving skills	Imipramine acutely impaired lateral position control that diminished after repeated dosing
Imipramine, alprazolam	Weissman et al. (1992)	25	60–85	HAM-D	Equivalent efficacy
Imipramine	Gentsch et al. (1989)	19 depressed patients 11 normal controls	28–72 22–64	HAM-D	No difference in mean density (B_{max}) and affinity (K_d) values between patients and controls or between time points tested. Findings did not support hypothesis that number of ^{3}H-IMI binding sites is a marker for depression
Imipramine	Slotkin et al. (1989)	18	60–80 25–45	Measurement of uptake of radiolabeled serotonin into platelets	Depression in both age groups associated with decreased number of IMI binding sites. Elderly subjects exhibited small but significant reduction in platelet serotonin uptake

Drug	Reference	N	Age	Scale	Results
Imipramine	Schneider et al. (1988a)	39	Mean 73	NA	Results provide preliminary evidence for relative specificity of platelet ^{3}H-IMI binding as marker for primary major depression compared with secondary depression in medically ill elderly patients
Imipramine	Georgotas et al. (1987b)	37	55–71	HAM-D	^{3}H-clonidine and ^{3}H-IMI binding measured in depressed patients; no significant correlation between binding and severity of depression before treatment; significant negative correlation between dissociation constant of binding sites and HAM-D scores
Imipramine, fluvoxamine	Wakelin (1986)	45	60–71	?	Equal efficacy; more confusion with imipramine
Imipramine, mianserin	Eklund et al. (1985)	50	60–90	HAM-D, CGI, GDS, VAS, TESS	No significant efficacy difference between the two drugs; significantly greater number of side effects in group receiving IMI
Imipramine, amitriptyline, desipramine, nortriptyline, ECT	Meyers & Mei-Tal (1985)	70	60–91 Mean 72.6	NA	Significant improvement in 15 of 24 subjects receiving HCAs; 16 of 17 receiving ECT responded; 11 of 15 receiving an antidepressant followed by ECT responded; conclusion: ECT highly beneficial treatment
Imipramine, doxepin	Neshkes et al. (1985)	36	55–81	HAM-D, BP	Equal efficacy; greater orthostatic decrease in BP with imipramine
Imipramine	Severson et al. (1985)	23 post-mortem	4(17–40), 16(41–70), 3(71–100) Mean 67.7	NA	Aging associated with increase in density of specific binding sites for ^{3}H-IMI in postmortem specimens of human hypothalamus, frontal cortex, and partial cortex; *in vitro* regulation of ^{3}H-IMI binding by sodium was impaired with age in hypothalamic homogenates.

(continued)

Table 9.2. *(continued)*

Drugs	Studies	N	(Age range; mean)	Outcome Scales	Results
Imipramine, nomifensine	Cohn et al. (1984)	63	≥60	HAM-D, CGI, BPRS, HSCL	Nomifensine and imipramine superior to placebo; lab and physical exam (including ECGs) showed no clinically significant changes associated with either drug; more rapid improvement and fewer side effects with nomifensine
Imipramine, nomifensine	Merideth et al. (1984)	61	≥60	HAM-D, BDI, Covi, Raskin, CGI, BPRS, HSCL, side effects	Among nomifensine-treated subjects, 75% rated as improved at end of therapy compared with 6% of imipramine-treated subjects and 20% of subjects receiving placebo; sedating and cholinergic effects frequent in group receiving nomifensine
Imipramine, alprazolam	Rothblum et al. (1982)	18	60–85	HAM-D, Raskin	Good compliance and response with drugs in elderly patients; brief role transitions preceded onset of depression
Imipramine, trazodone	Hayes et al. (1983)	54	60–90	ECG	ECG effects evaluated at drug-free baseline and weekly thereafter in subjects receiving imipramine or trazodone; 18 were crossed-over from placebo group; imipramine increased heart rate and was associated with more isolated ECG complications; trazodone and placebo had no adverse effects on ECG
Imipramine or doxepin vs. psychodynamic group therapy or cognitive behavior group therapy	Jarvik et al. (1982, 1983)	58	55–80	HAM-D	Remission rate of 12% in patients receiving group psychotherapy, 45% in patients receiving imipramine or doxepin; little or no benefit in 36% of patients

Drugs	Reference	N	Age	Measures	Comments
Imipramine, nortriptyline, perphenazine	Bjerre et al. (1981)	15	62–79	HAM-D, plasma levels	Dose changes may result in unpredictable changes in plasma drug levels during imipramine therapy; therapy control by monitoring plasma drug levels may be difficult; additional therapy with perphenazine in subjects receiving imipramine or nortriptyline caused rise in plasma imipramine levels, particularly desipramine metabolite levels
Imipramine, nortriptyline	Thayssen et al. (1981)	19	62–78	Heart rate, blood pressure, systolic time intervals, ECG, 24-hr ECG	Imipramine limited by orthostatic hypotension reaction at subtherapeutic plasma levels; nortriptyline at therapeutic levels did not significantly influence orthostatic BP; nortriptyline caused moderate changes in systolic time intervals, an effect not seen with imipramine, but most subjects did not achieve therapeutic plasma drug levels because of BP reactions.
Imipramine, trazodone	Gerner et al. (1980)	34	60–90	HAM-D, BDI, TESS, visual integration, Wechsler, Guild	Imipramine and trazodone similarly efficacious but fewer side effects with trazodone than imipramine suggesting the utility of trazodone in geriatric populations (especially vulnerable to cardiovascular and anticholinergic side effects)
Imipramine, maprotiline	Middleton (1975)	28	65–83	GAS, target symptoms scale, VAS, adverse reactions	Trial unable to show significant difference between the two groups in terms of efficacy and onset of action, possibly due to small number of patients in trial
Imipramine, Gerovital-H3	Zung et al. (1974)	30	61–77	ASI, CGI, DSI, SAS, SDS	Trial of 30 geriatric patients receiving IMI, Gerovital-H3, or placebo; Gerovital-H3 superior

(continued)

Table 9.2. *(continued)*

Drugs	Studies	N	(Age range; mean)	Outcome Scales	Results
			MAPROTILINE		
Maprotiline, mianserin	Schifano et al. (1990)	48	>65	GDS, HSCL, CGI	Comparing efficacy of mianserin with maprotiline, side effects similar in two treatment groups; mianserin somewhat more effective; both drugs somewhat safer than first generation HCAs
Maprotiline, amitriptyline	Koncevoj et al. (1989)	38	Mean 67 (AMI) Mean 61 (MPT)	HAM-D, BPRS, CGI, EEG, ECG, gerontopsychiatric interview	No severe adverse reactions found; results suggest side effects can be minimized with careful monitoring for cardiovascular effects and adequate activity regimen
Maprotiline	Tollefson et al. (1989)	10	Mean 65.7	HAM-D, serum drug concentration	Assessed pharmacokinetic properties of maprotiline, indicating that maprotiline was well tolerated: significantly improved depressive symptoms in 7 subjects
Maprotiline, doxepin, desipramine	Kushnir (1988)	1	102	Clinical observation	Maprotiline most effective of the three—no adverse effects; doxepin caused sedation, desipramine caused hallucinations
Maprotiline, mianserin, nomifensine	Siegfried et al. (1986)	71	67–83	?	Maprotiline least effective
Maprotiline, zimeldine	Nystroem & Haellstroem (1985)	75	20–59	CPRS	Both drugs improved depression: maprotiline in subjects with few prior episodes and few years since first episode; zimeldine most effective in subjects with several previous episodes
Maprotiline, doxepin	Gwirtsman et al. (1983)	38	>65	?	Maprotiline superior to doxepin

Drugs	Reference	N	Age	Measures	Outcome
Maprotiline, imipramine	Middleton (1975)	28	65–83	GAS, target symptoms scale, VAS, adverse reactions	No significant difference between the two groups in efficacy and onset of actions, possibly due to small number of patients in trial
NORTRIPTYLINE					
Nortriptyline, paroxetine	Mamo et al. (2002)	42	>60	Postural sway measures	No change in postural sway observed with either agent
Nortriptyline, paroxetine	Solai et al. (2002)	66	>60	Measure of CPY2D6 activity	Both nortriptyline and paroxetine inhibit CPY2D6; paroxetine significantly more extensive inhibitor
Nortriptyline, paroxetine	Bump et al. (2001)	116	72.5	HAM-D, MMSE, GAS, MATTIS	Equal efficacy in prevention of recurrence and relapse
Nortriptyline, perphenazine	Meyers et al. (2001)	28	71.8	HAM-D, Barnes atathisia, Simpson Angus, AIMS	No difference in efficacy when perphenazine added to nortriptyline treatment of psychotic depression
Nortriptyline, paroxetine	Mulsant et al. (2001)	116	72	HAM-D, side-effect scale	No difference in efficacy in acute treatments; nortriptyline had higher discontinuation rate
Nortriptyline, citalopram	Navarro et al. (2001)	58	69.7	HDRS, side-effect scale	Nortriptyline had higher remission rate among moderate to severe patients and higher dropout rate secondary to autonomic side effects
Nortriptyline	Weintraub (2001)	10	>65	CGI–I	7 out of 10 patients responded to addition or substitution of nortriptyline after failing SSRI monotherapy
Nortriptyline, sertraline	Bondareff et al. (2000)	210	67.8	ADS, MMSE, POMS, Q-LES-Q, HAM-D, WAIS	Sertraline equal in efficacy; similar in safety profile, and more efficacious in individuals over 70
Nortriptyline, sertraline	Finkel et al. (1999)	76	>70	HAM-D, CBI	Greater efficacy for sertraline
Nortriptyline, paroxetine	Mamo et al. (2000)	62	71.6	EPS	No significant difference in change in EPS

(continued)

Table 9.2. *(continued)*

Drugs	Studies	N	(Age range; mean)	Outcome Scales	Results
Nortriptyline, sertraline	Oslin et al. (2000)	97	83.1	MMSE, PSMS, HAM-D	Better efficacy for nortriptyline but equal to sertraline in tolerability
Nortriptyline, sertraline	Nobler et al. (2000)	20	67	HAM-D	Equal efficacy; responders showed reduced cerebral blood flow in frontal and anterior temporal regions
Nortriptyline, paroxetine	Pollock et al. (2000a)	96	68.3	HAM-D	Variations in alleles for serotonin transporter gene promoter region correlate with response to paroxetine not to nortriptyline
Nortriptyline, paroxetine	Pollock et al (2000b)	17	53—65	Platelet release products	Reduced levels of platelet–release factors for paroxetine but not nortriptyline, suggesting that platelet aggregation in ischemic heart disease may be inhibited by paroxetine which may positively impact on mortality from IHD in these patients
Nortriptyline	Streim et al. (2000)	69	79.5	MMSE, CIRS, PSMS, HAM-D, CGI, GDS, plasma level	Depressions that occur with dementia may represent a treatment-relevant condition with different relation between plasma level and response
Nortriptyline, paroxetine	Weber et al. (2000)	32	74	Weights, BMI	No differential weight change
Nortriptyline, paroxetine	Green et al. (1999)	80	75	HAM-D	Sleep deprivation added to antidepressants produces a rapid response
Nortriptyline	Marracini et al. (1999)	37	N/A	Asberg side-effect scale	Side effects primarily related to residual depression rather than nortriptyline
Nortriptyline, paroxetine	Mulsant et al. (1999)	80	75	HAM-D, MMSE	Equal efficacy and tolerability observed in 6-week treatment trial

Treatment	Study	N	Age	Measures	Results
Nortriptyline, interpersonal therapy, placebo	Reynolds et al. (1999a)	180	60–91	HAM-D, BDI, GAS, BAS, interpersonal support measures, sleep measures	Older patients (70+) had excellent short-term but brittle long-term response; combined medication and psychotherapy may represent best long-term treatment
Nortriptyline, interpersonal therapy	Reynolds et al. (1999b)	80	>50	HAM-D, BDI, GAS, side-effect profile, vital signs	Nortriptyline, but not interpersonal therapy; superior to placebo in bereaved patients; combination treatment had greater efficacy and a higher completion rate
Nortriptyline	Reynolds et al. (1999c)	187	67	HAM-D, BDI, GAS, side-effect scale	Combined nortriptyline and interpersonal therapy superior to therapy and placebo, with significant trend to superior efficacy over nortriptyline monotherapy
Nortriptyline, paroxetine	Walters (1999)	40	77.5	HAM-D, MMSE, DRS, plasma levels	Paroxetine equal in efficacy to nortriptyline in delaying and preventing relapse in recovered patients
Nortriptyline	Miller et al. (1998)	50	>60	ECG, HR, PR interval, QT interval	Nortriptyline associated with increased PR interval, HR, QRS duration and CTc, which persisted after 1 year; patients with preexisting cardiac disease did not show significantly worse ECG changed than noncardiac patients and showed no long term ECG worsening
Nortriptyline	Reynolds et al. (1997)	40	N/A	Sleep latency and maintenance, time in slow-wave sleep, time in REM sleep, total delta wave count, delta sleep ratio	Patients on maintenance nortriptyline took longer to fall asleep, did not maintain sleep better than placebo but showed enhanced delta-wave production in first NREM period and increased REM activity throughout night

(continued)

Table 9.2. *(continued)*

Drugs	Studies	N	(Age range; mean)	Outcome Scales	Results
Nortriptyline, adjunct lorazepam, interpersonal therapy	Buysse et al. (1997)	119	68	HAM-D, BDI, GAS, sleep measures	Lorazepam, useful for treating anxiety in elderly depressed patients, did not slow antidepressant response
Nortriptyline, moclobemide	Kin et al. (1997)	95	71	DST	DST-positive patients had better nortriptyline response; DST-negative patients had better moclobemide response
Nortriptyline (BL 80–120 ng/ml)	Reynolds et al. (1996a)	148	60–91	HAM-D	78.4% remission; elderly patients responded more slowly than mid- to late-life patients; 15.5% relapse rate on maintenance treatment
Nortriptyline, adjunct lithium, adjunct perphenazine, adjunct paroxetine	Reynolds et al. (1996b)	158	68.3	HAM-D, BDI, GAS, PAS, RSQI, PSS	Worse response and remission rates in adjunctive medication patients
Nortriptyline, sertraline	Finkel & Richter (1995)	76	70+	HAM-D	Slightly greater efficacy for sertraline; more side effects with nortriptyline
Nortriptyline, paroxetine	Laghrissi-Thode (1995)	20	57–69	Postural sway	No difference in body sway parameters between nortriptyline and paroxetine
Nortriptyline, sertraline	McEntee et al. (1995)	208	Mean age 68	HAM-D	Equal efficacy
Nortriptyline, moclobemide	Nair et al. (1995)	109	60+	NA	Nortriptyline had a higher remission rate than moclobemide and placebo, moclobemide had a higher remission rate than placebo

Drug	Reference	N	Age	Measures	Results/Comments
Nortriptyline	Pollock et al. (1994)	26	60–80	NA	During maintenance therapy: increased triglycerides and very low density lipoproteins; elevated heart rate, decreased creatinine clearance
Nortriptyline	Reynolds et al. (1994)	32	60–78	HAM-D	80% remission in recurrent depressive episodes
Nortriptyline, fluoxetine	Roose et al. (1994)	66	Mean 71.5	HAM-D	Nortriptyline superior for melancholic patients
Nortriptyline, fluoxetine	Rothschild (1994)	1	73	Case report	Patient previously treatment resistant; attained full remission with combination
Nortriptyline	Rosen et al. (1993)	26	Mean 71.5	HAM-D	79% complained of anticholinergic side effects (bethanechol effective in reducing them)
Nortriptyline, desipramine, fluoxetine	Brymer & Winograd (1992)	103	Mean 81	?	Relative efficacy not reported; fluoxetine associated with weight loss
Nortriptyline	Miller et al. (1991)	45	60–79	HAM-D, illness burden scale, side effects	Efficacious and well tolerated; acute side effects declined by 50% and may have been somatic symptoms of depression
Nortriptyline	Dietch & Fine (1990)	10	72–95	Serial ECGs, plasma NT levels	Lack of clinically adverse cardiac changes suggest HCAs present little risk in patients with first-degree atrioventricular hemiblock; patients with bundle-branch and bifascicular block at greater risk but can be treated with HCAs
Nortriptyline	Hoff et al. (1990)	9	58–84	HAM-D measured verbal, logical, and visual memories; concentration speed (pre- and posttherapy)	Three measures of verbal learning and memory decreased

(continued)

Table 9.2. *(continued)*

Drugs	Studies	N	(Age range; mean)	Outcome Scales	Results
Nortriptyline	Katz et al. (1990)	21	NA	GDS, cumulative illness rating scale, physical self-maintenance scale	Significant difference between drug and placebo. Incidence of adverse events (34%) required early termination of therapy; high levels of self-care disability and low levels of serum albumin associated with decreased therapeutic response
Nortriptyline, phenelzine	Georgotas et al. (1989b)	26	≥65	RDC, HAM-D	More severely depressed subjects took longer to respond; those with endogenous depression responded more quickly.
Nortriptyline, phenelzine	Georgotas & McCue (1989a)	41	>55	RDC, HAM-D	Subjects with more prior episodes of depression had greater risk of relapsing
Nortriptyline, phenelzine	Georgotas & McCue (1989b)	100	?55	NA	Addition of 2 weeks to study period produced 15% increase in response; one-third of subjects who had not responded by week 9 responded when kept on medication for 12 weeks
Nortriptyline	Katz et al. (1989)	22	NA	NT plasma levels, a₁-acid glycoprotein, *trans* metabolite, *cis* metabolite	No difference in nortriptyline kinetics, compared with previously reported findings for younger, healthier subjects
Nortriptyline	Koenig et al. (1989)	41	≥65	MMSE, GDS, MADRS, CGI	Study halted at midpoint if medical illness prevented 80% of eligible patients from participating; major or minor medical constraints present in over 90% of patients

Drug	Reference	N	Age	Measures	Results/Comments
10-hydroxynortriptyline	McCue et al. (1989a)	64	55–77	HAM-D Plasma NT Plasma 10-OH-NT	Results suggest no relation between levels of 10-OH-NT and clinical response; plasma levels of E-OH-NT were low and did not correlate with other reported side effects
Nortriptyline 10-hydroxynortriptyline	McCue et al. (1989b)	31	55–77	ECG, PR interval, QT, interval, HAM-D	No consistent correlations between changes in ECG and treatment
Nortriptyline	Reynolds et al. (1989)	27	NA	HAM-D, MMSE, NT plasma level	Mean survival without recurrence 21.3 months; this pilot experience with maintenance nortriptyline in late-life depression more favorable than outcome reported in more naturalistic settings
Nortriptyline, phenelzine	Georgotas et al. (1988)	60	55–77	HAM-D	Assessment of subjects' maintenance phase outcomes: either drug could be used in continuation therapy with low risk of relapse
Nortriptyline, 10-hydroxynortriptyline	Schneider et al. (1988b)	21	60–83	ECG, plasma levels of NT, E-OH-NT, and 10-OH-NT	10-OH-NT concentrations contributed substantially to intercardiac conduction delay associated with nortriptyline treatment in subjects; nortriptyline alone associated with modest increases in PR interval and QRS duration
Nortriptyline, ECT	Stack et al. (1988)	17	61–78	HAM-D, BDI	Evaluated utility of AM PSOP in predicting clinical response to treatment with nortriptyline or ECT: AM PSOP showed significant inverse correlation with percent change in HAM-D scores. In subjects receiving nortriptyline, PSOP correlated significantly with percent change in HAM-D scores; similar association seen in subjects receiving ECT

(continued)

Table 9.2. *(continued)*

Drugs	Studies	N	(Age range; mean)	Outcome Scales	Results
10-hydroxynortriptyline	Young et al. (1988)	37	≥60	Plasma levels of NT metabolite, HAM-D	Suggested association between high plasma E-10-OH-NT and poor therapeutic response
Nortriptyline	Zubenko et al. (1988)	14	NA	HAM-D, MMSE	Subjects with progressive cognitive impairment had increased platelet membrane fluidity—an abnormality previously found by investigation in approximately 50% of AD patients.
Nortriptyline, phenelzine	Georgotas et al. (1987a)	75	?55	RDC, HAM-D	Significantly greater mean orthostatic fall in systolic BP in patients treated with nortriptyline or phenelzine compared with placebo subjects; no significant difference between nortriptyline and phenelzine
Nortriptyline, phenelzine	Georgotas et al. (1987b)	14	?55	HAM-D	Analysis of 3H-clonidine and ^{3}H-imipramine binding showed significant negative correlation between dissociation constant of binding sites and scores on HAM-D; no significant difference between groups; no significant relation between binding and severity of depression or between receptor data from responders and nonresponders to antidepressant treatment
Nortriptyline, phenelzine	Georgotas et al. (1987c)	42	55–82	RDC Newcastle Diagnostic Scale DSM-111	Consistent with findings that subtype of depression does not predict antidepressant response

Drug	Study	N	Age	Measure	Results
Nortriptyline, phenelzine	Georgotas et al. (1987d)	44	55–82	ECG	Nortriptyline produced significant increases in both heart rate and PR intervals; phenelzine significantly decreased QT interval; no pathological ECG changes
Nortriptyline, phenelzine	Georgotas et al. (1987e)	75	?55	NT plasma levels, platelet MAO inhibition HAM-D	Nortriptyline and phenelzine more effective than placebo in treating depressed mood, guilt feelings, suicidal ideation, agitation, loss of energy, diurnal variation of mood; nortriptyline better than phenelzine and placebo in improving middle/late insomnia
Nortriptyline	Kumar et al. (1987)	13	60–78 Mean 67	HAM-D	No difference between geriatric and younger ECGsubjects in plasma levels and elimination halflife of nortriptyline; antidepressant effects of nortriptyline similar in geriatric and younger subjects; geriatric patients had few subjective side effects with nortriptyline
Nortriptyline, ECT	Reynolds et al. (1987)	16	NA	HAM-D, MMSE, 2 dementia scales	Treatment response of elderly patients with mixed depression and cognitive impairment similar to that of cognitively intact depressed elderly patients
Nortriptyline	Young et al. (1987)	16	Mean 76.4	Plasma NT levels + E-10-OH-NT concentrations determined by high-performance liquid chromatography	Renal function one determinant of plasma E-10-OHNT in subjects treated with nortriptyline
Nortriptyline, phenelzine	Georgotas et al. (1986a)	47	55–76	RDC, HAM-D	Both drugs well tolerated: Late-life depression can be treated despite common misconceptions about depression being a natural consequence of aging.
Nortriptyline, phenelzine	Georgotas et al. (1986b)	72	58–82	DST	No correlation between baseline DST and treatment response to antidepressants; no practical value of DST as indicator of impending recovery from major depression in elderly patients; failure of DST results to normalize may have prognostic significance

(continued)

Table 9.2. *(continued)*

Drugs	Studies	N	(Age range; mean)	Outcome Scales	Results
Nortriptyline, interpersonal psychotherapy	Schneider et al. (1986a)	34	?60	HAM-D, B_{max}	Studied platelet ^{3}H-imipramine binding (B_{max}) relative to family history and clinical response in depressed elderly patients. B_{max} of relatives of depressed subjects with positive family history for depression lower than that of controls or subjects without family history; good clinical response to either nortriptyline or psychotherapy linked to low B_{max}
Nortriptyline	Schneider et al. (1986b)	10	?60	B_DDI, HAM-D	Investigated predictive value of PSOP in subjects about to receive 16 weeks of nortriptyline or interpersonal psychotherapy: significant correlation between PSOP and improvement in Beck and HAM-D scores; both groups responded equally to treatment; in group receiving nortriptyline, PSOP correlated more strongly with improvement in Beck scores.
Nortriptyline, amitriptyline, desipramine, imipramine, ECT	Meyers & Mei-Tal (1985)	70	60–91 Mean 72.6	NA	Significant improvement in 15 of 24 subjects receiving HCAs; 16 of 17 receiving ECT responded; 11 of 15 receiving an antidepressant followed by ECT responded; conclusion: ECT is highly beneficial treatment
Nortriptyline	Young et al. (1985)	18	61–88	ECG	Plasma E-10-OH-NT and NT distinguished the group with conduction/repolarization effects; plasma nortriptyline, age, drug dose, and baseline ECG did not.
Nortriptyline	Georgotas et al. (1984)	30	60–81	DST, RDC, Newcastle diagnostic scales, clinical observation	Great majority (83.3%) of patients diagnosed with endogenous depression were nonsuppressors; only 16.7% of patients with nonendogenous depression were; DST tended to normalize clinical recovery

Drug(s)	Reference	N	Age	Measures	Comments
Nortriptyline, imipramine, perphenazine	Bjerre et al. (1981)	15	62–79	HAM-D, plasma levels	Dose changes may result in unpredictable changes in plasma drug levels during imipramine therapy; control by monitoring plasma drug levels may be difficult; addition of perphenazine in subjects receiving imipramine or nortriptyline caused rise in plasma imipramine levels, particularly desipramine metabolite levels
Nortriptyline	Dawling et al. (1981)	10	72–90 Mean 82	Plasma concentrations of NT	Plasma nortriptyline concentration used to predict daily dose required to achieve steady-state concentration within 50–150 mg/L range: prescribed mean 50 mg daily (range 20–100 mg)
Nortriptyline, imipramine	Thayssen et al. (1981)	19	62–78	Heart rate, blood pressure, ECG, 24-hr ECG	Imipramine limited by orthostatic hypotension at subtherapeutic plasma levels; no significant influence of nortriptyline on orthostatic BP therapeutic levels; nortriptyline caused moderate changes in systolic time intervals, an effect not seen with imipramine but most subjects did not achieve therapeutic plasma drug levels because of BP reactions
Nortriptyline	Dawling et al. (1980)	20 geriatric patients 17 young volunteers	68–100 mean 81 20–35 mean 25.5	Plasma drug concentrations	Plasma nortriptyline half-life longer and clearance slower in elderly patients than in young volunteers. Age not correlated with either variable in both groups. No gender difference in nortriptyline pharmacokinetics.
Nortriptyline	Sorensen et al. (1978)	34	5(30–55) 3(55–60) 4(60–65) 7(65–70) 5(70–75) 4(75–80) 2(80–84) 2(85–86)	Plasma drug levels	Cautious dose policy led to low plasma nortriptyline levels, followed by dose increase in about 40% of patients; general outcome about 20% failure; outcome same or better for patients over 65.

(continued)

Table 9.2. *(continued)*

Drugs	Studies	N	(Age range; mean)	Outcome Scales	Results
Nortriptyline (10 mg tid) Fluphenazine (0–5 mg tid) Promazine (50 mg tid)	Brodie et al. (1975)	62	?65	Physician's clinical rating scale, patient's VAS	For mixed depression/anxiety, fluphenazine and nortriptyline superior to promazine in relieving symptoms of anxiety associated with lower incidence of side effects.
Nortriptyline	Kernohan et al. (1967)	84	NA	Motor discrimination and memory ability, student interviewer ratings, nurse's aide observation scale, inpatient multidimensional psychiatric rating scale	Patients receiving nortriptyline improved in self-care and maintained a better level of adjustment; side effects reversible and not serious.
TRIMIPRAMINE					
Trimipramine, fluoxetine	Wolf et al. (2001)	41	68.7	Sleep study	Early antidepressant effects independent of REM suppression

ASI, Anxiety Status Inventory; BDI, Beck Depression Inventory; BPRS, Brief Psychiatric Rating Scale; CGI, Clinical Global Impressions Scale; Covi, Covi Anxiety Scale; CPRS, Comprehensive Psychiatric Rating Scale; DSI, Depression Status Inventory; DST, dexamethasone suppression test; ECG, electrocardiogram; ECT, electroconvulsive therapy; EEG, electroencephalogram; GAS, Global Assessment Scale; GDS, Geriatric Depression Scale; GH, growth hormone; Guild, Guild Memory Scale; HAM-D, Hamilton Rating Scale for Depression; HSCL, Hopkins Symptom Checklist; LEEDS, LEEDS Rating Scale; MADRS, Montgomery-Asberg Depression Rating Scale; MAO, monoamine oxidase; MAOI, monoamine oxidase inhibitor; MMSE, Mini-Mental State Exam; MPT, maprotiline; NA, not available (not given in reference); NE, norepinephrine; OH-DMI, hydroxydesipramine; 10-OH-NT, 10-hydroxynortriptyline; PH, phenelzine; POMS, Profile of Mood States; PRL, prolactin; PSOP, pretreatment systolic orthostatic blood pressure; Raskin, Raskin Depression Scale; RDC, Research Diagnostic Criteria; SAS, Self-Rating Anxiety Scale; SCL-58, Symptom Checklist-58 items; SD, standard deviation; SDS, Zung Self-Rating Depression Scale; TESS, Treatment Emergent Symptom Scale; VAS, Visual Analogue Scale; Wechsler, Wechsler Memory Scale. Based on Salzman, C. Pharmacological treatment of depression in elderly patients. In: Schneider, LS, Reynolds, CF, Lebowitz, BD, Friedholt, AJ, eds. *Diagnosis and Treatment of Depression in Late Life*, Washington, DC: American Psychiatric Press, 1994, with permission.

Secondary Amines

Secondary amines, particularly nortriptyline and desipramine, are preferable to tertiary amines for older patients because metabolism of secondary amines is less complex and their side effects are milder; these tricyclics include desipramine, nortriptyline, protriptyline, amoxapine, and maprotiline. Nortriptyline and desipramine in particular have two advantages for geriatric patients. First, clinical and research experience with their use in the elderly is extensive. Second, information on plasma levels is available and can help clinicians determine the most effective antidepressant TCA dosage for each elderly patient.

Nortriptyline. Considered as the "gold-standard" antidepressant by geriatric clinicians and researchers, this secondary-amine TCA is effective for a broad range of late-life depressive syndromes. Nortriptyline is the only TCA with a "therapeutic window." The ability to measure plasma levels of nortriptyline is a necessary prerequisite for its use in older patients. Nortriptyline plasma levels above 150 ng/ml are associated with a lower response rate than levels between 50 to 150 ng/ml. In many elderly patients, the therapeutic window is 60–260 ng/mL and may occur at low nortriptyline dosages, although some geriatric patients may require dosages comparable to those of younger adults.[21] Nortriptyline may be particularly useful for the treatment of elderly patients who fail to respond to an adequate trial of other antidepressants such as an SSRI.[22] Nortriptyline continues to be useful for frail elderly nursing home patients despite the side effects associated with TCAs; therapeutic blood levels may be lower for this population.[23]

In 50% of nortriptyline-treated elderly patients, side effects decline during the acute-treatment phase, suggesting that many physical complaints attributed to nortriptyline may, in fact, be somatic symptoms of depression or that elderly patients may be habituated to nortriptyline adverse effects. Like desipramine, nortriptyline is less sedating and less anticholinergic than tertiary amine antidepressants. It also produces less frequent and less severe blood pressure reduction than other TCAs. Overall, nortriptyline is well tolerated by depressed elderly patients. Nonetheless, in one inpatient setting, nortriptyline could not be used in 7% of geriatric patients, and side effects necessitated discontinuation in 9% of those who started treatment.[21]

Desipramine. This drug has the least severe anticholinergic side effects of any TCA, and thus may be somewhat better tolerated by patients sensitive to these effects. Desipramine produces little sedation; in some patients, it may be stimulating and produce or exacerbate agitation.

Protriptyline. One of the least sedating and most stimulating of the TCAs, protriptyline, is, however, associated with orthostatic hypotension, cardiovascular toxicity, and moderately intense anticholinergic side effects. Although it may be useful on occasion for the withdrawn, motorically retarded, or apathetic geriatric patient, its extremely long elimination half-life (140 hr) may expose the older person to long periods of toxicity. Because of the risk of toxicity and the sparse clinical and research experience with this drug, protriptyline is not recommended for geriatric patients.

Amoxapine. Amoxapine is a structurally atypical secondary amine with a therapeutic and side-effect profile resembling that of nortriptyline. Because one of the metabolites of amoxapine blocks dopamine neurotransmission, typical extrapyramidal symptoms (similar to those produced by neuroleptics) may result. Older patients may be especially sensitive to amoxapine-induced dopamine blockade because of an age-related decline in CNS dopamine neurotransmission. High doses of amoxapine have also been associated with grand mal seizures. The risk of tardive dyskinesia and the overall high side-effect profile of amoxapine has limited its use in geriatric depression.

Tertiary Amines

As a group, tertiary amines are effective antidepressants although their usefulness in older patients is limited by the high incidence and severity of side effects. Because this group of antidepressants may be especially toxic in older patients, plasma-level monitoring is recommended whenever possible to ensure use of the lowest necessary therapeutic dose. However, with the exception of imipramine, the relation between blood level and tertiary amine antidepressant efficacy is not consistent. Expert Consensus Guidelines in late-life depression do not recommend using these antidepressants[2]

Amitriptyline. Although associated with a 60% response rate in elderly patients,[24] amitriptyline has strong sedating effects, frequently causes anticholinergic side effects in older people, and is especially likely to produce a CNS anticholinergic syndrome. Even though low doses and frequent monitoring of plasma levels can reduce anticholinergic reactions, amitriptyline is not recommended for antidepressant use in older depressed patients.

Imipramine. Imipramine is an effective antidepressant for older patients. Although its anticholinergic side effects are somewhat less severe than those of amitriptyline, imipramine frequently causes orthostatic hypotension. It is, however, less sedating than amitriptyline. Four studies reported the efficacy of imipramine in elderly patients.[25–28] In each, imipramine was effective but was associated with the development of significant anticholinergic and other side effects.

Doxepin. Like amitriptyline, doxepin has strong anticholinergic and sedating side effects. In low doses, however, it may be well tolerated by some elderly patients. Although favorable response to doxepin is associated with high plasma levels of both doxepin and its metabolite desmethyldoxepin, the relation between plasma level and efficacy of doxepin has not been firmly established. Doxepin has strong antihistamine (H_2) properties that may be useful for depressed older patients with peptic ulcer or gastritis but concerns about sedation and anticholinergic side effects limit its use for the elderly.

Trimipramine. This drug has been thought to be useful in older patients whose depression includes symptoms of excitement, hostility, anxiety, agitation, motor retardation, and emotional withdrawal.[29] It has strong sedating and anticholinergic side effects, comparable to those of amitriptyline and doxepin. Like doxepin, trimipramine has strong H_2-blocking properties, which may benefit patients with ulcers. Because its effect on norepinephrine presynaptic reuptake is weak, trimipramine is a relatively weak antagonist of guanethidine-like antihypertensive agents. Lack of research experience in geriatric patients and strong sedative and anticholinergic effects limit the use of trimipramine in the elderly.

Clomipramine. Clomipramine, a chlorinated derivative of imipramine, is a tertiary amine TCA with strong anticholinergic and antihistaminic properties. It is not commonly used in late-life depression because of the frequency and severity of its side effects. It may have some use in treating elderly patients with severe obsessive-compulsive disorder (see Chapter 16).

Dosage and Administration

Some antidepressants exhibit an approximate correlation between the plasma level of the drug and its clinical effect. Imipramine and desipramine have a sigmoidal relation between drug plasma levels and antidepressant efficacy. Patients improve as plasma drug levels increase—imipramine up to 200 ng/mL and desipramine up to 115 ng/mL, but there is no additional benefit to higher plasma levels.[15,16] Nortriptyline, in contrast, achieves optimal clinical efficacy within a "therapeutic window" of plasma levels of 60 to 150 ng/mL. At levels higher or lower than this range, efficacy declines ("inverted-U" correlation).

As noted, geriatric patients require plasma levels of nortriptyline and desipramine comparable to those of younger adults. However, many geriatric patients develop higher antidepressant plasma levels than younger adults while receiving comparable daily dosages. For this reason, 10 mg of nortriptyline or desipramine at bedtime is often given as the starting dosage. If the patient tolerates this initial dose without change in blood pressure and pulse rate or development of sedation, then the dosage should be increased by 10 or 25 mg every 2 to 4 days. Baseline blood pressure should be determined before drug treatment begins, and blood pressure should be checked before and after each dosage increment. The clinical effect, which may not appear for 3 to 5 weeks, is often noted at dosages of 50 to 75 mg of nortriptyline and 100 to 150 mg of desipramine. Because an occasional patient may require higher doses of antidepressants to attain therapeutic plasma levels, the plasma level should be determined before changing to another antidepressant.

The onset of antidepressant response occurs within four weeks in the majority of depressed geriatric patients. However, improvement proceeds more slowly than in younger adults and complete remission may not occur before 9 to 12 weeks of treatment[1,2]; in younger adults, 6 weeks usually suffice. Medical illness in a depressed person can be associated with poor antidepressant treatment outcome.[21,30] Depressed elderly patients with active physical illness often have poor prognosis.

Side Effects

Common TCA side effects hazardous in elderly patients are orthostatic hypotension, sedation, cardiac toxicity, and anticholinergic reactions.

Orthostatic Hypotension

For elderly patients, orthostatic hypotension is a potentially serious side effect of most TCAs, although frequency and severity vary among TCAs (see Table 9.1). Orthostatic hypotension results from blockade of peripheral alpha-adrenergic receptors in a manner similar to that induced by neuroleptic drugs (see Chapter 9). Orthostatic hypotension is often a reason for drug discontinuation because it can cause falls, fractures, strokes, or heart attacks.[31] Patients with preexisting orthostatic hypotension are at risk of falling and sustaining head injuries or fractures of the hip, humerus, or other bones. Nortriptyline is less likely to cause orthostatic hypotension than imipramine[30] and can be used safely in most patients who fail to tolerate imipramine. Falls and hip fractures are more likely to occur with the use of TCAs than with SSRIs and other new antidepressants, although all antidepressants carry risk of falls in the frail elderly nursing home patient.[31,32]

Heart failure appears to be a risk factor for imipramine-induced orthostatic hypotension in depressed patients. Approximately 50% of depressed patients with heart failure develop significant orthostatic hypotension when treated with imipramine[33] whereas only 8% of medically healthy depressed patients develop this side effect. Elderly depressed patients with heart failure may be at risk for imipramine-induced orthostatic hypotension, which has been reported in 4% of nondepressed heart failure patients who receive imipramine for arrhythmias.[34,35]

Although orthostatic hypotension is an important cause of falls in elderly patients on TCAs, other causes of falls should be considered as well. Gait instability, increased body sway, poor recognition of topographic relationships, and impaired attention increase the probability of falling. TCAs may impair cognitive function mainly through their anticholinergic action and thus increase the risk of falls.[36]

Sedation

The degree of sedation produced by each TCA varies considerably (see Table 9.1). In the early stages of antidepressant treatment, these sedative side effects may be useful in relieving the insomnia associated with depression.[37] As the older patient becomes less depressed, however, sedation usually is less desirable: therapeutic nighttime sedation commonly leads to unwanted morning hangover or next-day drowsiness because of the prolonged elimination half-life of antidepressants in older persons. The less-sedating antidepressants are therefore preferred. If necessary, trazodone or zolpidem may be used to improve sleep until the insomnia of depression remits (see Chapter 18). However, use of sedating drugs is not a recommended routine practice in geriatric depression.

Cardiac Toxicity

Cardiotoxicity is the most serious side effect of TCA treatment in older patients. The quinidine-like effects of TCAs stabilize abnormal cardiac rhythms at low plasma drug levels. However, at higher plasma levels, these effects interfere with cardiac conduction. Serious conduction alterations, including right and left bundle-branch block or partial or complete atrioventricular (AV) block, occur at high or toxic plasma levels and are reflected in the ECG as prolonged PR, QRS, and QT intervals and T-wave flattening or inversion.[33]

Patients with preexisting conduction defects have the highest risk. The risk for second-degree AV block is greater in patients with a preexisting bundle-branch block (9%) than in those with normal electrocardiograms (0.7%).[38,39] For this reason, TCAs should not be prescribed for patients with bundle-branch blocks. In addition, TCAs should not be routinely prescribed for patients with ventricular arrhythmias. Even for elderly patients without cardiac disease, pretreatment ECGs are strongly recommended, and frequent ECG monitoring during the course of treatment is important. If a TCA prolongs the PR or QRS interval, the medication may be continued under the supervision of a cardiologist.

TCAs have type IA antiarrhythmic properties. Type I antiarrhythmics increase mortality in postmyocardial infarction patients.[40] Although these findings raise concern, whether or not TCAs increase mortality in depressed patients with ischemic heart disease is unclear.

In addition to direct cardiotoxicity, TCAs may indirectly lead to adverse cardiac effects. For example, nortriptyline leads to weight gain in 15 to 20% of elderly patients, elevates the heart rate by an average of 15 beats per minute, and increases triglyceride and low-density lipoprotein blood levels, although it does not influence overall cholesterol levels.[41] These metabolic changes might increase the risk for vascular disease.

Sudden and unexpected deaths of children receiving desipramine have been reported, raising concern about the risk of cardiotoxicity for older patients from TCAs in general and desipramine in particular. Evidence for reduced heart-rate variability is associated with increased vulnerability to serious arrhythmias.[42] A comparison of nortriptyline and paroxetine in patients with comorbid major depressive disorder and ischemic heart disease demonstrates that both agents are effective antidepressants but that nortriptyline is associated with sustained increases in heart rate and reduced heart-rate variability.[43] Because heart-rate variability diminishes in depression,[44] depressed elderly patients may already be at risk for cardiac death. However, parasympathetic input to the heart declines significantly with aging,[45] suggesting that TCAs may have a more pronounced effect on the heart of younger patients in whom parasympathetic control of the heart is most active. Furthermore, TCAs are potent suppressors of ventricular arrhythmias.[46] Further study is needed to determine the clinical significance of antidepressant-induced reduction in heart-rate variability and its relation to cardiotoxicity in elderly patients.

Anticholinergic Toxicity

TCAs produce anticholinergic side effects of varying frequency and intensity. The tertiary amine antidepressants (particularly amitriptyline, clomipramine, and doxepin) have strong anticholinergic properties whereas these properties in the secondary amine antidepressants (nortriptyline, amoxapine, and maprotiline) are moderate. Although desipramine induces relatively weaker anticholinergic toxicity in older patients, these effects may still be intense, particularly in frail or debilitated patients. Regardless of the relative intensity of anticholinergic properties of any specific antidepressant, anticholinergic side effects depend on individual sensitivity as well as the dosage and the plasma level of each drug. Anticholinergic side effects are typically subdivided into those that affect the periphery and those that affect the CNS.

Peripheral Anticholinergic Reactions. Peripheral anticholinergic side effects of antidepressants can cause complications or reduce treatment adherence. Dry mouth (xerostomia), the most frequent of these side effects, may lead to loss of porcelain dental fillings, malfitting dentures, parotitis, and *Candida* infection. In an effort to reduce the discomfort caused by dry mouth, elderly patients sometimes eat less and become malnourished. Patients also may increase their water intake to the point of water intoxication. Dry mouth may be ameliorated by the use of sugarless candies, saliva substitutes, and petroleum jelly or other commercial jellies applied to the gums. The peripheral cholinergic agonist bethanechol (10 mg three times daily) may reduce subjective complaints of anticholinergic side effects.[47]

Constipation, often occurring naturally as people age, is also a common side effect of TCAs. In its milder form, constipation, like dry mouth, may lead to poor adherence to the drug regimen. Mild drug-induced constipation may respond to bran and high-fiber diets; adding bethanechol is occasionally helpful. More severe constipation can progress to paralytic ileus, which should be treated by reducing the antidepressant dosage or using a less anticholinergic drug. Regular use of laxatives should be discouraged in older patients.

Urinary retention is another common peripheral anticholinergic side effect in older persons. In a mild form, initiating urination is difficult. In serious cases, however, urine retention can predispose to bladder infections that may ascend to the kidneys. Elderly men with prostatic hypertrophy are at especially high risk for this complication. Retention may be complete, requiring immediate catheterization, or partial, leading to increased residual urine and eventually to urinary tract infections. The clinician should ask the patient frequently about difficulties in initiating urination. If such symptoms develop, a urinalysis and urine culture should be obtained to identify a possible urinary tract infection. Bladder catheterization should be considered for all patients with suspected partial urinary retention who receive TCAs.

The anticholinergic mydriatic action of TCAs can precipitate or exacerbate narrow-angle glaucoma, which is relatively common in elderly patients because of cataract formation. Adjustment in dosage of topical medication for the treatment of glaucoma may be necessary in older patients who are being treated with TCAs. Patients with wide-angle glaucoma are better able to tolerate the anticholinergic side effects of TCAs than those with narrow-angle glaucoma.

CNS Anticholinergic Syndrome. CNS anticholinergic syndrome may be produced by any drug that blocks CNS acetylcholine receptors. Old people are predisposed to CNS anticholinergic side effects because acetylcholine neurotransmission in the brain decreases with advanced age. In addition, age-related alterations in the metabolism of antidepressants may result in higher plasma levels, and lead to severe and long-lasting CNS anticholinergic effects.

Characteristics of CNS anticholinergic syndrome include increased anxiety, agitation, confusion, restlessness, and disorientation. As the syndrome becomes more severe, assaultiveness, paranoia, and visual hallucinations may occur; the most extreme manifestations are stupor and coma.

Severe symptoms of CNS anticholinergic syndrome can be misdiagnosed as psychosis-related agitation, and the neuroleptic drugs often used to treat these disorders may worsen the patient's condition. Rather than prescribing neuroleptics, the physician should discontinue use of antidepressants.

Physostigmine has been used to reverse CNS anticholinergic syndrome in young patients. However, because this drug increases acetylcholine levels by blocking its metabolism, symptoms of cholinergic excess such as heart block, seizures, and increased salivary secretions with bronchoconstriction may result. Because experience in using physostigmine to treat CNS anticholinergic syndrome in older people is very limited, it should be administered with extreme caution and only under carefully controlled, medically supervised conditions. The dose of physostigmine is 0.1 mg, administered subcutaneously or by very slow intravenous drip. A safer alternative to physostigmine is cholinesterase inhibitors. However, lack of research studies limits the use of these agents in patients with CNS anticholinergic syndrome.

Memory Disturbance

Some elderly patients who receive TCAs complain of forgetfulness. Because memory complaints are common in normal aging, the older patient, the family, or the physician may have difficulty distinguishing normal recent-memory impairment from memory loss secondary to drug effects. Nortriptyline studies have shown little evidence of clinically significant impairment in memory or other neuropsychological function.[48] However, discontinuation of this TCA can lead to subjective experience of improved memory; no memory improvement is documented by objective tests. Approximately 35% of patients above 40 years of age experience memory problems when treated with amitriptyline, although this side effect occurs in only 2% of younger patients.[49] Memory disturbance with this tricyclic appears to be confined to recall of recently memorized verbal information; patients can still recognize such information when it is presented to them. Unassisted recall of recently learned visual material and long-term memory are not affected.

Memory dysfunction induced by TCAs may result, in part, from a CNS effect on the cholinergic pathways related to memory function. The pattern of memory impairment induced by TCAs antidepressants is similar to that observed after administration of the antimuscarinic drug scopolamine. Cholinergic (muscarinic M_1) receptors in the brain are particularly sensitive to the aging process. Based on the assumption that the anticholinergic effect of tricyclic antidepressants contributes to memory dysfunction, use of drugs with a low anticholinergic profile is recommended for depressed geriatric patients. Patients with cognitive impairment and those with depression associated with Alzheimer's disease (AD) are at particularly high risk of additional memory problems. Slow introduction of the antidepressant and frequent assessment of memory function are important for these patients. Discontinuation of the TCA results in restoration of memory function[48] although depression may reappear.

Weight Gain and Hormonal Regulation

TCAs do not appear to increase weight in depressed elderly individuals.[49] Successful antidepressant treatment is associated with a reestablishment of premorbid weight in the elderly.[50] Treatment of late-life depression with TCAs may be associated with an alteration in blood glucose regulation. Nortriptyline may worsen glycemic control[51,52] although improvement of depression has a beneficial effect on glucose regulation.

Treatment of Mild Depressive States

Should a geriatric patient with a relatively mild depression be treated with an antidepressant? Elderly persons often manifest apathy, anhedonia, restriction and diminution of interests, reduced activities and energy, pessimism, and, in some cases, reduced concentration. These patients sometimes say that they have lived long enough, that nothing seems meaningful, or that there is no reason for them to continue trying because they can no longer be useful. Mild apathetic mood states may occur in the context of a medical illness, disability, or interpersonal loss, or even in the absence of an obvious precipitant. Early stage dementia may explain some aspects of this syndrome (e.g., reduced memory, apathy, irritability, restriction of interests and activities). Similarly, debilitation due to severe medical illness may present with some of these behavioral changes. Elderly patients frequently offer rationalizations, e.g., they see their symptoms as a natural consequence of old age, when in fact these symptoms are part of depression. If depressive ideation is present, this syndrome should be identified as depression that is either primary or related to a neurological or medical illness.

Most elderly patients with mild depressive syndromes are treated with SSRIs, bupropion or SNRIs because of their favorable side-effect profile (see Chapter 10). TCAs may be considered for mild depression or dysphoric states of these patients only after SSRIs or other newer agents fail. The decision to administer a trial of TCAs to a geriatric patient in a mild depressive state raises at least two questions: (1) Is the discomfort or behavioral change severe enough to justify even the mild risks of TCAs? (2) Does the patient belong in a high-risk group for treatment with TCAs? Psychotherapy and increased socialization and activities are helpful in mild depression and should be used in addition to treatment with TCAs or as a therapeutic alternative where the risks of drug treatment outweigh the benefits.

Treatment of Bereavement-Related Depression

For elderly persons, bereavement is a common occurrence; the annual incidence of spousal death is 1.6% for older men and 3% for older women.[53] Approximately 16% of individuals whose spouses die can be found to be depressed throughout the first year.[54] SSRIs as well as other newer antidepressants are effective treatments for severe bereavement states. Nortriptyline is also effective in bereavement-related depression, with improvement occurring after a median treatment interval of 6.4 weeks.[55] Because grieving is associated with increased depression and anxiety, psychotherapy should also be considered[56] in conjunction with pharmacotherapy.

Monoamine Oxidase Inhibitors

Monoamine oxidase inhibitors (MAOIs), like TCAs, are less commonly used in late-life depression. Side effects, drug interactions, and interactions with some food make these drugs more difficult to use than SSRIs and other antidepressants. Nevertheless, in some elderly patients, MAOIs produce a dramatic reversal of depressive symptoms with fewer and less severe side effects than TCAs. The older depressed patient who requires antidepressant treatment but has not responded to newer antidepressants or a TCA may be a candidate for a MAOI trial. This is particularly true if the depression is characterized by high degrees of anxiety and relatively few or only mild vegetative signs. Studies of MAOIs are summarized in Table 9.3.

In younger adults, MAOIs are particularly helpful in the treatment of "atypical" depression, characterized by dysphoric mood, anxiety, phobias, increased sensitivity in interpersonal relationships, and a "reverse" vegetative syndrome that

Table 9.3. Studies of Geriatric Depressed Populations Using Monoamine Oxidase Inhibitors(MAOIs)

Drug	Study	N	(Age range; mean)	Outcome Scales	Results
MOCLOBEMIDE					
Moclobemide, nortriptyline	Kin et al. (1997)	95	71	DST	DST positive patients had a better NT response, DST negative patients had a better MOC response
Moclobemide	Roth et al. (1996)	726	73.6	HAM-D, MMSE, SCAG, CGI, BG-P	Moclobemide showed equal efficacy to placebo, but was superior in demented patients
Moclobemide, nortriptyline	Nair et al. (1995)	10	≥60		Nortriptyline had a higher remission rate than moclobemide and placebo , moclobemide had a higher remission rate than placebo
PHENELZINE					
Phenelzine, nortriptyline	Georgotas et al. (1989a)	51	≥55	Plasma NT levels, platelet MAO inhibition, HAM-D	Maintenance therapy in elderly depressed patients: More subjects receiving phenelzine remained well compared with subjects receiving nortriptyline or placebo.
Phenelzine, nortriptyline	Georgotas et al. (1989b)	76	≥65	RDC, HAM-D	Factors affecting delay of antidepressant effect in responders: More severely depressed subjects took longer to respond; those with endogenous depression responded sooner to nortriptyline.
Phenelzine, nortriptyline	Georgotas & McCue (1989a)	41	≥55	HAM-D, RDC	Subjects with more prior episodes of depression had greater risk of relapse.
Phenelzine, nortriptyline	Georgotas & McCue (1989b)	100	≥55	NA	Addition of 2 weeks to study period produced 15% increase in response; 1/3 of subjects who had not responded by week 9 responded when kept on medication for 12 weeks

Phenelzine, nortriptyline	Georgotas et al. (1989a)	51	≥55	Plasma NT levels, platelet MAO inhibition, HAM-D	Maintenance therapy in elderly depressed patients: More subjects receiving phenelzine remained well compared with those receiving nortriptyline or placebo.
Phenelzine nortriptyline	Georgotas et al. (1988)	60	≥55	HAM-D	Follow-up of elderly patients who responded to nortriptyline or phenelzine; 70% remained well, 11 relapsed, 3 dropped out because of side effects, and 3 prematurely terminated therapy in good clinical condition; no significant difference between relapse rates for nortriptyline and phenelzine
Phenelzine, nortriptyline	Georgotas et al. (1987a)	75	≥55	RDC, HAM-D	Significantly greater mean orthostatic fall in systolic BP in patients treated with nortriptyline or phenelzine compared with placebo, no significant difference between the two drugs.
Phenelzine nortriptyline	Georgotas et al. (1987b)	10 (14 controls)	≥55	HAM-D	Analysis of H-clonidine and H-imipramine binding; significant negative correlation between dissociation constant of binding sites and scores on HAM-D; no significant relation between binding and severity of depression and no significant difference between receptor data from responders and nonresponders to antidepressant treatment
Phenelzine, nortriptyline	Georgotas et al. (1987c)	42	55–82	RDC, Newcastle Diagnostic Scale, DSM-III	Results consistent with finding that subtype of depression does not predict antidepressant response
Phenelzine, nortriptyline	Georgotas et al. (1987d)	44	55–82	ECG	Nortriptyline produced significant increases in both heart rate and PR interval; none was outside normal range. Phenelzine significantly decreased QT interval; no pathologic ECG changes; 75% of nortriptyline patients and 57% of phenelzine patients responded

(continued)

Table 9.3 *(continued)*

Drug	Study	N	(Age range; mean)	Outcome Scales	Results
Phenelzine, nortriptyline	Georgotas et al. (1987e)	75	≥55	NT plasma level, platelet MAO inhibition, HAM-D	Phenelzine and nortriptyline more effective than placebo in treating depressed mood, guilt feelings, suicidal ideation, agitation, loss of energy, and morning diurnal variation of mood; nortriptyline better than phenelzine and placebo in improving middle/late insomnia
Phenelzine, nortriptyline	Georgotas et al. (1986a)	47 (26 controls)	55–76	RDC, HAM-D	Late-life depression can be treated despite common misconceptions that it is a natural consequence of aging; both drugs well tolerated
Phenelzine, nortriptyline	Georgotas et al. (1986b)	72	58–82	DST	No correlation between DST and treatment response to antidepressants; DST had no practical value as indicator of impending recovery from major depression in elderly patients; however, failure of DST results to normalize may have prognostic significance
Phenelzine	Lazarus et al. (1986)	15	60–75	HAM-D	Efficacy and side effects of phenelzine examined in elderly patients with severe treatment-resistant depression: 3 responded, 4 responded partially; phenelzine may be an alternative antidepressant treatment for geriatric patients
Phenelzine	Georgotas et al. (1983a)	10	67–82	HAM-D, CGI, mental status questionnaire	Most subjects recovered from depression but no significant changes on cognitive measures over course of treatment period, and no changes on cognitive scores as result of treatment

Table 9.3. *(continued)*

Drug	Study	N	(Age range; mean)	Outcome Scales	Results
Phenelzine, nortriptyline	Georgotas et al. (1987e)	75	≥55	NT plasma level, platelet MAO inhibition, HAM-D	Phenelzine and nortriptyline more effective than placebo in treating depressed mood, guilt feelings, suicidal ideation, agitation, loss of energy, and morning diurnal variation of mood; nortriptyline better than phenelzine and placebo in improving middle/late insomnia
Phenelzine, nortriptyline	Georgotas et al. (1986a)	47 (26 controls)	55–76	RDC, HAM-D	Late-life depression can be treated despite common misconceptions that it is a natural consequence of aging; both drugs well tolerated
Phenelzine, nortriptyline	Georgotas et al. (1986b)	72	58–82	DST	No correlation between DST and treatment response to antidepressants; DST had no practical value as indicator of impending recovery from major depression in elderly patients; however, failure of DST results to normalize may have prognostic significance
Phenelzine	Lazarus et al. (1986)	15	60–75	HAM-D	Efficacy and side effects of phenelzine examined in elderly patients with severe treatment-resistant depression: 3 responded, 4 responded partially; phenelzine may be an alternative antidepressant treatment for geriatric patients
Phenelzine	Georgotas et al. (1983a)	10	67–82	HAM-D, CGI, mental status questionnaire	Most subjects recovered from depression but no significant changes on cognitive measures over course of treatment period, and no changes on cognitive scores as result of treatment

includes hypersomnia, weight gain, and worsening mood in the evening. Currently no corresponding data exist, however, on the efficacy of MAOIs in older persons with atypical depression. Evidence does suggest that MAOIs may be as effective as TCAs in treating depressed elderly patients.[57,58] No difference in response rates between melancholic and nonmelancholic depressed geriatric patients treated with phenelzine has been found.[58]

Several factors require attention for effective and safe use of MAOIs. Prior to treatment, elderly patients must have a medical evaluation, with special attention to pretreatment blood pressure, history of headaches, and ECG; MAOIs may decrease an already low blood pressure. History of intermittent headaches may interfere with early recognition of hypertensive crises; headache is usually the first sign of orthostatic crises. The patient's need for drugs that interact adversely with MAOIs should be identified. Elderly patients who cannot comply with a low tyramine diet should not receive MAOIs because a dangerous hypertensive crisis may result from a diet violation.

Clinical Pharmacology

Monoamine oxidase (MAO) is responsible for the intraneuronal metabolism of norepinephrine, dopamine, and serotonin in the brain. This enzyme occurs in two forms, MAO_A and MAO_B. MAO_A is partly responsible for metabolizing the mood-regulating neurotransmitters norepinephrine and serotonin; MAO_B metabolizes dopamine and phenylethylamine in the brain and the platelets. When MAOIs were first used, they were thought to counteract depression by decreasing the metabolism of norepinephrine and serotonin.[59] However, this is only a short-term effect that occurs within the first few days of treatment. MAOIs have complex effects on monoamine receptors, including downregulation of the beta- and alpha$_2$-noradrenergic receptors as well as the serotonin 5-HT1 and 5-HT2 receptors.[59] After three weeks of exposure to

MAOIs, brain monoamine concentrations return to pretreatment levels and the neuronal firing rate decreases. Which of these effects is directly related to the antidepressant action of MAOIs remains unclear.

Absorption

MAOIs are well absorbed by the gastrointestinal system. Although the mild anticholinergic effects of MAOIs may slightly reduce intestinal motility, this effect probably does not substantially influence absorption.

Hepatic Metabolism

Two chemically distinct classes of MAOIs are currently available for clinical use: hydrazines, represented by phenelzine, and nonhydrazines, represented by tranylcypromine, which is structurally similar to amphetamine. Both hydrazine and nonhydrazine MAOIs are inactivated by acetylation in the liver. This rate of acetylation is not influenced by aging.

MAO exists in platelets; measurement of platelet MAO activity is assumed to correlate roughly with enzyme levels in the brain. An 80% inhibition of platelet MAO activity during treatment with phenelzine is associated with a favorable antidepressant response, presumably reflecting an inhibition in CNS activity.[60] This degree of inhibition is achieved in approximately 90% of mixed-age patients receiving 60 mg of phenelzine daily. Geriatric patients who receive an average phenelzine dose of approximately 55 mg daily develop mean platelet MAO activity inhibition of approximately 85%.[61] It appears, therefore, that geriatric patients require only slightly lower dosages of phenelzine than younger adults to achieve the therapeutic 80% inhibition of platelet MAO activity that occurs early in treatment.

Tranylcypromine inhibits platelet MAO activity at doses considerably lower than those required for an antidepressant response. Measuring platelet MAO inhibition following administration of this drug therefore offers little help in adjusting dosage.

Platelet and brain MAO, particularly MAO$_B$ activity, increases with age.[62] Moreover, patients with late-onset depression and depression with reversible dementia,[63] as well as depression that occurs in the context of AD[64] may all have higher platelet MAO activity than geriatric patients with onset of depression in early life. It is unclear, however, whether geriatric patients with late-onset depression have a more favorable response to MAO$_B$ inhibitors than younger depressive patients, geriatric patients with early-onset depression, or patients with depression and dementia. The selective MAO$_B$ inhibitor *l*-deprenyl (Selegiline) has been shown to have mild efficacy in elderly patients, especially at dosages higher than 10 mg daily.[65] At these dosages selegiline is no longer selective and inhibits both MAO$_A$ and MAO$_B$, thus requiring low monoamine diet.

Side Effects

Use of MAOIs commonly results in weight gain and orthostatic hypotension in both old and young patients. Less frequent but nonetheless distressing side effects include dry mucous membranes, insomnia, overstimulation, and sexual dysfunction.

Orthostatic Hypotension

MAOIs frequently produce significant orthostatic hypotension in elderly patients. Unlike hypotension resulting from use of TCAs, MAOI-induced orthostatic hypotension develops gradually over 6 to 8 weeks. Although elderly patients may be able to tolerate MAOIs initially, they may also develop significant orthostatic hypotension within 2 or 3 months and be forced to discontinue using this class of drugs. Sudden decreases in blood pressure may result in falls, fractures, stroke, and myocardial infarction as well as confusion and disorientation. Because of their high sensitivity to orthostatic hypotension, elderly patients taking MAOIs should have their blood pressure monitored (supine, sitting, and standing positions) for several months after initiation of treatment. They should also be in-structed to get up slowly from a lying or seated position; should dizziness occur, they should sit down, wait a few seconds, and then slowly get up again.

MAOIs do not have an adverse effect on cardiac functions. Phenelzine either reduces heart rate or has no effect; it also reduces QT$_c$ and does not appear to impair cardiac conduction. Whether or not phenelzine has an adverse effect on myocardial performance is not known.

Anticholinergic-like Symptoms

MAOIs can produce an anticholinergic syndrome but MAOI-induced anticholinergic side effects are milder than those of TCAs. Dry mouth is the most common of these symptoms in older patients. MAOIs also cause urinary retention and constipation. Phenelzine is slightly more anticholinergic than tranylcypromine.

Sedation

Older patients treated with MAOIs sometimes experience sedation, which is an uncommon side effect in younger patients. With continued administration of MAOIs, most elderly patients develop tolerance to sedation.

Peripheral Neuropathy

MAOIs may cause peripheral neuropathy. In geriatric patients, this condition may present as a gradual weakness of the legs that eventually leads to gait disturbance and falls. Elderly patients taking MAOIs should be asked about paresthesias and be examined periodically for diminution of muscle strength as well as sensation of pain, touch, and vibration. Peripheral neuropathy can be prevented or reversed with vitamin B$_6$.

Exacerbation of Cognitive Dysfunction

MAOIs, like TCAs, may exacerbate memory loss and confusion in demented older people. For this reason, demented geriatric patients receiving MAOIs should have frequent mental status examinations, and MAOIs should be discontinued if confusion or worsened memory occurs.

MAOIs often stimulate the older patient. In addition to exacerbating the cognitive symptoms and signs of dementia, they may contribute to the development of restlessness, agitation, paranoia, and insomnia.

Hypertensive Crisis

Hypertensive crises have been observed in patients receiving MAOIs. Inhibition of MAO by these drugs in the intestine, liver, and blood vessels interferes with the metabolism of tyramine in food. Accumulation of tyramine, in turn, leads to release of catecholamines that dramatically raise blood pressure. MAOIs must not be used in conjunction with tyramine-rich food. Food that must be avoided includes all cheese (except cottage and cream cheese), yeast extract, caviar, sausage, herring, liver, avocado, chocolate, caffeine, red wine, and beer. A tyramine-free diet greatly decreases the incidence of hypertensive crises. Confused, forgetful, or poorly compliant patients should not receive MAOIs without diet supervision.

The recent development of a transdermal selegiline delivery system,[66] may be useful for elderly patients who cannot swallow pills. By circumventing the first-pass effect, transdermally administered selegiline has a modest effect on the intestinal and liver MAO but enters the CNS and inhibits CNS MAO. Thus transdermal selegiline may exert its therapeutic action at a low risk of hypertensive crisis following tyramine ingestion. Moclobemide, a selective and reversible MAO_A inhibitor not available in the United States, is infrequently associated with hypertensive crises even after substantial tyramine intake. Tyramine displaces moclobemide from its MAO_A binding sites in the gut, thereby deaminating ingested tyramine via intestinal MAO_A even in the presence of moclobemide. However, unlike moclobemide, tyramine does not cross the blood-brain barrier, and thus does not interfere with moclobemide inhibition of CNS MAO_A[69] (see Table 9.3).

Hypertensive crises may also be induced by certain drugs taken concomitantly with MAOIs. Catecholamine precursors (e.g., L-dopa or Sinemet, L-tryptophan or 5-hydroxytryptophan) and catecholamines with indirect sympathomimetic action (e.g., amphetamine or phenylephrine found in over-the-counter cold preparations) must not be used by patients taking MAOIs. These drugs can induce hypertensive crisis by increasing the amount of catecholamine released at CNS nerve endings or from the adrenals. Directly acting catecholamines such as norepinephrine, dopamine, or epinephrine (found in dental anesthesia preparations) should not be given to elderly patients taking MAOIs. MAOIs should be discontinued for 2 weeks or longer before either a tyramine-rich diet or drugs interacting with MAOIs are introduced.

Drug Interactions

In addition to interactions with sympathomimetic drugs, MAOIs may interact negatively with many other medications. The most important interaction is with meperidine (Demerol), which may lead to fatal elevations in body temperature (hyperpyrexia) in patients taking MAOIs because of increased serotonin release. Physicians managing postsurgical geriatric patients or those with chronic pain syndromes should be alert to this interaction and avoid meperidine. MAOIs also interfere with the detoxification of barbiturates and anticholinergic drugs and thus potentiate their effect.

Weight Gain

Some patients treated with MAOIs gain weight; whether older patients are particularly susceptible to this side effect is unclear. Because weight control is an important part of the clinical management of hypertension, hypercholesterolemia, and diabetes mellitus, MAOIs should be prescribed with caution. The patient's weight should be recorded before treatment begins and monitored throughout treatment.

Inhibition of Orgasm

Some patients receving MAOIs experience difficulty reaching orgasm; occasionally, male patients experience difficulty maintaining an erection. These effects seem to be dosage related and are reversible when the medication is reduced or discontinued. Because impaired sexual function can exacerbate feelings of worthlessness, sexually active older patients should be warned of this potential side effect.

Choice of MAOIs

No evidence exists for the therapeutic superiority of phenelzine or tranylcypromine. Although phenelzine is the most extensively investigated MAOI in older and younger adults, most clinicians are guided in their choice by their clinical familiarity with one or the other of these drugs.

Phenelzine

For elderly patients, the initial dose of phenelzine is 7.5 mg, with increases of 7.5 mg every 4 to 8 days, depending on side effects. In older patients, the therapeutic dosage range is 22.5 to 60 mg per day. Sedation, orthostatic hypotension, and dry mouth are the most frequent side effects and, in most cases, are not serious enough to warrant discontinuation. Phenelzine is less stimulating than tranylcypromine but may lead to lack of energy and weight gain.

Tranylcypromine

Tranylcypromine has stimulant properties and may be useful for withdrawn and apathetic patients. The initial dose for the older patient is 5 mg, with dosage increments of 5 mg every 3 to 4 days. Therapeutic effects occur at 15 to 30 mg/day. Tranylcypromine may result in less weight gain and more energy than phenelzine. However, tranylcypromine may cause agitation, nervousness, and insomnia.

Tranylcypromine may be prescribed in patients who fail to respond to phenelzine or develop side effects. A 15-day, phenelzine-free period is necessary to permit re-generation of MAO and other enzymes inhibited by phenelzine. Concomitant administration of phenelzine and tranylcypromine may lead to a hypertensive crisis and should be avoided. A 15-day, drug-free period is also necessary in patients changing from phenelzine to a TCA. Conversely, if a patient is taking an SSRI or a TCA and a trial of an MAOI is planned, the TCA or the SSRI should be discontinued for a time equal to 5 times the elimination half-life of the first drug before the MAOI is started. Seven weeks should be allowed for patients on fluoxetine because its active metabolite norfluoxetine has a long half-life (7–8 days). Addition of an MAOI in patients taking TCAs is associated with fewer hypertensive crises than the addition of a TCA in patients taking MAOIs.

Psychostimulants

Although not severely depressed, some elderly persons appear to loose their zest for life and become apathetic, withdrawn, and progressively disinterested in their surroundings. Elderly patients with chronic diseases may become discouraged and demoralized and stop participating in activities aimed at rehabilitation. Families often are the first to notice the development of apathy, while the patients themselves may remain unaware of it.

Psychostimulants enhance the release of and inhibit the reuptake of dopamine and norepinephrine. The stimulating action in these neurotransmitters is thought to be responsible for the generalized excitation in the brain that increases alertness. Psychostimulants are effective for depressed medically ill patients,[68] for apathetic nursing home patients,[69] and medically ill patients treated with stimulants.[67] However, these drugs are ineffective in treating major melancholic depression.[70] Studies of stimulants are summarized in Table 9.4.

Methylphenidate

In apathetic elderly patients, low doses of methylphenidate may increase motiva-

Table 9.4.   Use of Psychostimulants in Elderly Depressed Patients

Drug/Dose	Study	N	Age/Condition	Comments
METHYLPHENIDATE				
Methylphenidate 8-day trial (5–20 mg)	Wallace et al. (1995)	16	Mean 72.3; depressed medical or surgical inpatients	Dramatic decrease in depressive symptoms in 7/16; moderate improvement in additional 3; immediate effect in those receiving methylphenidate as first drug
Methylphenidate (1.25–5 mg)	Gurian & Rosowsky (1990)	2	91, 104; frail, depressed, medically ill	Significant and sustained decrease in apathy, anhedonia, fatigue, diminished appetite
Methylphenidate (2.5–20 mg)	Askinazi et al. (1986)	13	58–83; depressed, medically ill	7/13—definite improvement, 3—marked improvement, 2—moderate improvement 2—mild improvement, 6/7 responders were women
Methylphenidate (single dose, 20 mg)	Spar & LaRue (1985)	71	Mean 71.8; major depression	Response to methylphenidate predicted response to desipramine but not imipramine
Methylphenidate	Branconnier & Cole (1980)	56	Mildly depressed, mildly senile, poor	Significant improvement in depression, vigor, fatigue motivation
Methylphenidate (20 mg/d)	Katon & Raskind (1980)	3	73,82,85; depressed,	Rapid improvement for medically ill
Methylphenidate (10 mg/d)	Clark & Mankikar (1979)	88	Apathetic, poor motivation	28 markedly improved; 50% improved
Methylphenidate (10 mg/d)	Kaplitz (1975)	44	Depressed, withdrawn, apathetic	Patients became active
Methylphenidate (10–30 mg)	Jacobson (1958)	54	60–70, depressed	27 received methylphenidate, 2—marked improvement, 8—moderate improvement 12—minimal improvement, 5—worse
PEMOLINE				
Pemoline 37.5–75 mg	Gurevitch et al. (1991)	6	65–85; nonbipolar, nonpsychotic, depressed	Mild improvement in depression; significant improvement in energy
Pemoline (50–150 mg)	Gilbert et al. (1973)	78	60+; not depressed	Minimal improvement on depression ratings; improved "friendliness"

tion, attention, and sense of well-being. In such patients, the recommended starting dose is 2.5 to 5 mg .[70] If the drug is well tolerated, the dosage may be increased by 2.5 to 5 mg every 2 or 3 days until a total daily dosage of 20 mg is reached. Methylphenidate should be given in the morning; if given in the late afternoon, evening, or nighttime, it may cause insomnia.

Stimulants are usually well tolerated and pose little risk for habituation or nonmedical drug-seeking by older individuals. Most apathetic elderly patients develop little tolerance to stimulants and do not require significant dosage increases. The most common side effects of methylphenidate are tachycardia and a mild blood pressure increase. Under medically supervised conditions, stimulants are safe; once they experience the energizing effects of the agents, older patients should be encouraged to pursue their interests and establish an active lifestyle.

Modafinil

Modafinil is a new wakefulness-promoting agent shown to decrease daytime sleepiness associated with narcolepsy. It is not chemically related to amphetamine, methylphenidate, or phenylethylamine, and the mechanism of its action is not known. Preclinical studies suggest that modafinil-wakefulness is associated with altered levels of inhibitory GABA and the excitatory glutamate neurotransmitters in the anterior hypothalamus and adjacent areas. Unlike the wakefulness produced by psychostimulants, modafinil-induced wakefulness does not depend on dopamine- or norepinephrine-synaptic increase, although it binds weakly to the dopamine reuptake site. An intact dopamine reuptake transport system and intact alpha-1 adrenergic receptors are required for modafinil's action.

Recent findings suggest that modafinil may improve some cognitive functions, increase energy, and may even have some antidepressant action. In healthy young men, modafinil increases performance in digit span, visual recognition memory,

spatial planning, and reaction time. An anecdotal report of 10 patients with traumatic brain injury suggests that modafinil can increase attention and other cognitive functions.[71] It has been effective in reducing fatigue in patients with multiple sclerosis.[72] Finally, some evidence suggests that modafinil improves both cognition and some symptoms of depression.[73–76]

Although geriatric studies of modafinil have not been conducted, clinical experience suggests that this agent may be a useful adjunct in the treatment of depressed, apathetic, and debilitated elderly patients. Side effects include headache, nausea, anxiety, and insomnia. Modafinil is less likely to result in irritability, palpitations, and increased blood pressure than sympathomimetic amines. Dosages of 100 mg to 200 mg daily are appropriate for elderly patients.

Treatment of Psychotic Depression

Psychotic depression occurs in 3.6% of elderly depressives living in the community[77] and in 20 to 45% of hospitalized elderly depressives.[78] A severe illness with profound depressive symptoms, psychotic depression is accompanied by delusions and less frequently by hallucinations. Delusions occur in successive episodes of geriatric depression if the severity of episodes is high.[79,80] However, in geriatric patients, psychotic depression is not merely a consequence of severity of depression, since high percentages of severely depressed elderly patients do not develop delusions.[79,80] Because psychotic depression is associated with risk of suicide,[81,82] usually by violent means,[83] timely diagnosis and treatment are crucial.

Distinguishing depressive delusions from overvalued ideas of worthlessness and hopelessness is often difficult, although nondelusional depressed patients as a rule can recognize the exaggerated nature of their overvalued ideas even though they cannot stop their preoccupation with them. Depressive delusions can be distinguished from delusions of demented patients. The former usually present as organized ideas of hypochondriasis, nihilism, guilt, persecution, or jealousy; the latter are less systematized and less congruent with the affective disturbance.[84] However, geriatric depression with reversible dementia, usually called pseudodementia, is often a psychotic depression with a poor long-term outcome.[85] The dementia syndrome associated with psychotic depression initially subsides after effective antidepressant treatment. However, over time, a high percentage of affected patients develop irreversible dementia.

Elderly patients with psychotic depression respond poorly to acute treatment with TCAs alone,[82] a response not explained solely by the severity of depression.[86] In controlled studies of younger patients,[87] TCAs in combination with neuroleptics may be effective; however, this combination therapy is less efficacious in older patients.[88] The most frequently prescribed TCAs are nortriptyline or desipramine at plasma levels comparable to those of younger adults (60–150 ng/mL for nortriptyline; above 115 ng/mL for desipramine). Perphenazine, the neuroleptic that has been used in most studies of psychotic depression, can be effective at daily doses of approximately 32 mg.[87] However, perphenazine increases blood levels of TCAs predisposing elderly patients to potential toxicity.[89] Whether elderly patients can respond to lower doses of neuroleptics or whether other neuroleptics can be effective and better tolerated than perphenazine is unclear.

Limited experience is available on the use of SSRIs alone or in combination with atypical antipsychotic agents in psychotic depression[90] (see Chapter 10). However, the Expert Consensus Guidelines recommend SSRIs (citalopram, sertraline, or venlafaxine) in combination with atypical antipsychotics (risperidone or olanzapine) in geriatric psychotic depression.[2]

Although clinicians agree that psychotic depression requires combination drug therapy, such drug combinations may be poorly tolerated or inadequately efficacious for elderly patients. For this reason, electroconvulsive ECT is frequently the treatment of choice in psychotic depression (see Chapter 13). Comparison of actual ECT with the simulated version demonstrate benefit only of actual ECT in psychotic depression,[91] and some evidence suggests that bilateral ECT is more effective than unilateral ECT (see Chapter 13). While post-ECT recovered patients will require continuation antidepressant treatment,[92] there is no evidence that continuation treatment with both an antidepressant and an antipsychotic yields a lower relapse rate compared to antidepressant monotherapy. However, continuation treatment with nortriptyline and perphenazine after ECT-induced remission of geriatric psychotic depression offers similar protection from depressive relapse to nortriptyline alone but can lead to oral dyskinesia.[89]

Augmenting Strategies

Augmenting TCA treatment with a second medication for elderly patients whose depression only partially responds to treatment is sometimes useful. Unfortunately, an insufficient number of studies is available on the augmentation of antidepressant treatment in nonresponding or partially responding elderly patients. Drugs that have been used for younger populations include lithium carbonate, thyroid hormone, psychostimulants, and a combination of two classes of antidepressants. Lithium augmentation may be helpful for about half of depressed elderly patients who receive it but side effects are common; the efficacy of lithium augmentation is summarized in Table 9.5. Reducing lithium in order to diminish side effects, however, may result in recurrence of depression and subsequent lithium resistance.[93] No data support the use of thy-

Table 9.5. Lithium Augmentation of Tricyclic Treatment in Elderly Patients

Study	N	Age	Daily Dose	Results
Hardy et al. (1997)	9	69–85	Dose not given; BL 0.4 meq/I, side effects;	Lithium use associated with depressive episodes associated with life events not prevented by lithium; discontinuance may be associated with recurrence of depression
Reynolds et al. (1996)	39	68	600	64% response to lithium augmentation; 52% relapse when discontinued
Flint & Rifat (1994)	21	64–88	BL 0.5–1.0 mmol/L	No response in 13; complete response in 5; partial response in 3
Zimmer et al. (1991)	15	65–89	300–450 mg	For patients "resistant" to nortriptyline, adding lithium did *not* improve response in 12 of 13; 2 with partial response to lithium became complete responders
Van Marwijk et al. (1990)	51	64–88	30–150 mg	65% complete or partial response; 11% neurotoxicity
Finch & Katona (1989) (also in Katona & Finch, 1991)	9	63–93	Dose not given; BL 0.4–0.8	7 of 9 responded well
Lafferman et al. (1988)	14	61–82	100–300 mg	4 subjects added to treatment; 7 completely improved; 3 responded partially; 4 discontinued due to side effects
Kushnir (1986)	5	65–93	150–300 mg	Adding lithium produced "lasting remission in all"; low-dose lithium prevented serious side effects
Individual case reports: Schreiber & Shalev (1992) Hale (1987) Madakasira (1986) Pai et al. (1986) Pande & Max (1985) Weaver (1983)	10	65+	150–300 mg	Effective in 9 of 10; hypotension, tremor, muscle weakness most common but infrequent side effects

roid hormones or stimulants to augment TCA or MAOI antidepressant effects in the elderly. Stimulants, however, are sometimes added to increase daytime energy especially if the TCA has sedating properties. There is no literature support for combining a stimulant with an MAO inhibitor in geriatric depression.

Patients who have had a partial response to a TCA but do not respond to lithium augmentation may be treated by adding a second antidepressant. Expert consensus suggests adding an SSRI as a second line treatment.[2] There are no recommendations for augmentation of the therapeutic effect of MAO inhibitors in the elderly.

Although SSRIs are now rated by the Expert Consensus Guidelines as the first line of treatment for depression with comorbid medical condition, TCAs are rated as the first line of treatment for a patient with chronic nonmalignant pain[2] (see Chapter 11). TCAs may be used with other medications but should be monitored closely, especially when used with pain medications such as tramadol.[2] MAO inhibitors should not be combined with codeine, tramadol, or a TCA, and two TCAs should not be prescribed concomitantly.[2]

Clinical Vignettes

Case 9.1

Mr. A., a 75-year-old retired laundry worker, was hospitalized in a state of severe agitation manifesting as delusions about changes in his body—a rapid increase in the size of his nose, his skin becoming more flaccid, and his muscles wasting away. These symptoms had begun 1 month earlier when Mr. A. had given his entire life savings to one of his sons to help him pay off a gambling debt. Once the gambling debt was paid, the son moved to another state and refused further contact with the patient, who now had to struggle financially to support himself and his wife. Mr. A. grew progressively more despondent, developed a sleep and appetite disturbance, but denied any anger at his son. He had no prior history of depression.

Unmanageable at home, Mr. A. spent long hours at a mirror examining his nose, skin, and

muscles. When confronted with this irrational behavior, he became belligerent and assaultive. Despite treatment with citalopram, his condition grew progressively worse, and he finally required hospitalization.

In hospital, Mr. A. began a regimen of desipramine that was increased to a final dosage of 100 mg/day. Perphenazine also was begun and increased to a daily dosage of 12 mg. One week after Mr. A. was on a dosage of 100 mg plasma levels of desipramine were 120 ng/mL. Within 3 weeks, he showed a dramatic response: somatic delusions and preoccupations vanished entirely as did his sleep and appetite disturbance, and he was cheerful, optimistic, and realistic about plans for returning home. However, shortly after hospital discharge, he discontinued desipramine treatment. All his symptoms returned rapidly, and he was rehospitalized. This time he responded after 5 weeks to the same drug regimen. Once again, however, he discontinued use of desipramine, and for a third time his symptoms returned, leading again to rehospitalization.

The course of the third hospitalization differed from that of the first two. He did not respond to the regimen of desipramine and perphenazine after 4 weeks. Because of his progressive agitation, refusal to eat, weight loss, and persistent delusional thinking, ECT was begun. He responded rapidly, with complete symptom remission. Because of his history of psychotropic drug discontinuation, he received maintenance for the first 2 weeks, one treatment per week. During the next month, one ECT treatment was given every 2 weeks; later, one monthly ECT treatment was administered. The patient remained asymptomatic.

The case of Mr. A. illustrates the development of a psychotic depression in later life after an adverse life event in a person with no prior history of a mood disorder. His somatic delusions and their tenacity are characteristic of late-life depression. Drug discontinuation (noncompliance) is also a very common problem among older patients for many reasons, including denial of illness. Mr. A. claimed that he forgot he had been depressed and no longer understood the need for continuing medication.

Physicians should be aware of the tendency of older patients to deny having been ill and to discontinue medications once symptoms have abated. Some elderly patients may develop resistance to antidepressant medications in successive depressive episodes. This case shows that ECT may be therapeutic for drug-resistant depressions and useful as maintenance treatment in a noncompliant elderly patient.

Case 9.2

Mrs. B., a 65-year-old woman who appeared older than her age, was admitted to the hospital in a state of irritability, agitation, and belligerence, with marked speech pressure. A survivor of the Holocaust who had lost most of her family during World War II, Mrs. B. had a long history of psychiatric illness, with clearly documented episodes of psychosis at ages 20 and 50, and was considered to have chronic schizophrenia. At age 62 she suffered a stroke and was paralyzed on the left side. She was living alone at the time of hospital admission.

Because Mrs. B. had manic symptoms, initial therapy included a neuroleptic (risperidone, 1 mg two times a day) and an antimanic drug (lithium carbonate, 300 mg 3 times a day; plasma level 0.70 mEq/L). Within 9 days, her mania disappeared and she became depressed; symptoms included early morning insomnia, severe appetite disturbance, psychomotor retardation, anhedonia, and a pervasive sense of hopelessness and worthlessness. Mrs. B. refused to participate in ward activities and convinced the staff that she had reasons to be hopeless. Her symptoms did not abate even after discontinuing the neuroleptic. After 3 weeks, bupropion was given but had to be discontinued because of agitation. Then, nortriptyline therapy (10 mg at bedtime) began, with the dosage increased slowly to 75 mg and a steady state plasma level of 95 ng/mL.

After two weeks on nortriptyline and lithium, Mrs. B. became pleasant, but the nursing staff began to observe impaired short-term memory as well as moderate disorientation. These symptoms were unnoticed during her depression because she communicated little and was uncooperative. Reduced dosage of lithium and nortriptyline did not lead to cognitive improvement. The Mini Mental State Examination total score was 18, placing her in the range of mild-to-moderate dementia. Neurological examination revealed bilateral extensor plantar reflexes and anomia. Magnetic resonance imaging of the brain revealed an old infarct on the right hemisphere and lacunar lesions in the basal ganglia and the white matter, bilaterally. A diagnosis of vascular dementia was made, and it became apparent that living alone may have played a role in the exacerbation of her affective symptoms. Mrs. B. was discharged to an adult home on a regimen of nortriptyline 75 mg daily and lithium 300 mg three times a day and has remained well.

This case illustrates several typical problems of older depressed patients. Not infrequently, older patients have a longstanding prior psychiatric diagnosis that may mislead clinicians. When Mrs. B.'s past psychiatric history was reexamined, it became clear that, in fact, she had never been schizophrenic but probably had bipolar disorder since early life. Affective disturbances often increase in severity with advancing age, particularly when older people live alone.

The case of Mrs. B. also illustrates the diagnostic difficulties presented by coexisting dementia and depression. Not infrequently, depression or cognitive impairment induced by antidepressant drugs and mood stabilizers is mistaken for dementia. In the case of Mrs. B., however, the reverse was true. In addition to being depressed, she was also demented, but symptoms of dementia were obscured by her affective disturbance. Clinicians must remain alert to all aspects of the mental status examination of older patients, especially when symptoms are changing, resolving, or worsening.

Case 9.3

Mrs. C., a frail 76-year-old woman, was admitted to a psychiatric ward because of a pervasive sense of impending doom, hopelessness, and a wish to die. She paced the hospital floors in a frazzled, agitated state, incessantly moaning but unable to articulate her feelings or thoughts. She was uncooperative and persistently told the staff that she wanted to go home to die.

The patient was unable to tolerate paroxetine and was started on nortriptyline 10 mg at bedtime, with 10 mg increments every 2 days—a regimen on which her blood pressure and pulse remained stable. After she had taken 50 mg of nortriptyline, reaching a plasma level of 105 ng/mL, Mrs. C. had a dramatic response, becoming cheerful and optimistic but not hypomanic. She was discharged on the same dosage of nortriptyline and remained well.

The case of Mrs. C. illustrates several aspects of the agitated, depressed elderly patient who can be very difficult to manage in any treatment setting. Mrs. C.'s treatment was uncomplicated. Her case demonstrates that relatively small dosages of nortriptyline may lead to therapeutic plasma levels followed by antidepressant response. At a daily dosage of 50 mg, Mrs. C.'s plasma level of nortriptyline was in the therapeutic range, attesting to the altered pharmacokinetics of antidepressants in older patients: reduced clearance and altered volume of distribution presumably led to drug accumulation and therapeutic plasma levels at dosages lower than those required by young adult patients. It is important to emphasize, however, that many older patients require dosages comparable to those given to younger adults to achieve therapeutic plasma levels.

Case 9.4

Mr. D., a 68-year-old married tradesman, became increasingly depressed after his retirement and was hospitalized with severe middle insomnia and early morning awakening, anhedonia, delusions of guilt and persecution, a 30-lb weight loss, and psychomotor retardation.

Initially Mr. D. was treated with amitriptyline (100 mg at bedtime), thioridazine (100 mg twice a day) for his delusions of guilt, and biperiden (1 mg twice daily) to counteract possible extrapyramidal effects of thioridazine. He rapidly developed confusion and urinary hesitancy. Amitriptyline was discontinued and imipramine (100 mg a day) was started, without any significant change in his confusion. Imipramine was then discontinued, and he was treated with thioridazine in conjunction with biperiden. Two weeks later, Mr. D. was discharged from the hospital, no longer delusional but still feeling depressed and experiencing psychomotor retardation, early morning awakening, difficulty concentrating, and urinary hesitancy. In the evenings, he was frequently confused and forgetful, symptoms that frequently occur with dementia.

One month later, thioridazine and biperiden were tapered and then discontinued, and risperidone (2 mg daily) was started. Mr. D.'s concentration difficulties and nighttime symptoms gradually cleared but he remained depressed. A course of desipramine was started with a daily dosage of 25 mg and increased by 25 mg every 4 days to a total daily dose of 150 mg. Desipramine was maintained at 150 mg/day for 3 weeks. Since no clinical change occurred, desipramine was increased further to 200 mg per day, resulting in desipramine plasma levels of 130 ng/mL. Within 1 week after this increase, his mood brightened markedly, his sleep disturbance decreased, and his appetite returned to normal.

An ECG taken 2 weeks after recovery from depression revealed atrial flutter. Digoxin therapy was begun and desipramine therapy discontinued. Cardiac monitoring 1 week later revealed irregular AV-node conduction patterns, premature ventricular contractions (PVCs), and premature atrial contractions (PACs). Quinidine was added, and the PVCs and PACs subsided. When his depression rapidly returned, a cardiologist was consulted.

Venlafaxine treatment was added to risperidone (it had been successful previously), and

Mr. D.'s ECG was monitored very closely. After 3 weeks of treatment with venlafaxine (100 mg three times a day), Mr. D. began to improve and eventually recovered from his depression. He continued on this regimen for 6 months, at which time perphenazine was discontinued and venlafaxine was used at the same dosage as maintenance therapy. One year later, Mr. D. was still in remission and had no cardiac problems.

Mr. D. had a severe psychotic depression. Amitriptyline was initially selected because of its sedating effect. Thioridazine was prescribed in combination with amitriptyline to treat the psychotic depression syndrome. Biperiden was used to prevent potential extrapyramidal side effects of thioridazine. However, thioridazine possesses strong anticholinergic properties of its own and rarely leads to extrapyramidal side effects. The prophylactic use of biperiden was therefore unnecessary. Each of these drugs, alone or in combination, can produce severe anticholinergic symptoms in older patients, including a toxic confusional state. Mr. D.'s dementia-like symptoms were actually a CNS anticholinergic confusional state. Because of prolonged drug clearance in older people, several days are often required for these symptoms to subside following drug discontinuation.

Amitriptyline, a tertiary amine tricyclic antidepressant, should rarely be used in older patients and should not be prescribed in combination with thioridazine. Desipramine, a tricyclic antidepressant with less frequent and less severe anticholinergic effects, is less toxic than tricyclic antidepressants of the tertiary amine group. The therapeutic response to 200 mg per day after a lack of response to 150 mg per day attests to the need for high dosages in a few elderly patients. Most older patients require low dosages of tricyclics. However, like many older patients, Mr. D. developed cardiac side effects from the tricyclic antidepressants. Venlafaxine was selected because it has been shown to be effective in younger adults with severe, drug-resistant depressions. In addition, venlafaxine has few drug interactions and does not interfere with the use of quinidine.

The guidelines for continuation and maintenance treatment of geriatric psychotic depression are unclear. In Mr. D.'s case, continuation treatment with risperidone and venlafaxine and maintenance treatment with venlafaxine alone were effective. When elderly patients are exposed to neuroleptics for a long time, frequent examination is necessary to detect the onset of tardive dyskinesia. The dosages of antidepressants used for maintenance therapy should be the same as those used for acute treatment.

Case 9.5

Mrs. E. was a 70-year-old woman with a severe depression characterized by sadness, guilt, anxiety, loss of weight, and early morning awakening. She had experienced a previous episode of depression at the age of 47 and was successfully treated with ECT. SSRIs were not tolerated then, the current episode was treated with imipramine 75 mg daily, but severe breast engorgement necessitated discontinuation of treatment. Amoxapine (up to 100 mg daily) produced no benefit; and maprotiline (150 mg) led to headaches. When imipramine was tried for a second time, breast engorgement returned.

Therapy was begun with phenelzine (up to 45 mg per day) in combination with oxazepam (30 mg per day) for her anxiety and insomnia. After 2 weeks, when no change in her clinical status had occurred, the dosage of phenelzine was increased to 75 mg per day. At the higher dosage, Mrs. E. began to function better and her spirits improved. However, she began to have trouble falling asleep; her insomnia lessened when phenelzine was reduced to 45 mg per day. Treatment was maintained at 45 mg per day for several more weeks. The dosage was then reduced to 30 mg per day, but her anxiety recurred. She was returned to 45 mg a day and did well on that dosage.

The case of Mrs. E. illustrates the successful use of MAOIs in older patients. To avoid insomnia, phenelzine should be given in two dosages, one in the morning and the other in the early afternoon. The case of Mrs. E. demonstrates also the importance of using the lowest dosages of MAOIs that can induce and sustain remission of depression. Most older patients require a careful balance between therapeutic effects and side effects, i.e., a dosage that is therapeutically adequate but does not produce toxicity.

Case 9.6

Mrs. F., an 81-year-old married woman, first became depressed at the age of 68 years. Her depression was characterized by mild anhedonia, weight loss, and early morning insomnia, and her symptoms were related to environmental events as well as to psychological conflict. She had been treated with intensive psychotherapy for 5 years, resulting in substantial psychological insight but no improvement in her mood. During these 5 years she had been given

fluoxetine and sertraline, but both drugs were discontinued within 2 weeks because of restlessness. When she was 73 years old, doxepin therapy was started and increased to a total daily dose of 150 mg. After 3 weeks on doxepin, Mrs. F. began to improve and finally recovered.

Doxepin was prescribed at the same dosage for 6 months after recovery and was then discontinued gradually. For the next 3 years, Mrs. F. was free from depression. Just prior to a carefully planned and eagerly anticipated trip to Europe, she became depressed almost overnight. Doxepin therapy was again started, but when a daily dosage of 150 mg was reached, she became confused and disoriented. These symptoms quickly abated when the dosage of doxepin was lowered and recurred when raised. Her therapy was then changed to desipramine, and after 9 weeks of treatment with a daily dosage of 150 mg (plasma level of 120 ng/mL), her depression resolved without recurrence of confusion or disorientation. For the next 3 years, she continued to take desipramine at the same dosage. Although she had intermittent marital difficulties and was seen with her husband for brief psychotherapy, she was free of depression.

When Mrs. F. was 79 years old, her husband received an incorrect diagnosis of cancer. Within 24 hours of learning of this diagnosis, she became severely depressed. An 8-week trial of desipramine at a daily dosage of 150 mg (plasma levels of 130 ng/mL) failed to help her. She remained depressed, and despite her husband's favorable prognosis, her depression became more severe, and she developed delusions of guilt, psychomotor retardation, and suicidal ideation.

The rapid worsening of her depression and development of delusions and suicidal ideation led to hospitalization and treatment with ECT, six treatments administered unilaterally to the nondominant hemisphere. When Mrs. F. showed no response to these treatments, six bilateral treatments were administered. By the final treatment, she was no longer depressed, but she had substantial confusion and memory loss, requiring constant nursing supervision. ECT was discontinued. Continuation of treatment with nortriptyline (60 mg daily at plasma levels of 95 ng/mL) was prescribed, but her symptoms of depression gradually reappeared. Fluoxetine (10 mg daily) was added, and the dosage of nortriptyline was reduced to 30 mg. Two weeks later, her nortriptyline plasma level was 90 ng/mL. At this level, her mood brightened, and Mrs. F. began to evince interest in her surroundings; formerly an accomplished pianist, she began to play the piano in the hospital ward. Her blood pressure did not increase, nor did she have headaches or other symptoms of hypertension.

This case illustrates again the many complications that may occur in the treatment of depressed elderly patients. Mrs. F. had experienced multiple episodes of depression that increased in frequency and severity as she grew older. The course of depression with aging worsens in some geriatric patients. As Mrs. F. aged, she became unresponsive to tricyclic antidepressants, despite therapeutic doses, and distressing anticholinergic symptoms increased in severity.

Mrs. F.'s ECT treatment also illustrates problems that sometimes arise with elderly patients. Although many older people respond to nondominant unilateral ECT, occasionally response does not occur, especially when a low electrical stimulus is used, and bilateral treatment is necessary. However, as in Mrs. F.'s case, bilateral treatment can be accompanied by substantially increased likelihood of an organic confusional state.

The decision to combine an SSRI (fluoxetine) with a tricyclic antidepressant (nortriptyline) was a bold and relatively unusual decision in geriatric practice. Similar combinations have resulted in an early antidepressant response in younger adults and may even be effective in tricyclic nonresponders. Addition of SSRIs often increases the plasma levels of tricyclic antidepressants through inhibition of the IID6 mitochondrial P-450 cytochrome. When such combinations are prescribed, the dosage of tricyclic should be reduced by half, and plasma levels should be monitored to ensure that they are within the therapeutic window.

Mrs. F.'s experience also illustrates the frequent necessity for psychotherapeutic intervention as part of an overall program of antidepressant treatment. Although her symptoms were relieved by antidepressant drugs and ECT, the life stresses and concerns that contributed to Mrs. F.'s depression (or perhaps exacerbated her symptoms) required careful psychotherapy. A combination of psychotherapy and pharmacotherapy is often as necessary in older patients as with younger adults. For many patients, combination therapy may be more beneficial than either treatment alone.

Case 9.7

Mrs. G., an 81-year-old widowed retired schoolteacher, developed fatigue, mild somnolence, subjective difficulties in concentration, and anhedonia. The onset of symptoms was insidious.

Gradually, Mrs. G. reduced most of her activities. She stopped going to the senior citizen center, which she usually attended four times a week, asked her daughter to arrange for cooked meals to be delivered to her apartment, and gave up her subscription to the local chamber orchestra. She began taking one or two naps during the day, and her night sleep was interrupted. These behavioral changes occurred over a period of 10 to 12 months. Approximately 6 months before these changes, a good friend and bridge partner of Mrs. G. died of a heart attack in her sleep. Mrs. G. reported being distressed for some time by the death of her friend, and she gave up playing bridge. Mrs. G. reported 4 to 5 months of mild depression in her early 30s, after the birth of her second daughter. She recalled that she had asked her mother to stay with her for several weeks because she could not cope with the housework. The depressive syndrome remitted without treatment.

Mrs. G.'s medical history noted chronic hypothyroidism and mild hypertension; she was maintained on triiodothyronine 50 μg daily but did not require antihypertensive treatment. The only family member with a history of psychiatric illness was a maternal aunt whose midlife psychiatric syndrome responded to ECT. During a mental status examination, Mrs. G. appeared tired and requested shortening the examination if possible. She did not have depressed facies and denied feelings of sadness or anxiety, saying that lack of stamina was the reason for restricting her activities. Although she felt that recent changes in her behavior were undesirable, she thought they were the expected consequences of aging. She was not actively suicidal but indicated that it did not seem sensible to continue making plans for the future. Her cognitive functions were unimpaired. Physical examination was unremarkable as was a repeat of thyroid function tests, including thyrotropin blood levels.

Initially Mrs. G. was treated with psychotherapy. Although she appeared engaged, no significant change in her syndrome occurred after 4 months. At the encouragement of her therapist, she agreed to increase her activities, but a trial of methylphenidate increased to 15 mg daily over a period of 2 weeks led to unpleasant feelings of irritability, nervousness, and restlessness. Methylphenidate was discontinued after 4 weeks, and soon after, Mrs. G. fell and broke her humerus, which further restricted her activities and intensified her symptoms. Somnolence during the day increased, and her night sleep became more fitful with many awakenings. She had, however, no loss of appetite or weight. The night sleep disturbance, daytime somnolence and fatigue, history of snoring, and the observation that Mrs. G. was mildly overweight led to the suspicion of sleep apnea syndrome. Polysomnography did not support this diagnosis, however.

Finally, a trial of nortriptyline was begun, dosage was raised over a period of 2 weeks to a daily total of 60 mg. Blood levels (86 ng/mL) obtained 2 weeks after dosage were stabilized and appeared to be in the therapeutic range, although Mrs. G. experienced mildly dry mouth and mild constipation. Her symptoms began to improve after approximately 3 weeks of treatment. Two months later, she resumed most of her activities and became again the self-motivated, witty, and often authoritarian person she was known to be.

The case of Mrs. G. illustrates the diagnostic difficulty presented by geriatric depressive syndromes that do not fully meet DSM-IV criteria for major depression. The insidious onset, lack of energy, somnolence, and absence of profoundly depressed mood suggested either a medical illness, possibly hypothyroidism, or sleep apnea syndrome. The loss of a good friend who had a functional role in Mrs. G.'s life suggested an adjustment disorder. However, the increased severity of the syndrome, history of a previous depressive episode, and possible family history of depression pointed to the possibility of a depressive disorder. Even though the diagnosis of major depression cannot be firmly established in some geriatric patients, the severity of the syndrome justifies a trial of an antidepressant, especially when these drugs are not contraindicated for the patient.

Case 9.8

Mr. H., a 71-year-old retired policeman, was admitted to the coronary care unit of a general hospital for unstable angina. Two days later he suffered a subendocardial myocardial infarction. His cardiac status stabilized after 5 to 6 days, and he was able to move from the coronary care unit to the cardiac telemetry unit. However, soon after he moved, Mr. H. developed anxious and depressed mood, hopelessness, and severe preoccupation with his health that included complaints about symptoms that could not be justified by his cardiac condition. Within 5 days, his appetite decreased, his sleep was interrupted, and he became irritable and agitated, requiring restraints intermittently. Soon Mr. H.'s hypochondriacal preoccupation reached delusional proportions. He maintained that his heart was losing its ability to pump blood in his body and that his extremities were very cold and were gradually ''drying up.'' The consulting psychiatrist diagnosed delusional depression. There was no personal or family history of depression, and although Mr. H. had a history of alcohol abuse, he had been abstinent for 12 years prior to admission.

Mr. H. was initially treated with haloperidol (up to 3 mg daily). Treatment with a neuroleptic was chosen to reduce his agitation and delusions and permit further stabilization of his cardiac state before a tricyclic antidepressant was considered. At this point, Mr. H. was transferred to the psychiatry service. While on haloperidol, his agitation subsided, but he developed suicidal ideation. Eighteen days after his myocardial infarction, his angina was under control while on nitrates and a calcium channel blocker. Holter monitoring showed rare premature ventricular contractions. In consultation with a cardiologist, Mr. H. was started on bupropion but developed restlessness and severe insomnia. When bupropion was substituted by venlafaxine, he developed severe restlessness. This time venlafaxine was substituted by nortriptyline, 25 mg daily. One week later, Mr. H. developed left bundle-branch block (QRS: 1.15) and a first-degree atrioventricular block (PR: 26). A repeat of Holter monitoring showed increased premature ventricular contractions and a few runs of bigeminy. Approximately 1 week after discontinuation of nortriptyline while remaining on haloperidol 3 mg daily, Mr. H.'s atrioventricular block reversed (PR: 18), and the left bundle-branch block subsided (QRS: 0.95). Because depression and suicidal ideation persisted, Mr. H. was started on 7.5 mg of phenelzine, with dosage increased to 30 mg daily over a period of 9 days. Phenelzine was well tolerated; ECGs obtained every 3 days showed no change in cardiac function. Within 2 weeks of phenelzine treatment, his anxiety began to subside, and he soon had a complete remission. Although no change in blood pressure occurred when phenelzine was initially prescribed, 3 weeks later his blood pressure decreased from $145/85$ to $130/80$, with a standing blood pressure of 115/75, although he experienced no distress or symptoms of orthostatic hypotension.

Depression often develops in the context of medical hospitalization for an acute condition and is particularly common in patients suffering myocardial infarction. In this case, the patient developed psychotic depression with acute suicidal ideation. In such cases, ECT can offer dramatic relief of depressive symptoms and can reduce the mortality risk from suicide or agitation. However, ECT was not administered to Mr. H. because of its cardiac risk during the immediate postmyocardial infarction period. Mild dosages of neuroleptics, however, are usually tolerated well by patients with acute myocardial infarction, and these drugs may be used as an interim treatment until cardiac status is stabilized.

For delusional depression, a combination of an antidepressant and a neuroleptic can provide effective treatment. Bupropion was the antidepressant chosen during the first attempt at combination therapy because it has been found safe for cardiac patients. When bupropion was not tolerated, venlafaxine was chosen because it can be effective in severe and even drug-resistant depression. In a postmyocardial infarction patient, follow-up of cardiac status should include daily examination for precordial discomfort, ECG at least every other day, and Holter monitoring if there is evidence of arrhythmia. A cardiologist should also follow the patient closely.

MAOIs are a reasonable alternative in a post-myocardial infarction patient. Although the efficacy of MAOIs has not been adequately studied in delusional depression, clinical impression suggests that a combination of MAOIs and neuroleptics can lead to resolution of this syndrome. Although MAOIs have a minimal effect on cardiac conduction, their major disadvantage is that they preclude the use of sympathomimetic amines. Patients recovering from myocardial infarction may develop acute cardiac events requiring treatment with sympathomimetic amines (e.g., adrenaline in asystole or noradrenaline or dopamine in shock). Orthostatic hypotension is frequent in patients on MAOIs and develops after 3 to 4 weeks of treatment; continuous monitoring of blood pressure is essential for at least 10 weeks after the beginning of treatment.

Case 9.9

Mrs. I., a 76-year-old widow, was diagnosed with AD. Although her dementia was moderate, she was still able to function in her own home with a 24-hour companion. After a fall, she sprained her right ankle, and her mobility decreased for 2 to 3 weeks. During this time, Mrs. I. became apathetic, disinterested in television or socialization, and she developed insomnia and appetite loss. The diagnosis of depression was made and imipramine was begun, with dosage increased by 25 mg every other day up to 75 mg daily. After 6 days on imipramine 75 mg, Mrs. I. developed agitation, confusion, inability to sustain attention, and incoherent speech. Her symptoms were significantly worse at night; she appeared frightened and kept saying that her neighbors were coming to ``put her away.'' Her face was flushed, her skin dry, and her pulse was 120 per minute.

Mrs. I. was admitted to an acute psychiatric unit with a diagnosis of anticholinergic delirium. Imipramine was discontinued, a course of hydration was begun, and her vital signs were monitored closely. Mrs. I.'s pulse decreased to 95 per minute within 24 hours. Three days later, her confusion and agitation lessened, but the symptoms of depression were even more apparent. She gradually developed severe psychomotor retardation and began refusing to eat or drink. Treatment with paroxetine (10 mg daily) began and was increased to 20 mg daily in 3 days. A week later, before paroxetine had a chance to work, Mrs. I. required tube feeding. At this point, paroxetine was discontinued and unilateral ECT was begun. ECT was administered twice a week, and after eight treatments, Mrs. I.'s depression was in complete remission.

Elderly patients are sensitive to the anticholinergic effect of tricyclic antidepressants. Delirium, persistent sinus tachycardia, or urinary retention often lead to discontinuation of these drugs. When the diagnosis of anticholinergic delirium is in doubt, physostigmine 1 mg diluted in 10 mL of normal saline should be administered intravenously over a period of 5 to 7 minutes; the mental status of patients with anticholinergic delirium improves almost immediately. (However, physostigmine should be avoided in very old patients or patients with cardiac disease, as it may cause sinus brachycardia or transient sinus arrest.) Patients with bronchial asthma may develop bronchospasm after administration of physostigmine.

ECT is the treatment of choice in a rapidly worsening depressed elderly patient. ECT-induced memory dysfunction may be more severe and prolonged in demented patients than in nondemented ones. There is no evidence, however, that ECT worsens the course of dementia. Use of brief pulse stimulus, unilateral electrode placement using a high-energy electrical stimulus, and administration of ECT twice instead of three times weekly may reduce ECT-induced memory problems in demented patients.

Case 9.10

Mrs. J., a 103-year-old widowed female, asked her internist to arrange for her to see a psychiatrist because, in her words, ``I am depressed. I pity myself for being in such a state. I'm no good for anything.'' She dated the onset of her symptoms to a 2-week hospitalization for pneumonia and mild congestive heart failure 6 weeks earlier, and she noted a decrease in her appetite beginning 8 weeks earlier. She complained of sleep disturbance, absence of pleasure, lack of motivation, and fatigue that seemed to begin by noon and progress during the day. ``I have no desire to live, no ambition. I would take a pill now to die. It is not worth the struggle. I pray to die.''

First seen in her home, this thin, frail woman was seated comfortably on a cushioned chair, with her legs extended on an ottoman. She wore a pink lace bonnet, housecoat, and shoes. On a table next to her were a telephone, medicine bottles, magazines and newspapers, knitting bag, radio, and a pile of mail. She sat in a sunroom filled with plants and surrounded by windows. An oxygen tank was nearby.

Mrs. J. stated that she had never been depressed until her recent hospitalization. Following discharge, she developed periods of confusion, felt agitated, had decreased appetite, and awoke several times during the night. She reported feeling exhausted by noon each day, having periods of crying (which was unusual for her), and losing interest in her knitting and reading. Her medications at this time included furosemide (20 mg) and occasional use of triazolam (0.125 mg). Her symptoms were consistent with a diagnosis of major depression.

Because of her advanced age and unreliable supervision, cyclic antidepressants and MAOIs were considered potentially toxic. Although SSRIs may be safe, experience with these agents in very old patients is limited. Therefore, CNS stimulants were selected. A trial of a small amount of methylphenidate was begun.

Mrs. J. was started on 1.25 mg methylphenidate at noon daily (each 5 mg tablet broken into four quarters). One day after her first dose, she was more alert, less tired, and reported feeling better. Five days later, her appetite was better, her disposition cheery, she felt relieved to be free of the depressive thoughts, and she no longer wanted to die. Her granddaughter reported: ``My grandmother has improved significantly. She has coherent conversations now. There has been a great change in the last week.'' Her internist visited and found her vital signs and cardiac status to be unchanged and agreed to continue with the medication.

Home visits for psychotherapy were continued once a week for several weeks, at which point Mrs. J. suggested that she no longer needed regular visits and would be pleased to be called periodically ``just to check up.'' She was followed for 9 months with no recurrence of depressive symptoms and no untoward side effects of the methylphenidate. At this point, she was hospitalized with pneumonia and experienced a recurrence of depressive symptoms. Methylphenidate was increased to 2.5 mg

daily, and her symptoms remitted. She was placed in a nursing home and has recently celebrated her 105th birthday.

Case 9.11

Mrs. K., a 70-year-old married woman, had progressively declined in independent functioning over the three-year period since knee-replacement surgery. Previously physically active and socially outgoing, during the postsurgery years she had ceased activities that she had always enjoyed, such as her weekly bridge game, participation in an investors club, and dinner outings with friends. Her adult children reported that their mother had grown increasingly dependent on their father, seeming unable to make decisions without him. They noted that she appeared passive about significant events in her life and had become less involved with her grandchildren. Mrs. K. denied feelings of sadness, changes in sleep and appetite, or suicidal ideation. She did acknowledge fatigue, decreased interest in her earlier activities, and vague feelings of inadequacy, guilt, and worthlessness. She attributed these changes to ``growing old.''

After declining an invitation to her 7-year-old granddaughter's birthday party, her family urged her to see her family doctor for a physical evaluation. The examination and routine laboratory screen, including TSH, B_{12}, and RBC folate, were unremarkable and her physician diagnosed depression. He initiated sertraline at 25 mg per day, followed soon after by complaints of headache and nausea by the patient. Similarly, a trial of paroxetine was subsequently attempted but not tolerated. At this time, Mrs. K.'s symptoms were noted to worsen as she began to display episodic tearfulness and angry outbursts. She was referred to a psychiatrist for further treatment.

Bupropion-SR was initiated and titrated to a dose of 450 mg per day for 6 weeks. This medication was tolerated well but did not improve Mrs. K's depressive symptoms. Bupropion was discontinued and a mirtazapine trial was begun. Mirtazapine at a maximum daily dose of 45 mg led to somnolence and a weight gain of 12 lbs but an equivocal reduction of depressive symptoms.

At that point, mirtazapine was discontinued and a nortriptyline trial was begun. Over 2 weeks, nortriptyline was increased to a target daily dose of 1.2 mg/kg (75 mg daily), which led to a plasma level of 101 ng/ml at steady state (after 1 week on 75 mg). About 3 weeks after initiation of the nortriptyline trial, Mrs. K. began to experience renewed energy and increased her daily activities and social contacts. Her family noted that Mrs. K reached her pre-morbid functional level 10 weeks after starting nortriptyline therapy.

This case illustrates the continued usefulness of TCAs in those individuals who fail trials of SSRI and atypical antidepressants or who are unable to tolerate these medications. TCAs should be considered in the outpatient setting in individuals with significant and debilitating depression even if the severity of depression does not warrant hospitalization. Such patients should have baseline and follow-up EKGs in order to identify a preexisting or an emerging cardiac conduction defect.

Case 9.12

Mr. L., an 80-year old widower, developed severe symptoms of depression 4 months after his wife passed away after a long struggle with cancer. He had experienced at least one previous episode of major depression 25 years earlier following a business setback that had been treated successfully with doxepin. Throughout his adult life, Mr. L had battled alcohol dependence but had been alcohol-free 10 years prior to developing depression symptoms. He was otherwise in good health.

The patient initially presented with low mood and accompanying crying spells, restlessness, and social withdrawal. Neighbors in his apartment building grew more concerned when Mr. L began to appear unkempt and suffered a 15 lb weight loss. When questioned about his change in appearance, the patient became verbally abusive and began to accuse these neighbors of trying to steal from him and evict him from his apartment. The county crisis team was called and the patient was hospitalized.

Combination treatment with venlafaxine 112.5 mg daily and risperidone 1 mg was begun but interrupted when the patient voiced suicidal ideation and refused to eat. As Mr. L's physical state deteriorated, he was hospitalized; a court order was obtained and ECT, over objection, was initiated. The patient was free from paranoia and his mood symptoms remitted after 8 bilateral ECT treatments.

Following ECT, venlafaxine was restarted and titrated to a daily dose of 112.5 mg daily. Approximately 4 weeks later the patient again become sad and tearful and began to eat less. Nortriptyline was initiated and titrated to a dose of 60 mg po qd yielding a blood level of 76 ng/ml. Mr. L's depressive symptoms began to resolve again after 2 weeks on this nortriptyline dose. Arrangements were made for him to

have weekly interpersonal therapy aimed at addressing the loss of his wife and the accompanying social isolation. The patient remained on nortriptyline maintenance therapy, free of depressive symptoms for one year.

This case illustrates the value of tricyclic agents as continuation therapy in patients with severe depression, which frequently necessitates ECT. Mr. L had previously responded to a TCA agent but failed continuation therapy with venlafaxine. If depressive symptoms emerge following successful ECT, moving directly to nortriptyline is often warranted. Moreover, this patient's depressive symptoms arose in the context of a complicated clinical scenario involving bereavement that often necessitates psychotherapeutic intervention. Combination treatment pharmacotherapy and interpersonal psychotherapy has been shown to be most effective in the treatment of late-life depression.

Case 9.13

Mr. M., a 66- year-old married attorney who recently suffered a myocardial infarction and was admitted to a coronary care unit. The patient's multiple medical problems included diabetes, transient ischemic attacks, a 10-year history of angina, and a long history of non-compliance with his diabetes medications. His wife describes him as a "Type A personality"—highly competitive and quick-tempered. Nursing staff described Mr. M as a "nice guy" but demanding and sarcastic at times. He had a previous major depressive episode after the collapse of his first marriage 20 years earlier and had responded well to desipramine.

During his recuperation period following hospital discharge, the patient became depressed with prominent sadness, anhedonia, insomnia with early morning awakening, and loss of appetite. He refused to speak with friends by telephone or receive any visitors and declined to participate in the cardiac rehabilitation program prescribed for him. Mr. M described himself as hopeless and wondered aloud to his wife if he would be better off dead.

The patient visited his previous psychiatrist, who recalled the past positive response to a tricyclic agent. After consultation with a cardiologist, this psychiatrist initiated desipramine 3 weeks after the MI and gradually increased the dose to 100 mg daily. After 3 weeks on this dose, Mr. M. showed a dramatic improvement in mood and activity level. Desipramine raised his heart rate to 100–110 per minute, which was reduced to 90 per minute with atenolol 25 mg twice daily. By the 8th week on desipramine, the patient developed a right bundle-branch block with a QRS: 110 msec, without significant changes in the QTc. Following cardiology consultation, desipramine was stopped and replaced with paroxetine. Within one week, the bundle-branch block was reversed and his QRS interval returned to normal (QRS: 90). His resting heart rate returned to 70 beats per minute and atenolol was discontinued. The patient was maintained on paroxetine for 16 months without the return of depressive symptoms and further ECG changes were noted.

This case illustrates the potential hazards associated with the use of TCAs in postmyocardial infarction patients. AV block, arrhythmias, and persistently increased heart rate are risks inherent in treatment with TCAs. In contrast, SSRIs and bupropion have established cardiac safety and, unless compelling reasons require deciding otherwise, they may be the first agents to prescribe in depressed cardiac patients.

Case 9.14

Mrs. N, a 68-year-old housewife with a history of recurrent depression since her early 20s, experienced early depressive episodes characterized by depressed mood, severe anxiety, weight gain, lack of energy, panic attacks and severe anxiety, periods of insomnia alternating with hypersomnia, and excessive interpersonal sensitivity. During early episodes, she had failed to respond to successive trials of imipramine and nortriptyline at adequate plasma levels (190 ng/mL and 96 ng/mL respectively). During her early 30s she had required psychiatric hospitalization because of severe suicidal ideation, and responded to nine bilateral ECT treatments but began to experience symptoms of depression and anxiety two weeks afterward, despite continuation treatment with doxepin 150 mg daily. At this point, desipramine was discontinued and phenelzine was prescribed after a drug-free period of eight days. The depressive symptoms subsided rapidly and the patient was maintained on phenelzine 45–60 mg daily until the age of 67. Phenelzine was gradually tapered and discontinued on two occasions before elective surgery. On both occasions, Mrs. N. developed symptoms of depression and anxiety, which subsided when phenelzine was reintroduced.

During the past year, Mrs. N's chronic hypertension became difficult to manage. Despite use of diuretics, calcium channel blockers, ACE inhibitors, and beta-blockers, she had persistently high blood pressure interrupted by periods of orthostatic hypotension accompanied by dizziness. In consultation with her internist, phenel-

zine was tapered and discontinued. As in the past, Mrs. N developed symptoms of depression, only this time she experienced a melancholic syndrome with weight loss, psychomotor agitation and retardation, severe diurnal variation, and panic attacks occurring mainly in the morning. Sequential trials of paroxetine, citalopram, venlafaxine, and mirtazapine failed to alleviate her symptoms. Finally, phenelzine was started when Mrs. N developed suicidal ideation and did not consent to any other treatment trial except phenelzine. After a drug-free interval of 15 days, phenelzine, 60 mg daily, was introduced. Again, she responded promptly and became almost asymptomatic within six weeks.

Mrs. N's case illustrates the difficulty some patients experience in remaining well after discontinuation of MAOIs. Whether these patients represent a minority of depressed individuals who selectively respond to MAOIs or whether chronic use of MAOIs interferes with these patients' ability to respond to other agents remains unclear. In either case, MAOIs may need to be introduced earlier for depressed patients who fail other antidepressant trials especially if they have history of earlier response to MAOIs.

Case 9.15

Mrs. O., aged 66, had been healthy, active, and cheerful throughout her life until she suffered a mild stroke. Following a good physical recovery with no significant residual symptoms, she began to realize how serious this episode might have been and she became depressed. Fluoxetine 20 mg was started but had no therapeutic effect. Mirtazapine, which was initially helpful for both her mood and her sleep soon lost its effect.

Mrs. O. described her mood as wishing to withdraw (each morning she would think, ``Oh, God, another day to get through''), with frequent sighing, tearfulness, frequent thoughts of death. Despite being reassured that her physical health was excellent, she found herself focusing on many small physical symptoms, wondering if they were prodromes of another stroke. She noted that her thinking was not as sharp and that she had a great deal of difficulty concentrating (``I think there is something wrong with my brain''). Neuropsychologic tests, as well as office appraisal of her cognitive status, failed to find any cognitive dysfunction. In fact, she was alert, very bright, and had normal memory for a woman of her age.

Gradually it became apparent that Mrs. O.'s depression had a high component of anxiety. Benzodiazepines were helpful for sleep but had little effect on her mood. After unsuccessful trials of several nontricyclics, nortriptyline was begun at a dose of 10 mg and then raised to 20 mg. Mrs. O. experienced significant relief from both depression and anxiety but still felt ''I'm not all the way back yet.'' Fluoxetine, therefore, was restarted at 10 mg, together with nortriptyline. With this combination, she once again felt her old self: active, alert, and cheerful.

Patients who experience a cerebrovascular accident (CVAA) commonly experience a poststroke depression that may vary in degree of severity. Considerable anxiety about a recurrence is not surprising. Poststroke depression often responds well to treatments with TCAs and with SSRIs (see Ch Small). The treatment of Mrs. O. also illustrates the importance of trying successive antidepressants when a response is inadequate or incomplete. The combination of low doses of a TCA along with an SSRI antidepressant is often an effective combination when treatment with either drug alone is insufficient.

Case 9.16

Mr. P., a 72-year-old retired professional man, complained of a lack of purpose in his life. Although he continued to consult on a part-time basis, his days were mainly without meaningful structure or activity, as he defined it. He felt bored, lonely, and useless. The latter feeling revived concerns from his young adult life when he doubted his choice of profession and his usefulness to society. This theme also recurred in his marriage although, in fact, he had a long and stable loving relationship with his wife.

Like many older individuals, Mr. P. undertook a program of exercise, healthy eating, and adult education to occupy his time and improve his mood. Although each activity was successful in its own right, his mood did not improve and he sought psychiatric treatment. There were many issues for psychotherapy and Mr. P. readily agreed to a series of regular psychotherapeutic appointments, but his mood still did not improve. A program of treatment with antidepressant medications was initiated with several SSRIs that were either ineffective or produced significant sexual dysfunction (which was already a problem for this 72-year-old man).

With each medication failure, Mr. P.'s depression worsened and he soon had significant interrupted sleep, diminished appetite with weight loss, and energia and anhedonia. A trial of nortriptyline 10 mg was initiated. As the dose was gradually raised to 90 mg (blood level 90 hg/ml), Mr. P. began to feel substantially better. As his mood improved, themes in psychother-

apy shifted from past feelings of uselessness to planning for his current daytime activity. He became more actively involved in the community, began teaching in continuing education and English-as-a- second-language programs, and embarked on a program of creative writing—all of which helped his mood. He remained stable on a dose of 70 mg of nortriptyline (blood level 80), and occasional psychotherapeutic visits.

Treatment of Mr. P. illustrates the usefulness of TCAs for older individuals. Aside from mildly dry mouth and slight constipation (which he readily treated with over-the-counter medications), nortriptyline actually was better tolerated and more effective than SSRIs. The sexual dysfunction produced by SSRIs (and venlafaxine) may be particularly troublesome for elderly men who experience erectile dysfunction and diminished libido as a consequence of their age.

References

1. Salzman C, Wong E, and Wright BC. Treatment of depression in the elderly, 1996–2001: A literature review. *Biol Psychiatry* 2002;52:265–284.
2. Alexopoulos G, Katz IR, Reynolds RF III, et al. The Expert Consensus Guideline Series: Pharmacotherapy of depressive disorders in older patients. Postgraduate Medicine (Special Report) October 2001.
3. Plotkin DA, Gerson SG, Jarvik LF. Antidepressant drug treatment in the elderly. In: Meltzer HY, ed. *Psychopharmacology: the third generation of progress.* New York: Raven 1987;1149–1158.
4. Kitanaka I, Zavadil AP, Cutler NR, et al. Altered hydroxydesipramine concentrations in elderly depressed patients. *Clin Pharmacol Ther* 1982;31: 51–55.
5. Young RC, Alexopoulos GS, Shamoian CA, et al. Plasma 10-hydroxynortriptyline in elderly depressed patients. *Clin Pharmacol Ther* 1984;35:4: 540–544.
6. Young RC, Alexopoulos GS, Dhar AK, et al. Plasma 10-hydroxynortriptyline and renal function in elderly depressives. *Biol Psychiatry* 1987; 22:1283–1287.
7. Potter WZ, Rudorfer MV, Lane EA. Active metabolites of antidepressants: pharmacodynamics and relevant pharmacokinetics. In: Usdin E, Asberg M, Bertilsson, et al., eds. *Frontiers in biochemical and pharmacological research in depression.* Vol. 39. New York: Raven, 1984:373–390.
8. Schneider LS, Cooper TB, Suckow RF, et al. Relationship of hydroxynortriptyline to nortriptyline concentration and creatinine clearance in depressed elderly outpatients. *J Clin Psychopharmacol* 1990;10:333–337.
9. Mindel JS, Rubin MA, Kharlamb AB. The pupil response to E-10-hydroxynortriptyline in rabbit with ocular sympathetic paresis. *J Auton Nerv Syst* 1990;30:175–198.

10. Wagner A, Ekqvist B, Bertilsson L, et al. Weak binding of 10-hydroxynortriptyline to rat brain muscarinic acetylcholine receptors. *Life Sci* 1984;35:1379–1383.

11. Pollock BG, Everett G, Perel JM. Comparative cardiotoxicity of nortriptyline and its isomeric 10-hydroxynortriptyline. *Neuropsychopharmacology* 1992;6:1–10.

12. Young RC, Alexopoulos GS, Kent E, et al. Plasma 10-hydroxynortriptyline and ECG changes in elderly depressed patients. *Am J Psychiatry* 1985; 142:866–868.

13. Schneider LS. Monitoring hydroxymetabolites of nortriptyline. *N Engl J Med* 1986;314:989.

14. Kutchner SP, Reid K, Dubb JD, et al. Electrocardiogram changes and therapeutic desipramine and 2-hydroxydesipramine concentrations in elderly depressives. *Br J Psychiatry* 1986;148: 676–679.

15. Nelson JC, Athlasoy E, Mazure C, et al. Hydroxy desipramine in the elderly. *J Clin Psychopharmacol* 1988;8:428–433.

16. Nelson JC, Mazure CM, Jatlow PI. Desipramine treatment of major depression in patients 75 years of age. *J Clin Psychopharmacol* 1995;15: 99–105.

17. Murphy GM, Pollock BG, Kirshner M, et al. CYP2D6 Genotyping with oligonucleotide microarray and nortriptyline concentrations in geriatric depression. *Neuropsychopharmacology* 2001;25:737–743.

18. Charney DS, Menkes DB, Heninger GR. Receptor sensitivity and the mechanism of action of antidepressant treatment. Implications for the etiology and therapy of depression. *Arch Gen Psychiatry* 1981;38:1160–1180.

19. Gottfries CG. Amine metabolism in normal aging and in demented disorders. In: Roberts RJ, ed. *Biochemistry of dementia.* London: John Wiley & Sons, 1980:213–241.

20. Mann JJ, McBride PA, Stanley M. Aminergic receptor binding correlates of suicide: methodological issues. *Psychopharmacol Bull* 1986;22: 741–743.

21. Rosen J, Sweet K, Pollock BG, Mulsant BH. Nortriptyline in the hospitalized elderly. Tolerance and side effect reduction. *Psychopharmacol Bull* 1993;29:327–332.

22. Weintraub D. Nortriptyline in geriatric depression resistant to serotonin reuptake inhibitors: case series. *J Geriatr Psychiatry Neurol* 2001;14: 28–32.

23. Streim JE. Drug treatment of depression in frail elderly nursing home residents. *Am J Geriatr Psychiatry* 2000;8:150–159.

24. Robinson DS. Age–related factors affecting antidepressant drug metabolism and clinical response. In: Nandy K, ed. *Geriatric psychopharmacology.* New York: Elsevier/North Holland, 1979: 17–30.

25. Tignol J, Pujol-Domenech J, Chartres JP, et al. Double-blind study of the efficacy and safety of milnacipram and imipramine in elderly patients with major depressive episode. *Acta Psychiatry Scand* 1998;97:157–165.

26. Katona C. Reboxetine versus imipramine in the treatment of elderly patients with depressive disorders: a double-blind randomized trial. *J Affect Disord* 1999;55:203–213.

27. Schweizer E. Buspirone and imipramine for the treatment of major depression in the elderly. *J Clin Psychiatry* 1998;59:175–183.

28. Forlenza OV, Stoppe Jr A, Ferreira RC. Antidepressant efficacy of sertraline and imipramine for the treatment of major depression in elderly outpatients. *Sao Paulo Med J* 2000;118:99–104.

29. Lehmann HE, Kral VA, Ban TA, et al. The effects of trimipramine on geriatric patients. In: Lehmann HE, ed. *Trimipramine: a new antidepressant.* Montreal, Quebec: Psychopharmacology Research Association, 1964.

30. Thaysse P, Bjerre M, Kragh-Sørensen P, et al. Cardiovascular effects of imipramine and nortriptyline in elderly patients. *Psychopharmacology* 1981;74:360–364.

31. Liu B, Anderson G, Mittmann N, et al. Use of selective serotonin-reuptake inhibitors or tricyclic antidepressants and risk of hip fractures in elderly people. *Lancet* 1998;351:1303–1307.

32. Thapa PB, Gideon P, Cost TW, et al. Antidepressants and the risk of falls among nursing home residents. *N Engl J Med* 1998;339:875–882.

33. Glassman AH, Preud'homme XA. Review of the cardiovascular effects of tricyclic antidepressants. *J Clin Psychiatry* 1993;54(2 suppl):16–22.

34. Roose SP, Glassman AH, Siris SG, et al. Comparison of imipramine- and nortriptyline-induced orthostatic hypotension: a meaningful difference. *J Clin Psychopharmacol* 1981;1:316–319.

35. Glassman AH, Johnson LL, Giardina EGV, et al. The use of imipramine in depressed patients with congestive heart failure. *JAMA* 1983;250: 1997–2001.

36. Langhrisi-Thode F, Pollock BG, Miller M, et al. Comparative effects of sertraline and nortriptyline on body sway in older depressed patients. *Am J Geriatr Psychiatry* 1995;3:217–228.

37. Kantor SJ, Glassman AH. The use of tricyclic antidepressant drugs in geriatric patients. In: Eisdorfer C, Fann WE, eds. *Psychopharmacology of aging.* New York: Spectrum, 1980:99–118.

38. Roose SP, Glassman AH, Giardina EGV, et al. Tricyclic antidepressants in depressed patients with cardiac conduction disease. *Arch Gen Psychiatry* 1987;44:273–275.

39. Roose SP, Dalack GW. Treating the depressed patient with tricyclic antidepressants. *J Clin Psychiatry* 1992;53(9 suppl):25–31.

40. Glassman AH, Roose SP, Bigger JT Jr. The safety of tricyclic antidepressants in cardiac patients. Risk–benefit measures. *JAMA* 1993;2673–2675.

41. Pollock BG, Perel JM, Paradis CF, et al. Metabolic and physiologic consequences of nortriptyline treatment in the elderly. *Psychopharmacol Bull* 1994;30:145–151.

42. van Ravenswaaij-Arts CMA, Kollee LAA, Hopman JCW, et al. Heart rate variability. *Ann Intern Med* 1993;118:436–447.

43. Roose SP, Laghrissi-Thode F, Kennedy JS, et al. Comparison of paroxetine and nortriptyline in depressed patients with ischemic heart disease. *JAMA* 1998; 279: 287–291.

44. Roose SP, Dalack GW, Woodring S. Death, depression, and heart disease. *J Clin Psychiatry* 1991;52(suppl 6):34–39.

45. Korkushko OV, Shatilo VB, Plachinda YI, et al. Autonomic control of cardiac chronotropic function in man as a function of age: assessment by power spectral analysis of heart rate variability. *J Auton Nerv Syst* 1991;32:191–198.

46. Giardina EGV, Bigger JT Jr. Antiarrhythmic effect of imipramine hydrochloride in patients with ventricular premature complexes without psychological depression. *Am J Cardiol* 1982;50: 172–179.

47. Rosen J, Pollock BG, Altieri LP. Treatment of nortriptyline's side effects in elderly patients: a double blind study of bethanechol. *Am J Psychiatry* 1993;150:1249–1251.

48. Young RC, Mattis S, Alexopoulos GS, et al. Verbal memory and plasma drug considerations in elderly depressives treated with nortriptyline. *Psychopharmacol Bull* 1991;27:291–294.

49. Branconnier RJ, DeVitt DR, Cole JO, et al. Amitriptyline selectively disrupts verbal recall from secondary memory of the normal aged. *Neurobiol Aging* 1982;3:55–59.

50. Rigler SK, Webb MJ, Redford L, et al. Weight outcomes among antidepressant users in nursing facilities. *J Am Geriatr Soc* 2001;49:49–55.

51. Weber E, Stack J, Pollock BG, et al. Weight change in older depressed patients during acute pharmacotherapy with paroxetine and nortriptyline: A double-blind randomized trial. *Am J Geriatr Psychiatry* 1999;8:245–250.

52. Lustman PJ, Griffith LS, Clouse RE, et al. Effects of nortriptyline on depression and glycemic control in diabetes: results of a double-blind, placebo-controlled trial. *Psychosom Med* 1997;59: 241–250.

53. Eerdewegh VM, Clayton PJ. Bereavement. In: Michels P, ed. *Psychiatry*. Philadelphia: JB Lippincott, 1988.

54. Murrell SA, Norris F, Hutchins G. Distribution and desirability of life events in older adults: population and policy implications. *J Community Psychiatry* 1984;12:301–311.

55. Pasternak RE, Reynolds CF III, Schlernitzauer M, et al. Acute open-trial nortriptyline therapy of bereavement-related depression in late life. *J Clin Psychiatry* 1991;52:7:307–310.

56. Bruce ML, Kim K, Leaf PJ, et al. Depressive episodes and dysphoria resulting from conjugal bereavement in a prospective community sample. *Am J Psychiatry* 1990;147:608–611.

57. Georgotas A, McCue RE, Cooper T, et al. Clinical predictors of response to antidepressants in elderly patients. *Biol Psychiatry* 1987;22:733–740.

58. Georgotas A, McCue RE, Hapworth W, et al. Comparative efficacy and safety of MAOIs versus TCAs in treating depression in the elderly. *Biol Psychiatry* 1986;21:1155–1166.

59. Kurtz NM and Robinson DS. Monoamine oxidase inhibitors. In: A Georgotas and R Canao, eds. *Depression and mania*. New York: Elsevier, 1988:358–371.

60. Robinson DS, Nies A, Ravaris L, et al. Clinical pharmacology of phenelzine. *Arch Gen Psychiatry* 1978;35:629–635.

61. Georgotas A, McCue RE, Cooper T, et al. How effective and safe is continuation therapy in elderly depressed patients? *Arch Gen Psychiatry* 1988;45:929–932.

62. Robinson DS, Nies H. Demographic biologic and other variables affecting monoamine oxidase activity. *Schizophr Bull* 1980;6:298–307.

63. Alexopoulos GS, Lieberman KW, Young RC, et al. Platelet MAO activity and age at onset of depression in elderly depressed women. *Am J Psychiatry* 1984;141:1276–1278.

64. Alexopoulos GS, Young RC, Lieberman KW, et al. Platelet MAO activity in geriatric patients with depression and dementia. *Am J Psychiatry* 1987; 144:1480–1483.

65. Mendlewicz J, Youdim MB. L-deprenyl, a selective monoamine oxidase type B inhibitor, in the treatment of depression; a double blind evaluation. *Br J Psychiatry* 1983;142:508–511.

66. Bodkin JA, Amsterdam JD. Transdermal selegilene in major depression: a double-blind, placebo-controlled, parallel-group study in outpatients. *Am J Psychiatry* 2002;159:1869–1875.

67. Lotufo-Neto F, Trivedi M, Thase ME. Meta-analysis of the reversible inhibitors of monoamine oxidase type A moclobemide and brofaromine for the treatment of depression. *Neuropsychopharmacology* 1999;20:226–247.

68. Satel SL, Nelson JC. Stimulants in the treatment of depression: a critical overview. *J Clin Psychiatry* 1989;50:241–249.

69. Wallace AE, Kofoed LL, West AN. Double-blind, placebo-controlled trial of methylphenidate in older, depressed medically ill patients. *Am J Psychiatry* 1995;152:929–931.

70. Kaplitz SE. Withdrawn, apathetic geriatric patients responsive to methylphenidate. *J Am Geriatr Soc* 1975;23:271–276.

71. Teitelman E. Off-label uses of modafinil. *Am J Psychiatry* 2001; 158:970–971.

72. Zifko UA, Rupp M, Schwarz S, et al. Modafinil in treatment of fatigue in multiple sclerosis. Results of an open-label study. *J Neurol* 2002;249: 983–987.

73. Kaufman KR, Menza MA, Fitzsimmons A. Modafinil montherapy in depression. *Eur Psychiatry* 2002;17:167–169.

74. Menza MA, Kaufman KR, Castellanos A. Modafinil augmentation of antidepressant treatment of depression. *J Clin Psychiatry* 2000;61:378–381.

75. De Batiste C. Modafinil as adjunctive treatment of fatigue and hypersomnia in major depression. Annual Meeting of the American Psychiatric Association, New Orleans, LA, 2001.

76. Schwartz TL, Lees L, Beadle M, et al. Modafinil in the treatment of depression with severe comorbid medical illness. *Psychosomatic* 2002;336–337.

77. Kevin SL, Pahkala K. Delusional depression in the elderly. A community study. *Gerontol* 1989; 22:236–241.

78. Meyers BS. Geriatric delusional depression. *Clin Geriatr Med* 1992;8:299–308.

79. Baldwin RC. Delusional and non-delusional depression in late life. Evidence for distinct subtypes. *Br J Psychiatry* 1988;152:39–44.

80. Sands JR, Harrow M. Psychotic unipolar depression at followup: factors related to psychosis in the affective disorders. *Am J Psychiatry* 1994;151: 995–1000.

81. Roose SP, Glassman AH, Walsh T, et al. Depres-

sion, delusions, and suicide. *Am J Psychiatry* 1983; 140:1150–1162.

82. Alexopoulos GS, Young RC, Meyers BS. Outcome of geriatric delusional depression [Abstract]. American Psychiatric Association, Annual Meeting, New Orleans, LA, 1991.

83. Isometsa E, Henriksson M, Aro H, et al. Suicide in psychotic major depression. *J Affective Disord (Netherlands)* 1994;31:187–191.

84. Greenwald BS, Kramer-Ginsberg E, Marin DB, et al. Dementia with coexistent major depression. *Am J Psychiatry* 1989;146:1472–1478.

85. Alexopoulos GS, Meyers BS, Young RC, et al. The course of geriatric depression with "reversible dementia": a controlled study. *Am J Psychiatry* 1993;150:1693–1699.

86. Finlay-Jones R, Parker G. A consensus conference on psychotic depression. *Aust NZ J Psychiatry* 1993;27:581–589.

87. Spiker DG, Weiss JC, Dealy RS, et al. The pharmacological treatment of delusional depression. *Am J Psychiatry* 1985;142:430–436.

88. Meyers BS, Klimstra SA, Gabriele M, et al. Continuation treatment of delusional depression in older adults. *Am J Geriatr Psychiatry* 2001;9: 415–422.

89. Mulsant BH, Sweet RA, Rosen J, et al. A double-blind randomized comparison of nortriptyline plus perphenazine versus nortriptyline plus placebo in the treatment of psychotic depression of late life. *J Clin Psychiatry* 2001;62:597–604.

90. Zanardi R, Franchini L, Serretti A, et al. Venlafaxine versus fluvoxamine in the treatment of delusional depression: a pilot double-blind controlled study. *J Clin Psychiatry* 2000;61:26–29.

91. Clinical Research Centre. The Norwick Park ECT Trial: predictors of response to real and simulated ECT. *Br J Psychiatry* 1984;114:227–237.

92. Sackeim HA, Haskett RF, Mulsant BH, et al. Continuation pharmacotherapy in the prevention of relapse following electroconvulsive therapy. *JAMA* 2001;285:1299–1307.

93. Hardy BG, Shulman KI, Zucchero C, et al. Gradual discontinuation of lithium augmentation in elderly patients with unipolar depression. *J Clin Psychopharmacology* 1997;17:22–26.

Table 9.2 References

Altamura AC, Mauri MC, Colacurcio F, et al. Efficacy and tolerability of fluoxetine in the elderly: a double-blind study verus amitriptyline. *Int Clin Psychopharmacol* 1989a;4(suppl 1):103–106.

Altamura AC, Mauri MC, Rudas N, et al. Trazodone in late life depressive states: a double-blind multicenter study versus amitriptyline and mianserin. *Psychopharmacology* 1988;95(suppl):34–36.

Altamura AC, Percudani M, Guercetti G, et al. Clinical activity and tolerability of trazodone, mianserin, and amitriptyline in elderly subjects with major depression: a controlled multicenter trial. *Clin Neuropharmacol* 1989b;12(Suppl):s25–s33.

Ather SA, Ankier SI, Middleton RSW. A double-blind evaluation of trazodone in the treatment of depression in the elderly. *Br J Clin Practice* 1985; 39:192–199.

Bjerre M, Gram LF, Kragh-Sørensen P, et al. Dose-dependent kinetics of imipramine in elderly patients. *Psychopharmacology* 1981;75:354–357.

Blacker R, Shanks NJ, Chapman N, et al. The drug treatment of depression in general practice: a comparison of nocte administration of trazodone with mianserin, dothiepin and amitriptyline. *Psychopharmacology* 1988;95:18–24.

Bondareff W, Alpert M, Richter E, et al. Comparison of sertraline and nortriptyline in the treatment of major depressive disorder in late life. *Am J Psychiatry* 2000;157:729–736

Branconnier RJ, Cole JO, Ghazvinan S, et al. Treating the depressed elderly patient: the comparative pharmacology of mianserin and amitriptyline. *Adv Biochem Psychopharmacol* 1982;32: 195–212.

Brodie NH, McChie RL, O'Hara H, et al. Anxiety/depression in elderly patients. A double-blind comparative study of fluphenazine/nortriptyline and promazine. *Practitioner* 1975;215:660–664.

Brymer C, Winograd CH. Fluoxetine in elderly patients: is there cause for concern? *J Am Geriatr Soc* 1992;40:902–905.

Bump GM, Mulsant BH, Pollock BG, et al. Paroxetine versus nortriptyline in the the continuation and maintenance treatment of depression in the elderly. *Depress Anxiety* 2001;13:38–44.

Burch JE, Ahmed O, Hullin RP, et al. Antidepressive effect of amitriptyline treatment with plasma drug levels controlled within three different ranges. *Psychopharmacology* 1988;94:197–205.

Buysse DJ, Reynolds CF III, Houck PR, et al. Does lorazepam impair the antidepressant response to nortriptyline and psychotherapy? *J Clin Psychiatry* 1997;58:426–432.

Cohn CK, Shrivastava R, Mendels J, et al. Double-blind, multicenter comparison of sertraline and amitriptyline in elderly depressed patients. *J Clin Psychiatry* 1990;51:28–33.

Cohn JB, Varga L, Lyford A. A two-center double-blind study of nomifensine, imipramine and placebo in depressed geriatric outpatients. *J Clin Psychiatry* 1984;45(4 sec 2):68–72.

Cutler NR, Zavadil AP, Linnoila M, et al. Effects of chronic desipramine on plasma norepinephrine concentrations and cardiovascular parameters in elderly depressed women: a preliminary report. *Biol Res* 1984;19:549–556.

Dawling S, Crome P, Braithwaite R. Pharmacokinetics of single oral doses of nortriptyline in depressed elderly hospital patients and young healthy volunteers. *Clin Pharmacokinet* 1980;5: 394–401.

Dawling S, Crome P, Heyer EJ, et al. Nortriptyline therapy in elderly patients: dosage prediction from plasma concentration at 24 hrs. after a single 50 mg dose. *Br J Psychiatry* 1981;139:413–416.

Dietch JT, Fine M. The effect of nortriptyline in elderly patients with cardiac conduction disease. *J Clin Psychiatry* 1990;51:65–67.

Dinan TG, Barry S. Responses of growth hormone to desipramine in endogenous and non–endogenous depression. *Br J Psychiatry* 1990;156: 680–684.

Dunner DL, Cohn JB, Walshe T III, et al. Two combined, multicenter double-blind studies of paroxetine and doxepin in geriatric patients with major depression. *J Clin Psychiatry* 1992;160: 217–222.

Eklund K, Dunbar GC, Pinder RM, et al. Mianserin and imipramine in the treatment of elderly depressed patients. *Acta Psychiatr Scand* 1985; 72(suppl 320):54–59.

Fairweather DB, Kerr JS, Harrison DA, et al. A double-blind comparison of the effects of fluoxetine and amitriptyline on cognitive function in elderly depressed patients. *Human Psychopharmacology* 1993;8:41–47.

Feighner JP, Cohn JB. Double-blind comparative trials of fluoxetine and doxepin in geriatric patients with major depressive disorder. *J Clin Psychiatry* 1985;46:20–25.

Finkel SI, Richter EM. Double-blind comparison of sertraline and nortriptyline in late-life depression. Presented at the VIIIth Congress of the European College of Neuropsychopharmacology, Venice, Italy, October 1, 1995.

Finkel SI, Richter EM, Clary CM. Comparative efficacy and safety of sertraline versus nortriptyline in major depression in patients 70 and older. *Int Psychogeriatr* 1999;11:85–99.

Forlenza OV, Junior AS, Hirala ES, et al. Antidepressant efficacy of sertraline and imipramine for the treatment of major depression in elderly outpatients. *Sao Paolo Med J* 2000;118:99–104.

Gentsch C, Lichsteiner M, Gaspar M, et al. Platelet-sup-3H-imipramine binding sites in depressed patients and healthy controls: a comparison between morning and afternoon samples. *J Affect Disord* 1989;6:65–70.

Georgotas A, Stokes PE, Krakowski M, et al. Hypothalamic–pituitary–adrenocortical function in geriatric depression: diagnostic and treatment implications. *Biol Psychiatry.* 1984;19:685–93.

Georgotas A, McCue RE, Hapworth W, et al. Comparative efficacy and safety of MAOIs versus TCAs in treating depression in the elderly. *Biol Psychiatry* 1986a;21:1155–1166.

Georgotas A, Stokes PE, McCue RE, et al. The usefulness of DST in predicting response to antidepressants: a placebo-controlled study. *J Affect Disord* 1986b;11:22–28.

Georgotas A, McCue RE, Friedman E, et al. A placebo-controlled comparison of the effect of nortriptyline and phenelzine on orthostatic hypotension in elderly depressed patients. *J Clin Psychopharmacol* 1987a;7:413–416.

Georgotas A, Schweitzer J, McCue RE, et al. Clinical and treatment effects of 3H-clonidine and 3H-imipramine binding in elderly depressed patients. *Life Sciences* 1987b;40:2137–2143.

Georgotas A, McCue RE, Cooper T, et al. Clinical predictors of response to antidepressant in elderly patients. *Biol Psychiatry* 1987c;22:733–740.

Georgotas A, McCue RE, Friedman E, et al. Electrocardiographic effects of nortriptyline, phenelzine and placebo under optimal treatment conditions. *Am J Psychiatry* 1987d;144:798–801.

Georgotas A, McCue RE, Friedman E, et al. Response of depressive symptoms to nortriptyline, phenelzine and placebo. *Br J Psychiatry* 1987e;151: 102–106.

Georgotas A, McCue RE, Cooper TB, et al. How effective and safe is continuation therapy in elderly depressed patients? Factors affecting relapse rate. *Arch Gen Psychiatry* 1988;45:929–932.

Georgotas A, McCue RE. Relapse of depression in patients after effective continuation of therapy. *J Affective Disord* 1989a;17:159–164.

Georgotas A, McCue RE. The additional benefit of extending an antidepressant trial past seven weeks in the depressed elderly. *Int J Geriatr Psychiatry* 1989b;4(4):191–195.

Georgotas A, McCue RE, Cooper TB, et al. Factors affecting the delay of antidepressant effect in responders to nortriptyline and phenelzine. *Psychiatry Res* 1989b;28:1–9.

Geretsegger C, Stuppaeck CH, Mair M, et al. Multicenter double-blind study of paroxetine and amitriptyline in elderly depressed inpatients. *Psychopharmacology* 1995;119:277–281.

Gerner R, Estabrook W, Steuer K, et al. Treatment of geriatric depression with trazodone, imipramine and placebo: a double-blind study. *J Clin Psychiatry* 1980;41:216–220.

Goldstein SE, Birnbom F, Laliberte R. Nomifensine in the treatment of depressed geriatric patients. *J Clin Psychiatry* 1982;43:287–289.

Green TD, Reynolds CF III, Mulsant BF, et al. Accelerating antidepressant response in geriatric depression: a post hoc comparison of combined sleep deprivation and paroxetine versus monotherapy with paroxetine, nortriptyline, or placebo. *J Geriatr Psychiatry Neurol* 1999;12:67–71.

Guillibert E, Pelicier Y, Archambault JP. A double-blind, multicentre study of paroxetine versus clomipramine in depressed elderly patients. *Acta Psychiatr Scand* Suppl 1989;350:132–134.

Gwirtsman EH, Ahles S, Halaris A, et al. Therapeutic superiority of maprotiline versus doxepin in geriatric depression. *J Clin Psychiatry* 1983;44: 449–453.

Halikas J. Two combined, multicentre, doxepin–controlled, double-blind studies of paroxetine in geriatric depressed outpatients. Proceedings of the 5th World Congress of Biological Psychiatry, Florence, Italy, 1991.

Hayes RL, Garner RH, Fairbanks L, et al. ECG findings in geriatric depressives given trazodone, placebo or imipramine. *J Clin Psychiatry* 1983;44: 180–183.

Hoff AL, Shukla S, Helms PM, et al. The effects of nortriptyline on cognition in elderly depressed patients. *J Clin Psychopharmacol* 1990;10:231–232.

Høyberg OJ, Maragakis B, Mullin J, et al. A double-blind multicentre comparison of mirtazapine and amitriptyline in elderly depressed patients. *Acta Psychiatr Scand* 1996;93:184–190.

Hutchinson DR, Tong S, Moon CA, et al. Paroxetine in the treatment of elderly depressed patients in general practice: a double-blind comparison with amitriptyline. *Int Clin Psychopharmacol* 1992; 6(supp 4):43–51.

Jarvik LF, Mintz J, Steuer JL, et al. Treating geriatric depression: a twenty-six week interim analysis. *J Am Geriatr Soc* 1982;30:713–717.

Jarvik LF, Read SL, Mintz J, et al. Pretreatment of orthostatic hypotension in geriatric depression: predictor of response to imipramine and doxepin. *J Clin Psychopharmacol* 1983;3:368–372.

Katona CL, Hunter BN, Bray J. A double-blind comparison of the efficacy and safety of paroxetine and imipramine in the treatment of depression with dementia. *Int J Geriatr Psychiatry* 1998;13: 100–108.

Katona C, Bercoff E, Chiu E, et al. Reboxetine versus imipramine in the treatment of elderly patients with depressive disorders: a double-blind randomised trial. *J Affect Disord* 1999;55:203–213.

Katz IR, Simpson GM, Jethanandani V, et al. Steady state pharmacokinetics of nortriptyline in the frail elderly. *Neuropsychopharmacology* 1989;2: 229–236.

Katz IR, Simpson GM, Curlik SM, et al. Pharmacologic treatment of major depression for elderly patients in residential care settings. *J Clin Psychiatry* 1990;51(suppl):41–48.

Kernohan WJ, Chambers JL, Wilson WT, et al. Effects of nortriptyline on the mental and social adjustment of geriatric patients in residential care settings. *J Am Geriatr Soc* 1967;15:196–202.

Kin NM, Nair NP, Amin M, et al. The dexamethasone supression test and treatment outcome in elderly depressed patients participating in a placebo-controlled multicenter trial involving moclobemide and nortriptyline. *Biol Psychiatry* 1997; 42:925–931.

Koenig HG, Goli V, Shelp F, et al. Antidepressant use in elderly medical inpatients: lessons from an attempted clinical trial. *J Gen Intern Med* 1989;4: 498–505.

Koncevoj VA, Kolibas E, Psatnickij AN, et al. Comparison of the side effects of tricyclic and tetracyclic antidepressants in old age depression. *Activ Nerv Sup* 1989;31:288–289.

Kumar V, Smith RC, Reed K, et al. Plasma levels and effects of nortriptyline in geriatric depressed patients. *Acta Psychiatr Scand* 1987;75:20–28.

Kunik ME, Pollock BG, Perel JM, et al. Clomipramine in the elderly: tolerance and plasma levels. *J Geriatr Psychiatry Neurol* 1994;7:139–143.

Kushnir SL. Diagnosis and treatment of depression in a 102-year-old woman (letter). *JAMA* 1988;259: 2547.

Kutcher SP, Shulman KI, Reed K. Desipramine plasma concentrations and therapeutic response in elderly depressives: a naturalistic pilot study. *Can J Psychiatry* 1986;31:752–754.

Kyle CJ, Petersen HEH, Overo KF. Comparison of the tolerability and efficacy of citalopram and amitriptyline in elderly depressed patients treated in general practice. *Depress Anxiety* 1998; 8:147–153.

Laghrissi-Thode F, Pollock BG, Miller MC, et al. Double-blind comparison of paroxetine and nortriptyline on the postural stability of late-life depressed patients. *Psychopharmacol Bull* 1995; 31: 659–663.

Lakshmanan M, Mion LC, Frengley JD. Effective low dosage tricyclic antidepressant treatment for depressed geriatric rehabilitation patients: a double-blind study. *J Am Geriatr Soc* 1986;34:421–426.

Mamo DC, Sweet RA, Mulsant BH, et al. Effect of nortriptyline and paroxetine on extrapyramidal signs and symptoms: A prospective double-blind study in depressed elderly patients. *Am J Geriatr Psychiatry* 2000;8:226–231.

Mamo DC, Pollock BG, Mulsant B, et al. Effects of nortriptyline and paroxetine on postural sway in depressed elderly patients. *Am J Geriatr Psychiatry* 2002; 10:199–205.

Maraccini RL, Reynolds CF III, Houck PR, et al. A double-blind placebo-controlled assessment of nortriptyline's side-effects during 3-year maintenance treatment in elderly patients with recurrent major depression. *Int J Geriat Psychiatry* 1999; 14:1014–1018.

McCue RE, Georgotas A, Suckow RF, et al. 10-hydroxynortriptyline and treatment effects in elderly depressed patients. *J Neuropsychiatry Clin Neurosci* 1989a;1:176–180.

McCue RE, Georgotas A, Nagachandran N, et al. Plasma levels of nortriptyline and 10-hydroxynortriptyline and treatment-related electrocardiographic changes in the elderly depressed. *J Psychiatry Res* 1989b;23:73–79.

McEntee WJ, Coffey DJ, Bondareff W, et al. A double-blind comparison of sertraline and nortriptyline in the treatment of depressed geriatric outpatients. Poster presented at the 148th Annual Meeting of the American Psychiatric Association, Miami, FL, 1995.

Merideth CH, Feighner JP, Hendrickson G. A double-blind comparative evaluation of the efficacy and safety of nomifensine, imipramine, and placebo in depressed geriatric outpatients. *J Clin Psychiatry* 1984;45:73–77.

Meyers BS, Mei-Tal V. Empirical study on an inpatient psychogeriatric unit: biological treatment in patients with depressive illness. *Int J Psychiatry Med* 1985–1986;15:11–124.

Meyers BS, Klimstra SA, Gabriele M, et al. Continuation treatment of delusional depression in older adults. *Am J Geriatr Psychiatry*. 2001;9:415–422.

Middleton RWS. A comparison between maprotiline (ludiomil) and imipramine in the treatment of depressive illness in the elderly. *J Int Med Res* 1975;3(supp 2):79–83.

Miller MD, Pollock BG, Rifai AH, et al. Longitudinal analysis of nortriptyline side effects in elderly depressed patients. *J Geriatr Psychiatry Neurol* 1991; 4:226–230.

Miller MD, Curtiss EI, Marino L, et al. Long-term ECG changes in depressed elderly patients treated with nortriptyline: a double-blind randomized placebo controlled evaluation. *Am J Geriatr Psychiatry* 1998;6:59–66.

Mulsant BH, Pollock BG, Nebes RD, et al. A double-blind randomized comparison of nortriptyline and paroxetine in the treatment of depression: 6 week outcome. *J Clin Psychiatry* 1999;60(suppl 20):16–20.

Mulsant BH, Pollock BG, Nebes, R et al. A twelve-week, double-blind, randomized comparison of nortriptyline and paroxetine in older depressed inpatients and outpatients. *Am J Geriatr Psychiatry* 2001;9:406–414.

Nair NP, Amin M, Holm P, et al. Moclobemide and nortriptyline in elderly depressed patients. A randomized, multicentre trial against placebo. *J Affective Disord* 1995;33:1–9.

Navarro V, Gasto C, Torres X, et al Citalopram versus nortriptyline in late-life depression: a 12-week randomized single blind study. *Acta Psychiatr Scand* 2001;103:435–440.

Nelson JC, Price LH, Jatlow PI. Neuroleptic dose and

desipramine concentrations during combined treatment of unipolar delusional depression. *Am J Psychiatry* 1986;143:1151–1154.

Nelson JC, Atillasoy E, Mazure CM, et al. Hydroxydesipramine in the elderly. *J Clin Psychopharmacol* 1988;8:428–433.

Nelson JC, Mazure CM, Jatlow PI. Desipramine treatment of major depression in patients over 75 years of age. *J Clin Psychopharmacol* 1995;15: 99–105.

Neshkes RE, Gerner R, Jarvik LF, et al. Orthostatic effect of imipramine and doxepin in depressed geriatric outpatients. *J Clin Psychopharmacol* 1985; 5:102–106.

Nobler MS, Roose SP, Prohovnik I, et al. Regional cerebral blood flow in mood disorders V.: effects of antidepressant medication in late-life depression. *Am J Geriatr Psychiatry* 2000;8:289–296.

Nystroem C, Haellstroem T. Double-blind comparison between a serotonin and noradrenaline reuptake blocker in the treatment of depressed outpatients: clinical aspects. *Acta Psychiatr Scand* 1985;72:6–15.

Oslin DW, Streim JE, Katz IR, et al. Heuristic comparison of sertraline with nortriptyline for the treatment of depression in frail elderly patients. *Am J Geriatr Psychiatry* 2000;8:141–149.

Pelicier Y, Schaeffer P. A multi–centre, blind study to compare the efficacy and tolerability of paroxetine and clomipramine in elderly patients with reactive depression. *Encephale* 1993;19:257–261.

Petracca G, Teson A, Chemerinski E, et al. A double-blind placebo controlled study of clomipramine in depressed patients with Alzheimer's disease. *J Neuropsychiatry* 1996;8:270–275.

Pollock BG, Perel JM, Paradis CF, et al. Metabolic and physiologic consequences of nortriptyline treatment in the elderly. *Psychopharmacol Bull* 1994;30:145–150.

Pollock BG, Laghrissi-Thode F, Wagner W. Evaluation of platelet activation in depressed patients with ischemic heart disease after paroxetine or nortriptyline treatment. *J Clin Psychopharmacol* 2000a;20:137–140.

Pollock BG, Ferrell RE, Mulsant BH et al. Allelic variation in the serotonin transporter promoter affects onset of paroxetine treatment response in late-life depression. *Neuropsychopharmacology* 2000b;23:587–590.

Reynolds CF III, Perel JM, Kupfer DJ, et al. Open-trial response to antidepressant treatment in elderly patients with mixed depression and cognitive impairment. *Psychiatry Res* 1987;21:111–122.

Reynolds CF III, Perel JM, Frank E, et al. Open-trial maintenance pharmacotherapy in late-life depression: Survival analysis. *Psychiatry Res* 1989; 27:225–231.

Reynolds CF III, Frank E, Perel JM, et al. Treatment of consecutive episodes of major depression in the elderly. *Am J Psychiatry* 1994;151:1740–1743.

Reynolds CF III, Frank E, Kupfer DJ, et al. Treatment outcome in recurrent major depression: a post hoc comparison of elderly ("young old") and midlife patients. *Am J Psychiatry* 1996a;153: 1288–1292.

Reynolds CF III, Frank E, Perel JM, et al. High relapse rate after discontinuation of adjunctive medication for elderly patients with recurrent major depression. *Am J Psychiatry* 1996b;153: 1418–1422.

Reynolds CF, Buysse DJ, Brunner DP, et al. Maintenance nortriptyline effects on electroencephalopgraphic sleep in elderly patients with recurrent major depression: double-blind, placebo- and plasma-level–controlled evaluation. *Biol Psychiatry* 1997;42: 560–567.

Reynolds CF III, Frank E, Dew MA, et al. Treatment of 70+ year-olds with recurrent major depression: Excellent short-term but brittle long-term response. *Am J Geriatric Psychiatry* 1999a;7:64–69.

Reynolds CF III, Miller MD, Pasternak R et al. Treatment of bereavement-related major depressive episodes in later-life: a controlled study of acute and continuation treatment with nortriptyline and interpersonal psychotherapy. *Am J Psychiatry* 1999b;156:202–208.

Reynolds CF IIII, Frank E, Perel JM, et al. Nortriptyline and interpersonal psychotherapy as maintenance therapies for recurrent major depression. *JAMA* 1999c;281:39–45.

Roose SP, Glassman AH, Attia E, et al. Comparative efficacy of selective serotonin reuptake inhibitors and tricyclics in the treatment of melancholia. *Am J Psychiatry* 1994;151:1735–1739.

Rosen J, Pollock BG, Altieri LP, et al. Treatment of nortriptyline's side effects in elderly patients: a double-blind study of bethanechol. *Am J Psychiatry* 1993;150:1249–1251.

Rothblum ED, Sholomskas AJ, Berry C, et al. Issues in clinical trials with the depressed elderly. *J Am Geriatr Soc* 1982;30:694–699.

Rothschild BS. Fluoxetine-nortriptyline therapy of treatment-resistant major depression in a geriatric patient. *J Geriatr Psychiatry Neurol* 1994;7: 137–138.

Rouillon F. A double-blind, multicentre study comparing increasing doses of paroxetine (20–50 mg) and clomipramine (50–150 mg) in elderly patients with major depression. Proceedings of the 5th World Congress of Biological Psychiatry, Florence, Italy, 1991.

Samuelian JC. A dose titration study comparing the efficacy and tolerability of paroxetine and clomipramine in elderly outpatients with moderate depression. Proceedings of the 5th World Congress of Biological Psychiatry, Florence, Italy, 1991.

Sauvage P, Hassel L, Michel J-P. Double blind study of trazodone versus amitriptyline in a geriatric environment. *Psychologie Medicale* 1987;19: 1357–1364.

Schifano F, Garbin A, Renesto V, et al. A double-blind comparison of mianserin and maprotiline in depressed medically ill elderly people. *Acta Psychiatr Scand* 1990;81:289–294.

Schneider LS, Frederickson ER, Severson JA, et al. 3H-imipramine binding in depressed elderly: relationship to family history and clinical response. *Psychiatry Res* 1986a;19:257–266.

Schneider LS, Sloane RB, Staples FR, et al. Pretreatment orthostatic hypotension as a predictor of response to nortriptyline in geriatric depression. *J Clin Psychopharmacol* 1986b;6:172–176.

Schneider LS, Severson JA, Sloane RB, et al. Decreased platelet 3H-imipramine binding in primary major depression compared with depression secondary to medical illness in elderly outpatients. *J Affect Disord* 1988a;15:195–200.

Schneider LS, Cooper TB, Weverson JA, et al. Electrocardiographic changes with nortriptyline and 10-hydroxynortriptyline in elderly depressed outpatients. *J Clin Psychopharmacol* 1988b;8: 402–408.

Schweizer E, Rickels K, Hassman H, et al. Buspirone and imipramine for the treatment of major depression in the elderly. *J Clin Psychiatry* 1998; 59:175–183.

Severson JA, Marusann JO, Osterburg HH, et al. Elevated density of 3-H imipramine binding in aged human brain. *J Neurochem* 1985;45:1382–1389.

Siegfried K, O'Connolly M. Cognitive and psychomotor effects of different antidepressants in the treatment of old age depression. *Int Clin Psychopharmacol* 1986;1:231–243.

Slotkin TA, Whitmore WL, Barnes GA, et al. Reduced inhibitory effect of imipramine on radiolabeled serotonin uptake into platelets in geriatric depression. *Biol Psychiatry* 1989;25:687–691.

Solai LK, Pollock BG, Mulsant BH, et al. Effect of nortriptyline and paroxetine on CYP2D6 activity in depressed elderly patients. *J Clin Psychopharmacol* 2002;22:481–486.

Sørensen B, Kragh-Sørensen P, Larsen NE, et al. The practical significance of nortriptyline plasma control: a prospective evaluation under routine conditions in endogenous depression. *Psychopharmacology* 1978;59:35–39.

Spar JA, LaRue A. Acute response to methylphenidate as a predictor of outcome of treatment with TCAs in the elderly. *J Clin Psychiatry* 1985;46: 466–469.

Stack JA, Reynolds CF III, Perel JM, et al. Pretreatment systolic orthostatic blood pressure (PSOP) and treatment response in elderly depressed inpatients. *J Clin Psychopharmacol* 1988;8:116–120.

Streim JE, Oslin DW, Katz IR, et al. Drug treatment of depression in frail elderly nursing home residents. *Am J Geriatr Psychiatry* 2000;8:150–159.

Thayssen P, Bjerre M, Kragh-Sorensen P, et al. Cardiovascular effects of imipramine and nortriptyline in elderly patients. *Psychopharmacology* 1981;74: 360–364.

Tignol J, Pujol-Domenech J, Chartres JP, et al. Double-blind study of the efficacy and safety of milnacipran and imipramine in elderly patient with major depressive episode. *Acta Psychiatr Scand* 1998;97:157–165.

Tollefson G, Montague-Clouse J, Lesan T, et al. Pharmacokinetic properties of maprotiline in geriatric depression. *J Clin Psychopharmacol* 1989;9: 313–315.

van Laar MW, van Willigenburg APP, Volkerts ER. Acute and subchronic effects of nefazodone and imipramine on highway driving, cognitive functions, and daytime sleepiness in healthy adult and elderly subjects. *J Clin Psychopharmacol* 1995;15: 30–40.

Waite J, Grundy E, Arie T. A controlled trial of antidepressant medication in elderly inpatients. *Int Clin Psychopharmacol* 1986;1:113–126.

Wakelin JS. Fluvoxamine in the treatment of the older depressed patient; double-blind, placebo-controlled data. *Int Clin Psychopharmacol* 1986;1: 221–230.

Walters G, Reynolds CF III, Mulsant BH, et al. Continuation and maintenance pharmacotherapy in geriatric depression: An open-trial comparison of paroxetine and nortriptyline in patients older than 70 years. *J Clin Psychiatry* 1999;60(suppl 20): 21–25.

Weber E, Stack J, Pollock BG, et al. Weight change in older depressed patients during acute pharmacotherapy with paroxetine and nortriptyline: A double-blind randomized trial. *Am J Geriatr Psychiatry* 2000;8:245–250.

Weintraub D. Nortriptyline in geriatric depression resistant to serotonin reuptake inhibitors: case series. *J Geriatr Psychiatry Neurol* 2001;14:28–32.

Weissman MM, Prusoff B, Sholomskas AJ, et al. A double-blind clinical trial of alprazolam, imipramine, or placebo in the depressed elderly. *J Clin Psychopharmacol* 1992;12:175–182.

Wilkins JN, Spar JE, Carlson HE. Desipramine increased circulating growth hormone in elderly depressed patients: a pilot study. *Psychoneuroendocrinology* 1989;14:195–202.

Wolf R, Dykierek P, Gottaz WF, et al. Differential effects of trimipramine and fluoxetine on sleep in geriatric depression. *Pharmacopsychiatry* 2001; 34:60–65.

Young RC, Alexopoulos GS, Shamoian CA, et al. Plasma 10-hydroxynortriptyline and ECG changes in elderly depressed patients. *Am J Psychiatry* 1985;142:866–868.

Young RC, Alexopoulos GS, Dhar AK, et al. Plasma 10-hydroxynortriptyline and renal function in elderly depressives. *Biological Psychiatry* 1987;22: 1283–1287.

Young RC, Alexopoulos GS, Shindledecker R, et al. Plasma 10-hydroxynortriptyline and therapeutic response in geriatric depression. *Neuropsychopharm* 1988;1:213–215.

Zubenko GS, Reynolds CF III, Perel JM, et al. Platelet membrane fluidity and treatment response in cognitively–impaired, depressed elderly: Initial results. *Psychopharmacology* 1988;94:3347–3349.

Zung WWK, Gianturco D, Pfeiffer E, et al. Pharmacology of depression in the aged: evaluation of gerovital H3 as an antidepressant drug. *Psychosomatics* 1974;15:127–131.

Table 9.3 References

Ashford JW, Ford CV. Use of MAO inhibitors in elderly patients. *Am J Psychiatry* 1979;136: 1466–1467.

Georgotas A, Friedman E, McCarthy M, et al. Resistant geriatric depressions and therapeutic response to monoamine oxidase inhibitors. *Biol Psychiatry* 1983b;18:195–205.

Georgotas A, Mann J, Friedman E. Platelet monoamine oxidase inhibition as a potential indicator of favorable response to MAOIs in geriatric depressions. *Biol Psychiatry* 1981;16:997–1001.

Georgotas A, McCue RE. Relapse of depression in patients after effective continuation of therapy. *J Affective Disord* 1989a;17:159–164.

Georgotas A, McCue RE. The additional benefit of extending an antidepressant trial past seven weeks in the depressed elderly. *Int J Geriatr Psychiatry* 1989b;4:191–195.

Georgotas A, McCue RE, Cooper T, et al. Clinical predictors of response to antidepressant in elderly patients. *Biol Psychiatry* 1987c;22:733–740.

Georgotas A, McCue RE, Cooper TB. A placebo-controlled comparison of nortriptyline and phenelzine in maintenance therapy of elderly depressed patients. *Arch Gen Psychiatry* 1989a;46: 783–786.

Georgotas A, McCue RE, Cooper TB, et al. How effective and safe is continuation therapy in elderly patients? Factors affecting relapse rate. *Arch Gen Psychiatry* 1988;45:929–932.

Georgotas A, McCue RE, Cooper TB, et al. Factors affecting the delay of antidepressant effect in responders to nortriptyline and phenelzine. *Psychiatry Res* 1989b;28:1–9.

Georgotas A, McCue RE, Friedman E, et al. A placebo-controlled comparison of the effects of nortriptyline and phenelzine on orthostatic hypotension in elderly depressed patients. *J Clin Psychopharmacol* 1987a;7:413–416.

Georgotas A, McCue RE, Friedman E, et al. Electrocardiographic effects of nortriptyline, phenelzine and placebo under optimal treatment conditions. *Am J Psychiatry* 1987d;144:798–801.

Georgotas A, McCue RE, Friedman E, et al. Response of depressive symptoms to nortriptyline, phenelzine and placebo. *Br J Psychiatry* 1987e;151: 102–106.

Georgotas A, McCue RE, Hapworth W, et al. Comparative efficacy and safety of MAOIs versus TCAs in treating depression in the elderly. *Biol Psychiatry* 1986a;21:1155–1166.

Georgotas A, Reisberg B, Ferris S. First results on the effects of MAO inhibition on cognitive functioning in elderly depressed patients. *Arch Gerontol Geriatr* 1983a;2:249–254.

Georgotas A, Schweitzer J, McCue RE, et al. Clinical and treatment effects of 3H-clonidine and 3H-imipramine binding in elderly depressed patients. *Life Sci* 1987b;40:2137–2143.

Georgotas A, Stokes PE, McCue RE, et al. The usefulness of DST in predicting response to antidepressants: a placebo-controlled study. *J Affective Disord* 1986b;11:21–28.

Jenike MA. Monoamine oxidase inhibitors as treatment for depressed patients with primary degenerative dementia (Alzheimer's disease). *Am J Psychiatry* 1985;142:763.

Kin NMK, Nair NPV, Amin M, et al. The dexamethasone supression test and treatment outcome in elderly depressed patients participating in a placebo-controlled multicenter trial involving moclobemide and nortriptyline. *Biol Psychiatry* 1997; 42:925–931.

Lazarus LW, Groves L, Gierl B, et al. Efficacy of phenelzine in geriatric depression. *Biol Psychiatry* 1986;21:699–701.

Nair NP, Amin M, Holm P, et al. Moclobemide and Nortriptyline in elderly depressed patients. A randomized, multicentre trial against placebo. *J Affective Disord* 1995; 33:1–9.

Roth M, Mountjoy CQ, Amrein R. Moclobemide in elderly patients with cognitive decline and depression: an international double-blind, pla-cebo-controlled trial. *Br J Psychiatry* 1996;168: 149–157.

Sunderland T, Cohen RM, Molchan S, et al. High-dose seligiline in treatment-resistant older depressive patients. *Arch Gen Psychiatry* 1994;51:607.

Table 9.4 References

Askinazi C, Weintraub RJ, Karamouz N. Elderly depressed females as a possible subgroup of patients responsive to methylphenidate. *J Clin Psychiatry* 1986;47:467–469.

Branconnier R, Cole JO. The therapeutic role of methylphenidate in senile organic brain syndrome. In: Cole JO, Barrett J, eds. *Psychopathology in the aged.* New York: Raven, 1980:183–195.

Clark AN, Mankikar GD. *d*-Amphetamine in elderly patients refractory to rehabilitation procedures. *J Am Geriatr Soc* 1979;27:174–177.

Gilbert JG, Donnelly KJ. Effect of magnesium pemoline and methylphenidate on memory improvement and mood in normal aging subjects. *Int J Aging Hum Dev* 1973;4:35–51.

Gurevitch D, Bagne CA, Perl E, et al. A review of psychostimulants in elderly patients with refractory depression. In: JD Amsterdam, ed. *Advances in neuropsychiatry and psychopharmacology. Vol. 2: Refractory depression.* New York: Raven, 1991: 167–175.

Gurian B, Rosowsky E. Low-dose methylphenidate in the very old. *J Geriatr Psychiatry Neurol* 1990;3: 152–154.

Jacobson A. The use of Ritalin in psychotherapy of depressions of the aged. *Psychiatr Q* 1958;32: 474–483.

Kaplitz SE. Withdrawn, apathetic geriatric patients responsive to methylphenidate. *J Am Geriatr Soc* 1975;23:271–276.

Katon W, Raskind M. Treatment of depression in the medically ill elderly with methylphenidate. *Am J Psychiatry* 1980;137:963–965.

Spar JA, LaRue A. Acute response to methylphenidate as a predictor of outcome of treatment with TCAs in the elderly. *J Clin Psychiatry* 1985;46: 466–469.

Wallace AE, Kofoed LL, West AN. Double-blind, placebo-controlled trial of methylphenidate in older, depressed, medically ill patients. *Am J Psychiatry* 1995;152:929–931.

Table 9.5 References

Finch EJ, Katona CL. Lithium augmentation in the treatment of refractory depression in old age. *Int J Geriatr Psychiatry* 1989;4:41–46.

Flint AJ, Rifat SL. A prospective study of lithium augmentation in antidepressant–resistant geriatric depression. *J Clin Psychopharmacol* 1994;14: 353–356.

Hale AS, Procter AW, Bridges PK. Clomipramine, tryptophan and lithium in combination for resistant endogenous depression: seven case studies. *Br J Psychiatry* 1987;151:213–217.

Hardy BG, Shulman KI, Zucchero C. Gradual discontinuation of lithium augmentation in elderly patients with unipolar depression. *J Clin Psychopharmacology* 1997;17:22–26.

Katona CL, Finch EJ. Lithium augmentation for refractory depression in old age. In: Amsterdam JD, ed. *Advances in neuropsychiatry and psychopharmacology. Vol. 2: Refractory depression.* New York: Raven, 1991:177–184.

Kushnir SL. Lithium-antidepressant combinations in the treatment of depressed, physically ill geriatric patients. *Am J Psychiatry* 1986;142:378–379.

Lafferman J, Solomon K, Ruskin P. Lithium augmentation for treatment-resistant depression in the elderly. *J Geriatr Psychiatry Neurol* 1988;1:49–52.

Madakasira S. Low dose potency of lithium in antidepressant augmentation. *Psych J Univ Ottawa* 1986; 11:107–109.

Pai M, White AC, Deane AG. Lithium augmentation in the treatment of delusional depression. *Br J Psychiatry* 1986;148:736–738.

Pande AD, Max P. A lithium-tricyclic combination for treatment of depression. *Am J Psychiatry* 1985; 142:1228–1229.

Reynolds CF, Frank E, Perel JM, et al. High relapse rate after discontinuation of adjunctive medication for elderly patients with recurrent major depression. *Am J Psychiatry* 1996;153:1418–1422.

Schreiber S, Shalev A. Lithium augmentation for mianserin-resistant depression in the elderly. *Harefuah* 1992;123:250–251.

van Marwijk HW, Bekker FM, Nolen WA, et al. Lithium augmentation in geriatric depression. *J Affective Disord* 1990;20(4):217–233.

Weaver KEC. Lithium for delusional depression. *Am J Psychiatry* 1983;140:962–963.

Zimmer B, Rosen J, Thorton JE, et al. Adjunctive lithium carbonate in nortriptyline–resistant elderly depressed patients. *J Clin Psychopharmacol* 1991;11:254–256.

Supplemental Readings

General

Alexopoulos GS, Abrams RC, Young RC, Shamoian CA. Cornell scale for depression in dementia. *Biol Psychiatry* 1988;23:271–284.

Ananth JV, Sohn JH, Ban TA, et al. Doxepin in geriatric patients. *Curr Ther Res* 1979;25:133–138.

Austin LS, Arana GW, Melvin JA. Toxicity resulting from lithium augmentation of antidepressant treatment in elderly patients. *J Clin Psychiatry* 1990;51:344–345.

Baldessarini RJ. *Biomedical aspects of depression and its treatment.* Washington, DC: American Psychiatric Press, 1983.

Cole JO, ed. *Psychopathology in the aged.* New York: Raven, 1980.

Cole JO, Branconnier R, Salomon M, Dessain E. Tricyclic use in the cognitively impaired elderly. *J Clin Psychiatry* 1983;44:14–19.

Crook T, Cohen GD. *Physicians' guide to the diagnosis and treatment of depression in the elderly.* New Canaan, CT: Powley, 1983.

Cutler NR, Narang PK. Implications of dosing tricyclic antidepressants and benzodiazepines in geriatrics. *Psychiatr Clin North Am* 1984;7: 845–861.

Diehl DJ, Houck PR, Paradis C, et al. Pretreatment systolic orthostatic blood pressure and treatment response in geriatric depression: a revisit. *J Clin Psychopharmacol* 1993;13:189–193.

Eastwood MR, Stiasny S, Meier HM, et al. Mental illness and mortality. *Compr Psychiatry* 1982;23: 377–385.

Finkel SI. Efficacy and tolerability of antidepressant therapy in the old-old. *J Clin Psychiatry* 1996;57: 5:23–28.

Georgotas A. Relapse of depression in patients after effective continuation of therapy. *J Affect Disord* 1989;317:159–164.

Georgotas A. The additional benefit of extending and antidepressant trial past seven weeks in the depressed elderly. *Int J Geriatr Psychiatry* 1989;4: 191–195.

Georgotas A, McCue RE. Relapse of depressed patients after effective continuation therapy. *J Affective Disord* 1989;17:159–164.

Georgotas A, McCue RE. The additional benefit of extending an antidepressant trial past seven weeks in the depressed elderly. *Int J Geriatr Psychiatry* 1989;4:191–195.

Georgotas A, McCue RE, Reisberg B, et al. The effects of mood changes and antidepressants on the cognitive capacity of elderly depressed patients. *Int Psychogeriatr* 1989;1:135–143.

Gerner RH. Depression in the elderly. In: Kaplan OJ, ed. *Psychopathology of aging.* New York: Academic Press, 1979:97–148.

Gerner RH, Post RM, Bunney WE. Biological and behavioral effects of one night's sleep deprivation in depressed and normals. *J Psychiatr Res* 1979;15:21–40.

Good MI. The concern of drug automatism. *Am J Psychiatry* 1976;133:948–952.

Halaris A. Antidepressant drug therapy in the elderly: enhancing safety and compliance. *Int J Psychiatry Med* 1986;16:1986–1987.

Heninger GP. Lithium carbonate augmentation of antidepressant treatment. *Arch Gen Psychiatry* 1983;40:1335–1342.

Jarvik L. Antidepressant therapy for the geriatric patient. *J Clin Psychopharmacol* 1981;1:55S–61S.

Jarvik LF, Read SL, Mintz J, et al. Pretreatment orthostatic hypotension in geriatric depression. Predictor of response to imipramine and doxepin. *J Clin Psychopharmacol* 1983;3:368–372.

Kantor SJ, Glassman AH. The use of tricyclic antidepressant drugs in geriatric patients. In: Eisdorfer C, Fann WE, eds. *Psychopharmacology of aging.* New York: Spectrum, 1980:99–118.

Katz IR, Parmelee PA, Beaston-Wimmer P, et al. Association of antidepressants and other medications with mortality in the residential-care elderly. *J Geriatr Psychiatry Neurol* 1994;7:221–226.

Katz IR, Simpson GM, Curlik SM, et al. Pharmacologic treatment of major depression for elderly patients in residential care settings. *J Clin Psychiatry* 1990;51:41–48.

Klerman G, DiMascio A, Weissman M, et al. Therapy of depression by drugs and psychotherapy. *Am J Psychiatry* 1974;131:186–195.

Knegtering H, Eijok M, Huilsman A. Effects of antidepressants on cognitive functioning of elderly patients. A review. *Drugs Aging* 1994;5:192–199.

Lafferman J, Solomon K, Ruskin P. Lithium augmentation for treatment-resistant depression in the elderly. *J Geriatr Psychiatry Neurol* 1989;1:49–52.

Marin RS, Fogel BS, Hawkins J, et al. Apathy: a treatable syndrome. *J Neuropsychiatry Clin Neurosci* 1995;7:23–30.

Miller FT, Freilicher J. Comparison of TCAs and SSRIs in the treatment of major depression in hospitalized geriatric patients. *J Geriatr Psychiatry Neurol* 1995;8:173–176.

Meyers BS, Alpert S, Gabriele M, et al. State specificity of DST abnormalities in geriatric depression. *Biol Psychiatry* 1993;34:108–114.

Panzer MJ, Mellow AM. Antidepressant treatment of pathologic laughing or crying in elderly stroke patients. *J Geriatr Psychiatry Neurol* 1992;5:195–199.

Passeri M, Cucinotta D, Abate G, et al. Oral 5-methyltetrahydrofolic acid in senile organic mental disorders with depression: results of a double-blind multicenter study. *Aging Milano* 1993;5:63–71.

Peabody CA, Whiteford HA, Hollister LE. Antidepressants and the elderly. *J Am Geriatr Soc* 1986;34:869–874.

Preskorn SH. Recent pharmacologic advances in antidepressant therapy for the elderly. *Am J Med* 1993;94:2S–12S.

Prien RF. Somatic treatment of unipolar depressive disorder. In: Frances A, Hales RE, eds. *Review of psychiatry*. Vol. 7. Washington, DC: American Psychiatric Association, 1988:213–234.

Remick RA, Blasberg B, Patterson BD, et al. Clinical aspects of xerostomia. *J Clin Psychiatry* 1983;44:63–65.

Reynolds CF III. Treatment of depression in late life. *Am J Med* 1994;97:398–468.

Reynolds CF III, Frank E, Perel JM, et al. Combined pharmacotherapy and psychotherapy in the acute and continuation treatment of elderly patients with recurrent major depression: a preliminary report. *Am J Psychiatry* 1992;149:1687–1692.

Reynolds CF III, Frank E, Perel JM, et al. Treatment of consecutive episodes of major depression in the elderly. *Am J Psychiatry* 1994;151:1740–1743.

Roose SP, Glassman AH, Attia E, Woodring S. Comparative efficacy of selective serotonin reuptake inhibitors and tricyclics in the treatment of melancholia. *Am J Psychiatry* 1994;151:1735–1739.

Salzman C. A primer on geriatric psychopharmacology. *Am J Psychiatry* 1982;139:67–76.

Salzman C. Clinical guidelines for the use of antidepressant drugs in geriatric patients. *J Clin Psychiatry* 1985;46:38–44.

Salzman C. Treatment of the depressed elderly patient. In: Altman HJ, ed. *Alzheimer's disease and dementia: problems, prospects, and perspectives*. New York: Plenum, 1987:171–182.

Salzman C, Nevis–Olesen J. Psychopharmacological and somatic treatments. In: Birren JE, ed. *Handbook of mental health and aging*. New York: Academic Press, 1992.

Salzman C, Schneider LS, Alexopolous GS. Psychopharmacological treatment of depression in late life. In: Bloom FE, Kupfer DJ, eds. *Psychopharma-*

cology: the fourth generation of progress. New York: Raven, 1995:1471–1477.

Schneider LS, Olin JT. Efficacy of acute treatment for geriatric depression. *Int Psychogeriatr* 1995;7:25.

von Moltke LL, Greenblatt DJ, Shader RI. Clinical pharmacokinetics of antidepressants in the elderly. Therapeutic implications. *Clin Pharmacokinet* 1993;24:141–160.

Zusky PM. Adjunct low dose lithium carbonate in treatment-resistant depression: a placebo-controlled study. *J Clin Psychopharmacol* 1988;8:120–124.

Pharmacokinetics of Cyclic Antidepressants

Alexanderson B, Kantor SJ, Glassman AG, et al. Pharmacokinetics of nortriptyline in man after single and multiple oral doses. *Eur J Clin Pharmacol* 1972;4:196–200.

Cole JO, Branconnier R, Salomon M, Dessain E. Tricyclic use in the cognitively impaired elderly. *J Clin Psychiatry* 1983;44:14–19.

Cook BL, Helms PM, Smith RE, Tsai M. Unipolar depression in the elderly. Reoccurrence on discontinuation of tricyclic antidepressants. *J Affective Disord* 1986;10:91–94.

Cutler NR, Narang PK. Implications of dosing tricyclic antidepressants and benzodiazepines in geriatrics. *Psychiatr Clin North Am* 1984; 7:845–861.

Cutler NR, Zavadil AP, Eisdorfer C, et al. Concentrations of desipramine in elderly women. *Am J Psychiatry* 1981;138:1235–1237.

Dawling S, Crome P, Braithwaite RA. Pharmacokinetics of single oral doses of nortriptyline in depressed elderly hospital patients and healthy young volunteers. *Clin Pharmacokinet* 1980;5:394–401.

Dawling S, Crome P, Braithwaite RA, et al. Nortriptyline therapy in elderly patients; dosage prediction after single dose pharmacokinetic study. *Eur J Clin Pharmacol* 1980;18:149–150.

Friedel RO. The pharmacotherapy of depression in the elderly: pharmacokinetic considerations. In: Cole JO, Barrett JE, eds. *Psychopathology in the aged*. New York: Raven, 1980:157–166.

Friedel RO. Effects of age on the pharmacology of tricyclic antidepressants. In: Raskin S, Robinson DS, Levin J, eds. *Age and the pharmacology of psychoactive drugs*. New York: Elsevier/North Holland, 1981:125–132.

Glassman AH, Perel JM. Tricyclic blood levels and clinical outcome. In: Lipton MA, DiMascio A, Killam KF, eds. *Psychopharmacology: a generation of progress*. New York: Raven, 1978:917–923.

Hicks R, Davis JM. Pharmacokinetics in geriatric psychopharmacology. In: Eisdorfer C, Fann WE, eds. *Psychopharmacology of aging*. New York: Spectrum, 1980:169–212.

Hicks R, Dysken MW, Davis JM, et al. The pharmacokinetics of psychotropic medication in the elderly: a review. *J Clin Psychiatry* 1981;42:374–385.

Hrdina PD, Rovei V, Henry JF, et al. Comparison of single–dose pharmacokinetics of imipramine and maprotiline in the elderly. *Psychopharmacology* 1980;70:29–34.

Kantor SJ, Glassman AH. The use of tricyclic antidepressant drugs in geriatric patients. In: Eisdorfer C, Fann WE, eds. *Psychopharmacology of the aging*. New York: Spectrum, 1980:99–118.

Maguire K. The pharmacokinetics of mianserin in elderly depressed patients. *Psychiatry Res* 1983;8: 281–287.

Nies A, Robinson DS, Friedman MJ, et al. Relationship between age and tricyclic antidepressant plasma levels. *Am J Psychiatry* 1977;134:790–793.

Nutter D, Brunswick D. Relevancy of tricyclic antidepressant plasma levels. *Am J Psychiatry* 1981;138: 526–527.

Preskorn SH. Tricyclic antidepressant plasma level monitoring: over the dose-response approach. *J Clin Psychiatry* 1986;47(suppl):24–30.

Robinson DS. Age–related factors affecting antidepressant drug metabolism and clinical response. In: Nandy K, ed. *Geriatric psychopharmacology*. New York: Elsevier/North Holland, 1979:17–30.

Schildkraut JJ. Tricyclic antidepressants and the aging process: discussion of selected pharmacodynamic and pharmacokinetic issues. In: Raskin A, Robinson DS, Levine J, eds. *Age and the pharmacology of psychoactive drugs*. New York: Elsevier/North Holland, 1981:133–150.

Schneider LS, Cooper TB, Staples FR, Sloane B. Prediction of individual dosage of nortriptyline in depressed elderly outpatients. *J Clin Psychopharmacol* 1987;7:311–314.

Schulz P, Turner-Tamiyasu K, Smith G, et al. Amitriptyline disposition in young and elderly normal men. *Clin Pharm Ther* 1983;33:360–366.

Simpson GM, White KL, Boyd JL. Relationship between plasma antidepressant levels and clinical outcome for patients receiving imipramine. *Am J Psychiatry* 1982;139:358–360.

Cardiovascular Side Effects of Cyclic Antidepressants

Georgotas A, McCue RE, Friedman E, Cooper TB. Electrocardiographic effects of nortriptyline, phenelzine, and placebo under optimal treatment conditions. *Am J Psychiatry* 1987;144: 798–801.

Georgotas A, McCue RE, Friedman E, Cooper TB. A placebo-controlled comparison of the effect of nortriptyline and phenelzine on orthostatic hypotension in elderly depressed patients. *J Clin Psychopharmacol* 1987;7:413–416.

Glassman AH, Walsh T, Roose P, et al. Factors related to orthostatic hypotension associated with tricyclic antidepressants. *J Clin Psychiatry* 1982;43: 35–38.

Hayes RL, Gerner RH, Fairbanks L, et al. ECG findings in geriatric depressives given trazodone, placebo, or imipramine. *J Clin Psychiatry* 1983; 44: 180–183.

Himmelhoch JM. Cardiovascular effects of trazodone in humans. *J Clin Psychopharmacol* 1981;1: 765–815.

Risch SC, Groom G, Janowsky DS. Interfaces of Psychopharmacology and cardiology. *Int J Clin Psychiatry* 1981;42:23–34.

Roose SP, Glassman AH. Cardiovascular effects of tricyclic antidepressants in depressed patients. *J Clin Psychiatry* 1989;7:1–18.

Verrier RL. Autonomic substrates from arrhythmias. *Prog Cardiol* 1988;1:65–85.

Vohra J, Burrows GD, Sloman G. Assessment of cardiovascular side effects of therapeutic doses of tricyclic antidepressant drugs. *Aust NZ J Med* 1975; 5:7–11.

Cyclic Antidepressants

Amitriptyline

Branconnier RJ, Cole JO. Effects of acute administration of trazodone and amitriptyline on cognition, cardiovascular function and salivation in the normal geriatric patient. *J Clin Psychopharmacol* 1981; 1:82–88.

Branconnier RJ, DeVitt DR, Cole JO, et al. Amitriptyline selectively disrupts verbal recall from secondary memory of the normal aged. *Neurobiol Aging* 1982;3:55–59.

Jarvik LF, Kakkar PR. Aging and response to antidepressants. In: Jarvik LF, Greenblatt D, Harman D, eds. *Clinical pharmacology and the aged patient*. New York: Raven, 1981:49–77.

Lauritzen L, Bendsen BB, Vilmar T, et al. Post–stroke depression: combined treatment with imipramine or desipramine and mianserin. A controlled clinical study. *Psychopharmacology* (Berlin) 1994;114:119–122.

Monteleone P, Fabrazzo M. Blood levels of mianserin and amitriptyline and clinical response in aged depressed patients. *Pharmacopsychiatry* 1994; 27:238–241.

Schmider J, Deuschle M, Schweiger U, et al. Amitriptyline metabolism in elderly depressed patients and normal controls in relation to hypothalamic-pituitary-adrenal system function. *J Clin Psychopharmacol* 1995;15:250–258.

Schultz P, Turner-Tamiyasu T, Smith G, et al. Amitriptyline disposition in young and elderly normal men. *Clin Pharmacol Ther* 1983;33:360–366.

Clomipramine

Watson JU, Beaumont G, Poole P. Clomipramine and age: an interaction study. *J Int Med Res* 1980; 8:81–84.

Desipramine

Nelson JC, Mazure CM, Jatlow PI. Desipramine treatment of major depression in patients over 75 years of age. *J Clin Psychopharmacol* 1995;15: 99–105.

Veith EX, Lewis N, Lineras OA, et al. Sympathetic nervous system activity in major depression. Basal and desipramine-induced alterations in plasma norepinephrine kinetics. *Arch Gen Psychiatry* 1994;51:411–422.

Walsh BT, Elsa-Grace VG, Sloan RP, et al. Effect of desipramine on autonomic control of the heart.

J Am Acad Child Adolesc Psychiatry 1994;33:2: 191–197.

Doxepin

Ananth JV, Sohn JH, Ban TA, et al. Doxepin in geriatric patients. *Curr Ther Res* 1979;25:133–138.

Goldberg HL, Finnerty RJ, Cole JO. The effect of doxepin in the aged: interim report on memory changes and electrocardiographic findings. In: Mendels J, ed. *Sinequan: a monograph of recent clinical findings.* Amsterdam: Excerpta Medica, 1975: 65–69.

Roose SP, Delack GW, Glassman AH, et al. Is doxepin a safer tricyclic for the heart? *J Clin Psychiatry* 1991;52:338–341.

Imipramine

Roose SP, Glassman AH, Siris SG, et al. Comparison of imipramine and nortriptyline–induced orthostatic hypotension. *J Clin Psychopharmacol* 1981;1: 316–319.

Maprotiline

Ananth J, Ayd FJ. Maprotiline therapy: update 1980. In: Ayd FJ, ed. *Clinical depressions: diagnostic and therapeutic challenges.* Baltimore: Ayd Medical, 1980:203–215.

Hoffman BF, Wachsmith R. Maprotiline and seizures. *J Clin Psychiatry* 1982;43:117–118.

Nortriptyline

Chesrow EJ, Kaplitz SE, Breme JT, et al. Nortriptyline for the treatment of anxiety and depression in chronically ill geriatric patients. *J Am Geriatr Soc* 1964;12:271–277.

Georgotas A, McCue RE, Cooper TB. A placebo controlled comparison of nortriptyline and phenelzine in maintenance therapy of elderly depressed patients. *Arch Gen Psychiatry* 1989;76:783–786.

Georgotas A, McCue RE, Friedman E, Cooper TB. Response of depressive symptoms to nortriptyline, phenelzine and placebo. *Br J Psychiatry* 1987; 151:102–106.

Glassman AH, Walsh T, Roose SP, et al. Factors related to orthostatic hypotension associated with tricyclic antidepressants. *J Clin Psychiatry* 1982;43: 35–38.

Kanba S, Matsumoto K, Nibuya M, et al. Nortriptyline response in elderly depressed patients. *Biol Psychiatry* 1992;16:301–309.

Katz IR, Simpson GM, Jethanandani V, et al. Steady state pharmacokinetics of nortriptyline in the frail elderly. *Neuropsychopharmacology* 1989;2: 229–236.

Lazarus LW, Moberg PJ, Langsley PR, Lingam VR. Methylphenidate and nortriptyline in the treatment of poststroke depression: a retrospective comparison. *Arch Phys Med Rehabil* 1994;75: 403–406.

McCue RE, Georgotas A, Nagachandran N, et al.

Plasma levels of nortriptyline and 10-hydroxynortriptyline and treatment-related electrocardiographic changes in the elderly depressed. *J Psychiatr Res* 1989;23:73–79.

Meyers BS, Mattis S, Gabriele M, Kakuma T. Effects of nortriptyline on memory self-assessment and performance in recovered elderly depressives. *Psychopharmacol Bull* 1991;27:295–299.

Miller MD, Pollock BG, Rifai AH, et al. Longitudinal analysis of nortriptyline side effects in elderly depressed patients. *J Geriatr Psychiatry Neurol* 1991; 4:226–230.

Nair NP, Amin M, Holm P, et al. Moclobemide and nortriptyline in elderly depressed patients. A randomized multicentre trial against placebo. *J Affective Disord* 1995;33:1–9.

Reynolds CF III, Hoch CC, Buysse DJ, et al. Sleep in late-life recurrent depression. Changes during early continuation therapy with nortriptyline. *Neuropsychopharmacology* 1991;5:85–96.

Zimmer B, Rosen J, Thornton JE, et al. Adjunctive lithium carbonate in nortriptyline-resistant elderly depressed patients. *J Clin Psychopharmacol* 1991;11:254–256.

Monoamine Oxidase Inhibitors

Ashford W, Ford CV. Use of MAO inhibitors in elderly patients. *Am J Psychiatry* 1979;136: 1466–1467.

Bridge TP, Potkin S, Wise CD, et al. Monoamine oxidase and aging. In: Raskin A, Robinson DS, Levine J, eds. *Age and the pharmacology of psychoactive drugs.* New York: Elsevier/North Holland, 1981:79–90.

Bridge TP, Soldo BJ, Phelps BH, et al. Platelet monoamine oxidase activity: demographic characteristics contribute to enzyme activity variability. *J Gerontol* 1985;40:23–28.

Comfort A. Phenelzine therapy: the doctor, the patient, and the wine and cheese party. *J Oper Psychiatry* 1982;13:37–40.

Georgotas A, Friedman E, McCarthy M, et al. Resistant geriatric depressions and therapeutic response to monoamine oxidase inhibitors. *Biol Psychiatry* 1983;18:195–205.

Georgotas A, McCue RE, Cooper TB. A placebo-controlled comparison of nortriptyline and phenelzine in maintenance therapy of elderly depressed patients. *Arch Gen Psychiatry* 1989;46:783–786.

Georgotas A, McCue RE, Cooper TB, et al. Factors affecting the delay of antidepressant effect in responders to nortriptyline and phenelzine. *Psychiatry Res* 1989;28:1–9.

Georgotas A, McCue RE, Friedman E, Cooper TB. Response of depressive symptoms to nortriptyline, phenelzine and placebo. *Br J Psychiatry* 1987; 151:102–106.

Giese AA, Leibenluft E, Green S, Moriole LA. Phenelzine-associated inappropriate ADH secretion. *J Clin Psychopharmacol* 1989;9:309–310.

Jenike MA. The use of monoamine oxidase inhibitors in the treatment of elderly, depressed patients. *J Am Geriatr Soc* 1984;32:571–575.

Malcolm DE, Yu PH, Bowen RC, et al. Phenelzine reduces plasma vitamin B_6. *J Psychiatry Neurosci* 1994;19:332–334.

Meyer D, Halfin V. Toxicity secondary to meperidine in patients on monoamine oxidase inhibitors. *J Clin Psychopharmacol* 1981;1:319–321.

Nies A, Robinson DS, Ravaris CL, et al. Amines and monoamine oxidase in relationship to aging and depression in man. *Psychosom Med* 1971;33: 470–475.

O'Brien S, McKeon P, O'Regan M. A comparative study of the electrocardiographic effect of tranylopromine and amitriptyline when prescribed singly and in combination. *Int Clin Psychopharmacol* 1991;6:11–17.

Quitkin F, Rifkin A, Klein DF. Monoamine oxidase inhibitors: a review of antidepressant effectiveness. *Arch Gen Psychiatry* 1979;36:749–760.

Robinson DS. Changes in monoamine oxidase and monoamines with human development and aging. *Fed Proc* 1975;34:103–107.

Robinson DS. Monoamine oxidase inhibitors and the elderly. In: Raskin A, Robinson DS, Levine J, eds. *Age and the pharmacology of psychoactive drugs.* New York: Elsevier/North Holland, 1981:151–162.

Robinson DS. Monoamine oxidase inhibitors in the elderly. In: Eisdorfer C, Fann WE, eds. *Treatment of psychopathology in the aging.* New York: Springer-Verlag, 1982:1–7.

Robinson DS, Nies A, Davis JM, et al. Aging, monoamines and monoamine oxidase. *Lancet* 1972;1: 290–291.

Robinson DS, Nies A, Ravaris CL. The monoamine oxidase inhibitor phenelzine in the treatment of depressive anxiety states. *Arch Gen Psychiatry* 1973; 29:407–412.

Robinson DS, Sourkes JL, Nies A, et al. Monoamine metabolism in human brain. *Arch Gen Psychiatry* 1977;34:89–92.

Salzman C. Monoamine oxidase inhibitors and atypical antidepressants. *Clin Geriatr Med* 1992;8: 335–348.

Swartz C. Depression with non-auditory hallucinations. Success with phenelzine. *Psychosomatics* 1979;20:286–289.

Psychomotor Stimulants

Crook T. CNS stimulants: appraisal of use in geropsychiatric patients. *J Am Geriatr Soc* 1979;27: 476–477.

Johnson ML, Roberts MD, Ross AR, Witten CM. Methylphenidate in stroke patients with depression. *Am J Phys Med Rehabil* 1992;71:239–241,

Kaplitz SE. Withdrawn, apathetic geriatric patients responsive to methylphenidate. *J Am Geriatr Soc* 1975;13:271–276.

Lazarus LW, Winemiller DR, Lingam VR, et al. Efficacy and side effects of methylphenidate for poststroke depression. *J Clin Psychiatry* 1992;53: 447–449.

Masand P, Chaudhary P. Methylphenidate treatment of poststroke depression in a patient with global aphasia. *Ann Clin Psychiatry* 1994;6:271–274.

Masand P, Murray GB, Pickett P. Psychostimulants in post-stroke depression. *J Neuropsychiatry Clin Neurosci* 1991:3:23–27.

Rosenberg PB, Ahmed I, Hurwitz S. Methylphenidate in depressed medically ill patients. *J Clin Psychiatry* 1991;52:263–267.

Satel SL, Nelson JC. Stimulants in the treatment of depression: a critical overview. *J Clin Psychiatry* 1989;50:241–249.

Chapter 10

Treatment of Depression with New and Atypical Antidepressants

Carl Salzman

Gary W. Small

The past few decades have brought remarkable advances in the pharmacologic treatment of depression for both young and old adults. Until the mid-1980s, only tricyclic antidepressants (TCAs) and the monoamine oxidase inhibitor (MAOI) groups of antidepressants were available for clinical use. Although effective for the treatment of the depressed elderly patient, they produced frequent and significant side effects that often limited their usefulness.

Two TCA antidepressants, bupropion and trazodone, were introduced about two decades ago, but major changes in antidepressant prescribing patterns for elderly patients began with fluoxetine (Prozac), the first of a group of antidepressants, known as the selective serotonin reuptake inhibitors (SSRIs), with a new chemical structure and mode of pharmacologic activity. Following the introduction of fluoxetine, four more SSRIs—sertraline, paroxetine, fluvoxamine, and citalopram—were introduced and are now in wide clinical use. Recently a variant of the citalopram molecule, escitalopram, was also introduced for clinical use as the sixth SSRI antidepressant. In the early 1990s, three other new antidepressants, each with a unique chemical structure and mode of pharmacologic activity, were introduced for clinical practice: venlafax-

ine, nefazodone, and mirtazapine. Although these three drugs have not been studied as frequently in older depressed patients as in younger depressed patients, evidence from studies of young and middle-aged adults suggests therapeutic efficacy and a favorable side-effect profile for each.

During the past five years, increased research studies have specifically examined the effects of the SSRIs and these newer antidepressants in older persons.[1–5] This chapter reviews available controlled research data as well as clinical experience with these newer antidepressant agents for geriatric depression and suggests guidelines for their use.

Selective Serotonin Reuptake Inhibitors

As their name implies, SSRIs selectively inhibit the reuptake of the neurotransmitter serotonin into presynaptic terminals to enhance serotonergic neurotransmission.[6] Although the actual mechanism for the therapeutic effects of SSRIs is not known, this rapid increase of serotonin in the neuronal synaptic cleft is followed by a considerably slower resolution of depressive symptoms, suggesting additional, more complicated therapeutic mechanisms. Recent evidence also suggests that genetic variations among elderly patients may be partly responsible for differences in response to SSRIs in the following manner: differences in gene alleles for the protein that carries serotonin back into the presynaptic nerve ending ("the serotonin transporter") have been linked to differential therapeutic response: elderly individuals who possess the long genotype (*l*) respond to paroxetine significantly more rapidly than those possessing a short (*s*) allele, despite equivalent paroxetine concentrations.[7]

Clinical studies of elderly patients with major depression treated with SSRI antidepressants have increased in number as agents in this drug group have become preferred as the first-line antidepressant therapy for most elderly patients.[1,3] Among a group of experts in geriatric psychiatry, a high level of consensus was obtained that, at present, SSRIs are the antidepressants of first choice for all types of depression in older patients.[8] They are effective for the treatment of elderly patients with major depression[9] as well as for minor depression[10,11] and dysthymia.[12-15] They have been successfully prescribed for frail elderly nursing home residents, for patients whose depression is complicated by medical illness, and with safety to those considered "old-old" (over age 75).[11,16] SSRIs, like TCAs, have been given to depressed demented patients, resulting in decreased depression as well as modest cognitive improvement.[17,18] Easier administration, reduced need for dosage adjustment, less severe adverse effect profiles, and greater acceptance of SSRIs favor use of these agents over TCAs and other antidepressants with prominent side effects. It is not surprising, therefore, that a survey of antidepressant use among the elderly in Canada found that use of SSRI antidepressants increased from 9.6% in 1993 to 45.1% in 1997 and was projected to reach approximately 56% by 2000.[19]

Despite clinical recommendations favoring SSRIs, a recent review concludes that efficacy studies do not convincingly demonstrate therapeutic superiority of SSRIs over other classes of antidepressants.[20] These data show that in some studies of elderly patients, the magnitude of therapeutic response and difference from placebo response is surprisingly small, the range of response among SSRI recipients is large, and elderly depressed patients are often left with significant residual symptoms of depression. In addition, although mild therapeutic response may appear within a few weeks of starting treatment, as long as 3 months may be required for a full therapeutic response to develop with SSRI treatment. This prolonged response time period is similar to antidepressant treatment with TCAs and other antidepressants, suggesting that therapeutic response is delayed in older patients regardless of the type of antidepressant used for treatment. Some studies also suggest that SSRIs may be less efficacious than TCAs for severe melancholic depressions in elderly patients[21-24] as in younger adults. Furthermore, although SSRIs are also recommended as first-choice antidepressants because of a presumed better side effect profile, the difference in their side effects, even when compared with TCAs, is slight[20] and does not necessarily result in improved compliance.[25] Despite these shortcomings, it appears that most clinicians currently prescribe an SSRI as a first-choice antidepressant to virtually all elderly depressed patients.

Clinical Pharmacology

Although SSRIs are *therapeutically* similar, important *pharmacokinetic* differences exist among the drugs in this class of antidepressants. Rates of hepatic clearance differ from one drug to another, resulting in wide variations in elimination half-life. For example, fluoxetine and its active metabolite norfluoxetine, as well as citalopram and its enantiomer escitalopram, have relatively long elimination half-lives whereas the half-lives of sertraline, fluvoxamine, and paroxetine are shorter (Table 10.1). The elimination half-life of an SSRI, however, bears no relation to its therapeutic properties, and whether or not a prolonged half-life increases the risk of adverse effects in the elderly is not known.

Table 10.1.   Clinical Pharmacology of Serotonin Reuptake Inhibitors

Drug	Elimination Half-Life (hr)	Effect on CP450 Hepatic Enzymes	Recommended Elderly Daily Dose (mg)
Paroxetine	12–20	Strong inhibitor of 2D6	5–40
Fluvoxamine	15	Inhibits 1A2 and 3A4	25–200
Sertraline	25	Weak inhibitor of 2D6 and 3A4	12.5–150
Fluoxetine	85	Strong inhibitor of 2D6; moderate inhibitor of 3A4	5–60
Citalopram	52	No effect on enzymes	10–20
Escitalopram	45	No effect on enzymes	5–20

Longer half-life compounds have the advantage of high compliance and steady blood levels should a dose be missed whereas shorter half-life SSRIs have the advantage of dosage flexibility. Clearance of fluoxetine and norfluoxetine is delayed in older patients, resulting in higher plasma levels.[26] Fluvoxamine also shows an age effect, with half-life increasing from 15 to 23 hours and clearance reduced by 50%.[27] Clearance of the shorter half-life SSRI paroxetine is also delayed by age but as with fluoxetine, whether or not this prolongation suggests a particular therapeutic usefulness or vulnerability to side effects compared with the other SSRI medications is not clear. The metabolism and clearance of sertraline, however, does not seem to be affected by age; plasma levels are comparable to those seen in younger patients.[28] The pharmacokinetics of citalopram and escitalopram also are unaffected by aging.[29]

SSRI antidepressants may influence their own metabolism as well as the metabolism of other drugs by inhibiting isoenzymes within the hepatic cytochrome enzyme system. Fluoxetine, norfluoxetine, and paroxetine strongly inhibit the 2D6 isoenzyme, causing nonlinear changes in their own plasma levels with each increase in dose. Inhibition of 2D6 also increases blood levels of other drugs metabolized by this isoenzyme, most significantly TCAs

and cardiac antiarrythmics.[26,27] Sertraline is a less potent 2D6 inhibitor and fluvoxamine, citalopram, and escitalopram do not inhibit this isoenzyme (see Appendix B). Fluoxetine, norfluoxetine, and fluvoxamine are also potent inhibitors of the 3A4 isoenzyme, which metabolizes a large number of drugs including TCAs, neuroleptics, mood stabilizers, and benzodiazepines, as well as numerous medical drugs including steroids and antibiotics.[26] Inhibition of 3A4 may have potentially meaningful clinical consequences for the depressed elderly patient who is taking multiple medications. Citalopram and escitalopram do not inhibit any isoenzymes and thus lack pharmacokinetic interactions with other drugs metabolized by the hepatic cytochrome enzymes.

Side Effects

Despite a favorable clinical profile, SSRIs still produce significant side effects, although usually with less frequency and intensity than other antidepressants. The most striking differences between SSRIs and TCAs, for example, are the absence of orthostatic hypotension and significant anticholinergic effects as well as low cardiotoxity. Side-effect profiles for the SSRIs show greater similarities to each other than differences. The most common side effects are gastrointestinal, including nausea and appetite loss, although the latter "complaint" is welcomed by some diet-conscious older individuals. (Advising older patients to take their medicine with meals and a full glass of water sometimes reduces nausea.) Some patients gain weight when taking SSRIs.

Fluoxetine sometimes increases anxiety although development of anxiety or agitation from fluoxetine or any SSRI may occur in the context of effective antidepressant therapeutic response.[30] Although individual variation in response to SSRIs among elderly patients is high, fluoxetine may be especially stimulating, causing daytime restlessness and nighttime insomnia, whereas paroxetine appears to have greater sedating effects than other SSRIs.[31] Nonetheless, some patients are sedated by fluoxetine and made more active by paroxetine.

SSRIs generally do not cause cognitive impairment in older persons and may even improve cognitive performance,[32] although confusion has been reported occasionally in elderly patients.[33] Improved cognition can occur without antidepressant efficacy[34] and may vary among the SSRIs. For example, in a comparison of fluoxetine and sertraline in older depressed patients, although both drugs had equivalent antidepressant efficacy, patients treated with sertraline showed significant improvement in digit-symbol substitution and shopping-list tasks.[27]

As a class of antidepressants, SSRIs produce markedly less inhibition of central nervous system (CNS) cholinergic activity, which may account for less cognitive impairment. Among the SSRIs, however, paroxetine has been reported to block CNS muscarinic receptors[35] and it commonly produces mild anticholinergic side effects such as dry mouth. However, serum levels of paroxetine are not elevated in the elderly and its use has not been associated with significant anticholinergic side effects.[36]

SSRIs commonly produce sexual dysfunction (impaired orgasm, ejaculation, and arousal) in sexually active elders as in younger adults. Treatments for these side effects have not been reliable; substituting a non-SSRI antidepressant, such as nefazodone or bupropion, may be helpful. Viagra is helpful for some male patients, but it cannot be taken with nitrate medications commonly prescribed for older persons with cardiac diseases. SSRIs occasionally cause hyponatremia resulting from inappropriate antidiuretic hormone (ADH) secretion,[37] which is thought to reflect dysregulation of serotonergic control of ADH release or metabolism.[38,39,40] Sodium concentrations can fall precipitously and result in markedly impaired mental status. The sodium concentration of elderly patients with hyponatremia returns to normal within days to weeks of SSRI withdrawal.[41]

SSRIs do not affect cardiac function[42–44] and do not cause orthostatic hypotension. However, their use has been associated with increased risk of falls, especially in elderly women in nursing homes,[45] and may occasionally cause increased bruising because of disruption of platelet function. An association between SSRI use and increased gastrointestinal bleeding may also occur, especially among octogenarians[46] although this association is controversial.[47]

Elderly patients with a first episode of major depression in late life are at high risk of recurrence following discontinuation of maintenance antidepressant treatment.[48] Relapse of elderly depressed patients after discontinuation of SSRIs is therefore not surprising.[15] Clinical experience suggests, however, that *abrupt* discontinuation of SSRI treatment in elderly patients may produce withdrawal syndromes consisting of flu-like symptoms, dizziness, instability, and agitation. Based on reports from younger adult patients, SSRIs with shorter half-lives, such as paroxetine and fluvoxamine, are more likely to cause withdrawal than sertraline. Fluoxetine is less likely to cause withdrawal following abrupt discontinuation.[49]

In general, the appearance of side effects correlates with the dosage of SSRIs: low doses are less likely to produce serious side effects than higher doses. For these reasons, low starting doses of SSRIs are usually recommended for the elderly depressed patient, with gradual dosage increases. Initial sedation, agitation, or gastrointestinal upset sometimes disappears after a week or two of very low dosing, allowing for subsequent gradual dosage increases.

Choice of SSRI

Comparative research studies as well as clinical experience suggest equal antidepressant efficacy in the elderly for fluoxetine, sertraline, paroxetine, fluvoxamine, and citalopram (Table 10.2); less information is available on the efficacy of fluvoxamine. As yet no information is available on the efficacy of escitalopram for elderly patients. In rating tolerability and efficacy in older patients, the Expert Consensus Guidelines selected citalopram as a first-choice SSRI, followed by sertraline and paroxetine. These higher ratings are reflective of studies that have found these medications effective, well tolerated, and with limited drug interactions. Although the rating of paroxetine was not quite as high as that of citalopram and sertraline, it is the only SSRI with demonstrated efficacy for the frail, very old depressed patient.[11] Selection of a medication among these, therefore, is not based on differences in therapeutic response among elderly patients. Clinicians consequently must select among available SSRI antidepressants based on clinical judgment and, when available, history of past response or lack of response to an individual drug. In all likelihood, the starting dose and rate of dose increase will have more clinical impact than the differences among these drugs. Variations in drug response among older persons may be greater than meaningful differences among the available SSRI antidepressants.[50]

When an antidepressant drug is partially effective but the patient continues to suffer significant residual depressive symptoms, a second antidepressant is sometimes added in an effort to augment the first drug's therapeutic effect. This augmenting strategy for the elderly patient has been best studied with TCAs. Unfortunately, adequately controlled data on strategies to augment SSRI response in antidepressant-resistant elderly depressed patients are lacking. The Expert Consensus Guidelines recommends augmenting partial response to SSRIs by adding bupropion or lithium as well as a TCA. Lithium augmentation, however, is less effective in the elderly and may result in neurotoxicity despite therapeutic doses.[51] Side effects also tended to occur more frequently in patients receiving fluoxetine and lithium than in those taking lithium in combination with either phenelzine or nortriptyline.[52] Methylphenidate has also been used to augment SSRI response in the elderly.[53,54] If a patient has had little or no response to an SSRI given at an adequate dosage and for an adequate length of time, the expert guidelines recommend switching to venlafaxine-XR or bupropion-SR rather that prescribing a second augmenting medication.

Dosage and Administration

As clinical experience and research data regarding the safety and efficacy of SSRI antidepressants in the elderly accumulate, a recommended pattern of prescribing is beginning to emerge. The starting dose for the older patient should be at least half of the starting dose recommended for young and middle-aged adults—lower if possible (Table 10.1). The side effects after the first dose or two may inform the clinician about the possibility of unacceptable adverse reactions and the need to change to another SSRI. Mild side effects may disappear after a brief period of time if the starting dose remains low. Once the elderly patient has been stabilized on a starting dose, dosage may be increased gradually, if necessary, to a full adult daily recommended dose.

Although the usual geriatric maxim "Start low and go slow" is a useful prescribing guideline, wide variation in response to SSRIs among older patients sug-

Table 10.2. Double-Blind Controlled Studies of Selective Serotonin Reuptake Inhibitor (SSRI) Use in Elderly Patients

Study[a]	N[b]	Age/Mean Age	Dose (mg/day)	Results
			CITALOPRAM	
Gutierrez (2000)	24	—	10–40	Elimination half-life 30% longer in elderly, although pharmacokinetics and tolerability are similar to those observed in young subjects
Karlsson et al. (2000)	336	—	20–40	Antidepressant response of patients with and without mild to moderate dementia: well-tolerated and nonsedating for elderly depressed patients with or without dementia
Klysner et al. (2002)	121	65+	20–40	Long-term treatment prevented recurrence compared with placebo
Kyle et al (1998)	365	65+	20–40	Efficacy comparable to amitriptyline but better tolerated
Lavretsky & Kumar (2001)	10	79.8	—	Methylphenidate addition to citalopram produced rapid response by week 2 without significant side effects
Navarro et al. (2001)	58	60+	30–40	Nortriptyline more efficacious but citalopram better tolerated
Nyth et al. (1992)	149	76.7	10–30	Superior to placebo, especially in patients with dementia
			FLUOXETINE	
Ackerman et al. (2000)	262	60+	20	Superior to placebo on all outcome measures beginning at week 4
Altamura et al. (1989)	28	65+	20	Equally effective as amitriptyline but with fewer side effects
Bocksberger et al. (1993)		65+	50–200	Equal in efficacy to moclobemide
Evans et al. (1997)	62	80.4	—	Only modest response in medically ill patients

Study	N	Age	Dose	Results
Fairweather et al. (1993)	33	70	20	Equal in efficacy to amitriptyline; superior effects on attention, reaction time
Falk et al. (1989)	27	62+	20–60	Trend toward superior response to trazodone
Feighner et al. (1988)	136	60+	20–80	Equal in efficacy to imipramine, amitriptyline, or doxepin
Feighner & Cohn (1985)	64	61–90	20–80	Equal to doxepin
Giakas et al. (1993)	11	70	40	Fluoxetine superior to bupropion (27 vs. 0% in medically ill patients)
Goldstein et al. (1997)	671	20		No weight change
Heiligenstein et al. (1995)	261	60+		Fluoxetine markedly superior to placebo
Koran et al. (1995)	671	68		43% response; 28% remission by week 4; early responders did not always predict final response
La Pia et al. (1992)	20	60–80	20	Equal in efficacy to mianserin
Nobler et al. (1996)	23	mean 67	20–60	Effective for dysthymia
Orengo et al. (1996)	31	75	—	Significant improvement in depressive symptoms
Rahman et al. (1991)		64+	50–200	Equal in efficacy to dothiepin
Roose et al. (1994)	22	73	Variable	Nortriptyline superior to fluoxetine (67 vs. 22%) in cardiac patients; response rate better for melancholia
Schneider & Olin (1995)	367	67.9	20	Estrogen replacement therapy augmented fluoxetine response
Schone & Ludwig (1993)	54	65–85	20–60	Equally effective to paroxetine
Small et al. (1995)	671	67.7	20	Fluoxetine markedly superior to placebo but no response predictors identified
Tollefson & Holman (1993)	671	>60	20	Superior to placebo
Wakelin (1986)	33	60–71	150–300	Efficacy equal to imipramine and superior to placebo
Wolf et al. (2001)	41	72.2	20	Equally effective as trimipramine; fluoxetine increased proportion of REM sleep and lengthened REM latency

(continued)

Table 10.2. *(continued)*

Study[a]	N[b]	Age/Mean Age	Dose (mg/day)	Results
			FLUVOXAMINE	
Rahman et al. (1991)	52	64+	100–200	Equally effective as dothiepin; no significant differences in side effects of nausea, dizziness, headache, somnolence, and constipation in both groups
			PAROXETINE	
Bump et al. (2001)	38	70	—	Rates of relapse and recurrence over an 18-month period similar for paroxetine and nortriptyline
Burrows et al. (2002)	20	87.9	20	Equal in efficacy to placebo for minor depression in nursing home residents; better response in more severely symptomatic residents
Cassano et al. (2002)	242	65+	20–40	Efficacy comparable to fluoxetine
Dorman (1992)	29	65+	15–30	Equal in efficacy to mianserin
Dunner et al. (1992)	136	50+	10–40	Equal in efficacy to doxepin
Dunner et al. (1992)	272	68	23.4	Efficacy equal to doxepin in 2 separate studies; well tolerated with less sedation and anticholinergic effects
Geretsegger et al. (1995)	44	65+	20–30	Efficacy equal to amitriptyline but with fewer side effects
Geretsegger et al. (1994)	52	74		Paroxetine superior to fluoxetine
Green et al. (1999)	93	70	10–40	Therapeutic sleep deprivation (TSD) brought rapid response to paroxetine recipients, suggesting that TSD plus paroxetine may be twice as successful as conventional monotherapy in achieving rapid response
Guillibert et al. (1989)	79	60+	20–30	Efficacy equal to clomipramine but with fewer side effects

Study	N	Age	Dose	Findings
Hebenstreit et al. (1988)	14	65+	20–40	Effective antidepressant; no relation between plasma level and therapeutic efficacy or adverse events
Hutchinson et al. (1992)	58	72	30	Efficacy equal to amitriptyline but with fewer side effects
Hutchinson et al. (1991)	58	65+	20–30	Efficacy equal to amitriptyline but with fewer side effects
Joo et al. (2002)	104	>69	10–40	38% of patients had at least one fall, 53% of these during first 6 weeks of treatment; addition of bupropion to paroxetine significantly increases risk for falls by additional 28%
Katona et al. (1998)	198	60+	20–40	Efficacy comparable to imipramine in depression with dementia
Mamo et al. (2000)	19	71.3	—	Equally effective as nortriptyline in reducing extrapyramidal symptoms
Marar et al. (2002)	4	61–74	—	Does not impair water excretion
Mulsant et al. (2001)	116	Mean=73	10–20	Efficacy comparable to nortriptyline
Mulsant et al. (1999)	80	75	10–30	No significant differences in dropout rates between paroxetine and nortriptyline, even among inpatients or patients with melancholic depression
Pollock (2000)	95	—	—	More rapid response to paroxetine for patients with long serotonin transporter gene promoter polymorphism than for those with S-allele, despite equivalent paroxetine concentrations
Pollock et al. (1998)	31	73.2	20–30	Serum and anticholinergic levels significantly lower than for nortriptyline and did not correlate with paroxetine plasma levels
Schatzberg et al. (2002)	120	72.5	33.6	Equally effective as mirtazapine but more dropouts
Schone & Ludwig (1993)	54	65–85	20–40	Equal in efficacy to fluoxetine

(continued)

Table 10.2. (continued)

Study[a]	N[b]	Age/Mean Age	Dose (mg/day)	Results
Walters et al. (1999)	40	75	24.5	Efficacy comparable to nortriptyline and paroxetine in preventing or delaying relapse or recurrence, with 80–90% of patients remaining well
Weihs et al. (2000)	100	60+	10–40	Efficacy comparable to bupropion (sustained release)
Williams et al. (2000)	415	71	10–40	Effective for elderly patients with dysthymia and minor depression
SERTRALINE				
Arranz & Ros (1997)	1437	68	50–200	Effective antidepressant for patients with depression complicated by medical comorbidity, polypharmacy, and increased sensitivity to drug effects
Bondareff et al. (2000)	210	60+	50–150	Efficacy comparable to nortriptyline
Cohn et al. (1990)	120	65+	50–200	Efficacy equal to amitriptyline but with fewer side effects
Finkel et al. (1999)	75	70+	50–100	Efficacy better than fluoxetine
Finkel et al. (1999)	76	70+	50–150	Efficacy better than nortriptyline
Forlenza et al. (2001)	55	60+	50	Equal to imipramine but with fewer side effects
Hindmarch et al. (1990)	21	Not given	60–200	No impairment of psychomotor function
"Projecto Terceira Idade," São Paulo, Brazil (2000)	55	68	50	No significant difference between sertraline and imipramine; side-effect profile similar in the two groups
Lyketsos et al. (2000)	22	Mean = 77	25–125	Superior to placebo in patients with depression complicated by AD

Reference	N	Age	Dose	Comments
Magai et al. (2000)	31	88.4	50–100	Mood enhancement in frail nursing home residents with advanced dementia; placebo group also improved
Newhouse et al. (2000)	236	60+	50–100	Greater cognitive improvement compared with fluoxetine
Nobler et al. (2000)	20	68 (mean)	150 (max)	Equal to nortriptyline in efficacy; reduced regional cerebral blood flow in frontal regions, similar to responders to ECT
Oslin et al. (2000)	28	83	25–100	Less effective than nortriptyline for treating depression of elderly nursing home residents with chronic disabling medical and neurologic illnesses; may not be significantly better tolerated than TCAs
Oslin et al. (2003)	52	82	18.75–150	No difference in efficacy but venlafaxine-IR less well tolerated and possibly less safe than sertraline
Ronfeld et al. (1997)	22	> 65	200	Pharmacokinetic study: elimination half-life similar in elderly males and females; both similar to young females
Rosen et al. (2000)	12			Significant improvement in residents of long-term care facilities with minor depression, disability, and risk of morbidity
Schneider et al. (2001)	210	67	50–150	Estrogen replacement therapy may augment SSRI response in post-menopausal depressed women
Solai et al. (1997)	14	73	50	Sertraline did not significantly increase nortriptyline blood levels

[a] Complete reference citations at end of chapter.
[b] N, Number of subjects randomized to specific drug.

gests that it is not always appropriate for all older individuals. Citalopram and paroxetine, for example, have been initiated with a full daily therapeutic dose of 20 mg in research studies of patients over 80 years of age without increased side effects.[11] An occasional elderly patient may require more than the average adult daily dose although, in general, high doses are not recommended and have not proven especially therapeutic in this age group

A waiting period of 2 to 5 weeks is necessary when changing a patient from an SSRI to an MAOI, and 2 weeks are necessary when changing from an MAOI to an SSRI. SSRIs should never be used concomitantly with MAOIs. This combination may result in a "serotonin syndrome" consisting of hyperthermia, rigidity, myoclonus, autonomic instability, fluctuating vital signs, agitation, delirium, or coma.

Other Atypical Antidepressants

Other atypical antidepressants include bupropion, trazodone, venlafaxine, nefazodone, and mirtazapine. Although the mechanism of therapeutic effect differs among these drugs, each may play a role in treating the elderly depressed person (Table 10.3).

Bupropion

The antidepressant bupropion became available for therapeutic use before fluoxetine and the other SSRIs, but it has not been as widely prescribed for older patients as the SSRIs. It is not an SSRI and does not share a chemical structure or pharmacologic properties with other clinically available antidepressants. Bupropion has relatively weak effects on norepinephrine and serotonin reuptake, low affinity for the α-adrenergic receptor but mild dopamine reuptake-blocking properties. Despite knowledge of such complex pharmacologic effects, its mechanism for antidepressant action is not known. Bupropion's efficacy is compara-

ble to that of TCAs and SSRIs for the treatment of major depression.[55,56] Clinical experience, however, suggests that bupropion activates elderly patients whose depression is characterized by anergia, withdrawal, and excessive somnolence and lethargy although its antidepressant properties are not as reliable or predictable as the SSRIs or TCAs. Bupropion, like the SSRIs, does not cause anticholinergic, hypotensive, cardiovascular side effects, or cognitive impairment. However, it is stimulating and may cause agitation in some older patients. Other elderly patients do not tolerate side effects of bupropion such as nausea, nervousness, or insomnia; prescribing the last daily dose in the late afternoon rather than in the evening may avoid insomnia. Older patients may also be at increased risk for accumulation of bupropion and its metabolites, which have dopaminergic properties that may increase insomnia and agitation.[57] Seizures may occur with the use of very high doses (> 400 mg/day).

The use of bupropion for older individuals is associated with increased risk of falls; when it is used to augment the therapeutic effect of another antidepressant, such as an SSRI, increased risk of falls is also possible.[58] Rare parkinsonian symptoms have also been reported.[59]

Daily dosage of immediate-release bupropion for elderly patients ranges from 75 to 300 mg. A sustained release form of bupropion is available and has replaced the immediate-release preparation in prescribing popularity. This form of bupropion, however, is only available in 100, 150, and 200 mg doses. No studies with elderly subjects are available for dosage guidelines.

Trazodone

Trazodone, an antidepressant with a unique chemical profile, has been available for clinical use for nearly two decades. Its pharmacologic properties affect the serotonin neurotransmission system in complex ways, but it does not belong to the SSRI class of antidepressants. Al-

Table 10.3. Double-Blind Controlled Studies of Atypical Antidepressant Use in Elderly Patients

Study[a]	N[b]	Age	Dose (mg/day)	Results
			BUPROPION	
Branconnier et al. (1983)	63	—	150 or 450	Both doses equivalent to imipramine in antidepressant effect; higher dose achieves more rapid effect onset; no sedation or anticholinergic side effects
Joo et al. (2002)	104	> 69	171 (mean)	38% of patients had at least one fall, 53% of which occurred during the first 6 weeks of treatment; addition of bupropion to paroxetine significantly increases risk for falls by additional 28%
Sweet et al. (1995)	6	—	—	Clearance of bupropion decreases elimination half-life increases; elderly are at risk for accumulation of bupropion and its metabolites.
Weihs et al. (2000)	100	70	100–300	Bupropion and paroxetine equally efficacious and tolerable
			MIRTAZAPINE	
Hoyberg et al. (1996)	115	70.5	15–45	Mirtazapine and amitriptyline equally efficacious and well tolerated
Roose et al. (2003)	49	89.3	18.5	Rapidly dissolving tablet effective in very elderly nursing home residents
Schatzberg et al. (2002)	126	71.7	25.7	Faster onset of affect and reduced anxiety/somatization and sleep disturbance with paroxetine
			NEFAZODONE	
Van Laar et al. (1995)	12	—	200–400	Effective antidepressant but only minor effects on psychomotor performance at higher dose, which also produced mild cognitive and memory impairment

Table 10.3.   *(continued)*

Study[a]	N[b]	Age	Dose (mg/day)	Results
			TRAZODONE	
Altamura et al. (1988)	60–83	25	150	Efficacy equal to amitriptyline and mianserin but fewer side effects
Falk et al. (1989)	62+	13	50–400	Efficacy equal to fluoxetine
Gerner et al. (1980)	60–90	19	50–200	Efficacy equal to imipramine but with fewer side effects; more effective than placebo
Jarvik et al. (1982)	55–81	32	25–250	Efficacy equal to imipramine
Kane et al. (1983)	55–77	38	75–200	Efficacy equal to bupropion but more cardiovascular side effects
Scardigli & Jans (1982)	51–88	23	200–405	Slower onset of action than mianserin
			VENLAFAXINE	
Amore et al. (1997)	28	73	75–225	Venlafaxine safe and well tolerated with 75% improvement rate in patients who completed acute phase without relapse during continuation phase
Dierick (1996)	116	65+	25–150	1-year open study: two-thirds improved by 2 months; 80% much or very much improved after 1 year
Gastó et al. (2003)	68	71.4	75–300	Remission in 22/34 (71%); equal remission rate with nortriptyline
Khan et al. (1995)	58	65+	—	Effective well-tolerated medication over a 12-month period; headache, nausea, insomnia, dry mouth, and sweating most common side effects
Mahapatra & Hackett (1997)	92	74.5	50–150	Venlafaxine and dothiepin were equally effective
Oslin et al. (2003)	52	82	18.75–150	There was no difference in efficacy but venlafaxine-IR was less well tolerated and possibly less safe than sertraline
Zimmer et al. (1997)	18	65–86	50–250	No sustained changes in blood pressure

[a] Complete reference citations at end of chapter.
[b] N = number of subjects randomized to specific drug.

though several clinical trials indicate that trazodone has efficacy similar to that of TCAs, bupropion, and fluoxetine, accumulated clinical experience suggests that the therapeutic properties of trazodone are unpredictable and unreliable. Although some elderly patients respond very well to trazodone and may even respond to this drug after having failed to respond positively to virtually all other antidepressants, many others do not. It is difficult to determine, however, whether a negative response is due to an intrinsic lack of efficacy of the drug or problems with side effects that interfere with drug-taking compliance.

Trazodone is associated with several side effects that occur frequently and pose a special hazard for elderly patients. Orthostatic hypotension caused by α_1-adrenergic blockade[60] may lead to falls, fractures, and head trauma, although the orthostasis associated with the drug is less severe than that of TCAs. Trazodone may also worsen preexisting ventricular irritability or cause complete heart block[61,62]; elderly patients with cardiovascular disease thus run the risk of arrhythmias. This drug also has a strong sedating effect, and some elderly patients become overly sedated when treated with even small daily doses. However, trazodone's sedative property may be useful for treating some agitated demented patients[63]; (see Chapter 7). For other anxious or agitated depressed patients, sedation is advantageous, and trazodone at bedtime can be an effective soporific (see Chapter 11, 16).

Trazodone may cause memory impairment. Although less severe than that observed with TCAs,[64,65] this impairment may be exacerbated by alcohol or other drugs.[66] Demented elderly patients in particular may be sensitive to potential memory effects.

Use of trazodone by young and middle-aged adult males is linked to the occasional development of priapism. This nonerotic swelling of the penis is reversible with immediate discontinuation of the drug but has led to permanent impotence when present for more than 24 hours.

There are no reports of priapism occurring in elderly males, but that does not mean it may not occur. Older male patients prescribed trazodone should be warned about this side effect and/or observed for the development of penile swelling.

The initial dose of trazodone for elderly patients is 25 mg, which may be increased to as much as 400 mg daily. Its relatively short elimination half-life approximates 5 hours in young adults but is closer to 8 hours in elderly men.[67] Thus, in some elderly patients, multiple daily dosing may not be necessary.

Venlafaxine

After introduction of the SSRIs, venlafaxine was the next antidepressant released for therapeutic use. Its pharmacologic profile resembles that of TCAs, as both compounds inhibit the presynaptic reuptake of norepinephrine and serotonin. Although age does not affect its steady-state pharmacokinetic disposition, clearance of venlafaxine's major metabolite is 15% lower in people older than 60 years, perhaps because of the decreased renal function associated with aging.[68] Although double-blind controlled trials of venlafaxine in elderly depressed patients are not nearly as common as studies with SSRIs, available data indicate its safety and efficacy for patients aged 65 years and older.[69,70] Recent research with young adult patients also suggests that venlafaxine treatment is associated with higher rates of symptomatic remission than comparable antidepressants.[71] Unfortunately no corresponding remission data are available on elderly patients.

Unlike the TCAs, venlafaxine has no effect on muscarinic, histaminergic, and adrenergic receptors; it thus lacks anticholinergic, sedative, or orthostatic hypotensive side effects.[72] Clinically significant cardiac conduction abnormalities or arrhythmias have not been reported, although studies of the cardiovascular effects of venlafaxine in elderly patients with underlying cardiovascular disease have been reported. Because diastolic blood pressure may increase, especially with higher doses of venlafaxine ($>$ 300 mg/day), it is not recommended as a first choice antidepressant for older patients who suffer from hypertension. Despite these potential side effects, a recent review showed that 229 patients aged 65 years or older given venlafaxine for up to 1 year had no unexpected problems compared with young adult patients.[73]

Starting doses for venlafaxine should be extremely low (12.5 mg/day), and dosage increases should be slow and gradual. Dose adjustments may be required for patients with moderate to severe hepatic or renal disease.[73] Because of its short half-life, twice- or thrice-daily dosing is necessary. Average daily dosages for elderly patients range from 50 to 225 mg. An extended-release (XR) form of venlafaxine is now available and is prescribed more frequently than the immediate release (IR) form because its use is associated with fewer side effects. Venlafaxine XR, however, is only available in dosage forms of 100 or 150 mg. These doses may be too high for some elderly (especially the frail elderly) patients; dosage guidelines based on controlled research studies are lacking. For these reasons, clinicians begin treatment with low doses of the IR form of venlafaxine and then switch to the XR form when a daily dose of 100 mg is reached. However, a recent clinical trial with elderly patients reported safety and efficacy of venlafaxine XR at starting daily doses of 100 mg,[74] suggesting that starting treatment with the XR preparation may be safe and effective.

Nefazodone

Nefazodone, a selective 5-HT$_2$ receptor antagonist, also inhibits presynaptic reuptake of serotonin. Like its pharmacologic relative trazodone, nefazodone is a therapeutic antidepressant that causes considerable sedation. Although older patients have been included in prior controlled research trials of nefazodone, few published studies focus exclusively on elderly depressed patients.

Results from mixed-age studies suggest that older patients who have received nefazodone experience antidepressant efficacy similar to that produced by comparison TCAs. Nefazodone is sedating and may have potential therapeutic advantages of promoting sleep and anxiolytic effects. At low doses it does not impair highway-driving performance in elderly subjects, but may impair cognitive function and driving with increased dosages and prolonged use.[75] It does not have sexual side effects and is thus a reasonable alternative for an older patient complaining of sexual dysfunction from SSRI treatment. Nefazodone treatment should be initiated at half the young-adult dosage (50 mg twice daily), with slow titration upward. Healthy older patients who respond do so most often at doses of 200 to 400 mg daily. Nefazodone is a potent inhibitor of the hepatic cytochrome isoenzyme 3A4 within the P-450 enzyme system. Because this isoenzyme metabolizes many psychotropic drugs (e.g., benzodiazepines, tricyclics, carbamazepine) and medical medications (e.g., steroids, antibiotics), its use may be limited in elderly patients who are receiving multiple medications.

Mirtazapine

Mirtazapine, released for therapeutic use in the United States in 1996, has a unique chemical and pharmacologic profile that enhances presynaptic norepinephrine release and secondarily increases serotonin neurotransmission through effects on both serotonin receptors and norepinephrine heteroreceptors. Although mirtazapine has not been widely studied in elderly patients, available research and clinical experience suggest that it is an effective antidepressant with sedating properties.[76] This sedative effect can be useful for elderly depressed patients who have interrupted or shortened sleep.

Mirtazapine lacks other antidepressant side effects such as cardiotoxicity or orthostatic hypotension. However, its use is associated with significant weight gain in many patients. This may be a benefit to frail, undernourished, depressed elderly individuals but may be a hazard to those who are overweight. Recently a rapidly dissolving form of mirtazapine has become available. This orange-tasting preparation has similar antidepressant properties to the pill form[77] and is well accepted by depressed elderly nursing home residents.

Treatment Duration

Studies of maintenance antidepressant treatment[78,79] using TCAs indicate their usefulness in preventing recurrences of depression. Based on this information, the National Institute of Mental Health Consensus Development Conference on the Diagnosis and Treatment of Depression in Late Life[80] concluded that maintaining elderly patients on the antidepressant dose that was effective in treating the acute depressive episode is the best approach to long-term prevention of new episodes of unipolar depression. Unfortunately, because clinical trials of the newer antidepressants in elderly patients are brief in duration, lasting only 4 to 6 weeks, data from these studies do not provide information regarding maintenance use. One report directly addresses maintenance treatment and relapse: in a 44-week treatment study of major depression, only 13% of mixed-age patients receiving sertraline relapsed, compared with 46% of those receiving placebo.[81] Patient ages ranged from 19 to 78 years, but the effect of age on outcome was not reported. In another study, citalopram treatment over 48 weeks was well tolerated and found to decrease time to recurrence compared with placebo.[82]

Relapse rates among elderly patients who discontinue therapeutically effective SSRI and other nontricyclic medication are similar to those following discontinuation of TCAs. Most elderly patients relapse within the first 4 to 6 weeks of discontinuing treatment; the subsequent 4 months are also a period of relatively high risk. In general, because depression is a relapsing illness and because its consequences in older individuals may be severe, elderly patients should be advised to continue taking their antidepressants for extended periods of time—that is, at least 1 year after therapeutic effect and longer if the drug is well tolerated. As with any antidepressant, discontinuation should be extremely gradual and carefully monitored by a physician.

These limited studies, together with clinical experience, suggest that older people whose depression has been successfully treated with an SSRI or other new antidepressant should be maintained on the drug for a minimum of 1 year after recovery. This is especially true for older patients with multiple prior depressive episodes or for those whose late-life depression is severe.

Clinical Vignettes

Case 10.1

Mr. A., a 61-year-old screenwriter with an 8-year history of a transient tremor of the left arm and leg was eventually diagnosed as having Parkinson's disease and was treated with combination carbidopa and levodopa. Despite improvement, he developed leg cramps at the high dosages necessary to control his Parkinson's symptoms.

Eight months prior to his psychiatric evaluation, upon discontinuation of Mr. A.'s Parkinson's medication, the symptoms of Parkinson's recurred, and he became depressed. He complained of feelings of hopelessness and worthlessness, fatigue, and middle insomnia—symptoms accompanied by a diurnal mood variation. In addition to sad and anxious mood, he expressed discouragement, felt he was a burden to his wife, and was especially worried about his inability to write because of his motoric symptoms. He was not suicidal, had no passive thoughts of death, and presented no evidence of psychosis or cognitive impairment.

Mr. A. performed normally on tests of orientation, attention, comprehension, repetition, naming, word-list generation, constructions, memory, abstraction, and judgment. His motor examination did indicate prominent parkinsonism, with an asymmetric resting tremor most marked in the left hand and arm, increased tone in his limbs, and marked bradykinesia. MRI scanning was normal.

Mr. A.'s Parkinson's symptoms responded to multiple small doses of the combination carbidopa and levodopa increased to 10 $^{10}/_{100}$-mg tablets daily. Deprenyl 5 mg daily and pergolide 3.5 mg daily were added when symptoms reemerged. Despite the success in managing these motoric symptoms, the patient's depression persisted, and he was given fluoxetine 20 mg daily. Lack of response led to a dosage increase to 40 mg daily, and Mr. A.'s depression remitted after 2 weeks. Sadness, fatigue, and insomnia lessened markedly, and Mr. A. returned to his screenwriting, reporting a surge of energy and enthusiasm and full remission of his writer's block.

When depression occurs in a patient with Parkinson's disease, the clinician first needs to manage the motoric symptoms. Most antiparkinsonian agents are not potent antidepressants. Bromocriptine, a dopamine receptor agonist, may exert mild antidepressant effects and occasionally precipitates mania. The discovery of low concentrations of 5-hydroxyindoleacetic acid in the cerebrospinal fluid of depressed Parkinson's disease patients provides a rationale for using SSRIs to treat such patients. Unfortunately, not all patients respond, and occasionally SSRIs exacerbate motoric symptoms.[83] Patients resistant to antidepressant treatment may be given a course of electroconvulsive therapy, which often relieves both depression and motoric symptoms.

Case 10.2

Mrs. B., a 79-year-old woman with a 45-year history of bipolar disorder, was one of the first patients to receive lithium. She responded well, with few subsequent manic and depressive episodes except when she decided on her own to stop taking her medication. By her late 70s, however, exacerbations became more frequent, and she developed several chronic physical illnesses, including osteoporosis and resultant chronic pain. She also experienced seasonal mood swings and profile—depressed during the winter months and manic during the summer.

Two weeks before the Thanksgiving holiday, she became lethargic, lost interest in usual activities, and began sleeping through most of the day. She also ate little and lost several pounds in a week. Her lithium was kept at its usual dose and she was prescribed 20 mg of fluoxetine daily. After 2 days, her depression remitted. However, on the third day of treatment, she started spending money frivolously, gave away jewelry to acquaintances, and contacted a travel agent to plan a safari in Africa. Fluoxetine was discontinued but her depressive symptoms returned after several days; it was begun once again but at half the dose. After a week, she became euthymic and remained asymptomatic for the next 6 months, after which fluoxetine was discontinued. The following winter she was provided with phototherapy, which seemed to prevent a depressive episode that year.

Mrs. B.'s retardation and hypersomnia are not unusual presentations for patients with bipolar disorder during depressive episodes. A generally activating SSRI such as fluoxetine is a reasonable choice in such situations. However, the risk of precipitating mania is always present, even when patients are maintained on lithium. Nonpharmacologic approaches, such as electric light therapy, should be used when indicated, especially for elderly persons sensitive to medication side effects. This case also illustrates how small changes in antidepressant dosage can have a profound pharmacologic effect in elderly persons.

Case 10.3

Mr. C., a 78-year-old retired executive, was used to being extremely active and productive in his work. He had few friends, no hobbies, and a cordial but distant relationship with his wife. Following retirement he and his wife sold their comfortable home to move to a new city near his children and grandchildren. Neither he nor his wife had any social contacts in this new city.

It took Mr. C. one year to settle into his new living arrangement and establish relationships with doctors and family physicians, attorneys, and financial advisors. He was active, upbeat, and happy. But he now noticed a gradual decline in mood, energy, and interest. After reading the morning newspapers, he would go for a walk, but by 11:00 AM, faced an empty day. Although he created a schedule for himself that included reading, exercise, shopping, and exploring the new city, he very quickly became bored and progressively more dysphoric. His sleep became fragmented, and his wife reported a significant increase in irritability.

In an initial consultation, Mr. C also described considerable obsessive behavior. He was perfectionistic and highly organized, often counting and checking his work and his household chores. When traveling, he would pack several days in advance, often unpacking and repacking, and then would leave for the airport 2 to 3 hours ahead of the recommend times. Although he did not exhibit hand-washing, he became progressively more occupied with his health, which was, in fact, excellent and stable. In the consultation he was clearly sad, anhedonic, anergic, and apathetic. He spoke of pleasure only obtained with the grandchildren; otherwise life seemed pointless and potentially hopeless. He was not psychotic and not suicidal.

After consultation with his primary care physician, Mr. C. was prescribed a low dose of fluvoxamine (25 mg a day). This SSRI was chosen because of its reputed effectiveness in treating obsessive-compulsive symptoms along with its antidepressant properties. Indeed, Mr. C. rapidly reported an increase in mood and energy. He was most surprised and pleased, however, when he realized he was no longer counting, checking, or obsessing. He no longer packed far in advance of a trip and stopped going to the airport hours in advance.

Mr. C. also found his psychotherapeutic meetings with the prescribing clinician to be of great importance. He began to review early life experiences and then to examine his long work career. He came to realize his essential social isolation and virtual estrangement from his wife. As he discussed these matters, his mood further brightened, and his relationship with his wife grew significantly closer. All irritability disappeared.

Case 10.4

A 76-year old woman, Mrs. D., came for treatment complaining of anxiety and falling asleep. She went on to comment that she felt sad, and worried constantly, "What if something is wrong?" She had recently been experiencing difficulty making decisions, "even over trivial matters," although she had never previously experienced these difficulties. There was a family history of depression in her parents.

Mrs. D.'s primary care physician had previously prescribed alprazolam which she found too sedating; no antidepressants had ever been given. She agreed to begin treatment with citalopram 10 mg, and experienced GI upset and muscle twitching, especially when falling asleep. After one month she said: "I'm marginally better," although her side effects were beginning to disappear. The dose was raised to 20 mg a day, and two weeks later she reported

"I'm better." Her sleep had improved, and there were no further muscular jerks or spasms. She reported increased energy and an improved ability to focus and concentrate. She also noted, parenthetically, that she felt less anxious and less ruminative.

Mrs. D. has continued to take citalopram 20 mg for the past year. Her mood has remained stable and euthymic, although she has some difficulties "mobilizing" in the morning. She also reports vivid dreams that she sometimes confuses with reality on awakening. Recently she has noticed that her balance seems to be slightly impaired and she has fallen twice. She is also reporting difficulties sometimes finding the right word to express her thoughts.

SSRI antidepressants are well tolerated by the elderly, and are helpful for treating dysphoria characterized by mixed anxiety and depressive symptoms. There are side effects and potentially serious consequences of these medications in the older age group. Most significantly is a decline in balance. SSRIs have been reported to be associated with falls in nursing homes, and this patient's impaired balance may be an illustration of this side effect. SSRIs may also interfere with word-finding in patients of all ages, but it is especially troublesome in the elderly who may already suffer from this impairment.

References

1. Salzman C. Practical considerations for treatment of depression in elderly and very elderly long-term care patients. *J Clin Psychiatry* 1999;60 (suppl 20):30–33.
2. Salzman C. Mood disorders. In: CE Coffey, JL Cummings, eds. *The American Textbook of Geriatric Neuropsychiatry, Second Edition.* Washington, DC: American Psychiatric Press, 2000:313–328.
3. Salzman C. Management considerations for late-life depression. *J Clin Psychiatry* 2000;2(suppl 5): 33–36.
4. Salzman C, Satlin A, Burrows AB. Geriatric Psychopharmacology. In: AF Schatzberg, CB Nemeroff, eds. *Essentials of Clinical Psychopharmacology.* Washington, DC: American Psychiatric Press, 2001:637–658 .
5. McDonald WM, Salzman C, Schatzberg AF. Depression in the elderly. *Psychopharm Bull* 2002; 36(Suppl 2):112–122.
6. Finley PR. Selective serotonin reuptake inhibitors: pharmacologic profiles and potential therapeutic distinctions. *Ann Pharmacother* 1994;28: 1359–1369.
7. Pollock BG. Allelic variation in the serotonin transporter promoter affects onset of paroxetine treatment response in late-life depression. *Neuropsychopharmacology* 2000;23:587–590.

8. Alexopoulos GS, Katz IR, Reynolds CF III, et al. The Expert Consensus Guideline Series: Pharmacotherapy of depressive disorders in older patients. Postgraduate Medicine, October 2001.

9. Mittmann N, Herrmann N, Shulman KI, et al. The effectiveness of antidepressants in elderly depressed outpatients: a prospective case study series. *J Clin Psychiatry* 1999;60:690–697.

10. Rosen J, Mulsant BH, Pollock BG. Sertraline in the treatment of minor depression in nursing home residents: a pilot study. *Int J Geriatr Psychiatry* 2000;15:177–180.

11. Burrows AB, Salzman C, Satlin A, et al. A randomized, placebo-controlled trial of paroxetine in nursing home residents with non-major depression. *Depress Anxiety* 2002;15:102–110.

12. Cummings J, Small GW. Dealing with writer's block in an older man: depression, Parkinson's disease, or both? *Hosp Community Psychiatry* 1991; 42:19–24.

13. Williams JW, Barrett J, Oxman T, et al. Treatment of dysthymia and minor depression in primary care: A randomized controlled trial in older adults. *JAMA* 2000;284:1519–1526.

14. Nobler MS, Devanand DP, Kim MK, et al. Fluoxetine treatment of dysthymia in the elderly. *J Clin Psychiatry* 1996;57:254–256.

15. Devanand DP, Kim MK, Nobler MS. Fluoxetine discontinuation in elderly dysthymic patients. *Am J Geriatr Psychiatry* 1997;5:83–87.

16. Finkel SI. Efficacy and tolerability of antidepressant therapy in the old-old. *J Clin Psychiatry* 1996; 57(Suppl 5):23–28.

17. Karlsson I, Godderis J, de Mendonca Lima A, et al. A randomized, double-blind comparison of the efficacy and safety of citalopram compared to mianserin in elderly, depressed patients with or without mild to moderate dementia. *Int J Geriatr Psychiatry* 2000;15:295–305.

18. Nyth AL, Gottfries CG, Lyby K, et al. A controlled multicenter clinical study of citalopram and placebo in elderly depressed patients with and without concomitant dementia. *Acta Psychiatr Scand* 1992;86:138–146.

19. Mamdani MM, Parikh SV, Austin PC, et al. Use of antidepressants among elderly subjects: trends and contributing factors. *Am J Psychiatry* 2000;157:360–367.

20. Salzman C, Wong E, Wright CB. Drug and ECT treatment of depression in the elderly, 1996–2001: A literature review. *Biol Psychiatry* 2002;52:265–284.

21. Spier SA, Frontera MA. Unexpected deaths in depressed medical inpatients treated with fluoxetine. *J Clin Psychiatry* 1991;52:377–382.

22. Leinonen E, Koponen H, Leopola U. Delirium during fluoxetine treatment: a case report. *Ann Clin Psychiatry* 1993;5:255–257.

23. Small GW, Birkett M, Meyers BS, et al. Impact of physical illness on quality of life and antidepressant response in geriatric major depression. *J Am Geriatr Soc* 1996;44:1220–1225.

24. Trappler B, Cohen CI. Using fluoxetine in "very old" depressed nursing home residents. *Am J Geriatr Psychiatry* 1996;4:258–262.

25. Thompson C, Peveler RC, Stephenson D, et al. Compliance with antidepressant medication in the treatment of fluoxetine and a tricyclic antidepressant. *Am J Psychiatry* 2000;157:338–343.

26. Preskorn SH. Recent pharmacologic advances in antidepressant therapy for the elderly. *Am J Med* 1993;94(suppl 5A):2S–12S.

27. Newhouse PA, Richter EM. SSRIs in depressed elderly: a double-blind comparison of sertraline and fluoxetine in depressed geriatric outpatients. Presented at American College of Neuropsychopharmacology meeting; December 11–14, 1994; Puerto Rico.

28. Warrington SJ. Clinical implications of the pharmacology of sertraline. *Int Clin Psychopharmacol* 1991;6(suppl 2):11–21.

29. Gutierrez M, Abramowitz W. Steady-state pharmacokinetics of citalopram in young and elderly subjects. *Pharmacotherapy* 2000;20:1441–1447.

30. Small GW, Hamilton SL, Bystritsky A, et al. Clinical response predictors in a double-blind, placebo-controlled trial of fluoxetine for geriatric major depression. *Int Psychogeriatr* 1995; 7(suppl):41–53.

31. Dorman T. Sleep and paroxetine: a comparison with mianserin in elderly depressed patients. *Int J Clin Psychopharmacol* 1992;4:53–58.

32. Oxman TE. Antidepressants and cognitive impairment in the elderly. *J Clin Psychiatry* 1996; 57(suppl):38–44.

33. Tourjman S, Fontaine R. Fluvoxamine can induce confusion in the elderly. *J Clin Psychopharmacol* 1992;12:293.

34. Hindmarch I, Shillingford J, Shillingford C. The effects of sertraline on psychomotor performance in elderly volunteers. *J Clin Psychiatry* 1990;51(suppl):34–36.

35. Richelson E. Synaptic effects of antidepressants. *J Clin Psychopharmacol* 1996;16(suppl 2):1S–9S.

36. Pollock BG, Mulsant BH, Nebes R, et al. Serum anticholinergicity in elderly depressed patients treated with paroxetine or nortriptyline. *Am J Psychiatry* 1998;155:1110–1112.

37. Druckenbrod R, Mulsant BH. Fluoxetine-induced syndrome of inappropriate antidiuretic hormone secretion: a geriatric case report and a review of the literature. *J Geriatr Psychiatry Neurol* 1994;7:255–258.

38. Goldstein L, Barker M, Segall F, et al. Seizure and transient SIADH associated with sertraline. *Am J Psychiatry* 1996;153:732.

39. Marar IE, Towers AL, Mulsant BH, et al. Effect of paroxetine on·plasma vasopressin and water load testing in elderly individuals. *J Geriatr Psychiatry Neurol* 2000;13:212–216.

40. Levsky ME, Schwartz JB. Sertraline-induced hyponatremia in an older patient [letter]. *J Am Geriatr Soc* (1998);46:1582–1583.

41. Kirby D, Ames D. Hyponatremia and selective serotonin re-uptake inhibitors in elderly patients. *Int J Geriatr Psychiatry* 2001;16:484–493.

42. Strik JJ, Honig A, Lousberg R, et al. Cardiac side-effects of two selective serotonin reuptake inhibitors in middle-aged and elderly depressed patients. *Int Clin Psychopharmacol* 1998;13:263–267.

43. Roose SP, Glassman AH, Attia E, et al. Cardiovascular effects of fluoxetine in depressed patients with heart disease. *Am J Psychiatry* 1998;155: 660–665.

44. Roose SP, Laghrissi-Thode F, Kennedy JS, et al.

Comparison of paroxetine and nortriptyline in depressed patients with ischemic heart disease. *JAMA* 1998;279:287–291.

45. Ruthazer R, Lipsitz LA. Antidepressants and falls among elderly people living in long-term care. *Am J Public Health* 1993;83:746–749.

46. van Walraven C, Mamdani MM, Wells PS, et al. Inhibition of serotonin reuptake by antidepressants and upper gastrointestinal bleeding in elderly patients: retrospective cohort study. *BMJ* 2001;323:655–658.

47. Dunn NR, Pearce GL, Shakir SA. Association between SSRIs and upper gastrointestinal bleeding. SSRIs are no more likely than other drugs to cause such bleeding [letter]. *BMJ* 2000;320: 1405–1406.

48. Flint AJ, Rifat SL. Recurrence of first-episode geriatric depression after discontinuation of maintenance antidepressants. *Am J Psychiatry* 1999;156:943–945.

49. Preskorn S, Lane R, Magnus R. The SSRI withdrawal syndrome. *Eur Neuropsychopharm* 1996; 6(suppl):121.

50. Salzman C. Heterogeneity of SSRI response. *Harvard Rev Psychiatry* 1996;4:215–217.

51. Austin LS, Arana GW, Melvin JA. Toxicity resulting from lithium augmentation of antidepressant treatment in elderly patients. *J Clin Psychiatry* 1999;51:344–345.

52. Flint AJ, Rifat SL. A prospective study of lithium augmentation in antidepressant-resistant geriatric depression. *J Clin Psychopharmacol* 1994;14: 353–356.

53. Lavretsky H, Kumar A. Methylphenidate augmentation of citalopram in elderly depressed patients. *Am J Geriatr Psychiatry* 2001;9:298–303.

54. Lavretsky H, Kim MD, Reynolds CF. Combined treatment with methylphenidate and citalopram for accelerated response in the elderly: an open trial. *J Clin Psychiatry* 2003;64:1410–1414.

55. Branconnier RJ, Cole JO, Ghazvinian S, et al. Clinical pharmacology of bupropion and imipramine in elderly depressives. *J Clin Psychiatry* 1983;44:130–133.

56. Kane JM, Cole K, Sarantakos S, et al. Safety and efficacy of bupropion in elderly patients: Preliminary observations. *J Clin Psychiatry* 1983;44: 134–136.

57. Sweet RA, Pollock BG, Kirschner M, et al. Pharmacokinetics of single- and multiple-dose bupropion in elderly patients with depression. *J Clin Pharmacol* 1995;35:876–884.

58. Joo J, Lenze E, Mulsant B, et al. Risk factors for falls during treatment of late-life depression. *J Clin Psychiatry* 2002;63:936–941.

59. Szuba MP, Leuchter AF. Falling backward in two elderly patients taking bupropion. *J Clin Psychiatry* 1992;53:157–159.

60. Rudorfer MV, Potter WZ. Antidepressants: a comparative review of the clinical pharmacology and therapeutic use of the "newer" versus the "older" drugs. *Drugs* 1989;37:713–738.

61. Haria M, Fitton A, McTavish D. Trazodone: a review of its pharmacology, therapeutic use in depression and therapeutic potential in other disorders. *Drugs Aging* 1994;4:331–335.

62. Rausch JL, Pavlinac DM, Newman PE. Complete heart block following a single dose of trazodone. *Am J Psychiatry* 1984;151:1472–1473.

63. Schneider LS, Sobin PB. Non-neuroleptic treatment of behavioral symptoms and agitation in Alzheimer's disease and other dementia. *Psychopharmacol Bull* 1992;28:71–79.

64. Branconnier RJ, Cole JO. Effects of acute administration of trazodone and amitriptyline on cognition, cardiovascular function and salivation in the normal agitated patient. *J Clin Psychopharmacol* 1981;1:2–8.

65. Knegtering H, Eijck M, Huijsman A. Effects of antidepressants on cognitive functioning of elderly patients: a review. *Drugs Aging* 1994;5: 192–199.

66. Wesnes KA, Simpson PM, Christmas L, et al. The effects of moclobemide on cognition. *J Neural Transm* 1989;28(suppl):91–102.

67. Greenblatt DJ, Friedman H, Burstein ES, et al. Trazodone kinetics: effect of age, gender, and obesity. *Clin Pharmacol Ther* 1987;42:193–200.

68. Parker V, Paerg L, Maloney K, et al. Effect of age and sex on the pharmacokinetics of venlafaxine. *J Clin Pharmacol* 1990;30:832.

69. Khan A, Rudolph R, Baumel B, et al. Venlafaxine in depressed geriatric outpatients: an open-label clinical study. *Psychopharmacol Bull* 1995;31: 753–758.

70. Mahapatra SN, Hackett D. A randomized, double-blind, parallel group comparison of venlafaxine and dothiepin in geriatric patients with major depression. *Int J Clin Pract* 1997;51: 209–213.

71. Thase ME, Entsuah AR, Rudolph RL. Remission rates during treatment with venlafaxine or selective serotonin reuptake inhibitors. *Br J Psychiatry* 2001;178:234–241.

72. Muth EA, Moyer JA, Haskins JT, et al. Biochemical, neurophysiological, and behavioral effects of Wy-45,233 and other identified metabolites of the antidepressant venlafaxine. *Drug Dev Res* 1991;23:191–199.

73. Danjou P, Hackett D. Safety and tolerance profile of venlafaxine. *Int Clin Psychopharmacol* 1995; 10(suppl 2):15–20.

74. van Laar MW, van Willigenburg APP, Volkerts ER. Acute and subchronic effect of nefazodone and imipramine on highway driving, cognitive functions, and daytime sleepiness in healthy adult and elderly subjects. *J Clin Psychopharmacol* 1995;15:30–40.

75. Schatzberg AF, Kremer C, Rodrigues H, et al. Double-blind, randomized comparison of mirtazapine and paroxetine in elderly depressed patients. *Am J Geriatr Psychiatry* 2002;10:541–550.

76. Roose ST, Nelson JC, Salzman C, et al. Mirtazapine orally disintegrating tablets in depressed patients in the nursing home. *Curr Med Res Opin.* 2003;19:737–746.

77. Reynolds CF, Frank E, Perel JM, et al. Maintenance therapies for late-life recurrent major depression: research and review circa 1995. *Int Psychogeriatr* 1995;7(suppl);27–39.

78. Old Age Depression Interest Group. How long should the elderly take antidepressants? A double-blind placebo-controlled study of continuation/prophylaxis therapy with dothiepin. *Br J Psychiatry* 1993;162:175–182.

79. NIH Consensus Development Panel on Depression in Late Life. Diagnosis and treatment

of depression in late life. *JAMA* 1992;268: 1018–1024.

80. Doogan DP, Caillard V. Sertraline in the prevention of depression. *Br J Psychiatry* 1992;160: 217–222.

81. Klysner R, Bent-Hansen J, Hansen HL, et al. Efficacy of citalopram in the prevention of recurrent depression in elderly patients: placebo-controlled study of maintenance therapy. *Br J Psychiatry* 2002;181:29–35.

82. Leo RJ, Lichter DG, Hershey LA. Parkinsonism associated with fluoxetine and cimetidine: a case report. *J Geriatr Psychiatry Neurol* 1995;8:231–233.

Table 10.2 References

Ackerman DL, Greenland S, Bystritsky A, et al. Side effects and time course of response in a placebo-controlled trial of fluoxetine for the treatment of geriatric depression. *J Clin Psychopharmacol* 2000;20:658–665.

Altamura AC, De Novelis F, Guercetti, et al. Fluoxetine compared with amitriptyline in elderly depression: a controlled clinical trial. *Int J Clin Pharmacol Res* 1989;9:391–396.

Arranz FJ, Ros S. Effects of comorbidity and polypharmacy on the clinical usefulness of sertraline in elderly depressed patients: an open multicenter study. *J Affect Disord* 1997;46:285–291.

Bocksberger JP, Gachoud JP, Richard J, et al. Comparison of the efficacy of moclobemide and fluvoxamine in elderly patients with a severe depressive episode. *Eur Psychiatry* 1993;8:319–324.

Bondareff W, Alpert M, Friedhoff AJ, et al. Comparison of sertraline and nortriptyline in the treatment of major depression in late life. *Am J Psychiatry* 2000;157:729–736.

Bump GM, Mulsant BH, Pollock BG, et al. Paroxetine versus nortriptyline in the continuation and maintenance treatment of depression in the elderly. *Depress Anxiety* 2001;13:38–44.

Burrows AB, Salzman C, Satlin A, et al. A randomized, placebo-controlled trial of paroxetine in nursing home residents with non-major depression. *Depress Anxiety* 2002;15:102–110.

Cassano GB, Puca F, Scapicchio PL, et al. Paroxetine and fluoxetine effects on mood and cognitive functions in depressed non-demented elderly patients. *J Clin Psychiatry* 2002;63:396–402.

Cohn CK, Shrivastava R, Mendels J, et al. Double-blind, multicenter comparison of sertraline and amitriptyline in elderly depressed patients. *J Clin Psychiatry* 1990;5(suppl B):28–33.

Dorman T. Sleep and paroxetine: a comparison with mianserin in elderly depressed patients. *Int Clin Psychopharmacol* 1992;6(suppl 4):53–58.

Dunner DL, Cohn JB, Walshe T, et al. Two combined, multicenter double-blind studies of paroxetine and doxepin in geriatric patients with major depression. *J Clin Psychiatry* 1992;53(suppl 2):57–60.

Evans M, Hammond M, Wilson K, et al. Placebo-controlled treatment trial of fluoxetine for depression in elderly physically ill patients. *Int J Geriatr Psychiatry* 1997;12:817–824.

Fairweather DB, Kerr JS, Harrison DA, et al. A double-blind comparison of the effects of fluoxetine and amitriptyline on cognitive function in elderly depressed patients. *Hum Psychopharmacol* 1993;8: 41–47.

Falk WE, Rosenbaum JE, Otto MW, et al. Fluoxetine versus trazodone in depressed geriatric patients. *J Geriatr Psychiatry Neurol* 1989;2:208–214.

Feighner JP, Boyer WF, Meredith CH, Hendrickson G. An overview of fluoxetine in geriatric depression. *Br J Psychiatry* 1988;153(suppl 3):105–108.

Feighner JP, Cohn JB. Double-blind comparative trials of fluoxetine and doxepin in geriatric patients with major depressive disorder. *J Clin Psychiatry* 1985;46:20–25.

Finkel SI, Richter EM. Clary CM, et al. Comparative efficacy of sertraline vs. fluoxetine in patients age 70 or over with major depression. *Am J Geriatr Psychiatry* 1999;7:221–227.

Finkel SI, Richter EM. Clary CM. Comparative efficacy and safety of sertraline versus nortriptyline in major depression in patients 70 and older. *Int Psychogeriatr* 1999;11:85–99.

Forlenza OV, Junior AS, Hirala ES, et al. Antidepressant efficacy of sertraline and imipramine for the treatment of major depression in elderly outpatients. *Sao Paolo Med J* 2000;118:99–104.

Geretsegger C, Bohmer F, Ludwig M. Paroxetine in the elderly depressed patient: randomized comparison with fluoxetine of efficacy, cognitive and behavioral effects. *Int Clin Psychopharmacol* 1994; 9:25–29.

Geretsegger C, Stuppaeck CH, Mair M, et al. Multicenter double blind study of paroxetine and amitriptyline in elderly depressed inpatients. *Psychopharmacology* 1995;119:277–281.

Giakas WJ, Miller JL, Hensala JD, et al. Fluoxetine vs. bupropion in geriatric depression. Paper presented at the American Psychiatric Association annual meeting, San Francisco, CA, May 1993.

Goldstein DJ, Hamilton SH, Masica CM. Fluoxetine in medically stable, depressed geriatric patients: Effects on weight. *J Clin Psychopharmacol* 1997;17: 365–369.

Green TD, Reynolds CF III, Mulsant BH, et al. Accelerating antidepressant response in geriatric depression: a post hoc comparison of combined sleep deprivation and paroxetine versus monotherapy with paroxetine, nortriptyline, or placebo. *J Geriatric Psychiatry and Neurol* 1999;12: 67–71.

Guillibert E, Pelicier Y, Archambault JC, et al. A double-blind, multicentre study of paroxetine versus clomipramine in depressed elderly patients. *Acta Psychiatr Scand* 1989;80(suppl 350):132–134.

Gutierrez M, Abramowitz W. Steady-state pharmacokinetics of citalopram in young and elderly subjects. *Pharmacotherapy* 2000;20:1441–1447.

Hebenstreit GF, Fellerer K, Zochling R, et al. A pharmacokinetic dose titration study in adult and elderly depressed patients. *Acta Psychiatr Scand* 1988;80(suppl 350):81–84.

Heiligenstein JH, Ware JE, Beusterien KM, et al. Acute effects of fluoxetine versus placebo on functional health and well-being in late-life depression. *Int Psychogeriatr* 1995;7(suppl): 125–137.

Hindmarch I, Shillingford J, Shillingford C. The effects of sertraline on psychomotor performance in elderly volunteers. *J Clin Psychiatry* 1990; 51(suppl B):34–36.

Hutchinson DR, Tong S, Moon CAL, et al. A double blind study in general practice to compare the efficacy and tolerability of paroxetine and ami-triptyline in depressed elderly patients. *Br J Clin Res* 1991;2:43–57.

Hutchinson DR, Tong S, Moon CAL, et al. Paroxetine in the treatment of elderly depressed patients in general practice: a double-blind comparison with amitriptyline. *Int Clin Psychopharmacol* 1992;6(suppl 4):43–51.

Joo J, Lenze E, Mulsant B, et al. Risk factors for falls during treatment of late-life depression. *J Clin Psychiatry* 2002;63:936–941.

Karlsson I, Godderis J, de Mendonca Lima A, et al. A randomized, double-blind comparison of the efficacy and safety of citalopram compared to mianserin in elderly, depressed patients with or without mild to moderate dementia. *Int J Geriatr Psychiatry* 2000;15:295–305.

Katona CL, Hunter BN, Bray J. A double-blind comparison of the efficacy and safety of paroxetine and imipramine in the treatment of depression with dementia. *Int J Geriatr Psychiatry* 1998;13: 100–108.

Klysner R, Bent-Hansen K, Hansen HL, et al. Efficacy of citalopram in the prevention of recurrent depression in elderly patients: placebo-controlled study of maintenance therapy. *Br J Psychiatry* 2002;181:29–35.

Koran LM, Hamilton SH, Hertzman M, et al. Predicting response to fluoxetine in geriatric patients with major depression. *J Clin Psychopharmacol* 1995;15:421–427.

Kyle CJ, Petersen HE, Overo KF. Comparison of the tolerability and efficacy of citalopram and amitriptyline in elderly depressed patients treated in general practice. *Depress Anxiety* 1998;8:147–163.

La Pia S, Giorgio D, Ciriello R, et al. Evaluation of the efficacy, tolerability, and therapeutic profile of fluoxetine versus mianserin in the treatment of depressive disorders in the elderly. *Curr Ther Res* 1992;52:847–858.

Lavretsky H, Kumar A. Methylphenidate augmentation of citalopram in elderly depressed patients. *Am J Geriatr Psychiatry* 2001;9:298–303.

Lyketsos CG, Sheppart J-Me, Steele CD, et al. Randomized, placebo-controlled, double-blind clinical trial of sertraline in the treatment of depression complicating Alzheimer's disease: initial results from the Depression in Alzheimer's Disease Study. *Am J Psychiatry* 2000;157:1686–1689.

Magai C, Kennedy G, Cohen CI, et al. A controlled clinical trial of sertraline in the treatment of depression in nursing home patients with late-stage Alzheimer's disease. *Am J Geriatr Psychiatry* 2000;8:66–74.

Mahapatra SN, Hackett D. A randomized, double-blind, parallel-group comparison of venlafaxine and dothiepin in geriatric patients with major depression. *IJCP* 1997;51:209–213.

Mamo DC, Sweet RA, Mulsant BH, et al. Effect of nortriptyline and paroxetine on extrapyramidal signs and symptoms. *Am J Geriatr Psychiatry* 2000; 8:226–231.

Marar IE, Towers AL, Mulsant BH, et al. Effect of paroxetine on plasma vasopressin and water load testing in elderly individuals. *J Geriatr Psychiatry Neurol* 2000;13:212–216.

Mulsant BH, Pollock BG, Nebes RD, et al. A double-blind randomized comparison of nortriptyline and paroxetine in the treatment of late-life depression: 6-week outcome. *J Clin Psychiatry* 1999;60(suppl 20):16–20.

Mulsant BH, Pollock BG, Nebes RD, et al. A twelve-week, double-blind, randomized comparison of nortriptyline and paroxetine in older depressed inpatients and outpatients. *Am J Geriatr Psychiatry* 2001;9:406–414.

Navarro V, Gasto C, Torres X, et al. Citalopram versus nortriptyline in late-life depression: A 12-week randomized blind study. *Acta Psychiatry Scand* 2001;103:435–440.

Newhouse PA, Krishnan K, Doraiswamy P, et al. A double-blind comparison of sertraline and fluoxetine in depressed elderly outpatients. *J Clin Psychiatry* 2000;61:559–568.

Nobler MS. Regional cerebral blood flow in mood disorders, V.: Effects of antidepressant medication in late-life depression. *Am J Geriatr Psychiatry* 2000;8:289–296.

Nobler MS, Devanand DP, Kim MK, et al. Fluoxetine treatment of dysthymia in the elderly. *J Clin Psychiatry* 1996;57:254–256.

Nyth AL, Gottfries CG, Lyby K, et al. A controlled multicenter clinical study of citalopram and placebo in elderly depressed patients with and without concomitant dementia. *Acta Psychiatrica Scand* 1992;86:138–145.

Orengo CA, Kunik ME, Molinari V, et al. The use and tolerability of fluoxetine in geropsychiatric inpatients. *J Clin Psychiatry* 1996;57:12–16.

Oslin DW, Ten Have TR, Streim JE, et al. Probing the safety of medication in the frail elderly: evidence from a randomized clinical trial of sertraline and venlafaxine in depressed nursing home residents. *J Clin Psychiatry* 2003;64:875–882.

Oslin DW, Streim JE, Katz IR, et al. Heuristic comparison of sertraline with nortriptyline treatment of depression for the treatment of depression in frail elderly patients. *Am J Geriatr Psychiatry* 2000; 8:141–149.

Pollock BG. Allelic variation in the serotonin transporter promoter affects onset of paroxetine treatment response in late-life depression. *Neuropsychopharmacology* 2000;23:587–590.

Pollock BG, Mulsant BH, Nebes R, et al. Serum anticholinergicity in elderly depressed patients treated with paroxetine or nortriptyline. *Am J Psychiatry* 1998;155:1110–1112.

"Projecto Terceira Idade," Institute of Psychiatry, Hospital das Clínicas. Faculdade de Medicina, Universidade de São Paulo, São Paulo, Brazil. *Sao Paulo Med J* 2000;118:99–104.

Rahman MK, Akhtar MJ, Salva NC, et al. A double-blind, randomized comparison of fluvoxamine with dothiepin in the treatment of depression in elderly patients. *Br J Clin Pract* 1991;45:255–258.

Ronfeld RA, Tremaine LM, Wilner KD. Pharmacokinetics of sertraline and its N-demethyl metabolite in elderly and young male and female volunteers. *Clin Pharmacokinet* 1997;32(Suppl 1):22–30.

Roose SP, Glassman AH, Attia E, et al. Comparative efficacy of selective serotonin reuptake inhibitors and tricyclics in the treatment of melancholia. *Am J Psychiatry* 1994;151:1735–1739.

Rosen J, Mulsant BH, Pollock BG. Sertraline in the treatment of minor depression in nursing home residents: a pilot study. *Int J Geriatr Psychiatry* 2000;15:177–180.

Salzman C, Wong E, and Wright CB. Drug and ECT treatment of depression in the elderly, 1996–2001: A literature review. *Biol Psychiatry* 2002;52:265–284.

Schatzberg AF, Kremer C, Rodrigues HE, et al. Double-blind, randomized comparison of mirtazapine and paroxetine in elderly depressed patients. *Am J Geriatr Psychiatry* 2002;10:541–550.

Schneider LS, Small GW, Clary CM. Estrogen replacement therapy and antidepressant response to sertraline in older depressed women. *Am J Geriatric Psychiatry* 2001;9:393–399.

Schneider LS, Olin JT. Efficacy of acute treatment for geriatric depression. *Int Psychogeriatr* 1995; 7(suppl):7–25.

Schone W, Ludwig M. A double-blind study of paroxetine compared with fluoxetine in geriatric patients with major depression. *J Clin Psychopharmacol* 1993;13(suppl 2):34S–39S.

Small GW, Hamilton SH, Bystritsky A, et al. Clinical response predictors in a double-blind, placebo-controlled trial of fluoxetine for geriatric major depression. Fluoxetine Collaborative Study Group. *Int Psychogeriatr* 1995; 7(suppl):41–53.

Solai LK, Mulsant BH, Pollock BG, et al. Effect of sertraline on plasma nortriptyline levels in depressed elderly. *J Clin Psychiatry* 1997;58:440–443.

Tollefson GD, Holman SL. Analysis of the Hamilton Depression Rating Scale factors from a double-blind, placebo-controlled trial of fluoxetine in geriatric major depression. *Int Clin Psychopharmacol* 1993;8:253–259.

Wakelin JS. Fluvoxamine in the treatment of the older depressed patient; double-blind, placebo-controlled data. *Int Clin Psychopharmacol* 1986;1: 221–230.

Walters G, Reynolds CF III, Mulsant BH, et al. Continuation and maintenance Pharmacotherapy in geriatric depression: an open-trial comparison of paroxetine and nortriptyline in patients older than 70 years. *J Clin Psychiatry* 1999;60(suppl 20): 21–25.

Weihs KL, Settle ED, Batey SR, et al. Bupropion sustained release versus paroxetine for the treatment of depression in the elderly. *J Clin Psychiatry* 2000;61:196–202.

Williams JW, Barrett J, Oxman T, et al. Treatment of dysthymia and minor depression in primary care: A randomized controlled in older adults. *JAMA* 2000;284:1519–1526.

Wolf R, Dykierek P, Gattaz WF, et al. Differential effects of trimipramine and fluoxetine on sleep in geriatric depression. *Pharmacopsychiatry* 2001; 34:60–65.

Table 10.3 References

Altamura AC, De Novelis F, Guercetti, et al. Fluoxetine compared with amitriptyline in elderly depression: a controlled clinical trial. *Int J Clin Pharmacol Res* 1989;9:391–396.

Amore M, Ricci M, Zanardi R, et al. Long-term treatment of geropsychiatric depressed patients with venlafaxine. *J Affect Disorders* 1997;46:293–296.

Branconnier RJ, Cole JO, Ghazvinian S, et al. Clinical pharmacology of bupropion and imipramine in elderly depressives. *J Clin Psychiatry* 1983;44: 130–133.

Dierick M. An open-label evaluation of the long-term safety of oral venlafaxine in depressed elderly patients. *Ann Clin Psychiatry* 1996;8:169–178.

Falk WE, Rosenbaum JE, Otto MW, et al. Fluoxetine versus trazodone in depressed geriatric patients. *J Geriatr Psychiatry Neurol* 1989;2:208–214.

Gastó C, Navarro V, Marcos T, et al. Single-blind comparison of venlafaxine and nortriptyline in elderly major depression. *J Clin Psychopharmacology* 2003;23:21–26.

Gerner R, Estabrook W, Steuer J, Jarvik L. Treatment of geriatric depression with trazodone, imipramine, and placebo: a double-blind study. *J Clin Psychiatry* 1980;41:216–220.

Høyberg OF, Maragakis B, Millin K, et al. A double-blind multicenter comparison of mirtazapine and amitriptyline in elderly depressed patients. *Acta Psychiatr Scand* 93:184–190.

Jarvik LF, Mintz J, Steuer J, et al. Treating geriatric depression: a 26-week interim analysis. *J Am Geriatr Soc* 1982;2:713–717.

Joo J, Lenze E, Mulsant B, et al. Risk factors for falls during treatment of late-life depression. *J Clin Psychiatry* 2002;63:936–941.

Kane JM, Cole K, Sarantakos S, et al. Safety and efficacy of bupropion in elderly patients: preliminary observations. *J Clin Psychiatry* 1983;44: 134–136.

Khan A, Rudolph R, Baumel B, et al. Venlafaxine in depressed geriatric outpatients: an open-label clinical study. *Psychopharmacol Bull* 1995;31: 753–758.

Roose ST, Nelson JC, Salzman C, et al. Mirtazapine orally disintegrating tablets in depressed patients in the nursing home. *Curr Med Res Opin* 2003;19: 737–746.

Scardigli G, Jans G. Comparative double-blind study on efficacy and side-effects of trazodone, nomifensine, mianserin in elderly patients. In: Costa E, Racayni G, eds. *Typical and atypical antidepressants: clinical practice.* New York: Raven Press, 1982.

Schatzberg AF, Kremer C, Rodrigues HE, et al. Double-blind, randomized comparison of mirtazapine and paroxetine in elderly depressed patients. *Am J Geriatr Psychiatry* 2002;10:541–550.

Sweet RA, Pollock BG, Kirschner M, et al. Pharmacokinetics of single- and multiple-dose bupropion in elderly patients with depression. *J Clin Pharmacol* 1995;35:876–884.

Van Laar MW, van Willigenburg AP, Volkerts ER. Acute and subchronic effects of nefazodone and imipramine on highway driving, cognitive functions, and daytime sleepiness in healthy adult and elderly subjects. *J Clin Psychopharmacol* 1995;15: 30–40.

Zimmer B, Kant R, Zeiler D, et al. Antidepressant efficacy and cardiovascular safety of venlafaxine in young vs old patients with comorbid medical disorders. *Int J Psychiatry Med* 1997;27:353–364.

Supplemental Readings

General

Alexopoulos GS, Chester JG. Outcomes of geriatric depression. *Clin Geriatr Med* 1992;8:363–376.

Amar KA, Wilcock GK. Antidepressant medicines for the elderly: are we using them appropriately? *Gerontology* 1994;40:314–318.

Bodner RA, Lynch T, Lewis L, et al. Serotonin syndrome. *Neurology* 1995:45:219–223.

Bressler R, Katz MD. Drug therapy for geriatric depression. *Drugs Aging* 1993;3:195–219.

Brown SL, Salive ME, Guralnik JM, et al. Antidepressant use in the elderly: association with demographic characteristics, health-related factors, and health care utilization. *J Clin Epidemiol* 1995; 48:445–453.

Callahan CM, Nienaber NA, Hendrie HC, et al. Depression of elderly outpatients: primary care physicians' attitudes and practice patterns. *J Gen Intern Med* 1992;7:26–31.

Cassano GB, Musetti L, Soriani A, et al. The pharmacologic treatment of depression: drug selection criteria. *Pharmacopsychiatry* 1993;26:(suppl 1): 17–23.

Chiu HF. Antidepressants in the elderly. *Int J Clin Pract* 1997;51:369–374.

Christensen DD. Rational antidepressant selection in the elderly. *Geriatrics* 1995;50(suppl 1): S41–S50.

Cole MG, Elie M, McCusker J, et al. Feasibility and effectiveness of treatments for depression in elderly medical inpatients: a systematic review. *International Psychogeriatrics* 2000;12:453–461.

Conn DK, Goldman Z. Pattern of use of antidepressants in long-term care facilities for the elderly. *J Geriatr Psychiatry Neurol* 1992;5:228–232.

DasGupta K. Treatment of depression in elderly patients: recent advances. *Arch Fam Med* 1998;7: 274–280.

Dewan MJ, Huszonek J, Koss M, et al. The use of antidepressants in the elderly: 1986 and 1989. *J Geriatr Psychiatry Neurol* 1992;5:40–44.

Diehl DJ, Houck PR, Paradis C, et al. Pretreatment systolic orthostatic blood pressure and treatment response in geriatric depression: a revisit. *J Clin Psychopharmacol* 1993;13:189–193.

Drevets WC. Geriatric depression: brain imaging correlates and pharmacologic considerations. *J Clin Psychiatry* 1994;55(suppl A):71–81, discussion 82, 98–100.

Emslie G, Judge R. Tricyclic antidepressants and selective serotonin reuptake inhibitors: use during pregnancy, in children/adolescents and in the elderly. *Acta Psychiatr Scand Suppl* 2000;403: 26–34.

Finkel SI. Efficacy and tolerability of antidepressant therapy in the old-old. *J Clin Psychiatry* 1996; 57(suppl):23–28.

Flint AJ, Rifat SL. Anxious depression in elderly patients. Response to antidepressant treatment. *Am J Geriatr Psychiatry* 1997;5:107–115.

Flint AJ, Rifat SL. Two-year outcome of elderly patients with anxious depression. *Psychiatry Res* 1997;66:23–31.

Flint AJ. Choosing appropriate antidepressant therapy in the elderly. A risk-benefit assessment of available agents. *Drugs Aging* 1998;13:269–280.

Flint AJ, Rifat SL. Maintenance treatment for recurrent depression in late life. A four-year outcome study. *Am J Geriatr Psychiatry* 2000;8:112–116.

Gareri P, Falconi U, De Fazio P, et al. Conventional and new antidepressants drugs in the elderly. *Prog Neurobiol* 2000;61:353–396.

Garrard J, Dunham T, Makris L, et al. Longitudinal study of psychotropic drug use by elderly nursing home residents. *J Gerontol* 1992;47:M183–M188.

Govoni S, Racchi M, Masoero E, et al. Extrapyramidal symptoms and antidepressant drugs: neuropharmacological aspects of a frequent interaction in the elderly. *Mol Psychiatry* 2001;6:134–142.

Halaris A. Antidepressant drug therapy in the elderly: enhancing safety and compliance. *Int J Psychiatry Med* 1986–87;16:1–19.

Herr KA, Mobily PR, Smith C. Depression and the experience of chronic back pain: a study of related variables and age differences. *Clin J Pain* 1993;9:104–114.

Heston LL, Garrard J, Makris L, et al. Inadequate treatment of depressed nursing home elderly. *J Am Geriatr Soc* 1992;40:1117–1122.

Jenike MA. Psychiatric illness in the elderly: a review. *J Geriatr Psychiatry Neurol* 1996;9:57–82.

Katona C. Rationalizing antidepressants for elderly people. *Int Clin Psychopharmacol* 1995;10(suppl 1):37–40.

Katz IR. Drug treatment of depression in the frail elderly: discussion of the NIH Consensus Development Conference on the Diagnosis and Treatment of Depression in Late Life. *Psychopharmacol Bull* 1993;29:101–108.

Katz IR, Parmelee PA, Beaston-Wimmer P, et al. Association of antidepressants and other medications with mortality in the residential-care elderly. *J Geriatr Psychiatry Neurol* 1994;7:221–226.

Katz IR, Streim J, Parmelee P. Prevention of depression recurrences and complications in late life. *Prev Med* 1994;23:743–750.

Knegtering H, Eijck M, Huijsman A. Effects of antidepressants on cognitive functioning of elderly patients. A review. *Drugs Aging* 1994;5:192–199.

Leonard BE. Pharmacological differences of serotonin reuptake inhibitors and possible clinical relevance. *Drugs* 1992;43(suppl):3–9; discussion 9–10.

Little JT, Reynolds CF III, Dew FE, et al. How common is resistance to treatment in recurrent, nonpsychotic geriatric depression? *Am J Psychiatry* 1998;155:1035–1038.

Liu B, Anderson G, Mittmann N, et al. Use of selective serotonin-reuptake inhibitors of tricyclic antidepressants and risk of hip fractures in elderly people. *Lancet* 1998;351:1303–1307.

Meyers BS. Late-life delusional depression: acute and long-term treatment. *Int Psychogeriatr* 1995; 7(suppl):113–124.

Meyers BS, Klimstra SA, Gabriele M, et al. Continuation treatment of delusional depression in older adults. *Am J Geriatr Psychiatry* 2001;9:415–422.

Meyers BS, Alpert S, Gabriele M, et al. State specificity of DST abnormalities in geriatric depression. *Biol Psychiatry* 1993;34:108–114.

Montgomery SA. Efficacy and safety of the selective serotonin reuptake inhibitors in treating depression in elderly patients. *Int Clin Psychopharmacol* 1998;13(suppl 5):S49–S54.

Nemeroff CB. Evolutionary trends in the pharmacotherapeutic management of depression. *J Clin Psychiatry* 1994;55(suppl):3–15; discussion 16–17.

Nolan L, O'Malley K. Adverse effects of antidepressants in the elderly. *Drugs Aging* 1992;2:450–458.

Oslin DW, Katz IR, Edell WS, et al. Effects of alcohol consumption on the treatment of depression among elderly patients. *Am J Geriatr Psychiatry* 2000;8:215–220.

Petracca G, Teson A, Chemerinski E, et al. A double-blind placebo-controlled study of clomipramine in depressed patients with Alzheimer's disease. *J Neuropsychiatry Clin Neurosci* 1996;8:270–275.

Preskorn SH. Recent pharmacologic advances in antidepressant therapy for the elderly. *Am J Med* 1993;94:2S–12S.

Riesenman C. Antidepressant drug interactions and the cytochrome P450 system: a critical appraisal. *Pharmacotherapy* 1995;15:84S–99S.

Reynolds CF. Treatment of depression in special populations. *J Clin Psychiatry* 1992;53(suppl):45–53.

Reynolds CF. Treatment of depression in late life. *Am J Med* 1994;97:39S–46S.

Reynolds CF, Frank E, Kupfer DJ, et al. Treatment outcome in recurrent major depression: a post hoc comparison of elderly ("young old") and midlife patients. *Am J Psychiatry* 1996;153:1288–1292.

Rigler SK, Webb MJ, Redford L, et al. Weight outcomes among antidepressant users in nursing facilities. *J Am Geriatr Soc* 2001;49:49–55.

Rothchild AJ. The diagnosis and treatment of late-life depression. *J Clin Psychiatry* 1996;57(suppl):5–11.

Salzman C. Monoamine oxidase inhibitors and atypical antidepressants. *Clin Geriatr Med* 1992;8:335–348.

Salzman C. Pharmacologic treatment of depression in the elderly. *J Clin Psychiatry* 1993;54(suppl):23–28.

Salzman C. Depressive disorders and other emotional issues in the elderly: current issues. *Int Clin Psychopharmacol* 1997;12(supp 7):S37–S42.

Schatzberg AF. New indications for antidepressants. *J Clin Psychiatry* 2000;61(supp 11):9–17.

Schneider LS. Efficacy of treatment for geropsychiatric patients with severe mental illness. *Psychopharmacol Bull* 1993;29:501–524.

Schneider LS, Olin JT. Efficacy of acute treatment for geriatric depression. *Int Psychogeriatr* 1995;7(suppl):7–25.

Schweizer E. Buspirone and imipramine for the treatment of major depression in the elderly. *J Clin Psychiatry* 1998;59:175–183.

Seth R, Jennings AL, Bindman J, et al. Combination treatment with noradrenalin and serotonin reuptake inhibitors in resistant depression. *Br J Psychiatry* 1992;161:562–565.

Stokes PE. Current issues in the treatment of major depression. *J Clin Psychopharmacol* 1993;13(suppl):2S–9S.

Stoudemire A, Hill CD, Morris R, et al. Long-term outcome of treatment-resistant depression in older adults. *Am J Psychiatry* 1993;150:1539–1540.

Taylor IC, McConnell JG. Severe hyponatremia associated with selective serotonin reuptake inhibitors. *Scott Med J* 1995;40:147–148.

Thapa PB, Gideon P, Cost TW, et al. Antidepressants and the risk of falls among nursing home residents. *N Engl J Med* 1998;339:875–882.

Thompson M, Samuels S. Rhabdomyolysis with simvastatin and nefazodone. *Am J Psychiatry* 2002;159:1607

Volz HP, Muller H, Sturm Y, et al. Effect of initial treatment with antidepressants as a predictor of outcome after 8 weeks. *Psychiatry Res* 1995;58:107–115.

Weintraub D. Nortriptyline in geriatric depression resistant to serotonin reuptake inhibitors: case series. *J Geriatr Psychiatry Neurol* 2001;14:28–32.

Wells KB, Norquist G, Benjamin B, et al. Quality of antidepressant medications prescribed at discharge to depressed elderly patients in general medical hospitals before and after prospective payment system. *Gen Hosp Psychiatry* 1994;16:4–15.

Young RC, Kalayam B, Nambudiri DE, et al. Brain morphology and response to nortriptyline in geriatric depression. *Am J Geriatr Psychiatry* 1999;7:147–150.

Zisook S, Downs NS. Diagnosis and treatment of depression in late life. *J Clin Psychiatry* 1998;59(supp 4):80–91.

Pharmacokinetics

Ascher JA, Cole JO, Colin JN, et al. Bupropion: a review of its mechanism of antidepressant activity. *J Clin Psychiatry* 1995;56:395–401.

Baumann, P. Care of depression in the elderly: comparative pharmacokinetics of SSRIs. *Int Clin Psychopharmacology* 1998;13:S35–S43.

DeVane CL, Pollock BG. Pharmacokinetic considerations of antidepressant use in the elderly. *J Clin Psychiatry* 1999;60(supp 20):38–44.

De Vries MH, Raghoebar M, Mathlener IS, et al. Single and multiple oral dose fluvoxamine kinetics in young and elderly subjects. *Ther Drug Monit* 1992;14:493–498.

Franklin M. Determination of nefazodone and its metabolites in plasma by high-performance liquid chromatography with coulometric detection. *J Pharm Biomed Anal* 1993;11:1109–1113.

Ghose K. The pharmacokinetics of paroxetine in elderly depressed patients. *Acta Psychiatr Scand* 1988;80(supp 350):87–88.

Gutierrez M, Abramowitz W. Steady-state pharmokinetics of citalopram in young and elderly subjects. *Pharmacotherapy* 2000;20:1441–1447.

Harris MG, Benfield P. Fluoxetine. A review of its pharmacodynamic and pharmacokinetic properties, and therapeutic use in older patients with depressive illness. *Drugs Aging* 1995;6:64–84.

Lantz MS, Buchalter E, Giambanco V. St. John's wort and antidepressant drug interactions in the elderly. *J Geriatr Psychiatry Neurol* 1999;12:7–10.

Marathe PH, Salazar DE, Greene DS, et al. Absorption and presystemic metabolism of nefazodone administered at different regions in the gastrointestinal tract of humans. *Pharm Res* 1995;12:1716–1721.

Mayol RF, Cole CA, Luke GM, et al. Characterization of the metabolites of the antidepressant drug nefazodone in human urine and plasma. *Drug Metab Dispos* 1994;22:304–311.

Murdoch D, McTavish D. Sertraline. A review of its pharmacodynamic and pharmacokinetic properties, and therapeutic potential in depression and obsessive-compulsive disorder. *Drugs* 1992;44: 604–624.

Norman TR. Pharmacokinetic aspects of antidepressant treatment in the elderly. *Prog Neuropsychopharmacol Biol Psychiatry* 1993;17:329–344.

Otani K, Yasui N, Kaneko S, et al. Trazodone treatment increases plasma prolactin concentrations in depressed patients. *Int Clin Psychopharm* 1995; 10:115–117.

Perry PJ, Yates WR, Williams RD, et al. Testosterone therapy in late-life major depression in males. *J Clin Psychiatry* 2002;63:1096–1101.

Perucca E, Gatti G, Spina E. Clinical pharmacokinetics of fluvoxamine. *Clin Pharmacokinet* 1994; 27:175–190.

Renshaw PF, Guimaraes AR, Fava M, et al. Accumulation of fluoxetine and norfluoxetine in human brain during therapeutic administration. *Am J Psychiatry* 1992;149:1592–1594.

von Moltke LL, Greenblatt DJ, Shader RI. Clinical pharmacokinetics of antidepressants in the elderly. Therapeutic implications. *Clin Pharmacokinet* 1993;24:141–160.

Yasui N, Otani K, Kaneko S, et al. Inhibition of trazodone metabolism by thioridazine in humans. *Ther Drug Monit* 1995;17:333–335.

Selective Serotonin Reuptake Inhibitors

Menting JE, Honig A, Verhey FR, et al. Selective serotonin reuptake inhibitors (SSRIs) in the treatment of elderly depressed patients: a qualitative analysis of the literature on their efficacy and side-effects. *Int Clin Psychopharmacology* 1996;11: 165–175.

Newhouse PA. Use of serotonin selective reuptake inhibitors in geriatric depression. *J Clin Psychiatry* 1996;57(suppl):12–22.

Skerritt U, Evans R, Montgomery SA. Selective serotonin reuptake inhibitors in older patients. *Drugs Aging* 1997;10:209–218.

Wallace AE, Kofoed LL, West AN. Double-blind, placebo-controlled trial of methylphenidate in older, depressed, medically ill patients. *Am J Psychiatry* 1995;152:929–931.

Citalopram

Gottfries CG. Scandinavian experience with citalopram in the elderly. *Int Clin Psychopharmacol* 1996; 11(supp 1):41–44.

Klysner R, Bent-Hansen J, Hansen HL, et al. Efficacy of citalopram in the prevention of recurrent depression in elderly patients: placebo-controlled study of maintenance therapy. *Br J Psychiatry* 2002;181:29–35.

Ragneskog H, Eriksson S, Karlsson I, et al. Long-term treatment of elderly individuals with emotional disturbances: an open study with citalopram. *Int Psychogeriatr* 1996;8:659–668.

Fluoxetine

Ahmed I, Dagincourt PG, Miller LG, et al. Possible interaction between fluoxetine and pimozide

causing sinus bradycardia. *Can J Psychiatry* 1993; 38:62–63.

Brymer C, Winograd CH. Fluoxetine in elderly patients: is there cause for concern? *J Am Geriatr Soc* 1992;40:902–905.

Connolly VM, Gallagher A, Kesson CM. A study of fluoxetine in obese elderly patients with type 2 diabetes. *Diabetic Med* 1995;12:416–418.

Devanand DP, Kim MK, Nobler MS. Fluoxetine discontinuation in elderly dysthymic patients. *Am J Geriatr Psychiatry* 1997;5:83–87.

Grimsley SR, Jann MW. Paroxetine, sertraline, and fluvoxamine: new selective serotonin reuptake inhibitors. *Clin Pharm* 1992;11:930–957.

Heiligenstein JH, Ware JE Jr, Beusterien KM, et al. Acute effects of fluoxetine versus placebo on functional health and well-being in late-life depression. *Int Psychogeriatr* 1995;7(suppl): 125–137.

Hon D. Mania during fluoxetine treatment for recurrent depression. *Am J Psychiatry* 1989;146: 1638–1639.

Kasantikul D. Reversible delirium after discontinuation of fluoxetine. *J Med Assoc Thai* 1995;78: 53–54.

Mallick R, Chen J, Entsuah AR, et al. Depression-free days as a summary measure of the temporal pattern of response and remission in the treatment of major depression: a comparison of venlafaxine, selective serotonin reuptake inhibitors, and placebo. *J Clin Psychiatry* 2003;64:321–330.

Mander A, McCausland M, Workman B, et al. Fluoxetine induced dyskinesia. *Aust NZ J Psychiatry* 1994;28:328–330.

Pillans PI, Coulter DM. Fluoxetine and hyponatremia—a potential hazard in the elderly. *NZ Med J* 1994;107:85–86.

Smith DM, Levitte SS. Association of fluoxetine and return of sexual potency in three elderly men. *J Clin Psychiatry* 1993;54:317–319.

Young SJ. Panic associated with combining fluoxetine and bupropion [Letter]. *J Clin Psychiatry* 1996:57:177–178.

Fluvoxamine

Mallick R, Chen J, Entsuah AR, et al. Depression-free days as a summary measure of the temporal pattern of response and remission in the treatment of major depression: a comparison of venlafaxine, selective serotonin reuptake inhibitors, and placebo. *J Clin Psychiatry* 2003;64:321–330.

Wilde MI, Plosker GL, Benfield P. Fluvoxamine. An updated review of its pharmacology, and therapeutic use in depressive illness. *Drugs* 1993;46: 895–924.

Paroxetine

Bayer AJ, Roberts NA, Allen EA, et al. The pharmacokinetics of paroxetine in the elderly. *Acta Psychiatr Scand* 1988;80(suppl 350):85–86.

Caley CF, Weber SS. Paroxetine: a selective serotonin reuptake inhibiting antidepressant. *Ann Pharmacother* 1993;27:1212–1222.

Doraisway PM, Khan ZM, Donahue RM. Quality of

life in geriatric depression: a comparison of re-mitters, partial responders, and nonresponders. *Am J Geriatr Psychiatry* 2001;9:423–428.

Dunner DL. An overview of paroxetine in the elderly. *Gerontology* 1994;40(suppl):21–27.

Dunner DL, Dunbar GC. Optimal dose regimen for paroxetine. *J Clin Psychiatry* 1992;53(suppl): 21–26.

Grimsley SR, Jann MW. Paroxetine, sertraline, and fluvoxamine: new selective serotonin reuptake inhibitors. *Clin Pharm* 1992;11:930–957.

Holliday SM, Plosker GL. Paroxetine. A review of its pharmacology, therapeutic use in depression and therapeutic potential in diabetic neuropathy. *Drugs Aging* 1993;3:278–299.

Jenner PN. Paroxetine: an overview of dosage, tolerability, and safety. *Int Clin Psychopharm* 1992; 6(suppl 4):69–80.

Mallick R, Chen J, Entsuah AR, et al. Depression-free days as a summary measure of the temporal pattern of response and remission in the treatment of major depression: a comparison of venlafaxine, selective serotonin reuptake inhibitors, and placebo. *J Clin Psychiatry* 2003;64:321–330.

Nebes RD, Pollock BG, Mulsant BH, et al. Cognitive effects of paroxetine in older depressed patients. *J Clin Psychiatry* 1999;60(supp 20):26–29.

Nemeroff CB. The clinical pharmacology and use of paroxetine, a new selective serotonin reuptake inhibitor. *Pharmacotherapy* 1994;14:127–138.

Reynolds CF. Paroxetine treatment of depression in late life. *Psychopharmacol Bull* 2003;37(supp 1): 123–134.

Walters G, Reynolds CF, Mulsant BH, et al. Continuation and maintenance Pharmacotherapy in geriatric depression: an open-trial comparison of paroxetine and nortriptyline in patients older than 70 years. *J Clin Psychiatry* 1999;60(supp 20): 21–25.

Weber E, Stack J, Pollock BG, et al. Weight change in older depressed patients during acute Pharmacotherapy with paroxetine and nortriptyline: a double-blind randomized trial. *Am J Geriatr Psychiatry* 2000;8:245–250.

Sertraline

Arranz FJ, Ros S. Effects of comorbidity and polypharmacy on the clinical usefulness of sertraline in elderly depressed patients: an open multicentre study. *J Affect Disord* 1997;46:285–291.

Forlenza OV, Almeida OP, Stoppe A, et al. Antidepressant efficacy and safety of low-dose sertraline and standard-dose imipramine for the treatment of depression in older adults: results from a double-blind, randomized, controlled clinical trial. *Intl Psychogeriatr* 2001;13:75–84.

Grimsley SR, Jann MW. Paroxetine, sertraline, and fluvoxamine: new selective serotonin reuptake inhibitors. *Clin Pharm* 1992;11:930–957.

Oslin DW, Streim JE, Katz IR, et al. Heuristic comparison of sertraline with nortriptyline for the treatment of depression in frail elderly patients. *Am J Geriatr Psychiatry* 2000;8:141–149.

Other Antidepressants

Bupropion

Ascher JA, Cole JO, Colin JN, et al. Bupropion: a review of its mechanism of antidepressant activity. *J Clin Psychiatry* 1995;56:395–401.

Balon R. Bupropion and nightmares [Letter]. *Am J Psychiatry* 1996;153:579–580.

Doraisway PM, Khan ZM, Donahue RM. Quality of life in geriatric depression: a comparison of re-mitters, partial responders, and nonresponders. *Am J Geriatr Psychiatry* 2001;9:423–428.

Popli AP, Tanquary J, Lamparella V, et al. Bupropion and anticonvulsant drug interactions. *Ann Clin Psychiatry* 1995;7:99–101.

Preskorn SH. Comparison of the tolerability of bupropion, fluoxetine, imipramine, nefazodone, paroxetine, sertraline, and venlafaxine. *J Clin Psychiatry* 1995;56(suppl 6):12–21.

Steffens DC, Doraisway PM, McQuoid DR. Bupropion in the naturalistic treatment of elderly patients with major depression. *Int J Geriatr Psychiatry* 2001;16:862–865.

Szuba MP, Leuchter AF. Falling backward in two elderly patients taking bupropion. *J Clin Psychiatry* 1992;53:157–159.

Young SJ. Panic associated with combining fluoxetine and bupropion [Letter]. *J Clin Psychiatry* 1996;57:177–178.

Zisook S, Shuchter SR, Pedrelli P, et al. Bupropion sustained release for bereavement: results of an open trial. *J Clin Psychiatry* 2001;62:227–230.

Milnacipran

Tignol J, Pujol-Domenech J, Chartres JP, et al. Double-blind study of the efficacy and safety of milnacipran and imipramine in elderly patients with major depressive episode. *Acta Psychiatr Scand* 1998;97:157–165.

Mirtazapine

Halikas JA. Org 3770 (mirtazapine) versus trazodone: a placebo controlled trial in depressed elderly patients. *Hum Psychopharmacol* 1995;10: S125–S133.

Hoyberg OJ, Maragakis B, Mullin J, et al. A double-blind multicentre comparison of mirtazapine and amitriptyline in elderly depressed patients. *Acta Psychiatr Scand* 1996;93:184–190.

Nefazadone

Fawcett J, Marcus RN, Anton SF, et al. Response of anxiety and agitation symptoms during nefazodone treatment of major depression. *J Clin Psychiatry* 1995;56(suppl 6):37–42.

Goldberg RJ. Nefazodone and venlafaxine: two new agents for the treatment of depression. *J Fam Pract* 1995;41:591–594.

Goldberg, RJ. Antidepressant use in the elderly. Current status of nefazodone, venlafaxine and moclobemide. *Drugs Aging* 1996;11:119–131.

Preskorn SH. Comparison of the tolerability of bupropion, fluoxetine, imipramine, nefazodone, paroxetine, sertraline, and venlafaxine. *J Clin Psychiatry* 1995;56(suppl 6):12–21.

Rickels K, Robinson DS, Schweizer E, et al. Nefazodone: aspects of efficacy. *J Clin Psychiatry* 1995; 56(suppl 6):43–46.

Saiz-Ruiz J, Ibanez A, Diaz-Marsa M, et al. Nefazodone in the treatment of elderly patients with depressive disorders: a prospective, observational study. *CNS Drugs* 2002;16:635–643.

Simonson W. Use of nefazodone for depression in the elderly in long-term care settings. *Consult Pharm* 1997;12:67–71.

Taylor DP, Carter RB, Eison AS, et al. Pharmacology and neurochemistry of nefazodone, a novel antidepressant drug. *J Clin Psychiatry* 1995;56(suppl 6):3–11.

Ware JC, Rose FV, McBrayer RH. The acute effects of nefazodone, trazodone and buspirone on sleep and sleep-related penile tumescence in normal subjects. *Sleep* 1994;17:544–550.

Reboxetine

Katona C. Reboxetine versus imipramine in the treatment of elderly patients with depressive disorders: a double-blind randomized trail. *J Affect Disord* 1999;55:203–213.

Trazodone

Halikas JA. Org 3770 (mirtazapine) versus trazodone: a placebo controlled trial in depressed elderly patients. *Hum Psychopharmacol* 1995;10: S125–S133.

Hayashi T, Yokota N, Takahashi T, et al. Benefits of trazodone and mianserin for patients with late-life chronic schizophrenia and tardive dyskinesia: an add-on, double-blind, placebo-controlled study. *Int Clin Psychopharmacology* 1997;12:199–205.

Lance R, Albo M, Costabile RA, et al. Oral trazodone as empirical therapy for erectile dysfunction: a retrospective review. *Urology* 1995;46:117–120.

Serra-Mestres J, Shapleske J, Tym E. Treatment of palilalia with trazodone [Letter]. *Am J Psychiatry* 1996;153:580–581.

Tejera CA, Saravay SM. Treatment of organic personality syndrome with low-dose trazodone [Letter]. *J Clin Psychiatry* 1995;56:374–375.

Van Bemmel AL, Beersma DG, Van den Hoofdakker RH. Changes in EEG power density of non-REM sleep in depressed patients during treatment with trazodone. *J Affective Disord* 1995;35:11–19.

Ware JC, Rose FV, McBrayer RH. The acute effects of nefazodone, trazodone and buspirone on sleep and sleep-related penile tumescence in normal subjects. *Sleep* 1994;17:544–550.

Venlafaxine

Clerc GE, Ruimy P, Verdeau-Pailles J, et al. A double-blind comparison of venlafaxine and fluoxetine in patients hospitalized for major depression and melancholia. *Int Clin Psychopharm* 1994;9: 139–143.

Goldberg RJ. Nefazodone and venlafaxine: two new agents for the treatment of depression. *J Fam Pract* 1995;41:591–594.

Goldberg RJ. Antidepressant use in the elderly. Current status of nefazodone, venlafaxine and moclobemide. *Drugs Aging* 1997;11:119–131.

Goodnick PJ. Treatment of chronic fatigue syndrome with venlafaxine [Letter]. *Am J Psychiatry* 1996;153:294.

Khan A, Fabre LF, Rudolph R. Venlafaxine in depressed outpatients. *Psychopharmacol Bull* 1991; 27:141–144.

Mallick R, Chen J, Entsuah AR, et al. Depression-free days as a summary measure of the temporal pattern of response and remission in the treatment of major depression: a comparison of venlafaxine, selective serotonin reuptake inhibitors, and placebo. *J Clin Psychiatry* 2003;64:321–330.

Morton WA, Sonne SC, Verga MA. Venlafaxine: a structurally unique and novel antidepressant. *Ann Pharmacother* 1995;29:387–395.

Preskorn SH. Comparison of the tolerability of bupropion, fluoxetine, imipramine, nefazodone, paroxetine, sertraline, and venlafaxine. *J Clin Psychiatry* 1995;56(suppl 6):12–21.

Staab JP, Evans DL. Efficacy of venlafaxine in geriatric depression. *Depress Anxiety* 2000;12(supp 1): 63–68.

Zimmer B, Kant R, Zeiler D, et al. Antidepressant efficacy and cardiovascular safety of venlafaxine in young vs old patients with comorbid medical disorders. *Int J Psychiatry Med* 1997;27:353–364.

Chapter 11

Treatment of Late-Life Depression Associated with Medical Illness

Carl Salzman

Steven P. Roose

Anjan Chatterjee

Serious medical illness, as well as disability, both acute and chronic, is common in late life. Depressive symptoms are frequently associated with many disorders and, if lasting, constitute a depressive disorder. Any serious and disabling disorder such as Parkinson's disease, cancer, or cardiovascular disease places an elderly patient at a higher risk for developing depression. Depression may also serve as a risk and/or prodrome for illness such as dementia, pancreatic cancer, and ischemic heart disease. In addition, depression (as well as just sadness) increases the risk of mortality associated with serious illness[1,2] and increases morbidity because it delays healing. Depression also impairs daily functioning of nondemented individuals 65 and older.[3]

Comorbidity of Depression with Medical Illness

The relation between depression and medical illness in the elderly has been commonly observed in clinical settings and increasingly reported in research literature (see Chapter 8). Regardless of an individual's age, four basic themes concerning depression and medical illness are evident: (1) depression is very common in medical illness; (2) comorbidity with depression hinders recovery and worsens prognosis; (3) medical illness is a risk factor for depression because of psychosocial stressors, functional impairment, and other biological mechanisms; and (4) depression may figure prominently as a risk factor in the onset and affect the course of medical illness.[4]

Recognition of the increased likelihood of comorbid depression and medical illness in late life has resulted in epidemiologic, clinical, and research data that are likely to increase the probability that depression will be diagnosed and treated in elderly patients who are medically ill. The fact that few depressed older adults receive effective treatment in primary care settings has prompted the development of programs to enhance collaborative care for late-life depression.[5] Diagnostic criteria for comorbid depression have been sharpened,[6] and treatment approaches developed with particular reference to cardiovascular disease, cancer, stroke, Parkinson's disease, and dementia.[7] In turn, the unmet treatment needs of the depressed medically ill elderly individual have been defined,[8] and outcome studies have been systematically reviewed.[7,9]

Recommendations for antidepressant treatments associated with medical illnesses are mainly derived from studies of mixed-age individuals, some of whom are elderly but many may be in their 50s or even younger. Although these recommendations may be suitable for older and very old individuals, clinicians must remain aware of special characteristics of the elderly that may require adjustment of drug selection, dose, timing of dose administration, as well as drug side effects more common among older persons. These factors include: increased (sometimes decreased) central nervous system (CNS) sensitivity to medications with a greater likelihood of side effects (as discussed in Chapter 4); altered pharmacokinetics and the need for dosage adjustments (as discussed in Chapter 5); increased probability of side effects from drug interactions due to the higher rate of polypharmacy in older individuals (see Chapter 2 and Appendix C).

This chapter considers six common categories of late-life medical illness: cardiac disease, hypertension, stroke, cancer, Parkinson's disease, and dementia. Although the number of older individuals with HIV/AIDS is increasing, virtually all recommendations for treating comorbid depression with HIV/AIDS are derived from studies and clinical observations of significantly younger individuals[7] and will not be addressed in this chapter.

Cardiovascular Disease

Depression is frequently present in patients with cardiovascular disease: 1 in 5 patients has major depression at the time of cardiac catheterization[10-12] or following myocardial infarction (MI);[13-15] one-third of patients who are initially free of depression following an acute MI experience a depressive episode within a year;[16] and follow-up studies of depression in the post-MI population document that depression tends to follow a chronic course during the first year after MI.[14,17,18] In patients with congestive heart failure, estimates of the prevalence of major depression range from 17 to 37%.[19]

Compelling evidence suggests that depression, regardless of patient age, is an independent risk factor that contributes to the development of ischemic heart disease (IHD) and increases cardiac mortality.[20] Presence of depression increases cardiovascular morbidity and mortality from IHD three to fourfold[21]; it increases disability as well.[22] These increased risks occur in individuals with IHD who have experienced MI as well as those who have not, regardless of age.

Physiological Mechanisms

Recent studies of platelet function and heart-rate variability measured in normal controls, patients with depression, and patients with IHD suggest possible physiological mechanisms underlying the association between depression, vascular disease, and sudden cardiac death.[23] When injury to blood vessel endothelia occurs, as in patients with atherosclerosis, a physical site develops at which platelets can aggregate and cause ischemia.

Depressed patients without medical illness have increased platelet activation and responsiveness compared to age- and gender-matched normal controls.[24] Despite aspirin therapy, patients with IHD and depression have statistically significant increases in measures of platelet activity (PF4 and BTG) compared to both nondepressed IHD patients and normal controls.[25]

Although the mechanism by which depression increases platelet activation is still under investigation, attention now focuses on sympathoadrenal hyperactivity, presumably secondary to hypothalamic pituitary hyperactivity. Elevated plasma cortisol is associated with coronary artery disease (CAD) and may indirectly promote vascular damage by inducing hypercholesterolemia and hypertension.[26] Direct effects of catecholamines on the heart and blood vessels further contribute to vascular injury. In addition, because human platelets contain adrenergic and serotonergic receptors, either increased circulating levels of catecholamines or increased platelet 5HT2 binding sites may lead to increased platelet activation.

Insulin resistance may also be an important mechanism implicating depression as a risk factor for vascular disease.[27] The hypercortisolia associated with depression can induce hyperglycemia, which leads directly to insulin resistance. Furthermore, increased plasma cortisol, as well as other hormone abnormalities associated with depression—specifically decreased secretion of growth hormone and sex steroids—lead to increased visceral fat that subsequently leads to insulin resistance. Once established, insulin resistance promotes hypertension through multiple mechanisms that include: (1) increased renal tubular reabsorption of sodium; (2) increased sympathetic activity; and (3) proliferation of vascular smooth muscle. Independent of its stimulation of insulin resistance, visceral fat further promotes vascular damage by activating hepatic secretion of tumor necrosis factor, ultimately leading to an inflammatory process now recognized as a critical component in the pathogenesis of atherosclerosis.

Impact of Depression on Cardiovascular Disease

Depression increases the risk that patients with CAD will experience a cardiac event following diagnostic cardiac catheterization[28,29] and is a risk factor for cardiac mortality and medical morbidity following an acute MI[15,30-32] in patients with unstable angina[33] and with transplanted heart.[34]

Depression is not only associated with increased risk of developing symptomatic vascular disease and increased mortality risk in patients with IHD; it is also associated with increased risk of sudden cardiovascular death in depressed patients presumably free of cardiac disease.[35] Depression can also double the risk of a first MI,[21] and is associated with significantly increased risk of developing heart failure post-MI.[36] Sudden cardiac death is presumed to result from an arrhythmic event; measurements of heart-rate variability in depressed patients show abnormalities interpreted to reflect increased vulnerability to fatal arrhythmias. Heart-rate variability (HRV) results from the moment-to-moment interplay between sympathetic and parasympathetic input on the cardiac pacemaker. HRV is decreased in depression and is increased by some antidepressants.

Approximately 40% of patients of all ages with acute MI experience major or minor depression within a few weeks after MI.[13,14,37,38] Depression significantly increases the risk of dying within 6 months of having an MI.[15] In addition to increased risk of cardiac mortality, depression significantly increases morbidity. Depressed post-MI patients also take longer to return to work than nondepressed patients. They are also more likely to drop out of exercise programs and cardiac rehabilitation programs or to be noncompliant with medical regimens; for example, depressed patients with CAD are less likely to comply with low-dose aspirin therapy than their nondepressed counterparts.[39] Post-MI depression also is associated with increased health care costs due to increased physician outpatient visits and hospital readmissions.[40,41] Another risk factor for cardiac illness that persists in depressed post-MI patients is smoking; depressed smokers are 40% less likely to stop smoking than nondepressed smokers.[42] The poor participation of depressed patients in rehabilitation, medical treatments, or change in lifestyle habits makes the treatment of depression compelling, especially in the elderly.

Treatment Associated with Cardiovascular Disease

Antidepressant treatment of depression following MI may decrease mortality and morbidity and improve quality of life.[31] Unfortunately, depression following MI is often inadequately treated.[40] Although tricyclic antidepressants (TCAs) and selective serotonin reuptake inhibitors (SSRIs) are effective for treating depression in patients with IHD, recent evidence clearly demonstrates the superior safety of at least two SSRIs (sertraline and paroxetine) for patients with coronary heart disease (CHD) *and* IHD[21,43] as well as post-MI depression.

Cardiovascular Effects of Tricyclic Antidepressants

The effects of a therapeutic plasma level of a TCA on cardiovascular function have been extensively studied in depressed patients of all ages, both with and without cardiovascular disease.[44] TCAs routinely increase heart rate by 11%, induce orthostatic hypotension that can result in falls and serious injuries, and slow cardiac conduction, which can result in 2-1 atrioventricular block in patients with preexisting bundle-branch block. TCAs do not routinely have an adverse effect on ventricular function even in patients with severe left ventricular impairment.

Like other 1A antiarrhythmic compounds, such as quinidine and moricizine, TCAs also induce significant antiarrhythmic activity by increasing the initial inward sodium current of the Purkinje fiber and reducing intraventricular conduction velocity. This antiarrhythmic effect at therapeutic plasma levels is responsible for extremely high plasma levels that cause ventricular arrhythmias and heart block as well as the high rate of mortality after TCA overdose. Elderly patients are at higher risk for fatal arrhythmia or heart block because elevated plasma levels may result from inappropriate dosing, drug interactions, age-related alterations in TCA metabolism, or a combination of all three factors (see Chapters 2 and 5). Consequently, TCAs are relatively contraindicated in elderly patients with IHD.[45]

Cardiovascular Effects of SSRI Antidepressants

SSRIs have largely replaced TCAs because of their more favorable side effect profile. They do not have adverse cardiovascular effects in patients with congestive heart failure, dysrhythmia, stable IHD, and even in patients after MI.[43,46] SSRIs do not slow cardiac conduction or cause orthostatic hypotension. Although heart rate may be slightly decreased (1–3 bpm), the clinical significance of this finding is not known. In contrast to TCAs, SSRIs, if taken alone, are only rarely lethal in overdose.[47]

SSRIs interfere with serotonin accumulation in platelets and SSRI treatment (but not TCA treatment) normalizes elevated indices of platelet activation and aggregation in patients with depression and IHD. The antiplatelet effect of the SSRIs is neither associated with antidepressant effect nor does resolution of depression immediately normalize increased platelet activity.[25]

The antiplatelet effect of SSRIs may reduce risk of future ischemic cardiovascular events. SSRI-treated patients have a significantly lower rate of MI than the non-SSRI-treated patients.[48] This lower MI rate may not simply be due to reduced psychiatric symptoms; for example, patients whose anxiety is reduced by anxiolytic medications do not have a reduced rate of MI.

Cardiovascular Effects of Other Antidepressants

Antidepressants other than SSRIs may also have deleterious cardiac effects. Although bupropion causes mild increase in supine diastolic blood pressure and orthostatic drop, neither of these findings is clinically significant. Bupropion does not alter heart rate, ejection fraction, or cardiac conduction.

Other antidepressant medications, particularly venlafaxine and mirtazapine, have not been specifically tested in depressed patients with IHD. Venlafaxine causes a slight increase in systolic and diastolic blood pressure when given in a dose greater than 300 mg/d and there is a 7–13% rate of sustained hypertension. Mirtazapine can cause significant weight gain, a cardiovascular risk factor. Furthermore, though neither medication has the type 1A antiarrhythmic properties characteristic of TCAs, both medications may increase norepinephrine activity and sympathetic tone. The effect on HRV of venlafaxine and mirtzaepine is unknown.

Concern about increased sympathetic tone, decreased HRV, and subsequent increased risk of ventricular fibrillation also extends to stimulants, frequently prescribed for older patients with medical illness and minor or major depression. Among older medically ill and nursing home residents, sudden cardiovascular increase in sympathetic tone that results in decreased HRV and sudden cardiac death is an effect that may go undetected in the clinical setting due to the high baseline rate of cardiac mortality.

For these reasons, elderly patients with IHD, CHF, or those who are post-MI should be treated with SSRI antidepressants as first-choice medications. TCAs are particularly hazardous in patients with CHF; the effect of bupropion, venlafaxine and mirtazepine have been less well studied in the elderly and should be used with caution in depressed elderly patients with preexisting heart disease.

Hypertension

Antihypertensives, such as reserpine, α-methyldopa, and propranolol can precipitate depression in susceptible patients or exacerbate already established depression. In addition, antihypertensives may have three potentially harmful interactions with TCAs. First, volume-depleting diuretics can exacerbate orthostatic hypotension caused by antidepressants. Second, most TCAs inhibit the uptake of guanethidine, bethanidine, and debrisoquine into presynaptic adrenergic synapses and interfere with their antihypertensive effect; they block the antihypertensive effect of clonidine as well. Third, the addition of TCAs to antihypertensive medication can lead to significant orthostatic hypotension that may result in falls.

The following considerations are relevant to the treatment of depressed hypertensive geriatric patients:

1. Use the lowest possible dosage of the mildest antihypertensive required for effective control of hypertension. Angiotensin-converting enzyme inhibitors and calcium channel blockers are commonly used antihypertensive treatments. Careful blood pressure monitoring and dosage adjustment are essential when antidepressants are given to patients receiving these drugs.

2. If depression develops in a patient receiving propranolol, α-methyldopa, or reserpine, substitute an antihypertensive less likely to cause depression, e.g., angiotensin-converting enzyme inhibitors.

3. If depression fails to improve after substituting another antihypertensive drug, add nortriptyline or a SSRI. A lower dosage of the antihypertensive drug may be necessary after antidepressant treatment has begun. Check for potential drug interactions (see Appendix C).

4. If a geriatric patient is being treated for mild hypertension with volume-depleting diuretics, evaluate the possibilities of decreasing the dosage or stopping the diuretic when antidepressant treatment begins.

5. Consider electroconvulsive therapy (ECT) for severely depressed hypertensive patients.

Stroke

Regardless of age, depression occurs in about 40% of patients with acute stroke and has been linked to poorer cognitive and physical recovery.[49] Stroke patients of all ages with major depression are eight times more likely to die within 15 months than nondepressed stroke patients.[50]

Risk Factors

In older individuals, depression is a risk factor for stroke: The rate of stroke is 2.3 to 2.7 times greater in persons 65 years and older with high versus low levels of depressive symptoms.[51] Approximately 30% of patients after stroke are depressed and depression is associated with a significantly higher mortality rate over the 10 years following the event.[50] Although a similar association between depression and mortality following MI can occur, poststroke depression may have different characteristics than post-MI depression. In patients after stroke, unlike patients after MI, both the volume and location of structural damage are critical to the development of depression; the highest rate of depression appears to occur in patients with left frontal and basal ganglia lesions. Thus, poststroke depression may be a consequence of structural damage to the brain, a paradigm that may also apply to depression concurrent with other neurologic syndromes such as Parkinson's disease.

Treatment

The presence of poststroke depression affects both recovery and mortality following the acute illness. Patients with major or minor depression diagnosed during initial acute hospitalization have a higher mortality rate than patients who were not depressed, even after controlling for other variables known to associate with poststroke mortality.[50] Although mortality is related to severity of the stroke, patients with major or minor depression are 8.1 times more likely to die over the subsequent 15 months following stroke than the nondepressed patients.

A significant and growing literature documents the effectiveness of antidepressant treatment for poststroke depression.[52,53] Depressed patients with stroke who are not treated for depression recover less frequently than those who are treated.[54]

TCAs have been the treatment of choice for poststroke depression, and most research studies support their therapeutic efficacy. Nortriptyline in particular[55] is effective and has been found to be superior to the SSRI fluoxetine for elderly patients;[56] a more recent study, however, supports the safety and efficacy of fluoxetine.[57]

SSRIs have come to be used with increased frequency because of their greater safety profile and the frequent concurrence of cerebrovascular and cardiac illness among geriatric patients.[58] Venlafaxine can also be an effective and safe treatment for poststroke depression.[59] A few elderly subjects may develop hypertension at doses above 150 mg/day, which may limit the available range of therapeutic doses for this population. SSRIs are also a useful treatment for the syndrome of pathological poststroke crying.

At present, clinical evidence supports treating elderly patients with poststroke depression with antidepressants if their medical condition allows. Nortriptyline and SSRIs are the antidepressants of first choice assuming no cardiovascular or other conditions contraindicate their use.

Parkinson's Disease and Depression

Idiopathic Parkinson's disease (PD), a neurodegenerative disorder of middle or late life, was first described by James Parkinson in his "Essay on the Shaking Palsy"[60]. PD affects approximately 107 per thousand persons across all age groups and prevalence increases with age.[61] Approximately half of depressed PD patients meet criteria for major depressive disorder. In some, the depression is persistent; in others, depressive symptoms fluctuate and may remit. Two-thirds of patients describe increased depression during "off" (akinetic) periods compared with mobile "on" periods.[62] Past history of depression is a risk factor for depression after parkinsonian symptoms develop, but no evidence exists that depression in PD is an independently inherited disorder.[62]

The prevalence of depression in patients with PD varies from 4 to 70%,[63] depending on sampling, diagnostic criteria, and instruments employed. Dysphoria, pessimism, irritability, sadness, and suicidal ideation are the most reliable indicators of depression in PD.[62] Although PD patients can experience suicidal ideation, rates of suicide are not higher in this population than in the general population.

Neuropathology

The pathology of PD is characterized by loss of pigmented neurons in the substantia nigra and other pigmented brainstem nuclei as well as presence in the remaining nigral cells of intracytoplasmic Lewy bodies.[64,65] The cause(s) of PD are unknown although current hypotheses favor the possibility of excitotoxic injury and environmental toxins as well as genetic factors in a significant minority of patients. Lewy bodies are the sine qua non of PD although their role in the pathogenesis of the disease is unknown. Three genes (Parkin, alpha-synuclein, and UCH-L1) and five genetic loci have been identified in a minority of patients with early-onset PD.[66]

Anatomic and neurochemical evidence suggests that depression is an endogenous feature of the disease. The diverse motor and nonmotor symptoms of PD are related to dysfunction in cortical-basal-ganglionic-thalamic loops.[67] Depressed patients with PD have increased neuronal loss in the dorsal raphe, in contrast to patients with psychosis, who have no specific neuropathological features.[68] In positron emission tomography (PET) studies comparing depressed with nondepressed PD patients and controls (matched by age and disease duration), a relative hypometabolism in the caudate and inferior orbital-frontal regions and in the medial frontal lobes occurrs in the depressed PD patients.[69,70]

Role of Neurotransmitters

Neurotransmitters such as serotonin, norepinephrine, and dopamine, all of which have been implicated in depression, have also been implicated in the pathogenesis of depression in PD. Dopamine deficiency has been suspected by some as the primary neurotransmitter associated with depression in PD because serotonergic neuronal damage is less pervasive and loss of neurons in the locus ceruleus (LC) does not correlate consistently with depression in PD patients.[71] Degeneration of dopamine neurons in the ventral tegmental area (VTA) has been postulated to predispose PD patients to depression.[72] In addition, decreased tyrosine-hydroxylase activity in the VTA (caused by degeneration of dopamine neurons) implies decreased dopaminergic output to cingulate, entorhinal, and frontal cortices—all areas of the brain linked to depression.[73] However, no correlations have been found between homovanillic acid (HVA), a dopamine metabolite, and depression in PD.[74–76]

Evidence has also been found for reduced peripheral and central metabolites of serotonin (5HT), which decreases depression.[74,77] Other evidence favoring 5HT as the causative neurotransmitter includes the finding of low levels of 5-HIAA in the cerebrospinal fluid of PD patients with depression although no correlation has been found between levels and severity of the depression.[74,75,78] In addition, degeneration of 5HT neurons of the dorsal raphe occurs[79] as well as abnormal binding of 5HT uptake sites;[80] transcranial sonography reveals greater disruption of brainstem dorsal raphe echogenicity in depressed than nondepressed PD patients.[81]

Decreased platelet-imipramine binding has also been described in depressed PD patients,[82,83] possibly implicating intrinsic neurochemical defects in norepinephrine in relation to the pathogenesis of depressive symptoms in this disease. Degeneration of norepinephrine-containing neurons of the LC[71,84,85] may also predispose PD patients to depression.

Treatment of Depression in Parkinson's Disease

Evaluating depression in the context of a motor disorder such as PD may be difficult because of the overlap of somatic symptoms of depression and the motor deficits of PD such as bradykinesia and flat affect.

Only a few double-blind placebo-controlled clinical trials assess the effects of antidepressants, specifically in the context of mood changes in PD.[86] Four double-blind randomized controlled trials using TCAs and one using bupropion have been conducted.[87–90] No randomized, blind, controlled trials using SSRIs exist.[91] A recent survey of 49 investigators from the Parkinson's Study Group assessing physician preferences for treatment found that 51% of physicians use SSRIs first, 41% TCAs first, and 8% "other" drugs first to treat depression in PD.[92,93]

Although TCAs or SSRIs are widely used in clinical practice, controlled clinical trials are necessary to prove the efficacy of SSRIs, specifically in parkinsonian depression. Use of TCAs for depression may affect memory because of their anticholinergic effects; other anticholinergic effects that must be monitored include urinary hesitance and blurry vision. TCAs may also cause orthostasis in elderly patients, requiring monitoring of blood pressure. SSRIs may be effective antidepressants although there is concern that they worsen PD by decreasing dopamine.[93] Studies of monoamine oxidase inhibitors (MAOIs) are few[94,95] and show only modest efficacy.[96]

Because dopamine agonists are commonly used to treat symptoms of PD and dopaminergic abnormalities may be involved in the pathophysiology of depression in PD, some investigators have looked at the use of drugs that enhance dopamine in the treatment of depression in PD. Bromocriptine, pramipexole, and pergolide have each been used to improve depressive symptoms in PD patients.[97,98] Whether symptom improvement is related to motor improvement provided by dopamine agonists or is the direct result of drug effect on depression remains unclear because symptoms may overlap and fluctuations in the severity of depression may be seen with the fluctuations of motor symptoms in PD.[99] Treatment of

the motor symptoms may sometimes improve the depression as well.[100] The pathophysiology of this "on-off" state may be related to catecholaminergic systems, and use of drugs that inhibit metabolism of catecholamines may also have beneficial effects on mood instability.[71]

Electroconvulsive therapy (ECT), another extremely useful treatment for major depression, has demonstrated proven efficacy as antidepressant therapy for patients with PD.[101] Although ECT treatment may cause loss of short-term memory, it may improve symptoms of PD, resulting in temporary reduction in dosage of antiparkinsonian medications.

Transcranial magnetic stimulation (TMS) can provide temporary relief of depression under experimental conditions.[102–104] No studies of TMS in the treatment of depression in PD are available, although it does appear to help the motor symptoms in some cases.[103]

When drug therapy is chosen for the treatment of depression, careful consideration must be given to potential drug interactions because adverse effects of polypharmacy in treatment of elderly depressed patients with PD are common. Concerns arise that SSRIs may actually worsen the motor symptoms.[92] Although a "serotonin syndrome" was described in the coadministration of seligiline with SSRIs,[92] safe coadministration of these drugs has also been reported.[105] Frequency of the 5HT syndrome has been estimated to be 0.24%, with 0.04% of patients experiencing symptoms considered serious. Because these data are derived from a survey, rather than a population-based sample, the true prevalence of this phenomenon may have been underestimated.[102]

Cancer

Incidence and prevalence of cancer is high among the elderly: approximately 60% of all cases occur in the geriatric population.[106] The prevalence of depression associated with cancer (in all age groups) ranges from 4.5% to 58%, with a mean prevalence of 22–29%.[107,108] Pancreatic cancer has the highest prevalence of depression (50%);[109] 71% of patients with pancreatic cancer have symptoms that could be considered depression or related to depression.[110]

Chronic depression may also be a risk factor for cancer.[111] In individuals over 65, social functioning, disease severity, and isolation may be more important precipitants of depression than the type of cancer.[112] Other factors that may increase the prevalence of depression and depressive symptoms are cancer chemotherapy and pain. Behavioral alterations in cancer patients may also represent a "sickness syndrome" that results from activation of inflammatory cytokines.[108]

Controversy exists regarding the use of antidepressants for the treatment of cancer in elderly individuals. Most studies do not focus exclusively on geriatric patients.[109] In studies of mixed-age patient samples, antidepressant therapy follows guidelines similar to treatment of non-comorbid depression, although cancer patients may be more susceptible to side effects.[7] Because of their better side effect profile, SSRIs may be preferred to TCAs and MAOIs. A metaanalysis of drug treatment in the elderly, however, showed no benefit of antidepressant drugs over placebo.[113] Some depressive symptoms may not be indications of a true major depressive disorder but, rather comprise a normal "reactive demoralization" that should be acknowledged and may respond to nonpharmacologic treatment.[114] The cancer patient may be better managed "through the consistent emotional support given by the oncologist with whom a trusting relationship has been nurtured."[107] When depressive symptoms are severe and last more than a week, however, antidepressants may be considered as part of an overall treatment program.

In lieu of research data to guide the clinician, all antidepressants should be considered. Selection among the various classes of antidepressants is based on the individual patient's symptoms, other medications (and potential drug interactions), and side effect profile of the antidepressant. SSRIs may be the first-line choice based on side effect profile. Although controlled studies of SSRIs in elderly cancer patients do not exist, lack of anticholinergic side effects, orthostatic hypotension, sedation, and cardiac toxicity suggests a preference for these medications. However, SSRIs are not without potential problems in this population. Four of the six available SSRIs inhibit one or more hepatic drug-metabolizing enzymes of the cytochrome P450 system. Inhibition of these enzymes may raise blood levels of other medications given to the elderly cancer patient, and cause unwanted adverse events. (A more detailed discussion of pharmacokinetic interaction is provided in Chapter 5, and specific drug interactions are presented in Appendix C.)

Despite the side effects that commonly occur, TCAs may be safely and effectively prescribed for depressed cancer patients.[107] No data are available regarding the use of MAO inhibitors, bupropion, venlafaxine, or nefazodone, in the treatment of depression associated with cancer.

Stimulants such as methylphenidate have also been used with considerable success to enhance the energy in physically depleted cancer patients, especially after chemotherapy. The dose of methylphenidate may vary, depending on the age and physical condition of the depressed elderly patient. Starting doses of 5 mg/d with gradual titration upward have been found effective in clinical practice, although no research studies are available to guide the clinician, in recommending average daily doses or in deciding how long to use an antidepressant.

From a practical and clinical perspective, elderly depressed cancer patients probably should remain on an antidepressant as long as it is effective and does not produce side effects or unwanted drug interactions. For this reason, antidepressants should be prescribed for depressed geriatric cancer patients only after careful consultation with the primary treating physician.

Treatment of Depression in Dementia

Depression and dementia commonly coexist (see Chapter 8); the relation between them is defined by the primary disorder. One form of the association between the two disorders is the well-known cognitive impairment of depression. Called "the dementia of depression," this coexistence has commonly been referred to as "pseudodementia,"[115] defined as "a number of conditions in which a clinical picture resembling organic dementia presents for attention, yet physical disease proves to be little if at all responsible."[116] The more preferred term is "depression-induced cognitive disorder," which refers to cognitive impairment secondary to a primary disorder and occurs most frequently in the elderly. Demonstrable cognitive impairment is present in 10 to 20% of depressed elderly patients. It includes impaired attention and recall but specific deficits such as aphasia, agraphia, acalculia are rarely present.[117] Recall is impaired in both depression-induced cognitive impairment and in irreversible dementia.[118] Depression-induced cognitive impairment may reflect additional structural brain disorder.[119]

In the second form of the relation between the disorders, dementia is primary with secondary development of depressive symptoms, usually early in the disorder when the patient recognizes progressive cognitive failure. As the dementia worsens, depressive symptoms are more difficult to identify. In clinical practice, a mixture of both forms of a dementia-depression is not unusual. However, elevated concentrations of CSF "tau protein" are present in Alzheimer's disease (AD) but not in late-life depression with cognitive impairment.[120] The tau protein may thus serve as a biomarker for AD and provide a means of differentiating patients whose cognitive impairment is secondary to AD and not depression.[120]

A third relation between depression and dementia is also possible. Recent evidence suggests that almost a five-fold increase in the risk of developing dementia over a 3-year period occurs among persons who originally present with depression-induced dementia.[121] This observation suggests that when elderly depressed patients also have significant cognitive impairment, they are at high risk for later dementia whether or not their impairment reverses with treatment.

Recent estimates of presence of depression in individuals with AD suggest major depression in 20 to 25% of cases, with other depressive syndromes affecting an additional 20 to 30%.[122] The depression may persist over at least 6 months[123] and may be more prevalent in mild to moderate dementia and less prevalent in less severe cases of the disorder.[124] Memory deficits may be severe in depressed individuals who are not demented as well as those who are: 70% of elderly depressed patients have deficits in memory and slowed cognition[119]—impairments that persist in approximately one-third of individuals even after successful treatment of depression.

Treating depression is particularly important in patients with AD because treatment might be associated with reversal of its consequences.[125] Depression in AD increases disability[126] as well as aggression,[127] is associated with earlier entry into nursing home[128], and slightly increased mortality,[129] as well as risk of suicide.[130] In view of these consequences of depression associated with dementia, it is disappointing that relatively little research has focused on this comorbid condition. A review of 11 studies found that antidepressants were effective for the treatment of depression; although TCAs were associated with diminished cognitive performance, this was not true of treatment with SSRIs.[125] A recent study confirms these observations, finding sertraline superior to placebo for treatment of major depression in AD although cognition did not improve.[122]

For clinicians wishing to treat a demented elderly patient who also is depressed, the following suggestions may be derived from the limited research data available:

1. Assuming no medical contraindications for use of an antidepressant, the demented patient's depressive symptoms should be treated with an antidepressant.
2. Because the only data available to guide the clinician are with SSRIs (especially sertraline and citalopram), these should be the first-choice drugs.
3. SSRI side effects in the geriatric population include tremor, restlessness, and sedation. Patients should probably be treated until their dementia progresses to the degree that communication and evaluation of affect are no longer possible.

For the elderly patient who is primarily depressed but reports a worsening of cognitive function, optimal antidepressant treatment is indicated. Guidelines for treatment of these patients follows the recommendations for treating all depressed elderly patients as described in Chapters 9, 10, 13, and 20.

References

1. Whooley MA, Browner WS. Association between depressive symptoms and mortality in older women. Study of Osteoporotic Fractures Research Group. *Arch Intern Med.* 1998;158: 2129–2135.
2. Cooper JK, Harris Y, McGready J. Sadness predicts death in older people. *J Aging Health.* 2002;4:509–526.
3. Wang L, van Belle G, Kukull WB, Larson EB. Predictors of functional change: a longitudinal study of nondemented people aged 65 and older. *J Am Geriatr Soc.* 2002;50:1525–1534.
4. Evans DL, Charney DS. Mood disorders and medical illness: a major public health problem. *Biol Psychiatry.* 2003;54:177–180.
5. Unutzer J, Katon W, Callahan CM, et al. Collaborative care management of late–life depression in the primary care setting: a randomized controlled trial. *JAMA.* 2002;288:2836–2845.
6. Koenig HG, George LK, Peterson BL, Pieper CF. Depression in medically ill hospitalized older adults: prevalence, characteristics, and course of symptoms according to six diagnostic schemes. *Am J Psychiatry* 1997;154:1376–1383.
7. Krishnan KR, Delong M, Kraemer H, et al. Comorbidity of depression with other medical diseases in the elderly. *Biol Psychiatry.* 2002;52: 559–588.
8. Charlson M, Peterson JC. Medical comorbidity and late life depression: what is known and what are the unmet needs? *Biol Psychiatry.* 2002; 52:226–235.
9. Cole MG. Public health models of mental health care for elderly populations. *Int Psychogeriatr* 2002 Mar;14(1):3–6.
10. Carney RM, Rich MW, teVelde AJ, et al. Major depressive disorders in coronary artery disease. *Am J Cardiol* 1987;60:1273–1275.
11. Hance M, Carney RM, Freedland KE, Skala J. Depression in patients with coronary heart disease: A twelve month follow–up. *Gen Hosp Psychiatry* 1995;18:61–65.
12. Gonzalez MB, Snyderman TB, Colket JT, et al. Depression in patients with coronary artery disease. *Depression* 1996;4:57–62.
13. Forrester AW, Lipsey JR, Teitelbaum ML, et al. Depression following myocardial infarction. *Int J Psychiatry Med* 1992;22:33–46.
14. Schleifer SJ, Macari–Hinson MM, Coyle DA, et al. The nature and course of depression following myocardial infarction. *Arch Int Med* 1989; 149:1785–1789.
15. Frasure–Smith N, Lesperance F, Talajic M. Depression following myocardial infarction: Impact on 6 month survival. *JAMA.* 1993;270: 1819–1825.
16. Lesperance F, Frasure–Smith N, Talajic M. Major depression before and after myocardial infarction: its nature and consequences. *Psychosom Med* 1996;58:99–110.
17. Stern JJ, Pascale L, Ackerman A. Life adjustment post myocardial infarction: Determining predictive variables. *Arch Intern Med* 1977;137: 1680–1685.
18. Travella JI, Forrester AW, Schultz SK, Robinson RG. Depression following myocardial infarction: A one year longitudinal study. *Int J Psychiatry Med* 1994;24:357–369.
19. Freedland KE, Rich MW, Skala JA, et al. Prevalence of depression in hospitalized patients with congestive heart failure. *Psychosom Med* 2003;65:119–128.
20. Rugulies R. Depression as a predictor for coronary heart disease. a review and meta–analysis. *Am J Prev Med* 2002;23:51–61.
21. Glassman, AH, O'Connor, CM, Califf, RM, et al. Sertraline treatment of major depression in patients with acute MI or unstable angina. *JAMA* 2002;288:701–709.
22. Ades PA, Savage PD, Tischler MD, et al. Deter-

minants of disability in older coronary patients. *Am Heart J* 2002;143:151–156.

23. Joynt KE, Whellan DJ, O'Connor CM. Depression and Cardiovascular Disease: Mechanisms of Interaction. *Biol Psychiatry* 2003;54:248–261.

24. Musselman DL, Evans DL, Nemeroff CB. The relationship of depression to cardiovascular disease: Epidemiology, biology, and treatment. *Arch Gen Psychiatry* 1998;55:580–592.

25. Pollock, B.G., Laghrissi–Thode, F. Wagner, W.R. Evaluation of platelet activation in depressed patients with ischemic heart disease after paroxetine or nortriptyline treatment. *J Clin Psychopharmacol* 2000;20:137–140.

26. Troxler, R.G., Sprague, E.A., Albanese, R.A., et al. The association of elevated plasma cortisol and early atherosclerosis as demonstrated by coronary angiography. *Atherosclerosis* 1977;26: 151–162.

27. Gold PW, Chrousos GP. The endocrinology of melancholic and atypical depression: relation to neurocircuitry and somatic consequences. *Proc Assoc Am Physicians* 1999;111:22–34.

28. Carney RM, Rich MW, Freedland KE, et al. Major depressive disorder predicts cardiac events in patients with coronary artery disease. *Psychosom Med* 1988;50:627–633.

29. Barefoot JC, Helms MJ, Mark DB, et al. Depression and long–term mortality risk in patients with coronary artery disease. *Am J Cardiol* 1996; 78:613–617.

30. Ahern DK, Gorkin L, Anderson JL, et al. Biobehavioral variables and mortality or Cardiac Arrhythmia Pilot Study (CAPS). *Am J Cardiol* 1990; 66:59–62.

31. Frasure–Smith N, Lespèrance F, Talajic M. Depression and 18 month prognosis after myocardial infarction. *Circulation* 1995;91:999–1005.

32. Ladwig KH, Kieser M, Konig J, et al. Affective disorders and survival after acute myocardial infarction. *Eur Heart J* 1991;12:959–964.

33. Lespérance F, Frasure–Smith N, Juneau M, Théroux P. Depression and 1–year prognosis in unstable angina. *Arch Intern Med* 2000;160: 1354–1360.

34. Dew MA, Kormos RL, Roth LH, et al. Early post–transplant medical compliance and mental health predict physical morbidity and mortality one to three years after heart transplantation. *J Heart Lung Transplant* 1999;18:549–562.

35. Malzberg B. Mortality among patients with involution melancholia. *Am J Psychiatry* 1937;93: 1231–1238.

36. Abramson J, Berger A, Krumholz HM, Vaccarino V. Depression and risk of heart failure among older persons with isolated systolic hypertension. *Arch Intern Med.* 2001;161:1725–1730.

37. Carney RM, Freedland KA, Jaffe AS. Insomnia and depression prior to myocardial infarction. *Psychosom Med* 1990;52:603–609.

38. Carney RM, Jaffe AS. Depression and myocardial infarction: The SADHART Trial. *JAMA* 2002;288:750–751.

39. Carney RM, Freedland KE, Eisen SA, et al. Major depression and medication adherence in elderly patients with coronary artery disease. *Health Psychol* 1995;14:88–90.

40. Luutonen S, Holm H, Salminen JK, et al. Inadequate treatment of depression after myocardial infarction. *Acta Psychiatr Scand* 2002;6:434–439.

41. Frasure–Smith N, Lesperance F, Gravel G, et al. Depression and health–care costs during the first year following myocardial infarction. *J Psychosom Res* 2000;48:471–478.

42. Glassman AH. Cigarette smoking and its comorbidity. *NIDA Res Monogr* 1997;172:52–60.

43. Roose SP, Laghrissi–Thode F, Kennedy JS, et al. Comparison of paroxetine and nortriptyline in depressed patients with ischemic heart disease. *JAMA* 1998a;279(4):287–291.

44. Roose SP, Glassman AH. Cardiovascular effects of TCAs in depressed patients with and without heart disease. *J Clin Psychiatry Monograph* 1989; 7:1–19.

45. Glassman AH, Roose SP, Bigger JT Jr. The safety of tricyclic antidepressants in cardiac patients. Risk–benefit considered. *JAMA* 1993; 269:2673–2675.

46. Roose SP, Glassman AH, Attia E, et al. Cardiovascular effects of fluoxetine in depressed patients with heart disease. *Amer J Psychiatry* 1998b;155:660–665.

47. Barbey, JT, Roose, SP. SSRI Safety in overdose. *J Clin Psychiatry* 1993;59(Suppl. 15):42–48.

48. Sauer WH, Berlin JA, Kimmel SE. Selective serotonin reuptake inhibitors and myocardial infarction. *Circulation* 2001;104:1894–1898.

49. Jorge RE, Robinson RG, Arndt S, et al. Mortality and poststroke depression: a placebo–controlled trial of antidepressants. *Am J Psychiatry* 2003;160:1823–1829.

50. Morris PL, Robinson RG, Andrzejewski P, et al. Association of depression with 10–year poststroke mortality. *Am J Psychiatry* 1993;150: 124–129.

51. Simonsick EM, Wallace RB, Blazer DG, et al. Depressive symptomatology and hypertension–associated morbidity and mortality in older adults. *Psychosom Med* 1995;57:427–435.

52. Whyte EM, Mulsant BH. Post stroke depression: epidemiology, pathophysiology, and biological treatment. *Biol Psychiatry* 2002;52: 253–264.

53. Robinson RG. Poststroke Depression: Prevalence, Diagnosis, Treatment, and Disease Progression. *Biol Psychiatry* 2003;54:376–387.

54. Gainotti G, Antonucci G, Marra C, et al. Relation between depression after stroke, antidepressant therapy, and functional recovery. *J Neurol Neurosurg Psychiatry* 2001;71:258–261.

55. Robinson RG. Treatment issues in poststroke depression. *Depress Anxiety* 1998;8(Suppl 1): 85–90.

56. Robinson RG, Schultz SK, Castillo C, et al. Nortriptyline versus fluoxetine in the treatment of depression and in short term recovery after stroke: A placebo–controlled, double–blind study. *Am J Psychiatry* 2000;157:351–359.

57. Fruehwald S, Gatterbauer E, Rehak P, Baumhackl U. Early fluoxetine treatment of post–stroke depression—a three–month double–blind placebo–controlled study with

an open–label long–term follow up. *J Neurol* 2003;250:347–351.

58. Cole MG, Elie LM, McCusker J, et al. Feasibility and effectiveness of treatments for post–stroke depression in elderly inpatients: systematic review. *J Geriatr Psychiatry Neurol.* 2001;14:37–41.

59. Staab JP, Evans DL. Efficacy of venlafaxine in geriatric depression. *Depress Anxiety.* 2000; 12(Suppl 1):63–68.

60. Parkinson J. *An essay on the shaking palsy.* London: Whittingham & Rowland 1817.

61. Mayeux R, Marder K, Cote LJ, et al. The frequency of idiopathic Parkinson's disease by age, ethnic group, and sex in northern Manhattan, 1988–1993. *Am J Epidemiol* 1995;142: 820–827.

62. Cummings JL. Depression and Parkinson's disease: a review. *Am J Psychiatry* 1992;149: 443–454.

63. de Rijk MC, Tzourio C, Breteler MM, et al. Prevalence of parkinsonism and Parkinson's disease in Europe: the EUROPARKINSON Collaborative Study. European Community Concerted Action on the Epidemiology of Parkinson's disease. *J Neurol Neurosurg Psychiatry* 1997;62:10–15.

64. Jellinger KA. The pathology of Parkinson's disease. *Adv Neurol* 2001;86:55–72.

65. Takahashi H, Wakabayashi K. The cellular pathology of Parkinson's disease. *Neuropathology* 2001;21:315–322.

66. Mouradian MM. Recent advances in the genetics and pathogenesis of Parkinson disease. *Neurology* 2002;58:179–185.

67. Alexander GE, DeLong MR, Strick PL. Parallel organization of functionally segregated circuits linking basal ganglia and cortex. *Ann Rev Neurosci* 1986;9:357–381.

68. Paulus W, Jellinger K. The neuropathologic basis of different clinical subgroups of Parkinson's disease. *N Neuropathol Exp Neurol* 1991;50: 743–755.

69. Mayberg HS, Starkstein SE, Sadzot B, et al. Selective hypometabolism in the inferior frontal lobe in depressed patients with Parkinson's disease. *Ann Neurol* 1990;28:57–64.

70. Ring HA, Bench CJ, Trimble MR, et al. Depression in Parkinson's disease. A positron emission study. *Br J Psychiatry* 1994;165:333–339.

71. Sandyk R, Fisher H. The relationship of serotonin metabolism secretion to the pathophysiology of tardive dyskinesia. *Int J Neurosci* 1989;48: 133–136.

72. Taylor AE, Saint–Cyr JA. Depression in Parkinson's disease: reconciling physiological and psychological perspectives. *J Neuropsychiatry Clin Neurosci* 1990;2:92–98.

73. Javoy–Agid F, Agid Y. Is the mesocortical dopaminergic system involved in Parkinson disease? *Neurology* 1980;30:1326–1330.

74. Mayeux R, Stern Y, Cote L, et al. Altered serotonin metabolism in depressed patients with Parkinson's disease. *Neurology* 1984;34:642–646.

75. Mayeux R, Stern Y, Sano M, et al. The relationship of serotonin to depression in Parkinson's disease. *Mov Disord* 1988;3:237–244.

76. Wolfe N, Katz DI, Albert ML, et al. Neuropsychological profile linked to low dopamine:

in Alzheimer's disease, major depression, and Parkinson's disease. *J Neurol Neurosurg Psychiatry* 1990;53:915–917.

77. Sano M, Stern Y, Williams J, et al. Coexisting dementia and depression in Parkinson's disease. *Arch Neurol* 1989;46:1284–1286.

78. Mayeux R, Stern Y, Williams JB, et al. Clinical and biochemical features of depression in Parkinson's disease. *Am J Psychiatry* 1986;143: 756–759.

79. Sano M, Stern Y, Cote L, et al. Depression in Parkinson's disease: a biochemical model. *J Neuropsychiatry Clin Neurosci* 1990;2:88–92.

80. Cash R, Raisman R, Ploska A, et al. High and low affinity [3H] imipramine binding sites in control and parkinsonian brains. *Eur J Pharmacol* 1985;117:71–80.

81. Becker T, Becker G, Seufert J, et al. Parkinson's disease and depression: evidence for an alteration of the basal limbic system detected by transcranial sonography. *J Neurol Neurosurg Psychiatry* 1997;63:590–596.

82. Langer SZ, Galzin AM, Poirier MF, et al. Association of [3H]–imipramine and [3H]–paroxetine binding with the 5HT transporter in brain and platelets: relevance to studies in depression. *J Recept Res* 1987;7:499–521.

83. Raisman R, Cash R, Agid Y. Parkinson's disease: decreased density of 3H–imipramine and 3H–paroxetine binding sites in putamen. *Neurology* 1986;36:556–560.

84. Chan–Palay V. Depression and dementia in Parkinson's disease. Catecholamine changes in the locus ceruleus, a basis for therapy. *Adv Neurol* 1993;60:438–446.

85. Chan–Palay V, Asan E. Alterations in catecholamine neurons of the locus coeruleus in senile dementia of the Alzheimer type and in Parkinson's disease with and without dementia and depression. *J Comp Neurol* 1989;287:373–392.

86. Poewe W, Seppi K. Treatment options for depression and psychosis in Parkinson's disease. *J Neurol* 2001;248(Suppl 3):III12–III21.

87. Strang RR. Imipramine in the treatment of parkinsonism. *Br Med J* 1965;2:33–34.

88. Laitinen L. Desipramine in the treatment of Parkinson's disease. *Acta Neurol Scand* 1969;45: 109–113.

89. Anderson G, Aabro E, Gulamann N, et al. Antidepressant treatment in Parkinson's disease: a controlled trial of the effect of nortriptyline in patients with Parkinson's disease treated with L–dopa. *Acta Neurol Scand* 1980;62:210–219.

90. Goetz CG, Tanner CM, Klawans HL. Bupropion in Parkinson's disease. *Neurology* 1984;34: 1092–1094.

91. Klaasen T, Verhey FR, Sneijders GH, et al. Treatment of depression in Parkinson's disease: a meta–analysis. *J Neuropsychiatry Clin Neurosci* 1995;7:281–286.

92. Richard IH, Kurlan R, Tanner C, et al. Serotonin syndrome and the combined use of deprenyl and an antidepressant in Parkinson's disease. Parkinson Study Group. *Neurology* 1997;48:1070–1077.

93. McDonald WM, Richard IH, DeLong MR. Prevalence, Etiology, and Treatment of Depression

in Parkinson's Disease. *Biol Psychiatry* 2003;54: 363–375.

94. Greenberg R, Meyers BS. Treatment of major depression and Parkinson's disease with combined phenelzine and amantadine. *Am J Psychiatry* 1985;142:273–274.

95. Hargrave R, Ashford JW. Phenelzine treatment of depression in Parkinson's disease. *Am J Psychiatry* 1992;149:1751–1752.

96. Steur EN, Ballering LA. Moclobemide and selegiline in the treatment of depression in Parkinson's disease. *J Neurol Neurosurg Psychiatry* 1997; 63:547.

97. Jouvent R, Abensour P, Bonnet AM, et al. Antiparkinsonian and antidepressant effects of high doses of bromocriptine. As independent comparison. *J Affect Disord* 1983;5:141–145.

98. Rektorova I, Rektor I, Hortova H. Depression in Parkinson's disease: an eight–month randomized, open–label, national, multi–centre comparative study of pramipexole and pergolide. *Parkinsonism Rel Disord* 2001;7:S68.

99. Friedenberg DL, Cummings JL. Parkinson's disease, depression, and the on–off phenomenon. *Psychosomatics* 1989;30:94–99.

100. Maricle RA, Nutt JC, Valentine RJ, et al. Dose–response relationships of levodopa with mood and anxiety in fluctuating Parkinson's disease: a double–blind, placebo–controlled study. *Neurology* 1995;45:1757–1760.

101. Burke WJ, Peterson J, Rubin EH. Electroconvulsive therapy in the treatment of combined depression and Parkinson's disease. *Psychosomatics* 1988;29:341–346.

102. George MS, Wasserman EM, Post RM. Transcranial magnetic stimulation: a neuropsychiatric tool for the 21st century. *J Neuropsychiatry Clin Neurosci* 1996;8:373–382.

103. Mally J, Stone TW. Improvement in Parkinsonian symptoms after repetitive transcranial magnetic stimulation. *J Neurol Sci* 1999;162: 179–184.

104. Tom T, Cummings JL. Depression in Parkinson's disease. Pharmacological characteristics and treatment. *Drugs Aging* 1998;12:55–74.

105. Waters CH. Fluoxetine and seligiline—lack of significant interaction. *Can J Neurol Sci* 1994; 21:259–261.

106. Ward H, Evans DL. Depression and Cancer. In: Nelson JC, ed. *Geriatric Psychopharmacolgy.* New York: Marcel Dekker, 1998:187–198.

107. Massie MJ, Holland JC. Depression and the cancer patient. *J Clin Psychiatry* 1990;51(Suppl): 12–19.

108. Raison CL, Miller AH. Depression in cancer: new developments regarding diagnosis and treatment. *Biol Psychiatry* 2003;54:283–294.

109. Petitto JM, Evans DL. Depression in cancer and HIV infection: research findings and implications of effective antidepressant treatment. *Depress Anxiety* 1998;8(suppl 1):80–84.

110. Green A, Austin C. Psychopathology of pancreatic cancer: a psychobiologic probe. *Psychosmoatics* 1993;34:208–221.

111. Penninx BW, Guralnik JM, Pahor M, et al. Chronically depressed mood and cancer risk in older persons. *J Natl Cancer Inst* 1998;90: 1888–1893.

112. Stommel M, Given BA, Given CW. Depression and functional status as predictors of death among cancer patients. *Cancer* 2002;94: 2719–2727.

113. Gill D, Hatcher S. Antidepressants for depression in medical illness. *Cochrame Database Sys Rev* 2000;CD001312.

114. Schuler US. Most patients depressed by cancer do not need drugs [Letter]. *BMJ* 2002;325: 1115.

115. Pearlson GD, Rabins PV, Kim WS, et al. Structural brain CT changes and cognitive deficits in elderly depressives with and without reversible dementia ('pseudodementia'). *Psychol Med* 1989;19:573–584.

116. Lishman WA. *Organic psychiatry, 2nd edition.* Oxford: Blackwell, 1987.

117. Baldwin R. Depressive disorders. In: Jacoby R and Oppenheimer C, eds. *Psychiatry in the elderly.* New York: Oxford University Press, 2002: 628–676.

118. McGuire MH, Rabins PV. Mood disorders. In: Coffey CE, Cummings JL, eds. *Textbook of geriatric psychiatry.* Washington: American Psychiatric Press, 1994:244–260.

119. Abas M, Sahakian B, Levy R. Neuropsychological deficits and CT scan changes in elderly depressives. *Psychol Med* 1990;20:507–520.

120. Buerger K, Zinkowski R, Teipel SJ, et al. Differentiation of geriatric major depression from Alzheimer's disease with CSF tau protein phosphorylated at threonine 231. *Am J Psychiatry* 2003;160:376–379.

121. Green RC, Cupples LA, Kurz A, et al. Depression as a risk factor for Alzheimer disease: the MIRAGE Study. *Arch Neuro.* 2003;60:753–759.

122. Lyketsos CG, DelCamppt L, Steinberg M, et al. Treating depression in Alzheimer disease. *Arch Gen Psychiatry* 2003;60:737–746.

123. Devanand DP, Jacobs DM, Tang MX, et al. The course of psychopathologic features in mild to moderate Alzheimer disease. *Arch Gen Psychiatry* 1997;54:257–263.

124. Lyketsos CG, Sheppard JM, Steele CD, et al. Randomized, placebo–controlled, double-blind clinical trial of sertraline in the treatment of depression complicating Alzheimer's disease: initial results from the Depression in Alzheimer's Disease study. *Am J Psychiatry* 2000; 157:1686–1689.

125. Lyketsos G, Olin J. Depression in Alzheimer's disease: overview and treatment. *Biol Psychiatry* 2002;51:243–252.

126. Gonzalez–Salvador T, Lyketsos CG, Baker A, et al. Quality of life in dementia patients in long–term care. *Int J Geriatr Psychiatry* 2000;15: 181–189.

127. Lyketsos CG, Steele C, Galik E, et al. Physical aggression in dementia patients and its relationship to depression. *Am J Psychiatry* 1999; 156:66–71.

128. Steele C, Rovner B, Chase GA, Folstein M. Psychiatric symptoms and nursing home placement of patients with Alzheimer's disease. *Am J Psychiatry* 1990;147:1049–1051.

129. Hoch CC, Reynolds CF, Houck PR, et al. Predicting mortality in mixed depression and de-

mentia using EEG sleep variables. *J Neuropsychiatry Clin Neurosci* 1989;1:366–371.

130. Rubio A, Vestner AL, Stewart JM, et al. Suicide and Alzheimer's pathology in the elderly: a case–control study. *Biol Psychiatry* 2001;49: 137–145.

Supplemental References

General

Beliles KE, Stoudemire A. Psychopharmacologic Treatment of Depression in the Medically Ill. *Psychosomatics* 1998; 39: S2–S19.

Iosifescu DV, Nierenberg AA, Alpert JE, et al. The impact of medical comorbidity on acute treatment in major depressive disorder. *Am J Psychiatry* 2003;160:2122–2127.

Zanardi R, Cusin C, Rossini D, et al. Comparison of response to fluvoxamine in nondemented elderly compared to younger patients affected by major depression. *J Clin Psychopharmacol* 2003;23: 535–539.

Cardiovascular

Anda R, Williamson D, Jones D, et al. Depressed affect, hopelessness, and the risk of ischemic heart disease in a cohort of U.S. adults [comment]. *Epidemiology* 1993; 4:285–294.

Appels AD, Barr FW, Bar J, et al. Inflammation, depressive symptomatology, and coronary artery disease. *Psychosom Med* 2000;62:601–605.

Aromaa A, Raitasalo R, Reunanen A, et al. Depression and cardiovascular diseases. *Acta Psychiatr Scand* 1994;377:77–82.

Bigger JT Jr. Implications of the cardiac arrhythmia suppression trial for antiarrhythmic drug treatment. *Am J Cardiol* 1990;65:3D–10D.

Blumenthal JA, Emery CF. Rehabilitation of patients following myocardial infarction. *J Consult Clin Psychol* 1988;56:374–381.

Bonnemeier H, Hartmann F, Uwe KH, et al. Course and prognostic implications of QT interval and QT interval variability after primary coronary angioplasty in acute myocardial infarction. *J Am Coll Cardiol* 2000;37:44–50.

Cardiac Arrhythmia Suppression Trial (CAST) Investigators. Preliminary report: effect of ecainide and flecainide on mortality in a randomized trial of arrhythmia suppression after myocardial infarction. *N Engl J Med* 1989;321:406–412.

Cardiac Arrhythmia Suppression Trial II Investigators. Effect of the antiarrhythmic agent moricizine on survival after myocardial infarction. *N Engl J Med* 1992;327:227–233.

Carney RM, Berkman LF, Blumenthal JA, et al. Heart rate variability and depression in patients with a recent acute myocardial infarction. *Psychosom Med* 2001;63:102.

Coplen SE, Antman EM, Berlin JA, et al. Efficacy and safety of quinidine therapy for maintenance of sinus rhythm after cardioversion: a meta–analysis of randomized control trials. *Circulation* 1990;82: 1106–1116.

Echt DS, Liebson PR, Mitchell LB, et al. Mortality and morbidity in patients receiving ecainide, flecainide, or placebo. The Cardiac Arrhythmia Suppression Trial. *N Engl J Med* 1991;324: 781–788.

Elming H, Holm E, Jun L, et al. The prognostic value of the QT interval and QT interval dispersion in all cause and cardiac mortality and morbidity in a population of Danish citizens. *Eur Heart J* 1998; 19:1391–1400.

Falk RH. Flecainide–induced ventricular tachycardia and fibrillation in patients treated for atrial fibrillation. *Ann Intern Med* 1989;111:107–111.

Ford DE, Mead LA, Change PP, et al. Depression is a risk factor for coronary artery disease in men. *Arch Intern Med* 1998;158:1422–1426.

Glassman A, O'Connor C, Harrison W. Sertraline treatment of major depression in patients with acute MI or unstable angina. Poster presented at American Psychiatric Association; May 9, 2001; New Orleans, LA.

Greenberg HM, Dwyer EM Jr, Hochman JS, et al. Interaction of ischemia and ecainide/flecainide treatment: a proposed mechanism for the increased mortality in CAST I. *Br Heart J* 1995;74: 631–635.

Hallstrom T, Lapidus L, Bengtsson C, et al. Psychosocial factors and risk of ischaemic heart disease and death in women: a twelve–year follow–up of participants in the population study of women in Gothenburg, Sweden. *J Psychosom Res* 1986;30: 451–459.

Kleiger RE, Miller JP, Bigger JT, Moss AJ. Decreased heart rate variability and its association with increased mortality after acute myocardial infarction. *Am J Cardiol* 1987;59:256–262.

Koenig HG, Meador KG, Cohen HJ, Blazer DG. Detection and treatment of major depression in older medically ill hospitalized patients. *Inter J of Psych in Med* 1988;18:17–31.

Lagrissi–Thode F, Wagner WR, Pollock BG, et al. Elevated platelet factor 4 and beta–thromboglobulin plasma levels in depressed patients with ischemic heart disease. *Biol Psychiatry* 1997;42: 290–295.

Mendes de Leon CF, Krumholz HM, Seeman TS, et al. Depression and risk of coronary heart disease in elderly men and women: *New Haven EPESE*, 1982–1991. Established Populations for the Epidemiologic Studies of the Elderly. *Arch Intern Med* 1998;158:2341–2348.

Molnar J, Rosenthal JE, Weiss JS, Somberg JC. QT interval dispersion in healthy subjects and survivors of sudden cardiac death: Circadian variation in a twenty–four hour assessment. *Am J Cardiol* 1997;79:1190–1193

Murakawa Y, Inoue H, Nozaki A, Sugimoto T. Role of sympathovagal interaction in diurnal variation of QT interval. *Am J Cardiol* 1992;69:339–343.

Musselman DL, Marzec UM, Manatunga A, et al. Platelet reactivity in depressed patients treated with paroxetine: preliminary findings. *Arch Gen Psychiatry* 2000;57:875–882.

Musselman DL, Tomer A, Manatunga AK, et al. Exaggerated platelet reactivity in major depression. *Am J Psychiatry* 1996;153:1212–1217.

Pearlson GD, Rabins PV, Koven S. High fatality rates of late–life depression associated with cardiovascular disease. *J Affect Disord* 1985;9:165–167.

Pomeranz B, Macaulay RJ, Caudill MA, et al. Assessment of autonomic function in humans by heart rate spectral analysis. *Am J Physiol* 1985;248(1 Pt 2):H151–H153.

Pratt LA, Ford DE, Crum RM, et al. Depression, psychotropic medication, and risk of myocardial infarction: prospective data from the Baltimore ECA follow–up. *Circulation* 1996;94:3123–3129.

Roose SP, Dalack GW, Glassman AH, et al. Cardiovascular effects of bupropion in depressed patients with heart disease. *Am J Psychiatry* 1991;148: 512–516.

Roose SP, Dalack GW, Woodring S. Death, depression, and heart disease. *J Clin Psychiatry* 1991; 52(suppl):34–39.

Selzer A, Wray HW. Quinidine syncope: paroxysmal ventricular fibrillation occurring during treatment of chronic atrial arrhythmias. *Circulation* 1964;10:17–26.

Shapiro PA, Lespérance F, Frasure–Smith N, et al. for the Sertraline Anti-Depressant Heart Attack Trial. An open–label preliminary trial of sertraline for treatment of major depression after acute myocardial infarction (the SADHAT Trial). *Am Heart J* 1999;137:1100–1106.

Vrotec B, Starc V, Starc R. Beat–to–beat QT interval variability in coronary patients. *J Electrocardiol* 2000;33:119–125.

Wassertheil–Smoller S, Applegate WB, Berge K, et al. Change in depresssion as a precursor of cardiovascular events. SHEP Cooperative Research Group (Systolic Hypertension in the Elderly Project). *Arch Intern Med* 1996;156:553–561.

Writing Committee for the ENRICHD Investigators: Effects of Treating Depression and Low Perceived Social Support on Clinical Events after Myocardial Infarction. *JAMA* 2003;289:3106–3116.

Yeragani VK. Major depression and long–term heart period variability. *Depress Anxiety* 2000;12:51–52.

Yeragani VK, Pohl R, Balon R, et al. Heart rate variability in patients with major depression. *Psychiatry Res* 1991;37:35–46.

Yeragani VK, Pohl R, Jampala VC, et al. Increased QT variability in patients with panic disorder and depression. *Psychiatry Res* 2000;93:225–235.

Stroke

Morris PLP, Robinson RG, Andrzejewski P, et al. Association of depression with 10–year poststroke mortality. *Am J Psychiatry* 2003;150:124–129.

Narushima K, Kosier JT, Robinson RG. Preventing poststroke depression: a 12–week double–blind treatment trial and 21–month follow–up. *J Nerv Ment Dis* 2002;190:296–303.

Narushima K, Chan K, Kosier JT, et al. Does cognitive recovery after treatment of poststroke depression last? A 2–year follow–up of cognitive function associated with poststroke depression. *Am J Psychiatry* 2003;160:1157–1162.

Robinson RG, Kubos KL, Starr LB, et al. Mood changes in stroke patients: relationship to lesion location. *Compr Psychiatry* 1983;24:555–566.

Tateno A, Kimuro M, Robinson RG. Phenomenological characteristics of poststroke depression: early–versus late–onset. *Am J Geriatr Psychiatry* 2002;10:575–582.

Cancer

Purohit DR, Navlakha PL, Modi RS, et al. The role of antidepressants in hospitalized cancer patients. *J Assoc Physicians India* 1978;26:245–248.

Rayner AV, O'Brien JG. Depression and medical illness. In: Ellison JM and Verma S, eds. *Depression in later life*. New York: Marcel Dekker, 2003: 133–154.

Van Heeringen K, Zivkov M. Pharmacological treatment of depression in cancer patients. A placebo–controlled study of mianserin. *Br J Psychiatry* 1996;169:440–443.

Dementia

Alexopoulos GS. Biological abnormalities in late–life depression. *J Geriatr Psychiatry* 1989;22: 25–34.

Evers MM, Samuels SC, Lantz M, et al. The prevalence, diagnosis and treatment of depression in dementia patients in chronic care facilities in the last six months of life. *Int J Geriatr Psychiatry* 2002; 17:464–472.

Gottfries CG, Karlsson I, Nyth AL. Treatment of depression in elderly patients with and without dementia disorders. *Int Clin Psychopharmacol* 1992;6(suppl 5):55–64.

Green RC, Cupples LA, Kurz A, et al. Depression as a risk factor for Alzheimer Disease: The Mirage Study. *Arch Neurol* 2003;60:753–759.

Greenwald BS, Kramer–Ginsberg E, Marin DB, et al. Dementia with coexistent major depression. *Am J Psychiatry* 1989;146:1472–1478.

Katz IR. Diagnosis and treatment of depression in patients with Alzheimer's disease and other dementias. *J Clin Psychiatry* 1998;59(Suppl 9): 38–44.

Kral V. The relationship between senile dementia, Alzheimer's type, and depression. *Can J Psychiatry* 1983;28:304–306.

Kral VA, Emery OB. Long–term follow–up of depressive pseudodementia of the aged. *Can J Psychiatry* 1989;34:445–446.

Lee HB, Lysetkos CG. Depression in Alzheimer's Disease: heterogeneity and related issues. *Biol Psychiatry* 2003;54:353–362.

Lishman WA. *Organic psychiatry: the psychological consequences of cerebral disorder*, 3rd edition. Oxford, England: Blackwell Scientific, 1987.

Lysetkos CG, Olin J. Depression in Alzheimer's Disease: Overview and treatment. *Biol Psychiatry* 2002;52:243–252.

Nyth AL, Gottfries CG, Lyby K, et al. A controlled multicenter clinical study of citalopram and placebo in elderly depressed patients with and without concomitant dementia. *Acta Psychiatr Scand* 1992;86:138–145.

Nyth AL, Gottfries CG. The clinical efficacy of citalopram in treatment of emotional disturbances in dementia disorders. A Nordic multicentre study. *Br J Psychiatry* 1990;157:894–101.

Pearlson GD, Ross CA, Lohr WD, et al. Association

between family history of affective disorder and the depressive syndrome of Alzheimer's disease. *Am J Psychaitry* 1990;147:452–456.

Post F. The significance of affective symptoms in old age. *Maudsley Monographs*, 10. London: Oxford University Press, 1962.

Rabins PV, Pearlson GD. Depression induced cognitive impairment. In: Burns A, Levy R, eds. *Dementia*. London: Chapman and Hall, 2000:789–798.

Reifler BV, Larson E, Teri L. Dementia of the Alzheimer's type and depression. *J Am Geriatr Soc* 1986; 34:855–859.

Reifler BV, Teri L, Raskind M, et al. Double–blind trial of imipramine in Alzheimer's disease patients with and without depression. *Am J Psychiatry* 1989;146:45–49.

ReynoldsCF, Kupfer DJ, Hoch CC, et al. Two–year follow–up of elderly patients with mixed depression and dementia. *J Am Geriatr Soc* 1986;34: 793–799.

Chapter 12

Diagnosis and Treatment of Late-Life Bipolar Disorder

Andrew Satlin

Benjamin Liptzin

Robert C. Young

Research on the psychopharmacology of bipolar disorder has expanded enormously over the last 5 years. Findings from randomized controlled trials of several anticonvulsants and atypical antipsychotics have put new therapeutic tools in the hands of clinicians. Unfortunately, the available research evidence includes a relatively small number of geriatric patients—a situation not uncommon in geriatric medicine. Without research-based guidelines, the geriatric psychiatrist must rely on the general principles of geriatric physiology and medicine, applied to the individual patient. This chapter aims to aid the clinician in that process. It begins with an overview of bipolar disorder in the elderly, continues with general principles for the pharmacologic treatment of the acute and maintenance phases of the manic and depressed poles of the illness, and concludes with more specific treatment guidelines.

Epidemiology

Bipolar disorder in later life is not rare. About 10% of all bipolar patients have onset of mania after the age of 50,[1] and mania accounts for 5% to 10% of psychiatric admissions over the age of 60.[2–5] However, the prevalence of bipolar disorder in the community decreases with age from 1.4% in young adults to 0.4% in those aged 45 to 64 and 0.1% in those older than 65.[6] The incidence of bipolar disorder presenting with depression in the elderly, as well as the percentage of depressive episodes in the elderly due to bipolar depression, are not known.

Clinical Presentation and Diagnosis

Diagnosis of the manic and depressive poles of bipolar disorder in the older person is based on the same criteria as those used to diagnose younger patients. Physiological aging and physical illness may temper some of the manifestations of mania in the elderly and may contribute to the lower rating scale scores found in some[7,8] but not all case series.[9] Clinical experience suggests that in the elderly euphoria is less likely to be part of the manic syndrome; irritability and dysphoria are more common. However, in research studies no consistent differences from younger patients appear in the degree of hyperactivity, euphoria, flight of ideas, expansiveness, or grandiosity, and these typical symptoms occur in approximately 60% of elderly manic patients.[2,4] Similarly, research provides inconsistent support for the clinical impression that elderly manic patients have more psychosis than younger manics. Some studies find no difference[8,10] whereas more recent studies are mixed: some find more frequent psychosis in late-onset patients,[9] others find delusions, hallucinations, and paranoia more frequent among early-onset patients.[11–13] Mixed presentations of mania and depression may be less common in late-onset patients.[12]

Older manic patients may present with a dementia or delirium syndrome.[14,15] They may exhibit such marked distractibility, reduced attention span, impaired concentration, disorientation, mixed or labile affect, and irritability that the diagnosis of mania is overlooked. As with depression presenting with dementia or delirium, identification of the underlying affective illness is important because treatment can result in improvement in cognitive function.[15] In an older patient presenting with this type of complicated clinical picture, history of a prior affective disorder or a family history of bipolar disorder may provide a clue to a treatable manic illness.

Alternatively, presentation with a dementia or delirium syndrome may reflect increased likelihood of an organic basis for late-onset mania. Symptoms suggestive of mania are sometimes noted in patients with dementia, but the frequency of syndromal mania in patients with dementia is unresolved.[12,17] In view of the association between late-onset mania and neurologic or medical conditions, a thorough medical evaluation should be part of the evaluation of late-onset mania. This evaluation should include a detailed medical and treatment history, physical and neurologic examination, laboratory tests for hematology and chemistry, chest x-ray, and brain imaging.

No published studies compare the depressive features of bipolar with unipolar depression in older individuals. As for younger patients, the diagnosis of bipolar depression depends upon a history of a prior manic, hypomanic, or mixed episode. An accurate diagnosis has important therapeutic implications because treatment of bipolar depression with antidepressant monotherapy can be associated with precipitating mania or worsening the overall course of disease. Since some elderly patients with bipolar disorder may have had atypical presentations of mania, or may have had their only manic episode in the distant past, a detailed history and careful review of old medical records is warranted. Furthermore, because bipolar depression often requires combination pharmacologic treatment, confirming the need for such therapy ensures that the risks of producing additive side effects, pharmacokinetic interactions, and reduced compliance are justified.

Course of Illness

Elderly patients with mania report diverse psychiatric histories. Some have had courses of illness typical of bipolar disorder, with recurrent cycles of mania and depression beginning at an early age and continuing throughout life. With age, cycling may increase in frequency or become chronic, and episodes may become more symptomatically severe.[18] Among other geriatric patients, the first manic episode tends to occur relatively late in life; 25% of manic patients over the age of 65 have their first manic episode after this age.[19] In some of these patients, late-life mania follows one or more prior episodes of depression with a latency of 10 to 20 years.[5,8,19–21] A smaller number of late-onset patients present with unipolar mania.[22–24] Case reports suggest that these patients often have neurologic or other medical illnesses that are identified as risk factors for mania,[25–27] but this tendency may reflect bias either in diagnosis or reporting. There are no longitudinal data to suggest how commonly these patients go on to develop typical cycling between mania and depression. Elderly patients with late-life mania have greater mortality and progression to dementia than patients with unipolar depression,[18,21] which may reflect the higher rates of medical illness, especially cerebrovascular disease, in this group.[28]

In younger and middle-aged adults, relapses into depression occur far more often than relapses into mania, and depression accounts for the majority of time spent with affective illness in most patients with bipolar disorder.[29] Whether this pattern of relapse into depression persists into late life is not yet known.

Etiology

Many studies have attempted to elucidate the etiologic factors associated with mania by comparing groups of early- and late-onset bipolar patients. Interpretation of these studies is made difficult by their use of different definitions of early and late onset as well as different methods for assessing potential predisposing factors. Nevertheless, data from these studies reveal, in general, that rates of positive family history of affective illness are higher in patients with early age of onset, suggesting a greater genetic contribution from early rather than late-onset bipolar disorder.[4,19,22,30–32]

Conversely, a variety of medical and neurologic conditions are more frequent among late-onset compared to early-onset patients. The association of mania and age-associated neurologic disorders is documented in many clinical studies.[2,5,8,9,19–21,28,33,34] Mania is more common in patients with traumatic brain injury, temporal lobe epilepsy, space-occupying lesions, stroke, and Huntington's disease; hypomania-like syndromes are frequent in multiple sclerosis.[16] Mania also may be associated with central nervous system (CNS) infections such as syphilis and human immunodeficiency virus. Brain imaging of manic patients over 60 without focal neurologic findings reveals greater cortical sulcal widening, subcortical hyperintensities, and ventricular-to-brain ratios than age-matched nonmanic controls.[8,33,34]

Manic symptoms also occur in the context of a variety of physical disorders and drugs. Estimates for the rate of these "secondary" manias among hospitalized elderly manic patients are in the range of 25%, which is probably much higher than the rate for secondary mania in younger populations.[19] Several causes of secondary mania exist. These include metabolic disturbances such as vitamin B_{12} deficiency; endocrine disorders such as hypothyroidism; infections; hemodialysis; use of such medications as corticosteroids, anticholinergics, L-dopa, psychostimulants, and sympathomimetics; and drugs of abuse (e.g., cocaine, amphetamines) or alcohol; hyperthyroidism may be a rare cause.[35]

Neurologic studies of the disinhibition syndrome and secondary mania as well as psychiatric studies of bipolar disorder in the elderly have developed overlapping pathogenetic concepts, both of which implicate involvement of the orbito-frontal and basal temporal cortices of the right hemisphere.[36–38] In older persons, a genetic predisposition to mood disorder may increase the risk that a heterogeneous group of brain changes and disorders will induce a manic syndrome, even though the genetic predisposition may be weaker than in early onset cases. Triggering of the syndrome by an accumulation of neurologic insults may account for the relatively late onset of bipolar disorder in many elderly patients and the long latency from first onset of affective illness to first appearance of mania in others.

Support for this hypothesis of the effects of predisposing factors and age on the development of bipolar disorder is further suggested by the finding of higher rates of childhood behavioral and substance use disorders in patients with onset of psychotic mania before age 21 compared with those with onset after age 30.[11] Together with studies comparing adult-onset with geriatric-onset bipolar disorder, these findings suggest that neurodevelopmental abnormalities and substance abuse in adolescent-onset bipolar disorder play a similar role in the development and course of illness as that of neurological abnormalities seen in late-onset bipolar disorder insofar as both sets of risk factors interact with genetic predisposition to determine age of onset, phenomenology, and response to treatment.

General Treatment Principles

The somatic therapies available for treating bipolar disorder in the elderly are the same as those for younger patients, and treatment is similarly divided: (1) symptomatic control of acute manic and depressive episodes, and (2) long-term continuation or maintenance therapy to sustain benefits and prevent relapse. Recently revised practice guidelines[39] provide evidence-based recommendations for the first-line treatment of acute manic or mixed episodes for both severe and less-ill patients, alternative and adjunctive treatments for patients who fail to respond to first-line treatment, maintenance regimens, and treatment of recurrences despite maintenance therapy. These guidelines offer minimal specific recommendations for treatment of geriatric patients, reflecting the paucity of controlled clinical study data for this population. In general, therefore, the clinician treating an elderly manic patient should modify treatment based on guidelines for younger patients by considering several types of data: general principles of geriatric psychopharmacology; the available, largely uncontrolled, or anecdotal literature on treatment of elderly patients with bipolar disorder; and findings about side effects and drug interactions from studies of medications such as the anticonvulsants, used by the elderly for other indications. In addition, treatment decisions should be based on the individual patient's clinical profile, past history of treatment responsiveness, medical conditions, and concomitant medications. Because these factors typically vary across a range of geriatric bipolar patients more than over a range of their younger counterparts, selection of the most appropriate treatment for an individual elderly bipolar patient especially those who are manic, may be less clear than for a younger patient.

Acute Treatment of Mania

Lithium, valproate, and olanzapine are approved in the United States as first-line monotherapy for the acute treatment of mania. Patients with only partial response, or those with more severe or mixed episodes, may require combination treatment with either lithium or valproate and an antipsychotic. When optimal doses of these medications are unsuccessful, options include addition of another first-line agent or a different anticonvulsant or antipsychotic, switching from one anticonvulsant or antipsychotic to another, or using ECT.

Although controlled studies of these regimens are not available for patients above the age of 65, available evidence suggests that lithium is often effective for acute treatment when it is tolerated.[40–42] The presence of neurologic disease may, however, predict lack of tolerability and/or lack of efficacy.[43] Several other factors may be associated with a diminished response to lithium; these include more than 10 previous manic episodes[44] posttraumatic mania (i.e., mania presumed due to head injury), rapid-cycling disease, mixed states, comorbid substance abuse, psychosis, hypothyroidism, and development of neurotoxicity.

Among neurologically normal elderly patients with predominantly manic rather than mixed presentations, lithium monotherapy may result in greater rates of improvement than valproate monotherapy, although patients who achieve valproate levels between 65 to 90 mcg/mL appear to do equally well.[42] Valproate may be preferred in other instances, e.g., when patients have psychiatric histories consistent with secondary mania, rapid cycling, or mixed affective states; when a patient has a history of nonresponse or intolerable side effects to lithium; when medical conditions increase the risk of lithium-induced toxicity; and when parenteral therapy is needed for elderly patients who refuse oral treatment.[45,46] Combinations of lithium and valproate in elderly manic patients may augment clinical effects or allow use of better-tolerated lower doses of both drugs.[47–52] Carbamazepine is also effective but is used as second-line treatment because of its small but significant risk of blood dyscrasia and cardiotoxic effects that may be problematic in elderly patients with preexisting cardiac disease.

Antipsychotics are often prescribed as adjuncts to other treatments for mania but may be used alone in patients who are unresponsive to, or cannot tolerate, lithium or anticonvulsants. Interest in the use of antipsychotics for treatment of bipolar disorder has increased with the introduction of atypical agents.[53] These are presumed to be less problematic for the affectively ill population for several reasons: they are less potentially neurotoxic in combination with lithium; they show a lower rate of neuromotor side effects to which patients with affective disorders may be especially vulnerable; they are more effective for deficit or depressive symptoms that otherwise could exacerbate the depressive pole of the illness while having relative rapid onset of action. Atypical antipsychotics compared with typical also are preferred treatments for the elderly because of their relatively greater safety.[54] Double-blind controlled studies of use of typical antipsychotics for acute mania include two studies with olanzapine and one with risperidone; all three found atypical antipsychotics superior to placebo or equivalent to lithium or typical antipsychotics.[55] Although these studies did not include substantial numbers of manic patients over the age of 65, some evidence suggests that in subgroups of patients older than 50, olanzapine leads to reductions in manic symptoms comparable to those seen with valproate and greater than with placebo.[56]

Acute Treatment of Bipolar Depression

Treatment of bipolar depression is difficult in all age groups. Unfortunately, no controlled treatment studies of bipolar depression in the elderly are available. One open-case series of 5 women with bipolar disorder, ranging in age from 65 to 85 who remained depressed after 3 months on combined lithium and valproate, found remission of symptoms with the addition of lamotrigine.[57] Current treatment guidelines suggest lithium or lamotrigine as first-line treatment for acute episodes of bipolar depression.[39] Use of antidepressants as monotherapy is not recommended because of the risk of inducing mania or accelerating cycling, although some clinicians will simultaneously start an antidepressant and lithium. More severely ill patients are often treated with ECT.

Breakthrough episodes of depression in patients already on a mood stabilizer should be treated by using the optimum dose of maintenance medication. If this approach is unsuccessful, addition of a second mood stabilizer can be at least as effective as the addition of an antidepressant,[29] although evidence also supports the addition of either bupropion or paroxetine.[39] Atypical antipsychotics may be of benefit but, thus far, results are clearest for their use in combination with antidepressants for acute treatment and with lithium or valproic acid for maintenance.[57]

Maintenance Treatment

Maintenance treatment is generally recommended following acute treatment of a single manic episode.[39] Older patients, like their younger counterparts, are susceptible to recurrent episodes of mania. Furthermore, patients whose recurrent bipolar illness developed early in life may, in fact, develop more severe and more frequent episodes as they age. Because the consequences of a severe manic episode may be very serious in the older patient, long-term preventive treatment is as important with older patients as with younger ones. Exceptions may be those patients whose acute episode of mania was clearly associated with a treatable organic cause that has been addressed and is unlikely to recur.

In general, if lithium or an anticonvulsant has been successful in treating the acute episode, the same medication should be used for maintenance.[39,57,58] If an antipsychotic was used adjunctively during the acute episode, discontinuation should be considered unless is evidence for persistent psychosis is evident. If an antipsychotic was used as monotherapy for the acute manic episode, maintenance therapy with the same agent may be tried.

Lithium has the best empirical evidence for efficacy in the acute treatment of both mania and depression in bipolar disorder and for prophylaxis against recurrence of both types of mood episodes, and therefore comes closest to meeting the criteria for a comprehensive mood stabilizer.[57] Placebo-controlled trials of maintenance treatment for bipolar disorder in the 1970s found lithium effective, but a study in younger and middle-aged adults suggest less successful outcomes.[59] Differences in patient selection and study design may account for these changes. Controlled studies of lithium maintenance in elderly patients are unavailable; the poor tolerability of lithium in some aged patients emphasizes the need for such controlled investigation. Clinical observation suggests that long-term lithium treatment is less effective in older patients than in younger ones, which may reflect the effect of neurologic disease on the efficacy and/or tolerability of lithium by this population. Conversely, switching elderly patients who have done well on lithium for many years to newer agents is not justified.[60] Recent evidence suggests that long-term lithium use may have neuroprotective and neurotrophic effects that warrant further investigation in the geriatric population.[61,62]

In the last decade, placebo-controlled comparisons of lithium and anticonvulsants for maintenance treatment have confirmed the efficacy of both.[63,64] Lamotrigine has recently been approved by the U.S. Food and Drug Administration for the long-term maintenance treatment of adults with bipolar disorder, in order to delay the time to recurrence of depression, mania, hypomania, and mixed episodes in patients treated for acute episodes with standard therapy. Both lithium and lamotrigine are better than placebo in delaying time to any mood episode: lamotrigine is superior to placebo for preventing of depressive episodes and lithium superior to placebo for preventing of mania, hypomania, and mixed episodes.[65]

Controlled studies of anticonvulsants for maintenance have not been conducted in the geriatric population, but the same considerations that may influence the choice for acute treatment, such as presence of predictors of poor response or intolerance to lithium, may apply. Among the anticonvulsants, more recently available drugs such as lamotrigine[66] and oxcarbamazepine[67] may prove to have tolerability advantages for geriatric patients.

The role of antipsychotic medication in maintenance treatment for bipolar disorder remains uncertain. Thus far, open-label studies using clozapine[68] and olanzapine[69] as adjunctive treatment in patients with inadequate responses to mood stabilizers suggest efficacy of continued atypical antipsychotic treatment for up to a year after resolution of the acute episode. Substantial data on patients over the age of 65 are not available.

Treatment with Lithium

Prescribing lithium to older patients requires knowledge and attention to age-related changes in the pharmacotherapy and therapeutic sensitivity of this mood stabilizer. The pharmacokinetic disposition of lithium decreases whereas the CNS sensitivity increases with advancing age.

Clinical Pharmacology

Use of lithium for older patients requires special precautions because of age-related alterations in the pharmacologic effects of all drugs on aging (see Chapters 4 and 5).

Absorption

The absorption of lithium is complete, rapid, and unaffected by the aging process.

Protein Binding

Because lithium is not bound to plasma proteins, pharmacologically active lithium levels are not influenced by variations in plasma protein levels secondary to aging, nutritional state, or physical illness.

Volume of Distribution

Lithium is water soluble and is distributed throughout total body water. Because total body water decreases with age as a result of the loss of skeletal muscle mass, particularly in women, the amount of water available as a diluent for lithium also decreases (see Chapter 5); that is, the volume of distribution decreases, and for any given dosage of lithium, its levels are higher in older patients (especially women) than in their younger counterparts.

Metabolism

Lithium does not undergo hepatic metabolism and is unaffected by alterations in enzyme activity that occur with age or disease.

Excretion

As people age, decrease in renal blood flow and loss of renal tubules and glomeruli reduce renal function, reflected in a 30 to 60% decrease in creatinine clearance. Renal function may also be impaired because of physiological illness, dehydration, or medications that alter renal blood flow or tubular or glomerular function. This age-related decline in renal function results in reduced lithium clearance, which prolongs the average elimination half-life beyond that found in young adults (18 to 20 hours) to as long as 34 hours in elderly patients.

Drug interactions

Lithium and sodium are in functional balance in the plasma; when sodium concentrations decline, lithium levels rise, with the consequent potential for toxicity. Thiazide diuretics thus can result in elevations of plasma lithium levels and produce lithium toxicity. Hyponatremia caused by diet or sweating also may significantly increase plasma lithium levels and produce early signs of lithium toxicity such as confusion. For patients who must be maintained on diuretics, loop diuretics such as furosemide appear to have little effect on lithium clearance. A potassium-sparing agent such as amiloride also does not usually require an adjustment of lithium dose.

Certain drugs that may be taken by older patients increase pituitary antidiuretic hormone (ADH) secretion, resulting in impaired water excretion and subsequent hyponatremia. These drugs include vasopressin, oxytocin, vincristine, cyclophosphamide, fluphenazine, clofibrate, carbamazepine, amitriptyline, thiothixene, aspirin, acetaminophen, narcotics, barbiturates, and haloperidol. If these drugs are prescribed for an older patient taking lithium, toxicity may be more likely because of low sodium concentrations. Lithium levels also can be increased by concomitant administration of nonsteroidal anti-inflammatory drugs, metronidazole, tetracyclines, angiotensin-converting enzyme inhibitors and beta-blockers,[70] and possibly by angiotensin receptor blockers.[71] Clinical state and lithium levels must be monitored closely in patients on these medications, with reduction in lithium dosage if warranted.

Conversely, large intakes of sodium, such as a meal of Asian food or foods prepared with monosodium glutamate or intravenous fluids, may temporarily increase sodium levels sufficiently to decrease plasma lithium levels. Although hourly changes in lithium levels are probably of no clinical consequence, long-term, high-sodium diets may lower lithium levels sufficiently for symptoms of mania to reappear. Similarly, substances that inhibit the effect of ADH, such as caffeine and other xanthines, may lead to lower lithium levels or to higher levels if suddenly discontinued.

Pretreatment Evaluation

Lithium's potential for producing neurologic, cardiovascular, renal, endocrine, and gastrointestinal side effects or for exacerbating preexisting conditions forms the basis for a pretreatment medical workup that evaluates function in these organ systems. This workup should include:

- Complete medical history, including use of other medications
- Complete physical examination
- Neurological examination
- Mental status examination
- Complete blood count
- Serum electrolyte levels
- Blood urea nitrogen/ Plasma creatinine level
- Thyroxine/Thyrotropin-stimulating hormone (TSH) level
- Urinalysis
- ECG

As part of the medical pretreatment evaluation, the clinician must determine whether or not the older patient takes other medications that may interact with lithium and whether the patient is on a special or low-salt diet that will elevate plasma lithium levels. Because fluid intake may be altered with lithium use, ascertaining a patient's pretreatment fluid intake and urinary frequency is also helpful.

Plasma creatinine level is a particularly important measure of renal function prior to initiating treatment with lithium. In younger patients, increased plasma creatinine levels during lithium treatment may reflect declining renal function. In older people, however, plasma creatinine may be an unreliable marker for declining renal function because lower values may

be due to loss of skeletal muscle tissue. A normal plasma creatinine level during lithium treatment in the older patient therefore may be found even with impaired renal function. For this reason, assessment of estimated 24-hour creatinine clearance (using the Cockcroft-Gault formula) should be considered part of the baseline pretreatment evaluation.

Any pretreatment tremor or lack of muscle coordination should be evaluated because these symptoms may be produced or, if already present, exacerbated by lithium. Careful pretreatment examination for evidence of dementia, memory loss, and confusion should also be performed because lithium may alter the mental status of elderly patients.

Dosage and Administration

The starting dose of lithium for acute treatment of an elderly manic patient is 75 to 300 mg per day. Doses of 75 mg can be obtained by using lithium concentrate and doses of 150 mg by breaking a 300-mg tablet in half. In physically healthy elderly patients, lithium dosage may be increased by increments of 75 to 300 mg every 4 to 5 days. Elderly patients who are frail, who have cardiovascular or renal disease, or who are already confused or demented may require smaller dosage increments. Plasma lithium levels should be checked after an increase in daily dosage. Blood for determining plasma lithium levels should be drawn approximately 10 to 12 hours after the last dose of the medication.

When beginning treatment with lithium, dosage must be adjusted frequently, according to the patient's clinical state. Some older patients can show benefits with plasma lithium levels of 0.4 to 0.6 mEq/L or even less. If no improvement occurs at those levels after 10 days and no significant side effects arise, the oral dose may be increased gradually until the mania begins to subside or side effects appear. Elderly patients exhibit more interindividual variability than younger patients, and therapeutic effect may require lithium levels in the range of 0.8 to 1.0 mEq/L.[42]

As mania subsides, the older patient characteristically becomes less agitated and less hyperactive and begins to sleep longer. These early changes in behavior suggest that dosage is sufficient. Plasma lithium levels should then be monitored every few days and the patient's clinical state monitored to assess whether response is adequate. The clinician should be alert to the possibility that lithium dosages that were adequately tolerated may be associated with side effects as the patient becomes euthymic. Lithium dose also may require adjustment when there is a change in renal function, or when an electrolyte imbalance occurs due to sweating, vomiting, diarrhea, infection, disease, or concomitant medications.

Optimal lithium concentrations for maintenance treatment of geriatric patients have not been tested. Although low concentrations in young patients are less effective for prophylaxis than levels above 0.8 mEq/L, tolerability is a special concern in the elderly, and clinicians often attempt to keep levels well below 1.0 mEq/L for maintenance treatment. For many older patients, blood lithium levels as low as 0.2 to 0.6 mEq/L may suffice, although mean levels for elderly patients followed in lithium clinics may be slightly above this range.[72]

The greater potential for lithium toxicity in older patients indicates the need for close monitoring of therapy in this population. Under stable maintenance conditions, plasma lithium levels should be monitored at least every 3 months. Because older patients are sometimes forgetful or may be taking many different medications (each with its own dosage schedule), nonadherence can be a problem. Close contact between physician, patient, and family/caregivers is important to ensure that plasma lithium levels are monitored and to assess recurrence of affective symptoms or development of side effects. In physically healthy older patients, ECGs and tests of thyroid function

and creatinine clearance should be done annually or semiannually if an older patient has cardiovascular, thyroid, or renal impairment.

Side Effects

Clinical experience suggests that side effects may occur in as many as 60% of patients taking lithium regardless of age, but the rate of moderate to severe side effects is higher in older patients (about 40%) than in younger ones. The frequency of acute toxicity, i.e., symptoms requiring intervention, is in the range of 10% to 20%. The side effect profile of lithium is the same for elderly and younger patients: side effects and toxicity are generally dose- and level-dependent. They also are affected by other patient-related and illness-related variables, including extreme old age, multiple medical illnesses, brain disease, and the use of other medications. The most prominent side effects are neurological, cardiovascular, renal, thyroid, and gastrointestinal.

Neurologic Side Effects

Use of lithium is associated with subjective reports of memory loss, cognitive dulling, and apathy. These side effects may be more frequent and severe in elderly patients than in younger adults due to the presence of overt or previously undetected neurodegenerative disorders.[73] At times, the effects of advanced age, length of illness, or underlying degenerative disorders on cognitive function may be difficult to distinguish from lithium side effects. Lithium-induced, mild confused states and forgetfulness may be erroneously attributed to the normal consequences of old age and may also be difficult to detect in manic patients with preexisting cognitive deficits. Mild confusion and forgetfulness may cause older patients either to forget to take lithium on schedule or to take too much and thereby increase the risk of further side effects.

Elderly patients are very susceptible to lithium-induced delirium. Confusion, forgetfulness, disorientation, and impaired consciousness may be the first and most common signs of lithium toxicity in the geriatric patients and may progress to other signs of neurotoxicity such as tremor, lethargy, ataxia, slurred speech, and eventually coma. These toxic effects may be evident at therapeutic dosages even when lithium blood levels are within the usual therapeutic range.

Tremor and ataxia from a variety of causes are common in older persons, and lithium may exacerbate these symptoms. Lithium produces a fine resting tremor that may be indistinguishable from the senile tremor seen with advanced age but is less coarse than the resting tremor of Parkinson's disease. Tremor should be treated by reducing lithium dosage if possible. Severe cases of lithium-induced tremor that interfere with motor coordination may be treated with propranolol. However, because propranolol can produce cardiovascular side effects or depression, dosages should be kept to a minimum, and switching to another antimanic agent may be a better option. Lithium-related ataxia is caused by cerebellar dysfunction and often is accompanied by lack of coordination, dysarthria, and nystagmus; it is particularly troublesome because it can lead to falls and fractures. Concomitant use of benzodiazepines increases the risk of ataxia and falls.

Development of neurotoxicity may be associated with factors that increase blood levels, such as the use of diuretics and anti-inflammatory drugs. However, since neurotoxicity is likely to be related to the concentration of lithium in neurons, factors that affect distribution of lithium between extracellular and intracellular compartments may be more relevant than blood level alone. Among these factors are: (1) genetic susceptibility to greater cellular uptake of lithium, implying unpredictable interindividual differences; (2) cerebral pathology that may increase the vulnerability of brain cells to lithium uptake or reduce their capacity for lithium removal; (3) concomitant neuroleptic treatment,

which may predispose to increased cellular uptake of lithium; (4) hyponatremia, which leads to increased cellular uptake of lithium; and (5) rapid dose increases, which may result in higher peak-blood levels, leading to rapid rises in brain concentration.

Presence of these factors may explain why some elderly patients have the following sequelae: prolonged periods of lithium-induced neurotoxicity, lasting up to 10 weeks after discontinuation of treatment; increased risk for extrapyramidal symptoms from lithium, including tremor, oculogyric crisis, akathisia, dystonia, and tardive dyskinesia; and myoclonus and periodic EEG changes resembling Creutzfeldt-Jakob disease. Lithium may also contribute to greater vulnerability of affectively disordered patients to the development of tardive dyskinesia.

If evidence of neurotoxicity appears during lithium treatment of an older patient, dosage should be reduced or the drug discontinued completely. A search for and correction or modification of any of the factors just described should be made before any attempt to reinstitute lithium treatment.

Cardiovascular Side Effects

Lithium commonly causes T-wave flattening or inversion on the ECG—changes that are not clinically significant and disappear within two weeks of drug discontinuation. However, because lithium can alter electrolyte balance, serum potassium levels should be checked if ECG changes occur. Lithium may also cause sinus node dysfunction (sick sinus syndrome), sinoatrial block, or junctional bradycardia—all of which can reduce blood flow to the brain and cause somnolence or syncope. Although such episodes may be intermittent and are most common in patients with underlying cardiac disease, and a 24-hour cardiac monitor may be required to document them.

Lithium also aggravates preexisting arrhythmias and conduction defects. Patients with preexisting ventricular irritability or arteriosclerotic heart disease may be at increased risk of ventricular tachyarrhythmias while taking lithium. Patients who develop hypercalcemia with lithium treatment may be at greatest risk.[74] Careful monitoring of cardiovascular function and of concomitant medications that can cause bradycardia is essential, as is regular questioning of the patient regarding palpitations, irregular pulse, or diminished consciousness.

Renal Side Effects

Lithium commonly impairs urine concentration by the kidneys—a side effect that may be present in one-third of elderly patients. In a small but undetermined proportion of these instances, severe nephrogenic diabetes insipidus may result in the output of up to 6 L per 24 hours of very dilute urine and the intake of many liters of fluid. Since renal concentration function may already be reduced in older patients, diabetes insipidus may present an additional hazard. If not reversed, the syndrome can lead to altered electrolyte balance accompanied by lethargy, confusion, or even coma. Nephrogenic diabetes insipidus is usually completely reversible when lithium is discontinued. The condition may also respond to addition of a thiazide diuretic.

In older patients, lithium-induced polyuria may be confused with urinary frequency resulting from urinary tract infection. To distinguish between these, a clean-catch urine specimen is necessary. A very dilute specimen suggests nephrogenic diabetes insipidus secondary to lithium use.

Lithium typically does not cause changes in glomerular filtration rate or creatinine clearance greater than those caused by age alone. Renal tubular function has remained stable in elderly patients treated continuously with lithium for an average of 20 years. In some patients, however, long-term lithium use is associated with pathological kidney conditions, including tubular atrophy, glomerular sclerosis, and interstitial fibrosis.

Whether or not these structural changes further impair renal functioning in the older patient is not known. The suggestion that these changes may be related to multiple daily doses more than to single daily-dose regimens has been presented. Most histopathological renal changes associated with lithium use occur in patients with histories of lithium intoxication, suggesting that avoiding high peak levels may reduce risk of kidney damage. Factors that increase cellular uptake of lithium may also contribute to lithium intoxication. In a very small number of patients, nephrotic syndrome accompanied by acute tubular necrosis and renal insufficiency has been observed.[75]

If a decline in renal function or significant polyuria occurs during treatment, 24-hour urinary creatinine clearance estimates calculated using the Cockcroft-Gault formula may be compared with baseline measures. Assessment of urine osmolality and urine-specific gravity may also be helpful in determining whether renal function has been impaired. Because lithium is itself excreted by the kidney, any unexplained rise in lithium level should prompt an evaluation of renal function in an elderly patient. One dose daily may be preferable to multiple doses in elderly patients with renal side effects, but further reductions in frequency should not be tried: clinical relapse increases threefold in patients taking lithium only every other day.[76]

Thyroid Side Effects

Approximately 8% of elderly patients receiving lithium for prolonged periods will develop hypothyroidism or, more likely, a benign, diffuse nontoxic goiter due to the inhibition by lithium of the release of triiodothyronine (T3) and thyroxin (T4).[41] Because T3 concentration diminishes with age, the risk of lithium-induced pathological changes in the thyroid of elderly patients increases.

Elevated plasma TSH levels have been reported in 32% of elderly patients on lithium.[72] An increased TSH level indicates that lithium dosage must be either reduced or discontinued or that thyroid replacement must be added. For older patients without evidence of hypothyroidism, the TSH level should be checked annually. Clinical evidence of decreased thyroid function or appearance of goiter in an elderly patient should prompt lithium discontinuation and reassessment of thyroid function. Alternatives to lithium should be considered; if lithium treatment is resumed, thyroid function should be checked every 3 to 6 months.

Lithium-induced hypothyroidism, more common in women than in men, is characterized by fatigue, weight gain, hair loss, coarse skin, hoarse voice, pretibial edema, and sensitivity to cold. In older patients, hypothyroidism may cause dementia or depression. Hypothyroidism may predispose to the development of other symptoms of lithium toxicity and may interfere with treatment response. Although lithium-induced hypothyroidism usually develops insidiously, rare cases that present with myxedema coma can occur in patients with preexisting hypothyroidism. If an elderly patient taking lithium becomes listless and apathetic, thyroid function should immediately be checked. Lithium-induced goiter is usually detected only when difficulties in swallowing develop (usually 1 to 2 years after lithium treatment begins). Unlike hypothyroidism, this condition occurs slightly more frequently in men than in women.

Less commonly, lithium use may be associated with hyperthyroidism, probably by predisposing to autoimmune thyroid disease. As with hypothyroidism, thyrotoxicosis is associated with longer-duration lithium treatment. The usual intervention is to reduce lithium dosage and to add antithyroid medication, with radioactive iodine administration reserved for patients who do not respond.

Gastrointestinal Side Effects

Gastric irritability, nausea, vomiting, diarrhea, and abdominal pain tend to develop early in the course of lithium treatment. Although these side effects are not more common in older people, they may be more troublesome for the older patient, especially those experiencing gastric irritability from other causes. Furthermore, severe vomiting or diarrhea may lead to electrolyte imbalance in a dehydrated, malnourished, or frail older patient.

In general, gastrointestinal symptoms can be reduced by lowering the dosage of lithium and prolonging the interval between dosage increases. Patients with gastrointestinal side effects may also be helped by extended-action lithium preparations or liquid lithium citrate.

Other Side Effects

Hypercalcemia and elevated levels of parathyroid hormone occur in 10 to 40% of patients on maintenance lithium, possibly due to parathyroid adenomas.[77] Elderly patients with obstructive lung disease may develop respiratory depression when taking lithium. On rare occasions, lithium produces psoriasis, although more commonly the drug is associated with exacerbation of a preexisting psoriatic condition.

Treatment with Anticonvulsants

Anticonvulsants are now used as mood-stabilizing medications for acute and maintenance treatment of young and middle-aged bipolar patients. Their use in older patients is also increasingly common but less well reported in research data; the best-studied drug is valproic acid.

Valproic acid

Valproic acid is an anticonvulsant medication that has been found effective for acute treatment and prophylaxis of bipolar disorder in nonelderly adults.[69,78–81] Unfortunately, the double-blind, placebo-controlled clinical trials that established the efficacy of valproate for treatment of bipolar disorder have been restricted to patients under age 65. A number of case reports, however, document the usefulness and safety of valproic acid, usually in the form of divalproex sodium, an equimolar compound of valproic acid and sodium valproate available in an enteric-coated form, for elderly patients with mania.[47–52,82–84] Most of these case reports describe the use of valproic acid in combination with lithium. Open-label studies in patients with behavioral disturbances or manic-like agitation associated with dementia generally suggest efficacy and confirm the safety of valproic acid in these elderly populations.[85–87]

Predictors of differential benefit from valproic acid compared to lithium have not been established among elderly patients. One retrospective report found that optimizing doses of lithium and valproate resulted in similar efficacy, although lithium seemed more efficacious in patients with classic manic presentations.[42] Valproic acid may be preferred for elderly patients who present with mixed states, histories of rapid cycling, many previous manic episodes, posttraumatic mania (these patients often respond poorly to lithium),[84] or evidence for other neurologic abnormalities, including abnormal EEGs.

Valproic acid should be considered first-line acute and prophylactic treatment for patients who cannot tolerate lithium or who are at risk of significant toxicity due to comorbid medical conditions or use of other medications. For example, valproic acid is preferred to lithium for the older patient with impaired renal function. It also may be an alternative to lithium treatment for elderly patients with cardiovascular disease requiring diuretic treatment. Lithium-treated patients who develop hypercalcemia are more likely to develop cardiac conduction abnormalities than normocalcemic patients. These conduction abnormalities are further reduced in patients taking anticonvulsants, suggesting that anticonvulsants may have antiarrhythmic effects and may therefore be safer in patients with cardiac pathology.[74] Clinical experience suggests that some patients who experience distressing cognitive effects from lithium may function better on valproic acid when its use has permitted discontinuation or reduced dose of lithium.

Older patients do not differ in clinically significant degree from their younger counterparts in valproic acid volume of distribution, clearance, or half-life for total drug. However, a decline in plasma-protein binding can occur with aging, resulting in an increase in the free fraction.[88] Because of decreased oxidative metabolism of free drug, unbound concentrations of valproic acid in older persons increase relative to dose, and this unbound concentration may reflect the drug concentration in the cerebrospinal fluid. Thus, total concentrations as measured in blood may be misleading and may need to be lower in older than in younger patients. For these reasons, the useful starting dose in older patients should be moderately lower than for younger patients, or about 125 mg once a day. Mean doses reported with successful treatment are in the range of 800 to 1000 mg/day, with total blood levels in the range of 50 to 100 mcg/ml.

In general, valproic acid is well tolerated in older patients.[89] The most commonly reported side effects are neurological symptoms (including tremor, sedation, and ataxia), asymptomatic serum hepatic transaminase elevations, alopecia, and increased appetite and weight gain. The initial sedative effect, which generally lasts only about a week, may be helpful for agitated and insomniac manic patients. Gastrointestinal complaints, e.g., anorexia, nausea, vomiting, dyspepsia, and diarrhea, are uncommon with the enteric-coated form. Serious hepatotoxicity, which can lead to liver failure and death, is rare, idiosyncratic, unrelated to dosage, and more common in children who take multiple anticonvulsants. Baseline liver function tests are essential, however, and the drug should not be given to anyone with liver dysfunction. Other infrequent but serious complications that have been reported include pancytopenia, sensorineural hearing loss, and truncal muscle weakness with ventilatory failure. Valproic acid also may cause inappropriate antidiuretic hormone secretion, and the resultant hyponatremia may lead to toxicity. Thus, pretreatment evaluation also should include a complete blood count and urinalysis. Because of its high degree of protein binding, valproic acid has the potential to interact adversely with other protein-bound drugs. It can, for example, increase the effect of warfarin; anticoagulated patients require close monitoring of prothrombin ratios.

Lamotrigine

Lamotrigine has been found effective and well tolerated for the acute treatment of bipolar depression,[90] but little evidence supports its efficacy as a monotherapy for the acute treatment of mania. In young patients, maintenance lamotrigine treatment delays time to recurrence of any mood episode in patients stabilized after an acute manic episode,[63] and it may be more effective than lithium in preventing depressive relapses.[65] These findings suggest that lamotrigine and lithium may be more effective as maintenance therapy when used in combination. The most common side effects associated with lamotrigine in bipolar maintenance studies were, in order of decreasing frequency from 14% to 7%, nausea, insomnia, somnolence, fatigue, and rash.

Controlled data on use of lamotrigine in elderly psychiatric patients are not available. Lamotrigine has an elimination half-life of over 30 hours, but since its metabolism is primarily by hepatic glucuronidation, drug levels are not greatly affected by aging. Elderly epileptic patients appear to tolerate lamotrigine better than carbamazepine, largely due to lower frequencies of somnolence and rash, which are the most significant side effects leading to treatment discontinuation with both anticonvulsants.[66,91] Nevertheless, serious rash occurs in 0.3% of adults, and factors predicting increased risk have not been

identified. Based on these considerations and the limited data for elderly patients with epilepsy, starting doses should probably be 25 mg per day, with gradual increases in 25 mg increments every 2 weeks to a maximum of 300 to 500 mg per day.

Combination therapy of lamotrigine with other anticonvulsants requires careful monitoring and dose adjustment. Concomitant treatment with carbamazepine or phenytoin increases the apparent clearance of lamotrigine and reduces the half-life by 50%; however, co-administration with valproic acid decreases clearance and doubles the half-life. Conversely, lamotrigine enhances the metabolism of valproic acid and reduces its levels. For these reasons, doses of lamotrigine should probably be more than halved when given together with valproic acid. The effects of aging on these drug interactions are not well studied.

Carbamazepine

Like valproic acid, the anticonvulsant drug carbamazepine may be particularly useful in the treatment and prevention of mania in young and middle-aged patients with rapidly recurring cycles of affective illness.[92] When taken alone, carbamazepine does not seem to be as effective as lithium for the acute treatment of mania. In combination with lithium, however, it is sometimes effective for patients whose manic symptoms are resistant to either lithium treatment alone or lithium combined with antipsychotics. In maintenance treatment, both drugs appear to have comparable efficacy,[93] although with longer-term use patients who tolerate lithium and avoid early relapse appear to do better on most outcome measures than patients maintained on carbamazepine.[64,94]

For elderly manic patients, fewer reports of carbamazepine use are available than of valproic acid use. Greater potential for hepatic and hematologic toxicity exists with carbamazepine. Structurally related to tricyclic antidepressants, it shares many of their toxicities, such as anticholinergic and cardiovascular side effects. In older women particularly it can cause bradyarrhythmia. Carbamazepine may potentiate the bradyarrhythmic effects of lithium by causing/exacerbating further sinus node dysfunction and slowed atrioventricular node and His bundle conduction. Other side effects include confusion, ataxia, and impaired water excretion leading to hyponatremia.

As with lithium-induced neurotoxicity, confusion, sedation, disorientation, ataxia, and memory loss secondary to carbamazepine administration may be more common in elderly patients than in younger adults. The most serious toxic effect of carbamazepine is depression of bone marrow function, which can result in leukopenia and potentially fatal infections, although this appears to be less common in older patients than in younger ones. Hypersensitivity reactions such as aseptic meningitis have been reported.

As with initiation of lithium and valproic acid therapy, a complete history and physical examination are essential prior to beginning carbamazepine. Pretreatment laboratory tests should include a complete blood count, platelet count, assessment of serum iron level, liver function tests, and urinalysis.

Initial doses of carbamazepine can be 100 mg (one half the available 200-mg tablet), taken with a meal. Dosage may be increased by 100 mg per day, in divided doses taken with meals, to a maximum dosage of 300 to 800 mg per day. The recommended therapeutic plasma levels are between 4 and 8 µg/mL, although some patients may require plasma levels between 8 and 12 µg/mL. Blood samples, which should be obtained weekly for the first 6 weeks and monthly thereafter, should be tested for hemoglobin level, platelet count, liver enzyme levels, and blood urea nitrogen level. Should hematologic or hepatic side effects appear, carbamazepine dosage must be reduced or discontinued.

Other Anticonvulsants

Oxcarbazepine is structurally similar to carbamazepine. Several comparisons with lithium or neuroleptics have found evidence for efficacy in the treatment of acute mania, although placebo-controlled trials and studies of prophylactic treatment have not been conducted. Comparisons in epileptic patients suggest a lower incidence of adverse effects than seen with carbamazepine. Lack of metabolism by and induction of CYP450 enzymes suggests that oxcarbazepine may be associated with fewer clinically significant drug interactions than carbamazepine and may therefore be safer in elderly patients on multiple medications.[67] However, excretion is correlated with total renal clearance, suggesting the need for increased caution in patients with severe renal impairment and use of lower doses in the elderly.[95]

Oxcarbazepine has not been studied in elderly psychiatric patients. Based on usual dosing for epilepsy, and taking into account age-related reductions in creatinine clearance, starting doses of oxcarbazepine for elderly manic patients should not exceed 150 mg twice daily, with daily increases of 300 mg weekly to a maximum of 900 to 1200 mg per day.

Topiramate has the advantage of not causing weight gain and has had apparent efficacy in open studies, but the only placebo-controlled study of mania was negative.[96] A case study of a 59-year-old woman with recurrent acute mania revealed that after discontinuation of lithium due to weight gain, she responded to topiramate after 3 weeks, when the dose had been increased to 600 mg per day.[97] Unlike valproate but like lamotrigine, plasma levels of topiramate increase gradually and use of loading doses is not appropriate. Treatment of acute mania may require an initial combination of topiramate with other antimanic drugs such as antipsychotics.

Treatment of Mania with Antipsychotics

Data on use of atypical antipsychotics for elderly manic patients remain limited to case reports and open-label series. Olanzapine has been approved as a first-line agent for this use by the Food and Drug Administration based on the results of controlled trials.[98,99] Clozapine and quetiapine have benefited elderly patients with bipolar disorder in uncontrolled studies.[100,101] Atypical antipsychotic agents have supplanted classical agents due to better tolerability.

Evidence is conflicting regarding the relative efficacy of olanzapine and valproic acid in the acute treatment of mania in adult patients.[80,102] Although both drugs are well tolerated, olanzapine-treated patients generally have more frequent adverse events, especially weight gain, dry mouth, increased appetite, and somnolence. For patients 50 years old and older with acute mania, controlled, 3-week trials of olanzapine, compared with placebo or divalproex in acute mania, found comparable reductions in symptoms with olanzapine and divalproex compared with placebo. These changes were similar to those found in younger patients and no numerically different patterns of treatment-emergent adverse events were found in the two active drug treatment groups.[56]

Clinical practice varies with regard to the use of antipsychotics. Atypical antipsychotic medications are generally preferred to conventional agents because of their more benign side-effect profile. Risks of extrapyramidal side effects, especially parkinsonism, with the use of antipsychotics such as haloperidol or thioridazine warrant avoiding these drugs for elderly patients.

In young patients, these atypical antipsychotics are often prescribed early in treatment to reduce marked agitation or hyperactivity quickly while dosages of lithium or an anticonvulsant are being titrated to therapeutic levels. Antipsychotics may then be withdrawn once the florid manifestations of illness are resolved, usually within 10 to 21 days, unless psychotic symptoms persist.

Unless severe psychopathology requires early use, some clinicians defer use of antipsychotics for elderly patients when possible, preferring to assess benefits and side effects of a single agent when feasible, but adding antipsychotic augmentation later in treatment for patients with persisting symptoms. Atypical agents are probably safer and more effective than benzodiazepines for geriatric patients, but no direct comparison data are available. Antipsychotics are also recommended for patients who experience recurrent symptoms while on maintenance therapy with lithium or anticonvulsants. Little evidence is available to support use of antipsychotics for long-term maintenance therapy, although such use may be necessary for patients with persistent psychotic symptoms or those who do not respond to or tolerate other agents.

Some elderly patients may have adverse cognitive effects when treated with antipsychotic medication, but most of the studies on which this conclusion is based were conducted with populations whose subjects had underlying cognitive disorders such as Alzheimer's disease and Parkinson's disease. Available studies suggest that atypical antipsychotic agents may induce fewer cognitive adverse effects than the typical agents, but the combination of different effects on dopaminergic, cholinergic, and histaminergic systems suggests that individual agents will have unpredictable effects in any given elderly individual, especially if the patient has an underlying neurologic disorder. Monitoring for adverse cognitive effects may be appropriate, but reports of cognitive dysfunction associated with mania in the elderly, including presentations of mania with delirium, may detract from the ability of such monitoring to isolate drug effects from disease effects and positive treatment effects.[54]

Data from a large population registry study found olanzapine use associated with a 3-fold increase in the odds of developing hyperlipidemia compared with use of conventional antipsychotics.[103] Although data for the elderly are not available, this population may be at greater risk of increased lipid levels because of additive effects with other cardiovascular risk factors.

Doses of antipsychotic medication for the elderly manic patient must be titrated according to the severity of the patient's clinical condition and emergence of adverse effects. Acute bipolar mania in elderly patients can be successfully treated with a mean modal olanzapine dose of 16 mg per day, suggesting that dosage with this drug may be no different than that for younger patients, although a starting dose of 5 mg is appropriate.[104] Risperidone dosage for elderly patients with a variety of psychotic disorders ranges from 1.6 to 3.8 mg per day, which may be only slightly lower than doses for younger patients.[105] Doses of more sedating atypical antipsychotics are generally lower for geriatric patients, similar to recommendations for the typical agents. Patients with refractory geriatric mania require clozapine doses ranging from 25 to 112.5 mg per day,[106] and appropriate quetiapine doses are probably in the range of 100 mg per day.[101]

Treatment with other Agents

Some clinical experience suggests that clonazepam, a benzodiazepine that until recently was used primarily as an anticonvulsant, may be of value as an adjunctive treatment in acute manic patients by providing nonspecific sedation. The few published case reports in younger patients do not clarify whether it has a specific antimanic action or any prophylactic effects. Because benzodiazepine toxicity is problematic in older patients (see Chapter 16), the risk/benefit ratio for clonazepam for treating mania in the elderly is not favorable.

Calcium channel blockers also have been tried as potential treatment for mania, and several case reports suggest that verapamil can be effective in younger patients. However, controlled trials have found them no better than placebo and

inferior to lithium. No case reports or studies of its effect in older patients are available. Verapamil can increase carbamazepine-induced neurotoxicity and can enhance lithium excretion. Severe bradyarrhythmia and possible neurotoxicity have been associated with the combination of verapamil and lithium.

Small studies describe antimanic benefit from tamoxifen citrate,[107] which acts on second-messenger pathways by inhibiting protein kinase C, and omega-3 fatty acids,[108] which act through neuronal signal transduction pathways; thus far, however, data on elderly patients are lacking. Targeting acetylcholinergic neurotransmission with choline augmentation or cholinesterase inhibition has also been reported beneficial in young adult patients in preliminary reports: Of 11 patients aged 20 to 54 with treatment-resistant bipolar disorder (partial or no response to both lithium and divalproex or other treatments) treated with donepezil 5 mg, 6 improved markedly within 6 weeks, five within 2 weeks, and three other patients improved slightly.[109] These findings support the growing impression that cholinesterase inhibitors may benefit psychiatric symptomatology in a variety of neuropsychiatric disorders.[110]

Electroconvulsive Therapy

Used most often for severe major depression, ECT (see Chapter 13) is a safe and often effective treatment for acute mania as well.[111,112] Treatment of elderly manic patients with ECT should be restricted to those who do not respond to, or are intolerant of, lithium, anticonvulsants, antipsychotics, or those whose manic symptoms are so severe that immediate resolution of the episode is urgent to prevent physical harm due to accidentally injurious behavior or failure to take fluids.

Electrode placement and antimanic efficacy of ECT has not been studied in geriatric patients. In depressed elderly individuals, unilateral nondominant ECT causes fewer cognitive side effects, which is important for older people. In younger manic patients, some evidence suggests an advantage for bilateral treatment, but the data are limited and conflicting, and high-dose unilateral treatment, which may have more efficacy than conventional unilateral ECT, was not studied.

The number of ECT treatments required for resolution of a manic episode varies from patient to patient. In general, the older patient's manic episodes should begin to resolve after 4 to 6 ECT treatments. During ECT, use of psychotropic medications requires scrutiny to minimize interaction with ECT medications and seizure induction. Once the acute manic episode subsides following ECT, maintenance treatment with lithium or anticonvulsants should be initiated. Occasionally, maintenance ECT may be required to keep the patient euthymic.

CLINICAL VIGNETTES

Case 12.1

Mr. A., a 78-year-old widowed male, presented with a feeling of elation and increased energy and subjective rapid thinking, reporting decreased need for sleep. He was unusually talkative with a grandiose mood on interview. This picture developed after he had been treated for one week with bupropion up to 75 mg/day for a major depressive episode.

His first episode of depression had been at age 48. He had no history of hypomania and no family history of mood disorder. Mr. A. had been treated on an ambulatory basis for 14 months for depressive symptoms that included low mood, anhedonia, loss of appetite, loss of energy, hypersomnia, and subjective cognitive inefficiency. During the latest episode he had been unable to tolerate SSRI treatment, complaining of nausea. He was the treated with nortiptyline alone and with lithium augmentation, but his depressive symptoms persisted. His past medical history included coronary artery disease.

Mr. A. cooperated with ambulatory care and discontinued bupropion as directed. Although he disliked some aspects of his manic state, he enjoyed the sense of increased cognitive efficiency and was reluctant to take lithium. He also received lorazepam 0.5 mg h.s. prn for insomnia, with minimal benefit, and hypomania persisted for several months. He eventually agreed to a trial of divalproex, and responded over several weeks at a plasma concentration of 70 µg/mL, achieving remission.

This case illustrates occurrence of manic episode in late life after longstanding recurrent unipolar major depression. For this patient, treatment with an antidepressant was temporally linked to the onset of mania. The relation between antidepressant treatment and manic states in late life bipolar disorders is not established and remains controversial in younger patients, as ``spontaneous'' shifts in polarity are known to occur in the absence of such treatment. Clinicians, however, should be alert to such state changes in elders. In such circumstances, antidepressant medication should be discontinued and initiation of mood stabilizer treatment should not be avoided.

Case 12.2

Mrs. B., a 68-year-old married woman, was admitted to the psychiatric inpatient service for a manic syndrome of 6 weeks duration. She had been elated, at times irritable, and expressed grandiose, religious, and paranoid delusional ideation. She was overactive and had lost 10 pounds. Prior to admission she was prescribed increased doses of antipsychotic; however, she was poorly adherent to treatment and her husband was unable to look after her safely at home. Her medical history was unremarkable except for osteoarthritis. On mental status examination, she demonstrated euphoric mood, irritability, restlessness, disheveled appearance, and a low attention span. Physical, neurologic, and laboratory examination were not contributory.

The patient had a 40-year psychiatric history with a schizaffective bipolar pattern and poor toleration of classical antipsychotic medication trials in recent years. Atypical antipsychotic medications, including risperidone and olanzapine, for manic presentations had been only partially helpful. Lithium, divalproex, and carbamazepine also were not beneficial at tolerated doses, and she had complained of tremor with lithium and sedation with the other agents. Improvement had occurred with ECT in an episode 5 years before.

The patient initially received olanzapine at 10–15 mg per day and lamotrigine was added and gradually titrated up to 75 mg per day, but Mrs. B. continued to be manic and psychotic and was hyperactive and eating irregularly, remaining at risk to herself and others due to these features and impulsiveness.

Medical reevaluation was unremarkable. The anticipated risk-benefit ratio for a trial of ECT was favorable, which Mrs. B.'s husband supported, but the patient refused. A court order for acute ECT was obtained. Lamotrigine was tapered off and the patient received 8 bilateral treatments over a period of 3 weeks. Mrs. B. responded rapidly with resolution of affective symptoms, increased insight, and markedly reduced delusional ideation. She tolerated the treatment adequately, with moderate confusion after the third treatment that resolved after completion of the ECT series. Olanzapine was continued, and she later agreed to continuation/maintenance ECT treatment on an ambulatory basis with psychiatric follow-up, to which she was adherent with her husband's support.

This case illustrates the potential role of ECT in management of manic episodes for geriatric patients. Mrs. B. was refractory to and/or did not tolerate many pharmacotherapeutic trials. This treatment preceded the emergence of high-dose unilateral ECT as a treatment option. The critical role of families and caregivers in supporting the management of an elderly patient with bipolar disorder is also illustrated.

Case 12.3

At the age of 44, Mr. C. experienced the first of many agitated depressions following treatment of hypertension with propranolol. During the next 16 years, he experienced four severe depressions of psychotic proportion, each of which was successfully treated with ECT. Although the patient had occasional brief periods of euphoria during these 16 years, he was never clinically manic. A brief trial of lithium during this period produced a severe tremor and was discontinued.

Between the ages of 60 and 65, Mr. C. developed angina, had one small inferior myocardial infarction followed by a large anterior wall infarction, and developed worsening congestive heart failure that was successfully treated with digoxin and furosemide, up to 160 mg/day. At age 65, Mr. C. suddenly found himself unsteady on his feet when he got out of bed one morning. After a few hours, he seemed to be his usual self, but over the next few months he occasionally thought he detected some dizziness or sometimes clumsiness with his hands when he was shaving. Over the next 2 years, additional similar episodes occurred.

At the age of 65, Mr. C. sold his business and planned an extensive trip abroad with his wife. However, before they were scheduled to leave, he became preoccupied with financial concerns and feelings of extreme guilt about past minor business errors. Over a period of 2 weeks, he became withdrawn, fearful, and agitated. When he began to express suicidal thoughts, he was hospitalized. On admission, his speech was rambling and tangential. He was hyperactive, sleeping very little, and was observed to have impaired memory. He was convinced that because of a plot against him, his conversations with hospital staff were being recorded by cameras and microphones behind hospital heating vents.

Mr. C.'s paranoid thinking resulted in irritable and agitated behavior, and a daily regimen of 8 mg of perphenazine was begun. When this treatment produced confusion and disorientation, an MRI scan was performed, revealing multiple 2-to 5-mm punctate lesions with evidence of cavitation in the pons, basal ganglia, and thalamus. Perphenazine was subsequently discontinued, and haloperidol was started at 0.5 mg twice daily. However, even at this dose, Mr. A. developed marked stiffness, bradykinesia, and a shuffling gait. Because of these toxic reactions to two different neuroleptics, lithium carbonate was begun.

After 2 days on 150 mg twice daily, Mr. C. had severe tremor and a marked increase in slurred speech, ataxia, disorientation, and confusion. With discontinuation of lithium, these symptoms partially resolved over the next 3 days, but forgetfulness persisted. In addition, Mr. C. became more tearful, affectively labile, irritable, and verbally abusive. Sodium divalproex was begun at 250 mg/day and gradually titrated up to 750 mg/day. Over a period of 3 weeks, he improved dramatically: His mood became euthymic, irritability resolved, and cognitive function returned to his baseline. Initially, liver function tests increased to twice the upper limit of normal, but they returned to baseline after 2 months and remained just below the upper limit of normal at subsequent determinations.

Mr. C.'s clinical course illustrates several important aspects of late-life mania and its treatment. Mania often appears with a long latency following more than three episodes of depression; patients with neurological disorders may be at greatest risk. Mania also may first appear in a mixed state with depressive symptoms, often after a stressful life circumstance. Paranoia and irritability may be the most prominent presenting symptoms of mania in later life, and valproic acid is useful in controlling both the agitation and the paranoia associated with mania. This case also demonstrates the greater potential for neurotoxicity from lithium in the presence of pathological changes in brain structure. When lithium is prescribed for such a patient, the confusion and disorientation that may result from lithium toxicity can be mistaken for signs of progressive dementia. These side effects may persist long after the lithium has been cleared from the body.

Case 12.4

Mr. D. first developed manic symptoms while serving in the infantry in North Africa during World War II. He recovered after a brief stay in an Army hospital and was able to return to active duty. After the war, he became a successful businessman in the United States, although every few years he became expansive, irritable, paranoid, and prone to making reckless business decisions, which led to frequent altercations with his partners. During some episodes, he would stay up all night cooking and taking baths. On one occasion, he abruptly left his wife and impulsively traveled to Europe alone. In an effort to control the anxiety and sleeplessness he experienced during these hypomanic episodes, Mr. D. began to abuse alcohol, although he was able to keep his alcohol use under reasonable control when he was euthymic.

In 1970, when Mr. D. developed a full manic syndrome that led him to pick a fight with a much younger man in a bar, lithium became available for use in the United States. With the initiation of lithium, his mania rapidly abated, and he noted a serenity of mood different from any he had ever felt. His business associates described him as ``mellow,'' a term never used in referring to Mr. D. in the past. On 900 mg/day, Mr. D. was free of manic symptoms for the next 10 years, although he had brief, mild depressions that did not require treatment. After remaining stable for this long period of time, Mr. D. decided on his own to stop taking lithium and lost contact with his psychiatrist, a decision that was influenced by his retirement. He felt that without the stresses of running his business, he would be less vulnerable to a recurrence of his illness. However, with more time on his hands and no other interests to fall back on, Mr. D.'s alcohol use increased and became more regular.

Over the next few years, Mr. D. developed hypertension and diabetes, both of which remained undetected because of his unwillingness to see his physician on a regular basis. At age 70, he became increasingly lethargic and noted an increase in thirst and urine volume. Eventually he developed a urinary tract infection, and in this context became acutely uremic, with confusion, signs of fluid overload, and nausea and vomiting. With hospitalization and treatment of his infection, he returned to a stable baseline but was noted to have a creatinine of 4.0. Conservative treatment with protein restriction controlled his chronic renal failure, but Mr. D. became depressed while in the hospital and was started on 20 mg/day of fluoxetine. Within a few weeks, he had returned home and was feeling well, but he soon shifted into a manic phase. Fluoxetine was discontinued, but Mr. D.'s manic symptoms continued to escalate. After discussion between his internist and psychiatrist, resumption of lithium treatment, which had been so effective in the past, was begun. Because of Mr. D.'s impaired renal function, he was started on lithium citrate, in liquid form, at a starting dose of 75 mg/day. On this dose, his lithium level was 0.4, and his irritability and paranoia diminished. His doctors also urged him to stop drinking, but he was only able to reduce his intake.

Even with his low lithium level, Mr. D.'s symptoms remained well controlled, and his only significant side effect was tremor. His physician prescribed propranolol, 40 mg twice daily, which reduced the tremor to a manageable degree and also lowered his blood pressure. Over the next 5 years, he had no recurrences of mania, but one episode of major depression occurred despite lithium prophylaxis. Because of Mr. D.'s previous shift into a manic state when treated with an antidepressant, this depressive episode was treated with ECT, and it resolved after four unilateral treatments. Lithium was continued during this treatment and afterward as maintenance.

Elderly manic patients who have had early onset of affective illness often pursue a unipolar manic course. As with Mr. D., mild depression develops only after beginning lithium much later in life, and with a first major depression only after a significant medical illness. Mr. D.'s illness was well controlled with lithium, even after the development of chronic renal failure. The use of very low-dose lithium for such a patient is not contraindicated as long as renal and cardiovascular functions are carefully and frequently monitored and levels are watched closely. Low therapeutic levels also are appropriate for the elderly patient, who is prone to develop side effects at levels of 0.8 to 1.0, commonly used for younger patients.

This case also illustrates the frequent comorbidity of bipolar disorder and alcohol abuse. Although alcohol abuse is often overlooked in the elderly, it may contribute to disturbances of sleep and to exacerbations of renal, hepatic, pulmonary, and cardiac disease, as well as to depression.

Case 12.5

Dr. E. had no past history or family history of affective illness. Trained as an internist, he worked for many years as a clinical instructor at his local medical school and maintained a large general practice. He only began to reduce his clinical hours at age 72. At age 75, while winding down his practice further, he was taking a long walk with his wife when both were hit by a car. Mrs. E. had extensive fractures and internal injuries. Dr. E. was thrown about 10 feet, and the back of his head struck the curb; he lost consciousness for 1 hour.

Four months later, Dr. E. again began spending more time at the office, developed a number of ideas for papers on the history of medicine and the changes in clinical practice during his lifetime, and started staying up until 3 AM, shifting from one writing project to another. Eventually, he developed a full-blown manic syndrome with grandiose delusions, euphoria, hyperactivity, religiosity, and auditory hallucinations. In the hospital, his symptoms resolved with 2 mg per day of risperidone. A neurologic examination, skull x-rays, and brain MRI were all normal. A sleep/awake EEG revealed only some left temporal slowing.

Over the next 6 months, Dr. E. had two additional brief manic episodes, one of them requiring hospitalization. Each time, he improved with risperidone dosage, increased to 3 mg/day, but at this dosage he developed a shuffling gait and cogwheel rigidity of both arms. During the following 6 months, he had another manic episode and a first depressive episode, with marked psychomotor retardation, prominent diurnal variation of mood, and suicidal thoughts. The depression was only partially responsive to sertraline, bupropion, and nortriptyline, and with each of these treatments Dr. E. became more irritable and paranoid. At this point, divalproex sodium was added, with dosage gradually increased to 750 mg per day, producing a level of 65 mg/L. Within 2 weeks, Dr. E. reported complete resolution of his depressive symptoms. In addition, he was no longer irritable and felt like his old self for the first time since his head injury. He remained asymptomatic on a combination of divalproex sodium and sertraline for the next year.

Mania following head injury is not uncommon, even in the absence of neurologic or radiologic evidence of brain changes. A typical bipolar presentation may follow. Elderly patients with mania secondary to head injury are more prone to neurotoxicity on lithium, and a rapidly cycling course often predicts a poor therapeutic response to this medication. For such patients, an antiepileptic medication such as divalproex sodium may be an appropriate first-line mood stabilizer.

Case 12.6

Mrs. F., a 74-year-old art critic for her local newspaper, had a long history of recurrent depressive episodes and had been treated with a variety of antidepressants and psychotherapy during the course of her life. At times, when she was not depressed, her family noted that she was increasingly active, intrusive into their affairs, belligerent, and somewhat overcontrolling. These behaviors were accompanied by increased spending sprees, social activity, and nearly nonstop talking into the early hours of the morning. It was noted that ``Mother could be exhausting.'' Each of these hypomanic episodes, however, would last no longer than a month and seemed not to interfere with the patient's life or the lives of those around her other than as an annoyance. She was never treated with lithium.

When she was 74 years of age, Mrs. F.'s husband of more than 50 years died, and she went to live with her daughter and son-in-law. After a brief period of mourning, Mrs. F. again became hypomanic. At this time, however, because the family became concerned that she might not be able to supervise the handling of her husband's estate adequately during this episode, psychiatric consultation was sought. At this consultation, she was talkative, buoyant, and, although expressing concern about her future, was surprisingly at ease. She did not cry about the loss of her husband and seemed unaware that her mood and behavior were unusual for a grieving widow. A diagnosis of recurrent depressions alternating with hypomania was made. Since she was physically healthy, free of cardiovascular or renal disease, and not taking other medications, she was started on a trial of lithium in an attempt to stabilize her behavior. Her hypomania resolved at 600 mg of lithium (blood level 0.75 mEq/L).

Mrs. F., however, was not happy with how she felt. She began reporting an exacerbation of a long-standing psoriatic condition and was especially distressed by a 10-pound weight gain. In addition, she reported that she did not feel ``sharp'' mentally. She no longer felt excitement at going to a new art exhibit, and her columns for the paper became dull. She attributed these changes to being on lithium and requested a change in medication from her psychiatrist. Divalproex sodium was begun, with dosage gradually increased to 100 mg/day to achieve a blood level of 60 to 70 mg/L, followed by lithium taper and discontinuation.

Although Mrs. F.'s mania remained well controlled and her cognitive slowing and dulling improved greatly, she now reported significant sedation from her new medication. She felt the need to go to bed by 8 o'clock in the evening and even started napping during the day. These changes interfered with her attendance at art exhibits and led her to miss several deadlines for her column. The divalproex sodium was discontinued, and carbamazepine begun. At a dose of 600 mg/day and a blood level of 6.2 mg/mL, her affective symptoms remained in remission, and her only side effect was mild dry mouth.

The case of Mrs. F. illustrates that elderly patients may experience the same cognitive slowing from lithium that younger patients often report. Lithium also may aggravate psoriasis, and its use is associated with weight gain. For patients who otherwise tolerate lithium and do well on it, management of psoriasis with topical treatments or ultraviolet light exposure is appropriate, but the combination of several different side effects from lithium makes a shift to alternative therapy appropriate. Generally, divalproex sodium will be the next choice, but side effects such as sedation are possible with this medication as well. Carbamazepine may be useful in such cases, with careful monitoring for hematological and hepatic toxicity.

Case 12.7

Mrs. G.'s first episode of affective illness occurred at age 42, shortly after her husband was killed in an airplane accident. Her older daughter was 16 at the time and recalls overactivity suggestive of hypomania, followed by a psychotic depression. Mrs. G. was hospitalized and improved with ECT. She then did well for 11 years, when she was rehospitalized for depression that again resolved with ECT. She was without symptoms for the next 15 years but then fell in the bathtub, suffering a fractured right arm and several broken ribs. She required hospitalization for an open reduction of the arm fracture and then spent 4 weeks in a rehab hospital. During this time, she required lorazepam for anxiety.

Two years later, Mrs. G. developed osteomyelitis and had a difficult recovery. She was fatigued and anxious, felt inadequate, and lost her confidence. She stopped going out of the house and made lists of how bad she was. She also developed suicidal ideation and olfactory hallucinations of urine or food cooking. Mrs. G. was hospitalized and improved again with ECT, but after discharge she developed rapid pressured speech, made 2-hour phone calls to peo-

ple she was only slightly acquainted with, and made plans to buy a house she could not afford. These symptoms improved with the use of lithium carbonate, but she developed tremors, slurred speech, and an unsteady gait. She was able to remain on lithium at a reduced dose with a blood level of 0.5.

Over the next 5 years, Mrs. G. began to exhibit mild forgetfulness. She was able to continue to live independently, but it was necessary for her daughter to take charge of paying her bills. She then became mildly depressed and was treated with paroxetine, 20 mg/day. Mild high blood pressure was noted, and hydrochlorothiazide was prescribed. After a week, Mrs. G. noted a severe tremor and began dropping plates and utensils while doing the dishes; her lithium level had increased to 0.9. With her lithium dosage reduced by half, the blood level dropped to 0.4 and the tremor mainly disappeared.

A year later, when Mrs. G. was taking a walk with her granddaughter, she failed to see a break in the sidewalk and fractured her ankle. Surgery was again required to repair the fracture, and after a long period of recovery, she still had troublesome pain. She bought nonprescription ibuprofen and increased its use to 1600 mg/day. Over the next 2 weeks, she again developed a significant tremor. In addition, she began to have diarrhea and felt too weak to leave the house. Thinking that her gastrointestinal symptoms might be due to the paroxetine, her psychiatrist discontinued this medication, but without change in Mrs. G.'s condition; in fact, she became more markedly inattentive and confused. Finally, a lithium level was obtained, with a result of 1.27. The psychiatrist questioned Mrs. G.'s daughter, who found the empty ibuprofen bottles in her mother's apartment. This medication was disposed of, and lithium was withheld for a week and then resumed at the previous dosage.

Lithium was an effective treatment for Mrs. G., but she suffered from a number of side effects. The possible contribution of lithium to the development of a gait disturbance and the occurrence of falling illustrate the increased susceptibility of older patients to lithium neurotoxicity and the consequent need for careful and frequent monitoring. Drug interactions also may be significant. As a general principle, lithium and thiazide diuretics should not be prescribed together because plasma lithium levels will be elevated and toxicity may result. However, with dosage adjustment, the combination may be tolerated.

This case also illustrates the potential hazards of over-the-counter medication. Nonsteroidal anti-inflammatories are now readily available without prescription and are associated with decreased lithium excretion and increased levels. Because elderly persons are frequent users of over-the-counter medications, asking about their use must be a regular part of patient treatment and maintenance.

Case 12.8

Ms. H. was a charming and active 76-year-old woman who had experienced numerous episodes of major depression throughout her life, each responding well to antidepressant treatment. In between episodes she had with abundant energy and a cheerful outgoing nature. Athletic, sociable, and adventurous, she traveled frequently and shared many activities with her extended family, taking particular joy in skiing with her grandchildren. Nevertheless, at times her family became concerned that her abundant good nature was becoming worrisome. First, a series of minor automobile accidents occurred that she admitted were due to her inattention, followed by a series of purchases at yard sales that were not excessive but were unnecessary. Finally, she decided to sell her home, which she loved, to purchase a larger and more expensive, albeit beautiful, single-family home. Unmarried and living alone, she planned to use space in this larger house as an art studio. Her children, concerned that she was hypomanic, tried to suggest to her that the usual goal for a woman her age was to sell a home and move into smaller rather than larger quarters, but she was unpersuaded and purchased the new house within 48 hours of first visiting it.

Ms. H.'s sleep was normal and undisturbed, with no evidence of pressured speech, flight of ideas, or other inappropriate behavior. She admitted that she was probably ''slightly high'' and had been for the prior year and a half since her last depression had lifted. Ms. H., as well as her clinician, was reluctant to begin treatment with mood stabilizers. Although her behavior may meet criteria for hypomania, it was not considered serious enough to begin treatment with mood-stabilizing drugs that might produce side effects. She agreed to be followed closely by her physician; her children also agreed to stay in close contact with her physician if her behaviors further escalated.

Ms. H. then did well without any medications. Her case illustrates a clinical decision not use medications although the clinical indication might be present. Balancing the therapeutic effect of a mood stabilizer with some of its side effects, such as sedation, cognitive impair-

ment, and diminished energy, is especially important in older individuals since they are more sensitive to these side effects of mood stabilizers. The close association between Ms. H. and her family and Ms. H. and the treating clinician made an ongoing appraisal of this balance possible and helped avoid the use of these medications.

References

1. Yassa R, Nair NPV, Iskandar H. Late-onset bipolar disorder. *Psychiatr Clin North Am* 1988;11: 117–131.
2. Glasser M, Rabins P. Mania in the elderly. *Age Ageing* 1984;13:210–213.
3. Regier DA, Boyd JH, Burke JD, et al. One-month prevalence of mental disorders in the United States. *Arch Gen Psychiatry* 1988;45: 977–986.
4. Yassa R, Nair V, Nastase C, et al. Prevalence of bipolar disorder in a psychogeriatric population. *J Affective Disord* 1988;14:197–201.
5. Snowdon J. A retrospective case-note study of bipolar disorder in old age. *Br J Psychiatry* 1991; 158:485–490.
6. Weissman MM, Leaf PJ, Tischler GL, et al. Affective disorders in five United States communities. *Psychol Med* 1988;18:141–153
7. Young RC, Falk JR. Age, manic psychopathology and treatment response. *Int J Ger Psychiatry* 1989;4:73–78.
8. Broadhead J, Jacoby R. Mania in old age: a first prospective study. *Int J Geriatr Psychiatry* 1990; 5:215–222.
9. Wylie ME, Mulsant BH, Pollock BG, et al. Age at onset in geriatric bipolar disorder: effects on clinical presentation and treatment outcomes in an inpatient sample. *Am J Geriatr Psychiatry* 1999;7:77–83.
10. Post F. *The clinical psychiatry of late life.* Oxford: Pergamon Press, 1965:79–82.
11. Carlson GA, Bromet EJ, Sievers S. Phenomenology and outcome of subjects with early and adult-onset psychotic mania. *Am J Psychiatry* 2000;157:213–219.
12. Schurhoff F, Bellivier F, Jouvent R, et al. Early and late onset bipolar disorders: two different forms of manic-depressive illness? *J Affective Disord* 2000;58:215–221.
13. Schulze TG, Muller DJ, Krauss H, et al. Further evidence for age of onset being an indicator for severity in bipolar disorder. *J Affective Disorders* 2002;68:343–345.
14. Casey DA, Fitzgerald BA. Mania and pseudodementia. *J Clin Psychiatry* 1988;49:73–74.
15. Weintraub D, Lippmann S. Delirious mania in the elderly. *Int J Geriat Psychiatry* 2001;16: 374–377.
16. Lyketsos CG, Corazzini K, Steele C. Mania in Alzheimer's disease. *J Neuropsychiatry Clin Neurosci* 1995;7:350–352.
17. Nilsson FM, Kessing LV, Sorensen TM, et al.

Enduring increased risk of developing depression and mania in patients with dementia. *J Neurol Neurosurg Psychiatry* 2002;73:40–44.

18. Dhingra U, Rabins PV. Mania in the elderly: a 5–7 year follow-up. *J Am Geriatr Soc* 1991;39: 581–583.

19. Stone K. Mania in the elderly. *Br J Psychiatry* 1989;155:220–224.

20. Shulman K, Post F. Bipolar affective disorder in old age. *Br J Psychiatry* 1980;136:26–32.

21. Shulman KI, Tohen M, Satlin A, et al. Mania compared with unipolar depression in old age. *Am J Psychiatry* 1992;149(3):341–345.

22. Taylor M, Abrams R. Manic states: a genetic study of early and late onset affective disorders. *Arch Gen Psychiatry* 1973;28:656–658.

23. Winokur G. The Iowa 500: heterogeneity and course in manic-depressive illness (bipolar). *Comp Psychiatry* 1975;16:125–131.

24. Shulman KI, Tohen M. Unipolar mania reconsidered: evidence from an elderly cohort. *Br J Psychiatry* 1994;164(4):547–549.

25. Summers WK. Mania with onset in the eighth decade: two cases and a review. *J Clin Psychiatry* 1983;44:141–143.

26. Charron M, Fortin L, Paquette I. De novo mania among elderly people. *Acta Psychiatr Scand* 1991;84(6):503–537.

27. Kellner MB, Neher F. A first episode of mania after age 80. *Can J Psychiatry* 1991;36(8): 607–608.

28. Tohen M, Shulman KI, Satlin A. First-episode mania in late life. *Am J Psychiatry* 1994;151(1): 130–132.

29. Ernst CL, Goldberg JF. Antidepressant properties of anticonvulsant drugs for bipolar disorder. *J Clin Psychopharmacol* 2003;23:182–192.

30. Mendlewicz S, Fieve R, Rainer J, et al. Manic depressive illness: a comparative study of patients with and without a family history. *Br J Psychiatry* 1972;120:523–530.

31. James NM. Early- and late-onset bipolar affective disorder. *Arch Gen Psychiatry* 1977;34: 715–717.

32. Carlson GA, Davenport YB, Jamison K. A comparison of outcome in adolescent- and late-onset bipolar manic-depressive illness. *Am J Psychiatry* 1977;134:919–922.

33. Young RC, Nambudiri DE, Jain H, et al. Brain computed tomography in geriatric manic disorder. *Biol Psychiatry* 1999;45:1063–1065.

34. McDonald WM, Krishnan KR, Doraiswamy PM, et al. Occurrence of subcortical hyperintensities in elderly subjects with mania. *Psychiatry Res* 1991;40(4):211–220.

35. Nath J, Sagar R. Late-onset bipolar disorder due to hyperthyroidism. *Acta Psychiatr Scand* 2001;104:72–75.

36. Starkstein SE, Boston JD, Robinson RG. Mechanism of mania after brain injury. *J Nerv Ment Dis* 1988;176:87–100.

37. Shulman KI. Disinhibition syndromes, secondary mania and bipolar disorder in old age. *J Affective Disorders* 1997;46:175–182.

38. Braun CMJ, Larocque C, Daigneault S, et al. Mania, pseudomania, depression, and pseudodepression resulting from focal unilateral cortical lesions. *Neuropsychiatry Neuropsychol Behav Neurol* 1999;12:35–51.

39. American Psychiatric Association. Practice guidelines for the treatment of patients with bipolar disorder (revision). *Am J Psychiatry* 2002;159:(April suppl).

40. Shulman KI, Mackenzie S, Hardy B. The clinical use of lithium carbonate in old age: a review. *Prog Neuropsychopharmacol Biol Psychiatry* 1987;11:159–164.

41. Foster JR. Use of lithium in elderly psychiatric patients: a review of the literature. *Lithium* 1992;3:77–93.

42. Chen ST, Altshuler LL, Melnyk KA, et al. Efficacy of lithium vs valproate in the treatment of mania in the elderly: a retrospective study. *J Clin Psychiatry* 1999;60:181–185.

43. Himmelhoch JM, Neil JF, May SJ, et al. Age, dementia, dyskinesias, and lithium response. *Am J Psychiatry* 1980;137:941–945.

44. Swann AC, Bowden CL, Calabrese JR, et al. Mania: differential effects of previous depressive and manic episodes on response to treatment. *Acta Psychiatr Scand* 2000;101:444–451.

45. Herbert PB, Nelson JC. Parenteral valproate for control of acute mania. *Am J Psychiatry* 2000; 157:1023–1024 (letter).

46. Regenold WT, Prasad M. Uses of intravenous valproate in geriatric psychiatry. *Am J Geriatr Psychiatry* 2001;9:306–308.

47. Risinger RC, Risby ED, Risch SC. Safety and efficacy of divalproex sodium in elderly bipolar patients [Letter]. *J Clin Psychiatry* 1994;55:215.

48. McFarland BH, Miller MR, Straumfjord AA. Valproate use in the older manic patient. *J Clin Psychiatry* 1990;51:479–481.

49. Noagiul S, Narayan M, Nelson JC. Divalproex treatment of mania in elderly patients. *Am J Geriatr Psychiatry* 1998;6:257–262.

50. Schneider AL, Wilcox CS. Divalproate augmentation in lithium-resistant rapid cycling mania in four geriatric patients. *J Affective Disord* 1998; 47:201–205.

51. Mordecai DJ, Sheikh JI, Glick ID. Divalproex for the treatment of geriatric bipolar disorder. *Int J Geriatr Psychiatry* 1999;14:494–496.

52. Goldberg JF, Sachs MH, Kocsis JH. Low-dose lithium augmentation of divalproex in geriatric mania. *J Clin Psychiatry* 2000;61:304.

53. Brambilla P, Barale F, Soares JC. Atypical antipsychotics and mood stabilization in bipolar disorder. *Psychopharmacology* 2003;166: 315–332.

54. Byerly MJ, Weber MT, Brooks DL, et al. Antipsychotic medications and the elderly: effects on cognition and implications for use. *Drugs Aging* 2001;18:45–61.

55. Malhi GS, Berk M. Pharmacotherapy of bipolar disorder: the role of atypical antipsychotics and experimental strategies. *Hum Psychopharmacol Clin Exp* 2002;17:407–412.

56. Beyer J, Siegal A, Kennedy J, et al. Olanzapine, divalproex and placebo treatment: non-head-to-head comparisons of older adult acute mania. Tenth Congress of the International Psychogeriatric Association 2001; *Abstract P-170*.

57. Keck PE, McElroy SL. Redefining mood stabilization. *J Affective Disord* 2003;73:163–169.
58. Robillard M, Conn D. Gabapentin use in geriatric patients with depression and bipolar illness. [Letter] *Can J Psychiatry - Revue Canadienne de Psychiatrie*, 2001;46(8):764.
59. Bowden CL, Calabrese JR, McElroy SL, et al. A randomized, placebo-controlled 12-month trial of divalproex and lithium in treatment of outpatients with bipolar I disorder. *Arch Gen Psychiatry* 2000;57:481–489.
60. Shulman KI, Rochon P, Sykora K, et al. Changing prescription patterns for lithium and valproic acid in old age: shifting practice without evidence. *Br Med J* 2003;326:960–961.
61. Manji HK, Moore GJ, Chen G. Lithium at 50: have the neuroprotective effects of this unique cation been overlooked? *Biol Psychiatry* 1999; 46:929–940.
62. Moore GJ, Bebchuk JM, Wilds IB, et al. Lithium-induced increase in human brain grey matter. *Lancet* 2000;356:1241–1242.
63. Calabrese JR, Shelton MD, Rapport DJ, et al. Long-term treatment of bipolar disorder with lamotrigine. *J Clin Psychiatry* 2002;63:18–22.
64. Hartong EGTM, Moleman P, Hoogduin CAL, et al. Prophylactic efficacy of lithium versus carbamazepine in treatment-naïve bipolar patients. *J Clin Psychiatry* 2003;64:144–151.
65. Bowden CL, Calabrese JR, Sachs G, et al. A placebo-controlled 18-month trial of lamotrigine and lithium maintenance treatment in recently manic or hypomanic patients with bipolar I disorder. *Arch Gen Psychiatry* 2003;60:392–400.
66. Brodie MJ, Overstall PW, Giorgi L, The UK Lamotrigine Elderly Study Group. Multicentre, double-blind, randomised comparison between lamotrigine and carbamazepine in elderly patients with newly diagnosed epilepsy. *Epilepsy Research* 1999;37:81–87.
67. Hellewell JSE. Oxcarbazepine (Trileptal) in the treatment of bipolar disorders: a review of efficacy and tolerability. *J Affective Disord* 2002; 72:S23–S34.
68. Suppes T, Webb A, Paul B, et al. Clinical outcome in a randomized 1-year trial of clozapine versus treatment as usual for patients with treatment-resistant illness and a history of mania. *Am J Psychiatry* 1999;156:1264–1266.
69. Vieta E, Reinares M, Corbella B, et al. Olanzapine as long-term adjunctive therapy in treatment-resistant bipolar disorder. *J Clin Psychopharmacol* 2001;21(5):469–473.
70. Tueth MJ, Murphy TK, Evans DL. Special considerations: use of lithium in children, adolescents, and elderly populations. *J Clin Psychiatry* 1998;59:66–73.
71. Blanche P, Raynaud E, Kerob D, et al. Lithium intoxication in an elderly patient after combined treatment with losartan [Letter]. *Eur J Clin Pharmacol* 1997;52:501.
72. Head L, Dening T. Lithium in the over-65s: who is taking it and who is monitoring it? A survey of older adults on lithium in the Cambridge Mental Health Services catchment area. *Int J Geriatr Psychiatry* 1998;13:164–171.
73. Van Gerpen MW, Johnson JE, Winstead DK. Mania in the geriatric patient population: a review of the literature. *Am J Geriatr Psychiatry* 1999;7:188–202.
74. Wolf ME, Moffat M, Ranade V, et al. Lithium, hypercalcemia, and arrhythmia [Letter]. *J Clin Psychopharmacol* 1998;18:420–423.
75. Tam VK, Green J, Schwieger J, et al. Nephrotic syndrome and renal insufficiency associated with lithium therapy. *Am J Kidney Dis* 1996; 27(5):715–720.
76. Jensen HV, Plenge P, Mellerup ET, et al. Lithium prophylaxis of manic-depressive disorder: daily lithium dosing schedule versus every second day. *Acta Psychiatr Scand* 1995;92(1):69–74.
77. Kingsbury SJ, Salzman C. Lithium's role in hyperparathyroidism and hypercalcemia. *Hosp Community Psychiatry* 1993;44:1047–1048
78. Pope HG, McElroy SL, Keck PE, et al. Valproate in the treatment of acute mania: a placebo-controlled study. *Arch Gen Psychiatry* 1991;48: 62–68.
79. Bowden CL, Brugger AM, Swann AC, et al. Efficacy of divalproex vs lithium and placebo in the treatment of mania. The Depakote Mania Study Group. *JAMA* 1994;271(12):918–924.
80. Zajecka JM, Weisler R, Sachs G, et al. A comparison of the efficacy, safety, and tolerability of divalproex sodium and olanzapine in the treatment of bipolar disorder. *J Clin Psychiatry* 2002; 63:1148–1155.
81. Macritchie K, Geddes JR, Scott J, et al. Valproate for acute mood episodes in bipolar disorder (Cochrane Review). In: *The Cochrane Library*, Issue 1, 2003. Oxford: Update Software.
82. Kando JC, Tohen M, Castillo J, et al. The use of valproate in an elderly population with affective symptoms. *J Clin Psychiatry* 1996;57: 238–240.
83. Mazure CM, Druss BG, Cellar JS. Valproate treatment of older psychotic patients with organic mental syndromes and behavioral dyscontrol. *J Am Geriatr Soc* 1992;40:914–916.
84. Yassa R, Cvejic J. Valproate in the treatment of posttraumatic bipolar disorder in a psychogeriatric patient. *J Geriatr Psychiatry Neurol* 1994; 7(1):55–57.
85. Lott AD, McElroy SL, Keys MA. Valproate in the treatment of behavioral agitation in elderly patients with dementia. *J Neuropsychiatry Clin Neurosci* 1995;7:314–319.
86. Tariot PN, Schneider LS, Katz IR. Anticonvulsant and other non-neuroleptic treatment of agitation in dementia. *J Geriatr Psychiatry Neurol* 1995;8(suppl 1):S28–S39.
87. Tariot PN, Schneider LS, Jacobo E, et al. Safety and tolerability of divalproex sodium in the treatment of signs and symptoms of mania in elderly patients with dementia: results of a double-blind, placebo-controlled trial. *Current Therapeutic Research* 2001;62:51–67.
88. Felix S, Sproule BA, Hardy BG, et al. Dose-related pharmacokinetics and pharmacodynamics of valproate in the elderly. *J Clin Psychopharmacol* 2003;23:471–476.
89. Puryear LJ, Kunik ME, Workman R. Tolerability of divalproex sodium in elderly psychiatric patients with mixed diagnoses. *J Geriatr Psychiatry Neurol* 1995;8:234–237.

90. Calabrese JR, Bowden CL, Sachs GS, et al. A double-blind placebo-controlled study of lamotrigine monotherapy in outpatients with bipolar I depression. *J Clin Psychiatry* 1999;60:79–88.

91. Giorgi L, Gomez G, O'Neill F, et al. The tolerability of lamotrigine in elderly patients with epilepsy. *Drugs Aging* 2001;18:621–630.

92. Ballenger JC, Post RM. Carbamazepine in manic-depressive illness: a new treatment. *Am J Psychiatry* 1980;137:782–790.

93. Dardennes R, Even C, Bange F, et al. Comparison of carbamazepine and lithium in prophylaxis of bipolar disorders: a meta-analysis. *Br J Psychiatry* 1995;166:378–381.

94. Greil W, Ludwig-Mayerhofer W, Erazo N, et al. Lithium versus carbamazepine in the maintenance treatment of bipolar disorders: a randomised study. *J Affective Disord* 1997;43: 151–161.

95. Grunze H, Walden J. Relevance of new and newly rediscovered anticonvulsants for atypical forms of bipolar disorder. *J Affective Disord* 2002; 72:S15–S21.

96. Suppes T. Review of the use of topiramate for treatment of bipolar disorders. *J Clin Psychopharmacol* 2002;22:599–609.

97. Pecuch PW, Erfurth A. Topiramate in the treatment of acute mania. [Letter] *J Clin Psychopharmacol* 2001;21:243–4.

98. Tohen M, Sanger TM, McElroy SL, et al. Olanzapine versus placebo in the treatment of acute mania. *Am J Psychiatry* 1999;156:702–709.

99. Tohen M, Jacobs TG, Grundy SL, et al. Efficacy of olanzapine in acute bipolar mania: a double-blind, placebo-controlled study. The Olanzapine HGGW Study Group. *Arch Gen Psychiatry* 2000;57:841–849.

100. Sajatovic M. Clozapine for elderly patients. *Psychiatric Annals* 1999;30:170–174

101. Yeung PP, Tariot PN, Schneider LS, et al. Quetiapine for elderly patients with psychotic disorders. *Psychiatric Annals* 1999;30:197–201.

102. Tohen M, Baker RW, Altshuler LL, et al. Olanzapine versus divalproex in the treatment of acute mania. *Am J Psychiatry* 2002;159: 1011–1017.

103. Koro CE, Fedder DO, L'Italien GJ, et al. An assessment of the independent effects of olanzapine and risperidone exposure on the risk of hyperlipidemia in schizophrenic patients. *Arch Gen Psychiatry* 2002;59:1021–1026.

104. Street JS, Tollefson GD, Tohen M, et al. Olanzapine for psychotic conditions in the elderly. *Psychiatric Annals* 1999;30:191–196.

105. Madhusoodanan S, Brenner R, Cohen CI. Risperidone for elderly patients with schizophrenia or schizoaffective disorder. *Psychiatric Annals* 1999;30:175–180.

106. Shulman RW, Singh A, Shulman KI. Treatment of elderly institutionalized bipolar patients with clozapine. *Psychopharmacol Bull* 1997;33: 113–118.

107. Bebchuk JM, Arfken CL, Dolan-Manji S, et al. A preliminary investigation of a protein kinase C inhibitor in the treatment of acute mania. *Arch Gen Psychiatry* 2000;57:95–97.

108. Stoll AL, Severus E, Freeman MP, et al. Omega-3 fatty acids in bipolar disorder. *Arch Gen Psychiatry* 1999;56:407–412.

109. Burt T, Sachs G, Demopoulos C. Donepezil in treatment-resistant bipolar disorder. *Biol Psychiatry* 1999;45:959–964.

110. Cummings JL. Cholinesterase inhibitors: expanding applications. *Lancet* 2001;357:1039.

111. Mukherjee S, Sackeim HA, Schnur DB. Electroconvulsive therapy of acute manic episodes. *Am J Psychiatry* 1994;151:169–176.

112. American Psychiatric Association. *The Practice of Electroconvulsive Therapy: Recommendations for Treatment, Training, and Privileging: A Task Force Report of the American Psychiatric Association, 2nd ed.* Washington, DC: American Psychiatric Press, 2001.

Supplemental Readings

Epidemiology

McDonald WM. Epidemiology, etiology, and treatment of geriatric mania. *J Clin Psychiatry* 2000; 61[suppl 13]:3–11.

Regier DA, Boyd JH, Burke JD, et al. One-month prevalence of mental disorders in the United States. *Arch Gen Psychiatry* 1988;45:977–986.

Weissman MM, Leaf PJ, Tischler GL, et al. Affective disorders in five United States communities. *Psychol Med* 1988;18:141–153

Yassa R, Nair V, Nastase C, et al. Prevalence of bipolar disorder in a psychogeriatric population. *J Affective Disord* 1988;14:197–201.

Clinical Presentation, Diagnosis, and Course

Benazzi F. Bipolar II depression in late life: prevalence and clinical features in 525 depressed outpatients. *J Affective Disord* 2001;66:13–18.

Broadhead J, Jacoby R. Mania in old age: a first prospective study. *Int J Geriatr Psychiatry* 1990;5: 215–222.

Carlson GA, Davenport YB, Jamison K. A comparison of outcome in adolescent- and late-onset bipolar manic-depressive illness. *Am J Psychiatry* 1977;134: 919–922.

Carlson GA, Bromet EJ, Sievers S. Phenomenology and outcome of subjects with early- and adult-onset psychotic mania. *Am J Psychiatry* 2000;157: 213–219.

Casey DA, Fitzgerald BA. Mania and pseudodementia. *J Clin Psychiatry* 1988;49:73–74.

Charron M, Fortin L, Paquette I. De novo mania among elderly people. *Acta Psychiatr Scand* 1991; 84(6):503–507.

Conlon P. Rapid cycling mood disorder in the elderly. *J Geriatr Psychiatry Neurol* 1989;2: 106–108.

Dhingra U, Rabins PV. Mania in the elderly: a 5–7 year follow-up. *J Am Geriatr Soc* 1991;39:581–583.

Glasser M, Rabins P. Mania in the elderly. *Age Ageing* 1984;13:210–213.

Gnam W, Flint AJ. New onset rapid-cycling bipolar

disorder in an 87-year-old woman. *Can J Psychiatry* 1993;38(5):324–326.

Hays JC, Krishnan KRR, George LK, et al. Age of first onset of bipolar disorder: demographic, family history, and psychosocial correlates. *Depression and Anxiety* 1998;7:76–82.

James NM. Early- and late-onset bipolar affective disorder. *Arch Gen Psychiatry* 1977; 34:715–717.

Kellner MB, Neher F. A first episode of mania after age 80. *Can J Psychiatry* 1991;36(8):607–608.

McDonald WM, Krishnan KR, Doraiswamy PM, et al. Occurrence of subcortical hyperintensities in elderly subjects with mania. *Psychiatry Res* 1991; 40(4):211–220.

Meeks S. Bipolar disorder in the latter half of life: symptom presentation, global functioning and age of onset. *J Affective Disord* 1999;52:161–167.

Mendlewicz S, Fieve R, Rainer J et al. Manic depressive illness: a comparative study of patients with and without a family history. *Br J Psychiatry* 1972; 120:523–530.

Moorhead SRJ, Young AH. Evidence for a late onset bipolar-I disorder sub-group after 50 years. *J Affective Disord* 2003;73:271–277.

Post F. *The clinical psychiatry of late life.* Oxford: Pergamon Press, 1965:79–82.

Roth M. The natural history of mental disorder in old age. *J Ment Sci* 1955;101:281–301.

Schulze TG, Muller DJ, Krauss H, et al. Further evidence for age of onset being an indicator for severity in bipolar disorder. *J Affective Disorders* 2002;68:343–345.

Schurhoff F, Bellivier F, Jouvent R, et al. Early and late onset bipolar disorders: two different forms of manic-depressive illness? *J Affective Disord* 2000; 58:215–21.

Shulman K, Post F. Bipolar affective disorder in old age. *Br J Psychiatry* 1980;136:26–32.

Shulman KI, Tohen M, Satlin A, et al. Mania compared with unipolar depression in old age. *Am J Psychiatry* 1992;149(3):341–345.

Shulman KI, Tohen M. Unipolar mania reconsidered: evidence from an elderly cohort. *Br J Psychiatry* 1994;164(4):547–549.

Snowdon J. A retrospective case-note study of bipolar disorder in old age. *Br J Psychiatry* 1991;158: 485–490.

Spicer CC, Hare EH, Slater E. Neurotic and psychotic forms of depressive illness: evidence from age-incidence in a national sample. *Br J Psychiatry* 1973;123:535–541.

Stone K. Mania in the elderly. *Br J Psychiatry* 1989; 155:220–224.

Summers WK. Mania with onset in the eighth decade: two cases and a review. *J Clin Psychiatry* 1983; 44:141–143.

Swann AC, Bowden CL, Calabrese JR, et al. Mania: differential effects of previous depressive and manic episodes on response to treatment. *Acta Psychiatr Scand* 2000;101:444–451.

Taylor M, Abrams R. Manic states: a genetic study of early and late onset affective disorders. *Arch Gen Psychiatry* 1973;28:656–658.

Tohen M, Shulman KI, Satlin A. First-episode mania in late life. *Am J Psychiatry* 1994;151(1):130–132.

Umapathy C, Mulsant BH, Pollock BG. Bipolar disorder in the elderly. *Psychiatric Annals* 2000;30: 473–480.

Van Gerpen MW, Johnson JE, Winstead DK. Mania in the geriatric patient population: a review of the literature. *Am J Geriatr Psychiatry* 1999;7: 188–202.

Winokur G. The Iowa 500: heterogeneity and course in manic-depressive illness (bipolar). *Comp Psychiatry* 1975;16:125–131.

Wylie ME, Mulsant BH, Pollock BG, et al. Age at onset in geriatric bipolar disorder: effects on clinical presentation and treatment outcomes in an inpatient sample. *Am J Geriatr Psychiatry* 1999;7: 77–83.

Yassa R, Nair NPV, Iskandar H. Late-onset bipolar disorder. *Psychiatr Clin North Am* 1988;11: 117–131.

Young RC, Falk JR. Age, manic psychopathology and treatment response. *Int J Geriatr Psychiatry* 1989; 4:73–78.

Young RC, Klerman GL. Mania in late life: focus on age at onset. *Am J Psychiatry* 1992;149:867–876.

Young RC, Nambudiri DE, Jain H, et al. Brain computed tomography in geriatric manic disorder. *Biol Psychiatry* 1999;45:1063–1065.

Etiology

Benazzi F. Mania associated with donepezil. [Letter] *Int J Geriatr Psychiatry* 1998;13:813–821.

Braun CMJ, Larocque C, Daigneault S, et al. Mania, pseudomania, depression, and pseudodepression resulting from focal unilateral cortical lesions. *Neuropsychiatr Neuropsychol Behav Neurol* 1999;12:35–51.

Cassidy F, Carroll BJ. Vascular risk factors in late onset mania. *Psychol Med* 2002;32:359–362.

Khouzam HR, Emery PE, Reaves B. Secondary mania in late life. *J Am Geriatr Soc* 1994;42(1):85–87.

Krauthammer C, Klerman GL. Secondary mania: manic syndromes associated with antecedent physical illnesses or drugs. *Arch Gen Psychiatry* 1978;35:1333–1339.

Lyketsos CG, Corazzini K, Steele C. Mania in Alzheimer's disease. *J Neuropsychiatry Clin Neurosci* 1995; 7:350–352.

Nath J, Sagar R. Late-onset bipolar disorder due to hyperthyroidism. *Acta Psychiatr Scand* 2001;104: 72–75.

Nilsson FM, Kessing LV, Sorensen TM, et al. Enduring increased risk of developing depression and mania in patients with dementia. *J Neurol Neurosurg Psychiatry* 2002;73:40–44.

Shulman KI. Disinhibition syndromes, secondary mania and bipolar disorder in old age. *J Affective Disorders* 1997;46:175–182.

Starkstein SE, Boston JD, Robinson RG. Mechanism of mania after brain injury. *J Nerv Ment Dis* 1988; 176:87–100.

Weilburg JB, Sachs G, Falk WE. Triazolam-induced brief episodes of secondary mania in a depressed patient. *J Clin Psychiatry* 1987;48:492–493.

Weintraub D, Lippmann S. Delirious mania in the elderly. *Int J Geriat Psychiatry* 2001;16:374–377.

Young RC, Moline M, Kleyman F. Hormone replacement therapy and late-life mania. *Am J Geriatr Psychiatry* 1997;5:179–181.

Treatment: Reviews

American Psychiatric Association. Practice guideline for the treatment of patients with bipolar disorder (revision). *Am J Psychiatry* 2002;159:(April suppl).

Brambilla P, Barale F, Soares JC. Atypical antipsychotics and mood stabilization in bipolar disorder. *Psychopharmacology* 2003;166:315–332.

Cassano GB, McElroy SL, Brady K, et al. Current issues in the identification and management of bipolar spectrum disorders in 'special populations.' *J Affective Disord* 2000;59:S69–S79.

Dardennes R, Even C, Bange F, et al. Comparison of carbamazepine and lithium in prophylaxis of bipolar disorders: a meta-analysis. *Br J Psychiatry* 1995;166:378–381.

Ernst CL, Goldberg JF. Antidepressant properties of anticonvulsant drugs for bipolar disorder. *J Clin Psychopharmacol* 2003;23:182–192.

Foster JR. Use of lithium in elderly psychiatric patients: a review of the literature. *Lithium* 1992;3: 77–93.

Grunze H, Walden J. Relevance of new and newly rediscovered anticonvulsants for atypical forms of bipolar disorder. *J Affective Disord* 2002;72: S15–S21.

Keck PE, McElroy SL. Redefining mood stabilization. *J Affective Disord* 2003; 73:163–169.

Keck PE, Nelson EB, McElroy SL. Advances in the pharmacologic treatment of bipolar depression. *Biol Psychiatry* 2003;53:671–679.

Macritchie K, Geddes JR, Scott J, t al. Valproate for acute mood episodes in bipolar disorder (Cochrane Review). In: *The Cochrane Library*, Issue 1, 2003. Oxford: Update Software.

Mirchandani IC, Young RC. Management of mania in the elderly: an update. *Ann Clin Psychiatry* 1993;5(1):67–77.

Sajatovic M. Treatment of bipolar disorder in older adults. *Int J Geriatr Psychiatry* 2002;17:865–873.

Shulman KI, Hermann N. The nature and management of mania in old age. *Psychiatr Clin No Am* 1999;22:649–665.

Shulman KI, Mackenzie S, Hardy B. The clinical use of lithium carbonate in old age: a review. *Prog Neuropsychopharmacol Biol Psychiatry* 1987;11: 159–164.

Snowdon J. The relevance of guidelines for treating mania in old age. *Int J Ger Psychiatry* 2000;15: 779–783.

Tariot PN, Schneider LS, Katz IR. Anticonvulsant and other non-neuroleptic treatment of agitation in dementia. *J Geriatr Psychiatry Neurol* 1995; 8(suppl 1):S28–S39.

Lithium

Abou-Saleh MT, Coppen A. The prognosis of depression in old age: the case for lithium therapy. *Br J Psychiatry* 1983;143:527–528.

Ahrens B, Grof P, Mo HJ, et al. Extended survival of patients on long-term lithium treatment. *Can J Psychiatry* 1995;40(5):241–246.

Bushey M, Tathey U, Bowers MB. Lithium treatment in a very elderly nursing home population. *Compr Psychiatry* 1983;24:392–396.

Coppen A, Abou-Saleh MT. Lithium therapy; from clinical trials to practical management. *Acta Psychiatr Scand* 1988;78:754–762.

Fielding S, Kerr S, Godber C. Lithium in the over-65s—a dedicated monitoring service leads to a better quality of treatment supervision. [Letter] *Int J Geriatr Psychiatry* 1999;14:985–987.

Griel W, Stoltzenburg MC, Mairhofer ML, et al. Lithium dosage in the elderly: a study with matched age groups. *J Affective Disord* 1985;9:1–4.

Head L, Dening T. Lithium in the over-65s: who is taking it and who is monitoring it? A survey of older adults on lithium in the Cambridge Mental Health Services catchment area. *Int J Geriatr Psychiatry* 1998;13:164–171.

Hewick DS, Newbury P, Hopwood S, et al. Age as a factor affecting lithium therapy. *Br J Clin Pharmacol* 1977;4:201–205.

Himmelhoch JM, Neil JF, May SJ, et al. Age, dementia, dyskinesias, and lithium response. *Am J Psychiatry* 1980;137:941–945.

Jefferson JW. Lithium and affective disorder in the elderly. *Compr Psychiatry* 1983;24:166–178.

Jefferson JW, Sen D. Manic depressive disorder and lithium over the decades: the very educational case of Mrs. L. *J Clin Psychiatry* 1994;55(8): 340–343.

Jensen HV, Plenge P, Mellerup ET, et al. Lithium prophylaxis of manic-depressive disorder: daily lithium dosing schedule versus every second day. *Acta Psychiatr Scand* 1995;92(1):69–74.

Kushnir SL. Lithium-antidepressant combinations in the treatment of depressed, physically ill geriatric patients. *Am J Psychiatry* 1986;143:378–379.

Manji HK, Moore GJ, Chen G. Lithium at 50: have the neuroprotective effects of this unique cation been overlooked? *Biol Psychiatry* 1999;46:929–940.

Moore GJ, Bebchuk JM, Wilds IB, et al. Lithium-induced increase in human brain grey matter. *Lancet* 2000;356(9237):1241–1242.

Murray N, Hopwood S, Balfour DJK, et al. The influence of age on lithium efficacy and side effects in outpatients. *Psychol Med* 1983;13:53–60.

Prien RF, Gershon S. Lithium. In: Crook T, Cohen G, eds. *Physicians' handbook on psychotherapeutic drug use in the aged.* New Canaan, CT: Powley, 1981:38–42.

Roose SP, Bone S, Eisdorfer C, et al. Lithium treatment in older patients. *Am J Psychiatry* 1979;136: 843–844.

Schaffer CB, Garvey MJ. Use of lithium in acutely manic elderly patients. *Clin Gerontol* 1984;3: 58–60.

Schou M. Lithium in psychiatric therapy and prophylaxis. *J Psychiatr Res* 1968;6:69–95.

Schou M. Lithium prophylaxis: myths and realities. *Am J Psychiatry* 1989;146:573–576.

Shulman KI, Mackenzie S, Hardy B: The clinical use of lithium carbonate in old age: a review. *Prog Neuropsychopharmacol Biol Psychiatry* 1987;11: 159–164.

Tueth MJ, Murphy TK, Evans DL. Special considerations: use of lithium in children, adolescents, and elderly populations. *J Clin Psychiatry* 1998; 59[suppl6]:66–73.

Vestergaard P, Schou M. The effect of age on lithium

dosage requirements. *Pharmacopsychiatry* 1984; 17:199–201.

Side Effects of Lithium

Abraham G, Waldron JJ, Lawson JS. Are the renal effects of lithium modified by frequency of administration? *Acta Psychiatr Scand* 1995;92(2): 115–118.

Ananth J, Ghadirian AM, Engelsmann F. Lithium and memory: a review. *Can J Psychiatry* 1987;32: 312–316.

Bakker JB, Pepplinkhuizen L. Cutaneous side-effects of lithium. In: Johnson FN, ed. *Handbook of lithium therapy*. Lancaster: MTP, 1980:372–377.

Barclay ML, Brownlie BE, Turner JG, et al. Lithium associated thyrotoxicosis: a report of 14 cases, with statistical analysis of incidence. *Clin Endocrinol* (Oxf) 1994;40(6):759–764.

Barkin JS. Excessive lithium reabsorption by the proximal tubules [Letter]. *Am J Psychiatry* 1994; 151(4):618–619.

Bell AJ, Cole A, Eccleston D, et al. Lithium neurotoxicity at normal therapeutic levels [see comments]. *Br J Psychiatry* 1993;162:689–692.

Bendz H, Aurell M, Balldin J, et al. Kidney damage in long-term lithium patients: a cross-sectional study of patients with 15 years or more on lithium. *Nephrol Dial Transplant* 1994;9(9): 1250–1254.

Chacko RC, Marsh BJ, Marmion J, et al. Lithium side effects in elderly bipolar outpatients. *Hillside J Clin Psychiatry* 1987;9(1):79–88.

Farag S, Watson RD, Honeybourne D. Symptomatic junctional bradycardia due to lithium intoxication in patient with previously normal electrocardiogram [Letter]. *Lancet* 1994;343(8909):1371.

Ghadirian AM, Annable L, Belanger MC, et al. A cross-sectional study of parkinsonism and tardive dyskinesia in lithium-treated affective disordered patients. *J Clin Psychiatry* 1996;57(1):22–28.

Hestbach J, Hansen HE, Amdisen A, et al. Chronic renal lesions following long-term treatment with lithium. *Kidney Int* 1977;12:205–213.

Hetmar O, Povlsen UJ, Ladefoged J, et al. Lithium: long-term effects on the kidney. A prospective follow-up study ten years after kidney biopsy. *Br J Psychiatry* 1991;158:53–58.

Holroyd S, Rabins PV. A retrospective chart review of lithium side effects in a geriatric outpatient population. *Am J Geriatr Psychiatry* 1994;2(4): 346–351.

Holroyd S, Smith D. Disabling parkinsonism due to lithium: a case report. *J Geriatr Psychiatry Neurol* 1995;8(2):118–119.

Hwang S, Tuason VB. Long-term maintenance lithium therapy and possible irreversible renal damage. *J Clin Psychiatry* 1980;41:11–19.

Kallner G, Petterson U. Renal, thyroid and parathyroid function during lithium treatment: laboratory tests in 207 people treated for 1–30 years. *Acta Psychiatr Scand* 1995;91(1):48–51.

Kehoe RF. A cross-sectional study of glomerular function in 740 unselected lithium patients. *Acta Psychiatr Scand* 1994;89(1):68–71.

Kingsbury SJ, Salzman C. Lithium's role in hyperpar-

athyroidism and hypercalcemia. *Hosp Community Psychiatry* 1993;44:1047–1048.

Miller F, Menninger J, Whitcup SM. Lithium-neuroleptic neurotoxicity in the elderly bipolar patient. *J Clin Psychopharmacol* 1986;6:176–178.

Mitchell JE, McKensie TB. Cardiac effects of lithium therapy in man: a review. *J Clin Psychiatry* 1982; 43:47–51.

Nambudiri DE, Meyers BS, Young RC. Delayed recovery from lithium neurotoxicity. *J Geriatr Psychiatry Neurol* 1991;4(1):40–43.

Povlsen UJ, Hetmar O, Ladefoged J, et al. Kidney functioning during lithium treatment: a prospective study of patients treated with lithium for up to ten years. *Acta Psychiatr Scand* 1992;85(1): 56–60.

Ramchandani D, Schindler BA. The lithium toxic patient in the medical hospital: diagnostic and management dilemmas. *Int J Psychiatry Med* 1993; 23(1):55–62.

Roose SP, Nurnberger J, Dunner D, et al. Cardiac sinus node dysfunction during lithium treatment. *Am J Psychiatry* 1979;136:804–806.

Santiago R, Rashkin MC. Lithium toxicity and myxedema coma in an elderly woman. *J Emerg Med* 1990;8:63–66.

Smith RE, Helms PM. Adverse effects of lithium therapy in the acutely ill elderly patient. *J Clin Psychiatry* 1982;43:94–99.

Smith SJM, Kocen RS. A Creutzfeldt-Jakob-like syndrome due to lithium toxicity. *J Neurol Neurosurg Psychiatry* 1988;51:120–123.

Steckler TL. Lithium- and carbamazepine-associated sinus node dysfunction: nine-year experience in a psychiatric hospital. *J Clin Psychopharmacol* 1994; 14(5):336–339.

Tam VK, Green J, Schwieger J, et al. Nephrotic syndrome and renal insufficiency associated with lithium therapy. *Am J Kidney Dis* 1996;27(5): 715–720.

Tyrer SP, Schacht RG, McCarthy MJ, et al. The effect of lithium on renal haemodynamic function. *Psychol Med* 1983;13:61–69.

van der Velde CL. Toxicity of lithium carbonate in elderly patients. *Am J Psychiatry* 1971;127: 1075–1077.

Wolf ME, Moffat M, Ranade V, et al. Lithium, hypercalcemia, and arrhythmia [Letter]. *J Clin Psychopharmacol* 1998;18:420–423.

Pharmacokinetics of Lithium

Caldwell HC, Westlake WJ, Schriver RC, et al. Steadystate lithium blood level fluctuations in man following administration of a lithium carbonate conventional and controlled-release dosage form. *J Clin Pharmacol* 1981;21:106–109.

Chaperon DJ, Cameron IR, White LB, et al. Observations on lithium deposition in the elderly. *J Am Geriatr Soc* 1982;30:651–655.

Hardy BG, Shulman KI, Mackenzie SE, et al. Pharmacokinetics of lithium in the elderly. *J Clin Psychopharmacol* 1987;7:153–158.

Mester R, Toren P, Mizrachi I, et al. Caffeine withdrawal increases lithium blood levels. *Biol Psychiatry* 1995;37(5):348–350.

Prien RF. Age-related changes in lithium pharmacokinetics. In: Raskin A, Robinson DS, Levine J, eds. *Age and the pharmacology of psychoactive drugs.* New York: Elsevier/North Holland, 1981:163–170.

Valproic Acid

Armon C, Brown E, Carwile S, et al. Sensorineural hearing loss: a reversible effect of valproic acid. *Neurology* 1990;40:1896–1898.

Bauer LA, Davis R, Wilensky A, et al. Valproic acid clearance: unbound fraction and diurnal variations in young and elderly adults. *Clin Pharmacol Ther* 1985;37:697–700.

Bowden CL, Brugger AM, Swann AC, et al. Efficacy of divalproex vs lithium and placebo in the treatment of mania. The Depakote Mania Study Group. *JAMA* 1994;271(12):918–924.

Bowden CL, Calabrese JR, McElroy SL, et al. A randomized, placebo-controlled 12-month trial of divalproex and lithium in treatment of outpatients with bipolar I disorder. *Arch Gen Psychiatry* 2000;57:481–489.

Bryson SM, Verma N, Scott PJW, et al. Pharmacokinetics of valproic acid in young and elderly subjects. *Br J Clin Psychiatry* 1983;16:104–105.

Cates M, Powers R. Concomitant rash and blood dyscrasias in geriatric psychiatry patients treated with carbamazepine. *Ann Pharmacother* 1998;32:884–887.

Chen ST, Altshuler LL, Melnyk KA, et al. Efficacy of lithium vs valproate in the treatment of mania in the elderly: a retrospective study. *J Clin Psychiatry* 1999;60:181–185.

Emrich HM, Dose M, von Zerssen D. The use of sodium valproate and of oxcarbamazepine in patients with affective disorders. *J Affective Disord* 1985;8:243–250.

Felix S, Sproule BA, Hardy BG, et al. Dose-related pharmacokinetics and pharmacodynamics of valproate in the elderly. *J Clin Psychopharmacol* 2003;23:471–478.

Goldberg JF, Sachs MH, Kocsis JH. Low-dose lithium augmentation of divalproex in geriatric mania. *J Clin Psychiatry* 2000;61:304.

Guthrie SK, Stoysich AM, Bader G, et al. Hypothesized interaction between valproic acid and warfarin [Letter]. *J Clin Psychopharmacol* 1995;15(2):138–139.

Herbert PB, Nelson JC. Parenteral valproate for control of acute mania. *Am J Psychiatry* 2000;157:1023–1024 (letter).

Horne M, Lindley SE. Divalproex sodium in the treatment of aggressive behavior and dysphoria in patients with organic brain syndromes [Letter]. *J Clin Psychiatry* 1995;56(9):430–431.

Ikeda K, Moriyasu H, Yasaka M, et al. Valproate related syndrome of inappropriate secretion of antidiuretic hormone (SIADH)–a case report. *Rinsho Shinkeigaku* 1994;34(9):911–913.

Kando JC, Tohen M, Castillo J, et al. The use of valproate in an elderly population with affective symptoms. *J Clin Psychiatry* 1996;57:238–240.

Lott AD, McElroy SL, Keys MA. Valproate in the treatment of behavioral agitation in elderly patients with dementia. *J Neuropsychiatry Clin Neurosci* 1995;7:314–319.

Mazure CM, Druss BG, Cellar JS. Valproate treatment of older psychotic patients with organic mental syndromes and behavioral dyscontrol. *J Am Geriatr Soc* 1992;40:914–916.

McElroy SL, Keck PE, Pope HG, et al. Valproate in the treatment of rapid cycling bipolar disorder. *J Clin Psychopharmacol* 1988;8:275–279.

McFarland BH, Miller MR, Straumfjord AA. Valproate use in the older manic patient. *J Clin Psychiatry* 1990;51:479–481.

Mellow AM, Solano-Lopez C, Davis S. Sodium valproate in the treatment of behavioral disturbance in dementia. *J Geriatr Psychiatry Neurol* 1993;6:205–209.

Mordecai DJ, Sheikh JI, Glick ID. Divalproex for the treatment of geriatric bipolar disorder. *Int J Geriatr Psychiatry* 1999;14:494–496.

Niedermier JA, Nasrallah HA. Clinical correlates of response to valproate in geriatric inpatients. *Ann Clin Psychiatry* 1998;10:165–168.

Noagiul S, Narayan M, Nelson JC. Divalproex treatment of mania in elderly patients. *Am J Geriatr Psychiatry* 1998;6:257–262.

Perucca E, Grimaldi R, Gatti G, et al. Pharmacokinetics of valproic acid in the elderly. *Br J Clin Pharmacol* 1984;17:665–669.

Pope HG Jr, McElroy SL, Keck PE Jr, et al. Valproate in the treatment of acute mania. A placebo-controlled study. *Arch Gen Psychiatry* 1991;48(1):62–68.

Pope HG Jr, McElroy SL, Satlin A, et al. Head injury, bipolar disorder, and response to valproate. *Compr Psychiatry* 1988;29:34–38.

Puryear LJ, Kunik ME, Workman R Jr. Tolerability of divalproex sodium in elderly psychiatric patients with mixed diagnoses. *J Geriatr Psychiatry Neurol* 1995;8(4):234–237.

Regenold WT, Prasad M. Uses of intravenous valproate in geriatric psychiatry. *Am J Geriatr Psychiatry* 2001;9:306–308.

Risinger RC, Risby ED, Risch SC. Safety and efficacy of divalproex sodium in elderly bipolar patients [Letter]. *J Clin Psychiatry* 1994;55(5):215.

Robinson D, Langer A, Casso D, et al. Pancytopenia and valproic acid–a possible association [Letter]. *J Am Geriatr Soc* 1995;43(2):198.

Schneider AL, Wilcox CS. Divalproate augmentation in lithium-resistant rapid cycling mania in four geriatric patients. *J Affective Disord* 1998;47:201–205.

Shulman KI, Rochon P, Sykora K, et al. Changing prescription patterns for lithium and valproic acid in old age: shifting practice without evidence. *Br Med J* 2003;326:960–961.

Stoll AL, Locke CA, Vuckovic A, et al. Lithium-associated cognitive and functional deficits reduced by a switch to divalproex sodium: a case series. *J Clin Psychiatry* 1996;57:356–359.

Tariot PN, Schneider LS, Jacobo E, et al. Safety and tolerability of divalproex sodium in the treatment of signs and symptoms of mania in elderly patients with dementia: results of a double-blind, placebo-controlled trial. *Current Therapeutic Research* 2001;62:51–67.

Trehan R, Clark CF. Valproic acid-induced truncal weakness and respiratory failure [Letter]. *Am J Psychiatry* 1993;150(8):1271.

Wils V, Goluke-Willemse G: Extrapyramidal syndrome due to valproate administration as an adjunct to lithium in an elderly manic patient (letter). *Int J Geriatr Psychiatry* 1997;12:272–273.

Yassa R, Cvejic J. Valproate in the treatment of post-traumatic bipolar disorder in a psychogeriatric patient. *J Geriatr Psychiatry Neurol* 1994;7(1): 55–57.

Zajecka JM, Weisler R, Sachs G, et al. A comparison of the efficacy, safety, and tolerability of divalproex sodium and olanzapine in the treatment of bipolar disorder. *J Clin Psychiatry* 2002;63: 1148–1155.

Lamotrigine

Bowden CL, Calabrese JR, Sachs G, et al. A placebo-controlled 18-month trial of lamotrigine and lithium maintenance treatment in recently manic or hypomanic patients with bipolar I disorder. *Arch Gen Psychiatry* 2003;60:392–400.

Brodie MJ, Overstall PW, Giorgi L, The UK Lamotrigine Elderly Study Group. Multicentre, double-blind, randomised comparison between lamotrigine and carbamazepine in elderly patients with newly diagnosed epilepsy. *Epilepsy Research* 1999;37:81–87.

Calabrese JR, Bowden CL, Sachs GS, et al. A double-blind placebo-controlled study of lamotrigine monotherapy in outpatients with bipolar I depression. *J Clin Psychiatry* 1999;60:79–88.

Calabrese JR, Shelton MD, Rapport DJ, et al. Long-term treatment of bipolar disorder with lamotrigine. *J Clin Psychiatry* 2002;63(suppl 10):18–22.

Giorgi L, Gomez G, O'Neill F, et al. The tolerability of lamotrigine in elderly patients with epilepsy. *Drugs Aging* 2001;18:621–630.

Carbamazepine

Ballenger JC, Post RM. Carbamazepine in manic-depressive illness: a new treatment. *Am J Psychiatry* 1980;137:782–790.

Greil W, Ludwig-Mayerhofer W, Erazo N, et al. Lithium versus carbamazepine in the maintenance treatment of bipolar disorders: a randomised study. *J Affective Disord* 1997;43:151–161.

Hartong EGTM, Moleman P, Hoogduin CAL, et al. Prophylactic efficacy of lithium versus carbamazepine in treatment-naïve bipolar patients. *J Clin Psychiatry* 2003;64:144–151.

Hemet C, Chassagne P, Levade MH, et al. Aseptic meningitis secondary to carbamazepine treatment of manic-depressive illness [Letter]. *Am J Psychiatry* 1994;151(9):1393.

Kasarskis EJ, Kuo C-S, Berger R, et al. Carbamazepine-induced cardiac dysfunction: characterization of two distinct clinical syndromes. *Arch Intern Med* 1992;152:186–191.

Okuma T, Inanaga K, Otsuki S, et al. A preliminary double-blind study of the efficacy of carbamazepine in prophylaxis of manic-depressive illness. *Psychopharmacology* 1981;73:95–96.

Post RM, Uhde TW, Ballenger JC, et al. Prophylactic efficacy of carbamazepine in manic-depressive illness. *Am J Psychiatry* 1983;140:1602–1604.

Price WA, Zimmer B. Lithium-carbamazepine neu-rotoxicity in the elderly. *J Am Geriatr Soc* 1985;33: 876–877.

Small JG, Klapper MH, Milstein V, et al. Carbamazepine compared with lithium in the treatment of mania. *Arch Gen Psychiatry* 1991;48(10):915–921.

Steckler TL. Lithium- and carbamazepine-associated sinus node dysfunction: nine-year experience in a psychiatric hospital. *J Clin Psychopharmacol* 1994; 14(5):336–339.

Yassa R, Iskandar H, Natase C, et al. Carbamazepine and hyponatremia in patients with affective disorder. *Am J Psychiatry* 1988;145:339–342.

Antipsychotics

Beyer J, Siegal A, Kennedy J, Kaiser C, et al. Olanzapine, divalproex and placebo treatment: non-head-to-head comparisons of older adult acute mania. Tenth Congress of the International Psychogeriatric Association 2001; *Abstract P-170.*

Byerly MJ, Weber MT, Brooks DL, et al. Antipsychotic medications and the elderly: effects on cognition and implications for use. *Drugs Aging* 2001;18:45–61.

Glassman AH, Bigger JT Jr. Antipsychotic drugs: prolonged QTc interval, torsade de pointes, and sudden death. *Am J Psychiatry* 2001;158:1774–1782.

Koro CE, Fedder DO, L'Italien GJ, et al. An assessment of the independent effects of olanzapine and risperidone exposure on the risk of hyperlipidemia in schizophrenic patients. *Arch Gen Psychiatry* 2002;59:1021–1026.

Madhusoodanan S, Brenner R, Cohen CI. Risperidone for elderly patients with schizophrenia or schizoaffective disorder. *Psychiatric Annals* 1999; 30:175–180.

Malhi GS, Berk M. Pharmacotherapy of bipolar disorder: the role of atypical antipsychotics and experimental strategies. *Hum Psychopharmacol Clin Exp* 2002;17:407–412.

Sajatovic M. Clozapine for elderly patients. *Psychiatric Annals* 1999;30:170–174.

Shulman RW, Singh A, Shulman KI. Treatment of elderly institutionalized bipolar patients with clozapine. *Psychopharmacol Bull* 1997;33:113–118.

Street JS, Tollefson GD, Tohen M, et al. Olanzapine for psychotic conditions in the elderly. *Psychiatric Annals* 1999;30:191–196.

Suppes T, Webb A, Paul B, et al. Clinical outcome in a randomized 1-year trial of clozapine versus treatment as usual for patients with treatment-resistant illness and a history of mania. *Am J Psychiatry* 1999;156:1264–1266.

Tohen M, Sanger TM, McElroy SL, et al. Olanzapine versus placebo in the treatment of acute mania. *Am J Psychiatry* 1999;156:702–709.

Tohen M, Jacobs TG, Grundy SL, et al. Efficacy of olanzapine in acute bipolar mania: a double-blind, placebo-controlled study. The Olanzapine HGGW Study Group. *Arch Gen Psychiatry* 2000;57: 841–849.

Tohen M, Baker RW, Altshuler LL, et al. Olanzapine versus divalproex in the treatment of acute mania. *Am J Psychiatry* 2002;159:1011–1017.

Vieta E, Reinares M, Corbella B, et al. Olanzapine as long-term adjunctive therapy in treatment-resistant bipolar disorder. *J Clin Psychopharmacol* 2001;21(5):469–473.

Yeung PP, Tariot PN, Schneider LS, et al. Quetiapine for elderly patients with psychotic disorders. *Psychiatric Annals* 1999;30:197–201.

Other Treatments

American Psychiatric Association. *The Practice of Electroconvulsive Therapy: Recommendations for Treatment, Training, and Privileging: A Task Force Report of the American Psychiatric Association, 2ⁿᵈ ed.* Washington, DC: American Psychiatric Press, 2001.

Aronson TA, Shukla S, Hirschowitz J. Clonazepam treatment of five lithium-refractory patients with bipolar disorder. *Am J Psychiatry* 1989;146:77–80.

Bebchuk JM, Arfken CL, Dolan-Manji S, et al. A preliminary investigation of a protein kinase C inhibitor in the treatment of acute mania. *Arch Gen Psychiatry* 2000;57:95–97.

Burt T, Sachs G, Demopoulos C. Donepezil in treatment-resistant bipolar disorder. *Biol Psychiatry* 1999;45:959–964.

Chouinard G, Young SN, Annable L. Antimanic effects of clonazepam. *Biol Psychiatry* 1983;18: 451–466.

Cummings JL. Cholinesterase inhibitors: expanding applications. *Lancet* 2001;357:1039.

Dubovsky SL, Franks RD, Murphy J. Calcium antagonists in mania; a double-blind study of verapamil. *Psychiatry Res* 1986;18:309–320.

Giannini AJ, Houser WL Jr, Loiselle RH, et al. Antimanic effects of verapamil. *Am J Psychiatry* 1984; 141:1602–1603.

Hardy MC, Lecrubier Y, Widlocher D. Efficacy of clonidine in 24 patients with acute mania. *Am J Psychiatry* 1986;143:1450–1453.

Hellewell JSE. Oxcarbazepine (Trileptal) in the treatment of bipolar disorders: a review of efficacy and tolerability. *J Affective Disord* 2002;72: S23–S34.

McCabe MS. ECT in the treatment of mania: a controlled study. *Am J Psychiatry* 1976;5:191–197.

Mukherjee S, Sackeim HA, Schnur DB. Electroconvulsive therapy of acute manic episodes. *Am J Psychiatry* 1994;151:169–176.

Pecuch PW, Erfurth A. Topiramate in the treatment of acute mania. [Letter] *J Clin Psychopharmacol* 2001;21:243–244.

Prien RF, Gelenberg AJ. Alternatives to lithium for preventive treatment of bipolar disorder. *Am J Psychiatry* 1989;146:840–848.

Robillard M, Conn D. Gabapentin use in geriatric patients with depression and bipolar illness. [Letter] *Can J Psychiatry - Revue Canadienne de Psychiatrie,* 2001;46(8):764.

Salzman C. Electroconvulsive therapy in the elderly patient. *Psychiatr Clin North Am* 1982;5:191–197.

Stoll AL, Severus E, Freeman MP, et al. Omega-3 fatty acids in bipolar disorder. *Arch Gen Psychiatry* 1999;56:407–412.

Suppes T. Review of the use of topiramate for treatment of bipolar disorders. *J Clin Psychopharmacol* 2002;22:599–609.

Drug Interactions

Blanche P, Raynaud E, Kerob D, et al. Lithium intoxication in an elderly patient after combined treatment with losartan [Letter]. *Eur J Clin Pharmacol* 1997;52:501.

Dubovsky SL, Franks RD, Allen S. Verapamil: a new antimanic drug with potential interactions with lithium. *J Clin Psychiatry* 1987;48:371–372.

Guthrie SK, Stoysich AM, Bader G, et al. Hypothesized interaction between valproic acid and warfarin [Letter]. *J Clin Psychopharmacol* 1995;15(2): 138–139.

MacCollum W. Interaction of lithium with phenytoin. *Br Med J* 1980;1:610–611.

McGennis A. Beware of lithium and tetracycline toxicity. *Br Med J* 1978;1:1183.

Price WA, Zimmer B. Lithium-carbamazepine neurotoxicity in the elderly. *J Am Geriatr Soc* 1985;33: 876–877.

Price WA, Shalley JE. Lithium-verapamil toxicity in the elderly. *J Am Geriatr Soc* 1987;35:177–179.

Steckler TL. Lithium- and carbamazepine-associated sinus node dysfunction: nine-year experience in a psychiatric hospital. *J Clin Psychopharmacol* 1994; 14(5):336–339.

Wright JM, Stokes EF, Sweeney VP. Isoniazid-induced carbamazepine toxicity and vice versa. *N Engl J Med* 1982;307:1325–1326.

Electroconvulsive Therapy in Late-Life Depression

Harold A. Sackeim

Electroconvulsive therapy (ECT) plays a significant role in the treatment of late-life depression and other psychiatric conditions in the elderly. Compared to pharmacologic treatments, ECT is administered to an especially high proportion of elderly patients. For example, a survey of practice in California between 1977 and 1983 indicates that the probability of receiving ECT increases markedly with patient age (Figure 1). Of 1.12 persons per 10,000 in the general adult population treated with ECT, 3.86 per 10,000 are aged 65 years or older;[1] treatment with ECT was constant over this period and the high percentage of elderly patients is noteworthy. A national survey of inpatient psychiatric facilities conducted by the National Institute of Mental Health (NIMH) also indicates that patients aged 61 and older comprise the largest age group to receive ECT in 1975 to 1980.[2] In the mid-1970s when use of ECT in the United States had declined, ECT treatment of inpatients aged 61 and over remained constant.[2] Use increased again during the 1980s; in 1986 the national estimate was that 15.6% of inpatients aged 65 or older with mood disorders received ECT, compared with only 3.4% of younger inpatients with mood disorders.[3]

Data from the most comprehensive national study of factors associated with inpatient use of ECT, published in 1998, estimated that nearly 10% of a sample of nearly 25,000 depressed inpatients received ECT during their hospital stay.[4] (Figure 2) Factors most strongly predicting ECT use were age, race, insurance status, and median income of the patient's home zip code. Older patients, Caucasians, and those with private insurance living in affluent areas were most likely to be treated with ECT. Diagnosis rather than age, however, is the primary indication for the use of ECT. The vast majority of patients treated with ECT in the United States were experiencing an episode of major depression, either unipolar or bipolar. The NIMH national diagnostic survey conducted in 1986 reveals that 84% of patients who receive ECT are diagnosed with a major mood disorder.[3] The primary factors leading to consideration of ECT, regardless of age, are (1) a history of inadequate response or intolerance to antidepressant medication or (2) a history of good ECT response during prior depressive episodes.[5-7] ECT is administered less frequently for schizophrenia[8] and mania.[9]

Among patients of all ages, ECT is more effective and more likely to produce symptom remission than antidepressant medication.[10-15] The extent to which ECT is used early or late in the course of antidepressant treatment varies markedly from country to country and, within the United States, varies considerably among localities and practitioners.[16,17] ECT is particularly beneficial when elderly depressed patients are also medically ill, psychotic, or suicidal. Thus, ECT is most frequently administered to geriatric patients when anti-

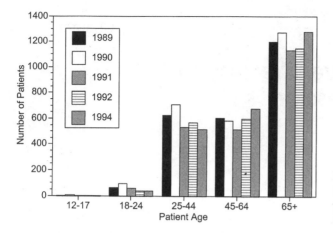

Figure 13.1. Patients treated with ECT in California, by age group and year; data for 1993 were unavailable.

depressant medications are too risky, have proven ineffective, or when ensuring a rapid or full clinical response is particularly important.

Indications for ECT

ECT is indicated for the acute treatment of depression as well as for maintenance treatment and prevention of relapse. Clinical outcome of ECT is more predictable in patients exhibiting particular characteristics of major depression. As with phar-

macologic treatment, duration of the depressive episode consistently correlates with a positive ECT response: patients (of all ages) with longer duration of illness respond less well.[18–24] This relation between duration of illness and treatment response may reflect the impact of depression in CNS functioning. Duration of a depressed state correlates with the extent of hippocampal atrophy associated with chronic depression. Because the hippocampus has an established role in regulating the hypothalamic–pituitary—adrenal

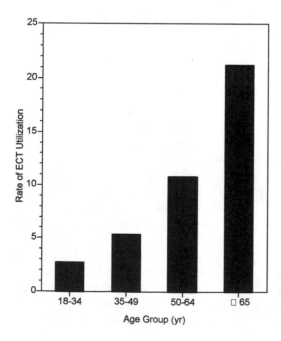

Figure 13.2. Rate of ECT utilization in a sample representative of inpatients in the US in 1993 with a diagnosis of recurrent, major depression. (From Olfson, et al. 1998.)[4]

(HPA) axis, the atrophic effects of depression may lead to increased vulnerability to stress and prolongation of the episode. Patients with hippocampal atrophy are especially resistant to antidepressant medications, particularly tricyclics. Poor response to antidepressants, in turn, predicts/correlates with inferior short-term response to ECT[18,25–27] as well as to other somatic treatments.[28,29] ECT is likely to be of greatest value when it is administered early in the course of a depressive episode and not as a last resort after all other treatments have failed.

Maintenance ECT, with treatments spaced over weekly to monthly intervals, is increasingly used for relapse prevention.[30–32] Unfortunately, continuation or maintenance ECT is commonly employed only after pharmacologic methods of relapse prevention have failed following successful ECT. At present, the vast majority of patients who respond to ECT are then treated with antidepressant medications despite evidence that failed medication regimens during the acute depressive episode are ineffective in preventing relapse following ECT.[24,26,30,33,34]

Efficacy

Overall, research observations and clinical experience indicate that ECT is particularly useful in the treatment of late-life depression. Prior to the introduction of ECT, elderly depressed individuals often exhibited chronic depression or died of intercurrent medical illnesses in psychiatric institutions.[35] A number of studies contrast the clinical outcome of depressed patients who received inadequate or no somatic treatment to that of patients who received ECT (Figure 3) While none of this work involves prospective, random-assignment designs, the findings are largely uniform. Contemporary ECT administered to elderly patients results in decreased chronicity, decreased morbidity, and possible decreased rates of mortality.[36–39]

Studies comparing ECT to other forms of antidepressant treatment[15,40] are relatively sparse. A metaanalysis of early comparative-age patient samples[11] reports that the average response rate to ECT is 20% higher when compared to tricyclic antidepressants (TCAs) and 45% higher when compared to monoamine oxidase inhibitors (MAOIs), although by modern standards, the pharmacologic treatments used were often suboptimal.[18,33,41,42] No study has ever found a pharmacologic regimen to be superior in antidepressant effects when compared to ECT. Rather, ECT consistently has had either equal or superior efficacy. In both young and elderly populations, ECT is superior to a standard antidepressant,[15] although the addition of lithium to an antidepressant results in more rapid onset of improvement compared to ECT in patients with treatment-resistant depression.[40,43,44]

Other differences between ECT and antidepressant treatments concern speed and quality of clinical response as well as residual symptoms. Residual symptomatology resulting from incomplete response to antidepressant medications may become chronic or lead to relapse.[45] Because remission is more likely following ECT, there is less chance of recurrence of chronic residual depressive symptoms.

Whether ECT reduces depressive symptoms more quickly than antidepressants in the elderly has not been adequately tested. Nonetheless, evidence suggests that no pharmacologic strategy results in as rapid symptomatic improvement as ECT.[10,12,13] Significant clinical improvement is usually seen within the first few treatments, with maximal gains seen by 3 weeks. This rapid improvement is less common with antidepressant medications.

Aging and Efficacy

The response rate to ECT is higher among older patients,[46–49] and a positive association is seen between patient age and degree of clinical improvement following

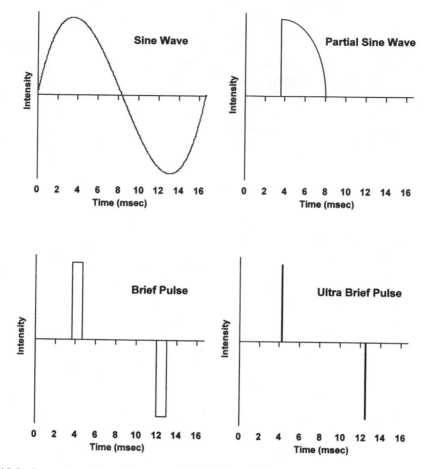

Figure 13.3. Examples of waveforms used in ECT. Top left: sine wave. Top right: chopped, rectified sine wave. Bottom left: brief pulse, square wave. Bottom right: ultra-brief pulse, square wave. (From Sackeim HA, Long J, Luber B, et al. Physical properties and quantification of the ECT stimulus: I. Basic principles. *Convuls Ther* 1994;10:93–123).

ECT.[46–49] Table 13.1 provides a selective summary of studies addressing the relation between patient age and ECT outcome. Older individuals, however, may have a diminished response to unilateral, as opposed to bilateral, ECT[50,51] and may require longer courses of treatment to achieve the same level of remission as younger patients.[52,53] ECT may also be effective in the very oldest depressed patients.[54–57]

Predictors of Response

Two factors correlate with response to ECT in the elderly: intensity of the electrical stimulus, and the patient's diagnosis.

The extent to which the intensity of the electroconvulsive stimulus exceeds the individual patient's seizure threshold determines the efficacy of right unilateral ECT and speed of response regardless of electrode placement.[58–62] Age is one of the more reliable predictors of seizure threshold[62–64]: the oldest patients generally have the highest thresholds, shortest seizure duration, and lowest EEG seizure amplitude.[60,65,66]

In addition to stimulus intensity, evidence shows that among depressed patients, those with psychotic or delusional depression respond especially well to ECT.[25,30,67–72] Although not definitively

Table 13.1.   Relation Between Patient Age and ECT Outcome: Selected Studies

Study[*]	Patients	Study Design	ECT Treatment	Results/Comments
Prudic et al. (2004)	347 patients with major depression treated at 7 hospitals in the New York metropolitan area	Prospective, naturalistic study of ECT practices and outcomes in community settings; evaluations before, immediately after, and monthly for 6 months following ECT	Modified ECT given 3 times/week; diverse electrode placement and dosing practices	Age, treated as a continuous variable, not related to symptom improvement or categorical clinical outcomes
O'Connor et al. (2001)	253 patients with major depression, treated openly with titrated (50% above seizure threshold) bilateral ECT	Prospective naturalistic acute phase study followed by double-blind continuation trial comparing nortriptyline and lithium with continuation ECT; acute response to ECT contrasted in 3 patient groups: young adult (<45 years), older adult (46 to 64 years) and elderly (65 years and older)	Modified ECT given 3 times/week; patients titrated at first session and treated afterward with suprathreshold intensity 50% above threshold	Lower remission (70%) in youngest age group than either older adults (89.8%) or elderly (90%); when these dimensions were treated as continuous variables, age was also related to outcome.
Sackeim et al. (2000)	80 inpatients with major depression randomized to 4 groups (right unilateral at 1.5, 2.5, or 6 times seizure threshold or bilateral ECT at 2.5 times seizure threshold); free of all medications except lorazepam (up to 3 mg/day PRN)	Double-blind, prospective study of effects of electrical dosage and electrode placement; patients evaluated before ECT and regularly during and after treatment course	Modified ECT given 3 times/week; patients randomized to 3 forms of right unilateral ECT (1.5, 2.5, or 6 × seizure threshold) or bilateral ECT (2.5 × ST)	High dosage right unilateral ECT (6 × threshold) and bilateral ECT (2.5 × threshold) equal in efficacy and superior to lower dosage right unilateral ECT; no age-related effects

(continued)

Table 13.1. (continued).

Study*	Patients	Study Design	ECT Treatment	Results/Comments
Tew et al. (1999)	268 patients with major depression, treated openly with suprathreshold unilateral or bilateral ECT; free of all medications except lorazepam (up to 3 mg/day PRN)	Prospective naturalistic acute phase study followed by double-blind continuation pharmacotherapy trial; acute response to ECT contrasted in 3 patient groups: adult (59 years and younger), young-old (60 to 74 years) and old-old (75 years and older)	Modified ECT given 3 times/week; patients titrated at first session and treated with suprathreshold intensity selected by treating psychiatrist	More physical illness and cognitive impairment in both older age groups than in adult group. Both older groups had shorter depressive episodes and were less likely to be medication resistant. The adult patients had a lower rate of ECT response (54%) than the young-old patients (73%), while the old-old patients had an intermediate rate of response (67%).
Sackeim et al. (1993)	96 inpatients with major depression randomized to 4 groups (unilateral or bilateral ECT at low- or high-stimulus intensity); free of all medications except lorazepam (up to 3 mg/day PRN); age range, 22–80; mean, 56.4	Double-blind, prospective study of effects of electrical dosage and electrode placement; patients evaluated before ECT and regularly during and after treatment course	Modified ECT given 3 times/week; patients titrated at first session and treated either at just above threshold or at 2.5 times initial seizure threshold	Electrical dosage determined unilateral ECT efficacy and speed of response for unilateral and bilateral ECT; no age-related effects seen.
Black et al. (1993)	423 depressed inpatients between 1970 and 1981	Retrospective chart review using multiple logistic regression to identify response predictors	Modified ECT given 3 times/week; bilateral, unilateral, mixed courses included	Patients rated as recovered (n = 295) older than those rated as unrecovered (n = 128)

Study	Sample	Method	Treatment	Results
Sackeim et al. (1987a, b)	52 inpatients with major depression randomized to unilateral or bilateral ECT; patients free of all medications except lorazepam (up to 3 mg/day PRN); age range, 25–83; mean, 61.3	Double-blind, prospective study comparing low-dose, titrated bilateral and unilateral ECT; patients evaluated before ECT and following treatments 1, 3, 5, 6 and every treatment thereafter	Bilateral or right unilateral modified ECT 3 times/week; patients titrated and treated at just above threshold	Low-dosage right unilateral ECT ineffective; regardless of ECT modality, age unrelated to clinical outcome
Coryell & Zimmerman (1984)	31 patients with unipolar depression selected prospectively	Prospective study of ECT response predictors; ratings made on HAM-D at weekly intervals by blind raters	Most treatments unilateral; most patients had at least 6 treatments; patients with fewer than 4 treatments excluded	Age independently associated with outcome on more than 1 of 3 outcome measures; superior outcome in older patients
Rich et al. (1984)	Data from 2 groups of patients pooled: 66 with major depressive episode or organic affective syndrome; antidepressant medications either stopped prior to ECT or held constant	Prospective study of response rate to conventional ECT by identifying point of maximal improvement; patients rated on HAM-D before first ECT and at 36–48 hours after each treatment	Modified ECT given 3 times/week; right unilateral ECT used >80% of patients; mean no. of treatments for each of 2 groups 8.6 and 8.3	Age associated with longer time to achieve response; study flawed by use of different rating scales and different ECT devices for 2 groups
Fraser & Glass (1980)	29 depressed (Feigner criteria) elderly (64–86 years) randomized to unilateral or bilateral ECT	Prospective, double-blind, randomized study; postictal recovery times, memory changes, and clinical improvement assessed by HAM-D	Modified ECT with twice-weekly treatment until patient well or ECT stopped	No age difference between good and moderate outcome groups
Heshe et al. (1978)	51 patients with endogenous depression randomized to unilateral or bilateral ECT	Prospective blind evaluations before ECT, at end of ECT, and 3 months after final treatment	Either modified unilateral (average 9.2 treatments) or bilateral ECT (average 8.5 treatments), twice weekly, number of treatments decided by treating clinician	In patients over 60, significantly better therapeutic effect from bilateral than unilateral treatment; regardless of modality, satisfactory results in 75% of patients >60 years and 96% of patients <60 years–a significant difference

(continued)

Table 13.1. (continued).

Study*	Patients	Study Design	ECT Treatment	Results/Comments
Herrington et al. (1974)	43 consecutive severely depressed patients (aged 25–69) randomized to ECT or l-tryptophan (up to 8 g/day); 40 patients included in efficacy analysis	Patients rated on day before treatment and weekly thereafter for 4 weeks	ECT given twice weekly for total of 6–8 treatments	Age unrelated to outcome
Strömgren (1974)	100 patients with endogenous unipolar or bipolar depression; aged 19–65; patients drug-free except for hypnotics and mild sedatives	Prospective, double-blind study contrasting unilateral and bilateral ECT	Minimum of 6 treatments given; duration of current individualized; average of 9 treatments given to younger patients, 8.7 to older patients	Of 53 patients aged 19–44, 17 were resistant; 7 of 47 aged 45–65 were resistant–a significant difference efficacy superior in older patients for both bilateral and unilateral ECT
Folstein et al. (1973)	118 consecutive patients who received ECT; diagnoses of schizophrenia, neurotic reactions, and affective disorders	Retrospective chart review: progress notes at time of discharge rated as to whether or not patient improved	Nature and duration of ECT not described	Improvement related to older age and shorter hospital stay; no significance tests provided; mean age of improved patients (n = 86) 50, compared with 31 inpatients rated not improved (n = 32)
Mendels (1965a, 1965b)	53 consecutive inpatients evaluated pre-ECT and 1 and 3 months post-ECT; age 21–76, mean 48.8	Prospective study: patients rated with HAM-D; evaluators not blind to treatment history	4–11 treatments (mean 6.4) with modified ECT	Superior outcome in patients over 50 at 3-month follow-up but not at 1-month follow-up
Carney et al. (1965)	129 depressed inpatients	Prospective study to establish predictive factors; patients scored for presence or absence of 35 features, followed up at 3 and 6 months post-ECT; outcome criteria defined	Patients received 3 or more treatments	Better response in endogenous depressives at 3 and 6 months (per factor analysis); in patients over 40, type of depression not associated with outcome

Study	Sample	Study design	ECT procedure	Findings
Nystrom (1964)	2 series of patients: 254 in Gothenburg series, 188 in Lund; most cases depressed but other diagnoses included	Prospective, blind evaluation; outcome criteria specified	Modified bilateral ECT at 2 treatments/week initially; average number in Lund series 6.9, 4.4 in Gothenberg	Lund series: positive association between age and degree of improvement in females; Gothenberg series: age <25 years negatively related to outcome
Greenblatt et al. (1962)	128 patients randomized to 4 treatment groups; diagnosis of schizophrenia, psychoneurotic and psychotic depressive reactions, involutional psychosis; 28 received ECT; age 16–70, mean 46	Prospective study compared ECT and antidepressant medications; explicit outcome criteria used	ECT modified by succinylcholine given 3/weekly for 3 weeks minimum, more at discretion of psychiatrist	Medications and ECT equally effective in youngest age group; ECT significantly more effective than medications in oldest age group
Ottoson (1960)	44 (18 males, 26 females) with endogenous depression; age 36–70, mean 55.8	Prospective study with blind raters; efficacy evaluated by outcome 1 week after 4th treatment, 1 week after end of ECT course, and total number of treatments required	Modified bilateral ECT with intervals between first 3 treatments of 2–4 days and between following treatments of 3–7 days; dose adjusted upward for age; patients divided into 2 groups: one received stimulus grossly above threshold, one moderately above threshold	Age not significantly related to efficacy; therapeutic response later in older patients
Hamilton & White (1960)	49 hospitalized male patients with severe depression; age range 21–69, mean 51.7	Patients assessed prospectively and 1 month after end of ECT	Usual course 6 treatments, maximum 10; 14 patients had second course	Age unrelated to Outcome
Roberts (1959a,b)	50 patients, women 41–60 years	Prospective study of predictors of ECT response; patients scored on clinical features prior to ECT and presence or absence of symptoms at 1 and 3 months post-ECT	Twice weekly modified ECT until maximum benefit; averaged between 7 and 8 treatments	Symptom scores at 1 month: significant inverse correlation with age (older women more improved); no correlation at 3 months

(continued)

Table 13.1. (continued).

Study*	Patients	Study Design	ECT Treatment	Results/Comments
Herzberg (1954)	227 cases selected from all patients who had received ECT; diagnoses of schizophrenia, manic depressive psychoses, involutional melancholia	Retrospective chart review of patients rated for initial response to ECT, continued response, no relapse after discharge	Nature and duration of ECT not described	Superior outcome or sustained improvement in patients in 4th decade compared with patients in other age groups
Hobson (1953)	150 patients at Maudsley Hospital; no diagnostic criteria used, but almost all cases were depressed; 127 included in analyses	Prospective study to identify predictors of ECT response; patients categorized as either free of symptoms or still having marked symptoms after ECT	Nature and number of ECT treatments not described	Age unrelated to outcome; several other predictors identified
Rickles & Polan (1948)	200 private patients treated with ECT; diverse diagnostic categories included schizophrenia	Retrospective study of why patients failed ECT; treatment considered failed when improvement not maintained for at least 1 year	Usual course 10–12 treatments; patients with schizophrenia also received 24–40 subcoma insulin shocks	Authors felt that ECT failed if patient was menopausal or postmenopausal; statistics not presented
Gold & Chiarello (1944)	121 consecutive male patients, 103 diagnosed as schizophrenic; age range 15–60	Prospective study of outcome predictors and outcome; patients placed in 1 of 4 categories from *much improved* to *no change*	Type and number of treatments not described	Superior clinical outcome in older age groups

* Complete reference citations at end of chapter.

established, it is also probable that, among patients who receive ECT, the elderly have a lower rate of comorbid Axis II pathology (e.g., personality disorders), which further contributes to a superior ECT response rate.[24,73]

ECT Treatment of Psychotic Depression

ECT is a primary treatment for patients with psychotic depression due to the severity of the disorder, the high rate of response to ECT, and relative poor rate of response to antidepressant monotherapy.[5,30] In mixed-age samples, approximately 30 to 40% of depressed patients who receive ECT present with psychotic depression.[27,67] This rate is likely higher among the elderly, who are more likely to present with psychotic depression than younger patients.[74,75]

Between 20 and 45% of hospitalized elderly depressed patients present with psychotic depression.[76–78] Typically, the elderly patient with psychotic features has severe depressive illness, although the overall severity of late-life depression does not invariably indicate psychosis. Identifying psychotic features in elderly depressed patients is essential because these individuals are at considerably high risk for suicide.[21,79,80]

Psychotic depression is often underrecognized, particularly in the elderly. A telltale sign of psychotic depression is found in the elderly patient who denies being depressed despite psychomotor retardation, anorexia, markedly diminished social interactions, or other symptoms of depression. Further complicating identification of psychotic depression is the need to distinguish between overvalued ideas (''near-delusional states'') and true delusions. Delusions are significantly more common than hallucinations in the geriatric patient with psychosis. In the elderly patient, greater difficulty also occurs in distinguishing between hypochondriasis and somatic delusions because of the common preoccupation with health in older people. Mood-incongruent delu-sions or hallucinations, whose content is inconsistent with depressive themes, are a consistent feature of psychotic depression. Some elderly patients, however, deny delusions, making diagnosis of psychotic depression more difficult. Since mood-incongruent features may be more common among younger depressed patients and/or those with bipolar depression, the presence of mood-incongruent psychotic features in an elderly patient should trigger consideration of possible bipolarity or an organic affective disorder.

Evidence that the manifestations of psychotic depression tend to be consistent from episode to episode suggests a trait-like quality.[81–83] Furthermore, psychotic depression appears to be inherited, with relatives sharing the same psychotic content.[84,85] Psychotic depression is more frequent in bipolar compared to unipolar depression.[75] However psychotic depression that appears as a first episode after age 50 is frequently unipolar in course. Compared with unipolar depression, the elderly bipolar patient with psychotic depression more frequently experiences psychomotor retardation and sleep disturbance.

Particularly difficult to treat, late-onset psychotic depression is not only subject to a relapsing course; it may lead to later development of dementia.[82,86] Distinguishing between delusions of dementia as opposed to psychotic depression may be problematic. In contrast to the delusions of psychotic depression, the patient with an organic psychotic affective disorder usually has delusions that are less systematized and less congruent with depressive themes whereas the delusions accompanying psychotic depression are usually highly organized and reflect unrealistic or bizarre ideas about somatic illness, nihilism, persecution, guilt, or jealousy. However, the elderly patient with psychotic depression is particularly subject to gross global cognitive deterioration (''pseudodementia''), which reverses with successful treatment of the mood disorder.[87] Evidence also suggests that such patients later develop a dementing illness.[88]

Elderly patients with psychotic depression respond less positively to pharmacologic treatment (particularly monotherapy) but more positively to ECT than nonpsychotic patients.[89] Specific delusions, in addition to vegetative or melancholic symptoms, predict favorable response,[19,70,90–93] as may psychomotor disturbance.[67,94] In elderly patients with psychotic depression, observation of early resolution of delusions, appetite and sleep disruption, with later improvement in subjective mood and feelings of self-worth is common. Certain delusional elements (bizarreness, effect on behavior, strength of delusional conviction, insight into delusional thoughts) may take longer to improve, with gradual recession during the course of ECT.

Traditionally, bilateral ECT has been the standard treatment for elderly pa-

tients with psychotic depression. However, recent experience suggests that high-dosage right unilateral ECT is at least as effective as bilateral ECT, with less long-term amnesia, which usually accompanies bilateral electrode placement. In the case of right unilateral ECT, high dosage is defined as treatment at least 6 times the seizure threshold. In the case of bilateral ECT, high dosage is defined as 2.5 times the seizure threshold (Figure 4).

The average number of ECT treatments given to patients of all ages in the United States in previous years for major depression was approximately 6; at present, the average is approximately 8 to 9 (possibly indicating increasing ECT treatment resistance) and the use of lower-intensity stimulation. Some depressed patients only begin to show clinical benefit after an extended ECT course, i.e., 10 to 12 treatments. Other elderly depressed patients with psychosis who do not im-

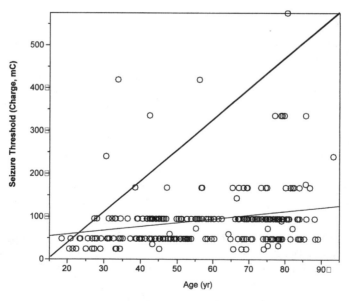

Figure 13.4. Initial seizure threshold as a function of age for 245 patients treated with right unilateral ECT (From Boylon LS, Haskett RF, Mulsant BH, et al. Determinants of seizure threshold in ECT: benzodiazepine use, anesthetic dosage, and other factors. *JECT* 2000;16:3–18). The line at the diagonal represents the dosage patients would receive based on age-based dosing, e.g., 50% of device output for 50-year-old. The lower line is the fit of the regression of age on seizure threshold. While there is a significant relationship (r = 0.19 for raw values), there is marked variability. Dosing based solely on age provides a poor approximation of dosing needs and results in the greatest over-dosing in the oldest age patients.

prove after a standard course of bilateral ECT may subsequently show rapid improvement with extended treatment. For the elderly patient with psychotic depression who shows slow or insufficient response to ECT, the addition of a neuroleptic, especially the newer second-generation antipsychotic drugs clozapine and risperidone, may augment treatment response.[95–99]

Medical Complications and Relative Contraindications

Rates of medical complications among elderly patients during the course of ECT range from 0 to 77% for one or more complications.[20,46,54,57,100–114] This wide variability reflects different definitions of "complication" as well as differences in the medical status of patient samples. Nonetheless, ECT-related medical complications are considerably more likely in the elderly, particularly in the oldest age subgroups, especially among patients with reexisting medical conditions.

ECT and Medical Illness Risks

The rate of ECT-associated mortality is very low among patients of all ages (estimated as about 1 per 10,000 mixed-aged patients treated), which is comparable to mortality rates from general anesthesia in minor surgery.[5,48,115] ECT may be a safer therapeutic treatment than the older TCA medications, particularly for the frail elderly.[5,47,116] Although there are no absolute medical contraindications for ECT,[5,117] risks for the elderly increase with the following conditions:

- space-occupying cerebral lesion
- recent intracerebral hemorrhage
- increased intracranial pressure
- recent myocardial infarction with instable cardiac function
- unstable vascular aneurysm or malformation
- pheochromocytoma

Cardiovascular Illness

Cardiovascular complications are the leading cause of mortality and significant morbidity with ECT, especially for geriatric patients.[5,100,118] The peripheral hemodynamic and cerebrovascular changes during and following the brief seizure are typically well tolerated, even in the frail elderly, despite their intensity. Prophylactic use of beta-adrenergic blocking agents, such as labetalol or esmolol, lessen the hypertensive and tachycardic effects of seizure induction.[119–124] Other agents that are similarly used include nitrates[125], hydralazine[126,127] calcium channel blockers,[128–132] diazoxide,[133] and ganglionic blockers (e.g., trimethaphan).[134] In recent years, a growing number of centers routinely use propofol as the anesthesia-induction agent, rather than methohexital or thiopental, partly because propofol results in less severe hemodynamic changes.[135–147]

Conservative clinical practice should guide the use of pharmacologic modifications of standard ECT in elderly patients. In 2001, an APA Task Force Report on ECT[5] recommended fully blocking the hemodynamic changes that accompany seizure induction for all treatments in patients who are unequivocally at increased risk for complications. In patients with unstable hypertension or cardiac conditions for whom ECT is not being considered an emergency treatment, clinicians should attempt to stabilize the medical condition before beginning ECT and closely monitor cardiovascular changes during initial treatments. If sustained hypertension and/or significant arrhythmia occur following seizure induction, prophylactic medication may be used for subsequent treatments.[100]

Cognitive Side Effects

Serious short- and long-term cognitive impairment is the primary side effect of ECT in the elderly, which argues against aggressive use in this population.[5,148,149] Prior to treatment, elderly depressed patients often exhibit deficits in acquiring information, which is mostly related to disturbances in attention and concentration as indicated by tests of immediate recall or recognition-of-item lists.[150–153]

Clinically, depressed elderly patients complain of pronounced problems with attention and concentration. ECT causes a new deficit in consolidation or retention so that newly learned information is rapidly forgotten[154] due to interrupted function of the medial temporal lobe.[155–161] During and following a course of ECT, elderly patients may also display retrograde amnesia (memory for events in the past, prior to receiving ECT). Deficits in the recall or recognition of both personal and general information are usually greatest for events that occurred closest to the treatment.[162–165] Both anterograde and retrograde amnesia are most marked for explicit or declarative memory, whereas no effect is expected on implicit or procedural memory.[166–168]

Patients vary considerably both in the severity of postictal cognitive changes and in speed of recovery. Specific postictal deficits may reflect a more intense form of the amnesia observed following the ECT course. For example, the disorientation with regard to identity, place, and time seen in the postictal state has been viewed as a form of rapidly shrinking retrograde amnesia (Figure 5).[169,170] Elderly patients often "age" with progressive recovery from disorientation. When first asked his or her age, the 80-year old patient frequently answers to being 20 years old; with repeated questioning, the correct age is eventually given, reflecting a remarkably rapid resolution of retrograde amnesia. Similarly, patients often revert to their mother tongue on awakening and only gradually return to English. Thus the severity of postictal disorientation predicts the degree of amnesia following termination of ECT.[169] Cognitive improvement after a course of ECT follows a sequential temporal pattern. Organic mental syndromes typically resolve within 2 to 10 days post-ECT.[171]

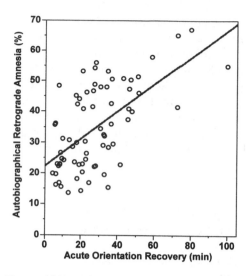

Figure 13.5. Relationship between the duration of acute postictal disorientation and retrograde amnesia for autobiographical information during the week following the ECT course. (From Sobin, et al. 1995, Reference 169.)

Recovery of cognitive function following a single ECT treatment is rapid, although in the immediate postictal period following ECT patients may manifest transient neurologic abnormalities, alterations of consciousness (disorientation, attentional dysfunction), sensorimotor abnormalities, and disturbance in the higher cognitive functions, particularly learning and memory.[148] Within several days following the course of ECT treatments, the cognitive functioning of an elderly patient slows or is typically unchanged. Occasionally immediate memory improves: change in clinical state is the critical predictor of the degree of subsequent improvements in cognition.[27,59,151,154] Following a typical course of ECT, patients of all ages often manifest a marked disturbance in their ability to retain information, reflecting ECT effects on impaired anterograde learning (the forming of new memories).[148] As the treatment series progresses, recovery of cognition in the elderly patient is often incomplete by the time of the next treatment,[20,110,170—173] causing progressive cognitive deterioration, and, in some elderly patients, an organic mental syndrome characterized by marked disorientation.[170,174] The development of a severe organic mental syndrome often results in interruption or premature termination of ECT since patients, relatives, and clinicians are unwilling to risk further deterioration of mental status functioning.[175]

Within days of ECT termination, elderly depressed patients often manifest superior cognitive performance relative to their pretreatment baseline. Intelligence test scores for all age groups, including the elderly, may even be higher shortly after ECT relative to scores in the untreated depressed state.[148,176] More than a week or two following the end of the ECT course, differences in the cognitive effects of bilateral and right unilateral electrode placements are difficult to discern in domains other than retrograde amnesia.[27,59,148,164,165] Early evidence of improved cognition following ECT is manifested in patients' activities. After a few treatments with ECT, elderly individuals may begin to read books, attend group meetings, and become capable of following complex instructions. However, despite this improvement in attention and concentration, elderly patients still may not retain information after a brief time period. This anterograde amnesia typically resolves within a few weeks of ECT termination.[59,148] It is doubtful that ECT alone ever causes a persistent deficit in anterograde amnesia.[59,177] Not infrequently, elderly inpatients will repeatedly request information about a pass for the weekend or an expected visit from a relative whereas memory for more remote events is intact. Patients may have difficulty recalling events that occurred during treatment, and months or, in rare instances, years prior to the ECT course.[178]

Retrograde amnesia gradually disappears so that over time more distant memories, seemingly "forgotten" immediately following the treatment course, subsequently return.[163,165,177,179] However, in some patients amnestic effects of ECT persist,[27,163,165] most likely due to a combination of retrograde and anterograde effects. Patients vary considerably in the degree of cognitive impairment, regardless of how ECT is administered.

Individual Correlates of Cognitive Dysfunction

Two key clinical questions arise regarding ECT-induced cognitive impairment: (1), are there signs during the ECT course that predict which patients will develop more severe and/or persistent short- and long-term cognitive deficits and (2), can we identify the patients most at risk for severe and/or persistent amnesia prior to the start of ECT?

Over the 70-year history of convulsive therapy, numerous investigations of the technical factors that influence the degree of cognitive side effects have been conducted. Surprisingly, only in the last few years has investigation focused on the patient factors that predict the variability in these deficits. Some patients will take twice or three times as long to reorient and be capable of leaving the recovery room; others will develop an organic mental syndrome, a continuous confusional state.[170,171] Although rapid improvement in global cognitive status immediately following termination of ECT will occur, patients with prolonged postictal disorientation are likely to develop the most severe and persistent retrograde amnesia.

A range of retrospective studies indicates that patient age and medical status are also predictors of the development of persistent confusion during the ECT course.[20,57,103,110,111,113,175,180] Older patients and those with compromised medical status are most at risk for prolonged confusion during the course of ECT. Older depressed patients experience more severe anterograde and retrograde amnesia immediately following the end of ECT relative to younger patients, with some differences persisting at one-month follow-up.[181] Elderly patients with preexisting cognitive impairment, even outside the context of frank neurologic disease, are at risk for more prolonged retrograde amnesia and require appropriate modification of ECT technique to lessen cognitive deficit (see Table 13.2). Global cognitive impairment seen in the depressed state also increases vulnerability for the amnestic effects of seizure induction. For example, elderly pseudodemented patients[87] often show dramatic improvement in global cognitive status during and following ECT but are at increased risk for more prolonged and deeper amnesia. Consequently, baseline cognitive impairment in the elderly depressed patient may denote a subgroup whose memory function is more fragile and likely to be affected by ECT.

Technical Administration

A variety of technical factors associated with ECT administration determine the degree and persistence of the cognitive side effects. These include the nature of electrical waveform, anatomic positioning of stimulating electrodes (electrode placement), electrical stimulus intensity, spacing or frequency of treatments, total number of treatments, duration of seizures, type and dosage of anesthetic agent, adequacy of oxygenation, and use of concomitant medications.[5,148] Table 13.2 summarizes the steps that can be taken to minimize cognitive side effects by altering ECT technique.

In recent years, sine wave stimulation has been replaced by standard brief-pulse stimulus, which dramatically reduces the acute cognitive side effects of ECT. (see Figure 6) Another recent modification, ultrabrief pulse stimulation, reduces adverse cognitive effects.[182–185] Ultrabrief pulse (0.3 ms) right unilateral ECT administered at 6 times initial seizure threshold is comparable in efficacy to standard pulse width (1.5 ms), bilateral (2.5 × ST), or right unilateral (6 × ST) ECT. In contrast, ultrabrief pulse (2.5 × ST) bilateral ECT lacks efficacy and has markedly inferior therapeutic effects than right unilateral ECT. Because ultrabrief right unilateral ECT (0.3 ms and 6 × ST) is highly effective and has a profoundly reduced side-effect profile, it is likely to become widely adopted as the "standard" ECT treatment.

Electrode Placement and Cognitive Dysfunction

Over the past 30 years, one of the most controversial aspects of ECT administration has been the anatomic positioning of stimulating electrodes, specifically the use of bilateral and right unilateral ECT. This debate has centered on possible differences in efficacy as well as experience suggesting that bilateral ECT accentuates long-term amnesia.[48,149,186,187] That bilateral ECT results in more profound acute and short-term cognitive impairment rather than right unilateral ECT is widely recognized.[148] In the immediate postictal period, the duration of disorientation will be considerably longer after bilateral relative to right unilateral ECT positioning.[59,169,170,188] During treatment and in the days following ECT termination, bilateral ECT will result in greater retrograde amnesia for personal and general information.[59,163–165] Anterograde amnesia—verbal memory in particular—will also be greater following bilateral ECT.[59,151,165,189] Compared to depressed patients treated with medications, patients treated with right unilateral ECT do not show greater retrograde amnesia for autobiographical information 6 months after the ECT course.[165]

Bilateral ECT is usually reserved for psychiatric or medical emergency or for medically high-risk patients for whom the number of treatments must be minimized. When bilateral ECT is administered, a switch to right unilateral ECT should be considered for patients exhibiting substantial clinical progress but unacceptable cognitive side effects. When right unilateral ECT is ineffective, increased stimulus dosage should be considered before a switch back to bilateral ECT.

Stimulus Dosing and Seizure Threshold

Three factors reliably predict seizure threshold: electrode placement, gender, and age.[60–62,190–192] In males relative to females, and in older patients, seizure threshold is higher with bilateral place-

Table 13.2. Treatment Technique Factors and Severity of Cognitive Side Effects

Treatment Factor	Effects on Cognitive Parameters	Methods to Reduce Cognitive Side Effects	References[a]
Stimulus waveform	Sine wave stimulation grossly increases cognitive side effects	Use square wave, brief pulse stimulation	Weiner et al. (1986) Daniel & Crovitz (1983a) Valentine et al. (1968)
Electrode placement	Standard bilateral (bifrontotemporal) ECT results in more widespread, severe, and persistent cognitive side effects	Switch to right unilateral ECT	McElhiney et al. (1995) Sackeim et al. (2000, 1993, 1996) Weiner et al. (1986) Daniel & Crovitz (1983b)
Stimulus dosage	Grossly suprathreshold stimulus intensity increases acute and short-term cognitive side effects	Adjust stimulus intensity to needs of individual patients by dosage titration	Sobin et al. (1995) Sackeim et al. (1993) Sackeim et al. (1986) Squire & Zouzounis (1986)
Number of treatments	Progressive cognitive decline with high-intensity treatments (sine wave, bilateral, or grossly suprathreshold)	Limit treatments to number necessary to achieve maximal clinical gains	Calev et al. (1991) Sackeim et al. (1986) Daniel & Crovitz (1983a) Fraser & Glass (1978, 1980)
Frequency of treatments	More frequent treatments (3–5 per week) result in greater cognitive deficits	Decrease frequency of ECT	Lerer et al. (1995) McAllister et al. (1987)
Oxygenation	Poor oxygenation can result in hypoxia and increased cognitive deficits	Pulse oximetry to monitor oxygen saturation and administer 100% O_2 prior to seizure induction	APA (2001, 1990) Holmberg (1953)
Concomitant medications	High anesthetic dose may increase cognitive effects, which some psychotropics can augment	Reduce anesthetic dose to produce light level of anesthesia; decrease or discontinue psychotropic dosage; discontinue lithium prior to ECT	Mukherjee (1993) APA (2001, 1990) Small & Milstein (1990) Miller et al. (1985)

Adapted from American Psychiatric Association Task Force on ECT. The practice of ECT: recommendations for treatment, training, and privileging. Washington, D.C.: American Psychiatric Press, 2001, with permission.
[a] Complete reference citations at end of chapter.

ment than with right unilateral electrode placement. However, the combined predictive power of these features is insufficient to base choice of electrical dosage on a formula.[5,192,193] Regardless of dosage choice, patients with the highest seizure thresholds are predominantly elderly males, especially those with cardiac disease.[194] The use of ultrabrief stimulation may partially redress this issue. Since this form of stimulation is considerably more efficient, seizure thresholds are much reduced, allowing greater effective range for dosing relative to threshold.

The efficacy of right unilateral ECT is especially sensitive to electrical dosage. When stimulus intensity is near the seizure threshold, right unilateral ECT lacks

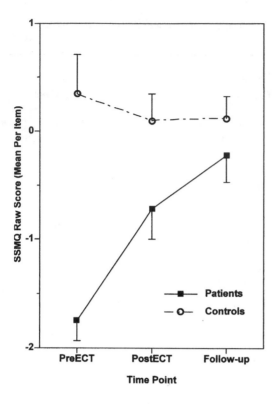

Figure 13.6. Score on the Squire Subjective Memory Questionnaire before and after the treatment course in ECT responders and nonresponders. Scores of '0' indicate no change in memory relative to before the episode of depression. (From Coleman EA, Sackeim HA, Prudic J, et al. Subjective memory complaints before and after convulsive therapy. *Biol Psychiatry* 1996;39:346–356).

therapeutic properties.[58,59] Since advanced age correlates with higher seizure threshold, older patients are less likely to benefit from standard electrical dosage.[60,62,190,191,195] The efficacy of right unilateral ECT improves with escalation of intensity of electrical stimulation relative to seizure threshold.[27,59] At markedly suprathreshold dosing (e.g., 6 times the initial seizure threshold), right unilateral ECT achieves an efficacy that is equivalent to that of robust forms of bilateral ECT (e.g., 2.5 times the initial seizure threshold).[27,59] Even at grossly suprathreshold stimulus intensities, right unilateral ECT retains significant advantages with respect to cognitive parameters.[27] The high sensitivity of geriatric patients to the cognitive side effects of bilateral ECT suggests that suprathreshold forms of right unilateral ECT should be routine in this population. Indeed, given the marked cognitive benefits of ultrabrief stimulation, optimal treatment might involve dose-titrated, ultrabrief stimulation, using markedly suprathreshold right unilateral ECT.

Efficacy, speed of response, and cognitive side effects of ECT depend on the degree to which the ECT stimulus exceeds the seizure threshold. Suprathreshold dosing will improve the efficacy of right unilateral ECT, enhance speed of clinical improvement with right unilateral and bilateral ECT, and will result in more severe acute and short-term cognitive impairment.[59,169,188,196]

Number and Schedule of Treatments

Cognitive effects of ECT are proportional to the frequency with which treatment is administered as well as to the total number of treatments given.[197–199] This is particularly true when the most intense form of ECT, suprathreshold, bilateral treatment is used. The most common schedule in the United States involves 3 treatments per week, whereas in England, 2 treatments per week is more common. The U.S. schedule results in more rapid improvement but increased short-term cognitive impairment.[198,200,201] Elderly patients may be more sensitive to the frequency and number of treatments.[20,110,172,188,202] Some clinicians reduce the frequency of treatment to twice weekly in elderly patients who show progressive clinical improvement but excessive cognitive deficit.

Concomitant Medications and Cognitive Effects

Evidence suggests that the dose of anesthetic agent may contribute to the severity of cognitive impairment during the postictal recovery period.[203] Not surprisingly, excessive anesthetic dose may result in prolonged postictal disorientation. For this reason, older patients should receive lower doses of anesthetic agents than younger patients. This is particularly important since the dose of the anesthetic may also alter seizure duration and intensity.[60,204]

A small dose of a muscarinic anticholinergic agent (0.4–0.8 mg atropine or 0.2–0.4 mg glycopyrrolate) is commonly administered intravenously in ECT, just prior to the anesthetic agent. The anticholinergic agent serves to block vagal outflow and limit the bradycardia produced by the ECT stimulus. This is especially necessary whenever the possibility of subconvulsive stimulation exists, or when patients are administered a β-blocker.[100] Atropine is preferred to glycopyrrolate since protection against bradycardia is less certain with glycopyrrolate. In addition, incidence of postictal nausea is also higher with glycopyrrate,[205,206] and glycopyrrolate holds no advantage with respect to cognitive effects during ECT.[205–211]

In sensitive elderly patients, a variety of psychotropic agents may intensify the adverse cognitive effects of ECT. Lithium carbonate, for example, causes acute confusion during ECT in approximately 1 in 15 patients; more rarely, status epilepticus occurs.[212–216] Lithium should be discontinued prior to the start of an ECT series, or it can be withheld the night and morning before an ECT treatment. In the elderly, concurrent use of benzodiazepines, neuroleptics, or other sedating psychotropic agents may increase cognitive side effects. Benzodiazepines and anticonvulsant medications may also interfere with efficacy by raising seizure threshold.[217,218]

ECT for Depressed Patients with Neurologic Disorders

Increasingly, ECT is used to treat psychiatric manifestations in a variety of patient populations with frank neurologic illness, including Parkinson's disease,[219–225] poststroke depression,[226–228] and to a lesser extent, dementing disorders.[229,230] Across a variety of neurologic disorders, ECT is effective in the treatment of primary or secondary mood disorders. In the case of Parkinson's disease, ECT frequently exerts beneficial effects on aspects of the movement disorder and has been used as a primary treatment for the neurologic condition. Duration of the antiparkinsonian effects is, however, unpredictable; some patients lose benefit within days, while others maintain improvement in the movement disorder for months or longer.[231] The role of continuation or maintenance ECT in sustaining improvement in the movement disorder is largely undocumented, although clinical experience indicates that such long-term treatment can be highly effective. Patients with Parkinson's disease who receive ECT may be at increased risk for prolonged confusion or delirium.[232,233] ECT is also effective in treating poststroke depression and major depression in the context of dementing illness,[229,230] although there is risk of increased severe cognitive side effects.

CLINICAL VIGNETTES

Case 13.1

Ms. A., a 71-year-old married retired schoolteacher, was seen in consultation regarding a serious chronic depression. Over the course of her adult life, she had suffered many such depressions that were always characterized by extreme anergia, anhedonia, and a sense of pointlessness. Ms. A. was never psychotic and never suicidal, but her diminished energy would often reach such severe proportions that she was unable to get out of bed for long periods during the day. She maintained her weight by forcing herself to eat, but no longer enjoyed the preparation or taste of food or, indeed, anything else. What was most striking to her was her subjective loss of interest in her grandchildren. Untreated, these depressive periods could last up to one year. Typically, however, although Ms. A. would begin to feel some symptomatic relief after a few months, a chronic pessimism and dysphoria persisted even in the absence of serious depressive symptoms (double depression).

Over the course of her life, Ms. A. had been treated with at least one antidepressant from each class of medication and had responded at least once to each. She had successful trials of imipramine, fluoxetine, venlafaxine; her response to monotherapy with nefazodone, mirtazapine, and bupropion was nontherapeutic. She never took an MAO inhibitor and never had lithium augmentation.

At the time she presented for evaluation, Ms. A. was in a state of profound melancholic, nonpsychotic depression. Out of desperation, she requested a consultation regarding ECT and agreed to a course of treatment. She initially received 2 bilateral treatments, and then was given 4 more treatments applied to the unilateral nondominant hemisphere on a thrice-weekly basis. Ms. A.'s response was rapid and dramatic. After the first 2 treatments, she no longer remained in bed and began actively to participate in family life. By the sixth treatment she proclaimed herself to be "back to normal." Based on evidence regarding high rates of relapse following ECT, Ms. A. was placed on a low dose of lithium carbonate (600 mg; blood level 0.4) for maintenance. She remained depression-free at one-year followup.

This case illustrates the importance of considering this most useful antidepressant treatment even for older patients who have had chronic depression over the course of a lifetime. Her treatment also illustrates the usefulness of post-ECT lithium maintenance to prevent relapse. Although Ms. A. experienced impairment of recent recall for the period during and prior to the ECT, she reported that this memory loss was a small price to pay for the dramatic improvement in her mood. Like other older patients whose depression has responded to ECT, she also indicated that the quality of the response to treatment was better than that from chemical antidepressants. She stated that her mood and thinking felt "clearer" following the ECT

during the memory loss. This is consistent with observations of clinicians experienced with use of ECT who have noted that some patients' response to ECT does seem to produce a better remission than chemical antidepressants, which may produce only a response or a partial response.

Case 13.2

Mr. B., a 76-year-old widowed attorney, developed a classical syndrome of severe major depression with melancholia. His first symptoms of depression appeared at the age of 73 after partial retirement from his law firm. Treatment with desipramine 85 mg daily (blood level of 140 ng/mL) led to dry mouth and mild urinary hesitancy; intravenous pyelogram revealed no significant residual urine. After approximately 4 weeks on desipramine, Mr. B.'s symptoms of depression remitted, although a feeling of "mild uneasiness" remained. He was able to return to work for a few hours a week and resumed most of his social activities. Approximately 3 months after the initial response, Mr. B.'s "uneasiness" intensified and became particularly prominent in the morning. Finally, depressed mood and feelings of hopelessness as well as insomnia and appetite loss developed over a period of 2 months despite maintenance therapy with desipramine together with supportive psychotherapy.

Severe exacerbation of his depressive symptoms followed some changes in Mr. B.'s law firm. Desipramine dosage was raised to a blood level of 182 ng/mL; later, thyroid augmentation was attempted with triiodothyronine (up to 50 mg daily) for 2 weeks. Because no change in his mental status occurred, triiodothyronine was discontinued, and lithium augmentation was attempted, with dosage gradually increased to 600 mg daily (blood level of 0.75 mEg/L). Depressive symptoms were ameliorated approximately 3 weeks after the introduction of lithium, but he developed tremor and unstable gait that required reducing the dosage to 300 mg daily (blood level of 0.44 mEg/L). Mr. B. remained partially symptomatic with mildly anxious and depressed mood, particularly in the morning, with early morning awakening and complaints of poor concentration.

Approximately 2 months after the improvement induced by lithium, Mr. B.'s depression worsened severely; suicidal ideation developed, and he was hospitalized in a geriatric psychiatry unit. Psychotropic drugs were discontinued, and 10 unilateral ECTs were administered, resulting in complete remission of his depression. Sertraline, 50 mg daily, was started immediately after the last ECT and increased to 75 mg 5 days later. This drug was chosen because the tricyclic antidepressant desipramine had failed to maintain Mr. B.'s remission. However, 3 weeks after the last ECT, Mr. B. began again to experience depressed mood, early morning awakening, and suicidal ideation. Sertraline was discontinued a week later, and three additional unilateral ECT treatments were administered, with excellent response. Although therapy with MAOIs was considered, maintenance ECT was chosen because his rapid development of suicidal ideation and lack of supervision after discharge placed him at risk. Compliance with MAO diet was also a concern, especially during the period after ECT when his memory was impaired. Maintenance ECT was given every 2 weeks during the first 2 months and then monthly. Nine months after completion of the initial ECT trial, Mr. B. was still asymptomatic.

Some depressed geriatric patients respond well to antidepressant treatment but cannot sustain remission despite continuation therapy with antidepressant drugs. Mr. B.'s major depression with onset in late life responded favorably to desipramine, desipramine combined with lithium, and a trial of ECT at various times. However, approximately 1 to 3 months after initial improvement, his depression returned, necessitating additional antidepressant treatment. Patients like Mr. B. often are difficult to treat, particularly if they cannot tolerate particular antidepressants or therapies. ECT is usually effective in such cases and should be considered, especially when the patient becomes disheartened by the repeated failures. The rollercoaster of hope and disappointment, coupled with the pessimism of the depressive syndrome, may cause the patient to give up and facilitate development of suicidal ideation.

Maintenance ECT needs further investigation. Many patients, however, remain in remission from depression while receiving ECT every 4 to 6 weeks. ECT appears to be a reasonable option for patients with severe depression who fail to remain in remission while on an adequate dosage of a heterocyclic antidepressant, a serotonin-reuptake inhibitor, or an MAOI. Only depressed patients who are able to tolerate and respond to a trial of ECT should be considered for maintenance ECT.

Case 13.3

Mrs. C., a 76-year-old widow, was diagnosed with Alzheimer's disease. Although her dementia was moderate, she was still able to function in her own home with a 24-hour companion.

After a fall, Mrs. C. sprained her right ankle, and her mobility decreased for 2 to 3 weeks. During this time, she became apathetic, lost interest in television or socialization, and developed insomnia and appetite loss. After a diagnosis of depression, imipramine was begun, with dosage increased by 25 mg every other day up to 75 mg daily. After 6 days on imipramine 75 mg, Mrs. C. developed agitation, confusion, inability to sustain her attention, and incoherent speech. Her symptoms were significantly worse at night; she appeared frightened and kept saying that her neighbors were coming to "put her away." Her face was flushed, her skin dry, and her pulse was 120 beats per minute.

Mrs. C. was admitted to an acute psychiatric unit with a diagnosis of anticholinergic delirium. Imipramine was discontinued, a course of hydration was begun, her vital signs were monitored closely, and her pulse decreased to 95 beats per minute within 24 hours. Three days later, her confusion and agitation lessened, but the symptoms of depression were even more apparent. She gradually developed severe psychomotor retardation and began refusing to eat or drink. Treatment with desipramine, 10 mg daily, began and was increased by 10 mg every 3 days. A week later, Mrs. C. required tube feeding. At 40 mg of desipramine daily, her pulse rate ranged between 100 and 110 beats per minute. At this point, desipramine was discontinued, and 5 days later unilateral ECT was begun. ECT was administered twice a week, and after a total of eight treatments, Mrs. C.'s depression was in complete remission.

Elderly patients are sensitive to the anticholinergic effect of heterocyclic antidepressants. Delirium, persistent sinus tachycardia, or urinary retention often lead to discontinuation of these drugs. When the diagnosis of anticholinergic delirium is in doubt, physostigmine 1 mg diluted in 10 mL of normal saline should be administered intravenously over 5 to 7 minutes. The mental status of patients with anticholinergic delirium improves almost immediately. However, physostigmine should be avoided for very old patients or those with cardiac disease because it may cause sinus brachycardia or transient sinus arrest. Patients with bronchial asthma may develop bronchospasm after administration of physostigmine.

ECT is the treatment of choice in a rapidly worsening depressed elderly patient. Although ECT-induced memory dysfunction may be more severe and prolonged in demented than in nondemented patients, there is no evidence that ECT worsens the course of dementia.

Acknowledgment. Preparation of this chapter was supported in part by grants MH35636, MH47739, MH55646, MH55716, MH59069, MH60884, and MH61609 and an award from the National Alliance for Research in Schizophrenia and Depression.

References

1. Kramer B. Use of ECT in California, 1977–1983. *Am J Psychiatry* 1985;142:1190–1192.
2. Thompson JW, Blaine JD. Use of ECT in the United States in 1975 and 1980. *Am J Psychiatry* 1987;144:557–562.
3. Thompson JW, Weiner RD, Myers CP. Use of ECT in the United States in 1975, 1980, and 1986. *Am J Psychiatry* 1994;151:1657–1661.
4. Olfson M, Marcus S, Sackeim HA, et al. Use of ECT for the inpatient treatment of recurrent major depression. *Am J Psychiatry* 1998;155:22–29.
5. American Psychiatric Association. *The Practice of ECT: Recommendations for Treatment, Training and Privileging.* Second Edition. Washington, D.C.: American Psychiatric Press, 2001.
6. American Psychiatric Association. Practice guideline for major depressive disorder in adults. *Am J Psychiatry* 1993;150:1–26.
7. American Psychiatric Association Task Force on ECT. The practice of ECT: Recommendations for treatment, training and privileging. *Convulsive Ther* 1990;6:85–120.
8. Sackeim HA. Electroconvulsive therapy and schizophrenia. In: Hirsch SR, Weinberger D, eds. *Schizophrenia.* Second Edition, Oxford: Blackwell, 2003:517–551.
9. Mukherjee S, Sackeim HA, Schnur DB. Electroconvulsive therapy of acute manic episodes: a review of 50 years' experience. *Am J Psychiatry* 1994;151:169–176.
10. Sackeim HA, Devanand DP, Nobler MS. Electroconvulsive therapy. In: Bloom F, Kupfer D, eds. *Psychopharmacology: The Fourth Generation of Progress.* New York: Raven, 1995:1123–1142.
11. Janicak P, Davis J, Gibbons R, et al. Efficacy of ECT: a meta-analysis. *Am J Psychiatry* 1985;142:297–302.
12. Segman RH, Shapira B, Gorfine M, Lerer B. Onset and time course of antidepressant action: psychopharmacological implications of a controlled trial of electroconvulsive therapy. *Psychopharmacology* (Berl) 1995;119:440–448.
13. Nobler MS, Sackeim HA, Moeller JR, et al. Quantifying the speed of symptomatic improvement with electroconvulsive therapy: comparison of alternative statistical methods. *Convuls Ther* 1997;13:208–221.
14. Rifkin A. ECT versus tricyclic antidepressants in depression: a review of the evidence. *J Clin Psychiatry* 1988;49:3–7.
15. Folkerts HW, Michael N, Tolle R, et al. Electroconvulsive therapy vs. paroxetine in treatment-resistant depression—a randomized study. *Acta Psychiatr Scand* 1997;96:334–342.
16. Hermann RC, Dorwart RA, Hoover CW, Brody J. Variation in ECT use in the United States. *Am J Psychiatry* 1995;152:869–875.
17. Hermann RC, Ettner SL, Dorwart RA, et al. Diagnoses of patients treated with ECT: a comparison of evidence-based standards with reported use. *Psychiatr Serv* 1999;50:1059–1065.
18. Prudic J, Haskett RF, Mulsant B, et al. Resistance to antidepressant medications and short-term clinical response to ECT. *Am J Psychiatry* 1996;153:985–992.
19. Hobson RF. Prognostic factors in ECT. *J Neurol Neurosurg Psychiatry* 1953;16:275–281.
20. Fraser R, Glass I. Unilateral and bilateral ECT in elderly patients. A comparative study. *Acta Psychiatr Scand* 1980;62:13–31.
21. Coryell W, Zimmerman M. Outcome following ECT for primary unipolar depression: a test of newly proposed response predictors. *Am J Psychiatry* 1984;141:862–867.
22. Black DW, Winokur G, Nasrallah A. Illness duration and acute response in major depression. *Convulsive Ther* 1989;5:338–343.
23. Kindler S, Shapira B, Hadjez J, et al. Factors influencing response to bilateral electroconvulsive therapy in major depression. *Convulsive Ther* 1991;7:245–254.
24. Prudic J, Olfson M, Marcus SC, et al. The effectiveness of electroconvulsive therapy in community settings. *Biol Psychiatry* 2004;55:301–312.
25. Prudic J, Sackeim HA, Devanand DP. Medication resistance and clinical response to electroconvulsive therapy. *Psychiatry Res* 1990;31:287–296.
26. Sackeim HA, Haskett RF, Mulsant BH, et al. Continuation pharmacotherapy in the prevention of relapse following electroconvulsive therapy: a randomized controlled trial. *JAMA* 2001;285:1299–1307.
27. Sackeim HA, Prudic J, Devanand DP, et al. A prospective, randomized, double-blind comparison of bilateral and right unilateral electroconvulsive therapy at different stimulus intensities. *Arch Gen Psychiatry* 2000;57:425–434.
28. Sackeim HA. The definition and meaning of treatment-resistant depression. *J Clin Psychiatry* 2001;62(Suppl 16):10–17.
29. Sackeim HA, Rush AJ, George MS, et al. Vagus nerve stimulation (VNS) for treatment-resistant depression: efficacy, side effects, and predictors of outcome. *Neuropsychopharmacology* 2001;25:713–728.
30. Sackeim HA. Continuation therapy following ECT: directions for future research. *Psychopharmacol Bull* 1994;30:501–521.
31. Clarke TB, Coffey CE, Hoffman GW, Weiner RD. Continuation therapy for depression using outpatient electroconvulsive therapy. *Convulsive Ther* 1989;5:330–337.
32. Decina P, Guthrie EB, Sackeim HA, Kahn D. Continuation ECT in the management of relapses of major affective episodes. *Acta Psychiatr Scand* 1987;75:559–562.
33. Sackeim HA, Prudic J, Devanand DP, et al. The impact of medication resistance and continuation pharmacotherapy on relapse following re-

sponse to electroconvulsive therapy in major depression. *J Clin Psychopharmacol* 1990;10: 96–104.

34. Prudic J, Olfson M, Sackeim HA. Electroconvulsive therapy practices in the community. *Psychol Med* 2001;31:929–934.

35. Post F. The management and nature of depressive illnesses in late life: a follow-through study. *Br J Psychiatry* 1972;121:393–404.

36. Philibert RA, Richards L, Lynch CF, Winokur G. Effect of ECT on mortality and clinical outcome in geriatric unipolar depression. *J Clin Psychiatry* 1995;56:390–394.

37. Avery D, Winokur G. Mortality in depressed patients treated with electroconvulsive therapy and antidepressants. *Arch Gen Psychiatry* 1976; 33:1029–1037.

38. Babigian H, Guttmacher L. Epidemiologic considerations in electroconvulsive therapy. *Arch Gen Psychiatry* 1984;41:246–253.

39. Wesner RB, Winokur G. The influence of age on the natural history of unipolar depression when treated with electroconvulsive therapy. *Eur Arch Psychiatry Neurol Sci* 1989;238:149–154.

40. Dinan TG, Barry S. A comparison of electroconvulsive therapy with a combined lithium and tricyclic combination among depressed tricyclic nonresponders. *Acta Psychiatr Scand* 1989;80:97–100.

41. Keller M, Lavori P, Klerman G, et al. Low levels and lack of predictors of somatotherapy and psychotherapy received by depressed patients. *Arch Gen Psychiatry* 1986;43:458–466.

42. Quitkin F. The importance of dosage in prescribing antidepressants. *Br J Psychiatry* 1985; 147:593–597.

43. Nemeroff CB. Augmentation strategies in patients with refractory depression. *Depress Anxiety* 1996–97;4:169–181.

44. Rouillon F, Gorwood P. The use of lithium to augment antidepressant medication. *J Clin Psychiatry* 1998;59(Suppl 5):32–39; discussion 40–41.

45. Paykel ES. Achieving gains beyond response. *Acta Psychiatr Scand Suppl* 2002;415:12–17.

46. Fraser RM. ECT and the elderly. In: Palmer RL, ed. *Electroconvulsive therapy: an appraisal.* New York: Oxford University, 1981:55–60.

47. Weiner RD. The role of electroconvulsive therapy in the treatment of depression in the elderly. *J Am Geriatr Soc* 1982;30:710–712.

48. Abrams R. *Electroconvulsive Therapy.* Fourth, New York: Oxford University Press, 2002.

49. Sackeim HA. The use of electroconvulsive therapy in late life depression. In: Schneider LS, Reynolds III CF, Liebowitz BD, Friedhoff AJ, eds. Diagnosis and Treatment of Depression in Late Life. Washington, D.C.: *American Psychiatric Press*, 1993:259–277.

50. Heshe J, Röder E, Theilgaard A. Unilateral and bilateral ECT. A psychiatric and psychological study of therapeutic effect and side effects. *Acta Psychiatr Scand Suppl* 1978;275:1–180.

51. Pettinati HM, Mathisen KS, Rosenberg J, Lynch JF. Meta-analytical approach to reconciling discrepancies in efficacy between bilateral and unilateral electroconvulsive therapy. *Convulsive Ther* 1986;2:7–17.

52. Ottosson JO. Experimental studies of the mode of action of electroconvulsive therapy. *Acta Psychiatr Scand Suppl* 1960;145:1–141.

53. Rich C, Spiker D, Jewell S, et al. The efficiency of ECT: I. Response rate in depressive episodes. *Psychiatry Res* 1984;11:167–176.

54. Alexopoulos G, Shamoian C, Lucas J, et al. Medical problems of geriatric psychiatric patients and younger controls during electroconvulsive therapy. *J Am Geriatr Soc* 1984;32: 651–654.

55. Cattan RA, Barry PP, Mead G, et al. Electroconvulsive therapy in octogenarians. *J Am Geriatr Soc* 1990;38:753–758.

56. Karlinsky H, Shulman K. The clinical use of electroconvulsive therapy in old age. *J Am Geriatr Soc* 1984;32:183–186.

57. Kramer B. Electroconvulsive therapy use in geriatric depression. *J Nerv Ment Dis* 1987;175: 233–235.

58. Sackeim HA, Decina P, Kanzler M, et al. Effects of electrode placement on the efficacy of titrated, low-dose ECT. *Am J Psychiatry* 1987;144: 1449–1455.

59. Sackeim HA, Prudic J, Devanand DP, et al. Effects of stimulus intensity and electrode placement on the efficacy and cognitive effects of electroconvulsive therapy. *N Engl J Med* 1993; 328:839–846.

60. Sackeim HA, Devanand DP, Prudic J. Stimulus intensity, seizure threshold, and seizure duration: impact on the efficacy and safety of electroconvulsive therapy. *Psychiatr Clin North Am* 1991;14:803–843.

61. Sackeim HA, Decina P, Portnoy S, et al. Studies of dosage, seizure threshold, and seizure duration in ECT. *Biol Psychiatry* 1987;22:249–268.

62. Sackeim HA, Decina P, Prohovnik I, Malitz S. Seizure threshold in electroconvulsive therapy. Effects of sex, age, electrode placement, and number of treatments. *Arch Gen Psychiatry* 1987; 44:355–360.

63. Watterson D. The effect of age, head resistance and other physical factors of the stimulus threshold of electrically induced convulsions. *J Neurol Neurosurg Psychiatry* 1945;8:121–125.

64. Weiner RD. ECT and seizure threshold: effects of stimulus wave form and electrode placement. *Biol Psychiatry* 1980;15:225–241.

65. Nobler MS, Sackeim HA, Solomou M, et al. EEG manifestations during ECT: effects of electrode placement and stimulus intensity. *Biol Psychiatry* 1993;34:321–330.

66. Krystal AD, Weiner RD, Coffey CE. The ictal EEG as a marker of adequate stimulus intensity with unilateral ECT. *J Neuropsychiatry Clin Neurosci* 1995;7:295–303.

67. Sobin C, Prudic J, Devanand DP, et al. Who responds to electroconvulsive therapy? A comparison of effective and ineffective forms of treatment. *Br J Psychiatry* 1996;169:322–328.

68. Petrides G, Fink M, Husain MM, et al. ECT remission rates in psychotic versus nonpsychotic depressed patients: a report from CORE. *J ECT* 2001;17:244–253.

69. Buchan H, Johnstone E, McPherson K, et al. Who benefits from electroconvulsive therapy? Combined results of the Leicester and

Northwick Park trials. *Br J Psychiatry* 1992;160: 355–359.

70. Nobler MS, Sackeim HA. Electroconvulsive therapy: Clinical and biological aspects. In: Goodnick PJ, eds. *Predictors of Response in Mood Disorders.* Washington, D.C.: American Psychiatric Press, 1996:177–198.

71. Wolfersdorf M, Barg T, Konig F, et al. Paroxetine as antidepressant in combined antidepressant-neuroleptic therapy in delusional depression: observation of clinical use. *Pharmacopsychiatry* 1995;28:56–60.

72. Mulsant BH, Haskett RF, Prudic J, et al. Low use of neuroleptic drugs in the treatment of psychotic major depression. *Am J Psychiatry* 1997;154:559–561.

73. Black DW, Winokur G, Nasrallah A. A multivariate analysis of the experience of 423 depressed inpatients treated with electroconvulsive therapy. *Convulsive Ther* 1993;9:112–120.

74. Parker G, Hadzi-Pavlovic D, Hickie I, et al. Psychotic depression: a review and clinical experience. *Aust N Z J Psychiatry* 1991;25:169–180.

75. Dubovsky SL. Challenges in conceptualizing psychotic mood disorders. *Bull Menninger Clin* 1994;58:197–214.

76. Nelson JC, Bowers MBJ. Delusional unipolar depression: description and drug response. *Arch Gen Psychiatry* 1978;35:1321–1328.

77. Avery D, Lubrano A. Depression treated with imipramine and ECT: the DeCarolis study reconsidered. *Am J Psychiatry* 1979;136:559–562.

78. Schatzberg AF, Rothschild AJ. Psychotic (delusional) major depression: should it be included as a distinct syndrome in DSM-IV? *Am J Psychiatry* 1992;149:733–745.

79. Spiker DG, Stein J, Rich CL. Delusional depression and electroconvulsive therapy: One year later. *Convulsive Ther* 1985;1:167–172.

80. Roose SP, Glassman AH, Walsh BT, et al. Depression, delusions, and suicide. *Am J Psychiatry* 1983;140:1159–1162.

81. Coryell W, Pfohl B, Zimmerman M. The clinical and neuroendocrine features of psychotic depression. *J Nerv Ment Dis* 1984;172:521–528.

82. Alexopoulus GS. Clinical and biological findings in late-onset depression. In: Tasman A, Goldfinger SM, Kaufman CA, eds. *American Psychiatric Press Review of Psychiatry* vol.9 Washington DC: American Psychiatric Press. 1990; 249–262.

83. Coryell W, Winokur G, Shea T, et al. The long-term stability of depressive subtypes. *Am J Psychiatry* 1994;151:199–204.

84. Aronson TA, Shukla S, Hoff A, Cook B. Proposed delusional depression subtypes: preliminary evidence from a retrospective study of phenomenology and treatment course. *J Affective Disord* 1988;14:69–74.

85. Kendler KS, Gruenberg AM, Tsuang MT. A DSM-III family study of the nonschizophrenic psychotic disorders. *Am J Psychiatry* 1986;143: 1098–1105.

86. Alexopoulos GS, Young RC, Shindledecker RD. Brain computed tomography findings in geriatric depression and primary degenerative dementia. *Biol Psychiatry* 1992;31:591–599.

87. Caine E. The neuropsychology of depression: The pseudodementia syndrome. In: Grant I, Adams KM, eds. *Neuropsychological Assessment of Neuropsychiatric disorders.* New York: Oxford University Press, 1986:221–243.

88. Mitchell AJ, Dening TR. Depression-related cognitive impairment: possibilities for its pharmacological treatment. *J Affect Disord* 1996;36: 79–87.

89. Parker G, Roy K, Hadzi-Pavlovic D, Pedic F. Psychotic (delusional) depression: a meta-analysis of physical treatments. *J Affect Disord* 1992;24: 17–24.

90. Mendels J. Electroconvulsive therapy and depression. II. Significance of endogenous and reactive syndromes. *Br J Psychiatry* 1965;111: 682–686.

91. Mendels J. Electroconvulsive therapy and depression. I. The prognostic significance of clinical factors. *Br J Psychiatry* 1965;111: 675–681.

92. Mendels J. Electroconvulsive therapy and depression. III. A method for prognosis. *Br J Psychiatry* 1965;111:687–690.

93. Hamilton M, White J. Factors related to the outcome of depression treated with ECT. *J Ment Sci* 1960;106:1031–1041.

94. Hickie I, Parsonage B, Parker G. Prediction of response to electroconvulsive therapy. Preliminary validation of a sign-based typology of depression. *Br J Psychiatry* 1990;157:65–71.

95. Benatov R, Sirota P, Megged S. Neuroleptic-resistant schizophrenia treated with clozapine and ECT. *Convuls Ther* 1996;12:117–121.

96. Bhatia SC, Bhatia SK, Gupta S. Concurrent administration of clozapine and ECT: a successful therapeutic strategy for a patient with treatment-resistant schizophrenia. *J ECT* 1998;14: 280–283.

97. Cardwell BA, Nakai B. Seizure activity in combined clozapine and ECT: a retrospective view. *Convuls Ther* 1995;11:110–113.

98. James DV, Gray NS. Elective combined electroconvulsive and clozapine therapy. *Int Clin Psychopharmacol* 1999;14:69–72.

99. Meltzer HY. Treatment of the neuroleptic-nonresponsive schizophrenic patient. *Schizophr Bull* 1992;18:515–542.

100. Zielinski RJ, Roose SP, Devanand DP, et al. Cardiovascular complications of ECT in depressed patients with cardiac disease. *Am J Psychiatry* 1993;150:904–909.

101. Rice EH, Sombrotto LB, Markowitz JC, Leon AC. Cardiovascular morbidity in high-risk patients during ECT. *Am J Psychiatry* 1994;151: 1637–1641.

102. Burd J, Kettl P. Incidence of asystole in electroconvulsive therapy in elderly patients. *Am J Geriatr Psychiatry* 1998;6:203–211.

103. Burke W, Rubin E, Zorumski C, Wetzel R. The safety of ECT in geriatric psychiatry. *J Am Geriatr Soc* 1987;35:516–521.

104. de Corle AJ, Kohn R. Electroconvulsive therapy and falls in the elderly. *J ECT* 2000;16:252–257.

105. Huuhka MJ, Seinela L, Reinikainen P, Leinonen EV. Cardiac arrhythmias induced by ECT in elderly psychiatric patients: Experience with 48-hour holter monitoring. *J ECT* 2003;19: 22–25.

106. Tomac TA, Rummans TA, Pileggi TS, Li H. Safety and efficacy of electroconvulsive therapy in patients over age 85. *Am J Geriatr Psychiatry* 1997;5:126–130.

107. Zorumski CF, Rubin EH, Burke WJ. Electroconvulsive therapy for the elderly: a review. *Hosp Community Psychiatry* 1988;39:643–647.

108. Zwil AS, Pelchat RJ. ECT in the treatment of patients with neurological and somatic disease. *Int J Psychiatry Med* 1994;24:1–29.

109. Braddock L, Cowen P, Elliott J, et al. Binding of yohimbine and imipramine to platelets in depressive illness. *Psychol Med* 1986;16:765–773.

110. Fraser R, Glass I. Recovery from ECT in elderly patients. *Br J Psychiatry* 1978;133:524–528.

111. Burke WJ, Rutherford J, Zorumski C, Reich T. Electroconvulsive therapy and the elderly. *Compr Psychiatry* 1985;26:480–486.

112. Burke WJ, Rubin EH, Zorumuski CF, et al. The safety of ECT in geriatric psychiatry. *Am J Geriatr Soc* 1987;35:516–521.

113. Gaspar D, Samarasinghe L. ECT in psychogeriatric practice—a study of risk factors, indications and outcome. *Compr Psychiatry* 1982;23:170–175.

114. Gerring J, Shields H. The identification and management of patients with a high risk for cardiac arrhythmias during modified ECT. *J Clin Psychiatry* 1982;43:140–143.

115. Abrams R. The mortality rate with ECT. *Convuls Ther* 1997;13:125–127.

116. Benbow SM. The role of electroconvulsive therapy in the treatment of depressive illness in old age. *Br J Psychiatry* 1989;155:147–152.

117. American Psychiatric Association. *The Practice of ECT: Recommendations for Treatment, Training and Privileging*. First Edition. Washington, D.C.: American Psychiatric Press, 1990.

118. Welch CA, Lambertus LJ. Cardiovascular effects of ECT. *Convulsive Ther* 1989;5:35–43.

119. Howie MB, Black HA, Zvara D, et al. Esmolol reduces autonomic hypersensitivity and length of seizures induced by electroconvulsive therapy. *Anesth Analg* 1990;71:384–388.

120. Kovac AL, Goto H, Pardo MP, Arakawa K. Comparison of two esmolol bolus doses on the haemodynamic response and seizure duration during electroconvulsive therapy. *Can J Anaesth* 1991;38:204–209.

121. McCall WV, Shelp FE, Weiner RD, et al. Effects of labetalol on hemodynamics and seizure duration during ECT. *Convulsive Ther* 1991;7:5–14.

122. Stoudemire A, Knos G, Gladson M, et al. Labetalol in the control of cardiovascular responses to electroconvulsive therapy in high-risk depressed medical patients. *J Clin Psychiatry* 1990;51:508–512.

123. Figiel GS, DeLeo B, Zorumski CF, et al. Combined use of labetalol and nifedipine in controlling the cardiovascular response from ECT. *J Geriatr Psychiatry Neurol* 1993;6:20–24.

124. Figiel GS, McDonald L, LaPlante R. Cardiovascular complications of ECT [letter; comment]. *Am J Psychiatry* 1994;151:790–791.

125. Ciraulo D, Lind L, Salzman C, et al. Sodium nitroprusside treatment of ECT-induced blood pressure elevations. *Am J Psychiatry* 1978;135:1105–1106.

126. Foster S, Ries R. Delayed hypertension with electroconvulsive therapy. *J Nerv Ment Dis* 1988;176:374–376.

127. Gaines GY III, Rees DI. Anesthetic considerations for electroconvulsive therapy. *South Med J* 1992;85:469–482.

128. Avramov MN, Stool LA, White PF, Husain MM. Effects of nicardipine and labetalol on the acute hemodynamic response to electroconvulsive therapy. *J Clin Anesth* 1998;10:394–400.

129. Antkiewicz-Michaluk L, Michaluk J, Romanska I, Vetulani J. The effect of calcium channel blockade during electroconvulsive treatment on cerebral cortical adrenoceptor subpopulations in the rat. *Pol J Pharmacol* 1993;45:197–200.

130. Ding Z, White PF. Anesthesia for electroconvulsive therapy. *Anesth Analg* 2002;94:1351–1364.

131. Wajima Z, Yoshikawa T, Ogura A, et al. Intravenous verapamil blunts hyperdynamic responses during electroconvulsive therapy without altering seizure activity. *Anesth Analg* 2002;95:400–402.

132. Wells DG, Davies GG, Rosewarne F. Attenuation of electroconvulsive therapy induced hypertension with sublingual nifedipine. *Anaesth Intensive Care* 1989;17:31–33.

133. Kraus R, Remick R. Diazoxide in the management of severe hypertension after electroconvulsive therapy. *Am J Psychiatry* 1982;139:504–505.

134. Petrides G, Fink M. Atrial fibrillation, anticoagulation, and electroconvulsive therapy. *Convuls Ther* 1996;12:91–98.

135. Avramov MN, Husain MM, White PF. The comparative effects of methohexital, propofol, and etomidate for electroconvulsive therapy. *Anesth Analg* 1995;81:596–602.

136. Boey WK, Lai FO. Comparison of propofol and thiopentone as anaesthetic agents for electroconvulsive therapy. *Anaesthesia* 1990;45:623–628.

137. Bone ME, Wilkins CJ, Lew JK. A comparison of propofol and methohexitone as anaesthetic agents for electroconvulsive therapy. *Eur J Anaesthesiol* 1988;5:279–286.

138. Dwyer R, McCaughey W, Lavery J, et al. Comparison of propofol and methohexitone as anaesthetic agents for electroconvulsive therapy. *Anaesthesia* 1988;43:459–462.

139. Kirkby KC, Beckett WG, Matters RM, King TE. Comparison of propofol and methohexitone in anaesthesia for ECT: effect on seizure duration and outcome. *Aust N Z J Psychiatry* 1995;29:299–303.

140. Fredman B, Husain MM, White PF. Anaesthesia for electroconvulsive therapy: use of propofol revisited. *Eur J Anaesthesiol* 1994;11:423–425.

141. Geretsegger C, Rochowanski E, Kartnig C, Unterrainer AF. Propofol and methohexital as anesthetic agents for electroconvulsive therapy (ECT): a comparison of seizure-quality measures and vital signs. *J ECT* 1998;14:28–35.

142. Hasan ZA, Woolley DE. Comparison of the effects of propofol and thiopental on the pattern

of maximal electroshock seizures in the rat. *Pharmacol Toxicol* 1994;74:50–53.

143. Lim SK, Lim WL, Elegbe EO. Comparison of propofol and methohexitone as an induction agent in anaesthesia for electroconvulsive therapy. *West Afr J Med* 1996;15:186–189.

144. Martensson B, Bartfai A, Hallen B, et al. A comparison of propofol and methohexital as anesthetic agents for ECT: effects on seizure duration, therapeutic outcome, and memory. *Biol Psychiatry* 1994;35:179–189.

145. Nguyen TT, Chhibber AK, Lustik SJ, et al. Effect of methohexitone and propofol with or without alfentanil on seizure duration and recovery in electroconvulsive therapy. *Br J Anaesth* 1997;79:801–803.

146. Saito S, Kadoi Y, Nara T, et al. The comparative effects of propofol versus thiopental on middle cerebral artery blood flow velocity during electroconvulsive therapy. *Anesth Analg* 2000;91: 1531–1536.

147. Zaidi NA, Khan FA. Comparison of thiopentone sodium and propofol for electro convulsive therapy (ECT). *J Pak Med Assoc* 2000;50: 60–63.

148. Sackeim HA. The cognitive effects of electroconvulsive therapy. In: Moos WH, Gamzu ER, Thal LJ, eds. *Cognitive Disorders: Pathophysiology and Treatment.* New York: Marcel Dekker, 1992: 183–228.

149. Sackeim HA. Memory and ECT: From polarization to reconciliation. *J ECT* 2000;16:87–96.

150. Sternberg DE, Jarvik ME. Memory function in depression: Improvement with antidepressant medication. *Arch Gen Psychiatry* 1976;33:219–224.

151. Steif B, Sackeim H, Portnoy S, et al. Effects of depression and ECT on anterograde memory. *Biol Psychiatry* 1986;21:921–930.

152. Sackeim HA, Steif BL. The neuropsychology of depression and mania. In: Georgotas A, Cancro R, eds. *Depression and Mania.* New York: Elsevier, 1988:265–289.

153. Zakzanis KK, Leach L, Kaplan E. On the nature and pattern of neurocognitive function in major depressive disorder. *Neuropsychiatry Neuropsychol Behav Neurol* 1998;11:111–119.

154. Cronholm B, Ottosson JO. The experience of memory function after electroconvulsive therapy. *Br J Psychiatry* 1963;109:251–258.

155. Nobler MS, Oquendo MA, Kegeles LS, et al. Decreased regional brain metabolism after ECT. *Am J Psychiatry* 2001;158:305–308.

156. Nobler MS, Sackeim HA, Prohovnik I, et al. Regional cerebral blood flow in mood disorders, III. Treatment and clinical response. *Arch Gen Psychiatry* 1994;51:884–897.

157. Sackeim HA. The anticonvulsant hypothesis of the mechanisms of action of ECT: current status. *J ECT* 1999;15:5–26.

158. Sackeim HA. Functional brain circuits in major depression and remission. *Arch Gen Psychiatry* 2001;58:649–650.

159. Sackeim HA, Decina P, Prohovnik I, et al. Anticonvulsant and antidepressant properties of electroconvulsive therapy: a proposed mechanism of action. *Biol Psychiatry* 1983;18:1301–1310.

160. Sackeim HA, Luber B, Katzman GP, et al. The effects of electroconvulsive therapy on quantitative electroencephalograms. Relationship to clinical outcome. *Arch Gen Psychiatry* 1996;53: 814–824.

161. Sackeim HA, Luber B, Moeller JR, et al. Electrophysiological correlates of the adverse cognitive effects of electroconvulsive therapy. *J ECT* 2000;16:110–120.

162. Squire L. Memory functions as affected by electroconvulsive therapy. *Ann NY Acad Sci* 1986; 462:307–314.

163. McElhiney MC, Moody BJ, Steif BL, et al. Autobiographical memory and mood: Effects of electroconvulsive therapy. *Neuropsychology* 1995;9:501–517.

164. Lisanby SH, Maddox JH, Prudic J, et al. The effects of electroconvulsive therapy on memory of autobiographical and public events. *Arch Gen Psychiatry* 2000;57:581–590.

165. Weiner RD, Rogers HJ, Davidson JR, Squire LR. Effects of stimulus parameters on cognitive side effects. *Ann NY Acad Sci* 1986;462:315–325.

166. Squire L, Cohen N, Zouzounis J. Preserved memory in retrograde amnesia: sparing of a recently acquired skill. *Neuropsychologia* 1984; 22:145–152.

167. Squire L, Shimamura A, Graf P. Independence of recognition memory and priming effects: a neuropsychological analysis. *J Exp Psychol Learn Mem Cogn* 1985;11:37–44.

168. Sackeim HA, Nobler MS, Prudic J, et al. Acute effects of electroconvulsive therapy on hemispatial neglect. *Neuropsychiatry, Neuropsychol and Behav Neurol* 1992;5:151–160.

169. Sobin C, Sackeim HA, Prudic J, et al. Predictors of retrograde amnesia following ECT. *Am J Psychiatry* 1995;152:995–1001.

170. Daniel W, Crovitz H. Disorientation during electroconvulsive therapy. Technical, theoretical, and neuropsychological issues. *Ann NY Acad Sci* 1986;462:293–306.

171. Summers W, Robins E, Reich T. The natural history of acute organic mental syndrome after bilateral electroconvulsive therapy. *Biol Psychiatry* 1979;14:905–912.

172. Daniel W, Crovitz H. Acute memory impairment following electroconvulsive therapy. 1. Effects of electrical stimulus waveform and number of treatments. *Acta Psychiatr Scand* 1983;67:1–7.

173. Calev A, Phil D, Cohen R, et al. Disorientation and bilateral moderately suprathreshold titrated ECT. *Convulsive Ther* 1991;7:99–110.

174. Figiel GS, Coffey CE, Djang WT, et al. Brain magnetic resonance imaging findings in ECT–induced delirium. *J Neuropsychiatry Clin Neurosci* 1990;2:53–58.

175. Miller M, Siris S, Gabriel A. Treatment delays in the course of electroconvulsive therapy. *Hosp Community Psychiatry* 1986;37:825–827.

176. Malloy F, Small I, Miller M, Milstein V. Changes in neuropsychological test performance after electroconvulsive therapy. *Biol Psychiatry* 1982; 17:61–67.

177. Squire L, Chace P. Memory functions six to nine months after electroconvulsive therapy. *Arch Gen Psychiatry* 1975;32:1557–1564.

178. Squire L. A stable impairment in remote memory following electroconvulsive therapy. *Neuropsychologia* 1975;13:51–58.

179. Weeks D, Freeman C, Kendell R. ECT: III: Enduring cognitive deficits? *Br J Psychiatry* 1980; 137:26–37.

180. Alexopoulous GS, Young RC, Abrams RC. ECT in the high–risk geriatric patient. *Convulsive Ther* 1989;5:75–87.

181. Zervas IM, Calev A, Jandorf L, et al. Age–dependent effects of electroconvulsive therapy on memory. *Convulsive Ther* 1993;9:39–42.

182. Valentine M, Keddie K, Dunne D. A comparison of techniques in electro–convulsive therapy. *Br J Psychiatry* 1968;114:989–996.

183. Cronholm B, Ottoson JO. Ultrabrief stimulus technique in electroconvulsive therapy. II. Comparative studies of therapeutic effects and memory disturbances in treatment of endogenous depression with the Elther ES electroshock apparatus and Siemens Konvulsator III. *J Nerv Ment Dis* 1963;137:268–276.

184. Cronholm B, Ottosson JO. Ultrabrief stimulus technique in electroconvulsive therapy. I. Influence on retrograde amnesia of treatments with the Elther ES electroshock apparatus, Siemens Konvulsator III and of lidocane–modified treatment. *J Nerv Ment Dis* 1963;137: 117–123.

185. Robin A, De Tissera S. A double–blind controlled comparison of the therapeutic effects of low and high energy electroconvulsive therapies. *Br J Psychiatry* 1982;141:357–366.

186. Kellner CH. Towards the modal ECT treatment. *J ECT* 2001;17:1–2.

187. Sackeim HA, Devanand DP, Lisanby SH, et al. Treatment of the modal patient: does one size fit nearly all? *J ECT* 2001;17:219–222.

188. Sackeim HA, Portnoy S, Neeley P, et al. Cognitive consequences of low–dosage electroconvulsive therapy. *Ann N Y Acad Sci* 1986;462: 326–340.

189. Daniel W, Crovitz H. Acute memory impairment following electroconvulsive therapy. 2. Effects of electrode placement. *Acta Psychiatr Scand* 1983;67:57–68.

190. Coffey CE, Lucke J, Weiner RD, et al. Seizure threshold in electroconvulsive therapy: I. Initial seizure threshold. *Biol Psychiatry* 1995;37: 713–720.

191. Enns M, Karvelas L. Electrical dose titration for electroconvulsive therapy: a comparison with dose prediction methods. *Convuls Ther* 1995; 11:86–93.

192. Colenda CC, McCall WV. A statistical model predicting the seizure threshold for right unilateral ECT in 106 patients. *Convuls Ther* 1996; 12:3–12.

193. Sackeim HA. Comments on the 'half–age' method of stimulus dosing. *Convuls Ther* 1997; 13:37–43.

194. Lisanby SH, Devanand DP, Nobler MS, et al. Exceptionally high seizure threshold: ECT device limitations. *Convuls Ther* 1996;12:156–164.

195. Coffey CE, Lucke J, Weiner RD, et al. Seizure threshold in electroconvulsive therapy (ECT) II. The anticonvulsant effect of ECT. *Biol Psychiatry* 1995;37:777–788.

196. Squire L, Zouzounis J. ECT and memory: brief pulse versus sine wave. *Am J Psychiatry* 1986;143: 596–601.

197. McAllister D, Perri M, Jordan R, et al. Effects of ECT given two vs. three times weekly. *Psychiatry Res* 1987;21:63–69.

198. Lerer B, Shapira B, Calev A, et al. Antidepressant and cognitive effects of twice–versus three–times–weekly ECT. *Am J Psychiatry* 1995; 152:564–570.

199. Sackeim HA, Prudic J, Olfson M, Fuller RB. Short– and long–term cognitive effects of electroconvulsive therapy in community settings. Submitted.

200. Lerer B, Shapira B. Optimum frequency of electroconvulsive therapy: Implications for practice and research [editorial]. *Convulsive Ther* 1986;2:141–144.

201. Shapira B, Calev A, Lerer B. Optimal use of electroconvulsive therapy: choosing a treatment schedule. *Psychiatr Clin North Am* 1991; 14:935–946.

202. Calev A, Nigal D, Shapira B, et al. Early and long–term effects of electroconvulsive therapy and depression on memory and other cognitive functions. *J Nerv Ment Dis* 1991;179: 526–533.

203. Miller A, Faber R, Hatch J, Alexander H. Factors affecting amnesia, seizure duration, and efficacy in ECT. *Am J Psychiatry* 1985;142: 692–696.

204. Krueger RB, Fama JM, Devanand DP, et al. Does ECT permanently alter seizure threshold? *Biol Psychiatry* 1993;33:272–276.

205. Kramer B, Allen R, Friedman B. Atropine and glycopyrrolate as ECT preanesthesia. *J Clin Psychiatry* 1986;47:199–200.

206. Swartz CM, Saheba NC. Comparison of atropine with glycopyrrolate for use in ECT. *Convulsive Ther* 1989;5:56–60.

207. Greenan J, Dewar M, Jones C. Intravenous glycopyrrolate and atropine at induction of anaesthesia: a comparison. *J R Soc Med* 1983;76: 369–371.

208. Kellway B, Simpson K, Smith R, Halsall P. Effects of atropine and glycopyrrolate on cognitive function following anaethesia and electroconvulsive therapy. *Int Clin Psychopharm* 1986; 1:296–302.

209. Simpson KH, Smith RJ, Davies LF. Comparison of the effects of atropine and glycopyrrolate on cognitive function following general anaesthesia. *Br J Anaesth* 1987;59:966–969.

210. Sommer BR, Satlin A, Friedman L, Cole JO. Glycopyrrolate versus atropine in post–ECT amnesia in the elderly. *J Geriatr Psychiatry Neurol* 1989;2:18–21.

211. Kramer BA. Anticholinergics and ECT. *Convulsive Ther* 1993;9:293–300.

212. Small JG, Kellams JJ, Milstein V, Small IF. Complications with electroconvulsive treatment combined with lithium. *Biol Psychiatry* 1980;15: 103–112.

213. Weiner RD, Volow MR, Gianturco DT, Cavenar JOJ. Seizures terminable and interminable with ECT. *Am J Psychiatry* 1980;137:1416–1418.

214. Milstein V, Small JG. Problems with lithium combined with ECT [letter]. *Am J Psychiatry* 1988;145:1178.

215. Small JG, Milstein V. Lithium interactions: lithium and electroconvulsive therapy. *J Clin Psychopharmacol* 1990;10:346–350.

216. Mukherjee S. Combined ECT and lithium therapy. *Convulsive Ther* 1993;9:274–284.

217. Pettinati HM, Stephens SM, Willis KM, Robin SE. Evidence for less improvement in depression in patients taking benzodiazepines during unilateral ECT. *Am J Psychiatry* 1990;147:1029–1035.

218. Greenberg RM, Pettinati HM. Benzodiazepines and electroconvulsive therapy. *Convulsive Ther* 1993;9:262–273.

219. Andersen K, Balldin J, Gottfries C, et al. A double–blind evaluation of electroconvulsive therapy in Parkinson's disease with "on–off" phenomena. *Acta Neurol Scand* 1987;76:191–199.

220. Balldin J, Edèn S, Granèrus A, et al. Electroconvulsive therapy in Parkinson's syndrome with "on–off" phenomena. *J Neural Transm* 1980;47:11–21.

221. Fromm G. Observations on the effect of electroshock treatment on patients with parkinsonism. *Bull Tulane Med Faculty* 1959;18:71–73.

222. Asnis G. Parkinson's disease, depression, and ECT: a review and case study. *Am J Psychiatry* 1977;134:191–195.

223. Douyon R, Serby M, Klutchko B, Rotrosen J. ECT and Parkinson's disease revisited: a "naturalistic" study. *Am J Psychiatry* 1989;146:1451–1455.

224. Faber R, Trimble MR. Electroconvulsive therapy in Parkinson's disease and other movement disorders. *Mov Disord* 1991;6:293–303.

225. Kellner CH, Beale MD, Pritchett JT, et al. Electroconvulsive therapy and Parkinson's disease: the case for further study. *Psychopharmacol Bull* 1994;30:495–500.

226. Murray G, Shea V, Conn D. Electroconvulsive therapy for poststroke depression. *J Clin Psychiatry* 1986;47:258–260.

227. Hsiao JK, Messenheimer JA, Evans DL. ECT and neurological disorders. *Convulsive Ther* 1987;3:121–136.

228. Gustafson Y, Nilsson I, Mattsson M, et al. Epidemiology and treatment of post–stroke depression. *Drugs Aging* 1995;7:298–309.

229. Price TR, McAllister TW. Safety and efficacy of ECT in depressed patients with dementia: A review of clinical experience. *Convulsive Ther* 1989;5:61–74.

230. Nelson JP, Rosenberg DR. ECT treatment of demented elderly patients with major depression: A retrospective study of efficacy and safety. *Convulsive Ther* 1991;7:157–165.

231. Pridmore S, Pollard C. Electroconvulsive therapy in Parkinson's disease: 30 month follow up *J Neurol Neurosurg Psychiatry* 1996;60:693.

232. Figiel GS, Hassen MA, Zorumski C, et al. ECT–induced delirium in depressed patients with Parkinson's disease. *J Neuropsychiatry Clin Neurosci* 1991;3:405–411.

233. Oh JJ, Rummans TA, O'Connor MK, Ahlskog JE. Cognitive impairment after ECT in patients with Parkinson's disease and psychiatric illness [letter]. *Am J Psychiatry* 1992;149:271.

Table 13.1 References

Black DW, Winokur G, Nasrallah A. A multivariate analysis of the experience of 423 depressed inpatients treated with electroconvulsive therapy. *Convulsive Ther* 1993;9:112–120.

Carney MWP, Roth M, Garside RF. The diagnosis of depressive syndromes and the prediction of ECT response. *Br J Psychiatry* 1965;111:659–674.

Coryell W, Zimmerman M. Outcome following ECT for primary unipolar depression: a test of newly proposed response predictors. *Am J Psychiatry* 1984;141:862–867.

Folstein M, Folstein S, McHugh PR. Clinical predictors of improvement after electroconvulsive therapy of patients with schizophrenia, neurotic reactions, and affective disorders. *Biol Psychiatry* 1973;7:147–152.

Fraser RM, Glass IB. Unilateral and bilateral ECT in elderly patients. A comparative study. *Acta Psychiatr Scand* 1980;62:13–31.

Gold L, Chiarello CJ. Prognostic value of clinical findings in cases treated with electroshock. *J Nerv Ment Dis* 1944;100:577–583.

Greenblatt M, Grosser GH, Wechsler H. A comparative study of selected antidepressant medications and EST. *Am J Psychiatry* 1962;119:144–153.

Hamilton M, White J. Factors related to outcome of depression treated with ECT. *J Ment Sci* 1960;106:1030–1040.

Herrington RN, Bruce A, Johnstone EC. Comparative trial of L–tryptophan and E.C.T. in severe depressive illness. *Lancet* 1974;2:731–734.

Herzberg F. Prognostic variables for electro–shock therapy. *J Gen Psychol* 1954;50:79–86.

Heshe J, Röder E, Theilgaard A. Unilateral and bilateral ECT. A psychiatric and psychological study of therapeutic effect and side effects. *Acta Psychiatr Scand Suppl* 1978;275:1–180.

Hobson RF. Prognostic factors in ECT. *J Neurol Neurosurg Psychiatry* 1953;16:275–281.

Mendels J. Electroconvulsive therapy and depression. I. The prognostic significance of clinical factors. *Br J Psychiatry* 1965a;111:675–681.

Mendels J. Electroconvulsive therapy and depression. II. Significance of endogenous and reactive syndromes. *Br J Psychiatry* 1965b;111:682–686.

Nystrom S. On relation between clinical factors and efficacy of ECT in depression. *Acta Psychiatr Neurol Scand Suppl* 1964;181:11–35.

O'Connor MK, Knapp R, Husain M, et al. The influence of age on the response of major depression to electroconvulsive therapy: a C.O.R.E. Report. *Am J Geriatr Psychiatry* 2001; 9:382–390.

Ottosson JO. Experimental studies of the mode of action of electroconvulsive therapy. *Acta Psychiatr Scand Suppl.* 1960;145:1–141.

Prudic J, Olfson M, Marcus SC, et al. The effectiveness of electroconvulsive therapy in community settings. *Biol Psychiatry* 2004;55:301–312.

Rich CL, Spiker DG, Jewell SW, et al. The efficiency of ECT: I. Response rate in depressive episodes. *Psychiatry Res* 1984;11:167–176.

Rickles NK, Polan CG. Causes of failure in treatment with electric shock: analysis of thirty–eight cases. *Arch Neurol Psychiatry* 1948;59:337–346.

Roberts JM. Prognostic factors in the electroshock treatment of depressive states. I. Clinical features from testing and examination. *J Ment Sci* 1959a; 105:693–702.

Roberts JM. Prognostic factors in the electroshock treatment of depressive states. II. The application of specific tests. *J Ment Sci* 1959b;105:703–713.

Sackeim HA, Decina P, Kanzler M, et al. Effects of electrode placement on the efficacy of titrated, low–dose ECT. *Am J Psychiatry* 1987a;144: 1449–1455.

Sackeim HA, Decina P, Prohovnik I, Malitz S. Seizure threshold in electroconvulsive therapy. Effects of sex, age, electrode placement, and number of treatments. *Arch Gen Psychiatry* 1987b;44:355–360.

Sackeim HA, Prudic J, Devanand DP, et al. Effects of stimulus intensity and electrode placement on the efficacy and cognitive effects of electroconvulsive therapy. *N Engl J Med.* 1993;328:839–846.

Sackeim HA, Luber B, Moeller JR, et al. Electrophysiological correlates of the adverse cognitive effects of electroconvulsive therapy. *J ECT* 2000;16: 110–120.

Strömgren LS. Unilateral versus bilateral electroconvulsive therapy. Investigations into the therapeutic effect in endogenous depression. *Acta Psychiatr Scand Suppl* 1973;240:8–65.

Tew JDJ, Mulsant BH, Haskett RF, et al. Acute efficacy of ECT in the treatment of major depression in the old–old. *Am J Psychiatry* 1999; 156: 1865–1870.

Table 13.2 References

American Psychiatric Association Task. *The Practice of ECT: Recommendations for Treatment, Training and Privileging.* First Edition. Washington, D.C.: American Psychiatric Press, 1990.

American Psychiatric Association. *The Practice of ECT: Recommendations for Treatment, Training and Privileging.* Second Edition. Washington, D.C.: American Psychiatric Press, 2001.

Calev A, Nigal D, Shapira B, et al. Early and long–term effects of electroconvulsive therapy and depression on memory and other cognitive functions. *J Nerv Ment Dis* 1991;179:526–533.

Daniel WF, Crovitz HF. Acute memory impairment following electroconvulsive therapy. 2. Effects of electrode placement. *Acta Psychiatr Scand* 1983b; 67:57–68.

Fraser RM, Glass IB. Recovery from ECT in elderly patients. *Br J Psychiatry* 1978;133:524–528.

Fraser RM, Glass IB. Unilateral and bilateral ECT in elderly patients. A comparative study. *Acta Psychiatr Scand* 1980;62:13–31.

Holmberg G. The influence of oxygen administration on electrically induced convulsions in man. *Acta Psychiatr Neurol Scand* 1953;28:365–386.

Lerer B, Shapira B, Calev A, et al. Antidepressant and cognitive effects of twice–versus three–times–weekly ECT. *Am J Psychiatry* 1995;152: 564–570.

McAllister DA, Perri MG, Jordan RC, et al. Effects of ECT given two vs. three times weekly. *Psychiatry Res* 1987;21:63–69.

McElhiney MC, Moody BJ, Steif BL, et al. Autobiographical memory and mood: Effects of electroconvulsive therapy. *Neuropsychology* 1995;9:501–517.

Miller AL, Faber RA, Hatch JP, Alexander HE. Factors affecting amnesia, seizure duration, and efficacy in ECT. *Am J Psychiatry* 1985;142:692–696.

Mukherjee S. Combined ECT and lithium therapy. *Convulsive Ther* 1993;9:274–284.

Sackeim HA, Luber B, Moeller JR, et al. Electrophysiological correlates of the adverse cognitive effects of electroconvulsive therapy. *J ECT* 2000;16: 110–120.

Sackeim HA, Prudic J, Devanand DP, et al. Effects of stimulus intensity and electrode placement on the efficacy and cognitive effects of electroconvulsive therapy. *N Engl J Med.* 1993;328:839–846.

Sackeim HA, Portnoy S, Neeley P. Cognitive consequences of low–dosage electroconvulsive therapy. *Ann N Y Acad Sci* 1986;462:326–340.

Small JG, Milstein V. Lithium interactions: lithium and electroconvulsive therapy. *J Clin Psychopharmacol* 1990;10:346–350.

Sobin C, Sackeim HA, Prudic J, et al. Predictors of retrograde amnesia following ECT. *Am J Psychiatry* 1995;152:995–1001.

Squire L, Zouzounis J. ECT and memory: brief pulse versus sine wave. *Am J Psychiatry* 1986;143: 596–601.

Valentine M, Keddie K, Dunne D. A comparison of techniques in electroconvulsive therapy. *Br J Psychiatry* 1968;114:989–996.

Weiner RD, Rogers HJ, Davidson JR, Squire LR. Effects of stimulus parameters on cognitive side effects. *Ann NY Acad Sci* 1986;462:315–325.

Supplemental Readings

General

Abou–Saleh MT, Phil M, Coppen AJ. Should tricyclic antidepressants or lithium be standard continuation treatment after ECT: An alternative view (A reply to Sackeim et al.) [letter]. *Convulsive Ther* 1989;5:183–184.

American Psychiatric Association Task Force on ECT. *Electroconvulsive Therapy, Task Force Report #14.* Washington, D.C.: American Psychiatric Association, 1978.

Andrade C, Gangadhar BN. When is an ECT responder, an ECT responder? [letter]. *Convulsive Ther* 1989;5:190–191.

Benbow SM. Management of depression in the elderly. *Br J Hosp Med* 1992;48:726–731.

Bracken P, Ryan M, Dunne D. Electroconvulsive therapy in the elderly. *Br J Psychiatry* 1987;150: 713.

Brandon S, Cowley P, McDonald C, et al. Electroconvulsive therapy: results in depressive illness from the Leicestershire trial. *Br Med J Clin Res* 1984; 288:22–25.

Branfield M. ECT for depression in elderly people. *Nurs Stand* 1992;6:24–27.

Carney MWP, Roth M, Garside RF. The diagnosis of depressive syndromes and the prediction of ECT response. *Br J Psychiatry* 1965;111:659–674.

Casey DA. Depression in the elderly. *South Med J* 1994;87:559–563.

Crow T. The scientific status of electro–convulsive therapy. *Psychol Med* 1979;9:401–408.

Crow TJ, Johnstone EC. Controlled trials of electroconvulsive therapy. *Ann NY Acd Sci* 1986;462: 12–29.

Depression Guideline Panel. Depression in Primary Care: Vol. 2. Treatment of Major Depression. Rockville, MD: U.S. Department of Health and Human Services, Public Health Service, Agency for Health Care Policy and Research, AHCPR. No. 93–0551, 1993.

Devons CA. Suicide in the elderly: how to identify and treat patients at risk. *Geriatrics* 1996;51: 67–72.

Ehrenberg R, Gullingsrud MJ. Electroconvulsive therapy in elderly patients. *Am J Psychiatry* 1955; 111:743–747.

Evans VL. Convulsive shock therapy in elderly patients—risks and results. *Am J Psychiatry* 1943;99: 531–533.

Farah A, Beale MD, Kellner CH. Risperidone and ECT combination therapy: a case series. *Convuls Ther* 1995;11:280–282.

Flint AJ, Rifat SL. The effect of sequential antidepressant treatment on geriatric depression. *J Affect Disord* 1996;36:95–105.

Georgotas A, Cooper T, Kim M, Hapworth W. The treatment of affective disorders in the elderly. *Psychopharmacol Bull* 1983;19:226–237.

Greenberg L, Fink M. Electroconvulsive therapy in the elderly. *Psychiatr Ann* 1990;20:99–101.

Greenberg L, Fink M. The use of electroconvulsive therapy in geriatric patients. *Clin Geriatr Med* 1992;8:349–354.

Gregory S, Shawcross C, Gill D. The Nottingham ECT Study. A double–blind comparison of bilateral, unilateral and simulated ECT in depressive illness. *Br J Psychiatry* 1985;146:520–524.

Hamilton M. Development of a rating scale for primary depressive illness. *Br J Soc Clin Psychol* 1967; 6:278–296.

Hamilton M. The effect of treatment on the melancholias (depressions). *Br J Psychiatry* 1982;140: 223–230.

Jenike MA. Treatment of affective illness in the elderly with drugs and electroconvulsive therapy. *J Geriatr Psychiatry* 1989;22:77–112; discussion 113–120.

Johnstone EC, Deakin JF, Lawler P, et al. The Northwick Park electroconvulsive therapy trial. *Lancet* 1980;1317–1320.

Kamholz BA, Mellow AM. Management of treatment resistance in the depressed geriatric patient. *Psychiatr Clin North Am* 1996;19:269–286.

Khan A, Cohen S, Stowell M, et al. Treatment op-

tions in severe psychotic depression. *Convulsive Ther* 1987;3:93–99.

Koenig HG. Treatment considerations for the depressed geriatric medical patient. *Drugs Aging* 1991;1:266–278.

Kral VA. Somatic therapies in older depressed patients. *J Gerontol* 1976;31:311–313.

Lambourn J, Gill D. A controlled comparison of simulated and real ECT. *Br J Psychiatry* 1978;133: 514–519.

Levy SD. Electroconvulsive therapy in the elderly. *Geriatrics* 1988;43:44–46.

Lovell HW. Electric shock therapy in the aging. *Geriatrics* 1948;3:285–293.

McCall WV, Reboussin DM, Weiner RD, Sackeim HA. Titrated moderately suprathreshold vs fixed high–dose right unilateral electroconvulsive therapy: acute antidepressant and cognitive effects. *Arch Gen Psychiatry* 2000;57:438–444.

Mendels J. Clinical management of the depressed geriatric patient: current therapeutic options. *Am J Med* 1993;94:13S–18S.

Mulsant BH, Rosen J, Thornton JE, Zubenko GS. A prospective naturalistic study of electroconvulsive therapy in late–life depression. *J Geriatr Psychiatry Neurol* 1991;4:3–13.

NIH. NIH consensus conference. Diagnosis and treatment of depression in late life. *JAMA* 1992; 268:1018–1024.

Norden DK, Siegler EL. Electroconvulsive therapy in the elderly. *Hosp Pract* (Off Ed) 1993;28: 59–60,65–68,71.

O'Brien DR. The effective agent in electroconvulsive therapy: convulsion or coma? *Med Hypotheses* 1989;28:277–280.

O'Connor MK, Knapp R, Husain M, et al. The influence of age on the response of major depression to electroconvulsive therapy: a C.O.R.E. Report. *Am J Geriatr Psychiatry* 2001;9:382–390.

Post F. Psychotherapy, electro–convulsive treatments, and long–term management of elderly depressives. *J Affective Disord* 1985;Suppl 1: S41–S45.

Prudic J, Sackeim H. Refractory depression and electroconvulsive therapy. In: Roose SP, Glassman AH, eds. *Treatment of Refractory Depression.* Washington, D.C.: American Psychiatric Press, 1990: 109–128.

Raskind M. Electroconvulsive therapy in the elderly. *J Am Geriatr Soc* 1984;32:177–178.

Rosenbach ML, Hermann RC, Dorwart RA. Use of electroconvulsive therapy in the Medicare population between 1987 and 1992. *Psychiatr Serv* 1997; 48:1537–1542.

Rothschild AJ. The diagnosis and treatment of late–life depression. *J Clin Psychiatry* 1996; 57(Suppl 5):5–11.

Sackeim HA, Prudic J, Devanand DP. Treatment of medication–resistant depression with electroconvulsive therapy. In: Tasman A, Goldfinger SM, Kaufmann CA, eds. *Annual Review of Psychiatry, Volume 9.* Washington, D.C.: American Psychiatric Press, 1990:91–115.

Sackeim HA. Optimizing unilateral electroconvulsive therapy. *Convulsive Ther* 1991;7:201–212.

Sackeim HA. The efficacy of electroconvulsive therapy in treatment of major depressive disorder. In: Fisher S, Greenberg RP, eds. *The Limits of Bio-*

logical Treatments for Psychological Distress: Comparisons with Psychotherapy and Placebo. Hillsdale, N.J.: Erlbaum, 1989:275–307.

Sackeim HA. The efficacy of electroconvulsive therapy: Discussion of Part I. *Ann N Y Acad Sci* 1986; 462:70–75.

Sackeim HA. The use of electroconvulsive therapy in late life depression. In: Schneider LS, Reynolds CF III, Liebowitz BD, Friedhoff AJ, eds. *Diagnosis and treatment of depression in late life.* Washington, DC: American Psychiatric Press, 1993: 259–277.

Salzman C, Wong E, Wright BC. Drug and ECT treatment of depression in the elderly, 1996–2001: A literature review. *Biol Psychiatry* 2002;52:265–284.

Salzman C. Electroconvulsive therapy in the elderly patient. *Psychiatr Clin North Am* 1982;5:191–197.

Schneider LS. Efficacy of treatment for geropsychiatric patients with severe mental illness. *Psychopharmacol Bull* 1993;29:501–524.

Sullivan MD, Ward NG, Laxton A. The woman who wanted electroconvulsive therapy and do–not–resuscitate status. Questions of competence on a medical–psychiatry unit. *Gen Hosp Psychiatry* 1992;14:204–209.

Tang WK, Ungvari GS. Efficacy of electroconvulsive therapy combined with antipsychotic medication in treatment–resistant schizophrenia: a prospective, open trial. *J ECT* 2002;18:90–94.

Thase ME, Rush AJ. Treatment–resistant depression. In: Bloom FE, Kupfer DJ, eds. *Psychopharmacology: the fourth generation of progress.* New York: Raven 1995:1081–1098.

The UK Review Group. Efficacy and safety of electroconvulsive therapy in depressive disorders: a systematic review and meta–analysis. *Lancet* 2003; 361:799–808.

Tomac TA, Rummans TA, Pileggi TS, Li H. Safety and efficacy of electroconvulsive therapy in patients over age 85. *Am J Geriatr Psychiatry* 1997;5: 126–130.

West E. Electric convulsion therapy in depression: a double–blind controlled trial. *Br Med J Clin Res* 1981;282:355–357.

Wolff GE, Garrett FH. Electric shock treatment in elderly mental patients. *Geriatrics* 1954;9: 316–318.

Zorumski CF, Rubin EH, Burke WJ. Electroconvulsive therapy for the elderly: a review. *Hosp Community Psychiatry* 1988;39:643–647.

Anesthesia

Boey WK, Lai FO. Comparison of propofol and thiopentone as anaesthetic agents for electroconvulsive therapy. *Anaesthesia* 1990;45:623–628.

Bone ME, Wilkins CJ, Lew JK. A comparison of propofol and methohexitone as anaesthetic agents for electroconvulsive therapy. *Eur J Anaesthesiol* 1988;5:279–286.

Cawley RH, Post F, Whitehead A. Barbiturate tolerance and psychological functioning in elderly depressed patients. *Psychol Med* 1973;3:39–52.

Ciraulo D, Lind L, Salzman C, et al. Sodium nitroprusside treatment of ECT–induced blood pressure elevations. *Am J Psychiatry* 1978;135: 1105–1106.

Dwyer R, McCaughey W, Lavery J, et al. Comparison of propofol and methohexitone as anaesthetic agents for electroconvulsive therapy. *Anaesthesia* 1988;43:459–462.

Gaines GY 3d, Rees DI. Electroconvulsive therapy and anesthetic considerations. *Anesth Analg* 1986; 65:1345–1356.

Greenan J, Dewar M, Jones CJ. Intravenous glycopyrrolate and atropine at induction of anaesthesia: a comparison. *J R Soc Med* 1983;76:369–371.

Ilivicky H, Caroff SN, Simone AF. Etomidate during ECT for elderly seizure–resistant patients. *Am J Psychiatry* 1995;152:957–958.

Kellway B, Simpson K, Smith R, Halsall P. Effects of atropine and glycopyrrolate on cognitive function following anaesthesia and electroconvulsive therapy. *Int Clin Psychopharm* 1986;1:296–302.

Kraus RP, Remick RA. Diazoxide in the management of severe hypertension after electroconvulsive therapy. *Am J Psychiatry* 1982;139:504–505.

Pitts FNJ, Desmarais G, Stewart W, Schaberg K. Induction of anesthesia in electroconvulsive therapy with methohexital and thiopental. *N Engl J Med* 1965;273:353–360.

Rouse EC. Propofol for electroconvulsive therapy. A comparison with methohexitone. Preliminary report. *Anaesthesia* 1988;43(Suppl):61–64.

Simpson KH, Smith RJ, Davies LF. Comparison of the effects of atropine and glycopyrrolate on cognitive function following general anaesthesia. *Br J Anaesth* 1987;59:966–969.

Sommer BR, Satlin A, Friedman L, Cole JO. Glycopyrrolate versus atropine in post–ECT amnesia in the elderly. *J Geriatr Psychiatry Neurol* 1989;2: 18–21.

Swartz CM. Obstruction of ECT seizure by submaximal hyperventilation: a case report. *Ann Clin Psychiatry* 1996;8:31–34.

Wells DG, Davies GG, Rosewarne F. Attenuation of electroconvulsive therapy–induced hypertension with sublingual nifedipine. *Anaesth Intensive Care* 1989;17:31–33.

Woodruff RA Jr, Pitts FN Jr, McClure JN Jr. The drug modification of ECT. I. Methohexital, thiopental, and preoxygenation. *Arch Gen Psychiatry* 1968; 18:605–611.

Concomitant Pharmacology

Bross R. Near fatality with combined ECT and reserpine. *Am J Psychiatry* 1957;113:933.

Foster MWJ, Gayle RFI. Chlorpromazine and reserpine as adjuncts in electroshock treatment. *South Med J* 1956;49:731–735.

Levin Y, Elizur A, Korczyn AD. Physostigmine improves ECT–induced memory disturbances. *Neurology* 1987;37:871–875.

Milstein V, Small JG. Problems with lithium combined with ECT. *Am J Psychiatry* 1988;145:1178.

Pritchett JT, Bernstein HJ, Kellner CH. Combined ECT and antidepressant drug therapy. *Convulsive Ther* 9:256–261.

Small JG, Kellams JJ, Milstein V, Small IF. Complications with electroconvulsive treatment combined with lithium. *Biol Psychiatry* 1980;15:103–112.

Small JG, Milstein V. Lithium interactions: lithium and electroconvulsive therapy. *J Clin Psychopharmacol* 1990;10:346–350.

Stern RA, Nevels CT, Shelhorse ME, et al. Antidepressant and memory effects of combined thyroid hormone treatment and electroconvulsive therapy: preliminary findings. *Biol Psychiatry* 1991;30:623–627.

Weiner RD, Whanger AD, Erwin CW, Wilson WP. Prolonged confusional state and EEG seizure activity following concurrent ECT and lithium use. *Am J Psychiatry* 1980;137:1452–1453.

Efficacy and ECT Technique

Abrams R. Stimulus titration and ECT dosing. *J ECT* 2002;18:3–9; discussion 14–15

Andrade C, Sudha S, Venkataraman BV. Herbal treatments for ECS–induced memory deficits: a review of research and a discussion on animal models. *J ECT* 2000;16:144–156.

Bailine SH, Rifkin A, Kayne E, et al. Comparison of bifrontal and bitemporal ECT for major depression. *Am J Psychiatry* 2000;157:121–123.

Blanch J, Martinez–Palli G, Navines R, et al. Comparative hemodynamic effects of urapidil and labetalol after electroconvulsive therapy. *J ECT* 2001; 17:275–279.

Bolwig T, Hertz M, Holm–Jensen J. Blood–brain barrier during electroshock seizures in the rat. *Eur J Clin Invest* 1977;7:95–100.

Bolwig T, Hertz M, Paulson O, et al. The permeability of the blood–brain barrier during electrically induced seizures in man. *Eur J Clin Invest* 1977; 7:87–93.

Bolwig TG, Hertz MM, Westergaard E. Acute hypertension causing blood–brain barrier breakdown during epileptic seizures. *Acta Neurol Scand* 1977; 56:335–342.

Bolwig TG. Blood–brain barrier studies with special reference to epileptic seizures. *Acta Psychiatr Scand* [Suppl] 1988;345:15–20.

Boylan LS, Devanand DP, Lisanby SH, et al. Focal Prefrontal Seizures Induced by Bilateral ECT. *J ECT* 2001;17:175–179.

Boylan LS, Haskett RF, Mulsant BH, et al. Determinants of seizure threshold in ECT: benzodiazepine use, anesthetic dosage, and other factors. *J ECT* 2000;16:3–18.

Casey DA, Davis MH. Obsessive–compulsive disorder responsive to electroconvulsive therapy in an elderly woman. *South Med J* 1994;87:862–864.

Castelli I, Steiner LA, Kaufmann MA, et al. Comparative effects of esmolol and labetalol to attenuate hyperdynamic states after electroconvulsive therapy. *Anesth Analg* 1995;80:557–561.

Coffey CE, Figiel GS, Weiner RD, Saunders WB. Caffeine augmentation of ECT. *Am J Psychiatry* 1990; 147:579–585.

Crow TJ, Johnstone EC. Controlled trials of electroconvulsive therapy. *Ann NY Acad Sci* 1986;462: 12–29.

Dannon PN, Iancu I, Hirschmann S, et al. Labetalol does not lengthen asystole during electroconvulsive therapy. *J ECT* 1998;14:245–250.

Decina P, Malitz S, Sackeim H, et al. Cardiac arrest during ECT modified by beta–adrenergic blockade. *Am J Psychiatry* 1984;141:298–300.

d'Elia G. Unilateral electroconvulsive therapy. *Acta Psychiatr Scand* [Suppl] 1970;215:1–98.

Delva NJ, Brunet D, Hawken ER, et al. Electrical dose and seizure threshold: relations to clinical outcome and cognitive effects in bifrontal, bitemporal, and right unilateral ECT. *J ECT* 2000;16: 361–369.

Drop L, Castelli I, Kaufmann M. Comparative doses and cost: esmolol versus labetalol during electroconvulsive therapy [letter]. *Anesth Analg* 1998;86: 916–917.

Frances A, Weiner RD, Coffey CE. ECT for an elderly man with psychotic depression and concurrent dementia. *Hosp Community Psychiatry* 1989;40: 237–238,242.

Heikman P, Kalska H, Katila H, et al. Right unilateral and bifrontal electroconvulsive therapy in the treatment of depression: a preliminary study. *J ECT* 2002;18:26–30.

Kellner CH, Monroe RRJ, Pritchett J, et al. Weekly ECT in geriatric depression. *Convulsive Ther* 1992;8:245–252.

Kelsey MC, Grossberg GT. Safety and efficacy of caffeine–augmented ECT in elderly depressives: a retrospective study. *J Geriatr Psychiatry Neurol* 1995;8:168–172.

Krystal AD, Weiner RD, McCall WV, et al. The effect of ECT stimulus dose and electrode placement on the ictal electroencephalogram: An intraindividual crossover study. *Biol Psychiatry* 1993;34: 759–767.

Lawson JS, Inglis J, Delva NJ, et al. Electrode placement in ECT: cognitive effects. *Psychol Med* 1990; 20:335–344.

Letemendia FJ, Delva NJ, Rodenburg M, et al. Therapeutic advantage of bifrontal electrode placement in ECT. *Psychol Med* 1993;23:349–360.

Lisanby SH, Morales O, Payne N, et al. New developments in electroconvulsive therapy and magnetic seizure therapy. *CNS Spectr* 2003;8:529–536.

Lisanby SH. Focal brain stimulation with repetitive transcranial magnetic stimulation (rTMS): implications for the neural circuitry of depression. *Psychol Med* 2003;33:7–13.

Maletzky B. Seizure duration and clinical effect in electroconvulsive therapy. *Compr Psychiatry* 1978; 19:541–550.

Meyers BS, Mei–Tal V. Empirical study on an inpatient psychogeriatric unit: biological treatment in patients with depressive illness. *Int J Psychiatry Med* 1986;15:111–124.

O'Connor C, Rothenberg D, Soble J, et al. The effect of esmolol pretreatment on the incidence of regional wall motion abnormalities during electroconvulsive therapy. *Anesth Analg* 1996;82: 143–147.

O'Shea B, Lynch T, Falvey J, O'Mahoney G. Electroconvulsive therapy and cognitive improvement in a very elderly depressed patient. *Br J Psychiatry* 1987;150:255–257.

Ottosson JO. Is unilateral nondominant ECT as efficient as bilateral ECT? A new look at the evidence. *Convulsive Ther* 1991;7:190–200.

Perera TD, Luber B, Nobler MS, et al. Seizure expression during electroconvulsive therapy: relationships with clinical outcome and cognitive side effects. *Neuropsychopharmacology* 2004;29: 813–825.

Petrides G, Fink M. Choosing a dosing strategy for electrical stimulation in ECT [letter; comment]. *J Clin Psychiatry* 1996;57:487–488.

Petrides G, Fink M. The 'half–age' stimulation strategy for ECT dosing. *Convuls Ther* 1996;12: 138–146.

Pettinati HM, Nilsen SM. Increased incidence of missed seizures during ECT in the elderly male. *Convulsive Ther* 1987;3:26–30.

Reynolds CF 3d, Perel JM, Kupfer DJ, et al. Open–trial response to antidepressant treatment in elderly patients with mixed depression and cognitive impairment. *Psychiatry Res* 1987;21: 111–122.

Rich CL, Spiker DG, Jewell SW, Neil JF. DSM–III, RDC, and ECT: depressive subtypes and immediate response. *J Clin Psychiatry* 1984;45:14–18.

Rifkin A. ECT versus tricyclic antidepressants in depression: a review of the evidence. *J Clin Psychiatry* 1988;49:3–7.

Roemer RA, Dubin WR, Jaffe R, et al. An efficacy study of single–versus double–seizure induction with ECT in major depression. *J Clin Psychiatry* 1990;51:473–478.

Sackeim HA, Long J, Luber B, et al. Physical properties and quantification of the ECT stimulus: I. Basic principles. *Convuls Ther* 1994;10:93–123.

Sackeim HA, Rush AJ. Melancholia and response to ECT. *Am J Psychiatry* 1995;152:1242–1243.

Sackeim HA. Are ECT devices underpowered? *Convulsive Ther* 1991;7:233–236.

Sackeim HA. ECT: twice or thrice a week? *Convulsive Ther* 1989;5:362–364.

Srinivasan TN, Suresh TR, Jayaram V, Fernandez MP. Nature and treatment of delusional parasitosis: a different experience in India. *Int J Dermatol* 1994;33:851–855.

Stack JA, Reynolds CF 3, Perel JM, et al. Pretreatment systolic orthostatic blood pressure (PSOP) and treatment response in elderly depressed inpatients. *J Clin Psychopharmacol* 1988;8:116–120.

Stoudemire A, Hill CD, Morris R, et al. Long–term affective and cognitive outcome in depressed older adults. *Am J Psychiatry* 1993;150:896–900.

Strömgren LS. Unilateral versus bilateral electroconvulsive therapy. Investigations into the therapeutic effect in endogenous depression. *Acta Psychiatr Scand* [Suppl] 1973;240:8–65.

Swartz CM, Larson G. ECT stimulus duration and its efficacy. *Ann Clin Psychiatry* 1989;1:147–152.

Tayek JA, Bistrian BR, Blackburn GL. Improved food intake and weight gain in adult patients following electroconvulsive therapy for depression. *J Am Diet Assoc* 1988;88:63–65.

Tew JDJ, Mulsant BH, Haskett RF, et al. Acute efficacy of ECT in the treatment of major depression in the old–old. *Am J Psychiatry* 1999;156: 1865–1870.

van Marwijk H, Bekker FM, Hop WC, et al. Electroconvulsive therapy in depressed elderly subjects; a retrospective study of efficacy and safety. *Ned Tijdschr Geneeskd* 1988;132:1396–1399.

Weiner RD. Treatment optimization with ECT. *Psychopharmacol Bull* 1994;30:313–320.

Zubenko GS, Mulsant BH, Rifai AH, et al. Impact of acute psychiatric inpatient treatment on major depression in late life and prediction of response. *Am J Psychiatry* 1994;151:987–994.

Zvara DA, Brooker RF, McCall WV, et al. The effect of esmolol on ST–segment depression and arrhythmias after electroconvulsive therapy. *Convuls Ther* 1997;13:165–174.

Mechanisms of Action

Ackermann R, Engel JJ, Baxter L. Positron emission tomography and autoradiographic studies of glucose utilization following electroconvulsive seizures in humans and rats. *Ann NY Acad Sci* 1986; 462:263–269.

D'Costa A, Breese CR, Boyd RL, et al. Attenuation of Fos–like immunoreactivity induced by a single electroconvulsive shock in brains of aging mice. *Brain Res* 1991;567:204–211.

Devanand DP, Dwork AJ, Hutchinson ER, et al. Does ECT alter brain structure? *Am J Psychiatry* 1994; 151:957–970.

Enns M, Peeling J, Sutherland GR. Hippocampal neurons are damaged by caffeine–augmented electroshock seizures. *Biol Psychiatry* 1996;40: 642–647.

Essman WB. Aging–related changes in retrograde amnesia for mice. *Gerontology* 1982;28:303–313.

Krueger RB, Fama JM, Devanand DP, et al. Does ECT permanently alter seizure threshold? *Biol Psychiatry* 1993;33:272–276.

Mann JJ, Manevitz AZ, Chen JS, et al. Acute effects of single and repeated electroconvulsive therapy on plasma catecholamines and blood pressure in major depressive disorder. *Psychiatry Res* 1990;34: 127–137.

McNamara MC, Miller AT Jr, Benignus VA, Davis JN. Age related changes in the effect of electroconvulsive shock (ECS) on the in vivo hydroxylation of tyrosine and tryptophan in rat brain. *Brain Res* 1977;131:313–320.

Mileusnic R, Veskov R, Rakić L. The effect of electroconvulsive shock on brain tubulin during development and aging. *Life Sci* 1986;38:1171–1178.

Nobler MS, Sackeim HA, Prohovnik I, et al. Regional cerebral blood flow in mood disorders, III. Treatment and clinical response. *Arch Gen Psychiatry* 1994;51:884–897.

Nutt DJ, Gleiter CH, Glue P. Neuropharmacological aspects of ECT: in search of the primary mechanism of action. *Convulsive Ther* 1989;5:250–260.

O'Brien DR. The effective agent in electroconvulsive therapy: convulsion or coma? *Med Hypotheses* 1989;28:277–280.

Oztas B, Kaya M, Camurcu S. Age related changes in the effect of electroconvulsive shock on the blood brain barrier permeability in rats. *Mech Ageing Dev* 1990;51:149–155.

Sackeim HA, Decina P, Prohovnik I, et al. Anticonvulsant and antidepressant properties of electroconvulsive therapy: a proposed mechanism of action. *Biol Psychiatry* 1983;18:1301–1310.

Sackeim HA, Devanand DP, Nobler MS. Electroconvulsive therapy. In: Bloom F, Kupfer D, eds. *Psychopharmacology: the fourth generation of progress.* New York: Raven, 1995:1123–1142.

Sackeim HA, Luber B, Katzman GP, et al. The effects of electroconvulsive therapy on quantitative electroencephalograms. Relationship to clinical outcome. *Arch Gen Psychiatry* 1996;53:814–824.

Sackeim HA. Central issues regarding the mechanisms of action of electroconvulsive therapy: directions for future research. *Psychopharmacol Bull* 1994;30:281–308.

Sackeim HA. Mechanisms of action of electroconvulsive therapy. In: Hales RE, Frances J, eds. *Annual review of psychiatry,* vol. 7. Washington, DC: American Psychiatric Press, 1988:436–457.

Scott AI. Which depressed patients will respond to electroconvulsive therapy? The search for biological predictors of recovery. *Br J Psychiatry* 1989; 154:8–17.

Siesjö BK, Ingvar M, Wieloch T. Cellular and molecular events underlying epileptic brain damage. *Ann NY Acad Sci* 1986;462:207–223.

Medical and Neurological Conditions

Ananth J, Samra D, Kolivakis T. Amelioration of drug–induced Parkinsonism by ECT. *Am J Psychiatry* 1979;136:1094.

Andersen K, Balldin J, Gottfries CG, et al. A double–blind evaluation of electroconvulsive therapy in Parkinson's disease with "on–off" phenomena. *Acta Neurol Scand* 1987;76:191–199.

Asnis G. Parkinson's disease, depression, and ECT: a review and case study. *Am J Psychiatry* 1977;134: 191–195.

Balldin J, Edën S, Granërus AK, et al. Electroconvulsive therapy in Parkinson's syndrome with "on–off" phenomenon. *J Neural Transm* 1980; 47:11–21.

Douyon R, Serby M, Klutchko B. ECT and Parkinson's disease revisited: a "naturalistic" study. *Am J Psychiatry* 1989;146:1451–1455.

Fall PA, Granerus AK. Maintenance ECT in Parkinson's disease. *J Neural Transm* 1999;106:737–741.

Fromm G. Observations on the effect of electroshock treatment on patients with parkinsonism. *Bull Tulane Med Faculty* 1959;18:71–73.

Goldstein MZ, Jensvold MF. ECT treatment of an elderly mentally retarded man. *Psychosomatics* 1989;30:104–106.

Goswami U, Dutta S, Kuruvilla K, et al. Electroconvulsive therapy in neuroleptic–induced parkinsonism. *Biol Psychiatry* 1989;26:234–238.

Hartmann SJ, Saldivia A. ECT in an elderly patient with skull defects and shrapnel. *Convulsive Ther* 1990;6:165–171.

Hay DP, Hay L, Blackwell B, Spiro HR. ECT and tardive dyskinesia. *J Geriatr Psychiatry Neurol* 1990;3:106–109.

Hay DP. Electroconvulsive therapy in the medically ill elderly. *Convulsive Ther* 1989;5:9–16.

Johnson J, Sims R, Gottlieb G. Differential diagnosis of dementia, delirium and depression. Implications for drug therapy. *Drugs Aging* 1994;5: 431–445.

Malek–Ahmadi P, Beceiro JR, McNeil BW, Weddige RL. Electroconvulsive therapy and chronic subdural hematoma. *Convulsive Ther* 1990;6:38–41.

Malek–Ahmadi P, Weddige RL. Tardive dyskinesia and electroconvulsive therapy. *Convulsive Ther* 1988;4:328–331.

Martin M, Figiel G, Mattingly G, et al. ECT–induced interictal delirium in patients with a history of a CVA. *J Geriatr Psychiatry Neurol* 1992; 5:149–155.

Murray GB, Shea V, Conn DK. Electroconvulsive therapy for poststroke depression. *J Clin Psychiatry* 1986;47:258–260.

Oh JJ, Rummans TA, O'Connor MK, Ahlskog JE. Cognitive impairment after ECT in patients with Parkinson's disease and psychiatric illness. *Am J Psychiatry* 1992;149:271.

Rasmussen KG, Zorumski CF, Jarvis MR. Electroconvulsive therapy in patients with cerebral palsy. *Convulsive Ther* 1993;9:205–208.

Warren AC, Holroyd S, Folstein MF. Major depression in Down's syndrome. *Br J Psychiatry* 1989; 155:202–205.

Zwil AS, Pelchat RJ. ECT in the treatment of patients with neurological and somatic disease. *Int J Psychiatry Med* 1994;24:1–29.

Medical Complications and Cognitive Effects

Andrade C, Sudha S, Venkataraman BV. Herbal treatments for ECS–induced memory deficits: a review of research and a discussion on animal models. *J ECT* 2000;16:144–156.

Andrade C, Suresh S, Krishnan J, Venkataraman BV. Effects of stimulus parameters on seizure duration and ECS–induced retrograde amnesia. *J ECT* 2002;18:31–37.

Bennett–Levy J, Powell GE. The subjective memory questionnaire (SMQ). An investigation into the self–reporting of 'real–life' memory skills. *Br J Soc Clin Psychol* 1980;19:177–188.

Blanch J, Martinez–Palli G, Navines R, et al. Comparative hemodynamic effects of urapidil and labetalol after electroconvulsive therapy. *J ECT* 2001; 17:275–279.

Bright–Long LE, Fink M. Reversible dementia and affective disorder: the Rip Van Winkle syndrome. *Convulsive Ther* 1993;9:209–216.

Broadbent DE, Cooper PF, Fitzgerald P, Parkes KR. The cogntive failures questionnaire (CFQ) and its correlates. *Br J Clin Psychol* 1982;21:1–16.

Calev A, Gaudino EA, Squires NK, et al. ECT and non–memory cognition: a review. *Br J Clin Psychol* 1995;34 (Pt 4):505–515.

Calev A, Kochav–lev E, Tubi N, et al. Change in attitude toward electroconvulsive therapy: Effects of treatment, time since treatment, and severity of depression. *Convulsive Ther* 1991;7:184–189.

Carney M, Sheffield B. The effects of pulse ECT in neurotic and endogenous depression. *Br J Psychiatry* 1974;125:91–94.

Castelli I, Steiner LA, Kaufmann MA, et al. Comparative effects of esmolol and labetalol to attenuate hyperdynamic states after electroconvulsive therapy. *Anesth Analg* 1995;80:557–561.

Coffey CE, Hoffman G, Weiner RD, Moossy JJ. Electroconvulsive therapy in a depressed patient with a functioning ventriculoatrial shunt. *Convulsive Ther* 1987;3:302–306.

Coffey CE, Weiner RD, Kalayjian R, Christison C. Electroconvulsive therapy in osteogenesis imperfecta: issues of muscular relaxation. *Convulsive Ther* 1986;2:207–211.

Coffey CE, Weiner RD, McCall WV, Heinz ER. Electroconvulsive therapy in multiple sclerosis: a magnetic resonance imaging study of the brain. *Convulsive Ther* 1987;3:137–144.

Coleman EA, Sackeim HA, Prudic J, et al. Subjective memory complaints before and after electroconvulsive therapy. *Biol Psychiatry* 1996;39:346–356.

Cronholm B, Ottosson JO. The experience of memory function after electroconvulsive therapy. *Br J Psychiatry* 1963;109:251–258.

Daniel WF, Crovitz HF, Weiner RD. Neuropsychological aspects of disorientation. *Cortex* 1987;23:169–187.

Dannon PN, Iancu I, Hirschmann S, et al. Labetalol does not lengthen asystole during electroconvulsive therapy. *J ECT* 1998;14:245–250.

Decina P, Malitz S, Sackeim H, et al. Cardiac arrest during ECT modified by beta–adrenergic blockade. *Am J Psychiatry* 1984;141:298–300.

Devanand DP, Briscoe KM, Sackeim HA, Prudic J. Clinical features and predictors of postictal excitement. *Convulsive Ther* 1989;5:140–146.

Devanand DP, Malitz S, Sackeim HA. ECT in a patient with aortic aneurysm. *J Clin Psychiatry* 1990;51:255–256.

Devanand DP, Sackeim HA, Decina P. ECT–induced myoclonus. *Convulsive Ther* 1986;2:289–292.

Devanand DP, Sackeim HA, Decina P. The development of mania and organic euphoria during ECT. *J Clin Psychiatry* 1988;49:69–71.

Donahue AB. Electroconvulsive therapy and memory loss: a personal journey. *J ECT* 2000;16:133–143.

Drop L, Castelli I, Kaufmann M. Comparative doses and cost: esmolol versus labetalol during electroconvulsive therapy [letter]. *Anesth Analg* 1998;86:916–917.

Durrant BW. Dental care in electroplexy. *Br J Psychiatry* 1966;112:1173–1176.

Faber R. Dental fracture during ECT. *Am J Psychiatry* 1983;140:1255–1256.

Fawver J, Milstein V. Asthma/emphysema complication of electroconvulsive therapy: a case study. *Convulsive Ther* 1985;1:61–64.

Fochtmann LJ. Animal studies of electroconvulsive therapy: foundations for future research. *Psychopharmacol Bull* 1994;30:321–444.

Freeman C, Weeks D, Kendell R. ECT: II: patients who complain. *Br J Psychiatry* 1980;137:17–25.

Frith C, Stevens M, Johnstone E, et al. Effects of ECT and depression on various aspects of memory. *Br J Psychiatry* 1983;142:610–617.

Grunhaus L, Shipley JE, Eiser A, et al. Shortened REM latency postECT is associated with rapid recurrence of depressive symptomatology. *Biol Psychiatry* 1994;36:214–222.

Guttmacher LB, Greenland P. Effects of electroconvulsive therapy on the electrocardiogram in geriatric patients with stable cardiovascular diseases. *Convulsive Ther* 1989;6:5–12.

Harsch HH. Atrial fibrillation, cardioversion, and electroconvulsive therapy. *Convulsive Ther* 1991;7:139–142.

Hinkin C, van G, WG,, Satz P. Actual versus self–reported cognitive dysfunction in HIV–1 infection: memory–metamemory dissociations. *J Clin Exp Neuropsychol* 1996;18:431–443.

Kaufman KR. Asystole with electroconvulsive therapy. *J Intern Med* 1994;235:275–277.

Khan A, Mirolo MH, Claypoole K, et al. Effects of low–dose TRH on cognitive deficits in the ECT postictal state. *Am J Psychiatry* 1994;151:1694–1696.

Khan A, Mirolo MH, Lai H, et al. ECT and TRH: cholinergic involvement in a cognitive deficit state. *Psychopharmacol Bull* 1993;29:345–352.

Krueger RB, Sackeim HA, Gamzu ER. Pharmacological treatment of the cognitive side effects of ECT: a review. *Psychopharmacol Bull* 1992;28:409–424.

Larrabee GJ, Levin HS. Memory self–ratings and objective test performance in a normal elderly sample. *J Clin Exp Neuropsychol* 1986;8:275–284.

Levin Y, Elizur A, Korczyn A. Physostigmine improves ECT–induced memory disturbances. *Neurology* 1987;37:871–875.

Liston EH, Salk JD. Hemodynamic responses to ECT after bilateral adrenalectomy. *Convulsive Ther* 1990;6:160–164.

Mattes JA, Pettinati HM, Stephens S, et al. A placebo–controlled evaluation of vasopressin for ECT–induced memory impairment. *Biol Psychiatry* 1990;27:289–303.

McCall WV, Reid S, Ford M. Electrocardiographic and cardiovascular effects of subconvulsive stimulation during titrated right unilateral ECT. *Convulsive Ther* 1994;10:25–33.

McCall WV. Asystole in electroconvulsive therapy: Report of four cases. *J Clin Psychiatry* 1996;57:199–203.

O'Connor C, Rothenberg D, Soble J, et al. The effect of esmolol pretreatment on the incidence of regional wall motion abnormalities during electroconvulsive therapy. *Anesth Analg* 1996;82:143–147.

Perera TD, Luber B, Nobler MS, et al. Seizure expression during electroconvulsive therapy: relationships with clinical outcome and cognitive side effects. *Neuropsychopharmacology* 2004;29:813–825.

Pettinati H, Rosenberg J. Memory self–ratings before and after electroconvulsive therapy: depression–versus ECT induced. *Biol Psychiatry* 1984;19:539–548.

Pettinati HM, Bonner KM. Cognitive functioning in depressed geriatric patients with a history of ECT. *Am J Psychiatry* 1984;141:49–52.

Pettinati HM, Tamburello TA, Ruetsch CR, Kaplan FN. Patient attitudes toward electroconvulsive therapy. *Psychopharmacol Bull* 1994;30:471–475.

Prudic J, Fitzsimons L, Nobler MS, Sackeim HA. Naloxone in the prevention of the adverse cognitive effects of ECT: a within–subject, placebo controlled study. *Neuropsychopharmacology* 1999;21:285–293.

Prudic J, Peyser S, Sackeim HA. Subjective memory complaints: a review of patient self–assessment of memory after electroconvulsive therapy. *J ECT* 2000;16:121–132.

Prudic J, Sackeim H, Decina P, et al. Acute effects of ECT on cardiovascular functioning: relations to patient and treatment variables. *Acta Psychiatr Scand* 1987;75:344–351.

Rabbitt P. Development of methods to measure changes in activities of daily living in the elderly. In: Corkin S, Davis KL, Growdon JH, Usdin E, Wurtman R, eds. *Alzheimer's disease: A report of progress in research.* New York: Raven, 1982:127–131.

Regestein QR, Lind LJ. Management of electroconvulsive treatment in an elderly woman with severe hypertension and cardiac arrhythmias. *Compr Psychiatry* 1980;21:288–291.

Rubin EH, Kinscherf DA, Figiel GS, Zorumski CF. The nature and time course of cognitive side effects during electroconvulsive therapy in the elderly. *J Geriatr Psychiatry Neurol* 1993;6:78–83.

Sackeim HA, Ross FR, Hopkins N, et al. Subjective side effects acutely following ECT: associations with treatment modality and clinical response. *Convulsive Ther* 1987;3:100–110.

Sackeim HA. Acute cognitive side effects of ECT. *Psychopharmacol Bull* 1986;22:482–484.

Shellenberger W, Miller M, Small I, et al. Follow-up study of memory deficits after ECT. *Can J Psychiatry* 1982;27:325–329.

Squire L, Cohen N. Memory and amnesia: resistance to disruption develops for years after learning. *Behav Neural Biol* 1979;25:115–125.

Squire L, Slater P. Electroconvulsive therapy and complaints of memory dysfunction: a prospective three-year follow-up study. *Br J Psychiatry* 1983;142:1–8.

Squire LR, Miller PL. Diminution of anterograde amnesia following electroconvulsive therapy. *Br J Psychiatry* 1974;125:490–495.

Squire LR, Zouzounis JA. Self-ratings of memory dysfunction: different findings in depression and amnesia. *J Clin Exp Neuropsychol* 1988;10:727–738.

Squire LR. A stable impairment in remote memory following electroconvulsive therapy. *Neuropsychologia* 1975;13:51–58.

Squire SR, Slater PC. Bilateral and unilateral ECT: effects on verbal and nonverbal memory. *Am J Psychiatry* 1978;135:1316–1320.

Stern RA, Nevels CT, Shelhorse ME, et al. Antidepressant and memory effects of combined thyroid hormone treatment and electroconvulsive therapy: preliminary findings. *Biol Psychiatry* 1991;30:623–627.

Stoudemire A, Hill CD, Morris R, et al. Cognitive outcome following tricyclic and electroconvulsive treatment of major depression in the elderly. *Am J Psychiatry* 1991;148:1336–1340.

Stoudemire A, Hill CD, Morris R. Improvement in depression-related cognitive dysfunction following ECT. *J Neuropsychiatry Clin Neurosci* 1995;7:31–34.

Webb MC, Coffey CE, Saunders WR, et al. Cardiovascular response to unilateral electroconvulsive therapy. *Biol Psychiatry* 1990;28:758–766.

Weiner RD, Coffey CE. Use of electroconvulsive therapy in patients with severe medical illness. In: Stoudemire A, Fogel B, eds. *Treatment of psychiatric disorders in medical–surgical patients.* New York: Grune & Stratton, 1987:113–134.

Weiner RD. Does ECT cause brain damage? *Behav Brain Sci* 1984;7:1–53.

Weiner RD. The persistence of electroconvulsive therapy–induced changes in the electroencephalogram. *J Nerv Ment Dis* 1980;168:224–228.

Zornetzer S. Retrograde amnesia and brain seizures in rodents: Electrophysiological and neuroanatomical analyses. In: Fink M, Kety S, McGaugh J, Williams TA, eds. *Psychobiology of Convulsive Therapy.* Washington, DC: V.H. Winston & Sons, 1974:99–128.

Zvara DA, Brooker RF, McCall WV, et al. The effect of esmolol on ST–segment depression and arrhythmias after electroconvulsive therapy. *Convuls Ther* 1997;13:165–174.

Post–ECT Treatment

Coppen A, Abou–Saleh MT, Milln P, et al. Lithium continuation therapy following electroconvulsive therapy. *Br J Psychiatry* 1981;139:284–287.

Imlah NW, Ryan E, Harrington JA. The influence of antidepressant drugs on the response to electroconvulsive therapy and on subsequent relapse rates. *Neuropsychopharmacology* 1965;4:438–442.

Karliner W, Wehrtheim H. Maintenance convulsive treatments. *Am J Psychiatry* 1965;121:1113–1115.

Kay DW, Fahy T, Garside RF. A 7–month double–blind trial of amitriptyline and diazepam in ECT–treated depressed patients. *Br J Psychiatry* 1970;117:667–671.

Loo H, Galinowski A, Bourdel MC, Poirier MF. Use of maintenance ECT for elderly depressed patients. *Am J Psychiatry* 1991;148:810.

Perry P, Tsuang MT. Treatment of unipolar depression following electroconvulsive therapy: relapse rate comparisons between lithium and tricyclic therapies following ECT. *J Affective Disord* 1979;1:123–129.

Petrides G, Dhossche D, Fink M, Francis A. Continuation ECT: relapse prevention in affective disorders. *Convulsive Ther* 1994;10:189–194.

Reynolds CF 3rd, Frank E, Perel JM, et al. Maintenance therapies for late–life recurrent major depression: research and review circa 1995. *Int Psychogeriatr* 1995;7(Suppl):27–39.

Seager CP, Bird RL. Imipramine with electrical treatment in depression: a controlled trial. *J Ment Sci* 1962;108:704–707.

Stevenson GH, Geoghegan JJ. Prophylactic electroshock. A five–year study. *Am J Psychiatry* 1951;107:743–748.

Thienhaus OJ, Margletta S, Bennett JA. A study of the clinical efficacy of maintenance ECT. *J Clin Psychiatry* 1990;51:141–144.

Psychotic Depression

Aronson TA, Shukla S, Gujavarty K, et al. Relapse in delusional depression: a retrospective study of the course of treatment. *Compr Psychiatry* 1988;29:12–21.

Baldwin RC. Delusional and non–delusional depression in late life. *Br J Psychiatry* 1988;152:39–44.

Coryell W, Leon A, Winokur G, et al. Importance of psychotic features to long–term course in major depressive disorder. *Am J Psychiatry* 1996;153: 483–489.

Coryell W, Winokur G, Shea T, et al. The long–term stability of depressive subtypes. *Am J Psychiatry* 1994;151:199–204.

Coryell W. Psychotic depression. *J Clin Psychiatry* 1996;57(Suppl)3:27–31.

Dubovsky SL. Challenges in conceptualizing psychotic mood disorders. *Bull Menninger Clin* 1994; 58:197–214.

Farah A, Beale MD, Kellner CH. Risperidone and ECT combination therapy: a case series. *Convuls Ther* 1995;11:280–282.

Fennig S, Craig TJ, Tanenberg–Karant M, et al. Medication treatment in first–admission patients with psychotic affective disorders: preliminary findings on research–facility diagnostic agreement and rehospitalization. *Ann Clin Psychiatry* 1995;7: 87–90.

Gatti F, Bellini L, Gasperini M, et al. Fluvoxamine alone in the treatment of delusional depression. *Am J Psychiatry* 1996;153:414–416.

Janicak PG, Pandey GN, Davis JM, et al. Response of psychotic and nonpsychotic depression to phenelzine. *Am J Psychiatry* 1988;145:93–95.

Jeste DV, Heaton SC, Paulsen JS, et al. Clinical and neuropsychological comparison of psychotic depression with nonpsychotic depression and schizophrenia. *Am J Psychiatry* 1996;153:490–496.

Khan A, Cohen S, Stowell M, et al. Treatment options in severe psychotic depression. *Convulsive Ther* 1987;3:93–99.

Lyness JM, Conwell Y, Nelson JC. Suicide attempts in elderly psychiatric inpatients. *J Am Geriatr Soc* 1992;40:320–324.

Meyers BS. Late–life delusional depression: acute and long–term treatment. *Int Psychogeriat* 1995; 7(Suppl):113–124.

Nelson JC, Mazure CM. Lithium augmentation in psychotic depression refractory to combined drug treatment. *Am J Psychiatry* 1986;143: 363–366.

Nelson JC, Price LH, Jatlow PI. Neuroleptic dose and desipramine concentrations during combined treatment of unipolar delusional depression. *Am J Psychiatry* 1986;143:1151–1154.

Rothschild AJ, Samson JA, Bessette MP, Carter–Campbell JT. Efficacy of the combination of fluoxetine and perphenazine in the treatment of psychotic depression. *J Clin Psychiatry* 1993;54: 338–342.

Rothschild AJ. Management of psychotic, treatment–resistant depression. *Psychiatr Clin North Am* 1996;19:237–252.

Simpson GM, El Sheshai A, Rady A, et al. Sertraline as monotherapy in the treatment of psychotic and nonpsychotic depression. *J Clin Psychiatry* 2003;64:959–965.

Spiker DG, Weiss JC, Dealy RS, et al. The pharmacological treatment of delusional depression. *Am J Psychiatry* 1985;142:430–436.

Tang WK, Ungvari GS. Efficacy of electroconvulsive therapy combined with antipsychotic medication in treatment–resistant schizophrenia: a prospective, open trial. *J ECT* 2002;18:90–94.

Surveys of Practice

Chiam PC. Depression of old age. *Singapore Med J* 1994;35:404–406.

Draper B. The elderly admitted to a general hospital psychiatry ward. *Aust NZ J Psychiatry* 1994;28: 288–297.

Jorm AF, Henderson AS. Use of private psychiatric services in Australia: an analysis of Medicare data. *Aust NZ J Psychiatry* 1989;23:461–468.

Kornhuber J, Weller M. Patient selection and remission rates with the current practice of electroconvulsive therapy in Germany. *Convulsive Ther* 1995; 11:104–109.

Lambourn J, Barrington PC. Electroconvulsive therapy in a sample British population in 1982. *Convulsive Ther* 1986;2:169–177.

Pike AL, Otegui J, Savi G, Fernandez M. ECT: changing in Uruguay. *Convulsive Ther* 1995;11:58–60.

Structural Imaging

Bergsholm P, Larsen JL, Rosendahl K, Holsten F. Electroconvulsive therapy and cerebral computed tomography. A prospective study. *Acta Psychiatr Scand* 1989;80:566–572.

Calloway SP, Dolan RJ, Jacoby RJ, Levy R. ECT and cerebral atrophy. A computed tomographic study. *Acta Psychiatr Scand* 1981;64:442–445.

Coffey CE. The role of structural brain imaging in ECT. *Psychopharmacol Bull* 1994;30:477–483.

Coffey CE, Figiel GS, Djang WT, et al. Leukoencephalopathy in elderly depressed patients referred for ECT. *Biol Psychiatry* 1988;24:143–161.

Coffey CE, Hinkle PE, Weiner RD, et al. Electroconvulsive therapy of depression in patients with white matter hyperintensity. *Biol Psychiatry* 1987; 22:629–636.

Coffey CE, Weiner RD, Djang WT, et al. Brain anatomic effects of electroconvulsive therapy. A prospective magnetic resonance imaging study. *Arch Gen Psychiatry* 1991;48:1013–1021.

Figiel GS, Coffey CE, Djang WT, et al. Brain magnetic resonance imaging findings in ECT-induced delirium. *J Neuropsychiatry Clin Neurosci* 1990;2:53–58.

Figiel GS, Coffey CE, Weiner RD. Brain magnetic resonance imaging in elderly depressed patients receiving electroconvulsive therapy. *Convulsive Ther* 1989;5:26–34.

Hickie I, Scott E, Mitchell P, et al. Subcortical hyperintensities on magnetic resonance imaging: clinical correlates and prognostic significance in patients with severe depression. *Biol Psychiatry* 1995; 37:151–160.

Scott AI, Douglas RH, Whitfield A, Kendell RE. Time course of cerebral magnetic resonance changes after electroconvulsive therapy. *Br J Psychiatry* 1990;156:551–553.

Treatment Resistance

Bonner D, Howard R. Treatment–resistant depression in the elderly. *Int Psychogeriatr* 1995; 7(Suppl):83–94.

Dinan TG, Barry S. A comparison of electroconvulsive therapy with a combined lithium and tricyclic combination among depressed tricyclic nonresponders. *Acta Psychiatr Scand* 1989;80:97–100.

Magni G, Fisman M, Helmes E. Clinical correlates of ECT–resistant depression in the elderly. *J Clin Psychiatry* 1988;49:405–407.

Phillips KA, Nierenberg AA. The assessment and treatment of refractory depression. *J Clin Psychiatry* 1994;55(Suppl):20–26.

Prudic J, Sackeim H. Refractory depression and electroconvulsive therapy. In: Roose SP, Glassman AH, eds. *Treatment of refractory depression.* Washington, DC: American Psychiatric Press, 1990:109–128.

Quitkin F. The importance of dosage in prescribing antidepressants. *Br J Psychiatry* 1985;147:593–597.

Rothschild AJ. Management of psychotic, treatment–resistant depression. *Psychiatr Clin North Am* 1996;19:237–252.

Shapira B, Kindleer S, Lerer B. Medication outcome in ECT–resistant depression. *Convulsive Ther* 1988;4:192–198.

Chapter 14

Response Prediction and Maintenance Treatment

George S. Alexopoulos

Darin M. Lerner

Carl Salzman

In 1994 a Consensus Conference on late-life depression sponsored by the National Institute of Mental Health called for increased research to elucidate, among many factors, the course of antidepressant treatment response as well as predictors of response in geriatric patients.[1] In the decade since this conference, significant research expansion on treatment of depression has contributed to increased data on the heterogeneity of drug response, course of illness, and predictors of response in the elderly population.

Antidepressants of all types are helpful in treating depression, although the degree of change in depressive symptoms may vary widely among elderly patients. Overall, antidepressants reduce depressive symptom severity nearly 50%, compared to 30% with placebo. Some clinical studies suggest that antidepressants have comparable efficacy[2,3]; other studies demonstrate the superiority of tricyclic antidepressants (TCAs) and monoamine oxidase inhibitors (MAOIs).[4,5] Still other investigations indicate the superiority of selective serotonin reuptake inhibitors (SSRIs), based primarily on an advantageous side effect profile.[6-8] Nonetheless, regardless of class of antidepressant used, only 12% of elderly patients are completely resistant to vigorous antidepressant treatment.[9] With appropriate treatment, remission rates can be as high as 88%.[10]

Clinical Correlates of Treatment Response and Prediction

Several clinical correlates of response to treatment for depression in geriatric patients are receiving increased attention at clinical and research levels. These include: early versus late response, response and dosage, response and the "old-old," placebo response in clinical trials, and treatment response and sleep patterns.

Although geriatric depression has a recovery rate comparable to that of depression occurring in younger adults, different clinical characteristics affect the rate of recovery in older and younger depressed patients, making prediction of time and degree of response difficult.[11] For example, some data suggest that advanced age and late age of onset[11,12] predict a slow recovery in elderly depressives whereas poor social support is a strong predictor of nonrecovery in younger depressed patients.[11-13] High severity of depression and self-rated medical burdens are also associated with poor or delayed antidepressant response among geriatric patients.[14] In contrast, another body of data suggests that memory impairment, medical burden, social support, risk factors for stroke, and number of previous episodes do not influence the treatment outcome of geriatric depression[15,16]; rather, these data suggest that early onset of improvement and absence of prefrontal (executive) dysfunction, demonstrated by neuropsychological testing and imaging, are predictors of favorable antidepressant response.

Two additional factors complicate predicting treatment response in the elderly. First, placebo response among depressed elderly patients is unusually high, making interpretation of data from clinical trials more difficult than with younger depressed populations. Second, response of the "oldest-old" (those over 80) are now being studied more assiduously because this fast-growing subgroup of elders may have different response patterns to antidepressant treatment.

Age and Early Versus Late Response

The overall response to antidepressants in depressed older individuals is similar to that seen in younger adults.[8] As a general rule, however, older patients may take longer to respond.[11–13] Supporting this contention is a recent metaanalysis of several large geriatric treatment studies suggesting that at least 6 weeks of treatment is necessary to achieve optimum therapeutic effect.[17] Further, evidence from a double-blind fluoxetine study shows that early response has only fair reliability in predicting final outcome in older depressed patients, and a considerable number of geriatric patients who remain depressed after 3 months of treatment may meet criteria for response or remission when followed for 6 months or longer.[18]

Other evidence, however, points in a different direction. Some recent studies suggest that depressed elders who show no evidence of improvement after 4 weeks of treatment are unlikely to respond later.[19] Further, lack of early change in depressive symptoms after the introduction of an antidepressasnt can predict a poor final outcome[20]; and predicting by week 6 who will not remit by week 12 has been shown to be highly accurate.[21] In addition, depressed geriatric patients who respond quickly to treatment are more likely to experience marked improvement or remission compared with those who do not experience early response.[22]

Response and Dosage

Response to antidepressant treatment may depend on clinical manifestations of the depressive episode. Patients with dementia or high pretreatment anxiety are slower to respond, whereas attempted suicide or need for hospitalization are associated with shorter time to response.[23] Nontricyclic antidepressants may have superior efficacy in geriatric depressed patients with comorbid anxiety.[24]

Disappointing rates of response in elderly depression may be due, in part, to inadequate intensity of treatment. Documentation shows that when antidepressants were administered to over 90% of depressed elderly individuals, more than half received less than recommended doses and full recovery occurred in only about one-third of patients.[25] Other studies reveal that a rate of adequate antidepressant use below 30%[26] and sometimes as low as 6%.[27] When TCAs are prescribed, they are commonly given at subtherapeutic doses.[28]

Response and the "Old-Old"

Although the definition of "old-old" varies, it is usually set, by consensus, at 80 years and older. Relatively few studies of antidepressants have been conducted in this age group,[29] although it is the fastest-growing segment in the US population. In general, the oldest of depressed patients can be safely and effectively treated with antidepressant medications, and even with electroconvulsive therapy.[30–32] TCAs, although associated with unwanted and potentially hazardous side effects in this population, are efficacious.[33] Studies also document the efficacy and safety of SSRIs for patients 80 years and over.[33–35] The rate of response in patients older than 75 does not differ from those of younger elderly patients.[36]

Placebo Response in Geriatric Antidepressant Trials

Depressed elders have a high placebo response. Based on a recent metaanalysis,[37] the overall placebo response rate of depressed elders is estimated to be 27.5%, although metaanalyses of earlier studies indicate response rates ranging from 20 to 80%.[38–40] Ten recent studies confirm a high placebo response rate in the elderly: a study of clomipramine[41] revealed a response rate of 30%; a study of moclobemide, 25%[42]; a fluoxetine trial, 31.6%[22]; a fluoxetine trial of depressed physically ill patients, 38%.[43] A second moclobemide study had a response rate of 11%[44]; a study of mirtazapine, 35%,[45] a citalopram study, 28%[46]; and a nortriptyline study in a residential care facility resulted in a low response rate of 9%.[47]

Two studies of subjects over the age of 75 years also showed high placebo response. In each of these studies—one with paroxetine[34] and one with citalopram[48]—the active drug was not found superior to the placebo because of the high placebo-response rate.

In general, placebo response is higher in studies of less depressed elderly patients, and drug response is significantly stronger than placebo response when severely depressed patients are studied. In many investigations, side effects to placebo are similar in type and incidence to those of the active drug.

High placebo response in late-life antidepressant studies has several possible causes. Some of the placebo responders may have been misnamed; these individuals may well have responded to the increased attention generated by participation in a research study. Work is underway to define more precisely the characteristics of geriatric placebo response in order to improve clinical trials. Despite a high placebo response rate, active antidepressant medication consistently outperforms placebo in the treatment of depressed elderly patients.[17] Adequate dose and duration of treatment is necessary for optimum therapeutic effect.

Sleep and Treatment Response

Sleep is typically disturbed in major depression and is most disturbed in older individuals. Frequent awakenings throughout the night, early morning awakening, and trouble falling asleep are common in late life as well as in late-life depression. Although sleep measures are not yet available as predictors of treatment response, an older depressed individual's response to one night of total sleep deprivation may correlate with antidepressant treatment response and may even accelerate the response.[49,50] A decrease in depressive symptoms after sleep recovery from a night of sleep deprivation (rather than a reduction of depressive symptoms immediately following the night of sleep deprivation) correlates highly with subsequent antidepressant response.[51] This correlation between sleep recovery and antidepressant response in turn correlates with decreased regional glucose metabolism in the right cingulate gyrus.[52,53]

Neurobiologic Correlates of Outcome and Prediction

Over the past decade, research on several neurobiologic correlates of geriatric depression has resulted in significant data on response prediction and treatment outcome. Most prominent among these is the role of executive function as well as its nether side, executive dysfunction.

Executive Function

Cognitive functions such as planning, organizing, initiating, sequencing, information processing, and working memory comprise executive function, which requires integrity of the frontal cortex (see also Chapter 8). Recent studies suggest that some aspects of executive dysfunction may lead to poor and/or slow antidepressant response.[54] For example, abnormal scores in tests of initiation/perseveration and response inhibition predict slow or poor response to TCAs and other antidepressants and a low remission rate in nondemented elderly patients with major depression treated with "adequate" dosages of various antidepressants.[55] Slow or poor antidepressant response is also associated with psychomotor retardation[19] as well as prolonged latency of the P300 auditory evoked potential[54]—all decrements revealing compromised integrity of frontal systems.

In addition to poor antidepressant response, abnormal scores in initiation/perseveration tasks is also associated with early relapse and recurrence of late-life depression in elderly patients treated with nortriptyline.[55] The relation of executive dysfunction to slow and unstable antidepressant response thus may be specific as neither memory impairment, nor disability, medical burden, social support, or number of previous episodes were found to influence the course of geriatric depression.[55]

Executive dysfunction is common and persistent in geriatric depression: tasks requiring inhibitory control and sustained effort are most compromised while tasks of selective and sustained attention are impaired in depression across ages.[15] While executive dysfunction improves when depression subsides, some degree of executive dysfunction persists even after remission of depression.[56] These observations suggest that executive dysfunction is a stable clinical characteristic in some depressed elderly patients that is accentuated during episodes of depression. The relation of executive dysfunction to the course of geriatric depression further suggests that the neurologic impairments underlying this dysfunction are integral to the mechanisms perpetuating the depressive syndrome.

Depressed elders with executive impairment often have white matter hyperintensities (WMH),[57,58] which, like executive dysfunction, predict chronicity of depressive symptoms.[59,60] Subcortical vascular abnormalities have a stronger impact on worsening prognosis of geriatric depression than family history of mood disorders.[61] Severe hyperintensities in subcortical gray matter regions have also been associated with poor response of depressed elderly patients to electroconvulsive therapy.[62]

The relation of executive dysfunction to the course of geriatric depression suggests two outcome trajectories. First, underlying neurologic impairments of executive function are integral to the mechanisms perpetuating the depressive syndrome; and second, abnormality in some executive functions is associated with poor, slow, unstable treatment response of geriatric depression.

Metabolic Changes in Frontostriatal Pathways

Functional neuroimaging studies reveal that metabolic changes in frontostriatal pathways controlling executive functions may also influence the degree of antidepressant response. Remission of depressed younger adults is associated with metabolic increases in dorsal cortical regions, including the dorsal anterior and posterior cingulate, the dorsolateral, and the inferior parietal cortex.[63,64] In contrast, during remission in older depressed adults, decreased metabolism in ventral limbic and paralimbic structures (such as the subgenual cingulate, the hippocampus, and hypothalamus) occurs.[52,64,65] In younger adults, persistence of elevated amygdala metabolism during remission of depression is associated with high risk for relapse, and reduced metabolism of the rostral anterior cingulate is associated with treatment resistance.[66] In contrast, for older depressed persons, increased cingulate metabolism is a predictor of antidepressant response[67] whereas disruption in the reciprocal regulation of dorsal cortical and ventral limbic regions may contribute to depressive symptoms.[66] Early and persistent metabolic alterations at the right cingulate gyrus, demonstrated through PET imaging, are associated with improvement of depression after antidepressant medication.[53]

Nervous System Function and Treatment Response

A growing number of identified age-related changes in central nervous system function have recently been associated with geriatric antidepressant response:

- Overall reduction in resting regional blood flow in frontal regions following successful ECT.[68]
- Low activation of the dorsal anterior cingulate following "paced-word activation" in severe geriatric depression.[69]
- Reduced hippocampal volumes (especially on the right) and reduced likelihood of remission after antidepressant treatment.[70]
- Rapid antidepressant response to some, but not all, antidepressants in cognitively intact elderly patients and presence of the apolipoprotein E ε4 genotype[71]—an association congruent with the correlation of this genotype, WMHs, and geriatric depression.[72]
- Association of executive dysfunction and poor remission rate with microstructural white matter abnormalities lateral to the anterior cingulate and at the level of the middle frontal gyrus in elderly patients with major depression[73]—abnormalities that may interfere with dorsal cortical-ventral limbic regulation.
- Correlation of antidepressant response and baseline folate levels: higher folate levels predict better treatment response, especially with SSRI antidepressants;[74] however, no data currently available indicate the usefulness of adding folic acid to SSRIs or other antidepressants to improve antidepressant response.
- Correlation of reduced cerebrospinal fluid levels of corticotrophin releasing factor with response to antidepressant treatment, thus implicating the hypothalamic-pituitary-adrenal stress axis in late-life depression and its treatment.[75,76]
- Association of normalization of the dexamethasone test, a biologic marker of HPA activity in major depression, with antidepressant response in 70% of elderly patients—a finding further supporting the relevance of the hormonal axis in late-life depression.[77]
- Possible contribution of genetic polymorphisms of the serotonin-transporter protein (which returns synaptic serotonin to the presynpatic nerve ending) to the variable initial response of elderly patients treated with a SSRI: those with a homozygous long gene respond significantly more rapidly than those possessing the short allele of the same gene.[78]

Prediction of Relapse, Recurrence, and Remission

Rates for relapse and recurrence of major depression in geriatric patients range from 15 to 19%,[79] which are comparable to those of mixed-age populations (21%).[80,81] In mixed-age populations, a history of 3 or more prior depressive episodes and a late age of onset are the strongest predictors of relapse and recurrence.[80,81] In geriatric populations, likelihood of relapse occurs in patients with a history of frequent episodes, concomitant medical illnesses, and high severity of depression.[79,82] Past history of myocardial infarction also predicts frequent relapses in depressed medical outpatients.[83]

Because depression is a relapsing and recurring illness, 50 to 80% of elderly patients who have had one depressive episode can expect a recurrence, and the recurrence rate increases with each successive episode.[84,85] This relatively high relapse rate may be partly ascribed to underdosing. More than half of treated elderly patients receive less than the recommended doses, which correlates with less than full recovery and subsequent relapse or recurrence.[25] Relapse is also more likely if adjunctive medications (e.g., lithium, a neuroleptic, or a second antidepressant) are discontinued during the acute treatment phase.[86] If elderly patients remain on maintenance medication, however, 70 to 90% can expect to remain well without recurrence for 18 months to 4 years.[87,88] Rates of relapse are significantly higher for elderly individuals who suffer from a psychotic depression regardless of full-dose maintenance medication.[89]

The number of depression-free days during a period of remission, as well as the global severity of illness while a patient is symptomatic, may correlate with relapse patterns. Milder symptoms are associated with more depression-free days, which in turn correlate with duration of remission. Elderly patients successfully treated with an active antidepressant, rather than placebo, have lower ratings of illness severity and a higher number of depression-free days.[90] As might be expected, discontinuation of antidepressant medication is associated with a high degree of relapse, especially in a first episode of depression, although most patients respond to reinstated treatment.[91] Therapeutic antidepressant blood levels are associated with fewer residual depressive symptoms.[92]

No consistent social predictors of response and remission have yet been identified.[93] Older age at onset is related to improved remission in some studies but not others.[80,81,94,95] An even lower possibility of remission is suggested in 4 geriatric-patient subgroups: elderly males, patients of both genders with coexisting medical illness, those with a history of antidepressant use, and patients with experience of severe adverse life events.[96–98] In one study, only 33% of elderly patients achieved remission, suggesting that depression is a chronic condition for many elderly individuals.[99]

Maintenance Treatment

Because depression may be a severely debilitating or potentially lethal illness, older unipolar patients who have had two or more depressive episodes should receive maintenance treatment with antide-

pressants. The dosage of a TCA used for maintenance therapy, as in the dosage of an SSRI, should be the same as that used during the acute treatment phase.

TCAs are effective in preventing relapse and recurrence of major depression in older patients as they do in younger adults.[86,100] For example, controlled treatment studies of mixed-age depressives show that imipramine continuation therapy (intended to prevent relapse during the first 4 to 6 months after recovery) and maintenance therapy (intended to prevent recurrence after 4 to 6 months from recovery) succeed in preventing relapse or recurrence in 50 to 80% of the population over 1 to 3 years.[101,102] In contrast, only 20% of placebo-treated patients remain well.[101]

Two controlled treatment studies of elderly depressives suggest that other antidepressant drugs may also offer protection from relapse.[103,104] Continuation treatment of outpatients with major depression in their mid-60s with nortriptyline or phenelzine leads to a relapse rate of only 16.7% and 20.0%, respectively;[105] an even lower relapse rate is seen in a controlled treatment study.[104] Successful maintenance treatment with nortriptyline depends on drug plasma levels; fewer residual depressive symptoms are found when plasma levels are 80 to 120 ng/ml.[92] Combining nortriptyline and psychotherapy may also represent the best long-term treatment.[106]

Maintenance treatment with phenelzine is highly effective in preventing recurrence with a recurrence rate of 13.3%.[107] Both nortriptyline and interpersonal therapy have been shown superior to placebo in preventing recurrence of late-life depression, but combination maintenance treatment using nortriptyline and interpersonal therapy is superior to either nortriptyline or therapy alone.[106]

Studies of maintenance treatment using SSRIs and other newer antidepressants do not provide as much information regarding maintenance use as studies of TCAs (see Chapter 9). In a 44-week treatment study of major depression, only 13% of mixed-age patients receiving sertraline relapsed, compared with 46% of those receiving placebo.[108] Another placebo-controlled study of maintenance therapy using citalopram to prevent recurring depression in elderly patients over a 48-week period was found to decrease time to recurrence compared with placebo.[109]

Relapse rates among elderly patients who discontinue therapeutically effective SSRI and other nontrycyclic medication are similar to those following discontinuation of TCAs. Most elderly patients relapse within the first 4 to 6 weeks of discontinuing treatment, and the subsequent 4 months are also a period of relatively high risk. In general, because depression is a relapsing illness and because its consequences in older individuals may be severe, elderly patients should be advised to continue taking their antidepressants for extended periods of time—that is, at least 1 year after therapeutic effect and longer if the drug is well tolerated. As with any antidepressant, discontinuation should be extremely gradual and carefully monitored by a physician.

The limited number of studies available, together with clinical experience, suggest that older people whose depression has been successfully treated with an SSRI or other new antidepressant should be maintained on the drug from a minimum of 1 year after recovery. This is especially true for older patients with multiple prior depressive episodes or for those whose late-life depression is severe.

Regardless of the particular medication used for maintenance, careful monitoring of dosages and plasma levels and appropriate adjustment are necessary as the patient ages. In the case of relapse or recurrence, a regimen similar to that used in the original depressive episode may lead to remission in 80% of depressed geriatric patients.[86]

Patients whose depression has responded only to ECT should be placed on maintenance dosages of an antidepressant and perhaps a mood stabilizer as well (see Chapter 13). Antidepressants that fail to produce remission should not be selected for maintenance treatment after ECT. Combinations of TCAs with mood stabilizers are more effective than TCAs alone in reducing relapse and recurrence for patients with drug-resistant depression who respond to ECT.[110] Older patients who have had relapses while on antidepressants or mood stabilizers or who cannot tolerate these drugs because of medical contraindications should be considered for maintenance ECT. For these patients, a single ECT treatment every 3 to 6 weeks may prevent recurrence of depression.

Conclusions

For the clinician treating a depressed elderly patient, the important concern is whether the patient will respond at all and whether the response, if present, will be sufficient to induce a remission of depressive symptoms. On the basis of current information, the following conclusions appear reasonable:

- If an elderly patient responds even partially to antidepressant treatment, the treatment should be continued in order to achieve fuller response or remission.
- If no clinically meaningful response occurs within 6 weeks, the treatment should be declared ineffective. At this point, the clinician has several choices. The simplest is to switch medications. Alternatively, or concomitantly with switching medications, the clinician may wish to evaluate the patient for the presence of executive dysfunction, dementia, or other neurologic or medical disease that might interfere with antidepressant treatment response.
- Side effects may also correlate with antidepressant treatment response in the geriatric patient. In one study, for example, headache correlates with good response but increased anxiety is associated with poor response.[111]

- Chronicity of depression may also be associated with an elderly patient's clinical characteristics: Continuing symptoms, presence of dementia, coexisting medical illness alone, or together, predict poor treatment response and symptom chronicity.[112]

Even with aggressive and effective treatment leading to symptomatic remission, relapse rates tend to be high in this population.[113]

References

1. Schneider, CF Reynolds, BD Lebowitz, A Friedhoff, eds. *Diagnosis and Treatment of Depression in Late Life: Results of the NIH Consensus Development Conference.* Washington, D.C.: American Psychiatric Press, 1994:181–244.
2. McCusker J, Cole M, Keller M, et al. Effectiveness of treatments of depression in older ambulatory patients. *Arch Intern Med* 1998;158: 705–712.
3. Gerson S, Belin TR, Kaufman A, et al. Pharmacological and psychological treatments for depressed older patients: a meta–analysis and overview of recent findings. *Harv Rev Psychiatry* 1999;7:1–28.
4. Mittmann N, Herrmann N, Shulman KI, et al. The effectiveness of antidepressants in elderly depressed outpatients: a prospective case series study. *J Clin Psychiatry* 1999;90:690–697.
5. Weintraub D. Nortriptyline in geriatric depression resistant to serotonin reuptake inhibitors: case series. *J Geriatr Psychiatry Neurol* 2001;14: 28–32.
6. Salzman C, Satlin A, and Burrows AB. Geriatric Psychopharmacology. In: AF Schatzberg, CB Nemeroff eds. *Essentials of Clinical Psychopharmacology.* Washington, D.C.: American Psychiatric Press, 2001:637–658.
7. Alexopoulos GS, Katz IR, Reynolds CF III, et al. The Expert Consensus Guideline Series: Pharmacotherapy of depressive disorders in older patients. *Postgraduate Medicine,* October 2001.
8. Salzman C, Wong E, Wright BC. Drug and ECT treatment of depression in the elderly, 1996–2001: a literature review. *Biol Psychiatry* 2002;52:265–284.
9. Little JT, Reynolds CF, Dew MA, et al. How common is resistance to treatment in recurrent, nonpsychotic geriatric depression? *Am J Psychiatry* 1998;155:1035–1038.
10. Thomas L, Mulsant BH, Solano FX, et al. Response speed and rate of remission in primary and specialty care of elderly patients with depression. *Am J Geriatr Psychiatry* 2002;10: 583–591.
11. Alexopoulos GS, Meyers BS, Young RC, et al. Recovery in geriatric depression. *Arch Gen Psychiatry* 1996;53:305–312.
12. Georgotas A, McCue RE. The additional benefit of extending an antidepressant trial past seven weeks in the depressed elderly. *Int J Geriatr Psychiatry* 1989;4:191–195.
13. Sackeim H: How long should antidepressant trials be in geriatric depression? In: Late–Life Depression: *Old Myths and New Data.* Annual Meeting of the American Psychiatric Association 2002.
14. Lenze EJ, Miller MD, Dew MA, et al. Subjective health measures and acute treatment outcomes in geriatric depression. *Int J Geriatr Psychiatry* 2001;16:1149–1155.
15. Lockwood KA, Alexopoulos GS, van Gorp WG. Executive dysfunction in geriatric depression. *Am J Psychiatry* 2000;159:1119–1126.
16. Miller MD, Lenze EJ, Dew MA, et al. Effect of cerebrovascular risk factors on depression treatment outcome in later life. *Am J Geriatr Psychiatry* 2002;10:592–598.
17. Wilson K, Mottram P, Sivanranthan A, Nightingale A. Antidepressants versus placebo for the depressed elderly (Cochrane Review). In: *The Cochrane Library,* Issue 3 2002. Oxford: Update Software.
18. Small GW, Hamilton SH, Bystritsky A, et al. Clinical response predictors in a double–blind, placebo–controlled trial of fluoxetine for geriatric major depression. Fluoxetine Collaborative Study Group. *Int Psychogeriatr* 1995; 7(Suppl):41–53.
19. Alexopoulos GS. Frontostriatal and limbic dysfunction in late–life depression. *Am J Geriatr Psychiatry* 2002;10:687–695.
20. Myers BS. Treatment and course of geriatric depression: questions raised by an evolving clinical science [editorial]. *Am J Geriatr Psychiatry* 2002;10:497–502.
21. Roose SP, Sackeim HA. Clinical trials in late–life depression: revisited [editorial]. *Am J Geriatr Psychiatry* 2002;10:503–505.
22. Tollefson G, Bosomworth J, Heiligenstein J, et al. A double–blind, placebo–controlled clinical trial of fluoxetine in geriatric patients with major depression. *Int Psychogeriatr* 1995;7: 89–104.
23. Flint AJ, Rifat SL. Effect of demographic and clinical variables on time to antidepressant response in geriatric depression. *Depress Anxiety* 1997;5:103–107.
24. Doraiswamy PM. Contemporary management of comorbid anxiety and depression in geriatric patients. *J Clin Psychiatry* 2001;62(Suppl 12):30–35.
25. Heeren TJ, Derksen P, van Heycop, et al. Treatment, outcome and predictors of response in elderly depressed inpatients. *Br J Psychitry* 1997; 170:436–440.
26. Unutzer J, Simon G, Belin TR, et al. Care for depression in HMO patients aged 65 and older. *J Am Geriatr Soc* 2000;48:871–878.
27. Mamdani M, Herrmann N, Austin P. Prevalence of antidepressant use among older people: population–based observations. *J Am Geriatr Soc* 1999;47:1350–1353.
28. Lawrenson RA, Tyrer F, Newson RB, et al. The treatment of depression in UK general practice: selective serotonin reuptake inhibitors

and tricyclic antidepressants compared. *J Affect Disord.* 2000;59:149–157.

29. Salzman C. Practical considerations for the treatment of depression in elderly and very elderly long–term care patients. *J Clin Psychiatry* 1999;60(Suppl 20):30–3.

30. Finkel SI. Efficacy and tolerability of antidepressant therapy in the old–old. *J Clin Psychiatry* 1996;57(Suppl 5):23–28.

31. Tomac TA, Rummans TA, Pileggi TS, et al. Safety and efficacy of electroconvulsive therapy in patients over age 85. *Am J Geriatr Psychiatry* 1997;5:126–130.

32. Manly DT, Oakley SP, Bloch, et al. Electroconvulsive therapy in old–old patients. *Am J Geriatr Psychiatry* 2000;8:232–236.

33. Oslin DW, Streim JE, Katz IR, et al. Heuristic comparison of sertraline with nortriptyline for the treatment of depression in frail elderly patients. *Am J Geriatr Psychiatry* 2000;8:141–149.

34. Burrows AB, Salzman C, Satlin A, et al. A randomized, placebo–controlled trial of paroxetine in nursing home residents with non–major depression. *Depress Anxiety* 2002;15:102–110.

35. Mulsant BH, Sweet RA, Rosen J, et al. A double–blind randomized comparison of nortriptyline plus perphenazine versus nortriptyline plus placebo in the treatment of psychotic depression of late–life. *J Clin Psychiatry* 2001;62: 597–604.

36. Gildengers AG, Houck PR, Mulsant BH, et al. Course and rate of antidepressant response in the very old. *J Affect Disord* 2002;69:177–184.

37. Mittmann N, Hermann N, Emerson TR, et al. The efficacy, safety and tolerability of antidepressants in late life depression. *J Affect Disord* 1997;46:191–217.

38. Klawansky S. Meta–analysis on the treatment of depression in late life. In: Schneider LS, Reynolds CF III, Lebowitz BD, Friedhoff AJ, eds. *Diagnosis and treatment of depression in late life.* Washington DC: APA Press, 1994:331–352.

39. Salzman C. Pharmacological treatment of depression in the elderly. *J Clin Psychiatry* 1993; 54(Suppl):23–28.

40. Schneider LS, Olin JT. Efficacy of acute treatment of geriatric depression. *Int Psychogeriatr* 1995;7(suppl):7–25.

41. Petracca G, Teson A, Chemerinski E, et al. A double–blind placebo–controlled study of clomipramine in depressed patients with Alzheimer's disease. *J Neuropsychiatry* 1996;8: 270–275.

42. Roth M, Mountjoy CO, Amrien R, et al. Moclobemide in elderly patients with cognitive decline and depression. *Br J Psychiatry* 1996;68: 149–157.

43. Evans M, Hammond M, Wilson K, et al. Placebo–controlled treatment trial of depression in elderly physically ill patients. *Int J Geriatr Psychiatry* 1997;12:817–824.

44. Nair NPV, Amin M, Holm P, et al. Moclobemide and nortriptyline in elderly depressed patients. A randomized, multicenter trial against placebo. *J Affect Disord* 1995;33:1–9.

45. Halikas J. Org 3770 (mirtazapine) versus trazodone: a placebo controlled trial in depressed elderly patients. *Hum Psychopharm* 1995;10: S125–S133.

46. Nyth A, Gottfries C, Lyby K, et al. A controlled multicenter clinical study of citalopram and placebo in elderly depressed patients with and without concomitant dementia. *Acta Psychiatr Scand* 1992;86:138–145.

47. Katz I, Simpson G, Curlik S, et al. Pharmacologic treatment of major depression for elderly patients in residential settings. *J Clin Psychiatry* 1990;51(suppl 7):41–47.

48. Roose S, Salzman C, Nelson CT, et al. *Citalopram treatment of elderly patients over the age of 75.* (Submitted for publication).

49. Bump GM, Reynolds CF, Smith G, et al. Accelerating response in geriatric depression: a pilot study combining sleep deprivation and paroxetine. *Depress Anxiety* 1997;6:113–118.

50. Green TD, Reynolds CF, Mulsant BH, et al. Accelerating antidepressant response in geriatric depression: a post hoc comparison of combined sleep deprivation and paroxetine versus monotherapy with paroxetine, nortriptyline, or placebo. *J Geriatr Psychiatry Neurol* 1999;12: 67–71.

51. Hernandez CR, Smith GS, Houck PR, et al. The clinical response to total sleep deprivation and recovery sleep in geriatric depression: potential indicators of antidepressant treatment outcome. *Psychiatry Res* 2000:97:41–49.

52. Smith GS, Reynolds CF III, Pollock B, et al. Cerebral metabolic response to combined total sleep deprivation and antidepressant response in geriatric depression. *Am J Psychiatry* 1999; 156:683–689.

53. Smith GS, Reynolds CF III, Houck PR, et al. Glucose metabolic response to total sleep deprivation, recovery sleep, and acute antidepressant treatment as functional neuroanatomic correlates of treatment outcome in geriatric depression. *Am J Geriatr Psychiatry* 2002;10: 561–567.

54. Kalayam B, Alexopoulos GS. Prefrontal dysfunction and treatment response in geriatric depression. *Arch Gen Psychiatry* 1999; 56: 713–718.

55. Alexopoulos GS, Meyers BS, Young RC, et al. Executive dysfunction and long–term outcomes of geriatric depression. *Arch Gen Psychiatry* 2000; 57:285–290.

56. Butters MA, Becker JT, Nebes RT, et al. Changes in cognitive function following treatment of late–life depression. *Am J Psychiatry* 2000; 157:1949–1954.

57. Lesser I, Boone KB, Mehringer CM, et al. Cognition and white matter hyperintensities in older depressed adults. *Am J Psychiatry* 1996; 153:1280–1287.

58. Boone KB, Miller BL, Lesser IM, et al. Neuropsychological correlates of white–matter lesions in healthy elderly subjects. *Arch Neurol* 1992; 49:549–554.

59. Coffey CE, Figiel GS, Djang WT, et al. Leukoencephalopathy in elderly depressed patients referred for ECT. *Biol Psychiatry* 1988; 24: 143–161.

60. Hickie I, Scott E, Mitchell P, et al. Subcortical hyperintensities on magnetic resonance imag-

ing: clinical correlates and prognostic significance in patients with severe depression. *Biol Psychiatry* 1995;37:151–160.

61. Baldwin RC. Poor prognosis of depression in elderly people: causes and actions. *Ann Med* 2000;32:252–256.

62. Steffens DC, Conway CR, Dombeck CB, et al. Severity of subcortical gray–matter hyperintensity predicts ECT response in geriatric depression. *J ECT* 2001; 158:405–415.

63. Drevets WC, Neuroimaging studies of mood disorders. *Biol Psychiatry* 2000;48:813–819.

64. Liotti M, Mayberg HS. The role of functional neuroimaging in the neuropsychology of depression. *J Clin Exp Neuropsychol* 2001;23: 121–136.

65. Drevets WC. Prefrontal cortical–amygdalar metabolism in major depression. *Ann N Y Acd Sci* 1999;877:614–637.

66. Mayberg HS, Brannan SK, Mahurin RK, et al. Cingulate function in depression: a potential predictor of treatment response. *Neuroreport* 1997;8:1057–1061.

67. Mayberg HS, Liotti M, Brannan SK, et al. Reciprocal limbic–cortical function and negative mood: converging PET findings in depression and normal sadness. *Am J Psychiatry* 1999;156: 675–682.

68. Nobler MS, Roose SP, Prohovnik I, et al. Regional cerebral blood flow in mood disorders, V.: effects of antidepressant medication in late–life depression. *Am J Geriatr Psychiatry* 2000;8:289–296.

69. de Asis JM, Stern E, Alexopoulos GS, et al. Hippocampal and anterior cingulate activation in patients with geriatric depression. *Am J Psychiatry* 2001;158:1321–1323.

70. Hsieh MH, McQuoid DR, Levy RM, et al. Hippocampal volume and antidepressant response in geriatric depression. *Int J Geriatr Psychiatry* 2002;17:519–525.

71. Murphy GM, Kremer C, Rodrigues H, et al. The apolipoprotein E ε4 allele and antidepressant efficacy in cognitively intact elderly depressed patients. *Biol Psychiatry* 2003;54:665–673.

72. Steffens DC, Trost WT, Payne ME, et al. Apolipoprotein E genotype and subcortical vascular lesions in older depressed patients and control subjects. *Biol Psychiatry* 2003;54:674–681.

73. Alexopoulos GS, Kiosses DN, Choi S, et al. Frontal white matter microstructure and treatment response of late–life depression: a preliminary study. *Am J Psychiatry* 2002;159: 1929–1932.

74. Alpert M, Silva RR, Pouget ER. Prediction of treatment response in geriatric depression from baseline folate level: interaction with an SSRI or a tricyclic antidepressant. *J Clin Psychopharmacol* 2003;23:309–313.

75. Heusser I, Bissette G, Dettling M, et al. Cerebrospinal fluid concentrations of corticotrophin–releasing hormone, vasopressin, and somatostatin in depressed patients and healthy controls: response to amitriptyline treatment. *Depress Anxiety* 1998;8:71–79.

76. Taylor MP, Reynolds CF, Frank E, et al. Which elderly depressed patients remain well on maintenance interpersonal psychotherapy alone?: Report from the Pittsburgh study of maintenance therapies in late–life depression. *Depress Anxiety* 1999;10:55–60.

77. Kin NM, Nair NP, Amin M, et al. The dexamethasone suppression test and treatment outcome in elderly depressed patients participating in a placebo–controlled multicenter trial involving moclobemide and nortriptyline. *Biol Psychiatry* 1997;42:925–931.

78. Pollock BG, Ferrell RE, Mulsant BH, et al. Allelic variation in the serotonin transporter promoter affects onset of paroxetine treatment response in late–life depression. *Neuropsychopharmacology* 2000;23:587–590.

79. Zis AP, Grof P, Webster M, et al. The cyclicity of affective disorders and its modifications by drugs. *Psychopharm Bull* 1980;16:47–50.

80. Keller MB, Klerman GL, Lavori PW, et al. Long–term outcome of episodes of major depression. *JAMA* 1984;252:788–792.

81. Keller MB, Lavori PW, Lewis CE, et al. Predictors of relapse in major depressive disorder. *JAMA* 1983;250:3299–3304.

82. Alexopoulos GS, Young RC, Abrams RC, et al. Chronicity and relapse in geriatric depression. *Biol Psychiatry* 1989;26:551–564.

83. Wells KB, Rogers W, Burman MA, et al. Course of depression in patients with hypertension, myocardial infarction or insulin–dependent diabetes. *Am J Psychiatry* 1983;150:632–638.

84. Prien RF. Somatic treatment of unipolar depressive disorder. In: A Francis, RE Hales, eds. *Review of psychiatry. Vol 7.* Washington, DC: American Psychiatric Association, 1988:213–234.

85. Alexopoulos GS. Clinical and biological findings in late–onset depression. In: Tasman A, Goldfinger SM, Kaufman CA, eds. *American Psychiatric Press review of psychiatry, vol 9.* Washington, DC: American Psychiatric Press, 1990: 244–262.

86. Reynolds CF III, Frank E, Kupfer DJ, et al. Treatment outcome in recurrent major depression: a post hoc comparison of elderly ("young old") and midlife patients. *Am J Psychiatry* 1996; 153:1288–1292.

87. Walters G, Reynolds CF, Mulsant BH, et al. Continuation and maintenance pharmacotherapy in geriatric depression: an open–trial comparison of paroxetine and nortriptyline in patients older than 70 years. *J Clin Psychiatry* 1999;60(Suppl 20):21–25.

88. Flint AJ, Rifat SL. Maintenance treatment for recurrent depression in late life. A four–year outcome study. *Am J Geriatr Psychiatr* 2000;8: 112–116.

89. Flint AJ, Rifat SL. Two–year outcome of psychotic depression in late life. *Am J Psychiatry* 1998;155:178–183.

90. Mallick R, Chen J, Entsuah AR, et al. Depression–free days as a summary measure of the temporal pattern of response and remission in the treatment of major depression: a comparison of venlafaxine, selective serotonin reuptake inhibitors, and placebo. *J Clin Psychiatry* 2003;64:321–330.

91. Flint AJ, Rifat SJ. Recurrence of first–episode geriatric depression after discontinuation of

maintenance antidepressants. *Am J Psychiatry* 1999;156:943–945.

92. Reynolds CF, Perel JM, Frank E, et al. Three–year outcomes of maintenance nortriptyline treatment in late–life depression: a study of two fixed plasma levels. *Am J Psychiatry* 1999; 156:1177–1181.

93. Angst J, Kupfer DJ, Rosenbaum JF. Recovery from depression: risk or reality? *Acta Psychiatr Scand* 1996;93:413–419.

94. Keitner GI, Ryan CE, Miller IW, et al. Recovery and major depression: factors associated with twelve–month outcome. *Am J Psychiatry* 1992; 149:93–99.

95. Murphy E. The prognosis of depression in old age. *Br J Psychiatry* 1983;142:111–119.

96. Baldwin R, Jolley DJ. The prognosis of depression in old age. *Br J Psychiatry* 1986;149: 574–583.

97. Brodaty H, Harris L, Peters K, et al. Prognosis of depression in the elderly: a comparison with younger patients. *Br J Psychiatry* 1993;163: 589–596.

98. Godber G, Rosenvinge H, Wilkinson E, et al. Depression in old age: prognosis after ECT. *Int J Geriatric Psychiatry* 1987;2:19–24.

99. Bosworth HB, McQuaid DR, George LK, et al. Time–to–remission from geriatric depression: psychosocial and clinical factors. *Am J Geriatr Psychiatry* 2002;10:551–559.

100. Reynolds CF III, Frank E, Perel JM, et al. Treatment of consecutive episodes of major depression in the elderly. *Am J Psychiatry* 1994;151: 1740–1743.

101. Frank E, Kupfer DJ, Perel J, et al. Three–year outcomes for maintenance therapies in recurrent depression. *Arch Gen Psychiatry* 1990;47: 1093–1099.

102. Montgomery SA, Dufour H, Brion S, et al. The prophylactic efficacy of fluoxetine in unipolar depression. *Br J Psychiatry* 1988;153(suppl 3): 69–76.

103. Georgotas A, McCue RE, Cooper TB. A placebo–controlled comparison of nortriptyline and phenelzine in maintenance therapy of elderly depressed patients. *Arch Gen Psychiatry* 1989;46:783–785.

104. Reynolds CE, Frank E, Perel JM, et al. Combined pharmacotherapy and psychotherapy in the acute and continuation treatment of elderly patients with recurrent major depression: a preliminary report. *Am J Psychiatry* 1992;149: 1687–1692.

105. Georgotas A, McCue RE, Cooper T, et al. How effective and safe is continuation therapy in elderly depressed patients? *Arch Gen Psychiatry* 1988;45:929–932.

106. Reynolds CF IIII, Frank E, Perel JM, et al. Nortriptyline and interpersonal psychotherapy as maintenance therapies for recurrent major depression. *JAMA* 1999;281:39–45.

107. Reynolds CF, Perel JM, Frank E, et al. Open trial maintenance pharmacotherapy in late life depression: survival analysis. *Psychiatry Res* 1989;27:225–231.

108. Doogan DP, Caillard V. Sertraline in the prevention of depression. *Br J Psychiatry* 1992;160: 217–222.

109. Klysner R, Bent–Hansen J, Hansen HL, et al. Efficacy of citalopram in the prevention of recurrent depression in elderly patients: placebo–controlled study of maintenance therapy. *Br J Psychiatry* 2002;181:29–35.

110. Sackeim HA, Haskett RF, Mulsant BH, et al. Continuation pharmacotherapy in the prevention of relapse following electroconvulsive therapy. *JAMA* 2001;285:1299–1307.

111. Ackerman DL, Greenland S, Bystritsky A, et al. Side effects and time course of response in a placebo–controlled trial of fluoxetine for the treatment of geriatric depression. *J Clin Psychopharmacol* 2000;20:658–665.

112. Alexopoulos GS, Chester JG. Outcomes of geriatric depression. *Clin Geriatr Med* 1992;8: 363–376.

113. Stoudemire A, Hill CD, Marquardt M, et al. Recovery and relapse in geriatric depression after treatment with antidepressants and ECT in a medical–psychiatric population. *Gen Hosp Psychiatry* 1998;20:170–174.

Supplemental Readings

Alexopoulos GS, Raue P, Arean P. Problem–solving therapy versus supportive therapy in geriatric major depression with executive dysfunction. *Am J Psychiatry* 2003;11:46–52.

Cahn DA, Malloy PF, Salloway S, et al. Subcortical hyperintensities on MRI and activities of daily living in geriatric depression. *J Neuropsychiatry Clin Neurosci* 1996;8:404–411.

Greenwald BS, Kramer–Ginsberg E, Krishnan KR, et al. MRI signal hyperintensities in geriatric depression. *Am J Psychiatry* 1996;153:1212–1215.

Greenwald BS, Kramer–Ginsberg E, Krishnan KR, et al. Neuroanatomic localization of magnetic resonance imaging signal hyperintensities in geriatric depression. *Stroke* 1998;29:613–617.

Heuser I, Bissette G, Dettling M, et al. Cerebrospinal fluid concentrations of corticotropin–releasing hormone, vasopressin, and somatostatin in depressed patients and healthy controls: response to amitriptyline treatment. *Depress Anxiety* 1998; 8:71–79.

Koran LM, Hamilton SH, Hertzman M, et al. Predicting response to fluoxetine in geriatric patients with major depression. *J Clin Psychopharmacol* 1995;15:421–427.

Kramer–Ginsberg E, Greenwald BS, Krishnan KR, et al. Neuropsychological functioning and MRI signal hyperintensities in geriatric depression. *Am J Psychiatry* 1999;156:438–444.

McDonald WM, Salzman C, Schatzberg AF. Depression in the elderly. *Psychopharmacol Bull* 2002; 36(suppl 2):112–122.

McIntyre IM, Norman TR. Platelet serotonin response to treatment in geriatric depression [letter]. *Biol Psychiatry* 1989;26:434–436.

Meyers BS, Alexopoulos GS. Geriatric depression. *Med Clin North Am* 1988;72:847–866.

Murata T, Kimura H, Omori M, et al. MRI white matter hyperintensities, (1)H–MR spectroscopy and cognitive function in geriatric depression: a comparison of early–and late–onset cases. *Int J Geriatr Psychiatry* 2001;16:1129–1135.

Oshima A, Higuchi T. Treatment guidelines for geriatric mood disorders. *Psychiatry Clin Neurosci* 1999;53(suppl):s55–s59.

Pollock BG. Adverse reactions of antidepressants in elderly patients. *J Clin Psychiatry* 1999;60(suppl 20):4–8.

Reynolds CF III, Frank E, Dew MA, et al. Treatment of 70+–year–olds with recurrent major depression: Excellent short–term but brittle long–term response. *Am J Geriatr Psychiatry* 1999;7:64–69.

Reynolds CF, Lebowitz BD. What are the best treatments for depression in old age? *Harv Ment Health Lett* 1999;15:8.

Reynolds CF III. Treatment of major depression in later life: a life cycle perspective. *Psychiatr Q* 1997; 68:221–246.

Reynolds CF, Buysse DJ, Brunner DP, et al. Maintenance nortriptyline effects on electroencephalographic sleep in elderly patients with recurrent major depression: double–blind, placebo–and plasma–level–controlled evaluation. *Biol Psychiatry* 1997;42:560–567.

Reynolds CF, Frank E, Perel JM, et al. High relapse rate after discontinuation of adjunctive medication for elderly patients with recurrent major depression. *Am J Psychiatry* 1996;153:1418–1422.

Roose SP, Suthers KM. Antidepressant response in late–life depression. *J Clin Psychiatry* 1998; 59(suppl 10):4–8.

Steffens DC, McQuoid DR, Krishnan KR. Partial response as a predictor of outcome in geriatric depression. *Am J Geriatr Psychiatry* 2003;11: 340–348.

Stoudemire A, Hill CD, Morris R, et al. Long–term outcome of treatment–resistant depression in older adults. *Am J Psychiatry* 1993;150:1539–1540.

Wilson K, Mottram P, Sivanranthan A, Nightingale A. Antidepressants versus placebo for the depressed elderly (Cochrane Review). In: *The Cochrane Library*, Issue 3 2002. Oxford: Update Software.

Wolf R, Dykierek P, Gattaz WF, et al. Differential effects of trimipramine and fluoxetine on sleep in geriatric depression. *Psychiatr Clin North Am* 1996;19:269–286.

Part V: Anxiety and Related Disorders (Panic, OCD, Phobias)

Chapter 15

Diagnosis of Anxiety and Anxiety-Related Disorders

Carl Salzman

Javaid I. Sheikh

Anxiety, a universal human condition, exists along a continuum ranging from normal mild apprehension to disabling emotional disorder. If not severe, the experience of anxiety can be helpful in the development of planning and coping behavior. In its more extreme form—characterized by dreaded anticipation of a known or unknown threat, fear, extreme worry, and preoccupation with the future—anxiety preoccupies and can so overwhelm a person that planning or coping behavior is impaired. At this degree of severity, anxiety is considered a symptom, and relief is usually sought.

Older people frequently have much to worry about: illness, financial security, social isolation, safety, accidents, and the approach of death—each or all of which may serve as focal points of reality around which anxiety may grow and develop. Just as often, however, pathological anxiety develops with no apparent cause, disabling an otherwise well-functioning older adult.

As a diagnostic category, anxiety symptoms can reach a severity and duration that defines them along a spectrum of disorders that includes general anxiety disorder, social anxiety disorder, posttraumatic stress disorder (PTSD) as well as related phobic, panic, and obsessive-compulsive disorders. However, DSM criteria used for diagnostic purposes do not take into consideration the unique and specific characteristics of old age relative to these disorders. For example, an elderly person living on the third floor of a walk-up building in a high-crime area who is realistically worried and anxious about falling and being mugged would be characterized as having a general anxiety disorder according to these criteria.[1]

Anxiety in old age, as either symptom or disorder, may also be characteristic of lifelong neurotic adaptation. Older patients for whom this is an accurate characterization may seem to worry more about realistic stress and concerns than the average person of the same age and situation, or they may seem constantly anxious about one or another future event, real or imagined. When one anxious concern is removed, conquered, or forgotten, another takes its place. Regardless of where the older person's anxiety falls along the diagnostic spectrum of disorders, the severity of the anxiety is invariably associated with poor physical health and inversely correlated with low socioeconomic status and level of education.[2] The development and severity of anxiety are also strongly correlated with depression, life stress events, and medical comorbidity.[3]

Epidemiology

The epidemiology of anxiety as a subjective experience as well as a diagnosable disorder has been recently reviewed.[4] Anxiety disorders are present in significant numbers of elderly patients although they are less common than affective disorders.[5] If the diagnostic category generalized anxiety disorder is more or less equivalent to the symptoms of anxiety, its onset and prevalence is actually quite low among older persons,[6,7] accounting for 0.7 to 4% of anxiety disorders in studies of elderly persons.[8] Phobias may be present in both older men and women,[9] and panic disorder has been recognized increasingly in late life (Table 15.1).[10]

Anxiety that coexists with depression, however, is significantly more common. Ranging from 27.5%[11] to 47.5%,[12] these high prevalence rates suggest that anxiety and depression appear together with sufficient frequency to constitute a new geriatric diagnostic category: mixed anxiety-depression.

Characteristics of Late-Life Anxiety

Anxiety in older people is characterized by cognitive, emotional, and physical symptoms: Decreased concentration, attention, and memory are common; and dizziness, feelings of impending faintness, heart attack, or of "going crazy" occur. Difficulty falling asleep is almost always present as well as alterations in appetite. Some people eat less when they are anxious; others eat more and continually. Anxiety in older patients may thus exacerbate already existing age-related sleep and appetite disturbances.

Distinguishing between anxiety as a diagnostic category worthy of psychiatric treatment in contrast to "worry," a normal mood state in older persons that does not necessarily require treatment, may be a matter of symptom intensity. Older individuals worry, as do their younger counterparts, only more so.[13] Health concerns predominate; older people worry less about finances and social events than college students.[14]

Severe anxiety may mimic symptoms of actual cardiovascular, endocrine, and neurologic disorders that commonly occur in older persons and may be misinterpreted by the older patient as signs of serious physical illness. For example, symptoms such as nausea, abdominal burning, belching, flatulence, constipation, or diarrhea—all common components of anxiety—may be mistaken for signs of gastrointestinal disease such as cancer; tightness in the chest, difficulty breathing, and tachycardia may be misinterpreted as early signs of a heart attack; and poor memory, poor attention, and poor concentration may be feared by the anxious older person as rapidly approaching Alzheimer's disease.

Preoccupation with the physical symptoms of anxiety, together with the conviction that such symptoms are part of an undiagnosed illness, lead to hypochondriasis,[15,16] which is common in late life. Although a persistent obsessional, unrealistic concern about health may have a variety of psychological roots, it can also be understood as the somatic expression of anxiety in a person who finds physical illness less threatening than emotional distress. However, some of these "psychogenic" complaints may actually be due to physical factors in nearly half of all older patients.[15,16] Older hypochondriacal patients are often agitated, intrusive, and unrelieved by reassurance from a physician. They may pace, wring their hands, and obsessively discuss their "illness," their symptoms, their helplessness, and their fear of impending inevitable doom.

Differential Diagnosis

Anxiety may arise from physical illness, drugs, and depression or other psychiatric syndromes. It may also develop from emotional or environmental concerns.

Physical Illness

Anxiety's somatic symptoms (e.g., respiratory restriction, palpitations, feeling shaky, dizziness, headache, chest pains) and signs (e.g., sighing and rapid breath-

Table 15.1.   Prevalence (%) of Anxiety Disorders in Elderly Subjects, Combined Age Groups, and Peak Prevalence in Three Studies

Study[a]	All Anxiety Disorders[b]			Phobic Disorders[b]			Panic Disorders[b]			Generalized Anxiety Disorders[b]			Obsessive-compulsive Disorder[b]		
	M	F	Total	M	F	Total	M	F	Total	M	F	Total	M	F	Total
Epidemiologic Catchment Area (1)[a]															
Subjects aged ≥65 years	3.6	6.8	5.5	2.9	6.1	4.8	0.0	0.2	0.1	—	—	—	0.7	0.9	0.8
Subjects of all ages	4.7	9.7	7.3	3.8	8.4	6.2	0.3	0.7	0.5	—	—	—	1.1	1.5	1.3
Peak	4.7	11.7	8.3	3.5	10.2	6.9	0.3	1.1	0.7	—	—	—	1.2	1.9	1.8
Edmonton (2)[a]															
Subjects aged ≥65 years															
In households	2.7	4.1	3.5	1.8	3.8	3.0	0.0	0.5	0.3	—	—	—	0.9	1.9	1.5
In institutions	1.4	7.1	5.0	0.0	1.6	1.0	0.0	1.6	1.0	—	—	—	1.4	4.7	3.5
Subjects of all ages	—	—	6.5	—	—	5.1	—	—	0.7	—	—	—	—	—	1.6
Peak	—	—	—	—	—	—	—	—	—	—	—	—	—	—	—
National Survey of Psychotherapeutic Drug Use (3)[a]															
Subjects aged ≥65 years	—	—	10.2	—	—	3.1[c]	—	—	—	—	—	7.1			
Subjects of all ages	6.1	12.9	9.9	1.8[c]	4.9[c]	3.5[c]	—	—	—	4.3	8.0	6.4			
Peak	—	—	11.3	—	—	4.6[c]	—	—	—	—	—	8.6			

From Flint AF. Epidemiology and comorbidity of anxiety disorders in the elderly. *Am J Psychiatry* 1994;151:640–649. With permission.

[a] Complete citations for references at end of chapter.

[b] M, males; F, females.

[c] Includes combined agoraphobia and panic.

ing, trembling, diarrhea, vomiting, coughing, rapid pulse, sweating) may be difficult to distinguish from similar clinical manifestations of various physical illnesses.[15] Several common illnesses in later life may present with anxiety as part of the clinical picture. These include:

- Cardiovascular diseases, particularly cardiac failure, mitral valve prolapse, and cardiac arrhythmias
- Respiratory distress, including chronic obstructive pulmonary disease, pulmonary embolus, and sleep apnea
- Endocrine disorders, especially thyroid and adrenal hyperactivity
- Neurologic illness
- Vitamin B_{12} deficiency

Medical causes of anxiety are presented in Table 15.2. Clinical disorders that produce anxiety-like symptoms can develop in virtually every system of the body. For example, nearly half of patients admitted to a cardiac care unit (regardless of age) are diagnosed with anxiety.[17] Symptoms of anxiety such as dread, weakness, bewilderment, dizziness, respiratory distress, and/or sweating may be initial

signals of a myocardial infarction in elderly persons.[18] Anxiety may commonly accompany late-life respiratory illness, particularly severe asthma and chronic obstructive pulmonary disease, and may be associated with endocrine disorders of the thyroid and parathyroid glands.[15]

Drugs

Medications commonly prescribed for the elderly may cause or exacerbate anxiety. Caffeine also commonly causes anxiety or increases preexisting anxiety syndromes. Other drugs with stimulant properties, such as over-the-counter cold preparations that contain phenylpropanolamine, may also heighten anxiety. Antidepressant drugs with stimulating properties, such as monoamine oxidase inhibitors, desipramine, protriptyline, and fluoxetine, are frequently associated with the development or worsening of anxiety.

Depression

Anxiety and depression often coexist or overlap in the same person, and distinguishing between them or determining which constellation of symptoms predom-

Table 15.2.   Medical Disorders Associated with Anxiety

Conditions producing trembling, tachycardia, or hyperexcitability

- Hypoglycemia
- Pheochromocytoma
- Hyperthyroidism

Conditions producing dread, bewilderment, weakness, dizziness, respiratory distress, or sweating

- Silent myocardial infarct
- Pulmonary embolism
- Small stroke or cerebral ischemic attack
- Excess intake of caffeine
- Sympathomimetic medications in nonprescription drugs
- Withdrawal symptoms of sedatives, hypnotics, or alcohol

From Salzman C, Lebowitz BD. *Anxiety in the elderly*. New York: Springer, 1991;49 with permission.

inates may be difficult. Feelings of loss, uselessness, and helplessness, as well as sleep and appetite disturbance and poor memory and concentration, may be associated with anxiety as well as depression. If asked, older patients may use the words "anxiety" and "depression" interchangeably to describe their subjective discomfort. In older people, anxiety disorders are almost always accompanied by symptoms of depression, and major depressive disorder is almost always accompanied by symptoms of anxiety; high comorbidity of anxiety and depression has been observed in hospitalized elderly males[19] and in outpatients.[20] Comorbid anxiety and depression are also common in geriatric medical patients. For example, 13% of geriatric patients with cancer suffer from a mixed anxiety-depressive syndrome, while 8% experience an anxiety disorder without depressive symptoms.[21]

Determining which disorder is primary may be a difficult clinical task, although some clues may be helpful. Predominantly anxious older people tend to feel and look apprehensive and express a feeling that "something must be done"—a heightened state of preparation for activity accompanied by increased sweating, tachycardia, dry mouth, restlessness, inability to concentrate, and trouble falling asleep. Some anxious older people may eat to calm themselves. In contrast, predominantly depressed older people usually move more slowly and appear listless, apathetic, and without energy. Rather than expressing a need for something to be done, they may repeat over and over "nothing can be done." These individuals also cannot concentrate, usually because of lack of interest and motivation rather than restlessness and distraction. Depressed older people tend to eat less and spend more time in bed, and they may experience sweating, tachycardia, and other signs of autonomic arousal.

In the recent past, making a clinical distinction between anxiety and depression was considered to have pragmatic value because antidepressants such as the tri-

cyclics (TCAs) had many undesirable side effects for the elderly whereas anxiolytics like benzodiazepines and buspirone were relatively well tolerated. However, since the introduction of selective serotonin reuptake inhibitors (SSRIs) and increasing evidence of their efficacy in the mixed-symptom picture of anxiety and depression, this issue does not seem to be as clinically relevant (see Chapter 16). Thus acceptance of a mixed-symptom picture reflects a recent philosophical shift in the inclusion of mixed anxiety-depression syndrome as a special category in the DSM-IV.

In summary, a mixed picture of anxiety and depression is very common among older patients in both medical and psychiatric settings. Evidence suggesting efficacy of antidepressants when both depression and anxiety are present make diagnostic attempts to separate anxiety and depression somewhat less relevant from a clinician's perspective.

Delirium and Dementia

Anxiety symptoms may be significant in patients with dementia,[22,23] although anxiety can interfere with cognitive test performance and may lead to an inaccurate appraisal of dementia severity.[20] The older patient with acute cognitive dysfunction (from delirium) or chronic cognitive impairment (from dementia) is almost always anxious and appears apprehensive and fearful; autonomic hyperarousal is not unusual. Also, for a demented patient, the degree of anxiety does not necessarily correlate with the severity of the dementia[24]; rather, it is usually proportionate to that patient's awareness of cognitive impairment. Thus anxiety is most severe in mild delirium and dementia whereas in extreme delirium or advanced dementia, anxiety may actually lessen.

Because agitation is also a regular feature of delirium and dementia, anxiety and agitation may overlap. Anxiety can exist without agitation and is distinguished from it by the objective presence of extreme motor restlessness and purposeless activity seen in the agitated individual, in contrast to the inner apprehension that defines anxiety as a subjective state.

Diagnostic Evaluation

The essential feature of anxiety is an unrealistic or excessive apprehensive expectation about realistic and unrealistic problems in one's life. For older people, these concerns center on health, finances, loss of spouse and friends, and misfortune that may befall children and grandchildren. The experience of anxiety is one of inner subjective dread, but external objective autonomic signs of hyperarousal are usually also present. These subjective symptoms and objective signs fall into several categories:

- Motoric tension
- Trembling
- Muscle tension or aches
- Restlessness
- Easy fatigability
- Tightness around head
- Lump in throat
- Autonomic hyperactivity
- Shortness of breath
- Palpitations
- Sweating
- Dry mouth
- Dizziness
- Nausea and diarrhea
- Flushes or chills
- Frequent urination
- Trouble swallowing
- Vigilance and scanning
- Feeling keyed up or on edge
- Exaggerated startle response
- Difficulty concentrating
- Trouble falling asleep or staying asleep
- Irritability

The anxious older person finds it difficult to enjoy activities or look forward to the future. If anxiety is prolonged, a subjective sense of demoralization, physical and emotional depletion, and depression develops.

The decision to treat the anxious older person pharmacologically depends on an appraisal of the severity of anxiety symptoms and the degree to which they interfere with function. When anxiety interferes with an older person's ability to cope with life or to obtain pleasure or when anxious symptoms themselves become incapacitating, treatment is necessary. Anxiety may also exacerbate physical illness or be the first presenting symptom of an unrecognized medical disorder.

In evaluating the anxious elderly person, therefore, the first task is to assess the impact of the anxiety symptoms on social and emotional functioning and on physical health. A careful interview and physical examination should search for any underlying cause of anxiety, particularly evidence of underlying cardiac or endocrine abnormalities. A mental status examination may reveal the presence of depression, delirium, and/or dementia. A careful review of concomitant medications, including over-the-counter preparations, is part of pretreatment evaluation. Anxiety rating scales as initial screening devices can be helpful in assessing severity of symptoms and can be used as instruments to document effectiveness of various psychological and pharmacologic therapeutic interventions. These scales are primarily of two kinds: observer-rated and self-rated. The most commonly used observer-rated scale is the Hamilton Anxiety Rating Scale (HARS)—a 14-item scale on which each item is rated on severity from none to very severe [0–4]; a rating of 18 or above suggests clinically significant anxiety. The Beck Anxiety Inventory—a 21-item inventory with rating on a severity scale of none to severe [0–3] is the most commonly used self-rated scale; a rating of 21 or above suggests clinically significant anxiety. This instrument can be useful in differentiating anxious older individuals from those who are not anxious; it is also sufficiently sensitive to measure change with treatment.[25,26]

Neurobiologic Mechanisms of Anxiety

Research in the last two decades postulates several neurobiologic mechanisms focused on functional neuroanatomical pathways, neurochemistry, and the neuroendocrinology of anxiety.[27] Although most preclinical and neuroimaging studies have explored anxiety in younger patients, newer diagnostic techniques shed light on neurobiologic mechanisms, diagnosis, and possible treatment of late-life anxiety as well. This section summarizes this literature and discusses its relevance to older patients in light of normal age-related changes in various neurotransmitter systems.

Functional Neuroanatomic Pathways

Several theoretic models involving functional neuroanatomic pathways have been implicated in the neurobiology of anxiety states.[28] One complex schema concerns the central role of a "behavioral inhibition system" in manifestations of anxiety that involve neuroanatomic structures of the septohippocampal system and noradrenergic, serotonergic, and GABAergic neurotransmitter systems.[29] A second model[30] proposes a neuroanatomic hypothesis for panic disorder, locating the acute panic attack in the brain stem, anticipatory anxiety in the limbic system, and phobic avoidance in the prefrontal cortex.

In a third and most recent model,[31,32] the amygdala (an almond-shaped structure in the medial temporal lobe) mediates fear and anxiety responses with extensive afferent and efferent connections to many other fear-related neuronal structures including hippocampus, locus ceruleus, thalamus, hypothalamus, and orbitofrontal cortex. At their core, these functional pathways may best be conceptualized as a central fear-response system, with the amygdala as a critical hub.[32,33] Efferent pathways of the central nucleus of the amygdala (CnA) project to several target areas in the brainstem and hypo-thalamus to mediate cognitive, physiological, emotional, and behavioral characteristics of anxiety.[31] Under normal circumstances, reciprocal connections of medial prefrontal cortex with amygdala exert an "executive inhibitory control" over affect and modulate autonomic and neuroendocrine function.[34,35] However, under threatening circumstances, an instinctive, quicker, and more primitive "fight, flight, or freeze" response with input from the thalamus is executed, bypassing the more cognitive cortical response. Although favoring survival during eons of evolution, an amygdala-centered response has insufficient inhibitory cortical influences. This unbalanced response appears to be the hallmark of pathological anxiety disorders, particularly panic disorder[36]; it is also present in PTSD and, to a lesser extent, in obsessive-compulsive disorder (OCD) and generalized anxiety disorder (GAD).

Neurochemistry of Anxiety

Several neurotransmitter systems have been implicated in anxiety disorders. These include the amino acid neurotransmitters gamma aminobutyric acid (GABA) and glutamate, as well as the monoamine transmitters norepinephrine and serotonin. GABA, an inhibitory neurotransmitter, plays a central role in anxiety. Circulating GABA binds to its receptor (the $GABA_A$ receptor) that changes the electrochemical gradient across the cell surface membrane, resulting in decreased neuronal firing.

Benzodiazepine receptors are present in many of these $GABA_A$ receptors and facilitate the binding of GABA to its receptor (all benzodiazepine receptors are associated with GABA but not all GABA receptors are associated with benzodiazepine receptors). Benzodiazepines may decrease anxiety, therefore, by enhancing GABA binding to the $GABA_A$ receptor. Inhibitory GABA input that occurs at many synapses throughout the cortex and subcortical areas serves to balance the ubiquitous stimulatory neurotransmitter gluta-mate. The role of glutamate in anxiety has not yet been clarified, but the numerous interactions of glutamate with other neu-rotransmitters, including the catechola-mines, suggest that it plays a major role.

Monoamine neurotransmitters also play a role in anxiety, both directly and indirectly, by modulating GABA and glu-tamate; for example, serotonin modulates both GABA and glutamate.[33] Norepi-nephrine, a catecholamine neurotrans-mitter arising from the locus ceruleus in the midbrain, may play a central role in the development of panic attacks as well in heightening anxiety. Yohimbine, for example, which increases norepineph-rine via antagonism of α_2 presynaptic autoreceptors, can induce panic in indi-viduals prone to panic disorders.[37,38] In addition to increased levels of mono-amine oxidase B, decreased noradrener-gic function in old age includes decreased numbers of locus ceruleus neurons and decreased norepinephrine content in many brain areas.[39] This decline in nora-drenergic function may also explain a milder symptomatology in older panic dis-order patients.[40]

Neuroendocrinology of Anxiety

The hypothalamic-pituitary-adrenal (HPA) axis also plays a central role in anxiety states, particularly posttraumatic stress and panic disorders.[41,42] Although the HPA axis can be activated acutely, in the stress of chronic anxiety states, such as PTSD (and depression), a chronic dysreg-ulation of this axis seems to occur.[41,43] Acute stress induces activation of HPA axis, causing increased levels of cortico-tropin-releasing hormone (CRF), which then stimulates production of adrenocor-ticotropic hormone, resulting in in-creased cortisol production. Increased levels of cortisol bring the system back to homeostasis via a negative feedback mech-anism. Long-term stress tends to dysregu-late this mechanism, potentially resulting in high levels of resting cortisol. Antide-pressant treatment can potentially nor-malize such HPA dysregulation.[33]

Despite the role of the HPA axis in anx-iety, a single neurobiologic substrate for geriatic anxiety is unlikely. Whether the aging brain per se may be associated with increased predisposition to develop anxi-ety symptoms, as it is for depressive symp-toms, is also unclear.

Panic Anxiety, Obsessive-Compulsive Disorders, Phobias

Extreme states of anxiety are sometimes associated with panic, OCD, and phobias. These spectrum disorders are less com-mon in old than in younger adults, but when they do occur they may prevent the elderly person from participating in the normal activities of daily life.

Panic Disorder (with and without Agoraphobia)

Individuals who experience a panic at-tack, regardless of age, are in an acute state of extreme autonomic hyperarousal and are usually convinced that they will die, "go crazy," or lose control of their behavior. Because panic attacks inevitably arise without warning, patients become continually anxious, anticipating the next panic attack ("anticipatory anxiety"). One coping mechanism is to avoid loca-tions or activities associated with past panic attacks, which leads to secondary phobic avoidance behavior (agorapho-bia). Late-onset agoraphobic fears may also arise from an episode of physical ill-ness.[2]

Panic attacks rarely develop for the first time in late life. When they do appear, particularly in conjunction with agora-phobia, they are often associated with a serious depressive or physical illness. The prevalence of spontaneous panic attacks, with or without secondary agoraphobia, in older people is extremely low.[2,44-46] Panic and agoraphobic symptoms in older patients whose symptoms began in early life may continue into later life, although clinical experience suggests that their frequency decreases in old age.[47] Older persons who experience frequent panic attacks typically have received inadequate or no treatment over the years.[48] Panic disorder in young people is often associated with a higher-than-average cardiovascular mortality rate in male patients, together with depression, alcohol abuse, and increased risk of suicide[49]; some patients with panic disorder may therefore not live into old age. On the basis of these observations, the decreased frequency of panic disorder in old age might be explained in part by increased mortality of persons with the disorder.[49] Ongoing studies suggest that late-onset panic disorder may also be characterized by fewer panic symptoms, less avoidance, and lower scores on somatization measures than with early-onset panic disorder in older populations.[44–46]

Obsessive-Compulsive Disorder

Like panic disorder, OCD, rarely develops for the first time in late life. Epidemiologic data for OCD suggest a 6-month prevalence rate of about 1.5% in the elderly[3] although relatively little is known about any special manifestations in this age group. Many elderly patients are assumed to have an earlier onset with continuation into old age. Older people who are depressed or chronically physically ill also commonly obsess about their health and have feelings of hopelessness and guilt.

Compulsive behavior, however, is very unusual in elderly patients. Some late-life obsessions have the quality of delusions—bizarre fixed thoughts that cannot be challenged by realistic appraisal. An individual's endless ruminations and obsessions are invariably accompanied by autonomic arousal and apprehension. Anxiety may increase as the older patient tries not to obsess, and anxiety may be overwhelming if compulsive rituals are not followed. Even when the behaviors or thoughts are

allowed free rein, patients with this disorder usually experience high levels of generalized anxiety.

Among the anxiety-spectrum disorders, OCD is considered the most resistant to treatment. However, introduction of SSRI antidepressants and more effective cognitive-behavioral techniques seem to improve prognosis.[50] Unfortunately, no specific studies of treatment in elderly patients with OCD are available.

Phobias

Characterizing the longitudinal course of particular phobias is difficult, primarily because so many specific stimuli can cause them and partly because individuals with one phobia may develop another at some point in the course of their affliction. Systematic studies of specific phobias in older persons are unavailable. However, in urban settings, fear of crime is particularly prevalent in the elderly population,[51] leading to "nocturnal neurosis" (a general fear of nighttime) in some cases.[52]

Phobic disorders are associated with high psychiatric and medical morbidity, and elderly people with phobias make frequent visits to family practitioners.[4] Older patients with phobias commonly do not seek psychiatric treatment.

In younger individuals, clinically significant improvement may be obtained in 75 to 85% of specific phobias treated with cognitive-behavior therapy. Such treatment consists of one 2- to 3-hour, office-based, therapist-assisted exposure session that focuses on only one specific phobic avoidance per behavioral session.[53] The effectiveness of this procedure in the elderly, however, is not known. Administration of low-dose benzodiazepines before medical or dental procedures (common sources of phobic behavior in elderly individuals) may help alleviate anxiety for very fearful patients and may produce better compliance with treatment.

Social Anxiety Disorder

The National Comorbidity Survey (NCS) suggests a one-year prevalence rate of

7.9% for the specific type of phobia termed social phobia.[54] This form of phobic disorder arises in young adulthood, is chronic and unremitting, and persists into old age.[6] Clinical experience suggests that common social phobia symptoms, such as fear of eating or writing in public, may be more bothersome to the elderly because of the presence of dentures or tremors; fear of speaking in public is relatively uncommon in older individuals. Elderly patients with social anxiety disorder commonly also suffer from other disorders, including other specific phobias, agoraphobia, major depression, dysthymia, and alcohol abuse.[55]

Posttraumatic Stress Disorder

Much of the information on PTSD in the elderly comes from descriptions of those who experienced war-related trauma and then survived into late life. The term "shellshock" from World War I and "combat neurosis" from World War II probably are describing PTSD.[56] Estimates of PTSD in elderly survivors of World War II range from 19 to 20%.[57–59] Korean war POWs have high rates of PTSD; 40 years posttrauma, 70% still report having symptoms of varying degrees of severity[60] that include intrusive memories, anxiety, and hyperarousal. Elderly holocaust survivors who experienced severe trauma when young indicate that symptoms can become chronic and continue into old age; despite good psychosocial adjustment, 65% of these symptoms fulfill the criteria for PTSD.[61,62] Exposure to trauma during the holocaust also predisposed victims to developing PTSD after recurrent trauma in late life.[63,64]

Elderly people do not appear to be more likely than younger persons to develop PTSD following trauma.[56] Recent reports document the development of PTSD for the first time in old age among survivors of natural disasters such as the Armenian and Japanese earthquakes.[65–67] Although the overall severity of PTSD seems similar in young and elderly survivors of earthquakes, older survivors report less re-experiencing but more symptoms of hyperarousal than their younger counterparts.

Conclusions

Anxiety and anxiety-related disorders may be somewhat less frequent in an individual's later years than in earlier life. Nevertheless, symptoms of anxiety, whether acute or chronic, alone or in combination with other disorders, can cause great suffering in older persons. Thoughtful and compassionate attention to the diagnosis and use of modern therapeutic techniques as well as effective available medications should now be standard procedure for all clinicians.

References

1. Shamoian CA. What is anxiety in the elderly? In: Salzman C, Lebowitz BD, eds. *Anxiety in the elderly.* New York: Springer, 1991:3–15.
2. Lindesay J. Phobic disorders in the elderly. *Br J Psychiatry* 1991;159:531–541.
3. Blazer D, George LK, Hughes D. The epidemiology of anxiety disorders. An age comparison. In: Salzman C, Lebowitz BD, eds. *Anxiety in the elderly.* New York: Springer, 1991:17–30.
4. Alwahabi F. Anxiety symptoms and generalized anxiety disorder in the elderly: a review. *Harv Rev Psychiatry* 2003;11:180–193.
5. Flint AJ. Epidemiology and comorbidity of anxiety disorders in the elderly. *Am J Psychiatry* 1994; 151:640–649.
6. Regier DA, Boyd JH, Burke JD, et al. One month prevalence of mental disorders in the United States. *Arch Gen Psychiatry* 1988;45:977–986.
7. Sheikh JI, Salzman C. Anxiety in the elderly: course and treatment. *Psychiatr Clin North Am* 1995;4:871–883.
8. Krasucki C, Howard R, Mann A. The relationship between anxiety disorders and age, *Int J Geriatr Psychiatry* 1998;13:79–99.
9. Sheikh JI. Anxiety and its disorders in old age. In: Birren JE, Sloane RB, Cohen G, eds. *Handbook of mental health and aging.* 2nd ed. 1992: 409–432.
10. Smith SSL, Colenda CC, Espelaid MA. Factors determining the level of anxiety state in geriatric primary care patients in a community dwelling. *Psychosomatics* 1994;35:50–58.
11. Lenze EJ, Mulsant BH, Shear MK, et al. Comorbid anxiety disorders in depressed elderly patients. *Am J Psychiatry* 2000;157:722–728.
12. Beekman AT, de Beurs E, van Balkom AJ, et al. Anxiety and depression in later life: co-occur-

rence and communality of risk factors. *Am J Psychiatry* 2000;157:89–95.

13. Diefenbach GJ, Stanley MA, Beck JG. Worry content reported by older adults with and without generalized anxiety disorder. *Aging Ment Health* 2001;5:269–274.

14. Powers CB, Wisocki PA, Whitbourne SK. Age differences and correlates of worrying in young and elderly adults. *Gerontologist* 1992;32:82–88.

15. Cohen GD. Anxiety and general medical conditions. In: Salzman C, Lebowitz BD, eds. *Anxiety in the elderly*. New York: Springer, 1991:47–62.

16. Sklar M. Gastrointestinal diseases in the aged. In: Reichel W, ed. *Clinical aspects of aging*. Baltimore: Williams & Wilkins, 1978.

17. Cassem NY, Hackett TP. The psychiatric consultation in a coronary care unit. *Ann Intern Med* 1971;75:9–14.

18. Gurland BJ, Meyers BS. In: Talbott JA, Hales RE, Yudofsky SC, eds. *Textbook of psychiatry*. Washington, DC: American Psychiatric Press, 1988:1117–1139.

19. Hyer L, Gonveia I, Harrison WR, et al. Depression, anxiety, paranoid reactions, hypochondriasis, and recognitive decline of later–life inpatients. *J Gerontol* 1987;42:92–94.

20. Alexopoulos GS. Anxiety and depression in the elderly. In: Salzman C, Lebowitz BD. *Anxiety in the elderly*. New York: Springer, 1991:63–77.

21. Derogatis LR, Morrow GR, Fetting J, et al. The prevalence of psychiatric disorders among cancer patients. *J Am Med Association* 1983;249:751–757.

22. Hocking LB, Koenig HG. Anxiety in medically ill older patients: a review and update. *Int J Psychiatry Med* 1995;25:221–238.

23. Mintzer JE, Brawman–Mintzer O. Agitation as a possible expression of generalized anxiety disorder in demented elderly patients: toward a treatment approach. *J Clin Psychiatry* 1996; 57(suppl 7):55–63.

24. Yesavage JA, Taylor B. Anxiety and dementia. In Salzman C, Lebowitz BD, eds. *Anxiety in the elderly*. New York: Springer, 1991:79–85.

25. Stanley MA, Beck JG, Zebb BJ. Psychometric properties of four anxiety measures in older adults. *Behav Res Ther* 1996;34:827–838.

26. Wetherell JL, Reynolds CA, Gatz M, Pedersen NL. Anxiety, cognitive performance, and cognitive decline in normal aging. *J Gerontol B Psychol Sci Soc Sci* 2002;57:P246–55.

27. Sunderland T, Lawlor BA, Martinez RA, et al. Anxiety in the elderly: neurobiologic and clinical interface. In Salzman C, Lebowitz BD, eds. *Anxiety in the elderly*. New York: Springer Publishing, 1991:105–129.

28. Wilson WH, and Matthew RJ. Cerebral blood flow and metabolism in anxiety disorders. In Hoehn–Saric R, McLeod DR, eds. *Biology of anxiety disorders*. Washington, DC: American Psychiatric Press, 1992:1–50.

29. Gray JA. A theory of anxiety: the role of the limbic system. *Encephale* 1983;9:161B–166B.

30. Gorman JM, Liebowitz MR, Fyer AJ, et al. A neuroanatomical hypothesis for panic disorder. *Am J Psychiatry* 1989;146:148–161.

31. Davis M. Neurobiology of fear responses: the role of the amygdala. *J Neuropsychiatry Clin Neurosci* 1997;9:382–402.

32. LeDoux J. Fear and the brain: where have we been, and where are we going? *Biol Psychiatry* 1998;44:1229–1238.

33. Ninan PT, Feigon SA, Knight B. Neurobiology and mechanisms of antidepressant treatment response in anxiety. *Psychopharmacology Bulletin* 2002;36(suppl 3):67–78.

34. Ninan PT. The functional neuroanatomy, neurochemistry, and pharmacology of anxiety. *J Clin Psychiatry* 1999;60(suppl 22):12–17.

35. Barkley RA. Behavioral inhibition, sustained attention, and executive functions: constructing a unifying theory of ADHD. *Psychol Bull* 1997;121:65–94.

36. Gorman JM, Kent JM, Sullivan GM, Coplan JD. Neuroanatomical hypothesis of panic disorder, revised. *Am J Psychiatry* 2000;157:493–505.

37. Gorman JM, Hirschfeld RMA, Ninan PT. New developments in the neurobiological basis of anxiety disorders. *Psychopharmacology Bulletin* 2002;36(suppl 2):49–67.

38. Charney DS, Heninger GR, Sternberg DE: Assessment of alpha–2 adrenergic autoreceptor function in humans: Effects of oral yohimbine. *Life Sci*, 30:2033–2041, 1982.

39. Sunderland T, Lawlor B, Martinez R, Molchan S: Anxiety in the elderly: Neurobiological and clinical interface. In: Salzman C, Lebowitz BD, eds. *Anxiety in the elderly*. New York: Springer Publishing, 1991.

40. Sheikh JI, Swales PJ, Carlson EB, Lindley SE. Aging and panic disorder: Phenomenology, comorbidity, and risk factors. *Am J Ger Psychiatry* 2004;2:102–109.

41. Heim C, Newport DJ, Heit S, et al. Pituitary–adrenal and autonomic responses to stress in women after sexual and physical abuse in childhood. *JAMA* 2000;284:592–597.

42. Bandelow B, Wedekind D, Pauls J, et al. Salivary cortisol in panic attacks. *Am J Psychiatry* 2000;157:454–456.

43. Musselman DM, Nemeroff CB. Neuroendocrinology of depression. *Clin Neurosci*. 1993;1:115–121.

44. Luchins DJ, Rose RP. Late-life onset of panic disorder with agoraphobia in three patients. *Am J Psychiatry* 1989;146:920–921.

45. Sheik JI, Taylor CB, King RJ, et al. Panic attacks and avoidance behavior in the elderly. Proceedings of the 141st annual scientific meeting of the American Psychiatric Association, Montreal, 1988.

46. Sheikh JI. Is late–onset panic disorder a distinct syndrome? Proceedings of the 146th annual scientific meeting of the American Psychiatric Association, San Francisco, 1993.

47. Flint AJ, Cook JM, Rabins PV. Why is panic disorder less frequent in late life? *Am J Geriatr Psychiatry* (in press).

48. Sheikh JI, King RJ, Taylor CB. Comparative phenomenology of early-onset versus late-onset panic attacks: a pilot survey. *Am J Psychiatry* 1991;148:1231–1233.

49. Coryell W. Mortality of anxiety disorders. In: Noyes R Jr, Roth M, Burrows GD, eds. *Handbook of anxiety*. Vol. 2: Classification, etiological fac-

tors and associated distubances. Amsterdam: Elsevier, 1988:311–320.

50. Rasmussen SA, Eisen JL, Pato MT. Current issues in the pharmacologic management of obsessive compulsive disorder. *J Clin Psychiatry* 1993; 54(suppl 6):4–9.

51. Clarke AH, Lewis MJ. Fear of crime among the elderly. *Br J Criminol* 1982;22:49–62.

52. Cohen CI. Nocturnal neurosis of the elderly: failure of agencies to cope with the problem. *J Am Geriatr Soc* 1976;24:86–88.

53. Ost LG. One-session treatment for specific phobias. *Behav Res Ther* 1989;27:1–7.

54. Kessler RC, McGonagle DK, Zhao S, et al. Lifetime and 12-month prevalence of DSM-III-R psychiatric disorders in the United States: results from the National Comorbidity Survey. *Arch Gen Psychiatry* 1994;51:8–19.

55. Judd LL. Social phobia: a clinical overview. *J Clin Psychiatry* 1994;55(suppl 6):5–9.

56. Weintraub D, and Ruskin PE. Posttraumatic stress disorder in the elderly: a review. *Harvard Rev Psychiatry* 1999;7:144–152.

57. Blake DD, Keane TM, Wine PR, et al. Prevalence of PTSD symptoms in combat veterans seeking medical treatment. *J Trauma Stress* 1990;3:15–27.

58. Rosen J, Fields RB, Hand AM, et al. Concurrent posttraumatic disorder in psychogeriatric patients. *J Geriatr Psychiatry Neurol* 1989;12:65–69.

59. Sutker PB, Allain AN Jr, Winstead DK. Psychopathology and psychiatric diagnoses of World War II Pacific theater prisoner of war survivors and combat veterans. *Am J Psychiatry* 1993;150: 240–245.

60. Kluznik JC, Speed N, Van Valkenberg, et al. Forty-year follow-up of United States prisoners of war. *Am J Psychiatry* 1986;143:1443–1446.

61. Kuch K, Cox BJ. Symptoms of PTSD in 124 survivors of the Holocaust. *Am J Psychiatry* 1992;149: 337–340.

62. Speed N, Engdahl B, Schwartz J, et al. Posttraumatic stress disorder as a consequence of the POW experience. *J Nerv Ment Dis* 1989;177: 147–153.

63. Danieli Y. As survivors age: an overview. *J Geriatr Psychiatry* 1997;30:935–940.

64. Baider L, Peretz T, Kaplan. Effect of the Holocaust on coping with cancer. *Soc Sci Med* 1992; 34:11–15.

65. van der Kolk BA. Psychopharmacological issues in post–traumatic stress disorder. *Hosp Community Psychiatry* 1983;34:683–691.

66. Goenjian AK, Najarian LM, Pynoos RS, et al. Posttraumatic stress disorder in elderly and younger adults after the 1988 earthquake in Armenia. *Am J Psychiatry* 1994;151:895–901.

67. Kato H, Asukai N, Miyake Y, et al. Post-traumatic symptoms among younger and elderly evacuees in the early stages following the 1995 Hanshin-Awaji earthquake in Japan. *Acta Psychiatr Scand* 1996;93:477–481.

Table 15.1 References

1. Regier DA, Boyd JH, Burke JD Jr, et al. One-month prevalence of mental disorders in the United States: based on five Epidemiologic Catchment Area site. *Arch Gen Psychiatry* 1988;45: 977–986.

2. Bland RC, Newman SC, Orn H. Prevalence of psychiatric disorders in the elderly in Edmonton. *Acta Psychiatr Scand Suppl* 1988;338:57–63.

3. Uhlenhuth EH, Balter MB, Mellinger GD, et al. Symptom checklist syndromes in the general population: correlations with psychotherapeutic drug use. *Arch Gen Psychiatry* 1983;40:1167–1173.

Supplemental Readings

Copeland JRM, Dewey ME, Wood N, et al. Range of mental illness among the elderly in the community: prevalence in Liverpool using the GMS–AGECAT package. *Br J Psychiatry* 1987;150: 815–823.

Copeland JRM, Gurland BJ, Dewey ME, et al. Is there more dementia, depression and neurosis in New York? A comparative diagnosis AGECAT. *Br J Psychiatry* 1987;151:466–473.

Crook T. Diagnosis and treatment of mixed anxiety–depression in the elderly. *J Clin Psychiatry* 1982;43:35–43.

Flint AJ. Epidemiology and comorbidity of anxiety disorders in the elderly. *Am J Psychiatry* 1994;151: 640–649.

Hershey LA, Kim KY. Diagnosis and treatment of anxiety in the elderly. *Rational Drug Ther* 1988; 22:1–6.

Lindesay J. Phobic disorders in the elderly. *Br J Psychiatry* 1991;159:531–541.

Lindesay J, Briggs K, Murphy E. The Guy's Age Concern Survey: prevalence rates of cognitive impairment, depression and anxiety in an urban elderly community. *Br J Psychiatry* 1989;155:317–329.

Nakra BRS, Grossberg GT. Management of anxiety in the elderly. *Comp Ther* 1986;12:53–60.

Sallis JF, Lichstein KL. Analysis and management of geriatric anxiety. *Int J Aging Hum Dev* 1982;15: 197–205.

Salzman C. Treatment of agitation, anxiety, and depression in dementia. *Psychopharmacol Bull* 1988;24:39–42.

Shader RI, Greenblatt DJ. Management of anxiety in the elderly: the balance between therapeutic and adverse effects. *J Clin Psychiatry* 1982;43:8–18.

Turnbull JM, Turnbull SK. Management of specific anxiety disorders in the elderly. *Geriatrics* 1985; 40:75–82.

Chapter 16

Treatment of Anxiety and Anxiety-Related Disorders

Carl Salzman

The decision to treat the anxious older patient pharmacologically depends on an appraisal of the severity of the anxiety symptoms and the degree to which they impair function. In both older and younger adult patients, anxiety commonly interferes with work, social, and interpersonal activities of daily living. In the older patient, anxiety may also interfere with cognitive function, exacerbate physical illnesses, and be an unrecognized consequence of a medical disorder.

Contemporary diagnosis of anxiety is no longer limited to a list of the subjective symptoms and objective signs of anxiety. The DSM classification system subdivides clinical anxiety disorders into acute and chronic categories, the latter being further subdivided into specific anxiety syndromes. As described in Chapter 15, these include: generalized anxiety disorder (the category describing the nonspecific but enduring experience of worry and apprehension), as well as the specific disorders, panic and phobic disorders, social anxiety disorder, obsessive-compulsive disorder, and posttraumatic stress disorder. In this chapter, treatment of each subtype of anxiety disorder is discussed individually although it is important to emphasize that among the various anxiety disorders considerable overlap of symptoms as well as treatments prevail.

Acute Anxiety and Generalized Anxiety Disorder

Treatment of the acutely or chronically anxious older patient with generalized anxiety disorder (GAD) is usually limited to symptomatic relief rather than a more lengthy psychotherapeutic exploration of underlying psychic predispositions to anxiety. As a general principle, treatment should not be undertaken until a thorough medical and psychological appraisal of the symptoms has been conducted. In some cases, life-maintenance needs, combined with a lack of resources, suggest social intervention rather than medical therapy. When anxiety is related to a clear precipitant, its identification and clarification and a discussion of alternative coping strategies may suffice as treatment. For some elderly patients, brief psychotherapy, cognitive-behavioral therapy, or relaxation training may offer significant reduction in anxiety symptoms.[1] If these approaches are ineffective or if anxiety symptoms are incapacitating, then antianxiety drugs may be an effective part of a treatment program.

Treatment with Benzodiazepines

Acute anxiety as well as generalized anxiety disorder in older patients is still treated with benzodiazepines, although alternative medications are available. Extensive laboratory studies of the pharmacokinetics and toxicity of benzodiazepines in the elderly have provided many relevant sources of prescribing information for clinicians. These studies, as a group, indicate that older persons differ from younger adults with regard to both the pharmacological disposition of benzodiazepines and the sensitivity of the central nervous system (CNS) to their effects. Clinical trials of benzodiazepines in the elderly are relatively sparse so that research and clinical experience from treating younger adults, still provide the major source of benzodiazepine-prescribing information for the geriatric population.[2]

Benzodiazepines are still used for many (if not most) acutely anxious elderly patients who require drugs as a component of their treatment for anxiety. The controversy that has accompanied their use shows no sign of abating and is especially active with regard to very old patients.[3–8] This controversy focuses on three concerns: (1) the potential abuse of benzodiazepines by elderly patients; (2) whether or not long-term use is appropriate in view of the development of dependence and withdrawal symptoms; and (3) side effects, particularly cognitive impairment. Conflicting opinions among clinicians regarding these concerns may leave elderly patients and their families bewildered when faced with the decision of whether or not to take a benzodiazepine for treatment of anxiety.

Although benzodiazepines belong to the sedative/hypnotic class of psychotropic drugs, they are among the safest drugs known, with virtually no lethal potential when taken alone, and with few significant drug interactions.[9,10] Despite causing side effects and drug dependency, they still represent a major pharmacological advance in the treatment of acute anxiety compared with previously available sedative/hypnotic drugs.[11] Nevertheless, concern has often been expressed regarding excessive or inappropriate prescription of these drugs for older patients,[5,6,12,13] leading the Health Care Financing Administration of the U.S. Department of Health and Human Services to establish benzodiazepine-prescribing

guidelines restricting their use in nursing homes.[14] These restrictions have decreased the use of benzodiazepines by elderly residents of nursing homes,[15–17] but the impact of physician education programs, which are also part of these guidelines, is not as clear.[18] One survey reports that a large proportion of physicians fail to adjust benzodiazepine dosage for advancing age[19]; a second survey suggests that benzodiazepine-prescribing regulations are associated with a reduction in both the number of elderly patients being prescribed a benzodiazepine and the number of prescriptions given to chronic users.[16]

It appears incontrovertible that benzodiazepine usage rates have been higher for older patients than for younger ones with corresponding symptoms of anxiety. Prescriptions filled by elderly patients reveal a disproportionately large percentage of all prescriptions for benzodiazepines.[7,8,20] Most have used benzodiazepines regularly for long periods, and they constitute the largest group of all long-term users.[7] The high usage pattern may be due, in part, to the higher incidence of multiple chronic physical ailments in this age group.[7] For example, in a recent survey of an older Canadian population, long-term continuous use of benzodiazepines was 19.8%.[21,22] Studies of usage patterns of benzodiazepines by elderly individuals are presented in Table 16.1.

Despite medical and governmental concern about overuse of benzodiazepines, more than half of older patients who take benzodiazepines consider them helpful,[21,24] and the frequency of benzodiazepine use in the elderly may not be declining significantly.[21,25,26] Of older outpatients surveyed, 70% take benzodiazepines only occasionally for symptomatic relief, and the vast majority keep benzodiazepines available at home for such occasional use.[23] Short-term use is likely to be associated with periods of acute stress such as illness, hospitalization, moving, or death of a loved one. The typical long-term benzodiazepine user is an older

Table 16.1. Use of Anxiolytics by Elderly Patients: Benzodiazepines

Study[a]	Results
Petrovic (2002)	Chronic elderly BZ users are typically widowed females with dysthymic disorder, anxiety, predisposition to alcohol dependence, and borderline disorder
van Dijk (2002)	Coprescribing of BZs in 53% of elderly TCA users and 57% of elderly SSRI users; during SSRI therapy, significantly more start BZ therapy than during TCA therapy
Zandstra (2002)	Long-term BZ users are older, have more severe history of mental health problems, use more psychotropic drugs, and see more specialists in hospital; also more likely to have diabetes, asthma, chronic obstructive pulmonary disease, hypertension, or serious skin disorder
Elliot (2001)	BZs prescribed to one-third of elderly hospital inpatients, often inappropriately
Fourrier (2001)	5-year prevalence rate of BZ use, 32%: associated with female gender, previous psychiatric disease, concomitant antidepressant use, multiple drug use, multiple chronic diseases, and poor self-perceived health
Svarstad (2001)	Nearly one-fourth of all nursing home residents were prescribed BZ before 1990 and nearly one-tenth had chronic BZ use; pattern declined only slightly (by 4%) after implementation of federal prescribing guidelines
Tu (2001)	Prevalence of BZ therapy for older people in Ontario steadily declined between 1993 and 1998; trend observed for dispensing relatively more short-acting BZs as well as replacing BZs with antidepressants
van Haaren (2001)	Triplicate prescription rules in New York state associated with significant decrease in nursing home BZ prescriptions without increased use of BZ substitutes
Batty (2000)	BZs inappropriately prescribed for 65% of prescriptions for elderly medical inpatients
Blazer (2000)	10-year longitudinal study: frequency of BZ use among elderly not declining significantly; continues to remain greater than in general population
Egan (2000)	12-month prevalence of long-term BZ use nearly 20% and seems to increase with age
Jorm (2000)	17–20% of older community residents use BZs; much use is long term
Llorente (2000)	Disproportionate prescription of BZs for older adults usually also suffering from co-morbid medical and psychiatric conditions
Mort (2000)	Long-acting BZs (as well as antidepressants) account for most potentially inappropriate psychotropic drug prescriptions for the elderly
Kirby (1999)	BZs used by 44% of elderly community-dwelling subjects with an anxiety disorder, 34% with depression, and 10% with dementia; four-fifths of older people using a psychotropic drug take a BZ
Gleason (1998)	10% of community-dwelling elderly reported taking a BZ as an anxiolytic, often at a lower dose than prescribed and usually PRN
Taylor (1998)	Among elderly BZ users for anxiety, 61% are long-term users, largest proportion concurrently depressed; no decrease in BZ use from 1983 to 1991
Monette (1997)	Physicians frequently prescribing long-acting BZs for elderly are often themselves older, likely to have received MDs before 1979, general practitioners, and practice in long-term care settings
Zisselman (1997)	For hospitalized patients, BZs used to treat symptoms rather than disorders e.g., preoperative relaxation (26%), pain (14%), nausea (12%), to aid intubation (12%), or facilitate a medical test (10%)
Manela (1996)	Elderly community-dwelling people with GAD report high BZ use
Copeland (1987)	Anxious depression in community dwellers

(continued)

Table 16.1. *(continued)*

Study[a]	Results
Verhaeghe (1996)	Elderly patients: 42% had taken a BZ in week prior to evaluation in ER; more women than men took BZs; 10% took more than one
Zisselman (1996)	Inpatient geriatric sample: 39.5% of depressed patients receive BZ as sole prescription for depression; 64% receive BZ not according to HCFA guidelines
McNutt (1994)	Use by more females than males; fewer blacks fill BZ prescriptions
Stewart (1994)	Outpatient use in surveys 1978–79, 1984–85: 13% and 6% of women, respectively, use BZs
Mayer-Oakes (1993)	Older BZ users likely to take 10 or more drugs, have trouble falling asleep, and to be depressed
Avorn (1992)	Nursing home residents: 6–13% receive BZ anxiolytics; residents judge them helpful
Woods (1995)	Regular BZ use by 13–22% of elderly; BZ prescriptions for elderly account for disproportionately large fraction of all BZ prescriptions; high BZ use in institutions and community samples
Antonijoan (1990)	Inpatients in geriatric hospitals in Spain: 84% of all psychotropic drugs are BZs
Busto (1990)	Elderly general hospital inpatients: 15% taking BZs on admission; 42% receive BZs during hospital stay; 80% still take BZs 5 months posthospitalization
King (1990)	Older long-term BZ users have mixed opinions about their medication: half want to discontinue, half do not
Lockwood (1990)	Elderly Australians: 8.8% take BZs, compared with 4.8% of entire population
Beers (1989)	Elderly general practice patients: 36.5% use BZs
Lyndon (1988)	Intermediate-care facility residents: 24% use BZs
Rodrigo (1988)	41% of patients receive BZs for at least 1 year over 70; median BZ use 5 years
Copeland (1987)	Anxious depression in community dwellers
Whitcup (1987)	Women acute-care inpatients: 18% dependent on BZs
Allen (1986)	Use by 40–50% of nursing home patients, 17% of outpatients
Foy (1986)	Elderly patients admitted to hospital: 50% with positive BZ urine screens
Magni (1986)	Geriatric hospital outpatients: 24% take BZs
Salzman (1979)	General hospital patients: use by 33%
Parry (1973)	Elderly living in community: use by 18%

[a] Complete reference citations at end of chapter.

patient who suffers from medical illness, may be depressed as well as anxious, and makes frequent visits to physicians.[9,27] Some of these patients may take benzodiazepines regularly for many years, following the dose originally prescribed, with no complaint of frequent or troublesome side effects. Indeed, many elderly chronic users of benzodiazepines are scrupulous about their dosing, and, if anything, they reduce their dose slightly over time.[9] Physicians who frequently prescribe benzodiazepines for their elderly patients are often themselves older.[28]

Pharmacokinetics of Benzodiazepines

Compared with other psychotropic drugs, the pharmacokinetics and bioavailability of benzodiazepines in elderly people have been particularly well studied. This knowledge plays a direct role in guiding prescribing practice; salient pharmacokinetic parameters have been reviewed[29] and are discussed below, as well as in Chapter 5, and summarized in Table 16.2.

Absorption

Gastrointestinal absorption of benzodiazepines is only slightly slower in older patients than in younger ones, although food or antacids in the stomach may delay absorption. Peak blood levels and onset of therapeutic effect can be expected anywhere from 45 minutes to 3 hours after the medication is taken.

Anxious elderly patients are usually treated with benzodiazepines orally; intravenous benzodiazepine use is reserved for the treatment of seizures. Intramuscular absorption of benzodiazepines is slow and irregular, and is not recommended.

Protein Binding

Benzodiazepines, like other psychotropic drugs, bind extensively to plasma albumin. In older people with reduced levels of plasma albumin, increased sedation with some benzodiazepines has occurred.

Volume of Distribution

In general, the volume of distribution (Vd) of most benzodiazepines tends to increase with age. For reasons that are not clear, the Vd of alprazolam specifically decreases in elderly men but remains unchanged in elderly women.

Metabolism

As people age, hepatic metabolism slows, prolonging the elimination half-life of long half-life benzodiazepine such as chlordiazepoxide, diazepam, clorazepate, prazepam and their active metabolite is prolonged.

In some cases, the elimination half-life in the elderly is twice as long (e.g., chlordi-

Table 16.2   Pharmacokinetic Studies of Benzodiazepines in the Elderly

Study	Results
Dorling (2001)	Loprazolam can prolong maximum blood level in elderly, but no difference between older and young recipients in elimination half-life; well tolerated by both young and old patients
Kaplan (1998)	Elimination half-life, time of maximum concentration, volume of distribution, and apparent clearance similar for elderly and young; no evidence of increased sensitivity to the pharmacodynamics of alprazolam in elderly
Herman (1996)	Half-life and volume of distribution of diazepam approximately twofold greater than in younger subjects; extensive accumulation of diazepam and its major metabolite, desmethyldiazepam, during chronic administration
Fleishaker (1992)	Like other long half-life BZs, adnazolam and its desmethyl metabolite half-lives prolonged by approximately 40% with reduced clearance
Dehlin (1991)	Mean elimination half-life of alprazolam in elderly: 11 hours
Bandera (1984)	Metabolism of diazepam or pro "nondiazepam-like compounds" prolonged in elderly compared with oxazepam-like compounds
Greenblatt (1983)	Old age associated with impaired capacity to oxidize alprazolam, more significantly in men than women; half-life significantly prolonged and total clearance reduced in elderly vs. young men
Salzman (1983)	Extensive accumulation of diazepam but not oxazepam; sedation prolonged with diazepam
Greenblatt (1979)	Lorazepam: elimination half-life not significantly different in elderly compared with young controls; no gender relationship; IM and oral administration in elderly as in the young leads to rapid and nearly complete absorption into systemic circulation.

azepoxide) or three times longer (e.g., diazepam) than in young adults. Because of delayed elimination, both the prescribed drug and its active metabolite may accumulate, leading to the potential for increased toxicity. Gender also plays a role in benzodiazepine pharmacokinetics. The clearance of alprazolam, for example, a benzodiazepine with an intermediate half-life, is also delayed in the elderly,[30] almost exclusively because the elimination half-life in elderly men is longer than in younger men or in women of any age.[29]

Short half-life benzodiazepines such as lorazepam and oxazepam undergo less complex hepatic metabolism. The primary metabolic pathway of these compounds is glucuronidation, which is not significantly affected by age. Short half-life benzodiazepine anxiolytics reach steady-state plasma levels substantially faster than the long half-life drugs, and elimination is more rapid without significant accumulation. However, triazolam is unique among the short half-life benzodiazepines because it is extensively metabolized by oxidation; thus it and its metabolites may accumulate in older individuals.

Pharmacodynamics of Benzodiazepines

As a group, older patients are more sensitive to the potential toxicity of anxiolytic drugs. Four factors may predispose the older person to this increased toxicity: age, comorbidity, polypharmacy, and noncompliance with prescribed drug-taking schedules. Merely being older than 65, however, does not guarantee a uniformity of drug response: some older people are exquisitely sensitive while others are no more sensitive to benzodiazepine effects than their younger counterparts.

Age

With advancing age and the increased sensitivity of the CNS to the effects of benzodiazepines, older patients are more likely to develop CNS toxicity to anxiolytic doses that are nontoxic in younger adults.

This increased sensitivity to side effects is not related to the half-life of benzodiazepines. However, because long half-life benzodiazepines remain in the body longer because of age-related pharmacokinetic changes, they are likely to produce prolonged side effects.

Increased sensitivity of older people to benzodiazepines is due to age-related alterations in the CNS γ-aminobutyric acid (GABA) receptors where these drugs exert their therapeutic effects (see Chapter 6). No data are available that indicate an age effect on either the number of receptors or the affinity of these receptors for benzodiazepines.[29] Nevertheless, recent studies[31] suggest that the aging CNS is increasingly sensitive to the effects of benzodiazepines. Three factors have been hypothesized for this increased sensitivity: (1) a higher benzodiazepine level in the CNS than in the blood in older people because of increased brain uptake of drug into the aging CNS; (2) a higher plasma benzodiazepine concentration in older people because of altered pharmacokinetics; or (3) a combination of both factors.[29]

Comorbidity

Physical or emotional illness concurrent with anxiety may predispose the older patient to increased anxiolytic drug toxicity. For example, any CNS disorder (stroke, Parkinson's disease, dementia) may increase sensitivity to these drugs. Any disorder that compromises protein binding, hepatic metabolism, or renal clearance may also secondarily increase CNS sensitivity because of altered drug disposition.

Polypharmacy

The third factor that may increase toxicity of anxiolytic drugs in older persons is the interaction with other medications taken concurrently. On average, approximately one-quarter of older persons living in the community take medication regularly, and older patients in a general hospital take an average of eight medications simultaneously.[32] Many of these drugs, especially those with properties affecting the CNS, may exacerbate the CNS side effects of benzodiazepines even at doses that would not be considered harmful in younger adult patients. Benzodiazepine metabolism may be affected by other drugs. Blood levels of benzodiazepine anxiolytics, for example, may increase when they are taken with other medications such as nefazodone or ketaconazole that inhibit the cytochrome P-450 enzyme system (specifically, the 3A4 isoenzyme; see Chapter 5 and Appendix B); their blood levels may drop when taken with other medications that induce this hepatic isoenzyme such as carbamazepine.[33]

Noncompliance

Noncompliance with drug-prescribing schedules is frequent among older patients. Whether a result of forgetfulness, confusion resulting from different medications and dosing schedules, fearfulness, or personal beliefs about medications, older patients commonly take either too much medication or too little as prescribed. In either case, overdosing or underdosing with anxiolytic drugs may lead to toxicity or inadequate treatment of anxiety symptoms. Noncompliance is discussed in greater detail in Chapter 2.

Selection of Benzodiazepines

Comparative studies of clinical efficacy have not revealed any one benzodiazepine as therapeutically superior to any other for treatment of anxiety symptoms. Rational guidelines, therefore, can be formulated for the selection and prescription of an appropriate drug for each individual elderly patient on the basis of the clinical pharmacology of each benzodiazepine in relation to that patient's clinical profile rather than differential efficacy. Since reduced clearance of long half-life benzodiazepines predisposes older individuals to prolonged side-effect risk and they are more susceptible to benzodiazepine side effects, only short half-life benzodiazepines should be used to treat anxious elderly patients whether for acute

or chronic anxiety. (An exception: for treatment of panic disorder, alprazolam or clonazepam are specifically indicated.)

Short and Intermediate Half-Life Benzodiazepines

Three short or intermediate half-life benzodiazepines are currently available for clinical anxiolytic use: oxazepam, lorazepam, and alprazolam. No data are available comparing the anxiolytic effects of these three compounds in older anxious patients. Clinical experience suggests that they are equally therapeutic assuming equivalent doses are given.

Oxazepam. Oxazepam, a metabolite of diazepam and desmethyldiazepam, has no active metabolites of its own, and its metabolism, distribution, and elimination are unaffected by the aging process. In dosages of 10 to 45 mg per day, oxazepam decreases anxiety, tension, irritability, agitation, and insomnia. It is also effective in the treatment of the restless chronically ill older patient as well as the anxious older outpatient. Oxazepam should be given at least three times per day, with a starting dose of 15 mg per day for most elderly patients.

Lorazepam. Lorazepam is a structural analogue of oxazepam but is ten times more potent. Like oxazepam, it has a short half-life (10 to 12 hours) and no active metabolites of its own; its distribution and elimination are not significantly affected by aging. Lorazepam is one of the more commonly prescribed benzodiazepines for older individuals for treatment of acute as well as chronic anxiety states. It also reduces agitation, wandering, and restlessness in elderly demented patients and has been useful in reducing anxiety associated with physical illness in older patients with heart disease or cancer. Lorazepam is also an effective hypnotic, although some elderly patients experience impaired short-term memory after its use; some elderly patients taking lorazepam also experience morning drowsiness. The starting dose for older patients should not exceed 0.5 mg; the suggested therapeutic dosage range is 0.5 to 1.0 mg given two or three times per day.

Alprazolam. A triazolobenzodiazepine with an intermediate half-life (12 to 15 hours) and two active metabolites, alprazolam is extremely potent, with antianxiety properties noted at doses as low as 0.25 mg. In young adults, alprazolam is approximately ten times more potent than diazepam, with 1.5 mg of alprazolam equivalent to 18.6 mg of diazepam. Alprazolam prolongs REM latency (the time between sleep onset and the first REM phase). Because reduced REM latency is associated with major depressive disorder, this alprazolam effect suggests potential antidepressant activity, although no such effects have yet been reported specifically in older patients.

Alprazolam is also used to treat panic disorder, although no studies have examined this therapeutic use in older patients. As noted, the clearance of alprazolam is delayed in elderly patients,[30] almost exclusively because of a prolonged elimination half-life in elderly men, compared with that in younger men or women of any age.[29] The therapeutic anxiolytic dose range for elderly people is 0.25 to 2.0 mg per day given in divided doses.

That short half-life benzodiazepines do not accumulate in the elderly has generally been accepted. However, triazolam, a benzodiazepine used exclusively as a bedtime hypnotic medication, accumulates significantly in elderly patients who receive this drug for the treatment of insomnia (see Chapter 18). Triazolam undergoes oxidative metabolism, which is affected by age, in contrast with lorazepam and oxazepam, which only undergo metabolism via glucuronidation. Although the metabolites are of no clinical significance, some observations[34] suggest that they may accumulate in the elderly after chronic use.[29] Triazolam use has been associated with impaired memory and is no longer prescribed to elderly patients.

Long Half-Life Benzodiazepines

Because of the complex hepatic metabolism and prolonged elimination half-life of long-acting benzodiazepines and their active metabolites, the elderly patient who develops sensitivity to the toxic effects of these drugs may continue to retain clinically significant amounts of active compounds for days to weeks after drug discontinuance. For this reason, long-acting benzodiazepines have a smaller margin of safety than the intermediate and short half-life drugs.

The long-acting drugs, however, have a prescribing advantage. Because of their gradual accumulation and slow elimination, long-acting benzodiazepines can be given on a once-a-day or even every-other-day basis. For the elderly patient who is forgetful or is taking several other medications during the day, each with its own dosage schedule, a once-a-day antianxiety drug may be an advantage. If one dose is missed inadvertently, the clinical effect is not likely to be compromised. On balance, the hazards of prolonged elimination outweigh the benefit of once-a-day dosing so that long half-life benzodiazepines are used less frequently than short half-life compounds for anxious elderly patients.

Chlordiazepoxide. The complex metabolic pathway of chlordiazepoxide creates several active metabolites, primarily desmethylchlordiazepoxide and desmethyldiazepam. Each compound has a relatively long elimination half-life that is further prolonged by the aging process. In older people, therefore, chlordiazepoxide is associated with increased drowsiness, apathy, and ataxia for hours or even days when taken by an older patient. Like other long-acting benzodiazepines, it is an effective antianxiety agent for the elderly but is prescribed infrequently. If used, the recommended dosages are 20 to 40 mg per day, with starting dosages of 5 to 10 mg daily.

Diazepam. Diazepam and one of its active metabolites, desmethyldiazepam, has an elimination half-life in older people of approximately 75 to 100 hours. Like chlordiazepoxide, it is effective in treating anxiety, insomnia, and agitation as well as an increased incidence of sedation in and a prolonged risk of side effects. Once widely prescribed, diazepam is no longer commonly given to elderly anxious patients. Because of its long duration of action, diazepam, if used, should be given to these patients once a day or once every other day. The initial dose is 2 mg; the therapeutic dosage range is 2 to 10 mg per day.

Clonazepam. Clonazepam is a high-potency, long half-life benzodiazepine with strong anticonvulsant properties. It is commonly given to younger adults for the treatment of anxiety, panic, and obsessive-compulsive disorders as well as other psychiatric disorders including mania, psychosis, and severe agitation. Because the aging process prolongs the half-life of this drug (considerably more than 100 hours), side effects may appear days or even weeks after it has been taken, making it undesirable for most older patients. It is also extremely sedating and can cause unsteadiness and falls at therapeutic doses. Should clonazepam be used, the anxiolytic dose range for older patients is 0.25 to 2 mg given once a day or once every other day.

Side Effects of Benzodiazepines

Elderly patients are especially vulnerable to the side effects of benzodiazepines.[35] In addition to dependence on these compounds, four types of side effects are common: sedation and cerebellar toxicity, and psychomotor and cognitive impairment—all of which commonly occur in older patients at doses lower than for young adults.

Sedation

Although sedation may be helpful at bedtime, it can impair the daytime functioning of older persons. Chronically sedated older people may become increasingly confused, belligerent, and agitated. If long-acting agents are taken in the evening, these effects may persist the next morning, producing a hangover and difficulty getting out of bed to begin the day's activities. Because sedation can activate or exacerbate symptoms of dementia, it is not unusual to see mildly forgetful older people become increasingly confused, disoriented, agitated, and forgetful when taking benzodiazepines. The behavioral consequences of severe sedation, which are usually worse at night, can include disinhibited inappropriate social behavior, agitation, and even assaultiveness. The effects are more pronounced in the very aged and in those who are demented, and they are increased by alcohol or any other CNS sedatives. Sedation may contribute to benzodiazepine respiratory depression and sleep apnea, conditions more common in older than younger individuals.

Falls

Benzodiazepine use by elderly patients is strongly associated with an increased risk of falls and hip fractures. Although originally thought to be a side effect limited to short half-life agents,[36] more recent observations suggest that falls and fractures may be associated with all benzodiazepines, regardless of elimination half-life times.[37] In addition to impaired balance and falls, benzodiazepines can cause ataxia, dysarthria, dyscoordination, and unsteadiness in older people, many of whom already have tremor or difficulties with coordination. Dosage is a more significant causative factor than half-life; higher doses are more likely to be associated with falls and unsteadiness than are lower ones (Table 16.3).[38]

Psychomotor Impairment

Benzodiazepine-induced psychomotor impairment in older patients is characterized by slowed reaction time, dimin-

Table 16.3.   Benzodiazepines and Falls in Elderly Patients[a]

Study	Results
Ensrud (2002)	Both long- and short-acting BZs increase risk of falls in elderly women
Frels (2002)	Previous fall, BZ use, and need for maximum assistance significant predictors of falling
Pierfitte (2001)	Hip fracture risk not increased by BZ use in case-controlled study; risk increases with use of 2 or more BZs; only lorazepam significantly associated with increased risk of hip fracture
Tromp (2001)	Previous falls, visual impairment, urinary incontinence, and BZ use strongest predictors of falls
Wang (2001a)	Elderly particularly vulnerable to falls immediately after initiating BZ therapy and after more than 1 month of continuous use; all BZ doses $\geq$3 mg/d; diazepam equivalent significantly increases risk by 50%; shorter half-life drugs no safer than longer half-life agents
Wang (2001b)	Zolpidem associated with nearly twice the risk of hip fracture
Passaro (2000)	BZs with short and very short half-life important risk factor for falls in elderly hospitalized patients
Ray (2000)	Risk of falls in nursing home residents increased by BZs, only slightly less with short half-life drugs; risk greatest in first 7 days of use
Schwab (2000)	40% of community-dwelling or nursing home residents with hip fractures have detectable BZ blood levels
Sgadari (2000)	Risk of femur fracture highest with long half-life drugs, especially in those over 85
Caramel (1998)	Accidental falls more likely in those 85 and older
Neutel (1996)	Risk of falls higher for men than women; history of alcohol abuse very strong risk factor for both
Wysowski (1996)	No increased risk of hip fracture with either short- or ultrashort-acting BZ hypnotics
Gales (1995)	BZ use more common in inpatients who had fallen
Herings (1995)	Increased risk of falls and femur fractures mainly dose-dependent and not associated with elimination half-life
Weintraub (1993)	BZ triplicate prescription policy in NY State not associated with dramatic declines in rate of hip fracture
Trewin (1992)	Only lorazepam associated with significant increase in incidence of falls; women fall more frequently than men
Grisso (1991)	Use of long and short half-life BZs correlates with risk of hip fracture but is not the only cause
Lord (1991a, 1991b)	No increase in risk of falls associated with BZ in elderly care facility (mean age >80)
Myers (1991)	Increased falls associated with sedative-hypnotic drugs (including BZs) only in nursing home elderly patients, not with rehabilitation patients with chronic illness
Ray (1989a)	Increased risk of falls and hip fractures associated with long but not short half-life BZs
Ray (1989b)	Risk of hip fracture increased with long half-life BZs but not short half-life drugs
Sorock (1988a,1988b)	BZ medication alone does not increase risk of accidental falls in elderly survey subjects; mean age 80

(continued)

Table 16.3. *(continued)*

Study	Results
Taggart (1988)	No increased risk of hip fractures in outpatients; mean age 83
Tinetti (1988)	Sample of >75 living at home; increased risk of falling with BZs, phenothiazines, antidepressants, and cardiac medications
Granek (1987)	Increased risk of falls in long-term care facilities associated with BZs and other psychotropic and medical drugs
Wells (1985)	No increased falls associated with antianxiety drugs in elderly residents of long-term care facilities
Sobel (1983)	Sedative-hypnotics increase risk of falling
Prudham (1981)	Increased falls of elderly taking tranquilizers in England

[a] Complete reference citations at end of chapter.

ished speed and accuracy of motoric tasks, and impaired hand-eye coordination. These side effects may become dangerous when the older person drives an automobile, uses a kitchen knife, or operates complicated machinery. Taken as a single dose, sporadically, or in combination with other sedative-hypnotics, benzodiazepines impair automobile driving by interfering with reaction time, judgment, tracking, and hand-eye coordination. Motor vehicle crashes in which one person sustains bodily injury appear to be more likely when the elderly driver has taken a long half-life benzodiazepine; in contrast, no increased risk occurs after initiation of treatment with a short half-life benzodiazepine.[39]

The effects on psychomotor performance of acute administration of benzodiazepines in elderly recipients have also been well observed in research studies.[7] The results of these observations (Table 16.4) may be summarized as follows:

1. Acute administration of a benzodiazepine produces combined decrements in a variety of laboratory measures of psychomotor performance that together suggest slower and less accurate performance.
2. Decrements have been observed with long, intermediate, and short half-life benzodiazepines.
3. Decrements in performance associated with short half-life drugs may be correlated with plasma drug level and associated with dose; at very low therapeutic doses, the decrement may be minimal in recipients under the age of 70.
4. Long half-life drugs administered in the evening may adversely affect performance the following morning; performance decrements with long half-life drugs may not appear until after two weeks of administration.

Despite these four observational generalizations, wide interindividual variation occurs in psychomotor performance following benzodiazepine administration in elderly recipients. Either these drugs do not have specific effects on the various types of behavior tested, or the various experimental procedures used are not sensitive in the elderly to the effects of benzodiazepines.[7] To add to the uncertainty, adequate data are not available to develop generalizations about the effect of long-term benzodiazepine use on measures of psychomotor performance, especially in those over the age of 80.

Cognitive Impairment

As a side effect of benzodiazepines, cognitive impairment is characterized by an-

Table 16.4. Performance Effects of Benzodiazepines (BZs) in Elderly Individuals in Studies with Young Controls

Study[a]	Drug Dose (mg/day)	Results
Paterniti (2002)	Most frequently used benzodiazepines: bromazepam 34.1% lorazepam 31.1% prazepam 10.2% oxazepam 7.2% chlorazepate 5.4%	2-year follow-up study: episodic and recurrent users have modestly lower cognitive scores than nonusers; long-term BZ use has no detectable effect on immediate and delayed verbal recall
Hanlon (1998)	BZs, not specified	Elderly benzodiazepine users at 3-year follow-up: higher number of memory errors than nonusers; short-term use not associated with greater memory impairment
Foy (1995)	BZs, not specified	BZ doses equivalent to 5 mg diazepam decrease cognitive performance
Rummans (1993)	BZs, not specified	Nonanxious geriatric patients dependent on BZs still show decreased memory
Salzman (1992)	Several BZs	Elderly nursing home residents show very significant increase in memory following BZ discontinuation
Hart (1991)	Alprazolam (0.75)	No effect on DSST
Kroboth (1990)	Alprazolam (0.75, 1.5, 4)	All doses decrease DSST
Satzger (1990)	Lorazepam (1)	Drug decreases verbal and visual memory
Pomara (1989)	Diazepam[b] (2.5, 10, at weekly intervals)	Recall unaffected by 2.5 mg; 10 mg decreases recall in young and elderly equally
Sunderland (1989)	Lorazepam (1)	Drug decreases psychomotor performance
Hinrichs (1987)	Diazepam[b] (0.2 mg/kg)	Impairments in attention, recall, and other higher cognitive functions not age-related
Nikaido (1987)	Diazepam (5, 10, 15)	Reaction time decreases with 10 mg; all psychomotor performance decreases with 15 mg
Pomara (1985)	Diazepam[b] (2.5)	Memory and psychomotor impairment in elderly only; increased sedation in elderly
Scharf (1985)	Clorazepate (7.5)	Memory not decreased in nonanxious geriatric subjects
Swift (1985)	Diazepam[b] (10)	Impairment in attention and coordination in both; memory not assessed
Castleden (1982)	Nitrazepam (10)	No psychomotor effects at 11 hours postdrug
Bonnet (1981)	Ketazolam (30)	Next-day balance performance impaired in elderly but not in young
Greenblatt (1981)	Flurazepam (15)	Self-rated sedation increases in young and elderly
Briggs (1980)	Temazepam[b] (20)	Psychomotor impairment: elderly > young

Adapted from Pomara N, Deptula D, Singh R, et al. Cognitive toxicity of benzodiazepines in the elderly. In: Salzman C, Lebowitz BL, eds. *Anxiety in the elderly.* New York: Springer Publishing, 1991:175–190.
[a] Complete citations at end of chapter.
[b] Placebo controlled.
DSST, Digital Symbol Substitution Test.

terograde amnesia, diminished short-term recall, increased forgetfulness, and decreased attention. Such cognitive impairment may resemble the early stages of a dementing illness as well as normal age-related reduction in cognitive function (Table 16.5). Single doses of benzodiazepines or short-term use may be associated with demonstrable reduction in memory and attention.[40,41] Research observations

Table 16.5.   Effect of Benzodiazepines on Cognition in the Elderly

Study	Results
Lagnaoui (2002)	Past BZ use associated with significant increase in risk of dementia although no such association between dementia and current BZ use
Paterniti (2002)	Chronic BZ users have significantly higher risk of cognitive decline on MMSE, DSST, and Trail-Making tests
Vignola (2000)	Elders with insomnia perform worse than good sleepers on attention and concentration measures; unmedicated insomniacs subjectively rated their own performance more negatively than medicated insomniacs and good sleepers
Gray (1999)	BZs, along with opioids, anticholinergics, and TCAs are the most likely of all drug classes to cause cognitive impairment in elderly
Rasmussen (1999)	Postoperative cognitive dysfunction in elderly patients after surgery not explained by BZ concentrations detected in the blood
Hanlon (1998)	Current BZ use, especially in recommended or higher doses, associated with worse memory among community-dwelling elderly
Pomara (1998)	Acute doses significantly impair total recall and increase intrusion errors regardless of dose; only chronic treatment with high dose increases intrusions and self-rated sedation; single-dose rechallenge after chronic treatment associated with significantly less impairment than initial challenge in memory tasks
Ried (1998)	BZ exposure adds significantly to prediction of reduced functional status; associated with the same degree of impairment as several chronic medical conditions
Sumner (1998)	BZs associated with increased amnestic properties in elderly in relation to their already decreasing cognitive function
Bertz (1997)	Psychomotor impairment greater for elderly than for young controls, with digit symbol substitution and card-sorting
Scharf (1985)	Clorazepate: No decreased memory in nonanxious geriatric subjects

suggest that these decrements may be more significant with the use of short half-life, high-potency benzodiazepines such as lorazepam[42,43] than with longer half-life, lower-potency agents.[35]

Some cognitively impaired older patients who take benzodiazepines for long periods of time may actually experience progressive increase in benzodiazepine-induced cognitive impairment. A recent four-year follow-up study of individuals 60 to 70 years old reports lower cognitive performance in those taking benzodiazepines than in nonusers.[44] When benzodiazepines are discontinued in elderly patients, very significant improvement in memory function can be observed.[45,46] These observations suggest that long-term benzodiazepine use may contribute to cognitive impairment in elderly people,

especially in those whose memory may already be impaired. Although this memory impairment may persist into the early drug-free period,[46] its reversibility should reassure those concerned about permanent benzodiazepine-induced cognitive impairments in the elderly. Elderly patients who take benzodiazepines on a regular basis and who experience progressive cognitive impairment should not be assumed to have a dementing illness until the benzodiazepines have been discontinued and cleared.

Although there is wide variability among elderly patients taking benzodiazepines, recall is impaired in a dose-dependent fashion. Clinical observations suggest a greater decrement among the very old and among those already cognitively impaired, and the presence of the apolipoprotein E4 allele (see Chapter 21) may increase vulnerability to acute benzodiazepine-induced cognitive impairment.[21,47]

Respiratory Depression

Benzodiazepines can cause respiratory depression or can exacerbate preexisting respiratory impairment. In elderly patients with chronic obstructive pulmonary disease (COPD), benzodiazepines may worsen respiratory efficiency and contribute to decreased oxygen levels. This side effect is unfortunate since elderly individuals who are struggling to breathe, such as those with COPD, are usually intensely anxious and require some form of anxiolytic treatment. Satisfactory substitutes for benzodiazepine treatment of anxiety associated with respiratory impairment have not yet been found; buspirone has been recommended based on limited clinical and research experience.

Urinary Incontinence

Although less common than impaired cognition, motor skills, or respiratory impairment, elderly individuals who take benzodiazepines are nearly one and a half times more likely to experience urinary incontinence that those who do not take them. Elderly patients who frequently get up at night to urinate may be more likely to fall.[48] Incontinence is more likely with long half-life drugs.

Dependence

Like other sedative/hypnotics, prolonged benzodiazepine use may result in physiological dependence. Rates of developing dependence as well as its intensity correlate with daily dose and duration of treatment. In general, the higher the dose, the shorter the period of treatment necessary to produce dependence. At therapeutic daily doses, clinically significant dependence may develop after several weeks of treatment. The higher the dose, the more intense the dependency. Abrupt benzodiazepine discontinuation in a dependent elderly person leads to a predictable withdrawal syndrome.

Dependence on benzodiazepines taken for legitimate medical reasons, however, does not lead to abuse in patients not otherwise substance abusers.[8,10,20] Additionally, elderly people are not more likely to become dependent on therapeutic doses of benzodiazepines than younger individuals. Nevertheless, concern has been expressed in numerous medical and lay publications about possible overprescription of benzodiazepines to elderly patients and the dependence that ensues.

Prescribing Guidelines for Benzodiazepines

It is clear that benzodiazepines are effective anxiolytic drugs which are associated with potentially significant side effects and development of dependence. Clinicians therefore must consider risk versus benefits of their use. Benzodiazepines are relatively safe, despite their side effects, compared with other drugs that may be used to treat anxiety. However, in order to reduce risks of side effects and dependence, clinicians should strive to use the lowest therapeutically effective doses of benzodiazepines and prescribe for the shortest period of time consistent with good medical practice. Short half-life benzodiazepines are usually recommended for older patients because they do not accumulate in the blood, are rapidly cleared from the circulation, and offer greater dosage flexibility. In the typical clinical situation, multiple daily doses of a short half-life compound are prescribed for a limited period. As sedative-hypnotics, benzodiazepines exacerbate the effects of alcohol, and vice versa, and should be prescribed cautiously with other sedating medications.

Some elderly people may require long-term treatment with benzodiazepines because of the chronicity and/or severity of their anxiety symptoms. Older people with chronic physical illness, pain, and secondary depressions who are anxious and have trouble sleeping often benefit from long-term benzodiazepine use without unusual toxicity. Clinical experience suggests that these patients typically are scrupulous about adhering to their prescribed dosage, rarely take their medications without medical supervision, and do not typically take additional medications without medical approval. Long-term elderly users will become dependent on their benzodiazepine medication and are at risk for withdrawal symptoms only if discontinuation is abrupt.

Short half-life benzodiazepines are likely to be associated with a clinically significant discontinuance compared with long half-life drugs, especially when the drugs are abruptly discontinued after prolonged therapeutic use. Discontinuance symptoms usually include a marked ''rebound'' increase in anxiety, insomnia, and physical restlessness; flu-like symptoms, unsteadiness and perceptual distortions may also occur. For some older patients, these rebound discontinuance symptoms are so uncomfortable that patients who experience them are reluctant to give up their use of benzodiazepines. All chronic benzodiazepine treatment should be closely supervised; large renewable prescriptions should be avoided, and frequent mental status examinations should be performed to assess whether the benzodiazepine use is associated with progressive cognitive impairment. Benzodiazepines may exacerbate confusion, disorientation, and agitation, and should not be given to elderly patients who are severely demented or confused.

Treatment with Nonbenzodiazepine Anxiolytics

Several classes of drugs other than the benzodiazepines are also used to treat the symptoms or subjective experience of anxiety in older patients, although they have been used less frequently and with less predictable response. These include buspirone, β-blockers, antidepressants, and neuroleptics. Meprobamate is also still used by some elderly patients.

Barbiturates and Meprobamate

Since the early decades of this century, barbiturates (such as phenobarbital) and since the mid-1950s, propanediol tranquilizers (such as meprobamate) have been widely used to treat patients with anxiety. Some older patients may still be taking these medications and find them effective antianxiety agents. In one survey, 1.3% of older people with an average age of 81 took meprobamate regularly for treatment of anxiety, and some had taken this drug regularly for more than 25 years.[49]

Barbiturates and propanediols are potentially hazardous for older people. They may produce psychological dependence and withdrawal seizures, can be lethal in overdose, and increase the hepatic metabolism of other drugs. Sensitivity to the sedating and disorienting properties of these drugs increases with age causing confusion, disorientation, and agitation. The drugs may be particularly toxic in the evening and may contribute to, cause, or exacerbate preexisting nighttime confusion and agitation. For these reasons, barbiturates and propanediols are no longer recommended and should not be used as part of the treatment of anxiety in the elderly.

Buspirone

Buspirone, an anxiolytic drug with serotonergic properties, differs from benzodiazepines in its effect on the central nervous system. Lacking sedative properties and a potential to induce a state of drug dependency, it has been recommended for the elderly. Studies of its effect on cognitive performance also suggest that, unlike benzodiazepines, buspirone does not affect reaction time, vigilance, psychomotor speed, or memory function.[50] Unfortunately only five studies document the efficacy of buspirone in anxious elderly patients (Table 16.6). These investigations demonstrate therapeutic equivalence of this drug with the benzodiazepines with less sedation. However, because clinical experience with buspir-

Table 16.6.   Studies of Buspirone Use in Elderly Patients

Studies[a]	N	Age	Dose (mg/day)	Results
Hart (1991)	60	68.5	15	No adverse effect on cognitive performance in normal elderly; 80% of octogenarians improved; mild and infrequent side effects
Levine (1989)	41	80+	15	
Robinson (1988)	605	70.8	15	Up to 65% reduction in HAM-A by 4 weeks; 41% experience side effects: dizziness, GI upset, sleeplessness, headache, vomiting
Singh (1988)	12	66–75	5–30	Average therapeutic dose 20 mg (dose-finding study); no muscle-relaxant properties; marked improvement in anxiety, loss of tension
Napoliello (1986)	677 outpatients	60–66	20	Effective anxiolytic; 10% worsened; predominant side effects: dizziness, headache, sleep disturbance, GI upset

[a] Complete reference citations at end of chapter.

one in the elderly anxious patients remains relatively scant, recommendations regarding indications or contraindications for its use continue to be tentative.

The onset of buspirone's antianxiety effect may be delayed by several weeks, limiting its usefulness for acute states of anxiety where immediate anxiolytic effect is necessary. However, buspirone may be preferred for the anxious elderly individual who has a history of present or past alcohol abuse for whom benzodiazepines would be contraindicated. Buspirone, unlike the benzodiazepines, does not interfere with respiratory function and may be preferred for treatment of the anxious elderly patient with respiratory impairment. Buspirone has also been reported as effective in controlling severe agitation and disruptive behavior and dementia (see Chapter 20); one case of tardive dyskinesia has been reported.[51]

β-Blockers

Information on the effects of β-blockers for the treatment of anxiety comes from their use in younger anxious patients, in mentally retarded patients, or in elderly patients with serious neurological dysfunction. As with younger patients, therapeutic doses of β-blockers in older patients may substantially improve disruptive behavior, but no clinical trials have been conducted to evaluate their use in anxious elderly outpatients who are otherwise free of neurological, emotional, or physical disease. The effect of β-blockers in reducing autonomic anxiety symptoms (e.g., sweating, tachycardia, palpitations) in young patients also suggests their use with older patients, but no research data or even clinical reports are available on their use for the control of such symptoms in anxious elderly.

Antidepressants

Antidepressants have been reported effective in treating generalized anxiety disorder in young adult outpatients and have demonstrated efficacy in the control of other anxiety spectrum disorders as well. As with β-blockers, however, research data or published clinical experience using either tricyclic antidepressants (TCAs) or monoamine oxidase inhibitors to treat anxiety in the elderly is limited. No data suggest that these antidepressants are especially useful for elderly anxious patients or more useful than a benzodiazepine. Owing to their anticholinergic properties, TCAs can impair cognitive function, and older patients may be more susceptible to this toxic effect because of age-related reductions in CNS acetylcholine (see Chapter 4).

Prescribing patterns for the treatment of GAD in young and middle-aged adults are beginning to shift from benzodiazepines toward increased use of selective serotonin reuptake inhibitors (SSRIs) and other newer antidepressants.[52,53] Emerging evidence also suggests that SSRIs and other newer antidepressants may have anxiolytic properties useful in treating GAD in older individuals,[23,54–57] although the shift away from benzodiazepines may not be as pronounced as in younger adults.[25,26] Since anxiety and depression are commonly experienced together in older patients,[58] increased use of the newer antidepressants is not surprising, especially since benzodiazepines may produce unwanted side effects in the elderly. Although the therapeutic efficacy of these antidepressants may not be as strong or as reliable as the benzodiazepines and response time may vary,[21] even mild symptoms of depression accompanying anxiety may predict a more favorable response of GAD to an antidepressant than to a benzodiazepine.[55] Venlafaxine, a norepinephrine and serotonin reuptake inhibitor, has also been reported to reduce modestly the "core" symptoms of GAD in two-thirds of recipients.[59–61]

Antihistamines

Antihistamines such as diphenhydramine or anxiolytics with antihistaminic properties such as hydroxyzine are sometimes taken for short-term management of acute anxiety. They are nonspecifically sedating, however, and may cause confusion, disorientation, and oversedation. When taken with drugs that have anticholinergic properties such as antidepressants or neuroleptics, they may cause severe agitation, confusion, and delirium. Currently no support exists for the long-term use of these drugs to treat GAD.

Neuroleptics

The therapeutic usefulness of neuroleptics for the treatment of subjective anxiety states, especially in the elderly, has never been demonstrated in controlled trials. However, because neuroleptics are effective for the treatment of severe agitation in elderly patients (see Chapter 7) some clinicians have observed effective anxiolytic effect from very low doses of atypical neuroleptics. Given the potential toxicity of neuroleptics (extrapyramidal movements, anticholinergic reactions, sedation), these compounds should be given to elderly patients with caution.

Anxiety Spectrum Disorders

The pharmacologic treatment of extreme anxiety states—panic and social anxiety disorder, phobias, obsessive-compulsive disorder, and posttraumatic stress disorder—focuses on benzodiazepines and antidepressants.

Panic and Phobic Disorders

Alprazolam and clonazepam are therapeutic for elderly patients with panic and phobic disorders. Both drugs block acute panic symptoms, thereby facilitating reduced phobic avoidance behavior. Anticipatory anxiety and the comorbid GAD that frequently accompany late-life panic and phobias are also sometimes relieved by their use, although other benzodiazepines are effective as well. The use of alprazolam or clonazepam for the older or very old patient with panic disorder has not been described in the literature, and no research studies currently guide the clinician in the use of these drugs.

General strategies and cautions that pertain to benzodiazepine use for anxiety disorders apply as well to their use for panic and phobic anxiety states. However, because higher benzodiazepine doses are usually required to treat these states effectively, the older patient treated with alprazolam or clonazepam is likely to experience considerable toxicity, which limits the therapeutic usefulness of these drugs.

SSRIs and other newer antidepressants are now considered the "first-line" treatment for young and middle-aged adults with panic or phobic disorders[62] and are commonly used to treat these disorders. However, neither studies nor published clinical experience currently guide the clinician who wishes to use these antidepressants for elderly patients with panic or phobic disorders. Although their use may be associated with fewer cognitive side effects or development of dependence than occurs with benzodiazepines, falls and drug interactions may be an increased risk for older patients (see Chapter 12). Cautious use is recommended.

Social Anxiety Disorder

This anxiety spectrum disorder is common in young and middle-aged adults but is rarely described in older people. Nonetheless, many older people are afraid to leave their homes, especially in bad weather, if they are frail, live in dangerous urban neighborhoods, or are isolated in a rural environment when unable to drive. In younger populations, SSRIs in particular and newer antidepressants in general are effective in the treatment of this potentially disabling syndrome. However, at this time, no research studies or published clinical reports can guide the clinician in treating elderly patients with symptoms of social anxiety disorder. The anxiety associated with these circumstances may be treated with judicious use of benzodiazepines or with antidepressants if the disorder is accompanied by depressive symptoms.

Obsessive-Compulsive Disorder

Several placebo-controlled studies demonstrate the effectiveness of the serotonergic TCA clomipramine[63–65] and the SSRIs fluoxetine, sertraline, and fluvoxamine[66–68] in alleviating symptoms of obsessive-compulsive disorder (OCD) in a relatively younger adult population. Case studies indicate that older persons with OCD can benefit from the same pharmacologic treatments found to be effective in younger patients.[54,69,70] In practice, because of the rather undesirable side-effect profile of clomipramine in the elderly (resulting from the blockade of muscarinic, histaminic, and α-adrenergic receptors), SSRIs are preferable first-choice antidepressants for this disorder.

As with other anxiety spectrum disorders, no research studies or published clinical descriptions for using these drugs in older patients are available. However, because of increased CNS sensitivity to the toxic effects of these drugs as well as altered pharmacokinetics in the older patient, side effects and drug interactions are more common (see Chapters 4 and 5). A trial of at least 10 to 12 weeks of a particular SSRI is indicated before one can deem it a failure and consider alternative strategies. For patients who do not respond to such a trial, switching to another SSRI, or addition of buspirone or clonazepam, may be considered.

Posttraumatic Stress Disorder

Although posttraumatic stress disorder (PTSD) can be a chronic disorder continuing into old age,[62] no research data or clinical guidelines for its treatment for the elderly are currently available. Pharmacologic management in younger and middle-aged adults is complicated, often requiring multiple medications. In general, antidepressants, especially the SSRIs, are at the center of any polypharmacy treatment program—a generalization that cannot be uniformly applied to older patients because of increased risk of drug interactions. Other medications that have been used to treat PTSD in younger age groups include β-blockers, anticonvulsants, and clonodine. Symptomatic antianxiety treatment with benzodiazepines may be helpful, although side effects and dependency are likely with long-term use.

Lacking data to guide the clinician in treating late-life PTSD, the following guidelines are suggested:

- All elderly patients with PTSD should have a medical screening evaluation.
- Pharmacotherapy should be considered part of a routine program that includes other forms of therapy. Older people require more time than their younger counterparts to work through a traumatic event.[71] Previous trauma may also impair the ability of the elderly to cope with late-life stress.[72] In general, psychopharmacologic treatment of elderly patients with PTSD is only modestly successful. The more severe the disorder, the lower the likelihood of response to medication.[73,74]

CLINICAL VIGNETTES

Case 16.1

Mr. A., a 69-year-old gentleman who sought psychiatric treatment for depression, had recently begun to notice increasingly impaired concentration at his office job and forgetfulness at home. His wife noted a significant decline in his usual jovial good spirits, with concomitant increased lethargy and decreased interest in social interactions. At home on evenings and weekends, Mr A. sat in his easy chair reading the newspapers or watching television—a change from his usual highly energetic pursuit of hobbies and interests. Most of his complaints focused on his apparent forgetfulness and a sense of hopelessness about being able to continue to work. Although he admitted to being sad, he did not have disturbed sleep or appetite or diminished physical energy. Mr. A. rarely drank alcohol and never took other sedative/hypnotic drugs. During his initial consultations, he was able to smile and joke and denied a sense of worthlessness, helplessness, or suicidality. He was fidgety and apprehensive.

After several office visits, a diagnosis of depression was made; there was no evidence of a dementing illness. Several antidepressants were tried, but each produced significant side effects, and each seemed to make Mr. A. feel more restless and apprehensive. He began to

experience difficulty falling asleep. Alprazolam 0.5 mg was added at bedtime and brought dramatic relief to his insomnia. Antidepressants were discontinued, and alprazolam 0.25 mg was started on a b.i.d. schedule in addition to his nighttime dose. Over the next several weeks, Mr. A.'s apprehension declined substantially. He was calmer at home and at work and gradually noticed that his concentration increased. His wife commented that his spirits were improving as well.

Mr. A. continued to use alprazolam at the same doses for several years with no dose escalation. He did not report a worsening of his memory or concentration.

Alprazolam was a helpful drug for Mr. A., and his response suggests that his symptoms, although initially considered depressive, were actually more likely to have been anxious. This confusion in diagnosis between anxiety and depression, or a mixture of the two classes of symptoms, is common in the elderly. Lacking specific discriminating diagnostic criteria or laboratory tests to distinguish between anxiety and depression, clinicians commonly select one of the diagnoses on the basis of the clinical evidence at hand and begin an empirical treatment trial. In Mr. A.'s case, the selection was incorrect: the antidepressants actually worsened his condition.

Mr. A. also illustrates the effect of anxiety on cognitive function, especially concentration and recall. Like depression, anxiety may produce a decrement in these functions, and in elderly patients, the impairment may be considered evidence of an emerging dementia. Such worries, of course, only worsen the anxiety. Despite the ability of benzodiazepines to impair concentration and recall, the results of Mr. A.'s treatment illustrate the opposite effect: reduced clinical anxiety resulted in improved cognitive function. It must be emphasized, however, that the doses of benzodiazepine prescribed in this case were low, and Mr. A. did not use other sedative/hypnotic agents. Consequently, he was an ideal older candidate for benzodiazepine treatment. Many older patients like Mr. A. can also benefit from benzodiazepines without serious side effects.

Mr A. and his psychiatrist elected to continue alprazolam treatment on a maintenance basis even though his symptoms had subsided. This decision was reached jointly (with his wife's concurrence) because of the nearly incapacitating severity of his prior anxiety. Since he was not likely to abuse or misuse the benzodiazepine, the ongoing treatment appeared to carry little risk. Mr A. and his wife, however, were informed of the physical dependence on alprazolam that had developed during the course of treatment and were warned never to discontinue the medication abruptly. Mr. A.'s physician was also informed of the chronic benzodiazepine treatment and concurred with the decision.

Mr. A. did not appear concerned about his dependence on a medication. He was prepared to take alprazolam for the rest of his life if it prevented a return of anxiety, and its use was not associated with significant side effects. He agreed to see his prescribing clinician frequently for assessment of his cognitive function, with a plan of very gradual dose reduction as he continued to age.

Case 16.2

In the course of a research study conducted in a nursing home, elderly residents who had been taking benzodiazepines on a chronic basis were asked to volunteer for a study of benzodiazepine discontinuation. Thirteen volunteered, and with their physicians' and families' permission, benzodiazepine medication was gradually discontinued. Memory testing conducted several weeks after benzodiazepine use had been completely discontinued revealed a dramatic improvement in memory (1) relative to functioning measured while on benzodiazepines and (2) compared with that of a group of residents in the same nursing home who continued chronic benzodiazepine use.

Subsequently, the investigator lunched with the subjects who had discontinued the medication to review their experience, and asked members of the group, "Aren't you glad you've discontinued the medication that was interfering with your memory function?" The answer was uniformly, "No." Somewhat surprised by this response, he embarked on a lively discussion with these research subjects, all of whom were quite articulate about their experience. In essence, they acknowledged that their memory had improved following benzodiazepine discontinuation, but the improvement was not significant or relevant to their daily functioning. As one resident wryly noted, "What's to remember?" When subjects were asked about taking benzodiazepines and feeling calm in the daytime or sleeping well at night versus not taking them and having intact memory but being anxious or having trouble sleeping, they unanimously chose the former—the benzodiazepines. Because the use of these medications did not impair long-term memory, the nursing home residents deemed the sacrifice of short-term recall considerably less important than the therapeutic advantage of reduced anxiety and improved nighttime sleep.

The results of this informal post-study discussion suggests that although chronic therapeutic benzodiazepine use in elderly patients interferes with memory function, usage may be experienced as helpful by the recipients themselves. These observations have been supported in some surveys of long-term benzodiazepine use by elderly patients. The discussion also highlights the importance of asking the older patient how the medication affects his or her life, rather than assuming that side effects are an indication for drug discontinuation.

The investigator learned more than was expected from this discontinuation study. Had only the data been examined, the conclusion would have strongly suggested that benzodiazepines interfere with memory and that the return of memory following discontinuation supports the current concern about overuse of medication in this population. Only after asking the subjects themselves did a fuller picture of usefulness versus toxicity of these drugs emerge.

Case 16.3

Mrs. B., a mentally alert 78-year-old widow living in her apartment in good physical health except for diabetes mellitus, was observed by family members to be gradually more forgetful and confused, particularly in the evening. At times she was unsure of the day of the week, and she occasionally forgot whether she had eaten dinner. The family also noticed that Mrs. B., who was generally good-natured and cheerful, was having occasional periods of irritability and anger. She seemed unaware of her emotional and behavioral changes and was unwilling to participate in family discussions about her altered functioning. Because no changes in physical health were apparent, her children assumed that their mother was now becoming progressively demented, and they began to consider nursing home placement. As part of these discussions they sought psychiatric consultation.

Careful history-taking revealed that the patient had experienced brief periods of anxiety 5 years earlier, when her husband died. Around the time of consultation she had sold her house and moved into an apartment. During the anxiety-filled period 5 years earlier, diazepam (5 mg two times a day) had been prescribed to alleviate acute stress, and the patient revealed that she had continued to take the diazepam intermittently from that time on. During the preceding 3 months, in fact, she had taken it regularly. She admitted that at times she could not remember whether or not she had taken one of the pills, so she took another.

Diazepam was discontinued, and approximately 2 weeks later, Mrs. B.'s evening behavior began to improve. She no longer seemed confused or forgetful, and her irritability vanished almost entirely.

This case illustrates several important clinical points. First, older patients may take medications that the family and physician do not know about. Second, among the side effects of benzodiazepines in the elderly are confusion, irritability, and memory loss. Third, these side effects are often worse in the evening. Fourth, a dose of benzodiazepine that may have been well tolerated when prescribed may become toxic as the patient grows older.

Case 16.4

Mr. C., a 68-year-old man in good physical health, was admitted to the psychiatric unit of a general hospital because of depressive symptoms. Although he had sustained several episodes of depression when very young, he had remained symptom-free until his retirement. Upon retiring, he sold a flourishing business for a price that he later considered to be unfairly low. He subsequently became depressed, self-critical, and doubtful of his own abilities.

The patient was started on antidepressant medication at low dosages, but he rapidly became agitated. Alprazolam, 0.5 mg four times a day, was added to the antidepressant treatment in an attempt to diminish his agitation. Three days after treatment with alprazolam was started, Mr. C. became extremely confused, forgetful, and aggressive. Careful neurological examination, including a computerized tomography scan, failed to disclose any neurological cause for this sudden change in behavior. Alprazolam was discontinued, and within a week the patient's confusion vanished.

This case illustrates the potential for dementia-like side effects of benzodiazepines when these drugs are prescribed for elderly patients. It is not clear why these symptoms emerged in this particular man, as the dosage prescribed was within the usual range for geriatric patients. Nevertheless, the case illustrates the necessity of considering benzodiazepine toxicity whenever an older patient who is taking these drugs has a sudden unexplained change in behavior.

Case 16.5

A 71-year-old woman who had retired from high school teaching 6 years prior to consultation, Mrs. D. led an active life with her husband and was involved in a number of creative writing projects. She and her husband were also active in the local senior citizens' society and were leaders in political efforts to increase state legislative funding for older people. Although generally physically healthy, Mrs. D. suffered from chronic asthma and from intermittent lower back pain. Her asthma was controlled with bronchodilator inhalation (epinephrine) and occasional oral theophylline. However, this medication made her feel anxious and occasionally agitated and sometimes interfered with her sleep. At times she would also experience lower back pains, making participation in some of her activities very difficult. She noted that her asthma medication sometimes exacerbated her lower back pain; at other times, however, no connection between treatment of one problem and her symptoms of the other was apparent.

Mrs. D.'s local physician prescribed oxazepam, 15 mg four times daily, and she found this treatment extremely helpful in several ways. First, it alleviated the stimulation and agitation caused by her asthma medication. Second, it helped diminish her lower back pain, although it did not abolish the discomfort. Third, it helped her fall asleep easily, and she remarked that she slept better when taking the medication than she had in several years. Fourth, in retrospect, Mrs. D. noted that she probably had been anxious, although she was unaware of the symptoms. Oxazepam treatment caused dramatic and sustained relief from the anxiety. She did not experience side effects from this dosage, although occasionally she reported some morning drowsiness.

This case illustrates the positive effects of benzodiazepines when used to treat anxiety produced by other medications. It also demonstrates the usefulness and the relative lack of side effects of a short-acting benzodiazepine for older patients. Finally, this case highlights the important fact that some older people may be unaware of emotional distress.

References

1. McCarthy PR, Katz IR, Foa EB. Cognitive behavioral treatment of anxiety in the elderly: a proposed model. In: Salzman C, Lebowitz BD, eds. *Anxiety in the elderly.* New York: Springer Publishing, 1991:197–214.
2. Salzman C. Pharmacologic treatment of the anxious elderly patient. In: Salzman C, Lebowitz BD, eds. *Anxiety in the elderly.* New York: Springer Publishing, 1991:149–174.

3. Griffiths RR. Commentary on review by Woods and Winger. Benzodiazepines: long-term use among patients is a concern and abuse among polydrug abusers is not trivial. *Psychopharmacology* 1995;118:116–117.

4. Lader M. Commentary on review by Woods and Winger. Current benzodiazepine issues. *Psychopharmacology* 1995;118:118.

5. Lader M, Morton S. Benzodiazepine problems. *Br J Addict* 1991;86:823–828.

6. Tyrer P. Current problems with the benzodiazepines. In: Wheatley D. *The Anxiolytic Jungle: Where Next?* Chichester, England: Wiley and Sons, 1990:24–36.

7. Woods JH, Winger G. Current benzodiazepine issues. *Psychopharmacology* 1995;118:107–115.

8. Woods J, Winger G. Rebuttal of comments by Griffiths, Lader, and Greenblatt to review by Woods and Winger. *Psychopharmacology* 1995; 118:120–121.

9. American Psychiatric Association Task Force Report. *Benzodiazepine dependence, toxicity, and abuse.* Washington, DC: American Psychiatric Press, 1990.

10. Salzman C. The benzodiazepine controversy: therapeutic effects versus dependence, withdrawal, and toxicity. *Harvard Rev Psychiatry* 1997; 4:279–282.

11. Lader RI, Greenblatt DJ, Balter MB. Appropriate use and regulatory control of benzodiazepines. *J Clin Pharmacol* 1991;31:781–784.

12. Zisselman MH, Rovner BW, Shmuely Y. Benzodiazepine use in the elderly prior to psychiatric hospitalization. *Psychosomatics* 1996;37:38–42.

13. Avorn J, Soumerai SB, Everitt DE, et al. A randomized trial of a program to reduce the use of psychoactive drugs in nursing homes. *N Engl J Med* 1992;327:168–173.

14. Health Care Financing Administration. The state operations manual (transmittal no. 250). Washington, DC: Health Care Financing Administration, 1992.

15. McNutt L-A, Boles FB, McAuliffe T, et al. Impact of regulation benzodiazepine prescribing to a low income elderly population, New York State. *J Clin Epidemiol* 1994;47:613–625.

16. Gilbert A, Quinttrell LN, Owen N. Use of benzodiazepines among residents of aged-care accommodation. *Community Health Stud* 1988;12: 394–399.

17. Salem-Schatz SR, Fields D. A randomized trial of a program to reduce the use of psychoactive drugs in nursing homes. *N Engl J Med* 1992;327: 168–173.

18. Larson DB, Lyons JS, Hohmann AA, et al. Psychotropics prescribed to the U.S. elderly in the early and mid-1980s: prescribing patterns of primary care practitioners, psychiatrists and other physicians. *Int J Geriatr Psychiatry* 1991;6:63–70.

19. Monette J, Tamblyn RM, McLeod MJ, et al. Do medical education and practice characteristics predict inappropriate prescribing of sedative-hypnotics for the elderly? *Acad Med* 1994;69(Oct suppl):S10–S12.

20. Woods JH, Katz JL, Winger G. Abuse liability of benzodiazepines. *Pharmacology* 1987;39:251–419.

21. Doraiswamy PM. Contemporary management of

22. comorbid anxiety and depression in geriatric patients. *J Clin Psychiatry* 2001;62(suppl 12):30–35.

22. Egan M. Moride Y, Wolfson C, et al. Long-term continuous use of benzodiazepines by older adults in Quebec: prevalence, incidence, and risk factors. *J Am Geriatr Soc* 2000;48:811–816.

23. Pinsker H, Suljaga-Petchel K. Use of benzodiazepines in primary-care geriatric patients. *J Am Geriatr Soc* 1984;32:595–598.

24. King MB, Gabe J, Williams P, et al. Long term use of benzodiazepines: the views of patients [see comments]. *Br J Gen Pract* 1990;40:194–196.

25. Manela M, Katona C, Livingston G. How common are the anxiety disorders in old age? *Int J Geriatr Psychiatry* 1996;11:65–70.

26. Copeland JRM, Davidson IA, Dewey ME. The prevalence and outcome of anxious depression in elderly people aged 65 and over living in the community. In: Racagni G, Smeraldi E, eds. *Anxious depression: assessment and treatment.* New York: Raven Press, 1987:43–47.

27. Llorente MD, David D, Golden AG, et al. Defining patterns of benzodiazepine use in older adults. *J Geriatr Psychiatry Neurol* 2000;13:150–160.

28. Monette J, Tamblyn RM, McLeod PJ, et al. Characteristics of physicians who frequently prescribe long-acting benzodiazepines for the elderly. *Eval Health Prof* 1997;20:115–130.

29. Greenblatt DJ, Shader RI. Benzodiazepines in the elderly: pharmacokinetics and drug sensitivity. In: Salzman C, Lebowitz BD, eds. *Anxiety in the elderly.* New York: Springer Publishing, 1991: 131–139.

30. Kroboth PD, Mcauley JW, Smith RB. Alprazolam in the elderly: pharmacokinetics and pharmacodynamics during multiple doses. *Psychopharmacology* 1990;100:477–484.

31. Greenblatt DJ, Harmartz JS, Shapiro L, et al. Sensitivity to triazolam in the elderly. *N Engl J Med* 1991;324:1691–1698.

32. Salzman C, van der Kolk BA. Psychotropic drugs and polypharmacy in elderly patients in a general hospital. *J Geriatr Psychiatry* 1979;12:167–176.

33. Watsky E, Salzman C. Psychotropic drug interactions. *Hosp Community Psychiatry* 1991; 42: 247–256.

34. Kanba S, Miyaoka H, Terada H, et al. Triazolam accumulation in the elderly after prolonged use [Letter to the editor]. *Am J Psychiatry* 1991;148: 1264–1265.

35. Mendelson WB. Medications in the treatment of sleep disorders. In: Meltzer HY, ed. *Psychopharmacology: the third generation of progress.* New York: Raven Press, 1987:1305–1311.

36. Ray WA, Griffin MR, Schaffner W, et al. Psychotropic drug use and the risk of hip fracture. *N Engl J Med* 1987;316:363–369.

37. Ray WA, Griffin MR, Downey M. Benzodiazepines of long- and short-elimination half-life and the risk of hip fracture. *JAMA* 1989;262: 3303–3307.

38. Herings RMC, Stricker BHC, de Boer A, et al. Benzodiazepines and the risk of falling leading to femur fractures. *Arch Intern Med* 1995;155: 1801–1807.

39. Hemmelgard B, Suisse S, Huang, et al. Benzodi-

azepine use and the risk of motor vehicle crash in the elderly. *JAMA* 1997;278:27–31.

40. Foy A, O'Connell D, Henry D, et al. Benzodiazepine use as a cause of cognitive impairment in elderly hospital inpatients. *J Gerontol* 1995;50A: M99–M106.

41. Foy A, Drinkwater V, March S, et al. Confusion after admission to hospital in elderly patients using benzodiazepines. *Br Med J* 1986;293:1072.

42. Satzger W, Engel RR, Ferguson E, et al. Effects of single doses of alpidem, lorazepam, and placebo in memory and attention in healthy young and elderly volunteers. *Pharmacopsychiatry* 1990; 23(suppl):114–119.

43. Scharf MB, Hirschowitz J, Woods M, et al. Lack of amnestic effects of clorazepate on geriatric recall. *J Clin Psychiatry* 1985;46:518–520.

44. Paterniti S, Dufouil C, and Alpérovitch A. Long-term benzodiazepine use and cognitive decline in the elderly: the epidemiology of vascular aging study. *J Clin Psychopharmacol* 2002;22: 285–293.

45. Salzman C, Fisher J, Nobel K, et al. Cognitive improvement following benzodiazepine discontinuation in elderly nursing home residents. *Int J Geriatr Psychiatry* 1992;7:89–93.

46. Rummans TA, Davis LJ, Morese RM, et al. Learning and memory impairment in older, detoxified, benzodiazepine-dependent patients. *Mayo Clin Proc* 1993;68:731–737.

47. Pomara N, Tun H, Deptua D, et al. ApoE-allele and susceptibility to drug-induced memory impairment in the elderly [letter]. *J Clin Psychopharmacol* 1998;18:179–181.

48. Landi F, Cesari M, Russo A, et al. Benzodiazepines and the risk of urinary incontinence in frail older persons living in the community. *Clin Pharmacol Ther* 2002;72:729–734.

49. Hale WE, May FE, Moore MT, et al. Meprobamate use in the elderly. *J Am Geriatr Soc* 1998;36: 1003–1005.

50. Hart RP, Colenda CC, Hamer RM. Effects of buspirone and alprazolam on the cognitive performance of normal elderly subjects. *Am J Psychiatry* 1991;148:73–77.

51. Strauss A. Oral dyskinesia associated with buspirone use in an elderly person. *J Clin Psychiatry* 1988;49:322–323.

52. Feighner JP. Overview of antidepressants currently used to treat anxiety disorders. *J Clin Psychiatry* 1999;60(suppl22):18–22.

53. Salzman C, Goldenberg I, Bruce SE, and Keller MB. Pharmacologic treatment of anxiety disorders in 1989 versus 1996: Results from the Harvard/Brown Anxiety Disorders Research Program. *J Clin Psychiatry* 2001;62:149–152.

54. Flint AJ. Management of anxiety in late life. *J Geriatric Psychiatry and Neurol* 1998;11:194–200.

55. Rickels K, Downing R, Schweizer E, et al. Antidepressants for the treatment of generalized anxiety disorder. A placebo–controlled comparison of imipramine, trazodone, and diazepam. *Arch Gen Psychiatry* 1993;50:884–895.

56. Khan RJ, McNair DM, Lipman RS, et al. Imipramine and chlordiazepoxide in depressive and anxiety disorders, II: efficacy in anxious outpatients. *Arch Gen Psychiatry* 1986;43:79–85.

57. Hoehn–Saric R, McLeod DR, Zimmerli WD. Differential effects of alprazolam and imipramine in generalized anxiety disorder: somatic versus psychic symptoms. *J Clin Psychiatry* 1988;49: 293–301.

58. Lenze EJ, Mulsant BH, Shear MK, et al. Comorbid anxiety disorders in depressed elderly patients. *Am J Psychiatry* 2000;157:722–728.

59. Ballenger JC. Clinical guidelines for establishing remission in patients with depression and anxiety. *J Clin Psychiatry* 1999(suppl 22):29–34.

60. Katz IR, Alexopoulos G, Reynolds CF, et al. Venlafaxine XR in late life GAD: pooled analysis of five randomized clinical trials. In: Proceedings of the 14th annual meeting of the American Association for Geriatric Psychiatry; Feb 24–27, 2001; San Francisco, Calif. Poster SUQ33:117.

61. Samuelian JC, Hackett D. A randomized, double-blind, parallel-group comparison of venlafaxine and clomipramine in outpatients with major depression. *Int J Geriatr Psychopharmacol* 2000;2:83–85.

62. Sheik JI, Cassidy EL. Treatment of anxiety disorders in the elderly: issues and strategies. *J Anxiety Disord* 2000;14:173–190.

63. Insel TR, Murphy DDL, Cohen RM, et al. Obsessive-compulsive disorder: a double-blind trial of clomipramine and clorgyline. *Arch Gen Psychiatry* 1983;40:605–612.

64. Thoren P, Asberg M, Cronholm B, et al. Clomipramine treatment of obsessive-compulsive disorder: I. A controlled clinical trial. *Arch Gen Psychiatry* 1980;37:1281–1285.

65. Volvaka J, Neziroglu F, Yaryura-Tobias JA. Clomipramine and imipramine in obsessive-compulsive disorder. *Psychiatry Res* 1985;14:85–93.

66. Chouinard G, Goodman W, Greist J, et al. Results of a double-blind placebo controlled trial of a new serotonin uptake inhibitor, sertraline, in the treatment of obsessive-compulsive disorder. *Psychopharmacol Bull* 1990;26:279–284.

67. Greist J, Chouinard G, DuBoff E, et al. Double-blind comparison of three doses of sertraline and placebo in the treatment of outpatients with obsessive–compulsive disorder. Poster presented at the Collegium Internationale Neuropsychopharmacologicum 18th Congress, Nice, 1992.

68. Jenike MA, Hyman S, Baer L, et al. A controlled trial of fluvoxamine in obsessive compulsive disorder: implications for a serotonergic theory. *Am J Psychiatry* 1990;147:1209–1215.

69. Calamari JE, Faber SD, Hitsman BL, et al. Treatment of obsessive-compulsive disorder in the elderly: a review and case example. *J Behav Ther Exp Psychiatry* 1994;25:94–104.

70. Austin LS, Zealberg JJ, Lydiard RB. Three cases of pharmacotherapy of obsessive-compulsive disorder in the elderly. *J Nerv Ment Dis* 1991;179: 634–635.

71. Massey BA. Victims or survivors: a three-part approach to working with older adults in disaster. *J Geriatry Psychiatry* 1997;30:193–202.

72. Weintraub D, and Ruskin PE. Posttraumatic stress disorder in the elderly: a review. *Harvard Rev Psychiatry* 1999;7(Sep):144–152.

73. Sadavoy J. Survivors: a review of the late-life effects of prior psychological trauma. *Am J Geriatr Psychiatry* 1997;5:287–301.

74. Davidson JR, Kudler HA, Saunders, et al. Predicting response to amitriptyline in posttraumatic stress disorder. *Am J Psychiatry* 1993;150: 1024–1029.

Table 16.1 References

Allen RM. Tranquilizers and sedative/hypnotics: appropriate use in the elderly. *Geriatrics.* 1986;4: 75–78, 81–83, 87–88.

Antonijoan RM, Barbanoj MJ, Torrent J, et al. Evaluation of psychotropic drug consumption related to psychological distress in the elderly: hospitalized vs. nonhospitalized. *Neuropsychobiology* 1990; 23:25–30.

Avorn J, Soumerai SB, Everitt DE, et al. A randomized trial of a program to reduce the use of psychoactive drugs in nursing homes. *N Engl J Med* 1992;327:168–173.

Batty GM, Oborne CA, Swift CG, et al. Development of an indicator to identify inappropriate use of benzodiazepines in elderly medical in-patients. *Int J Geriatr Psychiatry* 2000;15:892–896.

Beers MH, Dang H, Hasegawa J, et al. Influence of hospitalization on drug therapy in the elderly. *J Am Geriatr Soc* 1989;37:679–683.

Blazer D, Hybels C, Simonsic E, et al. Sedative, hypnotic and anxiety medication use in an aging cohort over ten years. *J Am Geriatr Soc* 2000;48: 1073–1079.

Busto U, Chow B, Silver I, et al. Benzodiazepine prescription and use patterns in the hospitalized elderly. *Clin Pharmacol Ther* 1990;47:162.

Copeland JRM, Davidson IA, Dewey ME. The prevalence and outcome of anxious depression in elderly people aged 65 and over living in the community. In: Racagni G, Smeraldi E, eds. *Anxious depression: assessment and treatment.* New York: Raven Press, 1987:43–47.

Egan M, Moride Y, Wolfson C, et al. Long-term continuous use of benzodiazepines by older adults in Quebec: prevalence, incidence, and risk factors. *Am J Geriatr Soc* 2000;48:811–816.

Elliott RA, Woodward MC, Oborne CA. Improving benzodiazepine prescribing for elderly hospital inpatients using audit and multidisciplinary feedback. *Intern Med J* 2001;31:529–535.

Fourrier A, Letenneur L, Dartigues JF, et al. Benzodiazepine use in an elderly community-dwelling population. Characteristics of users and factors associated with subsequent use. *Eur J Clin Pharmacol* 2001;57:419–425.

Foy A, Drinkwater V, March S, et al. Confusion after admission to hospital in elderly patients using benzodiazepines. *Br Med J* 1986;293:1072.

Gleason PP, Schulz R, Smith NL, et al. Correlates and prevalence of benzodiazepine use in community-dwelling elderly. *J Gen Intern Med* 1998; 13:243–250.

Jorm AF, Grayson D, Creasey H, et al. GA Long-term benzodiazepine use by elderly people living in the community. *Aust N Z J Public Health* 2000;24: 7–10.

King MB, Gabe J, Williams P, et al. Long term use of benzodiazepines: the views of patients. *Br J Gen Pract* 1990;40:194–196.

Kirby M, Denihan A, Bruce I, et al. Benzodiazepine use among the elderly in the community. *Int J Geriatr Psychiatry* 1999;14:280–284.

Lockwood A, Berbatis CG. Psychotropic drugs in Australia: consumption patterns. *Med J Aust* 1990: 153:1604–1611.

Llorente MD, David D, Golden AG, et al. Defining patterns of benzodiazepine use in older adults. *J Geriatr Psychiatry Neurol* 2000;13:150–160.

Lyndon RW, Russel JD. Benzodiazepine use in a rural general practice population. *Aust NZ J Psychiatry* 1988;22:293–298.

Magni G, Schifano F, Pastorello M, et al. Use of psychotropic drugs in general medical geriatric inpatients. Relationship with various parameters of psychological distress (evaluated 'in blind'). *Neuropsychobiology.* 1986;16:181–185.

Manela M, Katona C, Livingston G. How common are the anxiety disorders in old age: *Int J Geriatr Psychiatry* 1996;11:65–70.

Mayer–Oakes SA, Kelman G, Beers MH, et al. Benzodiazepine use in older, community-dwelling southern Californians: prevalence and clinical correlates. *Ann Pharmacother* 1993;27:416–421.

McNutt L-A, Boles FB, McAuliffe T, et al. Impact of regulation on benzodiazepine prescribing to a low income elderly population, New York State. *J Clin Epidemiol* 1994;47:613–625.

Monette J, Tamblyn RM, McLeod PJ et al. Characteristics of physicians who frequently prescribe long-acting benzodiazepines for the elderly. *Eval Health Prof* 1997;20:115–130.

Mort JR, Aparasu RR. Prescribing potentially inappropriate psychotropic medications to the ambulatory elderly. *Arch Intern Med* 2000;160: 2825–2831.

Parry HJ, Balter MB, Mellinger GD, et al. National patterns of psychotherapeutic drug use. *Arch Gen Psychiatry* 1973;28:769–783.

Petrovic M, Vandierendonck A, Mariman A, et al. Personality traits and socio-epidemiological status of hospitalised elderly benzodiazepine users. *Int J Geriatr Psychiatry* 2002;17:733–738.

Rodrigo EK, King MB, Williams P. Health of long term benzodiazepine users. *Br Med J* 1988;296: 603–606.

Salzman C, van der Kolk BA. Psychotropic drugs and polypharmacy in elderly patients in a general hospital. *J Geriatr Psychiatry* 1979;12:167–176.

Stewart RB, Marks RG, Padgett PD, et al. Benzodiazepine use in an ambulatory elderly population: a 14-year overview. *Clin Ther.* 1994;16:118–124.

Svarstad BL, Mount JK. Chronic benzodiazepine use in nursing homes: effects of federal guidelines, resident mix, and nurse staffing. *J Am Geriatr Soc* 2001;49:1673–1678.

Taylor S, McCracken CF, Wilson KC, et al. Extent and appropriateness of benzodiazepine use. Results from an elderly urban community. *Br J Psychiatry* 1998;173:433–438.

Tu K, Mamdani MM, Hux JE, et al. Progressive trends in the prevalence of benzodiazepine prescribing in older people in Ontario, Canada. *J Am Geriatr Soc* 2001;49:1341–1345.

van Dijk KN, de Vries CS, ter Huurne K, et al. Concomitant prescribing of benzodiazepines during antidepressant therapy in the elderly. *J Clin Epidemiol* 2002;55:1049–1053.

VanHaaren AM, Lapane KL, Hughes CM. Effect of

triplicate prescription policy on benzodiazepine administration in nursing home residents. *Pharmacotherapy* 2001;21:1159–1166.

Verhaeghe W, Mets T, Corne L. Benzodiazepine use among elderly patients presenting at the emergency room. *Arch Gerontol Geriatr* 1996;22:55–62.

Whitcup SM, Miller E. Unrecognized drug dependence in psychiatrically hospitalized elderly patients. *J Am Geriatr Soc* 1987;35:297–301.

Woods JH, Winger G. Current benzodiazepine issues. *Psychopharmacology* (Berl) 1995;118:107–115.

Zandstra SM, Furer JW, van de Lisdonk EH, et al. Differences in health status between long-term and short-term benzodiazepine users. *Br J Gen Pract* 2002;52:805–808.

Zisselman MH, Rovner BW, Yuen EJ, et al. Physician rationale for benzodiazepine prescriptions to elderly hospitalized patients. *Am J Geriatr Psychiatry* 1997;5:167–171.

Zisselman MH, Rovner BW, Shmuely Y. Benzodiazepine use in the elderly prior to psychiatric hospitalization. *Psychosomatics* 1996;37:38–42.

Table 16.2 References

Bandera R, Bollini P, Garattini S. Long-acting and short-acting benzodiazepines in the elderly: kinetic differences and clinical relevance. *Curr Med Res Opin* 1984;8(Suppl 4):94–107.

Dehlin O, Kullingsjo H, Liden A, et al. Pharmacokinetics of alprazolam in geriatric patients with neurotic depression. *Pharmacol Toxicol* 1991;68:121–124.

Dorling MC, Hindmarch I. Pharmacokinetic profile of loprazolam in 12 young and 12 elderly healthy volunteers. *Drugs Exp Clin Res* 2001;27:151–159.

Fleishaker JC, Hulst LK, Ekernas SA, et al. Pharmacokinetics and pharmacodynamics of adinazolam and N-desmethyladinazolam after oral and intravenous dosing in healthy young and elderly volunteers. *J Clin Psychopharmacol* 1992;12:403–414.

Greenblatt DJ, Divoll M, Abernethy DR, et al. Alprazolam kinetics in the elderly. Relation to antipyrine disposition. *Arch Gen Psychiatry* 1983;40:287–290.

Greenblatt DJ, Allen MD, Locniskar A, et al. Lorazepam kinetics in the elderly. In: *Clin Pharmacol Ther* 1979;26:103–113.

Herman RJ, Wilkinson GR. Disposition of diazepam in young and elderly subjects after acute and chronic dosing. *Br J Clin Pharmacol* 1996;42:147–155.

Kaplan GB, Greenblatt DJ, Ehrenberg BL, et al. Single-dose pharmacokinetics and pharmacodynamics of alprazolam in elderly and young subjects. *J Clin Pharmacol* 1998;38:14–21.

Salzman C, Shader RI, Greenblatt DJ, et al. Long v short half-life benzodiazepines in the elderly. Kinetics and clinical effects of diazepam and oxazepam. *Arch Gen Psychiatry* 1983;40:293–297.

Table 16.3 References

Caramel VM, Remarque EJ, Knook DL, et al. Benzodiazepine users aged 85 and older fall more often. *J Am Geriatr Soc* 1998;46:1178–1179.

Ensrud KE, Blackwell TL, Mangione CM, et al. Central nervous system-active medications and risk for falls in older women. *J Am Geriatr Soc* 2002;50:1629–1637.

Frels C, Williams P, Narayanan S, et al. Iatrogenic causes of falls in hospitalised elderly patients: a case-control study. *Postgrad Med J* 2002;78:487–489.

Gales BJ, Menard SM. Relationship between the administration of selected medications and falls in hospitalized elderly patients. *Ann Pharmacother* 1995;29:354–358.

Granek E, Baker SP, Abbey H, et al. Medications and diagnoses in relation to falls in a long-term care facility. *J Am Geriatr Soc* 1987;35:503–511.

Grisso JA, Kelsey JL, Strom BL. Risk factors for falls as a cause of hip fracture in women. The Northeast Hip Fracture Study Group. *N Engl J Med* 1991;324:1326–1331.

Herings RM, Stricker BH, de Boer A, et al. Benzodiazepines and the risk of falling leading to femur fractures. *Arch Intern Med* 1995;155:1801–1807.

Lord SR, Clark RD, Webster IW. Visual acuity and contrast sensitivity in relation to falls in an elderly population. *Age Ageing* 1991a;20:175–181.

Lord SR, Clark RD, Webster IW. Physiological factors associated with falls in an elderly population. *J Am Geriatr Soc* 1991b;39:1194–1200.

Myers AH, Baker SP, Van Natta ML, et al. Risk factors associated with falls and injuries among elderly institutionalized persons. *Am J Epidemiol* 1991;133:1179–1190.

Neutel CI, Hirdes JP, Maxwell CJ, et al. New evidence on benzodiazepine use and falls: the time factor. *Age Ageing* 1996;25:273–278.

Passaro A, Volpato S, Romagnoni F, et al. Benzodiazepines with different half-life and falling in a hospitalized population: The GIFA study. Gruppo Italiano di Farmacovigilanza nell'Anziano. *J Clin Epidemiol* 2000;53:1222–1229.

Pierfitte C, Macouillard G, Thicoipe M, et al. Benzodiazepines and hip fractures in elderly people: case-control study. *BMJ* 2001;322:704–708.

Prudham D, Evans JG. Factors associated with falls in the elderly: a community study. *Age Ageing* 1981;10:141–146.

Ray WA, Thapa PB, Gideon P. Benzodiazepines and the risk of falls in nursing home residents. *J Am Geriatr Soc* 2000;48:682–685.

Ray WA, Griffin MR, Downey W. Benzodiazepines of long and short elimination half-life and the risk of hip fracture. *JAMA* 1989;262:3303–3307.

Ray WA, Griffin MR, Schaffner W, et al. Psychotropic drug use and the risk of hip fracture. *N Engl J Med* 1987;316:363–369.

Schwab M, Roder F, Aleker T, et al. Psychotropic drug use, falls and hip fracture in the elderly. *Aging* (Milano) 2000;12:234–239.

Sgadari A, Lapane KL, Mor V, et al. Oxidative and nonoxidative benzodiazepines and the risk of femur fracture. The Systematic Assessment of Geriatric Drug Use Via Epidemiology Study Group. *J Clin Psychopharmacol* 2000;20:234–239.

Sobel KG, McCart GM. Drug use and accidental falls in an intermediate care facility. *Drug Intell Clin Pharm* 1983;17:539–542.

Sorock GS. Falls among the elderly: epidemiology and prevention. *Am J Prev Med* 1988a;4:282–288.

Sorock GS, Shimkin EE. Benzodiazepine sedatives and the risk of falling in a community-dwelling elderly cohort. *Arch Intern Med* 1988b;148: 2441–2444.

Taggart HM. Do drugs affect the risk of hip fracture in elderly women? *J Am Geriatr Soc* 1988;36: 1006–1010.

Tinetti ME, Speechley M, Ginter SF. Risk factors for falls among elderly persons living in the community. *N Engl J Med* 1988;319:1701–1707.

Trewin VF, Lawrence CJ, Veitch GB An investigation of the association of benzodiazepines and other hypnotics with the incidence of falls in the elderly. *J Clin Pharm Ther* 1992 17(Apr 2):129–133.

Tromp AM, Pluijm SM, Smit JH, et al. Fall-risk screening test: a prospective study on predictors for falls in community-dwelling elderly. *J Clin Epidemiol* 2001;54:837–844.

Wang PS, Bohn RL, Glynn RJ, et al. Hazardous benzodiazepine regimens in the elderly: effects of half-life, dosage, and duration on risk of hip fracture. *Am J Psychiatry* 2001a;158:892–898.

Wang PS, Bohn RL, Glynn RJ, et al. Zolpidem use and hip fractures in older people. *J Am Geriatr Soc* 2001b;49:1685–1690.

Weintraub M, Handy BM. Benzodiazepines and hip fracture: the New York State experience. In: *Clin Pharmacol Ther* 1993;54:252–256.

Wells BG, Middleton B, Lawrence G, et al. Factors associated with the elderly falling in intermediate care facilities. *Drug Intell Clin Pharm* 1985;19: 142–145.

Wysowski DK, Baum C, Ferguson WJ, et al. Sedative-hypnotic drugs and the risk of hip fracture. *J Clin Epidemiol* 1996;49:111–113.

Table 16.4 References

Bonnet MH, Kramer M. The interaction of age, performance and hypnotics in the sleep of insomniacs. *J Am Geriatr Soc* 1981;29:508–512.

Briggs RS, Castleden CM, Kraft CA. Improved hypnotic treatment using chlormethiazole and temazepam. *Br J Med* 1980;1:601–604.

Castleden CM, George CF, Marcer D, et al. Increased sensitivity to nitrazepam in old age. *Br J Med* 1982; 1:10–12.

Foy A, O'Connell D, Henry D, et al. Benzodiazepine use as a cause of cognitive impairment in elderly hospital inpatients. *J Gerontol* 1995;50A:M99–M106.

Greenblatt DJ, Divoll M, Harmatz JS. Kinetics and clinical effects of flurazepam in young and elderly non-insomniacs. *Clin Pharmacol Ther* 1981; 30:475–486.

Hanlon J, Horner R, Schmader K, et al. Benzodiazepine use and cognitive function among community-dwelling elderly. *Clin Pharmacol Ther* 1998; 64:684–692.

Hart RP, Colenda CC, Hamer RM. Effects of buspirone and alprazolam on the cognitive performance of normal elderly subjects. *Am J Psychiatry* 1991;148:73–77.

Hinrichs JV, Ghoneim MM. Diazepam, behavior, and aging. Increased sensitivity or lower baseline performance? *Psychopharmacology* 1987;92:100–105.

Kroboth PD, McAuley JW, Smith RB. Alprazolam in the elderly: pharmacokinetics and pharmacodynamics during multiple doses. *Psychopharmacology* 1990;100:477–484.

Nikaido AM, Ellinwood EH, Heatherly DG, et al. Differential CNS effects of diazepam in elderly adults. *Pharmacol Biochem Behav* 1987;27:273–281.

Paterniti S, Dufouil C, Alpérovitch A. Long-term benzodiazepine use and cognitive decline in the elderly: the epidemiology of vascular aging study. *J Clin Psychopharmacol* 2002;22:285–293.

Pomara N, Deptula D, Medel M, et al. Effects of diazepam on recall memory: relationship to aging, dose, and duration of treatment. *Psychopharmacol Bull* 1989;25:144–148.

Pomara N, Stanley B, Block R, et al. Increased sensitivity of the elderly to the central depressant effects of diazepam. *J Clin Psychiatry* 1985;46: 185–187.

Rummans TA, Davis LJ, Morse RM, et al. Learning and memory impairment in older, detoxified, benzodiazepine-dependent patients. *Mayo Clin Proc* 1993;68:731–737.

Salzman C, Fisher J, Nobel K, et al. Cognitive improvement following benzodiazepine discontinuation in elderly nursing home residents. *Int J Geriatr Psychiatry* 1992;7:89–93.

Satzger W, Engel E, Ferguson H, et al. Effects of single doses of alpidem, lorazepam, and placebo on memory and attention in healthy young and elderly volunteers. *Pharmacopsychiatry* 1009;23: 114–119.

Scharf MB, Hirschowitz J, Woods M, et al. Lack of amnestic effects of clorazepate on geriatric recall. *J Clin Psychiatry* 1985;46:518–520.

Sunderland T, Weingartner H, Cohen RM, et al. Low-dose oral lorazepam administration in Alzheimer subjects and age-matched controls. *Psychopharmacol Ser* (Berlin) 1989;99:129–133.

Swift CG, Ewen JM, Clarke P, et al. Responsiveness to oral diazepam in the elderly: relationship to total and free plasma concentrations. *Br J Clin Pharmacol* 1985;20:111–118.

Table 16.5 References

Bertz RJ, Kroboth PD, Kroboth FJ, et al. Alprazolam in young and elderly men: sensitivity and tolerance to psychomotor, sedative and memory effects. *J Pharmacol Exp Ther* 1997;281:1317–1329.

Gray SL, Lai KV, Larson EB. Drug-induced cognition disorders in the elderly: incidence, prevention and management. *Drug Saf* 1999;101–122.

Hanlon JT, Horner RD, Schmader KE, et al. Benzodiazepine use and cognitive function among community-dwelling elderly. *Clin Pharmacol Ther* 1998;64:684–692.

Lagnaoui R, Begaud B, Moore N, et al. Benzodiazepine use and risk of dementia: a nested case-control study. *J Clin Epidemiol* 2002;55:314–318.

Pomara N, Tun H, DaSilva D, et al. The acute and chronic performance effects of alprazolam and lorazepam in the elderly: relationship to duration of treatment and self-rated sedation. *Psychopharmacol Bull* 1998;34:139–153.

Paterniti S, Dufouil C, Alperovitch A. A long-term benzodiazepine use and cognitive decline in the elderly: the Epidemiology of Vascular Aging Study. *J Clin Psychopharmacol* 2002;22:285–293.

Rasmussen LS, Steentoft A, Rasmussen H, et al. Benzodiazepines and postoperative cognitive dysfunction in the elderly. ISPOCD Group. International Study of Postoperative Cognitive Dysfunction. *Br J Anaesth* 1999;83:585–589.

Ried LD, Johnson RE, Gettman DA. Benzodiazepine exposure and functional status in older people. *J Am Geriatr Soc* 1998;46:71–76.

Scharf MB, Hirschowitz J, Woods M, et al. Lack of amnestic effects of clorazepate on geriatric recall. *J Clin Psychiatry* 1985;46:518–520.

Sumner DD. Benzodiazepine-induced persisting amnestic disorder: are older adults at risk? *Arch Psychiatr Nurs.* 1998;12:119–125.

Vignola A, Lamoureux C, Bastien CH, et al. Effects of chronic insomnia and use of benzodiazepines on daytime performance in older adults. *J Gerontol B Psychol Sci Soc Sci* 2000;55:P54–P62.

Table 16.6 References

Hart RP, Colenda CC, Hamer RM. Effects of buspirone and alprazalom on the cognitive performance of normal elderly subjects. *Am J Psychiatry* 1991;148:73–77.

Levine S, Napoliello MJ, Domantay AG. Open study of buspirone in octogenarians with anxiety. *Hum Psychopharmacol* 1989;4:51–53.

Napoliello MJ. An interim multicentre report on 677 anxious geriatric outpatients treated with buspirone. *Br J Clin Pract* 1986;40:71–73.

Robinson D, Napoliello MJ. The safety and usefulness of buspirone as an anxiolytic in elderly versus young patients. *Clin Ther* 1988;10:740–746.

Singh AN, Beer M. A dose range finding study of buspirone in geriatric patients with symptoms of anxiety. *J Clin Psychopharmacol* 1988;8:67–68.

Supplemental Readings

General

Allen RM. Tranquilizers and sedative/hypnotics: appropriate use in the elderly. *Geriatrics* 1986;41:75–88.

Ayd FJ Jr. Tranquilizers and the ambulatory geriatric patient. *J Am Geriatr Soc* 1960;8:909–914.

Ban TA. *Psychopharmacology for the aged.* Basel: Karger, 1980.

Bannen DM, Resnick O. Lorazepam versus glutethimide as a sleep-inducing agent for the geriatric patient. *J Am Geriatr Soc* 1973;21:507–511.

Beardsley RS, Larson PB, Burns BJ, et al. Prescribing of psychotropics in elderly nursing home patients. *J Am Geriatr Soc* 1989;37:327–330.

Beers M, Avorn J, Soumerai SB, et al. Psychoactive medication use in intermediate-care facility residents. *JAMA* 1980;260:3016–3020.

Bonnet MH, Kramer M, Roth T. A dose-response study of the hypnotic effectiveness of alprazolam and diazepam in normal subjects. *Psychopharmacology* 1981;75:258–261.

Castleden CM, George CF, Marcer D, et al. Increased

sensitivity to nitrazepam in old age. *Br Med J* 1982;1:10–12.

Covington JS. Alleviating agitation, apprehension, and related symptoms in geriatric patients: a double blind comparison of a phenothiazine and benzodiazepine. *South Med J* 1975;68:719–724.

Crook T. Diagnosis and treatment of mixed anxiety-depression in the elderly. *J Clin Psychiatry* 1982;43:35–43.

Divoll M, Greenblatt DJ. Effect of age and sex on lorazepam protein binding. *J Pharm Pharmacol* 1982;34:122–123.

Divoll M, Greenblatt DJ, Abernethy DR, et al. Cimetidine impairs clearance of antipyrine and desmethyldiazepam in the elderly. *J Am Geriatr Soc* 1982;30:684–689.

Fancourt G, Castleden M. The use of benzodiazepines with particular reference to the elderly. *Br J Hosp Med* 1986;35:321–326.

Fillingham JM. Double-blind evaluation of temazepam, flurazepam, and placebo in geriatric insomniacs. *Clin Ther* 1982;4:369–380.

Greenblatt DJ, Allen MD, Shader RI. Toxicity of high-dose flurazepam in the elderly. *Clin Pharmacol Ther* 1977;21:355–361.

Greenblatt DJ, Locniskar A, Shader RI. Halazepam as a precursor of desmethyldiazepam: quantitation by electron-capture gas-liquid chromatography. *Psychopharmacology* 1983;80:178–180.

Greenblatt DJ, Shader RI, Abernethy DR. Current status of benzodiazepines. *N Engl J Med* 1983;309:410–412.

Harry TVA, Richards DS. Lorazepam—a study in psychomotor depression. *Br J Clin Pract* 1972;26:371–373.

Hershey LA, Kim KY. Diagnosis and treatment of anxiety in the elderly. *Rational Drug Ther* 1988;22:1–6.

King DJ. Benzodiazepines, amnesia and sedation: theoretical and clinical issues and controversies. *Human Psychopharmacol* 1992;7:79–87.

Lyndon RW, Russell JD. Benzodiazepine use in a rural general practice population. *Aust NZ J Psychiatry* 1988;22:293–298.

Nakra BRS, Grossberg GT. Management of anxiety in the elderly. *Compr Ther* 1986;12:53–60.

Reeves RL. Comparison of triazolam, flurazepam, and placebo as hypnotics in geriatric patients with insomnia. *J Clin Pharmacol* 1977;17:319–323.

Sallis JF, Lichstein KL. Analysis and management of geriatric anxiety. *Int J Aging Hum Dev* 1982;15:197–205.

Salzman C. Recent advances in geriatric psychopharmacology. *American Psychiatric Association: annual update in psychiatry.* Washington, DC: American Psychiatric Press, 1990.

Salzman C. Psychotropic drug use and polypharmacy in a general hospital. *Hosp Community Psychiatry* 1981;3:1–9.

Salzman C. Treatment of agitation, anxiety, and depression in dementia. *Psychopharmacol Bull* 1988;24:39–42.

Schweizer E, Case WG, Rickels K. Benzodiazepine dependence and withdrawal in elderly patients. *Am J Psychiatry* 1989;146:529–531.

Shader RI, Greenblatt DJ. Management of anxiety in the elderly: the balance between therapeutic and adverse effects. *J Clin Psychiatry* 1982;43:8–18.

Sizaret P, Versavel MC, Engel G, et al. Clinical investigation of lorazepam. *Psychol Med* 1974;6:591–598.

Turnbull JM, Turnbull SK. Management of specific anxiety disorders in the elderly. *Geriatrics* 1985; 40:75–82.

Verhaeghe W, Mets T, Corne L. Benzodiazepine use among elderly patients presenting at the emergency room. *Archives of Gerontology and Geriatrics* 1996;22:55–62.

Woo E, Proulx SM, Greenblatt DJ. Differential side effect profile of triazolam versus flurazepam in elderly patients undergoing rehabilitation therapy. *J Clin Pharmacol* 1991;31:168–173.

Benzodiazepine Use in the Elderly

Allen RM. Tranquilizers and sedative/hypnotics: appropriate use in the elderly. *Geriatrics* 1998;41: 75–88.

Ancill RJ, Carlyle WW. Benzodiazepine use and dependency in the elderly: striking a balance. In: Hallstrom C, ed. *Benzodiazepine dependence.* New York: Oxford University Press, 1993:238–251.

Burch EA Jr. Use and misuse of benzodiazepines in the elderly. *Psychiatr Med* 1990;8:97–105.

Cutler NR, Narang PK. Implications of dosing tricyclic antidepressants and benzodiazepines in geriatrics. *Psychiatr Clin North Am* 1984;7: 845–861.

Fancourt G, Goldstein M. The use of benzodiazepines with particular reference to the elderly. *Br J Hosp Med* 1986;35:321–326.

Fourrier A, Letenneur L, Dartigues JF, et al. Benzodiazepine use in an elderly community-dwelling population. Characteristics of users and factors associated with subsequent use. *Eur J Clin Pharmacol* 2001;57:419–425.

Hershey LA, Mihlay E. A controlled evaluation of two dose levels of oxazepam compared to placebo. *J New Drugs* 1986;6:124.

Jenike MA. Treating anxiety in elderly patients. *Geriatrics* 1983;38:115–119.

Kanowski S. Sleep disturbances and agitational states in the elderly. Therapeutic possibilities and limitations in West Germany. *Acta Psychiatry Scand* 1986(suppl 329):77–80.

King MB, Gabe J, Williams P, et al. Long term use of benzodiazepines: the views of patients. *Br J Gen Pract* 1990;40:194–196.

Larson EB, Kukull WA, Buchner D, et al. Adverse drug reaction associated with global cognitive impairment in elderly persons. *Ann Intern Med* 1987; 107:169–173.

Mayer-Oakes SA, Kelman G, Beers MH, et al. Benzodiazepine use in older, community-dwelling southern Californians: prevalence and clinical correlates. *Ann Pharmacother* 1993;27:416–421.

McNutt L-A, Boles FB, McAuliffe T, et al. Impact of regulation on benzodiazepine prescribing to a low income elderly population, New York State. *J Clin Epidemiol* 1994;47:613–625.

Monette J, Tamblyn RM, McLeod PJ, et al. Characteristics of physicians who frequently prescribe long-acting benzodiazepines for the elderly. *Eval Health Prof* 1997;20:115–130.

Nakra BRS, Grossberg GT. Management of anxiety in the elderly. *Compr Ther* 1986;12:53–60.

Petrie WM. Drug treatment of anxiety and agitation in the aged. *Psychopharmacol Bull* 1983;19: 238–246.

Sallis JF, Lichstein KL. Analysis and management of geriatric anxiety. *Int J Aging Hum Dev* 1982;15: 197–211.

Salzman C. The American Psychiatric Association Task Force report on benzodiazepine dependency, toxicity, and abuse. *J Psychiatr Res* 1990; 24:1(suppl):35–37.

Shader RI, Greenblatt DJ. Management of anxiety in the elderly: the balance between therapeutic and adverse effects. *J Clin Psychiatry* 1982;43:8–18.

Thompson TL, Moran MG, Nies AS. Psychotropic drug use in the elderly. Part I. *N Engl J Med* 1983; 308:137–138.

Tobias CR, Turns DM, Lippmann S, et al. Psychiatric disorder in the elderly. *Postgrad Med* 1988;83: 313–319.

Turnbull JM, Turnbull SK. Management of specific anxiety disorders in the elderly. *Geriatrics* 1985; 40:75–82.

Zandstra SM, Furer JW, van de Lisdonk EH, et al. Differences in health status between long-term and short-term benzodiazepine users. *Br J Gen Pract* 2002;52:805–808.

Zisselman MH, Rovner BW, Yuen EJ, et al. Physician rationale for benzodiazepine prescriptions to elderly hospitalized patients. *Am J Geriatr Psychiatry* 1997;5:167–171.

Zisselman MH, Rovner BW, Shmuely Y. Benzodiazepine use in the elderly prior to psychiatric hospitalization. *Psychosomatics* 1996;37:38–42.

Kinetics of Benzodiazepines

Alvan G, Siwers B, Vessman J. Pharmacokinetics of oxazepam in healthy volunteers. *Acta Pharmacol Toxicol* (Copenh) 1977;40:40–51.

Bareggu SR, Nielsen NP, Leva S, et al. Age-related multiple-dose pharmacokinetic and anxiolytic effects of delorazepam (chlordesmethyldiazepam). *Int J Clin Pharm Res* 1986;6:309–314.

Breimer DD. Pharmacokinetics and metabolism of various benzodiazepines used as hypnotics. *Br J Clin Pharmacol* 1979;8:7S–13S.

Carskadon MA, Seidel WF, Greenblatt DJ, et al. Daytime carryover of triazolam and flurazepam in elderly insomniacs. *Sleep* 1982;5:361–371.

Cook PJ, Huggett A, Graham-Pole R, et al. Hypnotic accumulation and hangover in elderly inpatients: a controlled double-blind study of temazepam and nitrazepam. *Br Med J* 1983;286:100–102.

Crome P, Gain R, Suri AC, et al. Temazepam in elderly women: single and multiple dose kinetics and effects on psychomotor performance. *Br J Clin Pharmacol* 1985;19:583.

Divoll M, Greenblatt DJ. Effect of age and sex on lorazepam protein binding. *J Pharm Pharmacol* 1982;34:122–123.

Epstein LJ. Anxiolytics, antidepressants and neuroleptics in the treatment of geriatric patients. In: Lipton MA, DiMascio A, Killam KF, eds. *Psychopharmacology: a generation of progress.* New York: Raven, 1978:1517–1523.

Greenblatt DJ. Reduced serum albumin concentration in the elderly: a report from the Boston Collaborative Drug Surveillance Program. *J Am Geriatr Soc* 1979;27:20–22.

Greenblatt DJ, Allen MD, Harmatz JS, et al. Diazepam disposition determinants. *Clin Pharmacol Ther* 1980;27:301–312.

Greenblatt DJ, Allen MD, Locniskar A, et al. Lorazepam kinetics in the elderly. *Clin Pharmacol Ther* 1979;26:103–113.

Greenblatt DJ, Divoll MD, Abernethy DR, et al. Antipyrine kinetics in the elderly: prediction of age-related changes in benzodiazepine oxidizing capacity. *J Pharmacol Exp Ther* 1982;220:120–126.

Greenblatt DJ, Divoll M, Abernethy DR. Alprazolam kinetics in the elderly; relation to antipyrine disposition. *Arch Gen Psychiatry* 1983;40:287–292.

Greenblatt DJ, Divoll M, Harmatz JS, et al. Kinetics and clinical effects of flurazepam in young and elderly noninsomniacs. *Clin Pharmacol Ther* 1981; 30;475–486.

Greenblatt DJ, Divoll M, Harmatz JS, et al. Oxazepam kinetics: effects of age and sex. *J Pharmacol Exp Ther* 1980;215:86–91.

Greenblatt DJ, Shader RI, Franke K, et al. Pharmacokinetics and bioavailability of intravenous, intramuscular, and oral lorazepam in humans. *J Pharm Sci* 1979;68:57–63.

Greenblatt DJ, Sellers EM, Koch–Weser J. Importance of protein binding for the interpretation of serum or plasma drug concentration. *J Clin Pharmacol* 1982;22:259–263.

Greenblatt DJ, Shader RI. Benzodiazepine kinetics in the elderly. In: Usdin E, ed. *Clinical Pharmacology in psychiatry*. New York: Elsevier/North Holland, 1981:173–181.

Greenblatt DJ, Shader RI. *Pharmacokinetic understanding of clinical drug effects in the elderly.* New York: Excerpta Medica, 1978:13–15.

Greenblatt DJ, Shader RI, Divoll M, et al. Benzodiazepines: a summary of pharmacokinetic properties. *Br J Clin Pharmacol* 1981;11:11S–16S.

Hoyumpa AMJ. Disposition and elimination of minor tranquilizers in the aged and in patients with liver disease. *South Med J* 1978;71:23–28.

Johnson RF, Schenker S, Roberts RK, et al. Plasma binding of benzodiazepines in humans. *J Pharm Sci* 1979;68:1320–1322.

Kanto J, Maenpaa M, Mantyla R, et al. Effect of age on the pharmacokinetics of diazepam given in conjunction with spinal anesthesia. *Anesthesiology* 1979;51:154–159.

Klotz U, Avant GR, Hoyumpa A, et al. Effects of age and liver disease on disposition and elimination of diazepam in adult man. *J Clin Invest* 1975;55: 347–359.

Klotz U, Müller–Seydlitz P. Altered elimination of desmethyldiazepam in the elderly. *Br J Clin Pharmacol* 1979;7:119–120.

Kraus JW, Desmond PV, Marshall JP, et al. Effects of aging and liver disease on disposition of lorazepam. *Clin Pharmacol Ther* 1978;24:411–419.

Macklon AF, Barton M, James O, et al. The effect of age on the pharmacokinetics of diazepam. *Clin Sci* 1980;59:479–483.

MacLeod SM, Giles HG, Bengert B, et al. Age- and gender-related differences in diazepam pharmacokinetics. *J Clin Pharmacol* 1979;15:15–19.

Ochs HR, Greenblatt DJ, Allen MD, et al. Effect of age and Billroth gastrectomy on absorption of desmethyldiazepam from clorazepate. *Clin Pharmacol Ther* 1979;26:449–456.

Ochs H, Greenblatt DJ, Divoll M, et al. Diazepam kinetics in relation to age and sex. *Pharmacology* 1981;23:24–30.

Roberts RK, Wilkinson GR, Branch RA, et al. Effect of age and parenchymal liver disease on the disposition and elimination of chlordiazepoxide (Librium). *Gastroenterology* 1978;75:479–485.

Salzman C, Shader RI, Greenblatt DJ, et al. Long versus short half-life benzodiazepines in the elderly: kinetics and clinical effects of diazepam and oxazepam. *Arch Gen Psychiatry* 1983;40: 293–297.

Shader RI, Georgotas A, Greenblatt DJ, et al. Impaired desmethyldiazepam from clorazepate by magnesium aluminum hydroxide. *Clin Pharmacol Ther* 1978;24:308–315.

Shader RI, Greenblatt DJ, Ciraulo DA, et al. Effect of age and sex on disposition of desmethyldiazepam formed from its precursor clorazepate. *Psychopharmacology* 1981;75:193–197.

Shader RI, Greenblatt DJ, Harmatz JS, et al. Absorption and distribution of chlordiazepoxide in young and elderly male volunteers. *J Clin Pharmacol* 1977;17:709–718.

Shull HJ, Wilkinson GR, Johnson R, et al. Normal disposition of oxazepam in acute viral hepatitis and cirrhosis. *Ann Intern Med* 1976;84:420–425.

Swift CG, Ewen JM, Clarke P, Stevenson IH. Responsiveness to oral diazepam in the elderly: relationship to total and free plasma concentrations. *Br J Clin Pharmacol* 1985;20:111–118.

van der Kleijn E, Vree TB, Baars AM, et al. Factors influencing the activity and fate of benzodiazepines in the elderly. *Br J Clin Pharmacol* 1981;11: 85S–98S.

Wilkinson GR. Effects of aging on the disposition of benzodiazepines in human beings: binding and distribution considerations. In: Raskin A, Robinson DS, Levine J, eds. *Age and the Pharmacology of psychoactive drugs.* New York: Elsevier/North Holland, 1981:3–15.

Alprazolam

Aden GC, Thein SG. Alprazolam compared to diazepam and placebo on the treatment of anxiety. *J Clin Psychiatry* 1980;41:245–248.

Pitts WM, Fann WE, Sajadi C, Snyder S. Alprazolam in older depressed inpatients. *J Clin Psychiatry* 1983;44:213–215.

Chlordiazepoxide

Beber CR. Treating anxiety and depression in the elderly. *J Fla Med Assoc* 1971;58:35–38.

Boston Collaborative Drug Surveillance Program. Clinical depression of the central nervous system due to diazepam and chlordiazepoxide in relation to cigarette smoking and age. *N Engl J Med* 1973;288:277.

Goldstein BJ. Double-blind comparison of tybamate and chlordiazepoxide in geriatric patients. *Psychosomatics* 1967;8:334–337.

Greenblatt DJ, Koch-Weser J. Clinical toxicity of

chlordiazepoxide and diazepam in relation to serum albumin concentration: a report from the Boston Collaborative Drug Surveillance Program. *Eur Clin Pharmacol* 1974;7:259–262.

Jones TH. Chlordiazepoxide (Librium) and the geriatric patient. *J Am Geriatr Soc* 1962;10:259–263.

Shader RI, Greenblatt DJ, Harmatz JS, et al. Absorption and disposition of chlordiazepoxide in young and elderly male volunteers. *J Clin Pharmacol* 1977;17:709–718.

Desmethyldiazepam

Salzman C, Shader RI, Greenblatt DJ, et al. Long versus short half-life benzodiazepines in the elderly: kinetics and clinical effects of diazepam and oxazepam. *Arch Gen Psychiatry* 1983;40: 293–297.

Diazepam

Chesrow EJ, Kaplitz SE, Breme JT, et al. Use of a new benzodiazepine derivative (Valium) in chronically ill and disturbed elderly patients. *J Am Geriatr Soc* 1962;10:667–670.

DeLemos GP, Clement WR, Nickels E. Effects of diazepam suspension in geriatric patients hospitalized for psychiatric illnesses. *J Am Geriatr Soc* 1965; 13:355–359.

Greenblatt DJ, Harmatz JS, Shader RI. Factors influencing diazepam pharmacokinetics: age, sex and liver disease. *J Clin Pharmacol* 1978;16:177–179.

Hinrichs JV, Ghoneim MM. Diazepam, behavior, and aging: increased sensitivity or lower baseline performance? *Psychopharmacology* 1987;92:100–105.

Hoyumpa AMJ. Disposition and elimination of minor tranquilizers in the aged and in patients with liver disease. *South Med J* 1978;71:23–28.

Kirven LE, Montero EF. Comparison of thioridazine and diazepam in the control of nonpsychotic symptoms associated with senility: double blind study. *J Am Geriatr Soc* 1973;21:546–551.

Lynch T, Power P, Prasad HC. Comparison of oral and rectal diazepam (Valium) in the treatment of insomnia associated with anxiety in the elderly. *J Irish Coll Physicians Surg* 1981;11:73–75.

Pomara N, Stanley B, Block R, et al. Increased sensitivity of the elderly to the central depressant effects of diazepam. *J Clin Psychiatry* 1985;46: 185–187.

Ray W, Blazer D, Schaffner W, et al. Reducing chronic diazepam prescribing in office practice: a controlled trial of educational visits. *JAMA* 1986;256:2536–2539.

Salzman C, Shader RI, Greenblatt DJ, et al. Long versus short–life benzodiazepines in the elderly: kinetics and clinical effects of diazepam and oxazepam. *Arch Gen Psychiatry* 1983;40: 293–297.

Lorazepam

Ancill RJ, Embury GD, MacEwan GGW, et al. Lorazepam in the elderly—a retrospective study of the side-effects in 20 patients. *J Psychopharmacol* 1987;2:126–127.

Curran HV, Allen D, Lader M. The effects of single doses of alpidem and lorazepam on memory and psychomotor performance in normal humans. *J Psychopharmacol* 1987;2:81–89.

Paes de Sousa M, Figuiera ML, et al. Lorazepam and clobazam in anxious elderly patients. In: *Clobazam: Royal Society of Medicine international congress and symposium.* Series No. 43. London: Academic Press and Royal Society of Medicine, 1981: 119–123.

Pinosky DG. Clinical assessment of the safety and efficacy of lorazepam, a new benzodiazepine derivative, in the treatment of anxiety. *J Clin Psychiatry* 1978;39:24–29.

Oxazepam

Ayd FS. Oxazepam: an overview. *Dis Nerv Syst* 1975; 36(suppl):14–15.

Chewrow EJ, Kaplitz SE, Vetra H, et al. Blind study of oxazepam in the management of geriatric patients with behavioral problems. *Clin Med* 1965; 72:1001–1005.

Debert R. Oxazepam in the treatment of anxiety in children and the elderly. *Acta Psychiatr Scand* 1977;274(suppl):104–110.

Koepke HH, Gold RL, Linden ME, et al. Multicenter controlled study of oxazepam in anxious elderly outpatients. *Psychosomatics* 1982;23:641–645.

Merlis S, Koepke HH. Use of oxazepam in elderly patients. *Dis Nerv Sys* 1975;36:27–29.

Sanders JF. Evaluation of oxazepam and placebo in emotionally disturbed aged patients. *Geriatrics* 1965;739–746.

Benzodiazepines and Memory

Angus WR, Romney DM. The effect of diazepam on patients' memory. *Clin Psychopharmacol* 1984;4: 203–206.

Barnet DB, Taylor Davies A, Desai N. Differential effect of diazepam on short term memory in subjects with high or low level anxiety. *Br J Clin Pharmacol* 1981;11:411–412.

Curran HV, Allen D, Lader M. The effects of single doses of alpidem and lorazepam on memory and psychomotor performance in normal humans. *J Psychopharmacol* 1987;2:81–89.

Hartley LR, Spencer J, Williamson J. Anxiety, diazepam and retrieval from semantic memory. *Psychopharmacology* 1982;76:291–293.

Lucki I, Rickels K, Geller AM. Chronic use of benzodiazepines and psychomotor and cognitive test performance. *Psychopharmacology* 1986;88:426–433.

Lucki I, Rickels K, Giesecke MA, et al. Differential effects of anxiolytic drugs, diazepam and buspirone, on memory function. *Br J Clin Pharmacol* 1987;23:207–211.

Pomara N, Stanley B, Block R, et al. Adverse effects of single therapeutic doses of diazepam on performance in normal geriatric subjects: relationship to plasma concentrations. *Psychopharmacology* 1984;84:342–346.

Pomara N, Stanley B, Block R, et al. Diazepam impairs performance in normal elderly subjects. *Psychopharmacol Bull* 1984;20:137–139.

Pomara N, Stanley B, Block R, et al. Increased sensitivity of the elderly to the central depressant effects of diazepam. *J Clin Psychiatry* 1985;46:185–187.

Falls Associated with Benzodiazepines

American Psychiatric Association Task Force on Benzodiazepine Dependency, Toxicity, and Abuse. Washington, DC: American Psychiatric Press, 1989.

Campbell JA, Borrie MU, Spears GF. Risk factors for falls in a prospective study of community-based people 70 years or older. *J Gerontol* 1989;44:112–117.

Gagnon MA, Langlois Y, Boghen DR, et al. Effects of halazepam and diazepam on the motor coordination of geriatric subjects. *Eur J Clin Pharmacol* 1977;11:443–448.

Granek E, Baker SP, Abbey H, et al. Medications and diagnoses in relation to falls in a long-term care facility. *J Am Geriatr Soc* 1987;35:503–511.

Sorock GS, Shimken EE. Benzodiazepine sedative and the risk of falling in a community-dwelling elderly cohort. *Arch Intern Med* 1988;148:2441–2444.

Tinetti ME, Speechley M. Prevention of falls among the elderly. *New Engl J Med* 1989;320:1055–1059.

Buspirone

Domantay AG, Napoliello MJ. Buspirone for elderly anxious patients: a review of clinical studies. *Fam Pract Recertification* 1989;11:17–23.

Levine S, Napoliello MJ. An open study of buspirone in octogenarians with anxiety. *Hum Psychopharmacol* 1989;4:51–53.

Napoliello MJ. An interim multicentre report on 677 anxious geriatric out-patients treated with buspirone. *Br J Clin Pract* 1986;40:71–73.

Robinson D, Napoliello MJ, Schenk J. The safety and usefulness of buspirone as an anxiolytic drug in elderly versus young patients. *Clin Ther* 1988;10:740–746.

Singh A, Beer M. A dose range-finding study of buspirone in geriatric patients with symptoms of anxiety [letter]. *J Clin Psychopharmacol* 1988;8:67–68.

Strauss A. Oral dyskinesia associated with buspirone use in an elderly woman. *J Clin Psychiatry* 1988;49:322–323.

Meprobamate

Hale WE, May FE, Moore MT, Stewart RB. Meprobamate use in the elderly. *J Am Geriatr Soc* 1988;36:1003–1005.

Part VI: Sleep Disorders

Chapter 17

The Impact of Age on Sleep and Sleep Disorders

J. Christian Gillin

Sonia Ancoli-Israel

Many people feel dissatisfied with their sleep as they age. Not surprisingly, the prevalence of insomnia and the use of sleeping pills increase among older persons, especially among women and individuals with multiple medical, psychiatric, and social problems. In addition, some elderly individuals experience difficulty staying awake during the day. Because it is not always clear whether these age-related changes in sleep and wakefulness reflect "normal aging" or pathology, elderly patients often have multifaceted difficulties with sleep and wakefulness that are affected by multiple factors. Each serious complaint should be evaluated with the goal of identifying treatable conditions. The clinician's task is to weigh the relative importance of the contributory conditions, correct the treatable disorders, and offer symptomatic relief whenever appropriate. The goal is to reduce morbidity and excess mortality and to improve the quality of life for the patient and family.

This chapter describes sleep mechanisms in the elderly and introduces the clinical evaluation of sleep complaints. Treatment of sleep disorders is discussed in Chapter 18.

Neurobiology and Chronobiology of Normal Sleep

Normal sleep consists of two major states: rapid eye movement (REM) sleep and nonrapid eye movement (NREM) sleep. In young adults, NREM sleep is further divided into four sleep stages on the basis of electroencephalogram (EEG) patterns (see Table 17.1 and Figure 17.1). Sleep normally begins with Stage 1, a brief transitional phase, before progressing successively into Stages 2 through 4. In the young adult, the first REM period usually begins about 70 to 100 minutes after the onset of sleep, a term referred to as REM latency (the elapsed time between the onset of sleep and the first REM period). Thereafter, NREM and REM sleep oscillate with a cycle length of roughly 90 minutes. The first REM period usually lasts about 15 minutes; successive REM periods in young people increase to about 25 to 40 minutes. Sleep stages 3 and 4, known as delta sleep (based on the amount of delta waves in EEG (30 or 60 seconds for Stages 3 and more than 60 seconds for Stage 4), occur mainly in the first NREM period of the night and the amount declines with each successive NREM period. Therefore, most delta sleep occurs in the first third of the night and most REM sleep occurs in the last third of the night.

The sleep-wake cycle is a prime example of a circadian rhythm in humans (see Table 17.2). The rhythm of sleep and wakefulness is governed by one or more internal biological "clocks" or oscillators, environmental stimuli, and a host of processes that promote or inhibit arousal.

Two principles are useful in understanding normal sleep. The first is homeo-

Table 17.1. Commonly Used Terms in Sleep Research

Delta wave	EEG pattern conventionally defined as $\geq$75 microvolts, $\geq$0.5 Hz or cycles per second wave; amplitude tends to decrease with normal aging
Non-REM sleep	Stages 1, 2, 3, and 4 sleep
REM latency	Time from onset of sleep to onset of REM sleep; declines from about 70–100 minutes in 20s to 55–70 minutes in elderly; short REM latency associated with narcolepsy, depression, and a variety of clinical conditions
REM sleep	Rapid eye movement sleep: characterized by low voltage, relatively fast frequency EEG, bursts of rapid eye movements, and loss of tone in major antigravity muscles; associated with dreaming
Sleep efficiency	Percentage of time in bed spent in sleep: usually above 90% in the young; decreases somewhat with age
Sleep latency	Time from "lights out" to onset of sleep
Stage 1 sleep	Brief transitional state of sleep between wakefulness and sleep; characterized by low-voltage, mixed-frequency EEG and slow eye movements
Stage 2 sleep	Usually about 45–75% of total sleep time; characterized by K-complexes and sleep spindles (12–14 per cycle rhythms) in EEG
Stages 3 & 4 sleep	Sometimes referred to as delta sleep (based on amount of delta waves in EEG); 20–50% of an epoch (i.e., 30 or 60 seconds) for stage 3, more than 50% for stage 4; amount per night declines from about 20–25% of total sleep time in teens to near zero in elderly
WASO	Wake time after sleep onset

static, i.e., the longer the duration of wakefulness prior to the sleep period, the greater the likelihood of sleep. The amount of Stages 3 and 4 sleeping as well as the amplitude and number of delta waves are directly related to the duration of wakefulness prior to sleep onset and have been used as an indirect index of the homeostatic process in the elderly. Changes in the homeostatic process can lead to sleep-related changes as well.[1] The second principle is circadian: optimal sleep duration and structure occur when sleep begins at a time appropriate for the individual, defined in biological terms as that phase and amplitude of the endogenous circadian oscillator governing sleep-wake propensity. Precise measurement of circadian phase, amplitude, and cycle length is difficult in humans but can be approximated by measurements of: (1) circadian rhythm of core body temperature or cortisol every 20 to 30 minutes, (2) circadian melatonin concentrations in blood or saliva under dim light condi-

tions, or (3) temperature, cortisol, and melatonin under dim-light, bed-rest conditions every 30 minutes while individuals remain awake in bed for 24 to 36 hours and eat meals of the same caloric value. This latter protocol (Aconstant routine) controls for the effects of exercise, eating, light, orthostasis, and other circadian factors.

The Circadian Oscillator and the Environment

Daily sleep tendency peaks at two times: the first and obvious one is during the usual nocturnal bedtime, which begins on the descending limb of the circadian temperature curve; the second is in midafternoon ("the siesta hour"), which occurs about 12 hours after the middle of the night sleep period. Afternoon sleepiness has traditionally been attributed to lunch. Recent findings, however, indicate that this "siesta hour" sleepiness depends on the normal, physiological circadian oscil-

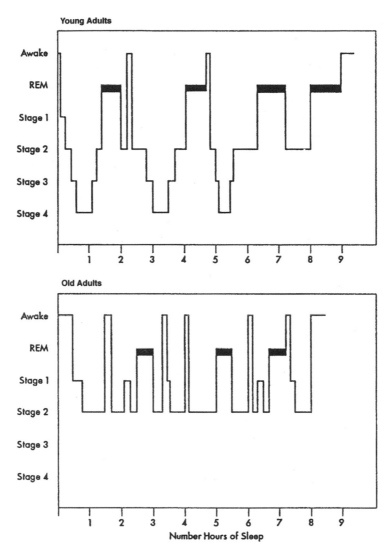

Figure 17.1. Sleep Stages in Young vs. Old. Reprinted with permission from Ancoli-Israel, S. *All I Want is a Good Night's Sleep.* Mosby Books, 1999.

Table 17.2.   Commonly Used Chronobiology Terms

Circadian rhythm	Biological rhythms with cycle length of about 24 hours; from Latin *circa dian* (about one day); examples include the sleep-wake cycle in man; temperature, cortisol, and psychological variation over the 24-hour day; characterized by exact cycle length, amplitude, and phase position
Phase position	Temporal relation between rhythms or between one rhythm and the environment, e.g., maximum daily temperature peak usually occurs in late afternoon
Phase-advanced rhythm	Patient retires and arises early
Phase-delayed rhythm	Patient retires and arises late
Zeitgebers	Time cues for social activities, meals, bright lights

lator rather than on food ingestion.[2] The propensity for afternoon sleep has practical implications. For example, napping during the midafternoon sleep-propensity period can be troublesome if individuals need to be alert; or it could be an advantage for the elderly with daytime sleepiness, or for the jet-lagged traveler who needs to catch up on sleep.

In the absence of cues about the time of day (*Zeitgebers,* time-givers), humans self-select a sleep-wake cycle of about 24.5 to 25 hours, which means that the average time between wake-up times is about 24.5 to 25 hours. For example, if a person lives in an experimental environment free of time cues and is allowed to go to bed and arise at will, that person will tend to go to sleep about 30 to 60 minutes later each "night" and to wake up about 30 to 60 minutes later each "morning." For this reason, shifts in the cycle of rest and activity are usually easier when the cycle is lengthened rather than shortened—in traveling west rather than east, for example—or when rotating from an afternoon to an evening rather than from an afternoon to a morning work shift.[3]

Effects of Light

Under normal conditions the circadian oscillator is "entrained" to the 24-hour environment by *Zeitgebers* such as social activities, meals, and especially environmental light. Information about light reaching the retina is conveyed to the suprachiasmatic nucleus (SCN) in the anterior hypothalamus. The SCN is an important biological clock or oscillator that maintains the circadian rhythm of sleep-wakefulness. Lesions of the SCN in rats, hamsters, and monkeys eliminate the normal 24-hour sleep-wake cycle,[4–6] and in these experimental animals, sleep and wakefulness are taken in short bouts evenly distributed over the 24-hour day.

In addition to synchronizing the circadian oscillator with the environment, light can also shift the phase position of the oscillator, i.e., the temporal relationship between rhythms or between one rhythm and the environment. Exposure to bright light (>1500 lux) in the evening (6 to 9 PM) tends to delay the phase position of the endogenous oscillator measured. For example, based on the nadir of the circadian temperature curve and the environment, one would go to bed later and wake up later. In contrast, exposure to bright light in the early morning (5 to 7 AM) tends to advance the phase, i.e., one would go to bed earlier and wake up earlier.[7,8] Because the cycle length of the endogenous clock is greater than 24 hours, it is easier to delay a phase than to advance it with administration of bright light. Furthermore, bright lights during daylight hours enhance the amplitude of the circadian rhythm, thereby demarcating the periods of both nocturnal sleep and daytime wakefulness. It is important to remember, however, that the use of bright lights to advance or delay the circadian rhythm has only recently been studied in older persons.[9–12]

Melatonin

Other effects of light have also been described. Exposure to bright light during the nocturnal hours inhibits the synthesis and release of melatonin, which is normally secreted by the pineal gland at night. The SCN probably times the onset and offset of melatonin release from the pineal gland under dark or dim light conditions. For individuals whose endogenous clock has been synchronized to the ambient light-dark cycle, melatonin secretion under dim light or dark conditions usually begins in the early evening and lasts about 10 to 12 hours. Therefore, the duration of melatonin secretion under normal day-to-day conditions varies directly with the photo period—for example, shortening in the spring and summer and increasing in the fall and winter. The amount of melatonin secreted per day tends to fall with normal aging and is significantly reduced by certain medications, including beta-blockers. Diminished nocturnal melatonin secretion has also been associated with mood and anxiety disorders and Alzheimer's disease.

The precise function of melatonin in humans is not known at this time; however, it may help to synchronize circadian rhythms. In a sense, melatonin may act as a period of darkness (a "dark pulse"), in contrast to a period of light (a "light pulse"). Administration of melatonin several hours prior to the sleep period appears to phase advance the clock; similarly, administration of melatonin at the end of the sleep period may delay the phase position of the endogenous clock.

Melatonin agonists are under investigation with the hope that they may have either hypnotic or phase-shifting effects. In the latter case, appropriate administration of a melatonin (M1) agonist could readjust the phase position of the endogenous circadian clock. If so, it may be possible to prevent or treat a range of circadian rhythm sleep disorders, including jet lag, phase-advance or phase-delay syndromes, non-24-hour sleep-wake disorders, or sleep-wake problems associated with shift work or total blindness.

Mood Effects

Bright light may have intrinsic alerting and mood-elevating effects. Studies report bright light to have antidepressant effects in winter depressions[13–15] that occur in some patients with major depressive disorder and bipolar depression,[16] as well as in premenstrual depression.[17]

Neurophysiologic Bases

The neurophysiologic underpinnings of sleep and wakefulness remain incompletely understood. The reticular activating system, arising within the brainstem, is necessary for behavioral and cortical EEG activation. Components of REM sleep itself are generated within the brainstem; that is, periodic episodes of rapid eye movements and muscle atonia occur in the brainstem between the upper brainstem (superior geniculate) and medulla.

NREM sleep, in contrast, is partially controlled by the basal forebrain, thalamus, and perhaps the hypothalamus and the area near the nucleus solitarius. However, no specific neuroanatomical "sleep center" has yet been identified with certainty for the entire constellation of either REM or NREM sleep, although components of sleep do appear to depend upon specific areas. For example, the muscle atonia of REM sleep can be abolished in cats by damage to the sublocus ceruleus, with the result that these animals walk about during REM sleep as if they were acting out their dreams. Whether or not this mechanism is responsible for the REM sleep behavior disorder that typically occurs in elderly men is not known. Also, cortical EEG delta waves may be suppressed by cholinergic neurons of the basal forebrain; lesions of the basal forebrain in animals significantly reduce total sleep time.

No specific "sleep neurotransmitter" has yet been accepted by the majority of investigators. Perhaps the greatest consensus is that cholinergic neurons, with their cell bodies in the lateral dorsal tegmental nucleus and the pedunculopontine tegmental groups in the dorsal tegmentum, are crucial for the initiation and maintenance of REM sleep. Serotonergic neurons and noradrenergic neurons originating in the dorsal raphe and locus ceruleus, respectively, apparently inhibit REM sleep or components of it (e.g., the pontine geniculate occipital "spikes" that precede and accompany REM sleep in cats). Histaminergic neurons, originating in the posterior hypothalamus, send neurons to the cortex that apparently help maintain arousal. Although some cholinergic neurons originating in the basal forebrain inhibit cortical EEG arousal, as mentioned, others, for which chemical identity has not been established, fire selectively during NREM sleep and may play an important role in the maintenance of this state of sleep.

Finally, a number of "sleep factors," or endogenous sleep-inducing compounds, have been postulated. These include adenosine, delta sleep-inducing peptide (DSIP), interleukin 1, tumor necrosis factor, prostaglandin D_2, and a variety of other substances. Of particular interest is the recent discovery of orexin (hypocretin), a neuropeptide originating in the lateral hypothalamus, with widespread projections in the brain tissue of narcoleptic patients that appears to be absent in the cerebrospinal fluid. Mice bred without orexin behave as it they were narcoleptic. Narcolepsy appears to result from a loss of orexin.

Normal Age-Related Changes in Sleep and Wakefulness

Age-related changes in sleep and wakefulness are important and sometimes profound. Sleep tends to be shallow, fragmented, and variable in duration in middle-aged and elderly adults compared with young adults. In addition, daytime sleepiness increases. Stages 1 and 2 sleep tend to increase while Stages 3 and 4 sleep decrease. By the age of 60 or 70, many individuals have little or no delta wave activity during sleep. Interestingly, men tend to lose delta sleep at an earlier age than women.[18] The loss of delta sleep results from a reduction in amplitude of the delta wave rather than only from a reduction in the number of slow (1–2 Hz) waves. Wakefulness after sleep onset (WASO) usually increases with aging, in part because older people are more easily aroused by either internal or external stimuli. The percentage of REM sleep does not change appreciably from early to late adulthood. Nevertheless, REM latency tends to decrease and length of the first REM period tends to increase with age.

Average total sleep time actually increases slightly after the age of about 65.[19] More strikingly, however, greater numbers of elderly individuals fall into either long-sleeping (9 hours) or short-sleeping (5 hours) subgroups. It is noteworthy that death rates are higher in long-sleeping and, possibly, in excessively short-sleeping individuals.[20,21] Speculation points to a physiological sleep disorder—sleep apnea—as a contributing element in the increased mortality in the long-sleeping group.[22,23] Reports of difficulty falling asleep tend to be more common with age. After the age of 65, about one in three women and one in five men report taking over 30 minutes to fall asleep.[24] Moreover—as people age, they tend to chose an "early-to-bed, early-to-rise" pattern of sleep-wakefulness (i.e., the circadian oscillator advances "good-night time," sleep onset, and sleep offset to an earlier hour; thus, this pattern reflects a "phase-advanced rhythm")—especially as compared to younger adults. Napping also increases with age, although it rarely accounts for a large proportion of total sleep time in healthy individuals.[25–27]

One theory of age-related changes affecting sleep suggests that aging is secondary to the deterioration of the neuroendocrine systems.[28] Decreases in growth hormone and cortisol secretion that may influence sleep in the aged, are not restricted to old age but decrease gradually throughout the adult lifespan.[29]

Although melatonin secretion at night apparently falls with aging, no convincing data have linked abnormal melatonin secretion with the pathogenesis of any disturbance of sleep, circadian rhythms, mood, or physical health. Nevertheless, reports of low melatonin secretion have been used to advocate administration of exogenous melatonin (0.3–10 mg by mouth) for disturbances of the sleep-wake cycle in the elderly, in shift work, or with jet lag.[30] Melatonin may shift the phase of the biological clock, acting as a Adark pulse. Unfortunately, neither the purity nor the safety of melatonin is regulated by the Federal Food and Drug Administration. Further research is needed to establish its efficacy and safety when exogenously administered.

In summary, the elderly tend to be more likely than the young to show objective disturbances of daytime alertness and of timing, initiation, maintenance, and depth of nocturnal sleep. Most sleep disturbance is due to medical burden rather than to aging itself.[31–33] However, in the individual patient with a sleep disorder, these problems reflect varying combinations of physiological changes associated with normal aging, primary or "intrinsic" sleep disorders arising within the individual, and secondary or "extrinsic" sleep disturbances in association with a variety of other conditions (environmental, psychological and psychiatric, medical, pharmacologic). For these reasons, chronic sleep disorders in the elderly tend to be multidetermined and multifaceted.

Napping Behaviors and Excessive Daytime Sleepiness

Sleep and wakefulness are part of the same 24-hour circadian cycle. Daytime behaviors affect sleep at night and visa versa. When nocturnal sleep is experimentally reduced, frequently interrupted, or disturbed, sleepiness the following day may increase. Furthermore, chronic sleep deprivation leads to a sleep debt that is not quickly repaid with a few hours or nights of sleep. Therefore, in older people, chronic daytime sleepiness is often a symptom of an underlying sleep disturbance. Much of the increased napping, daily fatigue, and daytime sleepiness seen in the elderly is secondary to the breakdown in the body's circadian rhythm, manifested in the advancement of the rhythm and decline in the rhythm amplitude.[34,35] Older individuals have a phase advance of about 90 minutes and reduced amplitude of about 30% in the body temperature rhythms as compared to younger adults.[7]

Over 80% of older individuals nap.[26] Although the elderly achieve the same total sleep time each day as the young, they spend more time in bed every day and must nap during the day in order to obtain the same amount of sleep time each day. Daytime sleepiness is more closely correlated with nocturnal sleep fragmentation than with sleep time. Numerous short arousals at night, sometimes not even consciously remembered, produce daytime sleepiness and subjectively unrefreshing sleep.

Daytime sleepiness can be objectively evaluated with the Multiple Sleep Latency Test (MSLT), a sleep laboratory test measuring the length of time required to fall asleep when instructed to sleep during four or five naps during the day (10 AM, 12 noon, 2 PM, 4 PM, and 6 PM).[36,37] Normal young individuals usually take at least 15 minutes, on average, to fall asleep, while older individuals typically fall asleep more quickly (8 to 12 minutes). Pathological daytime sleepiness is usually defined as an average sleep latency on the MSLT of 5 minutes or less.

A review of the epidemiology of sleep disorders in the elderly,[24] which found that many older people describe their sleep and daytime functioning as satisfactory but still report daytime sleepiness, concluded that the lack of complaint may reflect lowered expectations with advancing age—"I'm old therefore I'm supposed to be sleepy in the daytime"—rather than satisfactory sleep. Therefore, the clinician should carefully clarify both nocturnal and daytime sleep habits in the elderly, realizing that self-reports may be inaccurate if taken at face value without follow-up questions. Rather than asking only "Do you nap?" the clinician might also ask questions such as: "Do you find yourself falling asleep when you don't want to—for example, while driving, talking with friends or family, or watching an interesting television program?" or "Do you have to nap often in order to function well?"

Some age-related changes in sleep-wakefulness may result from changes in the circadian system.[38,39] For example, earlier bedtimes, difficulty falling asleep, shorter REM latency, sleep fragmentation, increased wakefulness and early morning awakening, and increased napping during the day are all consistent with the hypothesis that the endogenous cycle length (interval between sleep onset from one day to the next) of the endogenous circadian oscillator is shorter than normal in the elderly. Other hypotheses include: decreased amplitude of the circadian-oscillator cycle; a weaker signal from the oscillator; a relative loss of influence of *Zeitgebers* or other environmental influences on the oscillator; and other changes associated with aging, such as less daytime physical activity, less exposure to bright light, and blindness. It is also likely that inducing phase shifts in the circadian oscillator becomes increasingly difficult with age. This view is consistent with the assumption that elderly persons tolerate jet lag and shift-work less well than their younger counterparts.

Formal Evaluation of Sleep Disorders

Although the family physician may be the primary caregiver for most sleep complaints of older patients, psychiatrists and other mental health professionals, internists, pulmonologists, and ear, nose, and throat specialists also see many patients who complain of sleep disturbance. Table 17.3 provides a short glossary of some of the terms used with regard to sleep disorders. Evolving clinical experience and research during the past decade have stimulated developments in the practice of medicine focused on sleep disorders, and training programs have been established to train clinical specialists and technicians. Formal examinations have been instituted to verify the professional qualifications of sleep disorder specialists. In 2003, 620 accredited American Academy of Sleep Medicine (AASM) clinical sleep disorders centers and an estimated 1,800 nonaccredited centers operate in the United States.

Clinicians can initially evaluate most sleep complaints by relatively simple but systematic clinical methods, such as specific questions about sleep, medical and psychiatric history, mental status examination, and routine laboratory evaluations supplemented by sleep-wake diaries and interviews of bed partners (Table 17.4). Referral to a formal sleep disorders center, however, should be considered when strong clinical evidence suggests: (1) diagnosis of pathological excessive daytime sleepiness; (2) chronic, severe, intractable insomnia; certain organic conditions such as sleep apnea, REM sleep behavior disorder, or periodic leg movements (PLM) during sleep.

When evaluating the sleep disorder complaint, two issues are particularly important. The first question is: how long has the patient had the sleep disorder? Transient and short term insomnias, for example, usually occur in persons undergoing stress or other disruptions, such as jet lag, admission to a hospital, or acute pain. However, chronic hypersomnia, excessive daytime sleepiness, or insomnia (lasting for about 3 weeks or more) are frequently associated with psychiatric conditions, medical disorders, abuse of alcohol or sedatives, iatrogenic side effects of drugs, disturbances of the circadian sleep-wake cycle, sleep apnea, or PLM during sleep. By their nature, chronic sleep disorders may be complicated.

The second question in assessing a sleep disorder complaint is: does the patient suffer from any other disorders? That is, is the sleep disorder associated with another medical, psychiatric, or other problem that may cause or modify the disorder or affect treatment? If the sleep disorder appears to be caused by or affected by the primary diagnosis, treatment should generally be directed toward the underlying cause if possible, although adjunctive therapy directed toward the sleep problem often has a role in symptomatic relief.

Areas of specific interest in the sleep history include:

Table 17.3.   Selected Disorders and Terms Related to Clinical Sleep Disorders

Apnea index (AI)	Number of apneic events per hour of sleep; usually considered pathological if ≥5
Cataplexy	Sudden, brief loss of muscle tone; in waking state, usually triggered by emotional arousal (laughing, anger, surprise) involving either a few muscle groups (e.g., facial) or most of major antigravity muscles of the body; may be related to muscle atonia normally occurring during REM sleep; associated with narcolepsy
Enuresis	Bed wetting: Usually occurs in children, especially boys, in elderly may be associated with nocturnal confusion, certain medications, seizures, various neurologic, cardiovascular, genitourinary tract disorders
Hypopnea	50% or more reduction in respiratory depth for 10 seconds or more during sleep
Multiple sleep latency test (MSLT)	Objective method for determining daytime sleepiness; sleep latency and REM latency are determined for 4 or 5 naps (i.e., a 20-minute opportunity to sleep every 2 hours between 10 AM and 6 PM)
Periodic limb movements during sleep (PLMS)	Sleep-related periodic limb movements characterized by twitches of the big toe, ankle, or knee
PLMS index	Number of leg kicks per hour of sleep; usually considered pathological if ≥5
Polysomnography	Describes detailed, sleep-laboratory-based, clinical evaluation of patient with sleep disorder; may include measures of EEG, eye movements, muscle tone at chin and limbs, respiratory movements of chest and abdomen, oxygen saturation, ECG, nocturnal penile tumescence (NPT), esophageal pH, as indicated
REM sleep-behavior disorder	Clinical disorder characterized by augmented muscle tone and complex, often violent, dream-enacting behaviors during REM sleep; most often described in middle-aged men
Respiratory disturbance index (RDI)	Number of apneas and hypopneas per hour of sleep
Restless legs syndrome	Clinical disorder associated with discomfort in both legs when at rest or recumbent, usually described as tingling, pricking, or aching in thighs, accompanied by irresistible limb movements
Sleep apnea	Sleep-related breathing disorder characterized by at least 5 episodes of apnea per hour of sleep, each longer than 10 seconds
Somnambulism	Sleepwalking: Usually occurring in children, especially boys, during first non-REM period in association with stage 4 sleep; in adults may be associated with complex partial seizures, migraines, obstructive sleep apnea, or certain medications

1. Timing of sleep-wakefulness across the 24-hour period. When does the patient go to bed, go to sleep, wake up? Does the patient deliberately nap or have difficulty maintaining normal alertness during the day? Does the patient lead a relatively regular daily routine with sleep-wakefulness, exercise, relaxation, and work at the same times each day?

2. Quantitative aspects of sleep-wakefulness. How long does it take to fall asleep? How often, for how long, and when does the patient awaken after sleep onset? How much sleep does the patient obtain each day, both at night and by day? How long does the patient spend in bed each day? How much sleep does the patient need to feel

Table 17.4.   Office Evaluation of Chronic Sleep Complaints

1. Detailed history and review of the sleep complaint: predisposing, precipitating, and perpetuating factors
2. Review of difficulties falling asleep, maintaining sleep, and awakening early
3. Timing of sleep and wakefulness over the 24-hour day
4. Evidence of excessive daytime sleepiness and fatigue
5. Bedtime routines; sleep setting, preoccupations, anxiety; beliefs about sleep and sleep loss; fears about consequences of sleep loss; nightmares, enuresis, sleep-walking
6. Medical and neurologic history and examination, routine laboratory examinations
7. Use of prescription and nonprescription medications, alcohol, stimulants
8. Evidence of sleep-related breathing disorders: snoring, orthopnea, dyspnea; headaches, falling out of bed, nocturia; obesity, short fat neck, enlarged tonsils, narrow upper oral airway, foreshortened jaw (retrognathia).
9. Abnormal movements during sleep: "jerky legs," leg movements, myoclonus ("restless legs"), leg cramps, cold feet
10. Psychiatric history and examination, routine laboratory examinations
11. Social and occupational history, marital status, living conditions, financial and security concerns, physical activity
12. Sleep-wake diary for two weeks
13. Interview with bed partners or persons who observe patient during sleep
14. Tape recording of respiratory sounds during sleep to screen for sleep apnea
15. Review of daily activities and physical environment: timing of meals, light-dark exposure, emotional and physical stimulation, ambient temperature, noise levels
16. Especially for elderly, review:
    Cognition, orientation, confusion
    Ability to take care of activities of daily living
    Acute and chronic physical disorders
    Nocturia, enuresis, incontinence
    Vision and hearing
    Gait and mobility
    Orthopnea, paroxysmal nocturnal dyspnea, congestive heart failure
    Arthritis and painful conditions
    Depression, anxiety, bereavement
    Night wandering

comfortable? How active is the patient during the day?

3. Qualitative aspects of sleep-wakefulness. Is sleep refreshing? Is the patient alert, fatigued, or sleepy during the day?
4. Associated abnormal behavior. Is the patient troubled by sleepwalking? Enuresis? Sleep talking? Movements of the limbs or body? Nightmares? Panic attacks? Choking?
5. Sleep-associated respiratory difficulty. Does the patient snore or have sleep apnea, shortness of breath, or orthopnea?
6. Medications or other substances that affect sleep and wakefulness. Does the patient use stimulants, such as hypnotics/sedatives, caffeinated beverages, alcohol, or drugs with sedative or stimulating side-effects?
7. Expectations, concerns, and attitudes of the patient about sleep. Some patients may become either obsessed or phobic about certain aspects of sleep. For example, the harder many chronic insomniacs try to sleep, the more difficulty they have. Other patients may feel that something is wrong if they do not have 8 hours of sleep per day.
8. The sleep-wake environment, including the bed and bed partners. Are noise levels, daily lighting conditions, and situational aspects affecting sleep?

In addition, a bed partner or other individual who has observed the patient asleep may be able to verify details about sleep and lifestyle, as well as provide information about snoring, restless legs and nocturnal myoclonus, use of alcohol or other drugs of abuse, and personality characteristics. A sleep-wake diary for two weeks is also useful. If sleep apnea is suspected, a tape recorder at the bedside may provide evidence of snoring, gasping, and apnea.

Types of Sleep-Wake Disorders

The symptoms and signs of different sleep-wake disorders generally fall into four general categories: (1) insomnia, or subjective insufficient or unrefreshing sleep; (2) excessive daytime sleepiness, associated with pathological sleepiness or hypersomnia; (3) disorders of the circadian sleep-wake cycle, for example, associated with jet lag, shift-work, or abnormal timing of sleep and wakefulness, such as phase advance of the sleep period; and (4) parasomnias, which include abnormal behaviors during sleep, such as sleepwalking, nightmares, enuresis, night terrors, or nocturnal epilepsy.

The formal nosological classification of sleep-wake disorders is still evolving. Two major systems are currently in use (from early 1997–2002): the *Diagnostic and Statistical Manual of Mental Disorders, Fourth Edition (DSM-IV)*[40] and the *International Classification of Sleep Disorders (ICSD) Diagnostic and Coding Manual.*[41] The DSM-IV provides an abbreviated list of sleep disorders, which are organized into four major types according to the presumed etiology. These are (1) primary sleep disorders, which are believed to arise from endogenous abnormalities of the sleep-wake mechanisms, often complicated by conditioning factors, and include dyssomnias, characterized by abnormalities of the amount, quality, and timing of sleep, (e.g., primary insomnia and primary hypersomnia) and parasomnias; (2) sleep dis-

order related to another mental disorder, a classification identifying a sleep complaint sufficiently severe to warrant independent clinical attention even though it was one of the diagnostic criteria that establishes the diagnosis of the primary mental disorder; (3) sleep disorder due to a general medical condition, in which the sleep complaint arises directly from the physiological effects of a general medical condition on the sleep-wake system; and (4) substance-induced sleep disorder, a sleep complaint arising from the concurrent use or recent discontinuation of a substance or medication.

Although the DSM-IV system provides a simple conceptual nosology to guide clinicians toward a diagnosis, it is too restrictive in many common clinical situations. For example, it limits the use of primary insomnia and primary hypersomnia to disorders lasting at least one month and requires that the sleep disturbance cause clinically significant distress or impairment in social, occupational, or other important areas of function. This time restriction is not practical for many patients in the clinical setting. Neither patients nor clinicians should wait through a month of distress before making a diagnosis or initiating treatment.

The ICSD also proposed four categories of sleep disorders: (1) dyssomnias, defined as difficulty initiating or maintaining sleep or excessive sleepiness, which include intrinsic sleep disorders, i.e., those arising from within the body, extrinsic sleep disorders (i.e., those caused by factors outside the body), and circadian rhythm sleep disorders (i.e., those related to the timing of sleep within the 24-hour day); (2) parasomnias; (3) sleep disorders associated with medical/psychiatric disorders; and (4) proposed sleep disorders, which include those under consideration. A brief overview of sleep disorders based upon the first three categories of ICSD sleep disorders follows. Emphasis is on sleep disorders particularly common in the elderly.

Dyssomnias: Intrinsic Sleep Disorders

The diagnosis of insomnia is based upon the subjective complaint of difficulty in initiating or maintaining sleep or of nonrestorative sleep (not feeling well rested after sleep that is apparently adequate in amount).[42,43] Acute stress is probably the most common cause of transient and short-term insomnia, although patients with this condition are unlikely to come to the attention of a clinician.

Psychophysiological insomnia. Defined as a "disorder of somatized tension and learned sleep-preventing associations that results in a complaint of insomnia."[41,44] Many patients with chronic insomnia keep themselves awake with the frustration, anger, and anxiety associated with trying to sleep.

Narcolepsy. This disorder of excessive daytime sleepiness, is characterized by cataplexy, hypnogogic hallucinations, and sleep paralysis.[45,46] Since it usually begins during the teens and twenties, it is unlikely to be diagnosed for the first time in the elderly.

Obstructive sleep apnea. Characterized by repetitive episodes of upper airway obstruction that occur during sleep and temporarily stop the individual's breathing. This results in numerous interruptions of sleep continuity, hypoxemia, hypercapnia, bradycardia or tachycardia, and pulmonary and systemic hypertension. The condition may be associated with snoring, morning headaches, dry mouth upon awakening, excessive movements during the night, falling out of bed, enuresis, cognitive decline, personality changes, and complaints of either insomnia or, more frequently, hypersomnia and excessive daytime sleepiness.[47–55] The typical patient with clinical sleep apnea is a middle-aged male who is overweight or who has anatomic conditions narrowing his upper airway, but clinical sleep apnea should be considered in any elderly patient who complains of nonrestorative sleep.

Cessation of breathing for at least 10 seconds is usually defined as an apnea period; a reduction of 30 to 50% percent in respiratory depth for 10 seconds or more, accompanied by oxygen desaturation of an arousal, is a hypoapnea period. The number of apneas per hour of sleep is referred to as the Apnea Index (AI); the number of apneas plus hypopneas per hour of sleep is termed the Respiratory Disturbance Index (RDI) or Apnea-Hypopnea Index (AHI).

Sleep apnea is usually defined by either an AI greater than or equal to 5 or RDI greater than or equal to 10. Patients with full-blown sleep apnea actually may have several hundred apneic events per night, often without knowing it. Obstructive sleep apnea results from a complete closure of the upper airway during inspiration. It can be caused by bogginess or excessive pharyngeal mucosa and a large uvula, fatty infiltration of the base of the tongue, or collapse of the pharyngeal walls. The resulting decreased air passage compromises alveolar ventilation and causes blood oxygen desaturation and strenuous attempts at inspiration through the narrowed airway—all of which lighten and disrupt sleep. Hypercapnia, which results either from obstructive sleep apnea or from lung disease, reduces breathing without the presence of disruptive inspiratory efforts.

Snoring results from a partial narrowing of the airway caused by multiple factors such as inadequate muscle tone, large tonsils and adenoids, long soft palate, and flaccid tissue.[55] Snoring has been implicated not only in sleep apnea but also in angina pectoris, stroke, ischemic heart disease, and cerebral infarction, even in the absence of complete sleep apneas.[56–63] Loud snoring can be very disruptive, often causing the bed partner to move out of the bedroom. Since the prevalence of snoring increases with age, especially in women,[62] and since snoring can have serious medical consequences, the clinician must give serious attention to complaints of loud snoring.

Central sleep apnea. Associated with a decrease or cessation of breathing effort during sleep, usually with oxygen desaturation, frequent brief arousals from sleep during apnea, and bradytachycardia.[64]

Periodic limb movement disorder (PLMD). This condition, also known as nocturnal myoclonus, is characterized by periodic episodes of repetitive and stereotyped limb movements that occur during sleep, usually about every 20 to 40 seconds, involving the big toe, ankle, knee, and sometimes the hip. It is often associated with transient arousals in the EEG. A myoclonic index of 5 or more movements with arousals per hour of sleep is considered pathological. While patients are often unaware of these pathological leg movements or arousals, they may complain of either insomnia or excessive daytime sleepiness, cold feet, or restlessness during sleep.[65–68] This disorder may be particularly common in elderly people.

Restless legs syndrome. Associated with disagreeable sensations in the lower legs, feet, or thighs that occur in a recumbent or resting position and cause an almost irresistible urge to move the legs.[69] This condition usually accompanies PLMD and begins in middle age. It may be frequent in patients with uremia and rheumatoid arthritis or in pregnant women.

Dyssomnias: Extrinsic Sleep Disorders

Environmental sleep disorder. Associated with disturbing environmental factors such as noise, extremes of temperature, light, movement, or need to maintain vigilance.

Altitude insomnia. Associated with mountain sickness, which occurs upon attaining high altitude without adequate acclimatization.[70,71] It may be associated with pulmonary edema or periodic breathing during sleep.

Hypnotic dependent sleep disorder. Associated with tolerance to or withdrawal from hypnotic medications. Rebound insomnia—usually a brief period of transient insomnia upon abrupt discontinuation of hypnotics—is especially common with short-acting benzodiazepine such as triazolam or lorazepam.

Stimulant-dependent sleep disorder. This may occur with caffeinated beverages, amphetamines or cocaine, ephedrine, thyroid hormone, theophylline, fluoxetine, or other drugs with arousing properties.

Alcohol-dependent sleep disorder. This results from, in an effort to initiate sleep, repeated self-administration of ethanol in the late evening. In small amounts, alcohol does induce sleep, but sleep is difficult to maintain because of alcohol in the blood level falling during the course of the sleep period. Alcohol-induced gastric irritation or headache may also awaken the older person. In addition, alcohol may exacerbate sleep apnea or increase upper airway resistance during sleep. For these reasons, clinicians should always inquire about alcohol consumption when evaluating patients with sleep complaints. Tolerance develops with repeated nightly administration of alcohol, and the patient usually shows frequent awakening (particularly during REM sleep in the last half of the night), increased slow-wave sleep, and marked sleep disruption during withdrawal. This disorder should be distinguished from alcoholism.

Dyssomnias: Circadian Rhythm Sleep Disorders

Time zone change (jet lag) syndrome. This may be associated with difficulty initiating or maintaining sleep or with daytime sleepiness, impaired performance, and gastrointestinal disturbance following rapid transmeridian flights.[72,73] Individuals over the age of 50 appear to be more vulnerable to jet lag than younger persons.

Shift work sleep disorder. Related to unusual or changing work schedules, and can result in insomnia, chronic sleep debt, impaired performance, somatic complaints, poor morale, and excessive use of hypnotics, stimulants, and alcohol.[73-75] Older individuals appear to be more vulnerable than younger persons.

Delayed sleep phase syndrome. An apparently rare disorder in the elderly, the major sleep period is delayed in relation to normal bedtimes but is not inherently curtailed (if, for example, the patient sleeps from 3 AM to 11 AM).

Advanced sleep phase syndrome. The major sleep period is advanced in relation to normal clock time.[76] For example, the patient normally sleeps from 7–8 PM to 2–3 AM. This disorder appears to be more common in older than in younger people.[77]

Non-24-hour sleep-wake syndrome. This is is relatively rare. Patients tend to go to sleep 1 to 2 hours later each "night" and arise 1 to 2 hours later each "morning." Like the normal subject in a time-free environment, these "free-running" individuals live a day with a cycle length of about 24.5 to 26 hours. The condition tends to occur in socially or linguistically isolated individuals, the blind, and especially in the elderly.

Parasomnias

Sleep starts. Sometimes called hypnogogic jerks, are brief, sudden contractions of the legs or, less commonly, the arms and head associated with sleep onset.

Nocturnal leg cramps. Painful sensations of muscular tightness or tension, usually in the foot or calf, that occurs during sleep. They may be associated with prior vigorous exercise, pregnancy, diabetes, meta-

bolic disorders, neuromuscular disorders, arthritis, or Parkinson's disease. They may occur for the first time in the elderly.

Sleep-related painful erections. These may be associated with Peyronie's disease, although pathology is usually not known. This condition typically begins after the age of 40.

REM sleep behavior disorder. Described only recently, this disorder is characterized by intermittent loss of muscle atonia during REM sleep and by the appearance of elaborate motor activity associated with dreaming. The individual may run, leap, or punch as he "acts out" a dream, with risk of possible injury to self or others. The idiopathic form typically develops in the sixth or seventh decade in males. It has also been associated with withdrawal from alcohol or sedatives, during treatment with tricyclic antidepressants and biperiden, and various neurological disorders (including dementia), Parkinson's disease, subarachnoid hemorrhage, ischemic cerebrovascular disease, or degenerative disorders.

Sleep-related abnormal swallowing syndrome. Patients experience coughing, choking, and brief arousals during sleep as a result of inadequate swallowing of saliva. This condition appears to be relatively rare and to begin in middle age. Aspiration may result.

Medical/Psychiatric Sleep Disorders Associated with Mental Disorders

Sleep disorders associated with psychoses. These involve insomnia or, less commonly, excessive sleepiness. They occur in patients with schizophrenia, schizophreniform disorder, drug psychoses, delusional (paranoid) psychosis, or other psychotic disorders. The sleep disturbance is usually most severe during acute exacerbations of the psychosis, i.e., an acute florid psychotic break rather than a chronic psychotic state. Patients may show shortened and disrupted sleep, prolonged sleep latency, reduced amounts of delta sleep, shortened REM latency, variability of REM time, and increased REM density.

Sleep disturbance with depression. In the elderly, this usually involves severe depression associated with complaints of insomnia. Polygraphic sleep studies typically show state-dependent early morning awakening, shortened REM latency, decreased stage 4 sleep, increased REM density and REM percentage, poor sleep fragmentation, and loss of total sleep time.[78–80]

Age tends to exacerbate sleep disturbances in older depressives compared with age-matched controls and younger depressives. For example, REM latency is typically short in depressed persons as compared with normal, age-matched adults, but the differences between depressives and normal individuals increase with age. Similar trends have been described for sleep efficiency, delta sleep, and early morning awakening. Early morning awakening in a depressed older person may be difficult to distinguish from the lightened, shortened, and disrupted sleep that may be part of the normal, age-related phase-advance rhythm.

Sleep disturbances associated with anxiety disorders. Including anxiety and avoidance behaviors concerning sleep, prolonged sleep latency, fragmented and restless sleep, anxiety dreams, ruminative thinking, and autonomic symptoms such as sweating, shortness of breath, muscle tension, tachycardia, and dry mouth. These problems may occur in patients with anxiety disorders, posttraumatic stress disorder (PTSD), obsessive-compulsive disorder, and panic disorder. Panic attacks may occur during sleep itself, typically in the first 2 to 3 hours of sleep, usually lasting 8 to 10 minutes. Many elderly PTSD patients, including World War II veterans, have suffered from nightmares and in-

somnia for 50 to 60 years. Nefazodone, a sedating antidepressant, significantly improves subjective symptoms of nightmares and sleep disturbances as well as depressive and PTSD symptoms, as demonstrated in an open-label, 12-week trial.[81] Preliminary data also indicate that the alpha-1 adrenergic antagonist prazosin reduces nightmares in veterans with PTSD.[82]

Sleep disturbances associated with alcoholism. These disorders include insomnia, hypersomnia, circadian rhythms disturbances, and acute and subacute withdrawal syndromes. During heavy bouts of drinking, alcoholics may show hypersomnia induced by imbibing large amounts of alcohol or marked circadian disturbances of sleep-wakefulness, such as short bouts of sleep and wakefulness. During acute withdrawal, patients may occasionally show "terminal hypersomnia" in association with delirium tremens but, more commonly, marked agitation without sleep for several days. During prolonged withdrawal, patients with alcoholism show persistent objective and subjective sleep disturbances, including prolonged sleep latency, short total sleep time, reduced delta sleep, and loss of NREM sleep. These changes may persist for weeks to months—indeed, sometimes up to two years. Patients with primary alcoholism may show age-related sleep differences compared with normal controls.[83]

Medical/Psychiatric Sleep Disorders Associated with Neurologic Disorders

Cerebral degenerative disorders. Disorders such as Huntington's disease, torsion dystonia, musculorum deformans, hereditary progressive dystonia, olivopontocerebellar degeneration, and hereditary ataxias may be associated with insomnia, hypersomnia and excessive daytime sleepiness, circadian rhythm disturbances, and abnormal polysomnographic EEG features.

Sleep fragmentation is common, as is tonic or phasic limb contractions, periodic limb movements, and respiratory irregularities if the movement disorder affects the pharynx, larynx, or chest wall. Loss of delta sleep is also common and in some disorders, such as spinocerebellar degeneration, complete loss of REM sleep, muscle tone during REM sleep, or reduced REM sleep may occur.

Dementias. In the moderate to severe forms of Alzheimer's disease and other dementias, disturbed sleep at night and excessive sleepiness by day, including night wandering, disorientation, and confusion ("sundowning"), and accompanying problems of behavior management disrupt the life of family caregivers and are often major reasons for institutionalization.[84,85] Polygraphic features include sleep fragmentation, prolonged sleep latency, lowered sleep efficiency, and decreased total sleep time, delta sleep, and NREM sleep.

Parkinson's disease. Between 60% and 90% of patients with Parkinson's disease have sleep complaints. Insomnia is common, for example, secondary to pain in the legs and back, difficulties getting out of bed, turning in bed, inability to go to the bathroom, and vivid dreams and nightmares. Some sleep problems arise from the disease process itself: biochemical changes in the brain, dementia, bradykinesia and rigidity, tremor and respiratory disturbances associated with airway and respiratory movements. In addition, circadian rhythm disturbances are common, leading to nighttime insomnia and daytime sleepiness, or even to frank reversal of the circadian sleep-wake cycle. While drug treatment with low to moderate doses of dopamine agonists or antiparkinsonian agents may improve sleep by reducing rigidity and bradykinesia, they may also exacerbate or even create new sleep disturbances, such as those secondary to visual hallucinations associated with levodopa, nocturnal dystonia, choreic movements, and the on-off phenomenon.

Fatal familial insomnia. Only recently described, progressive disorder that begins with difficulty initiating sleep; it leads, within months, to total lack of sleep and later to spontaneous lapses from quiet wakefulness into a sleep state with enacted dreams (oneiric stupor). This fatal disorder usually begins in the fifth and sixth decades of life and affects men and women equally. The pathology involves severe bilateral loss of neurons in the anterior and dorsomedial thalamic nuclei. Additional symptoms include autonomic hyperactivity, pyrexia, excessive salivation, hyperhidrosis or anhidrosis, and cardiac and respiratory dysfunction, extreme body wasting, and infections. This rare disorder apparently results from a point mutation at codon 178 and a polymorphism on codon 129, on the prion gene on chromosome 20.

Medical/Psychiatric Sleep Disorders Associated with Other Medical Disorders

Nocturnal cardiac ischemia. Patients experience myocardial ischemia during sleep. Although specific prevalence is not known, clinical observation suggests that it is most common in males over the age of 45 and in postmenopausal females.

Chronic obstructive pulmonary disease (COPD). Patients typically have difficulty initiating sleep, frequent awakenings, shortness of breath, nocturnal cough, morning headaches, and unrefreshing sleep.[86] Some patients, ("blue-bloaters") are likely to experience more sleep-related hypoxemia than others who do not experience decreased oxygenation ("pink puffers"). Both central and obstructive sleep apnea may coexist with COPD-related sleep disturbances. Theophylline or other drugs used to treat COPD may exacerbate sleep difficulties in these patients.

Sleep related gastroesophageal reflux. Patients often awaken with a sour taste in the mouth and heartburn; the pain is caused by the regurgitation of gastric acid into the esophagus and pharynx. Among the complications are laryngopharyngitis, esophageal carcinoma, and pulmonary aspiration. In addition to medication, the patient may sleep better if the head is elevated by 3 to 6 inches. Other disorders of the gastrointestinal tract that awaken patients from sleep include peptic ulceration of the stomach and duodenum, carcinoma of the pancreas, and proctalgia fugax (a fleeting, lightning-like intense rectal spasm).

Fibrositis syndrome (fibromyalgia). This is typically associated with complaints of chronic, relapsing fatigue together with shallow, unrefreshing sleep and localized tenderness in different muscle groups (sometimes described as "trigger points").[87,88] No laboratory evidence of articular, nonarticular, or musculoskeletal and metabolic disease exists. Onset is usually in early adulthood, although the condition can develop in the elderly and is found much more frequently in women than men. Etiology is unknown. Polysomnographic recordings may show "alpha-delta" sleep (alpha [97.5–11Hz]) activity during NREM sleep, especially stages 3 and 4 sleep, and occasional PLMs.

Special Issues and Sleep-Wake Patterns in The Elderly

Mild to moderate sleep-related breathing disturbances increase with age, even in elderly persons without major sleep complaints. Incidence is higher in men than women, at least until the age of menopause, after which the rates in women increase and may approach that of men.

Sleep Apnea

Using the Apnea Index (AI) of more than 5 apneic episodes per hour as a cut-off criterion, prevalence rates range from 27 to 75 percent for older men and from 0 to 32 percent for older women.[24,89] In general, the severity of apnea in these older persons is mild—an average AI of about 13—compared with that seen in patients with clinical sleep apnea. However, older men and women with mild apnea have been reported to fall asleep at inappropriate times significantly more often than older persons without apnea. Furthermore, the incidence of sleep apnea and other sleep-related breathing disturbances is higher in individuals with dementia, hypertension, congestive heart failure, obesity, and other medical conditions.

Since increased mortality rates have been noted in both excessively short and long sleepers, sleep apnea may account for some excess deaths.[20–23] This is also consistent with evidence that excess deaths from all causes increases between 2 and 8:00 AM, specifically deaths related to ischemic heart disease in patients over 65.[90] Furthermore, in one prospective study of older community-dwelling patients, high respiratory distress indices (≥30) were associated with higher mortality rates and sleep apnea was associated with death at night.[91]

The clinical significance of relatively mild "subclinical" sleep apneas is not fully understood.[91] However, older individuals with symptomatic sleep apnea should be treated in the same fashion as younger patients with the same symptoms.[92,93] Clinicians should be aware that such disturbances may be associated with either insomnia or excessive daytime sleepiness. Furthermore, for some patients with sleep apnea, administration of hypnotics, alcohol, or other sedating medications is relatively contraindicated. The degree of risk is not known yet but reports indicate that benzodiazepines as well as alcohol may increase the severity of mild sleep apnea.[94,95] Therefore, clinicians should inquire about snoring, gasping, and other signs and symptoms of sleep apnea before administering a sleeping pill.

Sleep apnea, common in the elderly, is sometimes alleviated by weight loss, avoidance of sedatives, and breathing air under positive pressure through a comfortable face mask. Oxygen breathed at night may alleviate insomnia associated with apnea that is not accompanied by impeded inspiration. Pharyngoplasty, which tightens the pharyngeal mucosa and may also reduce the size of the uvula, or the use of a cervical collar to extend the neck, may relieve heavy snoring. Although tricyclic antidepressants are sometimes used to treat clinical sleep apnea in young adults, they may cause considerable toxicity in older people. Nevertheless, administration of low doses of a sedating antidepressant such as trazodone that gives the patient the needed aid to sleep may be a preferable alternative to the traditional sleeping pill, with its potentially harmful side effects.

Periodic Limb Movements

Also common in older individuals are periodic limb movements (PLM) during sleep with prevalence rates ranging from 25% to 60% in various studies of the healthy elderly.[66–68] Individuals with PLM are reported to sleep about an hour less per night than controls without the condition.[67,96,97] The prevalence of PLM is not higher in insomniac patients than those without insomnia. Complaints of excessive daytime sleepiness increase in individuals with PLM, probably consequent to the numerous sleep interruptions. The clinician may find it useful to talk with a bed partner, who will often describe kicking and leg twitches during sleep in individuals with PLM. Clonazepam, temazepam, and opiates have been reported to be useful in treating this disorder in young people but their use in the older patient has not been adequately studied.

Advanced Sleep Phase Syndrome

As noted, advanced sleep phase syndrome (ASPS) is more common in older people. People with ASPS get sleepy earlier in evening, around 8:00 PM. If they went to bed then, they would most likely sleep about 8 hours, waking at 4 AM. Most however, do not go to bed early even though tired, staying up until 10 to 11:00 PM; their bodies however still wake up at 4 AM. In this way, older people are essentially depriving themselves of sleep by not allowing enough time in bed to get sufficient sleep during the body's correct circadian phase.

Since light is such a strong *Zeitgeber,* appropriately timed exposure to bright light can influence phase and amplitude of the circadian timing system.[7] Specifically, bright light exposure in the evening delays the circadian rhythm, i.e., pushes the rhythm backward so that the individual is no longer sleepy early in the evening. Two hours of evening bright light exposure (of at least 2500 lux) have been found beneficial for sleep maintenance insomnia in healthy older individuals.[12]

Falls, Fractures, and Napping

Always a risk for the elderly, especially women, falls and fractures may be particularly likely to happen during the sleep period as the individual goes to the bathroom or walks about the house. Sedating medications, including hypnotics or drugs with hypotensive effects, increase the risk of falls.

While elective afternoon naps may be restorative for older people, especially very frail elderly persons, prolonged naps may actually interfere with falling asleep at bedtime. The clinician should evaluate the pros and cons of napping in the individual patient.

Circadian Factors and Blindness

In evaluating elderly patients with sleep-wake disorders, clinicians should consider factors that affect the circadian system. Living conditions or loss of sight or hearing may rob the elderly individual of circadian cues. For example, some normal elderly women and men experience only 45 minutes and 90 minutes of bright light per day, respectively; ambulatory AD patients living at home are exposed to only 30 minutes per day on average.[98,99] Chronically ill, institutionalized patients average less than 2 minutes of bright light per day. In a study of nursing home patients, one patient's wife wheeled him outside and exposed him to 11 minutes of bright light exposure, thus increasing the mean bright light exposure for the entire sample.[100]

Approximately 25% to 50% of fully blind individuals develop a "free-running" suprachiasmatic oscillator or circadian clock, since their endogenous oscillator is no longer synchronized to the outside world by light. Affected individuals who attempt to maintain a conventional sleep-wake pattern (10–11 PM to 6–7 AM sleep period) go in and out of phase with the circadian clock which goes around the 24-hour clock about every 3 weeks. Carefully timed administration of oral melatonin can synchronize the endogenous circadian clock with the exogenous 24-hour clock.[101]

Dementia and Sleep

Evidence demonstrates that dementia affects sleep differently than the normal aging process.[34] The sleep/wake rhythm in moderate to severe AD patients has been found to be extremely disturbed.[100,102,103] When compared to nondemented individuals, the waking EEG of dementia patients typically shows abundant, diffuse slow activity and decreased alpha frequency.[104] This slowing of EEG activity in dementia may cause difficulty in distinguishing wake from sleep and differentiating between sleep stages. Temporal asymmetry frequently appears in both the waking and REM sleep EEG.[105] Additionally, abnormalities in REM sleep measures (including REM percent and REM latency) are often found in AD patients and may present only in the more severe stages of the disease.[106]

Demented patients who are also depressed may suffer from even more serious sleep disturbances than those with dementia in the absence of depression. A polysomnographic study comparing AD patients with age-matched depressives found that the depressed patients had even more disturbed sleep than the demented patients.[107] In fact, elderly men and women with severe depression may appear to have symptoms of dementia.

In institutionalized elderly, sleep fragmentation can be extreme[102,103]; as noted, disturbed sleep (i.e., frequent awakenings, night wandering, wakefulness and confusion) is one of the most common symptoms leading to the institutionalization.[108] In addition, routine timing of meals, social activities, and bedtimes in nursing homes may not coincide with the circadian rhythm of all elderly residents and may, in fact contribute to the poor sleep of some. Nursing home residents are often neither asleep nor awake for a full hour throughout a 24-hour period[25,108,109]; rather, their sleep and wakefulness can be totally fragmented, similar to the sleep-wake patterns of animals with lesions of the SCN. Nonpharmacologic treatments of the circadian rhythms are being explored.[10,11,109–113]

Conclusion

The frequency of insomnia and excessive daytime sleepiness is greater in the older than in the younger population. In part, some of these changes may reflect normal age-related physiological trends, wherein sleep is more shallow and fragmented. However, much shallow and fragmented sleep in elderly patients results from an age-related increase in mild respiratory disturbance and PLM during sleep. In addition, sleep in older people is adversely affected by situational, medical, and psychological factors. Aging tends to increase the severity of the sleep disorders associated with depression and alcoholism. Furthermore, the aging process modifies the treatment options available to clinicians; for example, older patients tend to experience both the benefits and the side effects of sleeping medications at lower doses than younger patients. Sleep disorders associated with aging therefore require particular attention and knowledge on the part of the clinician.

ACKNOWLEDGMENT

Supported by: NIAAG08 415, NIH/NIMH 5 R01 MH38738-07, NBHLI 409301, VISN 22 MIRECC, GCRC M01 RR00827, and Veterans Affairs Research Service.

CLINICAL VIGNETTES

Case 17.1

Mr. A., a retired teacher in his late 60s was brought to a physician after the sudden onset of marked confusion and hallucinations at night upon surreptitiously using over-the-counter sleeping pills, which contained scopolamine, for the first time. Once the anticholinergic delirium cleared, the physician learned that the patient had suffered from chronic, unremitting insomnia for at least 15 years. Mr. A. was described as having always been a somewhat tense, ambitious individual who may have had a chronic low-grade depression. A heavy smoker since his late teens, he had experienced a marked, unproductive cough for many years, especially at night. Ten years before, he had undergone a right pneumonectomy for bronchial carcinoma, without evidence of recurrence or metastasis despite his continued smoking. He also had mild emphysema, peripheral arteriosclerosis, and well-controlled congestive heart failure.

His wife reported a gradual decline in Mr. A.'s cognitive abilities over the past 12 years or so but he was still socially appropriate, interested in current events, and capable of the normal activities of daily living. Because of his physical problems, he no longer exercised or walked for any distance on a regular basis. For his chronic cough, he used a codeine-containing cough medicine on a daily basis. He had also received barbiturates, chloral hydrate, chlordiazepoxide, diazepam, and trifluoperazine in low doses at various times to control his tension and insomnia, but none had been very helpful. He drank a cocktail at lunch and 2 to 3 cocktails at dinner each night.

He normally retired about 10 PM and arose about 8 AM, but reported difficulty sleeping in the middle and end of the night. His wife reported that he snored lightly at times during the night and appeared to be restless in his sleep. He had habitually napped for about an hour every afternoon since his mid 40s. Recently he had been seen dozing off briefly during the day on occasion. He expressed moderate to marked concern about his ''insomnia'' and inability to sleep well at night.

This patient illustrates the complexity of evaluating and managing the sleep complaints of many elderly individuals. To what extent does this patient suffer from insomnia, excessive daytime sleepiness, or both? Is he trying too hard to go to sleep? Does he suffer from a specific sleep disorder, such as a sleep related breathing disorder or periodic leg movements? The clinician must evaluate the relative importance of the many factors known to affect sleep and wakefulness, such as the patient's character traits, anxiety, mood disturbance, cognitive decline, cardiovascular and respiratory difficulties, the impact of multiple pharmacologic agents, use of cigarettes and alcohol, and lifestyle (including lack of exercise).

Case 17.2

Mr. B., a 68-year old bipolar patient, who had been well controlled on lithium for many years, volunteered to participate in a sleep laboratory study. During the medical and psychiatric history, he mentioned that he experienced difficulty staying awake while reading or watching television for the last year, even though he was motivated to stay awake and did not suffer from insomnia. His roommate confirmed that he did doze off frequently during the day and that he had been less physically active for the past year or so. Furthermore, the roommate reported that Mr. B. snored heavily and appeared to gasp and snort loudly at times during the night. Polysomnographic recordings revealed that the patient had a sleep apnea index of 25 apneic episodes per hour, a mean nocturnal oxygen saturation of 81%, and a mean MSL of 3.5 minutes, confirming the presumptive diagnosis of obstructive sleep apnea syndrome. Further history revealed that he had gained over 25 lbs during the past year, in part as a result of drinking many high caloric, caffeinated beverages consequent to polydipsia and lithium-induced polyuria.

Mr. B. illustrates the ease with which loss of energy and daytime sleepiness may be attributed erroneously to psychomotor retardation, depression, ''laziness,'' aging, a boring environment, sedating effects of drugs, obesity, or many other plausible factors and miss the most important diagnosis—sleep apnea.

Case 17.3

Mr. C., a 61-year old professional man complained of difficulty maintaining sleep for the past year. He associated this with anxiety about how he wanted to spend the remainder of his professional career and concerns that he no longer had the energy and creativity of his earlier years. His health was good and he denied past psychiatric difficulties.

Mr. C. said that his wife had complained about occasional snoring, but he denied daytime sleepiness. He was not using any medications but admitted to having 1 or 2 highballs each night at bedtime to help him sleep. Once he was persuaded to abandon the bedtime alcohol he reported that he slept much better. A neurological and mental status examination failed to reveal any evidence of dementia, which reassured the patient to some extent. Further progress resulted from several discussions with a physician about his future plans.

Mr. C. illustrates a number of common problems in older individuals that may contribute to insomnia: anxiety and concern about aging and possible dementia, reflections on career disappointments as retirement is anticipated, mild depression, and the role of alcohol as a self-medication for insomnia. Although alcohol may have sedative effects in some people, it is often counterproductive because of its short half-life, causing early morning insomnia. It also may induce or intensify sleep apnea by inhibiting the muscles of the upper airway which maintain patency, and may cause gastric irritation and nocturia. Mr. C. also benefited from the opportunity to talk with a clinician about age-related life issues such as these.

References

1. Buysse DJ, Monk TH, Reynolds CF, III, et al. Patterns of sleep episodes in young and elderly adults during a 36-hour constant routine. *Sleep* 1993;16:632–637.
2. Zulley J, Campbell SS. Napping behavior during "spontaneous internal desynchronization": sleep remains in synchrony with body temperature. *Hum Neurobiol* 1985;4:123–126.
3. Czeisler CA, Moore-Ede MC, Coleman RM. Rotating shift work schedules that disrupt sleep are improved by applying circadian princples. *Science* 1982;217:460–463.
4. Tobler I, Borbely AA, Groos G. The effect of sleep deprivation on sleep in rats with suprachiasmatic lesions. *Neurosci Lett* 1983;42:49–54.
5. Mistlberger RE, Bergmann BM, Waldenar W, et al. Recovery sleep following sleep deprivation in intact and suprachiasmatic nuclei lesioned rats. *Sleep* 1983;6:217–233.
6. Albers HE, Lydic R, Gander PH, et al. Role of the suprachiasmatic nuclei in the circadian timing system of the squirrel monkey. The generation of rhythmicity. *Brain Res* 1984;300: 275–284.
7. Czeisler CA, Kronauer RE, Allan JS, et al. Bright light induction of strong (type 0) resetting of the human circadian pacemaker. *Science* 1989; 244:1328–1332.
8. Drennan M, Kripke DF, Gillin JC. Bright light can delay human temperature rhythm independent of sleep. *Am J Physiol* 1989;257: 136–141.
9. Ancoli-Israel S, Jones DW, Hanger M, et al. Sleep in the nursing home. In: Kuna ST, Suratt PM, Remmers JE, eds. *Sleep and respiration in aging adults.* New York: Elsevier, 1991;10:77–84.
10. Satlin A, Volicer L, Ross V, et al. Bright light treatment of behavioral and sleep disturbances in patients with Alzheimer's disease. *Am J Psychiatry* 1992;149:1028–1032.
11. Okawa M, Hishikawa Y, Hozumi S, et al. Sleep-wake rhythm disorder and phototherapy in elderly patients with dementia. *Bio Psych* 1991;1: 837–840.
12. Campbell SS, Terman M, Lewy AJ, et al. Light treatment for sleep disorders: consensus report. V. Age-related disturbances. *J Biol Rhythms* 1995;10:151–154.
13. Rosenthal NE, Sack DA, Carpenter CJ, et al. Antidepressant effects of light in seasonal affective disorder. *Am J Psychiatry* 1985;142:163–170.
14. Lewy AJ, Sack RL, Singer CM, et al. Winter depression and the phase-shift hypothesis for bright light's therapeutic effects: history, theory, and experimental evidence. *J Biol Rhythms* 1988;3:121–134.
15. Lam RW, Kripke DF, Gillin JC. Phototherapy for depressive disorders: a review. *Can J Psychiatry* 1989;34:140–147.
16. Kripke DF, Mullaney DJ, Klauber MR, et al. Controlled trial of bright light for nonseasonal major depressive disorders. *Biol Psychiatry* 1992; 31:119–134.
17. Parry BL. Light therapy of premenstrual depression. In: Wetterberg L, ed. *Light and biological rhythms in man.* Stockholm: Pergamon Press, 1993:401–409.
18. Mourtazaev MS, Kemp B, Zwinderman AH, et al. Age and gender affect different characteristics of slow waves in the sleep EEG. *Sleep* 1995; 18:557–564.
19. Webb WB. Age-related changes in sleep. *Clin Geriatric Med* 1989;5:275–287.
20. Kripke DF, Simons RN, Garfinkel L, et al. Short and long sleep and sleeping pills: is increased mortality associated? *Arch Gen Psychiatry* 1979; 36:103–116.
21. Kripke DF, Garfinkel L, Wingard DL, et al. Mortality associated with sleep duration and insomnia. *Arch Gen Psychiatry* 2002;59:131–136.
22. Kripke DF, Ancoli-Israel S, Mason W, Messin S. Sleep related mortality and morbidity in the aged. In: Chase MH, Weitzman ED, eds. *Sleep*

disorders: Basic and clinical research. New York: Spectrum, 1983:415–429.

23. Kripke DF. Epidemiology of sleep apnea among the aged: is sleep apnea a fatal disorder? In: Guilleminault C, Lugaresi E, eds. *Sleep wake disorders: natural history, epidemiology, and long-term evolution.* New York: Raven, 1983:137–142.

24. Kripke DF, Ancoli-Israel S, Mason WJ, et al. Sleep apnea: Association with deviant sleep durations and increased mortality. Guilleminault C, Partinen M, eds. *Obstructive sleep apnea Syndrome.* New York: Raven Press, 1990:9–14.

25. Ancoli-Israel S. Epidemiology of sleep disorders. In: Roth TR, Roehrs TA, eds. *Clinics in Geriatric Medicine.* Philadelphia: W.B. Saunders, 1989:347–362.

26. Ancoli-Israel S, Parker L, Sinaee R, et al. Sleep fragmentation in patients from a nursing home. *J Gerontol* 1989;44:M18–M21.

27. Carskadon MA, Brown ED, Dement WC. Sleep fragmentation in the elderly: relationship to daytime sleep tendency. *Neurobiol Aging* 1982; 3:321–327.

28. Evans BD, Rogers AE. 24-hour sleep/wake patterns in healthy elderly persons. *Appl Nurs Res* 1994;7:75–83.

29. Dodt C, Theine K-J, Uthgenannt D, et al. Basal secretory activity of the hypothalamo-pituitary-adrenocortical axis is enhanced in healthy elderly. An assessment during undisturbed nighttime sleep. *Acta Endocrinol* (Copenh) 1994;131: 443–450.

30. Kern W, Dodt C, Born J, Fehm HL. Changes in cortisol and growth hormone secretion during nocturnal sleep in the course of aging. *J Gerontol A Biol Sci Med Sci* 1996;51:M3–M9.

31. Haimov I, Lavie P, Laudon M, et al. Melatonin replacement therapy of elderly insomniacs. *Sleep* 1995;18:598–603.

32. Schmitt FA, Phillips BA, Cook YR, et al. Self report on sleep symptoms in older adults: correlates of daytime sleepiness and health. *Sleep* 1996;19:59–64.

33. Hoch CC, Dew MA, Reynolds CF III, et al. A longitudinal study of laboratory- and diary-based sleep measures in healthy "old old" and "young old" volunteers. *Sleep* 1994;17: 489–496.

34. Monjan A, Foley D. Incidence of chronic insomnia associated with medical and psychosocial factors: an epidemiologic study among older persons. *J Sleep Res* 1996;25:108.

35. Bliwise DL. Review: Sleep in normal aging and dementia. *Sleep* 1993;16:40–81.

36. Vitiello MV. Sleep disorders and aging. *Curr Opin Psychiatry* (*Geriatric Psychiatry*) 1996;9: 284–289.

37. Carskadon MA, Dement WC, Mitler MM. Guidelines for the multiple sleep latency test (MSLT): a standard measure of sleepiness. *Sleep* 1986;9:519–524.

38. Monk TH. Circadian rhythm. In: Roth T, Roehrs TA, eds. *Clinics in geriatric medicine.* Philadelphia: WB Saunders, 1989:331–345.

39. Monk TH, Buysse DJ, Reynolds CF, Kupfer DJ, et al. Circadian temperature rhythms of older people. *Exp Gerontol* 1995;30:455–474.

40. APA Diagnostic and Statistical Manual of Mental Disorders (Edition IV). Washington D.C: American Psychiatric Association, 1994.

41. Thorpy MJ. *ICSD–International Classification of Sleep Disorders:Diagnostic and Coding Manual,* 1990.

42. Reynolds CF, Taska LS, Sewitch DE, et al. Persistent psychophysiologic insomnia: Preliminary research diagnostic criteria and EEG sleep data. *Am J Psychiatry* 1984;141:804–805.

43. Hauri P, Fisher J. Persistent psychophysiologic (learned) insomnia. *Sleep* 1986;9:38–53.

44. Reynolds CF, Buysse DJ, Kupfer DJ. Disordered sleep: developmental and biopyschosocial perspectives on the diagnosis and treatment of persistent insomnia. In: Kupfer DJ, Bloom eds. *American College of Neuropsychop Pharmacology: fourth generation of progress.* New York: Raven Press, 1995:1617–1629.

45. Fry JM, Brinley FJ, McCutchen C, et al. Narcolepsy and other neurological disorders of sleep. *Wake Up America: A National Sleep Alert* 1994: 252–273.

46. Guilleminault C. Narcolepsy Syndrome. In: Kryger MH, Roth T, Dement WC, eds. *Principles and practice of sleep medicine.* Philadelphia: W.B. Saunders Co. 1994:549–561.

47. Findley LJ, Barth JT, Powers DC, et al. Cognitive impairment in patients with obstructive sleep apnea and associated hypoxemia. *Chest* 1986;90:686–690.

48. Yesavage J, Bliwise D, Guilleminault C, et al. Preliminary communication: Intellectual deficit and sleep-related respiratory disturbance in the elderly. *Sleep* 1985;8:30–33.

49. Aldrich MS, Chauncey JB. Are morning headaches part of obstructive sleep apnea syndrome? *Arch Intern Med* 1990;150:1265–1267.

50. Bliwise DL, Tinkleberg J, Davies H, et al. Variation in dementia over time: overnight change in face-hand test (FHT) and sleep-related hypoxemia. *Gerontologist* 1985;25:116.

51. Guilleminault C, Eldridge F, Dement W. Insomnia with sleep apnea: a new syndrome. *Science* 1973;181:856–858.

52. Roehrs T, Conway W, Wittig R, et al. Sleep-wake complaints in patients with sleep-related respiratory disturbances. *Am Rev Respir Dis* 1985;132: 520–523.

53. Romaker AM, Ancoli-Israel S. The diagnosis of sleep–related breathing disorders. *Clin Chest Med* 1987;8:105–117.

54. Dement WC, Carskadon MA, Richardson G. Excessive daytime sleepiness in the sleep apnea syndrome. In: Guilleminault C, Dement WC, eds. *Sleep apnea syndromes.* New York: Alan R. Liss, 1978:23–46.

55. Fairbanks DNF. Snoring: an overview with historical perspectives. In: Fairbanks DNF, Fujita S, Ikematsu T, Simmons FB, eds. *Snoring and obstructive sleep apnea.* New York: Raven Press, 1987:1–18.

56. Koskenvuo M, Kaprio J, Partinen M, et al. Snoring as a risk factor for hypertension and angina pectoris. *Lancet* 1985:893–896.

57. Partinen M, Palomaki H. Snoring and cerebral infarction. *Lancet* 1985;2:1325–1326.

58. Koskenvuo M, Kaprio J, Heikkila K, et al. Snoring as a risk factor for ischaemic heart disease and stroke in men. *Br Med J* 1987;294:163–219.

59. Telakivi T, Partinen M, Koskenvuo M, et al. Snoring and cardiovascular disease. *Compr Ther* 1987;13:53–57.

60. Lugaresi E, Partinen M. Prevalence of snoring. In: Saunders NA, Sullivan C.E. eds. *Sleep and breathing*. New York: Marcel Dekker, 1994: 337–362.

61. Jennum P, Schultz-Larsen K, Davidsen M, et al. Snoring and risk of stroke and ischaemic heart disease in a 70-year old population. A 6-year follow-up study. *Int J Epidemiol* 1994;23: 1159–1164.

62. Martikainen K, Partinen N, Urponen H, et al. Natural evolution of snoring: a 5-year follow-up study. *Acta Neurol Scand* 1994;90:437–442.

63. Partinen M. Cerebrovascular impact of snoring and sleep apnea. In: Smirne S, Franceschi M, Ferini–Strambi L, eds. *Sleep in medical and neuropsychiatric disorders*. Milano: Masson S.p.A. 1988:51–55.

64. Olson LG, Strohl KP. Pathophysiology and treatment of central sleep apnea. *Chest* 1986; 90:154–155.

65. Ancoli-Israel S, Seifert AR, Lemon M. Thermal biofeedback and periodic movements in sleep: patient's subjective reports and a case study. *Biofeedback Self-Regulation* 1986;11:177–188.

66. Coleman RM, Pollak CP, Weitzman ED. Periodic movements in sleep (nocturnal myoclonus): relation to sleep disorders. *Ann Neurol* 1980;8:416–421.

67. Coleman R. Periodic movements in sleep (nocturnal myoclonus) and restless legs syndrome. In: Guilleminault C, ed. *Sleeping and waking disorders: indications and techniques*. Menlo Park: Addison-Wesley Publishing Co. 1982:265–296.

68. Coleman R, Bliwise DL, Sajben N, et al. Epidemiology of periodic movements during sleep. In: Guilleminault C, Lugaresi E, eds. *Sleep/wake disorders: natural history, edpidemiology, and long–term evolution*. New York: Raven Press, 1983:217–229.

69. Walters AS, Aldrich MS, Allen R, et al. Toward a better definition of the restless legs syndrome. *Movement Disorders* 1995;10:634–642.

70. White DP, Gleeson K, Pickett CK, et al. Altitude aclimatization: influence on periodic breathing and chemoresponsiveness during sleep. *Sleep* 1987;10:216–223.

71. Bauman JW, Boyle J. Sleep hypoxemia at high altitude. *N Engl J Med* 1980;302:813–814.

72. Evans JI, Christie GA, Lewis SA, et al. Sleep and time zone changes. A study in acute sleep reversal. *Arch Neurol* 1972;25:36–48.

73. Moore-Ede MC. Jet lag, shift work, and maladaption. *NIPS* 1986;1:156–160.

74. Fuller CA, Sulzman FM, Moore-Ede MC. Shift work and the jet lag syndrome: conflicts between environmental and body time. In: Johnson LC, Tepas DI, Colquhoun WP, Colligan MJ, eds. *The twenty-four hour workday: proceedings of a symposium on variations in work-sleep schedules*. Washington D.C. US DHHS (NIOSH), 1981: 305–320.

75. Czeisler CA, Johnson MP, Duffy JF, et al. Exposure to bright light and darkness to treat physiologic maladaption to night work. *N Engl J Med* 1990;322:1253–1259.

76. Lewy AJ, Sack RL. Phase typing and bright light therapy of chronobiologic sleep and mood disorders. In: Halaris A, ed. *Chronobiology and psychiatric disorders*. New York: Elsevier Science Publishing Co. 1987:181–206.

77. Myers BL, Badia P. Changes in circadian rhythms and sleep quality with aging: mechanisms and interventions. *Neurosci Biobehav Rev* 1996;19:553–557.

78. Gillin JC, Sitaram N, Wehr T, et al. Sleep and affective illness. In: Post RM, Ballenger J, eds. *Neurobiology of mood disorders*. Baltimore: William & Wilkins, 1984:157–189.

79. Gillin JC, Duncan WC, Murphy DL. Age related changes in sleep in depressed and normal subjects. *Psychiatry Res* 1981;4:73–81.

80. Knowles JB, Maclean AW. Age related changes in sleep in depressed and healthy subjects: a meta-analysis. *Neuropsychopharmacol* 1990;3: 251–260.

81. Gillin JC, Smith-Vaniz A, Schnierow B, et al. An open-label, 12 week clinical and sleep EEG study of nefazodone in chronic combat-related posttraumatic stress disorder. *J Clin Psychiat* 2001;62:789–796.

82. Raskind MA, Dobie DJ, Kanter ED, et al. The ₁-adrenergic antagonist prazosin amerliorates combat trauma nightmares in veterans with posttraumatic stress disorder: a report of 4 cases. *J Clin Psychiatry* 2000;61:129–133.

83. Gillin JC, Smith TL, Irwin M, et al. EEG sleep studies in "pure" primary alcoholism during subacute withdrawal: relationships to normal controls, age, and other clinical variables. *Biol Psychiatry* 1990;27:447–488.

84. Berry DTR, Webb WB. Sleep and cognitive functions in normal older adults. *J Gerontol* 1985;40:331–335.

85. Lowenstein RJ, Weingertner H, Gillin JC, et al. Disturbances of sleep and cognitive functioning of patients with dementia. *Neurobiol Aging* 1983;3:371–377.

86. Block AJ. Respiratory disorders during sleep. Part II. *Heart Lung* 1981;10:90–96.

87. Bird HA. Sleep in rheumatic diseases. *Intern Med* 1987;8:133–138.

88. Moldofsky H. Sleep and fibrositis syndrome. *Rheum Dis Clin North Am* 1989;15:91–103.

89. Ancoli-Israel S, Kripke DF, Klauber MR, et al. Sleep disordered breathing in community-dwelling elderly. *Sleep* 1991;14:486–495.

90. Mitler MM, Hajdukovic RM, Shafor R, et al. When people die. Cause of death versus time of death. *Am J Med* 1987;82:266–274.

91. Ancoli-Israel S, Kripke DF, Klauber MR, et al. Morbidity, mortality and sleep disordered breathing in community dwelling elderly. *Sleep* 1996;19:277–282.

92. Ingram F, Henke KG, Levin HS, et al. Sleep apnea and vigilance performance in a community-dwelling older sample. *Sleep* 1994;17: 248–252.

93. Ancoli-Israel S, Coy T. Are breathing disturbances in elderly equivalent to sleep apnea syndrome? *Sleep* 1994;17:77–83.

94. Mendelson WB, Garnett D, Gillin JC. Single case study: Flurazepam-induced respiratory changes. *J Nerv Ment Dis* 1981;169:261–264.

95. Block AJ, Dolly FR, Slayton PC. Does flurazepam ingestion affect breathing and oxygenation during sleep in patients with chronic obstructive lung disease? *Am Rev Respir Dis* 1983; 129:230–233.

96. Ancoli-Israel S, Kripke DF, Mason W, et al. Sleep apnea and periodic movements in an aging sample. *J Gerontology* 1985;40:419–425.

97. Ancoli-Israel S, Kripke DF, Klauber MR, et al. Periodic limb movements in sleep in community-dwelling elderly. *Sleep* 1991;14:496–500.

98. Campbell SS, Kripke DF, Gillin JC, et al. Exposure to light in healthy elderly subjects and Alzheimer's patients. *Physiol Behav* 1988;42:141–144.

99. Campbell SS, Gillin JC, Kripke DF, et al. Gender differences in the circadian temperature rhythms of healthy elderly subjects: relationships to sleep quality. *Sleep* 1989;12:529–536.

100. Ancoli-Israel S, Kripke DF. Now I lay me down to sleep: the problem of sleep fragmentation in elderly and demented residents of nursing homes. *Bull Clin Neurosci* 1989;54:127–132.

101. Sack RL, Brandes RW, Kendall AR, et al. Entrainment of free-running circadian rhythms by melatonin in blind people. *N Engl J Med* 2000;343:1070–1077.

102. Ancoli-Israel S, Klauber MR, Jones DW, et al. Variations in circadian rhythms of activity, sleep and light exposure related to severity of dementia in nursing home patients. *Sleep* 1997; 20:18–23.

103. Bliwise DL, Hughes M, McMahon PM, et al. Observed sleep/wakefulness and severity of dementia in an Alzheimer's disease special care unit. *J Gerontol* 1995;50A:M303–M306.

104. Prinz PN, Vitiello MV. Dominant occipital (alpha) rhythm frequency in early stage Alzheimer's disease and depression. *Electroencephalogr Clin Neuro* 1989;73:427–432.

105. Petit D, Montplaisir J, Lorrain D, et al. Temporal asymmetry in the awake and REM sleep EEG in mild to moderate Alzheimer's disease. *Sleep Res* 1992;21:305.

106. Reynolds CF, Kupfer DJ, Houck PR, et al. Reliable discrimination of elderly depressed and demented patients by electroencephalographic sleep data. *Arch Gen Psychiatry* 1988;45:258–264.

107. Reynolds CF, Hoch CC, Kupfer DJ, et al. Bedside differentiation of depressive pseudodementia from dementia. *Am J Psychiatry* 1988; 145:1099–1103.

108. Ancoli-Israel S, Parker L, Sinaee R, et al. Sleep fragmentation in patients from a nursing home. *J Gerontology* 1989;44:M18–M21.

109. Jacobs D, Ancoli-Israel S, Parker L, et al. 24-hour sleep/wake patterns in a nursing home population. *Psychol Aging* 1989;4:352–356.

110. Ancoli-Israel S, Kripke DF. Prevalent sleep problems in the aged. *Biofeedback Self Regul* 1991;16:349–359.

111. Monjan AA, Bliwise DL, Ancoli-Israel S, et al. Sleep and Aging. *Wake Up America: A National Sleep Alert* 1994:182–205.

112. Pollak CP, Perlick D. Sleep problems and institutionalization of the elderly. *J Geriatr Psychiatry Neurol* 1991;4:204–210.

112. Van Someren EJW, Mirmiran M, Swaab DF. Non-pharmacological treatment of sleep and wake disturbances in aging and Alzheimer's disease: chronobiological perspectives. *Behav Brain Res* 1993;57:235–253.

113. Lovell BB, Ancoli-Israel S, Gevirtz R. The effect of bright light treatment on agitated behavior in institutionalized elderly. *Psychiatry Res* 1995; 57:7–12.

Supplemental Readings

General

Bixler EO, Kales A, Soldatos CR, et al. Prevalence of sleep disorders: a survey of the Los Angeles Metropolitan Area. *Am J Psychiatry* 1979;136:1257–1262.

Bliwise DL, King AC, Harris RB, et al. Prevalence of self-reported poor sleep in a healthy population aged 50–65. *Soc Sci Med* 1992;34:49–55.

Coleman RM, Miles LE, Guilleminault C, et al. Sleep-wake disorders in the elderly: a polysomnographic analysis. *J Am Geriatr Soc* 1981;29:289–296.

Ehlers CL, Kupfer DJ. Effects of age on delta and REM sleep parameters. *EEG Clin Neurophysiol* 1989;72:118–125.

George LK. Social and economic factors related to psychiatric disorders in late life. In: Busse E, Blazer DG, eds. *Geriatric Psychiatry*. Washington, DC, American Psychiatric Press, 1989:203–234.

Globus G. A syndrome associated with sleeping late. *Psychosom Med* 1969;31:528–535.

Hartmann EL. *The sleeping pill*. New Haven, CT: Yale University Press, 1978.

Hauri P. *The sleep disorders: current concepts*. Kalamazoo, MI: Upjohn Co., 1977.

Hauri PJ. A cluster analysis of insomnia. *Sleep* 1983; 6:326–338.

Karacan I, Thornby JI, Arch M, et al. Prevalence of sleep disturbance in a primarily urban Florida county. *Soc Sci Med* 1976;10:239–244.

Kleitman M. *Sleep and wakefulness*. Chicago: University of Chicago Press, 1963.

Kryger MH, Roth T, Dement WC. *Principles and practice of sleep medicine*. Philadelphia: WB Saunders, 1989.

Kryger MH. Controversies in sleep medicine—melatonin. *Sleep* 1997;20:898.

Kupfer D. REM latency: a psychobiologic marker for primary depressive disease. *Biol Psychiatry* 1976; 11:159–174.

McGhie A, Russell SM. The subjective assessment of normal sleep patterns. *J Ment Sci* 1962;108:642–654.

Miles LE, Dement WC. Sleep and aging. *Sleep* 1980; 3:119–220.

Monane M. Insomnia in the elderly. *J Clin Psychiatry* 1992;53(suppl):23–28.

Moore-Ede MC, Sulzman FM, Fuller CA. *The clocks that time us.* Cambridge, MA: Harvard University Press, 1982:295–313.

Moran MG, Thompson TL, Nies AS. Sleep disorders in the elderly. *Am J Psychiatry* 1988;145: 1369–1378.

Regestein QR. Diagnosis and treatment of chronic insomnia. In: Gallon R, ed. *Psychosomatic treatment of illness.* New York: Elsevier/North Holland, 1982:107–141.

Regestein QR. *Sound sleep.* New York: Simon & Schuster, 1982.

Regestein QR. Sleep disorders in the medically ill. In: Fogel B, Stoudemise A, eds. *Principles of medical psychiatry.* Orlando, FL: Grune & Stratton, 1987:271–305.

Reynolds CF, Buysse DJ, Kupfer DJ. Treating insomnia in older adults: taking a long-term view. *JAMA* 1999;281:1034–1035.

Riedel BW, Lichstein KL, Dwyer WO. Sleep compression and sleep education for older insomniacs: self-help versus therapist guidance. *Psychol Aging* 1995;10:54–63.

Rodin J, McAvory G, Timko C. A longitudinal study of depressed mood and sleep disturbances in elderly adults. *J Gerontol* 1988;43:45–53.

Shorr RI, Robin DW. Rational use of benzodiazepines in the elderly. *Drugs Aging* 1994;4:9–20.

Vitiello MV, Prinz PN, Avery DH, et al. Sleep is undisturbed in elderly, depressed individuals who have not sought health care. *Biol Psychiatry* 1990;27: 431–440.

Williams RL, Karacan I, Hursch CJ. *EEG of human sleep: clinical applications.* New York: John Wiley & Sons, 1974.

Wooten V. Sleep disorders in geriatric patients. *Clin Geriatr Med* 1992;8:427–439.

Chronobiology

Campbell SS, Dawson D, Anderson MW. Alleviation of sleep maintenance insomnia with timed exposure to bright light. *J Am Geriatr Soc* 1995;41: 829–836.

Campbell SS, Terman M. Lewy AJ, et al. Light treatment for sleep disorders: consensus report, V: age-related disturbances. *J Biol Rhythms* 1995;10: 151–154.

Carrier J, Monk TH. Estimating the endogenous circadian temperature rhythm without keeping people awake. *J Biol Rhythms* 1997;12:266–277.

Gordon NP, Cleary PD, Parker CE, Czeisler CA. The prevalence and health impact of shift work. *Am J Public Health* 1986;76:1225–1228.

Harma MI, Hakola T, Akerstedt T, et al. Age and adjustment to night work. *Occup Environ Med* 1994;51:568–573.

Lam RW, Kripke DF, Gillin JC. Phototherapy for depressive disorders: a review. *Can J Psychiatry* 1989; 34:140–147.

Lingjaerde O, Bratlid T, Hansen T. Insomnia during the ''dark period'' in northern Norway: an explorative, controlled trial with light treatment. *Acta Psychiatr Scand* 1985;71:506–512.

Moldofsky H, Musisi S, Phillipson EA. Treatment of advanced sleep phase syndrome by phase advance chronotherapy. *Sleep* 1986;9:61–65.

Monk TH, Reynolds CF, Machen MA, et al. Daily social rhythms in the elderly and their relation to objectively recorded sleep. *Sleep* 1992;15: 322–329.

Monk TH, Reynolds CF, Kupfer DJ, et al. Differences over the life span in daily life-style regularity. *Chronobiol Int* 1997;14:295–306.

Prinz PN, Halter J, Benedetti C, et al. Circadian variation of plasma catecholamines in young and old men: relation to rapid eye movements and slow wave sleep. *J Clin Endocrinol Metal* 1979;49: 300–304.

Sloan EP, Flint AJ, Reinish L, et al. Circadian rhythms and psychiatric disorders in the elderly. *J Geriatr Psychiatry Neurol* 1996;9:164–170.

Vancauter E, Plat L, Leproult R, et al. Alterations of circadian rhythmicity and sleep in aging—endocrine consequences. *Horm Res* 1998;49:147–152.

Wessler R, Rubin M, Sollberger A. Circadian rhythm of activity and sleep-wakefulness in elderly institutionalized persons. *J Interdisc Cycle Res* 1976;7: 343–348.

Winget CM, DeRoshio CW, Markley CL, Holley DC. A review of human physiological and performance changes associated with desynchronosis of biological rhythms. *Aviat Space Environ Med* 1984;55:1085–1095.

Diagnosis of Sleep Disorders

American Psychiatric Association. *Diagnostic and statistical manual of mental disorders, 4th edition.* Washington, DC: American Psychiatric Association, 1994.

American Psychiatric Association. *Diagnostic and statistical manual of mental disorders, 3rd edition, rev.* Washington, DC: American Psychiatric Press, 1987.

Becker PM, Jamieson AO. Common sleep disorders in the elderly: diagnosis and treatment. *Geriatrics* 1992;47:41–42.

Buysse DJ, Reynolds CF III, Kupfer DJ, et al. Electroencephalographic sleep in depressive pseudodementia. *Arch Gen Psychiatry* 1988;45:568–575.

Diagnostic Classification Steering Committee. *International Classification of Sleep Disorders: Diagnostic and Coding Manual.* Rochester, MN: American Sleep Disorders Association, 1990.

Edinger JD, Hoelscher TF, Webb MD, et al. Polysomnographic assessment of DIMS: empirical evaluation of its diagnostic value. *Sleep* 1989;12: 315–322.

Gillin JC, Byerley WF. The diagnosis and management of insomnia. *N Engl J Med* 1990;322: 239–248.

Glassman JN, Darko DF, Gillin JC. Medication-induced somnambulism in patients with schizoaffective disorder. *J Clin Psychiatry* 1986;47: 523–524.

Jacobs EA, Reynolds CF III, Kupfer DJ, et al. The role of polysomnography in the differential diagnosis of chronic insomnia. *Am J Psychiatry* 1988; 145:346–349.

Kales A, Kales JD. *Evaluation and treatment of insomnia.* New York: Oxford University Press, 1984.

Mellman TA, Unde TW. Electroencephalographic sleep in panic disorder. *Arch Gen Psychiatry* 1989; 46:178–184.

Oswald I. Sudden bodily jerks on falling asleep. *Brain* 1959;82:92–103.

Puder E, Lacks P, Bertelson AD, Storandt M. Short-term stimulus control treatment of insomnia in older adults. *Behav Ther* 1983;14:424–429.

Reynolds CF, Kupfer DJ, Hoch CC, et al. Sleep deprivation as a probe in the elderly. *Arch Gen Psychiatry* 1987;44:983–990.

Roehrs T, Lineback W, Zorick F, Roth T. Relationship of psychopathology to insomnia in the elderly. *J Am Geriatr Soc* 1982;30:312–315.

Sanford JR. Tolerance of debility in elderly dependents by supporters at home: its significance for hospital practice. *Br Med J* 1975;3:471–473.

Dreams

Altshuler KZ, Barad M, Goldfarb AI. A survey of dreams in the aged. Part II: Noninstitutionalized subjects. *Arch Gen Psychiatry* 1963;8:33–37.

Barad M, Altshuler KZ, Goldfarb AI. A survey of dreams in aged persons. *Arch Gen Psychiatry* 1961; 4:419–424.

Kahn E, Fisher C, Lieberman L. Dream recall in the normal aged. *J Am Geriatr Soc* 1969;17:1121–1126.

Etiology of Sleep Disorders

Anlauf M, Hoersen H, Hampel R, et al. Comparative investigation of blood pressure, somatic side effects and manifest emotional state on treatment with clonidine and alpha-methyldopa. *Verh Dtsch Ges Inn Med* 1973;79:773–776.

Aschoff J. Survival value of diurnal rhythms. In: Edholm OG, ed. *The biology of survival.* London: Academic Press, 1964:79–98.

Cartwright RD. REM sleep during and after mood-disturbing events. *Arch Gen Psychiatry* 1983;40: 197–201.

Cartwright RD, Wood E. Adjustment disorders of sleep: the sleep effects of a major stressful event and its resolution. *Psychiatry Res* 1991;39: 199–209.

Feinberg I, Koresko RL, Heller N. EEG sleep patterns as a function of normal and pathological aging in man. *J Psychiatr Res* 1967;5:107–144.

Frankel BL, Patten BM, Gillin JC. Restless legs syndrome: sleep electroencephalographic and neurological findings. *JAMA* 1974;230:1302–1303.

Goldstein A, Kaizer S, Whitley O. Quantitative and qualitative difference associated with habituation to coffee. *Clin Pharmacol Ther* 1969;10:489–497.

Hench PK, Mitler MM. Fibromyalgia. I: Review of a common rheumatologic syndrome. *Postgrad Med* 1986;80:47–56.

Kales A, Soldatos CR, Cadieux R, et al. Propranolol in the treatment of narcolepsy. *Ann Intern Med* 1979;91:741–743.

Kales J, Tan T, Swearingen C, et al. Are over-the-counter sleep medications effective? *Ther Res Clin Exp* 1971;13:143–151.

Kantor HI, Michael CM, Shore H. Estrogen for older women. *Am J Obstet Gynecol* 1973;116:115–118.

Kostic VS, Susic V, Przedborski S, et al. Sleep EEG in depressed and nondepressed patients with Parkinson's disease. *J Neuropsychiatry Clin Neurosci* 1991;3:176–179.

Lugaresi E, Cirgnotta F, Coccagna G, Montagna P. Nocturnal myoclonus and restless legs syndrome. *Adv Neurol* 1986;43:295–306.

Martin PR, Lowenstein RJ, Kaye WH, et al. Sleep EEG in Korsakoff's psychosis and Alzheimer's disease. *Neurology* 1986;36:411–414.

Matthews BJ, Crutchfield MB. Painful nocturnal penile erections associated with rapid eye movement sleep. *Sleep* 1987;10:184–187.

Mendelson WB. *The use and misuse of sleeping pills.* New York: Plenum Press, 1980.

Menza MA, Rosen RC. Sleep in Parkinson's disease. The role of depression and anxiety. *Psychosomatics* 1995;36:262–266.

Moldofsky H, Scarisbrick P, England R, et al. Musculo-skeletal symptoms and non-REM sleep disturbance in patients with "fibrositis syndrome" and healthy subjects. *Psychosom Med* 1975;37: 341–351.

Muller JC, Pryor WW, Gibbons JE, et al. Depression and anxiety during rauwolfia therapy. *JAMA* 1955;159:836–839.

Newman AB, Enright PL, Manolio TA, et al. Sleep disturbance, psychosocial correlates, and cardiovascular disease in 5201 older adults: the Cardiovascular Health Study. *J Am Geriatr Soc* 1997;45: 1–7.

Nonaka K, Nakazawa Y, Kotori T. Effects of antibiotics minocycline and ampicillin on human sleep. *Brain Res* 1983;288:253–259.

Oswald I. Sudden bodily jerks on falling asleep. *Brain* 1959;82:92–93.

Prinz PN, Vitalian PP, Vitiello MV, et al. Sleep EEG and mental function changes in senile dementia of the Alzheimer's type. *Neurobiol Aging* 1982;3: 361–370.

Prinz PN, Peskind ER, Vitaliano PP, et al. Changes in the sleep and waking EEGs of nondemented and demented elderly subjects. *J Am Geriatr Soc* 1982;30:86–93.

Reynolds CF, Monk TH, Hoch CC, et al. EEG sleep in the healthy "old old": a comparison with the "young old" in visually scored and automated (period) measures. *J Gerontol A Biol Med Sci* 1991; 46:M39–M46.

Reynolds CF, Hoch CC, Buysse DJ, et al. EEG sleep in spousal bereavement and bereavement-related depression of late life. *Biol Psychiatry* 1992; 31:69–82.

Reynolds CF, Hoch CC, Buysse DJ, et al. REM sleep in successful, usual, and pathological aging: the Pittsburgh experience 1980–1991. *J Sleep Res* 1993;2:203–210.

Reynolds CF, Hoch CC, Buysse DJ, et al. Sleep after spousal bereavement: a study of recovery from stress. *Biol Psychiatry* 1993;34:791–797.

Roth T, Kramer M, Trinder J. The effect of noise during sleep on the sleep patterns of different age groups. *Can Psychiatr Assoc J* 1972;1:SS197–SS201.

Schenck CH, Bundlie SR, Ettinger MG, et al. Chronic behavioral disorders of human REM sleep: a new category of parasomnia. *Sleep* 1986; 9:293–308.

Schenck CH, Bundie SR, Patterson AL, Mahowald MW. Rapid eye movement sleep behavior disorder: a treatable parasomnia affecting older males. *JAMA* 1987;257:1786–1789.

Smirk H. Hypotensive action of methyldopa. *Br Med J* 1963;1:146–155.

Smith JW. Medical manifestations of alcoholism in the elderly. *Int J Addict* 1995;30:1749–1798.

Smith MC, Ellgring H, Oertel WH. Sleep disturbances in Parkinson's disease patients and spouses. *J Am Geriatr Soc* 1997;45:194–199.

Stocchi F, Barbato L, Nordero G. Sleep disorders in Parkinson's disease (review). *J Neurol* 1998; 245(suppl 1):S15–S18.

Tan A, Salgado M, Fahn S. Rapid eye movement sleep behavior disorder preceding Parkinson's disease with therapeutic response to levodopa. *Mov Disord* 1996;11:214–216.

Tomlinson BE, Blesser G, Roth M. Observations on the brains of demented old people. *J Neurol Sci* 1970;11:205–242.

van Hilten B, Hoff JI, Middelkoop HA, et al. Sleep disruption in Parkinson's disease. Assessment by continuous activity monitoring. *Arch Neurol* 1994; 51:922–928.

Weiner IH, Weiner HL. Nocturnal leg muscle leg cramps. *JAMA* 1980;244:2332–2333.

Wessler R, Rubin M, Sollberger A. Circadian rhythm of activity and sleep-wakefulness in elderly institutionalized persons. *J Interdisc Cycle Res* 1976;7: 343–348.

Wittig RM, Zorick FJ, Blumer D, et al. Disturbed sleep in patients complaining of chronic pain. *J Nerv Ment Dis* 1982;170:424–431.

Zaroslinsky JF, Browne RK, Almassy A. Placebo response in the evaluation of hypnotic drugs. *J Clin Pharmacol* 1969;9:91–98.

Physiology

Brendel DH, Reynolds CF, Jennings JR, et al. Sleep-stage physiology, mood, and vigilance responses to total sleep deprivation in healthy eighty year olds and twenty year olds. *Psychophysiology* 1990; 27:677–686.

Carlson HE, Gillin JC, Gorden P, Snyder F. Absence of sleep related growth hormone peaks in aged normal subjects and in acromegaly. *J Clin Endocrinol Metab* 1972;34:1102–1105.

Chase MH, Roth T. *Slow wave sleep: its measurement and significance.* Brain Information Service/Brain Research Institute, University of California. Los Angeles, 1990.

Inoue S, Schneider-Helmert D. *Sleep peptides: basic and clinical approaches.* Tokyo: Japan Scientific Societies Press, 1988.

Lydic R, Biebuyck JF. *Clinical physiology of sleep.* Baltimore: American Physiological Society, 1988.

Sleep Apnea

Ancoli-Israel S, Kripke DF, Mason W, et al. Sleep apnea and nocturnal myoclonus in a senior population. *Sleep* 1981;4:349–358.

Ancoli-Israel S, Klauber MR, Butters N, et al. Dementia in institutionalized elderly: relation to sleep apnea. *J Am Geriatr Soc* 1991;39:258–263.

Bassetti C, Aldrich MS, Chervin RD, et al. Sleep apnea in patients with transient ischemic attack and stroke: a prospective study of 59 patients. *Neurology* 1996;47:1167–1173.

Bixler EO, Vgontzas AN, Ten HT, et al. Effects of age on sleep apnea in men, I: prevalence and severity. *Am J Respir Crit Care Med* 1998;157: 144–148.

Dyken ME, Somers VK, Yamada T, et al. Investigating the relationship between stroke and obstructive sleep apnea. *Stroke* 1996;27:401–407.

He J, Kryger MH, Zorick FJ, et al. Mortality and apnea index in obstructive sleep apnea: experience in 385 male patients. *Chest* 1988;94:9–14.

Issa F, Sullivan C. Reversal of central sleep apnea using nasal CPAP. *Chest* 1986;90:165–171.

Kales A, Bixler EO, Cadieux RJ, et al. Sleep apnea in a hypertensive population. *Lancet* 1984;2: 1005–1008.

Kales A, Caldwell AB, Cadieux RJ, et al. Severe obstructive sleep apnea. II: Associated psychopathology and psychosocial consequences. *J Chron Dis* 1985;38:427–434.

Klink M, Quan SF. Prevalence of reported sleep disturbances in a general adult population and their relationship to obstructive airways diseases. *Chest* 1987;91:540–546.

Mohsenin V, Valor R. Sleep apnea in patients with hemispheric stroke. *Arch Phys Med Rehabil* 1995; 76:71–76.

Smallwood RG, Vitiello MV, Giblin EC, et al. Sleep apnea: relationship to age, sex, and Alzheimer's dementia. *Sleep* 1983;6:16–22.

Stone J, Morin CM, Hart RP, et al. Neuropsychological functioning in older insomniacs with or without obstructive sleep apnea. *Psychol Aging* 1994; 9:231–236.

Sullivan CE, Issa FG. Obstructive sleep apnea. *Clin Chest Med* 1985;6:633–650.

Williams RL, Karacan I, Hursch CJ. *EEG of human sleep: clinical applications.* New York: John Wiley & Sons, 1974.

Sleep Changes in Aging

Ancoli-Israel S. Sleep problems in older adults: putting myths to bed. *Geriatrics* 1997;52:20–30.

Baekeland F, Harmann E. Reported sleep characteristics: effects of age, sleep length, and psychiatric impairment. *Compr Psychiatry* 1971;12:141–147.

Ballinger C. Subjective sleep disturbance at the menopause. *J Psychosom Res* 1976;20:509–513.

Brezinova V. The number and duration of the episodes of the various EEG stages in young and older people. *Electroencephalogr Clin Neurophysiol* 1975;39:273–278.

Caraskadon MA, Dement WL. Sleep and sleepiness in the elderly. *J Geriatr Psychiatry* 1980;13: 135–151.

Cohen D, Eisdorfer C, Prinz P, et al. Sleep disturbances in the institutionalized aged. *J Am Geriatr Soc* 1983;31:79–82.

Feinberg I. Changes in sleep cycle patterns with age. *J Psychiatr Res* 1974;10:283–305.

Feinberg I, Braun M, Koresko R. Vertical eye-movement during REM sleep; effects of age and electrode placement. *Psychophysiology* 1969;5:556–561.

Feinberg I, Koresko RL, Heller N. EEG sleep patterns as a function of normal and pathological aging in man. *J Psychiatr Res* 1967;5:107–144.

Gaillard JM. Chronic primary insomnia: possible physiopathological involvement of slow-wave sleep deficiency. *Sleep* 1978;1:133–147.

Ganguli M, Reynolds CF, Gilby JE. Prevalence and persistence of sleep complaints in a rural older community sample: the MoVIES project. *J Am Geriatr Soc* 1996;44:778–784.

Gerard P, Collins K, Dore C, et al. Subjective characteristics of sleep in the elderly. *Age Ageing* 1978;7(suppl):55–63.

Hammond E. Some preliminary findings on physical complaints from a prospective study of 1,064,004 men and women. *Am J Public Health* 1964;54:11–23.

Hays JC, Blazer DG, Foley DJ. Risk of napping: excessive daytime sleepiness and mortality in an older community population. *J Am Geriatr Soc* 1996;44:693–698.

Hayward LB, Mant A, Eyland EA, et al. Neuropsychological functioning and sleep patterns in the elderly. *Med J Aust* 1992;157:51–52.

Hobson W, Pemberton J. *The health of the elderly at home*. London: Butterworth, 1955.

Johns M, Egan P, Gay J, et al. Sleep habits and symptoms in male medical and surgical patients. *Br Med J* 1970;2:509–512.

Hoch CC, Reynolds CF, Jennings JR, et al. Daytime sleepiness and performance among healthy 80 and 20 year olds. *Neurobiol Aging* 1992;13:353–356.

Johnson J, Clift A. Dependence of hypnotic drugs in general practice. *Br Med J* 1968;4:613–617.

Jouvet M. Neurophysiology of the states of sleep. *Physiol Rev* 1967;47:117–177.

Kahn E, Fisher C. The sleep characteristics of the normal aged male. *J Nerv Ment Dis* 1969;148:474–494.

Kahn E, Fisher C, Liberman L. The sleep characteristics of the human aged female. *Compr Psychiatry* 1970;11:274–278.

Kales A, Kales J, Bixler E. Insomnia: an approach to management and treatment. *Psychiatr Ann* 1974;4:28–44.

Kales A, Kales JD. Sleep disorders: recent findings in the diagnosis and treatment of disturbed sleep. *N Engl J Med* 1974;290:487–489.

Kales A, Wilson T, Kales J, et al. Measurements of all-night sleep in normal elderly persons: effects of aging. *J Am Geriatr Soc* 1967;15:405–414.

Kramer CJ, Kerkhof GA, Hofman WF, et al. Transitions from wakefulness to sleep at different time of day—old vs. young subjects. *Biol Rhythm Res* 1998;29:105–117.

Kutner NG, Schechtman KB, Ory MG, et al. Older adults' perceptions of their health and functioning in relation to sleep disturbance, falling, and urinary incontinence. FICSIT Group. *J Am Geriatr Soc* 1994;42:757–762.

Laird D. A survey of the sleep habits of 509 men of distinction. *Am Med J* 1931;26:271–274.

Maggi S, Langlois JA, Minicuci N, et al. Sleep complaints in community-dwelling older persons—prevalence, associated factors, and reported causes. *J Am Geriatr Soc* 1998;46:161–168.

Mant A, Eyland EA. Sleep patterns and problems in elderly general practice attenders: an Australian survey. *Community Health Stud* 1988;12:192–199.

Martin C, Zarcone V, LaBarber G, et al. Insomnia as presented to the private practice of a general physician. *Sleep Res* 1979;8:201.

McGhie A, Russel S. The subjective assessment of normal sleep patterns. *J Ment Sci* 1962;108:642–654.

Middelkoop HA, Smilde-van DD, Neven AK, et al. Subjective sleep characteristics of 1,485 males and females aged 50–93: effects of sex and age, and factors related to self-evaluated quality of sleep. *J Gerontol A Biol Sci Med Sci* 1996;51:M108–M115.

Morgan K, Healey DW, Healey PJ. Factors influencing persistent subjective insomnia in old age: a follow-up study of good and poor sleepers aged 65–74. *Age Ageing* 1989;18:117–122.

Morgan K. Hypnotic drugs, psychomotor performance and ageing. *J Sleep Res* 1994;3:1–15.

Morin C, Gramling S. Sleep patterns and aging: comparison of older adults with and without insomnia complaints. *Psychol Aging* 1989;4:290–294.

Myers BL, Badia P. Changes in circadian rhythm and sleep quality with aging: mechanisms and interventions. *Neurosci Biobehav Rev* 1995;19:553–571.

O'Connor A. *Sleep questionnaire responses related to age* [Master's thesis]. Miami, University of Florida, 1962.

Oliver-Martin R, Cendron H, Vallery-Masson J. Le sommeil chez les sujets ages: description et analyse de quelques données dans une population rurale. *Ann Med Psychol* (Paris) 1975;1:77–90.

Philip P, Dealberto MJ, Dartigues JF, et al. Prevalence and correlates of nocturnal desaturations in a sample of elderly people. *J Sleep Res* 1997;6:264–271.

Prinz P, Andrews-Kulis M, Storrie M, et al. Sleep waking pattern in normal aging and dementia. *Sleep Res* 1978;7:138.

Prinz PN. Sleep patterns in the healthy aged: relationship with intellectual function. *J Gerontol* 1977;32:279–286.

Prinz PN. Sleep changes with aging. In: Fann WE, Eisdorfer C, eds. *Psychopharmacology of aging*. New York: SP Medical, 1980:1–13.

Reynolds CF, Coble PA, Black RS, et al. Sleep disturbances in a series of elderly patients: polysomnographic findings. *J Am Geriatr Soc* 1979;28:164–170.

Roffwarg HP, Muzio JN, Dement WC. Ontogenetic development of the human sleep-dream cycle. *Science* 1966;152:604–619.

Rumble R, Morgan K. Hypnotics, sleep, and mortality in elderly people. *J Am Geriatr Soc* 1992;40:787–791.

Rye DB, Dihenia B, Weissman JD, et al. Presentation of narcolepsy after 40. *Neurology* 1998;50:459–465.

Schenck CH, Bundlie SR, Patterson AL, et al. Rapid eye movement sleep behavior disorder, a treatable parasomnia affecting older adults. *JAMA* 1987;257:1786–1789.

Stone WS. Sleep and aging in animals: relationships with circadian rhythms and memory. *Clin Geriatric Med* 1989;5:363–379.

Strauch I, Wollschlaeger M. Sleep behavior in the aged. In: Jovanovic U, ed. *The nature of sleep*. Stuttgart: Fisher, 1973:129–131.

Thornby K, Karacan I, Searle R. Subjective reports of sleep disturbance in a Houston metropolitan health survey. *Sleep Res* 1977;6:180.

Wauquier A, van Sweden B, Lagaay AM, et al. Ambulatory monitoring of sleep-wakefulness in health elderly males and females (greater than 88 years): the "senieur" protocol. *J Am Geriatr Soc* 1992;40:109–114.

Webb WB, Swinburne H. An observational study of sleep in the aged. *Percept Mot Skills* 1971;32:895–898.

Weiss H, Kasinoff B, Bailey M. An exploration of reported sleep disturbance. *J Nerv Ment Dis* 1962;134:528–534.

Welstein L, Dement W, Mitler M. Insomnia in the San Francisco Bay area: a continuing survey on complaints and remedies. *Sleep Res* 1979;8:222.

Wever R. The meaning of circadian periodicity for old people. *Verh Dtsch Ges Pathol* 1975;59:160–180.

Williams RL, Karacan I, Salis J. The electroencephalogram sleep patterns of middle-aged males. *J Nerv Ment Dis* 1972;154:22–30.

Zepelin H. A survey of age differences in sleep patterns and dream recall among well-educated men and women. *Sleep Res* 1973;2:81.

Zepelin H, McDonald CS. Age differences in autonomic variables during sleep. *J Gerontol A Biol Sci Med Sci* 1987;42:142–146.

Zepelin H, Mrgan LE. Correlates of sleep disturbances in retirees. *Sleep Research* 1981;10:120.

Chapter 18

Treatment of Insomnia in the Elderly

Charles F. Reynolds III

Quentin Regestein

Peter D. Nowell

Thomas C. Neylan

Sleep and sleep quality correlate with mental and physical wellbeing in the elderly. They are strong indicators of successful aging and adaptation in later life,[1] which manifests as good physical and mental health, active engagement in life (vitality), and adaptive response to stressors and setbacks (resilience).[2] A recent metanalysis of findings of normal aging in 41 published studies (combined N = 3293) examined the magnitude of change over the adult life span for four key sleep characteristics. Results reveal that waking frequency and duration increased with age and that nighttime sleep amount and the ability to initiate sleep decreased with age.[3] Most elderly people who adapt well typically enjoy stable high "sleep efficiency," that is, the percentage of time in bed actually spent sleeping (generally above 80% in "successful agers").[1] By contrast, failed adaptation is often associated with decrements in sleep continuity (e.g., prolonged time to fall asleep and increased wakefulness after sleep onset), in the deepest levels of sleep (slow-wave sleep), and REM sleep (e.g., in some neurodegenerative disorders such as Alzheimer's dementia).[1] Decreased REM sleep generation may indicate, liter-ally, brain failure and correlate with decreased life span.[4,5] Nevertheless, when the effects of comorbidities are discounted, insomnia per se is not associated with increased death rates.[5,6]

Examination of REM sleep parameters in the "old old" (those 75 and older) as compared to the "young old" (those 60 to 74)[7] found that subjective sleep complaints predict cognitive decline in middle-aged and older adults even after controlling for gender, length of follow-up interval, systemic diseases, and cognitive function at baseline, with a stronger association in men than in women.[8,9] Among persons aged 75 and older, sleep efficiency and subjective sleep quality decrease[6]; even with successful aging, the ability to sleep deeply and continuously diminishes, and the number of awakenings and length of daytime naps increases.[10] Earlier rise times and more beta EEG activity in healthy seniors has also been found.[11]

Older persons who suffer chronic illness show decreased sleep efficiency and are liable to experience subsequent worsening of sleep efficiency, as exemplified by those with arthritis.[12] Elderly people with the most objectively recorded "inefficient" sleep, based on sleep-laboratory measures, tend to share three characteristics: to have the least satisfactory subjective sleep quality, depression, and greater likelihood of having chronic medical illness.[13] These findings further indicate that sleep both reflects overall health and contributes to successful physical and mental adaptation in later life. In this context, estimating the prevalence of primary insomnia has been especially problematic due to the high number of "secondary insomnias"—sleep disturbance caused by a psychiatric or medical disorder potentially being attributed to "primary" causes (or to "normal aging"). Lifestyle factors such as obesity, physical inactivity and alcohol dependency, but not aging, were found to correlate with negative sleep quality in older adults. Medical problems such as musculoskeletal disorders and psychiatric illnesses also increase reports of insomnia.[14]

Insomnia complaints increase with age,[15] and are increasing more in women than in men.[16] When controlled for the effects of comorbidities, however, age per se does not increase the risk of insomnia,[13a] implying that insomnia results from other problems. For example, divorced, widowed, or separated individuals are more likely to report insomnia than are married persons; individuals from lower socioeconomic levels also report more insomnia.[15]

In a recent study from Germany,[17] severe insomnia was found more prevalent among women, the unemployed, those living alone after divorce or separation, and those in large cities but not more frequently in the elderly (aged 65 years and over). The majority of subjects had chronic complaints, with 74% suffering from severe sleep problems for over a year's time. Consultations with general physicians, medication usage, medical tests, and hospitalizations were greater among severe insomniacs compared to subjects who had no sleep complaints. Quality of life was rated bad in 22% and good in 28% of severe insomniacs, compared to 3% (bad) and 68% (good) in subjects with no sleep complaints. Despite this, only 55% of severe insomniacs had ever discussed their sleep problem with a doctor and the proportion that consulted their doctors specifically regarding sleep problems in the prior 12 months was even lower (36%). The vast majority (73%)

were not taking hypnotic or sedative medications. Thus, sleep disorders like insomnia have a significant impact on a person's quality of life and consumption of health care but are poorly recognized and associated with reluctance to seek treatment.[17]

Insomnia complaints vary over the life cycle. For example: 15% of young adults report occasional episodes of transient insomnia, 16% report recurrent episodes of transient insomnia, and 9% report chronic insomnia.[18,19] Follow-up studies of this population over 2 to 7 years reveal that half of those with occasional episodes of transient insomnia develop recurrent or persistent insomnia.[18,19] Of mixed-age patients diagnosed with chronic insomnia, most still suffer from insomnia 24 months later.[20] Similarly, approximately two of three rural elderly subjects who reported insomnia symptoms continue to report them at 2-year follow-up.[21] Deterioration in health, persistent sleep disturbance, and lack of formal support services predict persisting depressive symptoms in a sample of 1,885 adults aged 65 and older.[22]

The increased disease burden of the elderly underlies much insomnia and includes common conditions such as gastroesophageal reflux disease, hypertension, diabetes, Parkinson's disease, alcoholism, dementia and prostate disorders.[23–26] Even when optimally treated, residual symptoms of such conditions potentially disrupt sleep. Disease treatments also risk increased insomnia: medication such as beta-blockers, systemic antibronchiospastics, antidepressants, or sympathomimetic nasal decongestants may worsen sleep quality, as may certain treatments, such as renal dialysis. Even continuous positive airway pressure treatments, intended to relieve sleep disturbance, can worsen subjective sleep in anxious or phobic patients.

In one study, insomnia in women predicted subsequent depression but not mortality. In men, insomnia predicted mortality but after adjustment for risk factors, this association was not statistically significant: men with depression at baseline had an adjusted total death rate 1.9

times higher than in the nondepressed men.[27] However, other researchers have found that a report of insomnia in mixed-age samples was not associated with mortality.[28]

Van Sommeren[29] has recently provided a useful overview of circadian factors in sleep changes with old age. A question remains as to whether melatonin levels may be lower in older adults, in particular those with sleep difficulties. However, in general older people with age-related sleep maintenance problems do not have lower melatonin levels than older people reporting normal sleep, but subgroups may be found.[30-32]

Dijk et al.[32] propose that the circadian pacemaker and sleep homeostasis play pivotal roles in vigilance-state control. Age-related changes in the human circadian pacemaker, as well as sleep homeostatic mechanisms, contribute to the hallmarks of age-related changes in sleep, that is, earlier wake time and reduced sleep consolidation. Assessments of circadian parameters in healthy young persons (approximately 20 to 30 years old) and older people (approximately 65 to 75 years old)—in the absence of the confounding effects of sleep, changes in posture, and light exposure—demonstrate that an earlier wake time in older people is accompanied by about a one-hour advance of the rhythms of core body temperature and melatonin.

Insomnia/sleep quality symptoms in the elderly might also be due to other sleep disorders, including periodic limb movement disorder[32] and sleep apnea.[33] Furthermore, if excessive daytime sleepiness is a symptom present during an insomnia evaluation, rather than or in addition to fatigue, then that should be a warning sign to the clinician to consider diagnoses other than arousal-based primary insomnia in the elderly.[34]

Insomia Complaints and Use of Medications

Insomnia—the inability to fall asleep or to remain asleep despite the need to do so—is the most common sleep complaint, and chronic (primary) insomnia is among the most prevalent sleep disorders across the life cycle but especially among older people. One in three adults reports insomnia at least occasionally within a 1-year period[35,36]; approximately 1 in 10 adults reports chronic insomnia and considers it a serious problem.[36,37] Nevertheless, only a minority of patients with insomnia visits health care providers specifically for their sleep complaints.[38] Instead, between 10 and 20% of patients with insomnia use nonprescription drugs, aspirin, or alcohol for sleep difficulties.[37] Sleeping pills are used by 5% of the population; about 0.5% uses them for over 1 year.[37] Sleeping-pill use is especially prevalent in the elderly who, although they constitute about 12% of the population, account for 35 to 40% of sedative hypnotic consumption in the United States.[36,37,39] In 1990, the National Commission on Sleep Disorders Research estimated that direct costs of insomnia totaled $15.4 billion, of which the elderly may account for disproportionately less expense, because much of these costs result from loss of productivity in the work place and other employer-borne expense.[40] An additional $70 million is spent on over-the-counter (OTC) sleep medications. Sleep problems are common in the very old and are associated with female gender, depression, pain, and sedative hypnotic use.[41]

Approximately one-third of elderly people take prescription hypnotics,[37] many of them daily. As old people become progressively more infirm or require institutional care, their use of sedative-hypnotics increases. About 20 to 40% of patients in intermediate care facilities, one-third of general hospital inpatients,[42,43] and most elderly patients in longer-term facilities regularly receive such drugs.[44]

Treating Insomnia in Later Life

Before a physician prescribes any medication for insomnia for an elderly patient, he or she should first prescribe a program of improved sleep hygiene[45] and other nonpharmacological therapies approaches such as exercise. Underlying causes of disturbed sleep should be identified and treated, so that hypnotic drugs are not used to mask problems that potentially may be relieved. (For general reviews of insomnia treatment in the elderly, refer to references 46–48.)

Treatment of Underlying Illness

Physical and psychiatric illness worsens sleep quality. Cardiac disease, chronic pain, impaired respiration, or undiagnosed depression often underlie undiagnosed insomnia. Sleeplessness, in turn, aggravates physical and emotional disorders. Treatment of these primary disorders may improve sleep, and improved sleep may hasten healing.

Some empirical treatments developed for primary insomnia might be applied to secondary insomnias. Psychological treatment of insomnia has focused on primary insomnia (i.e., having a psychological origin), while secondary insomnia, although more common, has received very little attention as a result of the belief that it would be refractory to treatment. However, self-report assessments of older adults with secondary insomnia reveal that relaxation and stimulus control significantly decrease night wake time and increase sleep efficiency.[49] Similarly, the sleep of older adults with comorbid insomnia improves with cognitive behavioral treatment (CBT) or with home-based audio relaxation treatment (HART).[50] Although not as effective as in-person CBT, home interventions may have utility as a first-line, low-cost treatment.

Sleep Chart

Collecting data from a two-week log, or diary of information, indicating the patient's patterns of bedtime and rise time, timing and quantity of meals, use of caffeine or exercise, use of medications (prescribed and OTC), and self-report of the duration and quality of sleep each day is often useful. The elderly person charts when he or she turned out the light and tried to sleep, estimates sleep hours at night and time of rising, and when daytime naps were taken. Since insomnia is a subjective complaint, this chart can both record the dimensions of disrupted sleep and measure treatment progress. Although sleep charts are likely to underestimate sleep (compared with a polygraphic recording), they accurately document the subjective problems that motivate clinic visits, and the daily charting maintains the patient's cooperation in the insomnia treatment. Observations about loud snoring, abnormal behaviors during sleep (e.g., leg twitching or confusional or combative episodes), and the quality and quantity of daytime alertness should also be sought from the patient's spouse or bed partner.

Regular Rising Times

The circadian sleep/wake cycle is controlled by body clocks. Falling asleep is governed by an oscillator that also controls the body-temperature rhythm. On the basis of much animal experimentation, conclusions were that the human cycle length shortened with advanced age.[51] More recent observation of healthy elderly under time cue-free conditions suggests that human cycle length remains constant throughout the life span, a few minutes longer than 24 hours.[52] Under normal conditions, the sleep/wake cycle will be reinforced by a regular sleep schedule. Some older persons find difficulty remaining out of bed until a bedtime appropriate to a regularly predictable 24-hour sleep/wake schedule. This may result from a morning arising time that occurs too early, based on the inability to generate sleep enough to continue until normal arising time.[53] Some evidence suggests that evening bright-light treatment may push bedtime to a more appropriate later clock time, but this has not been clearly established for the elderly.[54,55]

The patient and clinician are left to decide whether bright-light treatment is worth trying. Special light boxes that emit very bright light are available. Should the patient feel unable to meet the purchase cost, other light sources may be tried. Very bright light (two unshaded 150-watt light bulbs directly in the visual field in front of some reading material) either in the late evening or for a period that interrupts the first half of the sleep period will reset the body clocks for later sleep times.[1] In general, however, we have found no trials on which to base conclusions for the effectiveness of this bright-light therapy for insomnia, with the review specifically in primary insomnia in elderly.[54]

Cardinali et al.[56] reported that melatonin treatment for elderly insomniacs, led to decreased sleep latency and increased sleep efficiency. This effect was particularly marked in Alzheimer's disease (AD) patients. In addition, melatonin administration may synchronize the sleep-wake cycle in blind people and in individuals suffering from delayed sleep phase syndrome or jet lag. Urinary levels of 6-sulphatoxymelatonin decrease with age and in chronic diseases like AD or coronary heart disease. The effect of melatonin on sleep may be the consequence of increasing sleep propensity (by inducing a fall in body temperature) and of a synchronizing effect on the circadian clock. Although some support for melatonin use exists, the concern that the FDA has not regulated it, as well as the potential for circadian disruption, is appropriate.

Restriction of In-Bed Times

Elderly people commonly spend 8 to 9½ hours in bed daily,[57,58] although 24-hour polygraphic studies suggest that total sleep times are much shorter.[59] The hours spent in bed fruitlessly trying to sleep may worsen overall sleep quality[55] because older persons develop relatively less "sleep pressure."[53] Thus daytime naps may induce earlier rising times,[60] as if naps consume some of a fixed 24-hour ra-

tion of sleep allotted to the individual and prolonged in-bed hours may foster a conditioned association between bed and frustrated wakefulness rather than between bed and sleep. In general, patients with insomnia sleep better and experience less daytime fatigue when their in-bed times are restricted and they spend less time in bed awake.[6] In this context, however, a recent negative study[61] compared the efficacy of sleep restriction therapy combined with sleep hygiene, nap modification of sleep restriction therapy combined with sleep hygiene, and sleep hygiene alone as treatments for insomnia in 39 community-dwelling men and women 55 years and older. Although subjects appeared to follow restriction on instructions through follow-up, the authors found few between-group differences in treatment efficacy.

Avoidance of Irregular Naps

On average, 70-year-olds are twice as likely to nap as 50-year-olds, and six times more likely to nap than 30-year-olds.[62] Like afternoon siestas in many countries, naps may be part of an older person's regular sleep schedule. Naps for old people may also retrace the developmental pattern back to childhood sleep patterns.[63] Casual and irregular naps that are unnecessary to fulfill sleep needs, however, are often associated with light sleep[64] and may impair the regular sleep/wake cycle. Naps most often occur after lunch or in midafternoon, but if elderly individuals can avoid napping by engaging in mental or physical activity, nocturnal sleep may improve.

Additional evidence[65] suggests that daily habits such as short naps and taking appropriate exercise in the evenings contributed to good sleep, and that sleep health is related to the activities of daily living (ADL) of the elderly. Monk et al.[60] found that healthy seniors were able to adopt a napping regimen involving a 90-minute siesta each day between 1:30 PM and 3:00 PM, achieving about one hour of actual sleep per nap. Although some negative consequences for nocturnal sleep in terms of reduced sleep efficiency and earlier wake times obtained, some positive consequences were seen in terms of objective evening performance, and, in the diary study, 24-hour sleep totals. Subjective alertness measures and performance measures showed no reliable effects and circadian phase parameters appeared unchanged. Subjective experience of wellness appears to correlate with regular, mid-afternoon napping in older adults.

Exercise

Physical fitness improves sleep quality of the elderly,[66–68] possibly because higher metabolic rate, greater vigor, and improved mood are associated with exercise. Individuals averaging 70 years of age with depressive disorders showed an unusually high improved long-term sleep quality on the Pittsburgh Sleep Quality Index after a 10-week interactive health education program.[68] Exercise programs for the elderly, however, must be sufficiently convenient and enjoyable to sustain motivation. Gentle repetitive urging, combined with instruction about relevance and importance for health and wellbeing as well as finding fitness programs at convenient places can motivate the reluctant older insomniac to begin a systematic exercise program.

Initial evaluation of cardiac behavior at high activity rates, maximal oxygen uptake, muscular strength, and endurance and body composition should be followed by discussion of what exercise is convenient and enjoyable. Design of the exercise program considers the details of cost, location, equipment, frequency, and intensity of activity. Increased strength, muscle mass, and walking speed improve even in the nonagenarian,[69] as do self-concept and sleep quality. For the substantial number of elderly whose insomnia results from depression, a systematic exercise program may provide relief as effectively as antidepressant medication.[70] Treatments by individually adjusted doses of sertraline, or by a 16-week program of exercise 3 times

a week (stationary bicycle or brisk walking) or both modalities combined showed statistically indistinguishable improvements on Hamilton and Beck depression measures. Reexamination 6 months after the experiment ended revealed that relapse rates in the medication and combination treatment groups were 38% and 30% respectively, compared with 8% in the exercise group.[71]

Hot Baths

A systematic review[72] found that a warm evening bath facilitates nighttime sleep for the healthy elderly with insomnia: artificially raising body temperature with hot baths stimulates deep sleep.[73] Elderly insomniac women who soaked in a hot bath 1½ hours prior to bedtime had significantly increased slow-wave sleep.[74] Many insomnia patients find relief through hot soaks for 20 to 30 minutes shortly before bedtime. Water should be hot (about 41°C, 106°F), and the individual should submerge as much as possible below the neck; large fraction of, but not all, insomnia patients react favorably, sleeping more soundly. Whether the baths are comfortable or uncomfortable seems not to correlate with effect on sleep quality. Older patients should stand up and exit the bath slowly, because orthostatic decrease in blood pressure is common in older people.

Relaxation Techniques

Many relaxation procedures have been used to help insomnia patients shift from evening activity to nighttime sleep. Relaxation procedures may especially help people when tension and ruminations delay sleep onset. During middle-of-the night awakenings, relaxation procedures with the eyes closed probably help more than most other activities insomnia patients engage in, such as reading or watching television.

No specific relaxation technique is more effective than any other. Perhaps the easiest for an older person to use is the "relaxation response.[75]"A comfortable prone position is assumed, with arms and legs uncrossed and eyes closed, and the word "one" is repeated silently to oneself with each breath exhalation. The relaxation technique should be practiced outside the bedroom daily until a sense of relaxation becomes learned. This relaxation technique should be used at the beginning of the night or it should be practiced on nights when the patient feels he or she can fall asleep. This prevents development of a conditioned connection between relaxing and lying awake.

Bladder Training

With age, the nocturnal proportion of daily urine volume becomes greater,[76] bringing with it increased nocturia.[77] Nocturia risk factors include caffeine and alcohol use, prostatism, diabetes, sleep apnea, stroke sequelae and neurodegenerative disease. Nocturia of at least two voids may be found in the majority of older people,[78] but only about one-third of them find it bothersome.[79] Since the length of time required to fall back to sleep after awakening increases with age, preventing nocturnal urination may improve sleep. Behavioral techniques may relieve nocturia. Pelvic floor exercises (Kegel exercises) may increase bladder capacity and diminish urgency but must be done repeatedly (e.g., sets of 10 to 30 ten-second contractions daily). Bladder training gradually raises the threshold for the urinary reflex by progressively delaying the interval between the urge to urinate and the act. Training occurs during the day, with time increments empirically worked out with the patient. An initial delay of 15 minutes is usually easy to achieve, and this can be increased progressively to 90 minutes over a 6-week period. Drinking additional water in the morning while maintaining the delay interval, as well as evening fluid restriction, complements the training.

Other Measures

A regular evening routine prior to a regular bedtime helps people fall asleep. Although not studied in older people, some evidence suggests that evening television watching lessens sleep quality among insomnia patients,[80] whereas a malt cereal drink at bedtime may induce longer, less broken sleep.[81]

Commercially available prerecorded voices and sounds are also intended to help induce sleep. A conditioned connection between using such devices and falling asleep presumably develops in some patients who use them nightly. Whether or not they are helpful specifically to older people is not known. Tape-recorded directions guiding imagery through a peaceful scenario helps some insomnia patients.

Drugs That Can Disrupt Sleep

Caffeine

Because the stimulant actions of caffeine last 12 to 20 hours after ingestion,[82] caffeine disturbs sleep in older persons, resulting in delayed sleep onset, lighter sleep, diminished restfulness, and increased morning drowsiness.

Nicotine

Nicotine diminishes sleep quality. Smokers experience lighter sleep than nonsmokers,[83] and their sleep may significantly improve within a week after they stop smoking[84] although some sleep restlessly during the first few days of withdrawal. Decrease in total sleep time correlates with the number of cigarettes smoked; the more cigarettes one smokes, the less one sleeps. Lung disease induced by smoking increases the risk of sleep apnea. To the elderly smoker who says that the physical damage incurred by smoking over decades has already occurred, one can reply that at least sleep may improve if cigarette smoking stops. Much evidence exists to optimize the clinical approach to smokers. Specific approaches have been described for smokers who wish to quit, who wish to quit but not now, or those who do not wish to quit.[85]

Alcohol

The effect of alcohol on sleep varies considerably; it may be helpful to some and injurious to others. Although many elderly people use alcohol in the evenings to fall asleep, alcohol can also cause or exacerbate insomnia in the older person. Even a small amount of alcohol, such as a glass of wine with supper, can cause wakefulness in the middle of the night. After alcohol ingestion, sleep may be lighter, and body movements and body temperature may increase later in the night. Since alcohol suppresses upper airway function during sleep, it worsens sleep apnea, a common disorder among the elderly.

Alcoholic older people experience impaired sleep during both drinking and dry periods. In the advanced stages of alcoholism, poor sleep occurs with frequent awakenings and altered time of sleep stages. Even years after alcohol withdrawal, alcoholics have more disrupted sleep than others.

Nonprescription drugs

About 11% of Americans between the ages 65 and 79 use OTC drugs to help them sleep,[37] although there is no evidence that these drugs (in comparison with placebo pills) improve their sleep; placebos, however, do help about a third of insomnia patients.[86] Older people use disproportionately high amounts of OTC sleep medications because they are readily available. Diphenhydramine, a frequently used OTC antihistamine commonly used as a hypnotic for older persons, induces more sleepiness than actual sleep.[87]

Although seemingly safe and modestly effective, the anticholinergic effects of OTC hypnotics such as scopolamine, diphenhydramine, and other sedatives may induce cognitive impairment or aggravate preexisting cognitive loss in the elderly. Anticholinergic drugs potentially aggravate tachyarrhythmias, constipation, and prostate disorders. Other drugs commonly taken by older people, such as nasal decongestants and appetite suppressants, have prolonged central stimulant effect and may also interfere with sleep.

Prescription drugs

Compared with the population at large, older people use a disproportionately high percentage of prescription drugs, many of which disrupt sleep. Drugs that affect neurotransmitter function (e.g., beta-blockers, beta-agonists, methysergide, stimulating antidepressants, thyroid and steroid hormones) disrupt sleep regulation. Side effects of antiarrhythmics and antibronchospastics can cause severe sleep disturbance. Some drugs disrupt sleep by more indirect mechanisms. For example, diuretics may interrupt sleep by worsening restless legs syndrome. Some antibiotics may interfere with sleep by inducing stomach pain or interfering with central nervous system protein synthesis.[88]

Although sometimes helpful for brief periods, all sedating and hypnotic drugs can distort the normal circadian sleep rhythms. Chronic use of hypnotic drugs generally neither produces sustained rapid onset of nocturnal sleep nor reduces intervening wakefulness.[89] After chronic use of hypnotics, some patients actually sleep less than before the drugs were used, a phenomenon known as sleeping pill insomnia.[90] Use of sedative drugs during the day may lessen the older person's energy and alertness and blunt the amplitude of the normal day/night wake/sleep cycle.

Pharmacologic Treatment of Late-Life Insomnia

Treatment of chronic insomnia must be conducted in relation to the natural history of the illness.[91] Most drug trials have involved only an acute intervention (i.e., several days to several weeks) and its immediate results. Clinicians, therefore, have little systemic information to judge the widespread daily use of medication to relieve insomnia.[92] No information from randomized, placebo-controlled trials is available on the efficacy of acute interventions beyond 35 days. Similarly, no randomized, placebo-controlled studies have addressed the efficacy of maintenance interventions, e.g., low-dose anxiolytic or antidepressant medication on a nightly basis for 1 year. In general, behavioral interventions may have a more durable impact than pharmacologic treatments on outcome over a long period of time[93]; however, studies are still needed to resolve the issue of chronic efficacy for both pharmacologic and behavioral intervention, and no direct comparisons between the two treatment approaches are available.

In controlled research studies of nongeriatric adults with chronic insomnia, two general conclusions regarding treatment efficacy that may be relevant for the elderly emerge[91]:

1. Subjective symptoms and objective signs of chronic insomnia respond to acute behavioral and pharmacologic interventions. Both types of intervention typically reduce sleep onset latency by 15 to 30 minutes from pretreatment levels, and the number of awakenings decreases by 1 to 3 per night. Pharmacologic agents are more therapeutic during the acute phase of treatment, whereas behavioral interventions appear to produce more sustained effects. No direct comparisons of long-term efficacy between pharmacologic and behavior treatment are available; widespread daily use suggests that hypnotic drugs are prized more by patients than by their doctors.[94]

2. Of the interventions reviewed, benzodiazepines, antidepressants, melatonin, zaleplon and zolpidem are effective pharmacologic agents; stimulus control, sleep restriction, exercise, relaxation strategies, and cognitive behavior therapy are effective behavioral interventions for acute management.

As noted, most research studies of chronic insomnia in elderly patients are

of short-term treatment. Overall, these studies—constituting a total of 1,082 elderly patients, including 516 psychogeriatric inpatients or residents of nursing homes—suggest short-term efficacy of zolpidem, triazolam, temazepam, zopiclone, flurazepam, and quazepam but not chloral hydrate (Table 18.1). These key findings do not differ qualitatively from those in studies of nongeriatric adults with a diagnosis of primary insomnia.

Principles/Recommendations for Treatment

If concomitant or underlying medical/psychiatric problems can be identified, the goals of treatment are to remove these underlying problems, restore daytime energy, improve quality of life (i.e., ability to cope and feeling of well-being), prevent progression of transient to chronic sleep impairment, and prevent recurrence of insomnia. Six basic principles characterize rational pharmacotherapy for insomnia for the geriatric patient: (1) use of the lowest effective dose, (2) intermittent dosing, (3) short-term use (i.e., hypnotic medication should not be used on a regular basis for more than 3 to 4 weeks), (4) limited use of sedative-hypnotics (two to four) times weekly, (5) gradual discontinuation, and (6) monitoring for aggravation of sleep impairment (rebound) following drug discontinuation. In addition, because minimizing carryover daytime sedation is usually desirable, agents with shorter elimination half-lives are generally preferred. Alcohol and OTC agents are minimally effective, further impair sleep quality, and adversely affect next-day performance. Many primary care physicians are confronted by elderly patients who do not wish to discontinue hypnotics; in such cases, treatment can be made contingent upon increasing compliance with sleep hygiene and adherence to an exercise regimen.

Table 18.1.   Placebo-Controlled Studies of Pharmacotherapy for Chronic Insomnia in the Elderly

Study[a]	N	Age	Agent/Dose (mg)	Duration	Measures[b]	Results
BROTIZOLAM						
Mauielak et al. (1989)	36	60–72	Brotizolam 0.25 Flurazepam 15	2 weeks	Questionnaire Mutliple sleep-latency test Neuropsychological tests	Rebound insomnia with brotizolam; both drugs increased daytime sleepiness; only placebo-treated group sleeping better at end of treatment than at baseline
CHLORAL HYDRATE						
Piccione et al. (1980)	27	70 (60–94)	Chloral hydrate 250–500 Triazolam 0.25–0.50	5 days	Patient self-report	Both doses of triazolam, but not chloral hydrate, better than placebo
DIAZEPAM						
Viukari & Miettinen (1984)	20	76 (1.3)	Diazepam 5 Probmethazine 25 Propiomazine 25	3 weeks	Staff observation Psychomotor tests	Both diazepam and propiomazine prolonged sleep; no rebound insomnia; no effect on psychomotor skills
Elie & Deschenes (1983)	30	75 (1.8) (60–93)	Flurazepam 15 Zopiclone 5,7.5, 10	3 weeks	Self-report	Response to zopiclone (7.5–10 mg) comparable to flurazepam response; no clinically significant side effects.
Frost & DeLucchi (1979)	6	(67–82)	Flurazepam 15	15 nights	Polysomnography	Increased TST, continuity
MELATONIN						
Garfinkel et al. (1995)	12	76 (±12)	Melatonin 2	3 weeks	Wrist actigraphy	Sleep efficiency: melatonin > placebo
Haimov et al. (1995)	51	75.1	Melatonin 2	7 nights	Wrist actigraphy	Improved sleep efficiency

PROMETHAZINE

Study	N	Age	Medication/dose	Duration	Method	Results
Viukari & Miettinen (1984)	20	76 (1.3)	Promethazine 25 Propiomazine 25 Diazepam 5	3 weeks	Staff observation Psychomotor tests	Both diazepam and propiomazine prolonged sleep; no rebound insomnia; no effect on psychomotor skills
Martinez & Serna (1982)	41	Aged 65 and older	Quazepam 15	5 days	Questionnaire EEG	Quazepam better than placebo in increasing quantity and quality of sleep
Caldwell (1982)	57	(60–81)	Quazepam 15	5 days	Questionnaire, physician global evaluation	Quazepam better than placebo for sleep quantity and quality; no serious adverse effects

TEMAZEPAM

Study	N	Age	Medication/dose	Duration	Method	Results
Vgontzas et al. (1994)	8	67 (1.4)	Temazepam 7.5	7 nights	Polysomnography	Decreased total wake time
Nakra et al. (1992)	45	72.2 (±4.4)	Temazepam 15–30 Triazolam 0.125–0.25	1 day	Neuropsychological testing	Impaired performance on social learning task for both high-dose medication groups
Meuleman et al. (1987)	17 nursing-home residents	78.1 (11) (56–97)	Temazepam 15 Diphenhydramine 50	5 days	Self-report Observe, sleep diary Psychomotor tests	Shorter sleep latency and longer sleep duration with diphenhydramine; poorer performance on psychomotor tests with both agents
Fillingim (1982)	75 "convalescent home residents"	81	Temazepam 30 Flurazepam 30	4 days	Patient self-report	Comparable efficacy; less drug hangover with temazepam

TRIAZOLAM

Study	N	Age	Medication/dose	Duration	Method	Results
Elie et al. (1990)	48	76 (1.3) (60–90)	Triazolam 0.125–0.25 Zopiclone 5–7.5	3 weeks	Self-report	Both better than placebo over 3 weeks
Mouret et al. (1990)	10	68.1 (10)	Triazolam 0.25 Zopiclone 7.5	15 days	Polysomnography	Improved sleep with both; decreased slow-wave sleep with triazolam, increased with zopiclone
Roehrs et al. (1985)	22	67 (6.6)	Triazolam 0.125	2 days	Polysomnography	Increased total sleep time

(continued)

Table 18.1. *(continued)*

Study[a]	N	Age	Agent/Dose (mg)	Duration	Measures[b]	Results
Carskadon et al. (1982)	13	(64–79)	Triazolam 0.25 Flurazepam 15	3 nights	Polysomnography MSLT POMS	Worsened MSLT with flurazepam; improved with triazolam; improved POMS with flurazepam; worsened POMS with triazolam
Piccione et al. (1980)	27	70 (60–94)	Triazolam 0.25–50 Chloral hydrate 250–500	5 days	Patient self-report	Both doses of triazolam, but not chloral hydrate, better than placebo
ZOPICLONE						
Elie et al. (1990)	48	76 (1.3) (60–90)	Zopiclone 5–7.5 Triazolam 0.125–0.25	3 weeks	Self-report	Both better than placebo over 3 weeks
Mouret et al. (1990)	10	68.1 (10)	Zopiclone 7.5 Triazolam .25	15 days	Polysomnography	Improved sleep with both; decreased slow-wave sleep with triazolam, increased with zopiclone
Elie & Deschenes (1983)	30	75 (1.8) (60–93)	Zopiclone 5, 7.5, 10 Flurazepam 15	3 weeks	Self-report	Zopiclone response (7.5–10 mg) comparable to flurazepam; no clinically significant side effects
ZOLPIDEM						
Kummer et al. (1993)	14	67.8 (2.2) (59–85)	Zolpidem 20	179	Polysomnography	Improved continuity and total sleep time
Roger et al. (1993)	221 inpatients	58–98	Zolpidem 5–10 Triazolam 0–25	3 weeks	Questionnaire Visual analogue scale Clinician global impression	Improvement for both agents; confusion only in triazolam group; no rebound insomnia
Shaw et al. (1992)	119 inpatients	74.5 (0.9)	Zolpidem 10–20	3 weeks	Nursing observation	20 mg dose improved total duration of sleep; no withdrawal symptoms

[a] Complete reference citations at end of chapter.
[b] MSLT, multiple sleep latency est; POMS, principle of mood states.

Benzodiazepines and Related Compounds

Correct diagnosis of the cause of the sleep disturbance is the most important factor in deciding to prescribe sleeping medication for chronic insomnia in later life. Other important considerations include (1) review of the relative indications and contraindications for using antidepressant medication (e.g., trazodone, trimipramine, doxepin or other sedating agents), antipsychotic medication, or benzodiazepines and related compounds; (2) changes in metabolic rate; (3) effects on daytime alertness and performance; (4) other concurrent sedating medications or alcohol that might potentiate the sedative effects of sleeping pills; and (5) potential effects on borderline or clinically significant sleep apnea.

Sedative hypnotics, especially benzodiazepines, zolpidem, or zaleplon have become the most widely used drugs for the treatment of insomnia. Older sedative hypnotics, including the barbiturates, ethchlorvynol, ethionamide, glutethimide, and methprylon should not be used in the management of insomnia for the elderly. Chloral hydrate syrup should be reserved for patients who cannot swallow pills. Although little scientific support can be found for its use by the elderly, chloral hydrate quickly exerts an hypnotic effect, has a short elimination half-life (approximately 8 hours), and is less likely to induce dependence and distort sleep patterns than barbiturates. Its most common side effect is gastric irritation, which can be a particular problem for elderly persons who may experience stomach upset from other causes. Because chloral hydrate induces hepatic enzymes, it may also increase the rate of metabolism of other drugs (such as the anticoagulants, particularly dicumarol). In addition, by displacing other drugs such as diuretics from carrier proteins, it may increase their effects.

Benzodiazepines, zolpidem, or zaleplon are safer for the elderly patient than other hypnotics. They do not induce hepatic enzymes, are less lethal in overdose, and very rarely produce seizures except upon abrupt withdrawal.

Benzodiazepines, imidazophyridines (e.g., zolpidem), or cyclopyrrolones (e.g., zopiclone) are believed to work via gamma aminobutyric acid (GABA)-receptor modulation and can be classified by their affinity for subtypes of the GABA receptor, (i.e., GABA-1 or GABA-2). [86] Benzodiazepines may also be divided into pharmacologic categories, depending on their GABA-receptor affinity, the rate at which they are metabolized, the presence or absence of active metabolites, and the duration of their action. Long- and intermediate-half-life benzodiazepine hypnotics have a complicated metabolic pathway and a prolonged effect. Therefore they accumulate, producing chronically high blood levels, particularly in the elderly (see Chapter 16). Flurazepam and quazepam have the longest elimination half-lives (36 to 120 hours) as well as active metabolites that accumulate in the plasma and lead to daytime sleepiness, cognitive impairment, lack of coordination, and worsening of depression. Benzodiazepines with intermediate elimination half-lives (10 to 24 hours) and no active metabolites (such as temazepam and estazolam), are less likely to be associated with excessive daytime sleepiness than agents with longer elimination half-lives. Drugs with very short elimination half-lives (2 to 5 hours) include triazolam and zolpidem. Although these agents may be useful for older patients who have difficulty falling asleep, they may be less useful for those with early morning awakening. Benzodiazepines with shorter elimination half-lives or zolpidem, which lack active metabolites and do not accumulate, are thus the hypnotic drugs of choice for elderly patients with transient or chronic primary insomnia.

Side Effects of Benzodiazepine Hypnotics

Benzodiazepines are most often the drugs of choice for insomnia in older persons; however, age-related pharmacokinetic changes predispose elderly patients to benzodiazepine side effects (see Chapter 16). This increased susceptibility is intensified in demented patients and those experiencing reduced plasma protein binding and renal failure.[95] Benzodiazepines produce adverse events such as memory impairment, falls, and excessive sleepiness; accidents may occur at higher doses or when the parent compound and active metabolites accumulate in the body.[96]

Chronic use of benzodiazepines carries the additional risk of physical dependence, withdrawal, and rebound insomnia.[97] Questions of long-term efficacy and concerns over risk of physical dependence led the FDA to establish guidelines discouraging the use of benzodiazepine hypnotics beyond 4 weeks, regardless of patient age.[98]

All sedating drugs, including benzodiazepine hypnotics, also adversely affect motor function and coordination. These hangover effects are worse in the morning than the afternoon and after higher doses, as might be expected. Because elderly infirm patients may be much more susceptible to developing these effects, falls with consequent fractures may occur when next-day sedation further worsens compromised motor competence.

When older patients gradually withdraw from long-term benzodiazepine treatment, disturbed sleep sometimes (but not always) occurs. Abrupt discontinuance of short or intermediate half-life benzodiazepine hypnotics commonly leads to rebound insomnia.[99] For example, rebound awakening may also occur several hours after the ultrashort half-life benzodiazepine triazolam is taken, necessitating a second dose to obtain a full night's sleep. Clinical experience suggests that older nursing home residents who take triazolam frequently take a second dose in the middle of the night. Because rebound awakening and rebound insomnia are so distressing to the older person, chronic nightly use of benzodiazepine hypnotics ensues, leading to increasingly severe symptoms of cognitive and motor impairment.

Older people who experience rebound insomnia, even following low-dose benzodiazepine hypnotic treatment, may have difficulty giving up use of the drug.[100] In addition, short half-life benzodiazepine hypnotics may produce anxiety, depression, confusion, and increased levels of somatized tension.[101-105] A triazolam syndrome, consisting of reversible delirium, anterograde amnesia, and automatic movements, has been reported,[106] though a report by the Institute of Medicine did not find evidence to support a unique adverse-effect profile for triazolam. Intermediate-acting drugs may be used, but some nursing homes avoid all hypnotic drugs.[107] Some investigators wonder whether sleeping pills are ever justified for the elderly,[101] suggesting a maximum of 20 doses per month for not more than 3 months. Others suggest doses two to three times weekly[102] or even one to two times weekly at the most.[93] Slight risks of increased mortality associated with sleeping pill use have also been found.[28]

Current recommendations for use of benzodiazepine hypnotics are for low doses of short or intermediate half-life agents without active metabolites, such as triazolam (0.125 mg), lorazepam (0.5 to 2.0 mg), temazepam (7.5 mg), zaleplon (5 mg), or zolpidem (5 mg). Patients are instructed to take the medication within 30 minutes of bedtime. A very small percentage of elderly patients, typically those with mood and/or anxiety disorders, seem to need these medications chronically, often as adjuncts to maintenance antidepressant treatment. Most geriatric patients, however, do not need increased dosages over time. Table 18.2 summarizes recommended doses and other salient pharmacokinetic properties of these and other widely used agents.

A recent review[108] and a placebo-controlled trial,[109] reveal that zaleplon, the newest benzodiazepine receptor agonist, has the shortest half-life of available agents. It is effective in improving sleep latency, duration, and sleep quality in older persons and does not appear to

Table 18.2. Commonly Prescribed Agents for Treating Insomnia

Medication (Trade Name)	Usual Geriatric Therapeutic Dose (mg)	Time for Onset (min)	$T1/2_{\beta\infty}$ (hr)[a]	Active Metabolite
Chloral hydrate[b]	500–2000	30–60	4–8	Yes
Clonazepam[c]	0.25–1	20–60	19–60	No
Clorazepate	3.75–7.5	30–60	6–8[d] 48–96[e]	Yes
Estazolam	0.5–1	15–30	8–24	No
Lorazepam[c]	0.25–1	30–60	8–24	No
Oxozepam	10–15	30–60	2.8–5.7	No
Quazepam	7.5	20–45	15–40[d] 39–120[e]	Yes
Temazepam	7.5–15	45–60	3–25	No
Triazolam	0.125	15–30	1.5–5	No
Haloperidol[b,c]	0.25–2	60	20	No
Trazodone[b,c]	25–100	30–60	5–9	No
Zolpidem[b]	5	30	1.5–4.5	No

References for data at end of chapter.
[a] Terminal elimination half-life.
[b] Nonbenzodiazepine.
[c] Used as hypnotic not indicated by FDA.
[d] Parent compound.
[e] Active metabolite.

cause rebound insomnia, residual sedation, or adversely affect psychomotor function.

Melatonin

Melatonin is a hormone and antioxidant produced by the pineal gland. The melatonin replacement hypothesis states that the well-evidenced age-related decline may contribute to insomnia and that replacement with physiological doses of melatonin improves sleep.

A recent review[110] examined evidence for the efficacy of melatonin in elderly insomniacs derived from studies and case reports; these show a trend toward its efficacy: sleep quality improved, and in patients with AD, sundowning was reduced. Melatonin in doses ranging from 0.5 to 6 mg before bedtime decreased sleep latency significantly. Other measures of sleep quality (sleep efficiency, total sleep time and wake time during sleep) also improved, although subjective sleep quality did not improve. No early-morning sleepi-

ness occurred. These studies suggest that melatonin is most effective in elderly insomniacs who chronically use benzodiazepines and/or with documented low melatonin levels during sleep. Conclusions suggest that for geriatric patients who suffer from insomnia low doses of melatonin improve initial sleep quality in selected elderly insomniacs, but larger randomized controlled trials, with less strict inclusion criteria are necessary to yield evidence of effectiveness (i.e., clinical and subjective relevance), before widespread use can be advocated.

Pharmacotherapy of Insomnia for Patients with Dementia

Sleep disturbances remain common among demented residents in nursing homes in a recent review[26] and observations.[111] Sleep onset latency is prolonged and the patients experience frequent wake bouts after sleep onset. The diminished ability of sustained sleep may be influenced by the prolonged time in bed.

A variety of pharmacologic treatments of insomnia have been used for patients with dementia. The effect of several different classes of psychoactive agents—butabarbital (50–100 mg), thioridazine (25 mg), flurazepam (15 mg), chloral hydrate (500 mg), lorazepam (2 mg), oxazepam (30 mg), temazepam (15 mg), and hydroxyzine (50–200 mg)—on sleep show that compared with placebo, active compounds are associated with increased sleep time but with variable effects on sleep onset time.[112–116] Among these drugs, low-dose thioridazine has been shown superior to the benzodiazepine nitrazepam (which increases daytime memory impairment, incontinence, and daytime sleepiness, and diminishes activities of daily living); in contrast, the benzodiazepine (flurazepam) can decrease motor performance.[117] Because of its side-effect profile, however, thioridazine is usually not recommended for elderly patients.

Additional side effects have been noted with other drugs used by older persons with dementia. Short-acting benzodiazepines may induce next-day paradoxical effects such as anxiety, agitation, and paranoia; upon withdrawal, they induce rebound insomnia. Significant withdrawal insomnia has been reported with chloral hydrate.[120]

Benzodiazepines may promote oropharyngeal collapse during respiration. Since sleep-disordered breathing occurs in demented patients, as well as in approximately 25% of community-residing elderly,[118] an interaction between sleep-disordered breathing and benzodiazepine sedative-hypnotic agents may worsen respiration. Impaired respiration, in turn, may worsen cognitive impairment. Cognitive impairment and impaired recent recall may improve following drug withdrawal, but this may occur after a period of aggravated confusion.

Pharmacotherapy of Sleep Impairment in Late-Life Depression

Major depressive episodes are associated with disrupted sleep. EEG disturbances include decreased sleep continuity and early morning awakening, shortened first non-REM (NREM) sleep period (REM latency), and diminished delta wave production during the first NREM sleep period.[119] Shortly after the start of antidepressant therapy in older persons the first periods of NREM sleep lengthen and production of slow waves increases during the first NREM sleep period.[120] Short-term as well as maintenance antidepressant treatment may significantly affect sleep in the elderly. Since depression itself usually worsens sleep, antidepressant treatment improves subjective sleep quality, both acutely and chronically, when prescribed as maintenance therapy. In addition to improving quality of life, long-term improvement of subjective sleep quality helps prevent relapse and recurrence of late-life depression.[121] Specifically, recurrence of major depressive episodes during maintenance antidepressant therapy is associated with lower-phase REM-activity counts during early maintenance therapy. Improvement in subjective sleep quality is also associated with a lower rate of recurrent depressive episodes in elderly patients, regardless of whether they are treated by maintenance antidepressant medication or interpersonal psychotherapy.

Antidepressants in the Treatment of Chronic Insomnia

Tertiary tricyclic antidepressants such as trimipramine, amitriptyline, and doxepin can produce subjective improvements in sleep quality and quantity as well as objective improvements as measured by polysomnography in the absence of a mood disorder.[122] These compounds, however, may exert troublesome anticholinergic side effects that potentially worsen glaucoma, tachyarrhythmias, constipation, cognition and prostatism. They may also cause orthostatic hypotension. Elderly patients are more sensitive to these side effects; usefulness of tertiary tricyclic antidepressants for sleep improvement depends on the clinical profile of such conditions.

Nevertheless, their use for the geriatric population as hypnotics has dramatically increased recently.[123] This increase in tricyclic prescription for sleep may be due to concern about benzodiazepine dependence, which has led to a 30% reduction in benzodiazepine hypnotic prescriptions.[123]

Serotonin-specific antidepressants, such as trazodone and nefazodone, may relieve sleep disturbances that accompany depression.[124–126] They have fewer side effects compared with tertiary amine antidepressants.[127,128] Although no studies of these drugs have been conducted on insomnia unassociated with depression, clinical experience with trazodone suggests that it is a very useful medication for sleep disorders in the elderly whether or not depression is present. The starting dose is 25 mg at bedtime, which may be increased as needed; doses above 100 to 150 mg are usually not necessary. Trazodone is well tolerated, and dosage escalation is usually not necessary. Detailed study of next-day function, however, has not been done. Blood pressure should be monitored during trazodone therapy because of orthostatic hypotension. Priapism has not been observed in elderly males taking the low doses (25 to 150 mg) typically used.

Behavioral Treatments of Chronic Primary Insomnia

Stimulus-control therapy,[129] a set of instructional procedures designed to curtail sleep-incompatible behaviors and to stabilize sleep-wake schedules, may be useful for elderly people. Instructions specify:

1. Go to bed only when sleepy.
2. Use the bed and bedroom only for sleep and sex (i.e., no reading, television watching, eating, or working during the day or night).
3. Leave the bed and go into another room if unable to sleep for 15 to 20 minutes and return only when sleepy again.
4. Arise in the morning at the same time regardless of the amount of sleep the previous night.
5. Do not nap during the day.

Sleep-restriction therapy consists of limiting the time spent in bed to actual sleeping.[107] This method may use the homeostatic regulation of sleep to allow a sleep debt (from limiting time in bed) to facilitate sleep initiation and maintenance and to delay final bedtime until a circadian time that comports more with sleep. The allowable time in bed is increased incrementally over time as long as the desired sleep efficiency is maintained. The efficacy of this approach has been demonstrated in a randomized clinical trial with elderly individuals.[130]

Other behavioral techniques also may be helpful for the elderly. Relaxation therapies, designed to alleviate somatic or cognitive arousal that interfere with sleep, consist of techniques such as progressive muscular relaxation, autogenic training, and biofeedback.[131] Sleep hygiene education is concerned with health practices such as diet, exercise, and substance use as well as with environmental factors such as light, noise, and temperature that may be either detrimental or beneficial to sleep.[131,132] Cognitive-behavioral treatment (CBT) for insomnia that may be of particular value for older persons targets maladaptive cognitions that perpetuate insomnia.[93] CBT for insomnia is also efficacious in mixed-age/older adults.[133–135]

Conclusion

Since primary insomnia in later life is often chronic and relapsing, clinicians and researchers need to take a long-term view of its management. More data are needed, particularly to find preventive strategies and longer-term efficacy of behavioral and pharmacologic approaches, whether prescribed singly or in combination. Sleep-restriction therapy, cognitive behavioral therapy, and selected antidepressant medications have been promising interventions in long-term efficacy studies. In addition to efficacy (both short and chronic), systematic evaluation of side effects and safety, ease of application, cost, and applicability to special populations such as the institutionalized elderly is needed.

CLINICAL VIGNETTES

Case 18.1

Mr. A., a 69-year-old, white, married male with no known personal or family history of psychiatric disorder, presented with a 2-year history of sleep-onset and sleep-maintenance insomnia resulting in daytime fatigue and decreased concentration. Referred by a pulmonary sleep specialist who found no abnormalities on an ambulatory sleep polysomnogram other than frequent awakenings, he reported being exquisitely sensitive to environmental noise and no longer able to sleep with his spouse because the light sound of her breathing kept him awake.

Mr. A. explained that his sleep problems began when the retail store he had managed for many years was purchased by a large firm with an announced intent to reduce the work force. He then would lie awake at night preoccupied with both job-related stress and his new sleep problems. Although he denied feeling depressed, his wife reported that he seemed unhappy and more irritable; he scored 11 on a 17-item Hamilton depression scale (nondepressed range = 0–7). He agreed to a trial of paroxetine (10 mg nightly), which improved his sleep continuity and daytime energy and decreased his irritability.

Case 18.2

Dr. B., a 68-year-old retired married grandfather, was troubled by frequent early morning awakenings and reduced daytime energy since his retirement three years before. He was physically healthy, took no regular medication, walked three miles daily, and adhered to a stable sleep-wake schedule. He denied feeling depressed or having any change in his weight or appetite and claimed to be happy in retirement, with time to read novels and take adult education classes.

Careful questioning revealed that he drank three to four glasses of wine each evening "to enjoy life and protect my coronary arteries at the same time!" Prior to retirement, Dr. B. drank very infrequently because he was accustomed to working several hours each evening. He reduced his alcohol intake, which resulted in improved sleep maintenance. He also enrolled in several more classes and returned to his previous habit of working several hours each evening.

Case 18.3*

Mr. C., a 75-year-old white married male, presented with a 5–10 year history of worsening restless sleep, daytime fatigue and sleepiness. He had difficulty falling asleep because he ruminated about problems of the day and could not find a comfortable position for his legs. He awoke frequently during the night and returned to sleep with difficulty. He felt an inner sense of restlessness that was relieved only by getting out of bed and walking for a few minutes. Once asleep, he would have vivid dreams, often related to his experiences as a prisoner of war in World War II. While memories of his POW experience were vague, he did recall prolonged periods of exposure to cold during long marches, accompanied by a profound sense of helplessness. He described a several-year period following his return from World War II of recurrent, distressing dreams about this experience, social avoidance, loss of pleasure, and a feeling of detachment from others that accompanied his restless sleep.

These symptoms gradually subsided in midlife as he became immersed in his work and family, although the distressing dreams and hypervigilance began to return as he entered his retirement years. His wife confirmed that his sleep was restless, and for the past few years she had slept in another room because, on occasion, he would hit her unknowingly during his sleep, in addition to making loud snoring noises. One night she noted that his legs twitched in a recurring pattern (she was able to count to 9 between regular leg twitches). She was not sure whether or not he stopped breathing for short periods during his sleep because it had been several years since they had slept together.

On awakening in the morning, Mr. C. felt low energy, fatigue, and sleepiness, as if he had been fighting throughout the night. When active during the day, he would not fall asleep; if left in an unstimulating setting, however, like watching the news, he would drift off to sleep. He denied episodes of cataplexy (loss of mus-

---

* Adapted from Nofzinger EA, Reynolds CF. Sleep impairment and daytime sleepiness in later life. *Am J Psychiatry* 1996;153(7):941–943, with permission.

cle tone during sudden emotional stimulation, leading to temporary bilateral paresis, falls, and other mishaps), hypnagogic hallucinations, or sleep paralysis. He described having some difficulty concentrating during the daytime, memory difficulties, and on one occasion being frightened by falling asleep briefly while driving. For that reason, he relinquished driving to family members when possible.

Initial Assessment

Not unusual in late-life, Mr. C.'s sleep disorder has clinical features suggesting a multifactor sleep/wake disturbance. Complaints include nighttime insomnia as well as daytime sleepiness and give clues as to the presence of a parasomnia (i.e., partial arousal from sleep, often with accompanying behavioral disturbances). The differential diagnosis and order of further assessment of this man's complaints are guided by (a) which sleep disorders, if present, would have the most significant impact on his life, including medical morbidity as well as death related to vigilance impairment, for instance, a motor vehicle accident, and (b) which sleep-disorder treatment would significantly enhance the quality of his life.

Given these guidelines, sleep apnea syndrome is the primary diagnosis to be considered for any elderly patient who complains of daytime sleepiness. This primary sleep disorder is characterized by daytime sleepiness and loud snoring. Repetitive apneas (often hundreds of times during a night's sleep) are brought about by collapse of upper airway muscles with partial or total obstruction of the upper airway. The loud snoring results from inspiratory efforts to overcome the obstruction and leads to arousals necessary to restore airway muscle tonus. Sleep apnea syndrome is associated with significant medical morbidity (e.g., systemic hypertension, congestive heart failure, cardiac arrhythmias, impaired executive function, cognitive dysfunction). In addition to the associated medical comorbidity, the subsequent daytime sleepiness caused by repetitive partial arousals related to apneic events during sleep may lead to life-threatening accidents or near-miss driving events as this patient experienced. Mr. C.'s risk factors for sleep apnea include male gender, advanced age, history of loud snoring, and significant daytime sleepiness. Since subjective complaints can poorly reflect objective measures of sleep apnea, the clinician is advised to maintain a low threshold for referring patients to a sleep evaluation center to assess sleep apnea.

Mr. C.'s clinical history also suggests a diagnosis of restless legs syndrome (RLS) and/or periodic limb movement disorder (PLMD). The clinical complaint of a sense of restlessness in the legs that occurs on retiring is classic for RLS. Nearly 70–80% of patients with RLS also manifest the related condition PLMD that involves repetitive twitches, especially in the legs. Screening for PLMD should be done in a sleep evaluation center. Sleep-laboratory testing documents the presence and extent of myoclonic activity in the lower extremities during sleep and the arousals from sleep associated with them.

The history of Mr. C.'s wife sleeping in another room to avoid being hit by her husband raises the clinical suspicion of a parasomnia (a sleep-related behavior disorder) such as sleepwalking or REM-sleep behavior disorder. In these conditions the normal muscle atonia of REM sleep is absent, allowing patients to engage in dream-enacting behavior. Not uncommonly, patients with PLMD will intermittently kick their bed partners as a result of involuntary movements of the larger limbs. For Mr. C., a former POW who also reported recurrent traumatic dreams of a threatening event, a diagnosis of posttraumatic stress disorder should be considered. Such patients are known to have increased incidence of PLMD as well as dream-enacting behaviors related to the traumatic experience.[40] Elderly individuals appear at increased risk for the emergence of both traumatic dreams and sleep-related behaviors that may not have been present during prior adult years. This propensity is most likely related to the age-related alterations in sleep integrity seen in this population.

Finally, the most likely cause of Mr. C.'s daytime sleepiness is disrupted nocturnal sleep from multiple factors, such as sleep apnea syndrome, RLS, PLMD, and recurrent traumatic dreams with subsequent chronic sleep deprivation. Further diagnostic testing was indicated to clarify the diagnosis and to guide treatment interventions.

Sleep Laboratory (Polysomnographic) Studies

The initial sleep study of 2 nights consisted of a recording montage that monitored electroencephalographic sleep staging, respiratory effort and airflow, oximetry, heart rate, periodic limb movements of the lower legs, and sleep-related behaviors via audiovisual recording. Sleep staging and sleep continuity measures from the 2 nights revealed severe difficulty initiating sleep, multiple prolonged awakenings, absence of slow-wave (deep) sleep, generalized reduction of REM sleep, and preservation of normal muscle atonia during REM sleep. Apnea measures showed 35 apneic events per hour of sleep (normal, ≤5), with related drops in oxyhemoglobin saturation to less than 85% for 25% of the night. The limb monitors showed 54 arousals per hour of sleep (normal is considered ≤5 events per hour of sleep in middle age), independent of apneic arousals. Audiovisual recording revealed no abnormal behaviors during sleep.

Sleep Study Interpretation

The sleep study confirmed the reports of Mr. C. and his wife of severe sleep disturbance, evidenced by prolonged time before sleep onset and lack of deep sleep. The frequency of apneic events and of the associated oxyhemoglobin desaturation confirmed that sleep apnea syndrome was an important cause of his excessive daytime sleepiness. The high frequency of PLMs and history of restless legs prior to sleep onset confirmed diagnoses of RLS and PLMD. The persistence of muscle atonia during REM sleep ruled out REM-sleep behavior disorder, while the audiovisual monitoring revealed no complex behaviors related to NREM sleep partial arousals. Parasomnias, if present, would need to be established by clinical reports in longitudinal follow-up with the patient.

Treatment Plan and Followup

The initial step in treatment was initiation of nasal CPAP (continuous positive airway pressure) therapy to relieve the sleep apnea syndrome. Nasal CPAP works by providing a pneumatic ``splint'' in the form of positive airway pressure to maintain airway patency during sleep and thereby prevent airway collapse leading to apnea. The success of this therapy was documented by a decrease to four apneic events per hour of sleep and maintenance of oxyhemoglobin saturations above 85% for 98% of the night. Despite this success, Mr. C. continued to suffer from difficulty initiating sleep, discontinuous sleep throughout the night, and significant daytime sleepiness.

The second step in treatment, therefore, was amelioration of both RLS and PLMD by treatment with clonazepam (1 mg orally before sleep). The rationale for benzodiazepine therapy in this context was to suppress the arousals associated with PLMs. Clonazepam is used widely for this purpose because its intermediate elimination half-life allows it to provide ``coverage'' for 6 to 8 hours. However, given the comorbid sleep apnea syndrome and the possibility that initiation of a benzodiazepine might exacerbate the sleep apnea, medication was begun during polysomnographic recording. During this study, apnea severity did not increase despite a reduction of PLMs to five events per hour of sleep and significant improvements in sleep continuity.

During the next 6 months, Mr. C. noted dramatic improvements in sleep continuity, daytime alertness and performance, and general well-being during combined treatment with nasal CPAP and clonazepam. Eventually, however, he reported increasing daytime sleepiness and sleep continuity disturbances, which were interpreted as resulting from adaptation to the effects of clonazepam. Increasing the dosage of the medication helped only temporarily. Therefore, the treatment of RLS and PLMD was changed from clonazepam to L-dopa/carbidopa, which produced profound clinical improvements in the RLS and PLMD symptoms. L-dopa/carbidopa (initial dosage $^{25}/_{100}$ mg with upward titrations according to clinical response) has considerable benefit in the treatment of PLMD and RLS, suggesting involvement of the dopaminergic system in the pathophysiology of these disorders, although in large part, their pathophysiology has not been clearly defined.

Over 3 years of follow-up on this regimen, Mr. C. noted persistent improvements in his ability to fall asleep, stay asleep, and maintain alertness and performance during the daytime. His frightening recurrent nightmares abated. During this time, however, he suffered a heart attack, which led to coronary artery bypass surgery. For approximately 3 months postoperatively, Mr. C took oxycodone and acetaminophen for relief of pain, and he found that he did not require the L-dopa during that period. He was advised to discontinue the L-dopa/carbidopa as long as he was taking the oxycodone, because of the known therapeutic effects of narcotics on RLS and PLMD. Upon discontinuing the oxycodone, however, he noted the reemergence of RLS and PLMD, leading him to reinitiate treatment, successfully, with L-dopa/carbidopa.

Summary

This case illustrates several fundamental principles in the DSM-IV nosology of sleep disorders: (1) the importance of making an etiological diagnosis of sleep impairment; (2) the coexistence of multiple etiological factors in the same patient (not uncommon in older patients, in whom sleep impairments are most prevalent); (3) the availability of specific, effective treatments for specific conditions; and (4) the need to take a long-term approach to the management of many sleep disorders. Working through sleep-disorder complaints systematically will help to achieve success in therapy, even in complex cases like that of Mr. C. Referral to specialized sleep disorders centers should be considered for patients with a primary complaint of excessive daytime sleepiness (to rule out sleep apnea syndrome or narcolepsy) or in cases of persistent insomnia when there is clinical concern about sleep-disordered breathing, nocturnal myoclonus, or failure to respond to usual care.

Case 18.4

Mrs. D., an 82-year-old retired musician, had a long history of sleep onset and sleep maintenance insomnia. She had tried multiple treatments for insomnia including biofeedback, meditation, sleep hygiene, and several trials of hypnotic medication. Her family physician was concerned that Mrs. D. was addicted to clonazepam, as she was using clonazepam 2 mg each night, which was twice the prescribed dose, and was said to have slurred speech during the day. Mrs. D.'s chief complaint was a profound sense of restlessness in her legs anytime she was in bed. She frequently paced about her house at night to avoid this extremely unpleasant sensation and desperately wanted some relief. A polysomnogram revealed frequent awakenings, absent slow-wave sleep, an apnea index of 7, and an average of 48 PLMs per hour of sleep, associated with brief EEG arousal. She was slowly tapered off clonazepam and was treated with a combination of L-dopa/carbidopa and codeine for a diagnosis of RLS, resulting in substantial improvement in sleep continuity and daytime alertness.

References

1. Reynolds CF, Hoch CC, Buysse DJ, et al. REM sleep in successful, usual, and pathological aging: the Pittsburgh experience 1980–1991. *J Sleep Res* 1993;2:203–210.
2. Rowe JW, Kahn RL. Human aging: usual and successful. *Science* 1987;237:143–149.
3. Floyd JA, Medler SM, Ager JW, et al.. Age-related changes in initiation and maintenance of sleep: a meta-analysis. *Res Nurs Health* 2000;23:106–117.
4. Hoch CC, Reynolds CF, Houck PR, et al. Predicting mortality in mixed depression and dementia using EEG sleep variables. *J Neuropsychiatr Clin Neurosci* 1989;1:366–371.
5. Hoch CC, Reynolds CF, Buysse DJ, et al. Two-year survival in patients with mixed symptoms of depression and cognitive impairment. *Am J Geriatr Psychiatry* 1993;1:59–66.
6. Hoch CC, Dew MA, Reynolds CF, et al. A longitudinal study of laboratory- and diary-based sleep measures in healthy "old old" and "young old" volunteers. *Sleep* 1994;17:489–496.
7. Vegni C, Ktonas P, Giganti F, et al. The organi-

zation of rapid eye movement activity during rapid eye movement sleep is further impaired in very old human subjects. *Neuroscience Letters* 2001;297:58–60.
8. Jelicic M, Bosma H, Ponds RW, et al. Subjective sleep problems in later life as predictors of cognitive decline. Report from the Maastricht Ageing Study (MAAS). *Int J Geriatr Psychiatry* 2002;17:73–77.
9. Cricco M, Simonsick EM, Foley DJ. The impact of insomnia on cognitive functioning in older adults. *J Am Geriatr Soc* 2001;49:1185–1189.
10. Park YM, Matsumoto K, Shinkoda H, et al. Age and gender difference in habitual sleep-wake rhythm. *Psychiatry Clin Neurosci* 2001;55:201–202.
11. Prinz PN, Bailey SL, Woods DL. Sleep impairments in healthy seniors: roles of stress, cortisol, and interleukin-1 beta. *Chronobiol International* 2000;17:391–404.
12. Jordan JM, Bernard SL, Callahan LF, et al. Self-reported arthritis-related disruptions in sleep and daily life and the use of medical, complementary, and self-care strategies for arthritis: the National Survey of Self-care and Aging. *Arch Fam Med* 2000;9:143–149.
13. Dew MA, Reynolds CF, Monk TH, et al. Psychosocial correlates and sequelae of EEG sleep in healthy elders. *J Gerontol* 1994;49:P8–P18.
14. Janson C, Lindberg E, Gislason T, et al. Insomnia in men: A 10-year prospective population based study. *Sleep* 2001;24:425–430.
15. Morin CM, Gramling SE. Sleep patterns and aging: comparison of older adults with and without insomnia complaints. *Psychol Aging* 1989;4:290–294.
16. Karacan I, Williams RL. Sleep disorders in the elderly. *Am Fam Physician* 1983;27:143–152.
17. Hajak G, SINE Study Group. Study of Insomnia in Europe. Epidemiology of severe insomnia and its consequences in Germany. *Eur Arch Psychiatr Neurosci* 2002;251:49–56.
18. Angst J, Vollrath M, Koch R. The Zurich study: VII. Insomnia: symptoms, classification and prevalence. *Eur Arch Psychiatr Neurosci* 1989;238:285–293.
19. Vollrath M, Wicki W, Angst J. The Zurich study: VIII. Insomnia: association with depression, anxiety, somatic syndromes, and course of insomnia. *Eur Arch Psychiatr Neurosci* 1989;239:113–124.
20. Mendelson WB. Long-term follow-up of chronic insomnia. *Sleep* 1995;18:698–701.
21. Ganguli M, Reynolds CF, Gilby JE. Prevalence and persistence of sleep complaints in a rural elderly community sample: the MoVIES project. *J Am Geriatr Soc* 1996;44:778–784.
22. Kennedy GJ, Kelman HR, Thomas C. Persistence and remission of depressive symptoms in late life. *Am J Psychiatry* 1991;148:174–178.
23. Raiha I, Impivaaca O, Seppala M, et al. Determinants of symptoms suggestive of gastro-esophageal reflux disease in the elderly. *Su J Gastroenteral* 1993;28:1011–1014.
24. Gislason T, Almquist M. Somatic diseases and sleep complaints: an epidemiological study of 3,201 Swedish men. *Acta Med Scand* 1987;22:475–481.

25. Karlson KH, Larsen JP, Trondberg E, et al. Influence of clinical and demographic variables on quality of life in patients with Parkinson's disease. *J Neural Neurosurg Psychiatry* 1999;66: 431–435.

26. Boeve BR, Silber MH, Ferman TJ. Current management of sleep disturbances in dementia. *Curr Neurol Neurosci Rep* 2002;2:169–177.

27. Mallon L, Broman, JE, Hetta J. Relationship between insomnia, depression, and mortality: a 12-year follow-up of older adults in the community. *Int Psychogeriatrics* 200;12:295–306.

28. Kripke DF, Garfinkel L, Wingard DL, et al. Mortality associated with sleep duration and insomnia. *Arch Gen Psychiatr* 2002;59:131–136.

29. Van Someren EJ. Circadian and sleep disturbances in the elderly. *Experi Gerontol* 200;35: 1229–1237.

30. Baskett JJ, Wood PC, Broad JB, et al. Melatonin in older people with age-related sleep maintenance problems: a comparison with age matched normal sleepers. *Sleep* 2001;24: 418–424.

31. Dijk DJ, Duffy JF, Czeisler CA. Contribution of circadian physiology and sleep homeostasis to age-related changes in human sleep. *Chronobiol Internat* 2000;17:285–311.

32. Gehrman PS. Long-term follow-up of periodic limb movements in sleep in older adults. *Sleep* 2002;25:340–343.

33. Grandjean CK, Gibbons SW. Assessing ambulatory geriatric sleep complaints. *Nurse Practitioner* 2002;25:25–32.

34. Ohayon MM, Vecchierini MF. Daytime sleepiness and cognitive impairment in the elderly population. *Arch Int Medicine* 2002;162:201–208.

35. Ford DE, Kamerow DB. Epidemiologic study of sleep disturbances and psychiatric disorders. *JAMA* 1989;262:1479–1484.

36. Balter MB, Uhlenhuth EH. New epidemiologic findings about insomnia and its treatment. *J Clin Psychiatry* 1992;53:34–39; discussion 40–42.

37. Mellinger GD, Balter MB, Uhlenhuth EH. Insomnia and its treatment. *Arch Gen Psychiatry* 1985;42:225–232.

38. Gallup Organization. *Sleep in America.* Princeton, NJ: Gallup Organization, 1991.

39. Pollak CP, Perlick D, Linsner JP, et al. Sleep problems in the community elderly as predictors of death and nursing home placement. *J Community Health* 1990;15:123–135.

40. National Commission on Sleep Disorders. *Wake up America: a national sleep alert.* Washington, DC: National Commission on Sleep Disorders, 1993.

41. Giron MS, Forsell Y, Bernsten C, et al. Sleep problems in a very old population: drug use and clinical correlates. *J Gerontol Series A Biol Sci & Med Sci* 2002;57:M236–M240

42. Beers M, Avorn J, Soumerai SB, et al. Psychoactive medication use in intermediate care facility residents. *JAMA* 1988;260:3016–3020.

43. Salzman C, van der Kolk B. Psychotropic drugs and polypharmacy in elderly patients in a general hospital. *J Geriatr Psychiatry* 1979;12: 167–176.

44. U.S. Public Health Service. *Physicians' drug prescribing patterns in skilled nursing facilities.* Washington, DC: Department of Health, Education, and Welfare, 1976.

45. Zarcone VP. Sleep Hygiene. In: Kryger MH, Roth T, Dement WC, eds. *Principles and Practice at Sleep Hygiene,* 3rd ed. Philadelphia: Sanders, 2000:657–661.

46. Ring D. Management of chronic insomnia in the elderly. *Clin Excell Nurse Pract* 2002;5:13–16.

47. Schneider DL. Insomnia. Safe and effective therapy for sleep problems in the older patient. *Geriatrics* 2002;57:24–26.

48. Shochat TL. Sleep disorders in the elderly. *Cur Treat Options in Neurol* 2001;3:19–36.

49. Lichstein KL, Wilson NM, Johnson CT. Psychological treatment of secondary insomnia. *Psychology & Aging* 2000;15:232–240.

50. Rybarczyk BL. Efficacy of two behavioral treatment programs for comorbid geriatric insomnia. *Psychol Aging* 2002;17:288–298.

51. Moore-Ede MC, Sulzman FM, Fuller CA. *The clocks that time us.* Harvard University Press, Cambridge MA, 1982:49–50.

52. Czeizler CA, Duffy JF, Shanahan TL, et al. Stability, precision and near-24-hour period of the human circadian pacemaker. *Science* 1999;284: 2177–2181.

53. Dijk DJ, Duffy JF, Czeisler CA. Age-related increase in awakenings: impaired consolidation of nonREM sleep at all circadian phases. *Sleep* 2001;24:565–577.

54. Montgomery P, Dennis J. Bright light therapy for sleep problems in adults aged 60 +. *Cochrane Database Syst Rev* 2002;CD03403.

55. Surner AG Murphy DJ, Campbell SS. Failure of timed bright light exposure to alleviate age-related sleep maintenance insomnia. *J Am Geriat Soc* 2002;50:617–623.

56. Cardinali DP, Brusco LI, Lloret SP, Furio AM. Melatonin in sleep disorders and jet-lag. *Neuro Endocrinol Lett* 2002;23(suppl 1):9–13.

57. Stromba-Badiale M, Ceretti A, Forni G. Aspects of sleep in the aged and very aged individual. *Minerva Med* 1979;70:2551–2554.

58. Webb WB, Swinburne H. An observational study of sleep of the aged. *Percept Mot Skills* 1971;32:895–898.

59. Regestein QR, Morris J. Daily sleep patterns observed among institutionalized elderly patients. *J Am Geriatr Soc* 1987;35:767–772.

60. Monk TH, Buysse DJ, Carrier J, et al. Effects of afternoon "siesta" naps on sleep, alertness, performance and circadian rhythms in the elderly. *Sleep* 2001;24:680–687.

61. Friedman L, Benson K, Noda A, et al. An actigraphic comparison of sleep restriction and sleep hygiene treatments for insomnia in older adults. *J Geriatr Psychiatry Neurol* 2000;13:17–27.

62. Tune GS. Sleep and wakefulness in 509 normal adults. *Br J Med Psychol* 1969;42:75–79.

63. Regestein QR. Insomnia and sleep disturbances in the aged. *J Geriatr Psychiatry* 1980;13: 153–171.

64. Evans FJ, Cook MR, Cohen HD, et al. Appeti

tive and replacement naps: EEG and behavior. *Science* 1977;197:687–688.

65. Arakawa M, Tanaka H, Toguchi H, et al. Comparative study on sleep health and lifestyle of the elderly in the urban areas and suburbs of Okinawa. *Psychiatry Clin Neurosci* 2002;56:245–246.

66. Sherril DL, Kotchou K, Quan SF. Association of physical activity and human sleep disorders. *Arch Intern Med* 1998;58:1894–1898.

67. Van Someren EJ, Lijzenga C, Mirmiran M, et al. Long-term fitness training improves the circadian rest-activity rhythm in healthy elderly males. *J Biol Rhythms* 1997;12:146–156.

68. Singh NA, Clements KM, Fiaterone MA. A randomized controlled trial of the effect of exercise on sleep. *Sleep* 1997;20:95–101.

69. Fiatrone MA, Marks EC, Ryan ND, et al. High intensity strength training in nonagenarians. *JAMA* 1990;263:3029–3034.

70. Blumenthal JA, Babyak MA, Moore KA et al. Effects of exercise training on older patients with major depression. *Arch Int Med* 1999;159:2349–2356.

71. Babyak M, Blumenthal JA, Jerman S, et al. Exercise treatment for major depression: maintenance of therapeutic benefit at 10 months. *Psychosom Med* 2000;62:633–638.

72. Liao W. Effects of passive body heating on body temperature and sleep regulation in the elderly: a systematic review. *Int J Nur Studies* 2002;39:803.

73. Horne JA, Reid AJ. Nighttime sleep EEG changes following body heating in a warm bath. *Electroencephalogr Clin Neurophysiol* 1985;60:154–157.

74. Dorsey CM, Lukos SE, Tiedren MH, et al. Effects of passive body heating on the sleep of older female insomniacs. *J. Geriatr Psychiatry Neurol* 1996;9:93–90.

75. Jacobs GD. Clinical applications of the relaxation response and mind-body interventions. *J Altern Complement Med* 2001;7(suppl 1):S93–S101.

76. Miller M. Nocturnal polyuria in older people: pathophysiology and clinical implications. *J Am Geriat Soc* 2000;48:1321–1329.

77. Schatzl G, Temml C, Schmilbauer J, et al. Cross-sectional study of nocturia in both sexes: Analysis of a voluntary health-screening project. *Urology* 2000;56:71–75.

78. Hale WE, Perkins LL, May FE, et al. Symptom prevalence in the elderly: an evaluation of age, sex, disease and medication use. *J Am Geriatr Soc* 1986;34:333–340.

79. Mortensen S, Nordling J Munkgaard S, et al. Elderly males and females do differ in urinary symptoms and bother. *Br J Urol* 1997;80(suppl 2):21(abstract).

80. Saletu B, Gruenberger J, Anderer P. Evening television and sleep. *Med Welt* 1983;34:866–870.

81. Brezinova V. Sleep after a bedtime beverage. *Br Med J* 1972;2:431–433.

82. Hollingsworth HL. The influence of caffeine on mental and motor efficiency. *Arch Psychol* 1912;20:1–166.

83. Wetter DW, Young TB. The relation between cigarettes smoking and sleep disturbance. *Prev Med* 1994;23:328–334.

84. Soldatos CR, Kales JD, Scharf MB, et al. Cigarette smoking associated with sleep difficulty. *Science* 1980;207:551–553.

85. Rigotti, NA. Treatment of tobacco use and dependence. *N Engl J Med* 2002;346:506–512.

86. Nicolis FB, Silvestri LG. Hypnotic activity of placebo in relation to severity of insomnia: a quantitative evaluation. *Clin Pharmacol Ther* 1967;8:841–848.

87. Roehrs TA, Tietz EI, Zorick FJ, Roth T. Daytime sleepiness and antihistamines. *Sleep* 1984;7:137–141.

88. Honuka K, Nakazawa Y, Kotori T. Effects of antibiotics minocycline and ampicillin on human sleep. *Brain Res* 1983;288:253–259.

89. Kales A, Bixler EO, Tan TJ, et al. Chronic hypnotic drug use. *JAMA* 1974;227:513–517.

90. Williams RL. Sleeping pill insomnia. *J Clin Psychiatry* 1980;41:153–154.

91. Nowell PD, Buysse DJ, Morin CM, Kupfer DJ. Effective treatments for selected DSM-IV sleep disorders. In: Gorman J, ed. *Psychotherapies and drugs that work: a review of the outcome studies.* New York: Oxford University Press, 1996.

92. Busto UE, Sproule BS, Knight K, et al. Use of prescription and nonprescription hypnotics in a Canadian elderly population. *Can J Clin Pharmacol* 2001;8:213–221.

93. Morin CM, Culbert JP, Schwartz SM. Nonpharmacological interventions for insomnia: a meta-analysis of treatment efficacy. *Am J Psychiatry* 1994;151:1172–1180.

94. Mah L, Upshur RE. Long term benzodiazepine use for insomnia in patients over the age of 60: discordance of patient and physician response. *BMC Fam Pract* 2002;3:9(electronic source).

95. Greenblatt DJ. Pharmacology of benzodiazepine hypnotics. *J Clin Psychiatr* 1992;(53 suppl):7–13.

96. Cook PJ. Benzodiazepine hypnotics in the elderly. *Acta Psychiatr Scand Suppl* 1986;74:149–158.

97. Linsen SM, Zitman FG, Breteler MH. Defining benzodiazepine dependence: the confusion persists. *Eur Psychiatry* 1995;10:306–311.

98. National Institute of Health. Drugs and insomnia. *NIH Consensus Development Conference. National Institutes of Health Consensus Development Conference Summary* 1984;4:1–9.

99. Kales A, Kales JD. *Evaluation and treatment of insomnia.* New York: Oxford University Press, 1984:263–265.

100. Schneider-Helmert D. Why low-dose benzodiazepine insomniacs can't escape their sleeping pills. *Acta Psychiatr Scand* 1988;78:706–711.

101. Reynolds CF, Kupfer DJ, Hoch CC, Sewitch DE. Sleeping pills for the elderly: are they ever justified? *J Clin Psychiatry* 1985;46:9–12.

102. Short-acting benzodiazepines: to prescribe or not to prescribe? [Editorial]. *Union Med Can* 1987;116:29.

103. Gaillard JM. Place of benzodiazepines in the treatment of sleep disturbances. *Rev Med Suisse Romande* 1987;107:717–720.

104. Kales A, Soldatos CR, Bixler EO, Kales JD. Early

morning insomnia with rapidly eliminated benzodiazepines. *Science* 1983;220:95–97.

105. Bayer AJ, Bayer EM, Pathy MSJ, et al. A double blind controlled study of chlormethiazole and triazolam as hypnotics in the elderly. *Acta Psychiatr Scand* 1986;73(suppl 329):104–111.

106. Patterson JF. Triazolam syndrome in the elderly. *South Med J* 1987;80:1425–1426.

107. Spielman AJ, Saskin P, Thorpy MJ. Treatment of chronic insomnia by restriction of time in bed. *Sleep* 1987;10:45–56.

108. Ancoli-Israel S. Insomnia in the elderly: a review for the primary care practitioner. *Sleep* 2000;23(suppl 1):S23–S30

109. Hedner J, Yaeche R, Emilien G, et al. Zaleplon shortens subjective sleep latency and improves subjective sleep quality in elderly patients with insomnia. The Zaleplon Clinical Investigator Study Group. *Int J Geriatr Psychiatry* 2000;15: 704–712.

110. Olde RM, Rigaud AS. Melatonin in elderly patients with insomnia. A systematic review. *Zeitschrift fur Gerontologie und Geriatrie* 2001;34: 491–497.

111. Fetveit A, Bjorvatn B. Sleep disturbances among nursing home residents. *Int J Ger Psychiatry* 2002;17:604–609.

112. Reynolds CF, Hoch CC, Monk TH. Sleep and chronobiologic disturbances in late-life. In: Busse E, Blazer DG, eds. *Handbook of geriatric psychiatry*. Washington, DC: American Psychiatric Press, 1989:475–488.

113. Stotsky BA, Cole JO, Tang YT. Sodium butabarbital as an hypnotic agent for age to psychiatric patients with sleep disorders. *J Am Geriatr Soc* 1971;19:860–870.

114. Linnoila M, Viukari M. Efficacy and side effects of nitrazepam and thioridazine as sleeping aids in psychogeriatric inpatients. *Br J Psychiatr* 1976;128:566–569.

115. Linnoila M, Viukari M, Lamminsivu U, Auvinen J. Efficacy and side effects of lorazepam, oxazepam, and temazepam as sleeping aids in psychogeriatric inpatients. *Int Pharmacopsychiatry* 1980;15:129–135.

116. Linnoila M, Viukari M, Numminen A. Efficacy and side effects of chloral hydrate and tryptophan as sleeping aids in psychogeriatric patients. *Int Pharmacopsychiatry* 1980;15:124–128.

117. Viukari M, Linnoila M, Aalto U. Efficacy and side effects of flurazepam, fosazepam, and nitrazepam sleeping aids in psychogeriatric patients. *Acta Psychiatr Scand* 1978;57:27–35.

118. Ancoli-Israel S, Kripke DJ, Klauber MR, et al. Sleep-disordered breathing in community-dwelling elderly. *Sleep* 1991;14:486–495.

119. Reynolds CF, Kupfer DJ. Sleep research in affective illness: state of the art circa 1987 (state-of-the-art review). *Sleep* 1987;10:199–215.

120. Reynolds CF, Hoch CC, Buysse DJ, et al. Sleep in late-life recurrent depression: changes during early continuation therapy with nortriptyline. *Neuropsychopharmacology* 1991;5:85–96.

121. Buysse DJ, Reynolds CF, Hoch CC, et al. Longitudinal effects of nortriptyline on EEG sleep and the likelihood of recurrence in elderly depressed patients. *Neuropsychopharmacology* 1996; 14:243–252.

122. Hohagen F, Montero RF, Weiss E, et al. Treatment of primary insomnia with trimipramine: an alternative to benzodiazepine hypnotics? *Eur Arch Psychiatry Clin Neurosc* 1994;244:65–72.

123. Walsh JK, Engelhardt CL. Trends in the pharmacologic treatment of insomnia. *J Clin Psychiatry* 1992;53:10–17; discussion 18.

124. Dunbar GC, Claghorn JL, Kiev A, et al. A comparison of paroxetine and placebo in depressed outpatients. *Acta Psychiatr Scand* 1993; 87:302–305.

125. Parrino L, Spaggiari MC, Boselli M, et al. Clinical and polysomnographic effects of trazodone CR in chronic insomnia associated with dysthymia. *Psychopharmacology* 1994;116:389–395.

126. Saletu-Zyhlarz GM, Abu-Bakr MH, Anderer P, et al. Insomnia in depression: differences in objective and subjective sleep and awakening quality to normal controls and acute effects of trazodone. *Prog Neuro Psychopharmacology Biol Psychiatry* 2002;26:249–260.

127. Hindmarch I. A review of the psychomotor effects of paroxetine. *Int Clin Psychopharmacol* 1992;6(suppl 4):65–67.

128. Kerr JS, Fairweather DB, Mahendran R, Hindmarch I. The effects of paroxetine, alone and in combination with alcohol on psychomotor performance and cognitive function in the elderly. *Int Clin Psychopharmacol* 1992;7:101–108.

129. Bootzin RR, Perlis ML. Nonpharmacologic treatments of insomnia. *J Clin Psychiatry* 1992; 53:37–41.

130. Friedman L, Bliwise DL, Yesavage JA, Salom SR. A preliminary study comparing sleep restriction and relaxation treatments for insomnia in older adults. *J Gerontol* 1991;46:1–8.

131. Hauri P. Treating psychophysiologic insomnia with biofeedback. *Arch Gen Psychiatry* 1981;38: 752–758.

132. Borkovec TD, Fowles DC. Controlled investigation of the effects of progressive and hypnotic relaxation on insomnia. *J Abnorm Psychol* 1973; 82:153–158.

133. Edinger JD, Wohlgemuth WK, Radtke RA, et al. Does cognitive-behavioral insomnia therapy alter dysfunctional beliefs about sleep? *Sleep* 2001;24:591–599.

134. Espie CA, Inglis SJ, Harvey L. Predicting clinically significant response to cognitive behavior therapy for chronic insomnia in general medical practice: analysis of outcome data at 12 months posttreatment. *J Consult Clin Psych* 2001;69:58–66.

135. Espie CA, Inglis SJ, Tessier S, et al. The clinical effectiveness of cognitive behavior therapy for chronic insomnia: implementation and evaluation of a sleep clinic in general medical practice. *Behavior Research & Therapy* 2001b;39: 45–60.

Table 18.1 References

Caldwell JR. Short-term quazepam treatment of insomnia in geriatric patients. *Pharmatherapeutica* 1982;3:278–282.

Carskadon MA, Seidel WF, Greenblatt DJ, Dement WC. Daytime carryover of triazolam and flurazepam in elderly insomniacs. *Sleep* 1982;5: 361–371.

Elie R, Frenay M, Le Morvan P, Bourgovin J. Efficacy and safety of zopiclone and triazolam in the treatment of geriatric insomniacs. *Int Clin Psychopharmacol* 1990;5(suppl 2):39–46.

Elie R, Deschenes JP. Efficacy and tolerance of zopiclone in insomniac geriatric patients. *Pharmacology* 1983;27(suppl 2):179–187.

Fillingim JM. Double-blind evaluation of temazepam, flurazepam, and placebo in geriatric insomniacs. *Clin Ther* 1982;4:369–380.

Frost JD, DeLucchi MR. Insomnia in the elderly: treatment with flurazepam hydrochloride. *J Am Geriatr Soc* 1979;27:541–546.

Garfinkel D, Laudon M, Nof D, Zisapel N. Improvement of sleep quality in elderly people by controlled-release melatonin. *Lancet* 1995;346: 541–544.

Haimov I, Lavie P, Laudon M, et al. Melatonin replacement therapy of elderly insomniacs. *Sleep* 1995;18:598–603.

Kummer J, Guendel L, Linden J, et al. Long-term polysomnographic study of the efficacy and safety of zolpidem in elderly psychiatric inpatients with insomnia. *J Int Med Res* 1993;21: 171–184.

Mamelak M, Csima A, Buck L, Price V. A comparative study on the effects of brotizolam and flurazepam on sleep and performance in the elderly. *J Clin Psychopharmacol* 1989;9:260–267.

Martinez HT, Serna CT. Short-term treatment with quazepam of insomnia in geriatric patients. *Clin Ther* 1982;5:174–178.

Meuleman JR, Nelson RC, Clark RL Jr. Evaluation of temazepam and diphenhydramine as hypnotics in a nursing–home population. *Drug Intell Clin Pharm* 1987;21:716–720.

Mouret J, Ruel D, Maillard F. Zopiclone versus triazolam in insomniac geriatric patients: a specific increase in delta sleep with zopiclone. *Int Clin Psychopharmacol* 1990;5(suppl 2):47–55.

Nakra BR, Gfeller JD, Hassan R. A double-blind comparison of the effects of temazepam and triazolam on residual, daytime performance in elderly insomniacs. *Int Psychogeriatr* 1992;4:45–53.

Piccione P, Zorick F, Lutz T, et al. The efficacy of triazolam and chloral hydrate in geriatric insomniacs. *J Int Med Res* 1980;8:361–367.

Roehrs T, Zorick F, Wittig R, Roth T. Efficacy of a reduced triazolam dose in elderly insomniacs. *Neurobiol Aging* 1985;6:293–296.

Roger M, Attali P, Coquelin JP. Multicenter, double-blind, controlled comparison of zolpidem and triazolam in elderly patients with insomnia. *Clin Ther* 1993;15:127–136.

Shaw SH, Curson H, Coquelin JP. A double-blind, comparative study of zolpidem and placebo in the treatment of insomnia in elderly psychiatric in-patients [published erratum appears in *J Int Med Res* 1992 Nov;20(6): following 494]. *J Int Med Res* 1992;20:150–161.

Vgontzas AN, Kales A, Bixler EO, Myers DC. Temazepam 7.5 mg: effects on sleep in elderly insomniacs. *Eur J Clin Pharmacol* 1994;46:209–213.

Viukari M, Miettinen P. Diazepam, promethazine and propiomazine as hypnotics in elderly inpatients. *Neuropsychobiology* 1984;12:134–137.

Table 18.2 References

American Hospital Formulary Service Drug Information, 1996;1536:1694–1718.

Bezchlibnuk-Butler KZ, Jeffries JJ, eds. *Clinical handbook of psychotropic drugs*, 5th ed. Seattle: Hogrefe and Huber, 1995.

Farney RJ, Walker JM. Office management of common sleep-wake disorders. *Med Clin North Am* 1995;79:391–414.

Garzone PD, Kroboth PD. Pharmacokinetics of the newer benzodiazepines. *Clin Pharmacokinet* 1989; 16:337–364.

Greenblatt DJ. Benzodiazepine hypnotics: sorting the pharmacokinetic facts. *J Clin Psychiatry* 1991; (suppl 52):4–10.

Greenblatt DJ. Pharmacology of benzodiazepine hypnotics. *J Clin Psychiatry* 1992;(suppl 53):7–13.

Supplemental Readings

General

American Psychiatric Association. *Diagnostic and statistical manual of mental disorders* (DSM-IV). Washington, DC: American Psychiatric Association, 1994.

Bliwise NG, Bliwise DL, Dement WC. Age and psychopathology in insomnia. *Clinics in Gerontology* 1985;4:3–9.

Bliwise DL. Sleep in normal aging and dementia. *Sleep* 1993;16:40–81.

Buysse DJ, Reynolds CF, Hauri PJ, et al. Diagnostic concordance for sleep disorders using proposed DSM-IV categories: a report from the APA/ NIMH DSM-IV field trial. *Am J Psychiatry* 1994; 151:1351–1360.

Buysse DJ, Reynolds CF, Kupfer DJ, et al. Clinical diagnoses in 216 insomnia patients using ICSD, and proposed DSM-IV and ICD-10 categories: a report from the APA/NIMH DSM-IV field trials. *Sleep* 1994;17:630–637.

Cartwright RD. Rapid eye movement sleep characteristics during and after mood-disturbing events. *Arch Gen Psychiatry* 1983;40:197–201.

Chenier MC. Review and analysis of caregiver burden and nursing home placement. *Geriatr Nurs* 1997;18:121–126,

Cohen S, Wills TA. Stress, social support, and the buffering hypothesis. *Psychol Bull* 1985;98: 310–357.

Cohen-Mansfield J, Werner P, Freedman L. Sleep and agitation in agitated nursing home residents: an observational study. *Sleep* 1995;18:674–680.

Cooke KM, Kreydatus MA, Atherton A, et al. The effects of evening light exposure on the sleep of elderly women expressing sleep complaints. *J Behav Med* 1998;21:103–114.

Dealberto MJ, Pajot N, Courbon D, et al. Breathing disorders during sleep and cognitive performance in an older community sample: the EVA study. *J Am Geriatr Soc* 1996;44:1287–1294.

Eaton WM, Badawi M, Melton B. Prodromes and precursors: epidemiologic data for primary prevention of disorders with slow onset. *Am J Psychiatry* 1995;152:967–972.

Englert S, Linden M. Differences in self-reported sleep complaints in elderly persons living in the community who do or do not take sleep medications. *J Clin Psychiatry* 1998;59:137–144.

Foley DJ, Monjan AA, Brown SL, et al. Sleep complaints among elderly persons: an epidemiologic study of three communities. *Sleep* 1995;18: 425–432.

Grad RM. Benzodiazepines for insomnia in community-dwelling elderly: a review of benefit and risk. *J Fam Pract* 1995;41:473–481.

Hauri P, Fisher J. Persistent psychophysiologic (learned) insomnia. *Sleep* 1986;9:38–53.

Hay DP, Bertz RJ. Conspectus. Psychopharmacologic treatment of insomnia in adults and the elderly. *Compr Ther* 1989;15:3–6.

Jenike MA. Psychoactive drugs in the elderly: antipsychotics and anxiolytics. *Geriatrics* 1988;43:53–57.

Karacan I, Thornby JI, Anch M, et al. Prevalence of sleep disturbance in a primarily urban Florida county. *Soc Sci Med* 1976;10:239–244.

Kuppermann M, Lubeck DP, Mazonson PD, et al. Sleep problems and their correlates in a working population. *J Gen Intern Med* 1995;10:25–32.

Lader M. The use of hypnotics and anxiolytics in the elderly. *Int Clin Psychopharmacol* 1986;1:273–283.

Lasagna L. The Halcion story: trial by media. *Lancet* 1980;1:815–816.

McCall WV. Management of primary sleep disorders among elderly persons. *Psychiatr Serv* 1995;46: 49–55.

Mendelson WB. Pharmacotherapy of insomnia. *Psychiatr Clin North Am* 1987;10:555–563.

Monane M. Insomnia in the elderly. *J Clin Psychiatry* 1992;53:23–28.

Nakra BR, Grossberg GT, Peck B. Insomnia in the elderly. *Am Fam Physician* 1991;43:477–483.

Prigerson HG, Frank E, Reynolds CF, et al. Protective psychosocial factors in depression among spousally bereaved elders. *Am J Geriatr Psychiatry* 1993; 1:296–309.

Prinz PN, Vitiello MV, Raskind MA, Thorpy MJ. Geriatrics: sleep disorders and aging. *N Engl J Med* 1990;323:520–526.

Reite M, Buysse D, Reynolds C, Mendelson W. The use of polysomnography in the evaluation of insomnia. *Sleep* 1995;18:58–70.

Reynolds CF, Buysse DJ, Kupfer DJ. Disordered sleep: developmental and biopsychosocial perspectives on the diagnosis and treatment of persistent insomnia. In: Kupfer DJ, Bloom F, eds. *American College of Neuropsychopharmacology: fourth generation of progress.* New York: Raven Press, 1995: 1617–1629.

Reynolds CF, Hoch CC, Buysse DJ, et al. Electroencephalographic sleep in spousal bereavement and bereavement-related depression of late life. *Biol Psychiatry* 1992;31:69–82.

Reynolds CF, Hoch CC, Buysse DJ, et al. Sleep after spousal bereavement: a study of recovery from stress. *Biol Psychiatry* 1993;34:791–797.

Reynolds CF, Monk TH, Hoch CC, et al. Electroencephalographic sleep in the healthy "old old": a comparison with the "young old" in visually scored and automated measures. *J Gerontol* 1991; 46:M39–M46.

Roehrs T, Lineback W, Zorick F, et al. Relationship of psychopathology to insomnia in the elderly. *J Am Geriatr Soc* 1982;30:312–315.

Rosen J, Reynolds CF, Yeager AL, et al. Sleep disturbance in survivors of the Nazi holocaust. *Am J Psychiatry* 1991;148:62–66.

Ross RJ, Ball WA, Dinges DF, et al. Motor dysfunction during sleep in posttraumatic stress disorder. *Sleep* 1994;17:723–732.

Ross RJ, Ball WA, Sullivan KA, Caroff SN. Sleep disturbance as the hallmark of post-traumatic stress disorder. *Am J Psychiatry* 1989;146:697–707.

Shorr RI, Robin DW. Rational use of benzodiazepines in the elderly. *Drugs Aging* 1994;4:9–20.

Strollo PJ, Rogers RM. Obstructive sleep apnea. *N Engl J Med* 1996;334:99–104.

Wauquier A, van Sweden B, Lagaay AM, et al. Clinical investigation: ambulatory monitoring of sleep–wakefulness patterns in healthy elderly males and females (>88 years): the "senieur" protocol. *J Am Geriatr Soc* 1992;40:109–114.

Williams RL, Karacan I. *Pharmacology of sleep.* New York: John Wiley & Sons, 1976.

Yehuda S, Carasso RL. DSIP—a tool for investigating the sleep onset mechanism: a review. *Int J Neurosci* 1988;38:345–353.

Youngstedt SD, Kripke DF, Elliott JA. Melatonin excretion is not related to sleep in the elderly. *J Pineal Res* 1998;24:142–145.

Etiology of Sleep Disorders

Aschoff J. Survival value of diurnal rhythms. In: Edholm OG, ed. *The biology of survival.* London: Academic Press, 1964:79–98.

Giubilei F, Iannilli M, Vitale E, et al. Sleep patterns in acute ischemic stroke. *Acta Neurol Scand* 1992; 86:567–571.

Good DC, Henkle JQ, Gelber D, et al. Sleep-disordered breathing and poor functional outcome after stroke. *Stroke* 1996;27:252–259.

Hoch CC, Dew MA, Reynolds CF, et al. Longitudinal changes in diary- and laboratory-based sleep measures in healthy "old old" and "young old" subjects: a three year follow-up. *Sleep* 1997;20: 192–202.

Hyyppa MT, Kronholm E. Quality of sleep and chronic illnesses. *J Clin Epidemiol* 1989;42:633–638.

Kales J, Tan T, Swearingen C, et al. Are over-the-counter sleep medications effective? *Ther Res Clin Exp* 1971;13:143–151.

Kantor HI, Michael CM, Shore H. Estrogen for older women. *Am J Obstet Gynecol* 1973;116:115–118.

Schenck CH, Bundlie SR, Patterson AL, et al. Rapid eye movement sleep behavior disorder. A treatable parasomnia affecting older adults. *JAMA* 1987;257:1786–1789.

Wessler R, Rubin M, Sollberger A. Circadian rhythm of activity and sleep-wakefulness in elderly institutionalized persons. *J Interdisc Cycle Res* 1976;7: 343–348.

Whitney CW, Enright PL, Newman AB, et al. Correlates of daytime sleepiness in 4578 elderly persons—the cardiovascular health study. *Sleep* 1998;21:27–36.

Williams DC. Periodic limb movements of sleep and

the restless legs syndrome. *Va Med Q* 1996;123: 260–265.

Treatment of Sleep Disorders

Adam K, Oswald I. Can a rapidly-eliminated hypnotic cause daytime anxiety? *Pharmacopsychiatry* 1989; 22:115–119.

Bachman DL. Sleep disorders with aging: evaluation and treatment. *Geriatrics* 1992;47:53–56.

Balter MB, Baner ML. Patterns of prescribing and use of hypnotic drugs in the United States. In: Clift A, ed. *Sleep disturbance and hypnotic drug dependence.* Amsterdam: Excerpta Medica, 1975: 274.

Berg S, Dehlin O, Falkheden T, et al. Long-term study of hypnotic medication in geriatric patients. A study of dixyrazine, nitrazepam and amylobarbitone. *Scand J Soc Med Suppl* 1977;14:85–96.

Bliwise DL. Dementia. In: Kryger MH, Roth T, Dement WC, eds. *Principles and practice of sleep medicine,* 2nd ed. Philadelphia: WB Saunders, 1994: 790.

Bliwise DL, Friedman L, Nekich JC, et al. Prediction of outcome in behaviorally based insomnia treatments. *J Behav Ther Exp Psychiatry* 1995;26:17–23.

Consensus Development Conference. *Diagnosis and Treatment of Sleep Disorders in Late Life.* Bethesda, MD, National Institutes of Health, 1990.

Derbez R, Grauer H. A sleep study with investigation of a new hypnotic compound in a geriatric population. *Can Med Assoc J* 1967;97:1389–1393.

Edinger JD, Hoelscher TJ, Marsh GR, et al. A cognitive-behavioral therapy for sleep-maintenance insomnia in older adults. *Psychol Aging* 1992;7: 282–289.

Engle-Friedman M, Bootzin RR, Hazlewood L, et al. An evaluation of behavioral treatments for insomnia in the older adult. *J Clin Psychol* 1992;48: 77–90.

Folks DG, Burke WJ. Psychotherapeutic agents in older adults. Sedative hypnotics and sleep. *Clin Geriatr Med* 1998;14:67–86.

Forsell Y, Winblad B. Psychiatric disturbances and the use of psychotropic drugs in a population of nonagenarians. *Int J Geriatr Psychiatry* 1997;12: 533–536.

Gottlieb GL. Sleep disorders and their management. Special considerations in the elderly. *Am J Med* 1990;88:29S–33S.

Kales A, Bixler EO, Kales JD, et al. Comparative effectiveness of nine hypnotic drugs: sleep laboratory studies. *J Clin Pharmacol* 1977;17:207–213.

Kripke D, Simons R. Average sleep, insomnia and sleeping pill use. *Sleep Res* 1976;5:110.

Kripke D, Simons R, Garfinkel L, et al. Short and long term sleep and sleeping pills. *Arch Gen Psychiatry* 1979;36:103–107.

Lichstein KL, Johnson RS. Relaxation for insomnia and hypnotic medication use in older women. *Psychol Aging* 1993;8:103–111.

Morin CM, Kowatch RA, Barry T, et al. Cognitive-behavior therapy for late-life insomnia. *J Consult Clin Psychol* 1993;61:137–146.

Morin CM, Colechi C, Stone J, et al. Behavioral and pharmacologic therapies for late-life insomnia:

a randomized controlled trial. *JAMA* 1999;281: 991–999.

Mulligan A, O'Grady C. Reducing night sedation in psychogeriatric wards. *Nurs Times* 1971;67: 1089–1091.

Nowell PD, Buysse DJ, Dew MA, et al. Paroxetine in the treatment of primary insomnia: preliminary clinical and EEG sleep data. *J Clin Psychiatry* 1995; 60:89–95.

Regestein QR. Specific effects of sedative/hypnotic drugs in the treatment of incapacitating insomnia. *Am J Med* 1987;83:909–916.

Satlin A, Volicer L, Ross V, et al. Bright light treatment of behavioral and sleep disturbances in patients with Alzheimer's disease. *Am J Psychiatry* 1992;149:1028–1032.

Seppala M, Hyyppa MT, Impivaara O, et al. Subjective quality of sleep and use of hypnotics in an elderly urban population. *Aging* (Milano) 1997; 9:327–334.

Wancata J, Benda N, Meise U, et al. Psychotropic drug intake in residents newly admitted to nursing homes. *Psychopharmacology* (Berl) 1997;134: 115–120.

Barbiturates

Cheymol G, Bernheim C, Besson J. Study of urinary excretion of butabarbitone in man in relation to the percentage of ideal body weight. *Br J Clin Pharmacol* 1979;7:303–309.

Benzodiazepines

Bandera R, Bollini P, Garattini S. Long-acting and short-acting benzodiazepines in the elderly: kinetic differences and clinical relevance. *Curr Med Res Opin* 1984;8(suppl 4):94–107.

Buchsbaum DG, Boling P, Groh M. Residents underdocumenting in elderly patients' records of prescriptions for benzodiazepines. *J Med Educ* 1987; 62:438–440.

Carskadon MA, Seidel WF, Greenblatt DJ, Dement WC. Daytime carryover of triazolam and flurazepam in elderly insomniacs. *Sleep* 1982;5: 361–371.

Church MW, Johnson LC. Mood and performance of poor sleepers during repeated use of flurazepam. *Psychopharmacology* 1979;61:309–316.

Cohn JB. Triazolam treatment of insomnia in depressed patients taking tricyclics. *J Clin Psychiatry* 1983;44:401–406.

Divoll M, Greenblatt DJ, Harmatz JS, et al. Effect of age and gender on disposition of temazepam. *J Pharm Sci* 1981;70:1104–1107.

Fillingham JM. Double-blind evaluation of the efficacy and safety of temazepam in outpatients with insomnia. *Br J Clin Pharmacol* 1979;8:73–77.

Greenblatt DJ, Allen MD, Shader RI. Toxicity of high-dose flurazepam in the elderly. *Clin Pharmacol Ther* 1977;24:355–361.

Greenblatt DJ, Divoll M, Harmatz JS, et al. Kinetics and clinical effects of flurazepam in young and elderly insomniacs. *Clin Pharmacol Ther* 1981;30: 475–486.

Kales A, Soldatos CR, Bixler EO, et al. Midazolam: dose-response studies of effectiveness and rebound insomnia. *Pharmacology* 1983;26:138–149.

Kesson C, Gray I, Lawson D. Benzodiazepine drugs in general medical patients. *Br Med J* 1976;1: 680–682.

Learoyd BM. Psychotropic drugs and the elderly patient. *Med J Aust* 1972;1:1131–1133.

Lucki I, Rickels K. The behavioral effects of benzodiazepines following long-term use. *Psychopharmacol Bull* 1986;22:424–433.

Martilla JK, Hammel RJ, Alexander B, et al. Potential untoward effects of long-term use of flurazepam in geriatric patients. *J Am Pharm Assoc* 1977;11: 692–695.

Mauro C, Sperlongano P. Controlled clinical evaluation of two triazole benzodiazepine hypnotics used the night before surgery. *Minerva Med* 1987; 78:1381–1384.

Mellman TA, Uhde TW. Withdrawal syndrome with gradual tapering of alprazolam. *Am J Psychiatry* 1986;143:1464–1466.

Merlis S, Koepke HH. The use of oxazepam in elderly patients. *Dis Nerv Syst* 1975;36:27–29.

Meyer BR. Benzodiazepines in the elderly. *Med Clin North Am* 1982;66:1017–1035.

Mitler MM. Evaluation of temazepam as a hypnotic. *Pharmacotherapy* 1981;1:3–13.

Oswald I, Adam K, Borrow W, et al. The effects of two hypnotics on sleep, subjective feelings, and skilled performances. In: Passouant P, Oswald I, eds. *Pharmacology of the states of alertness.* New York: Pergamon, 1979;51–63.

Patterson JF. Alprazolam dependency: use of clonazepam for withdrawal. *South Med J* 1988;81: 830–836.

Petursson H, Lader MH. Withdrawal from long–term benzodiazepine treatment. *Br Med J* 1981;283:643–645.

Poitras R. On episodes of anterograde amnesia associated with use of triazolam. *Union Med Can* 1980; 109:427–429.

Reeves RL. Comparison of triazolam, flurazepam, and placebo as hypnotics in geriatric patients with insomnia. *J Clin Pharmacol* 1977;17:319–323.

Rickels K. The clinical use of hypnotics: indications for use and the need for a variety of hypnotics. *Acta Psychiatr Scand Suppl* 1986;74:132–141.

Roth T, Hartse K, Saab PG, et al. The effects of flurazepam, lorazepam and triazolam on sleep and memory. *Psychopharmacology* 1980;70:231–237.

Roth T, Hartse KM, Zorick FJ, et al. The differential effects of short and long-acting benzodiazepines upon nocturnal sleep and daytime performance. *Drug Res* 1980;30:891–894.

Roth T, Piccione P, Salis P, et al. Effects of temazepam, flurazepam, and quinalbarbitone on sleep: psychomotor and cognitive function. *Br J Clin Pharmacol* 1979;8:47S–54S.

Roth T, Roehrs TA, Zorick FJ. Pharmacology and hypnotic efficacy of triazolam. *Pharmacotherapy* 1983;3:137–148.

Salzman C, Shader RI, Greenblatt DJ, et al. Long versus short half-life benzodiazepines in the elderly: kinetics and clinical effects of diazepam and oxazepam. *Arch Gen Psychiatry* 1983;40:293–297.

Scharf MB, Klosla N, Brocker N, Goff P. Differential amnestic properties of short- and long-acting benzodiazepines. *J Clin Psychiatry* 1984;45:51–53.

Schneider-Helmert D. Clouding of consciousness after use of the hypnotic midazolam. *Schweiz Med Wochenschr* 1985;115:247–249.

Slak S. Alprazolam withdrawal insomnia. *Psychol Rep* 1986;58:343–346.

Tien AY, Gujavarty K. Seizure following withdrawal from triazolam. *Am J Psychiatry* 1985;142: 1516–1517.

Tinetti ME, Speechley M, Ginter SF. Risk factors for falls among elderly persons living in the community. *N Engl J Med* 1988;319:1701–1707.

Tyrer P, Owen R, Dawling S. Gradual withdrawal of diazepam after long-term therapy. *Lancet* 1983; 1:1402–1406.

Chloral Hydrate

Kramer CH. Methaqualone and chloral hydrate: preliminary comparison in geriatric patients. *J Am Geriatr Soc* 1967;15:455–461.

Zolpidem

Fairweather DB, Kerr JS, Hindmarch I. The effects of acute and repeated doses of zolpidem on subjective sleep, psychomotor performance and cognitive function in elderly volunteers. *Eur J Clin Pharmacol* 1992;43:597–601.

Ganzoni E, Santoni JP, Chevillard V, et al. Zolpidem in insomnia: a 3-year post-marketing surveillance study in Switzerland. *J Int Med Res* 1995;23:61–73.

Hoehns JD, Perry PJ. Zolpidem: a nonbenzodiazepine hypnotic for treatment of insomnia [published erratum appears in *Clin Pharm* 1993 Dec; 12(12):881]. *Clin Pharm* 1993;12:814–828.

Scharf MB, Roth T, Vogel GW, Walsh JK. A multicenter, placebo-controlled study evaluating zolpidem in the treatment of chronic insomnia. *J Clin Psychiatry* 1994;55:192–199.

Sharpley AL, Cowen PJ. Effect of pharmacologic treatments on the sleep of depressed patients. *Biol Psychiatry* 1995;37:85–98.

Shaw SH, Curson H, Coquelin JP. A double-blind, comparative study of zolpidem and placebo in the treatment of insomnia in elderly psychiatric in–patients [published erratum appears in *J Int Med Res* 1992 Nov;20(6): following 494]. *J Int Med Res* 1992;20:150–161.

Caffeine, Smoking, and Alcohol

Brezinova V. Effect of caffeine on sleep: EEG study in late middle age. *Br J Clin Pharmacol* 1974;1: 203–208.

Henningfield JE. Pharmacologic basis and treatment of cigarette smoking. *J Clin Psychiatry* 1984;45: 24–34.

Part VII: Dementia and Memory Disorders

Chapter 19

Neurobiology of Alzheimer's Disease

George S. Zubenko

Alzheimer's disease (AD) is the most common cause of dementia in late life. A remarkable number of original reports addressing the neurobiology of this disorder have emerged during the past 10 years. Among the most stunning developments are the inroads that have been made in the biology of amyloid and the genetics of AD during this interval. Rather than catalogue these scientific contributions using an encyclopedic approach, this chapter reviews the progress made in major thematic areas of research on AD and attempts to assemble individual research findings into a more integrated picture of the etiopathogenesis of this disorder.

Neuropathology

The major histologic hallmarks of AD are senile plaques (SPs) and neurofibrillary tangles (NFTs). These aggregates of insoluble fibrillary proteins are distributed throughout the neocortex, hippocampus, and, to a lesser extent, subcortical regions in the brains of patients with this disorder.[1] Senile plaques are complex extracellular morphological lesions. Mature SPs have cores with aggregates of amyloid as their principal constituent[2,3] and are surrounded by dystrophic neurites and activated microglia (Fig. 19.1). These complex extracellular lesions can be visualized after staining with silver, thioflavin S, or with immunohistochemical methods that use antibodies against SP components. Among patients with AD, the density of SPs does not correlate with severity of cognitive impairment, suggesting that they reflect contributions made early in the disease process.[4–6]

Mature SPs appear to develop from diffuse forms that have less well defined ultrastructure and evolve with time into smaller, denser forms ("burnt out"). Diffuse plaques occur in the brains of older individuals without cognitive impairment as well as in locations of the brains of patients with AD, such as the cerebellum, where SPs and NFTs do not characteristically develop.[7,8] This observation suggests that the conversion of diffuse plaques to mature SPs involves events that may be prerequisite to the neurodegeneration that occurs in AD. Moreover, the apparent conversion of mature SPs into "burnt-out" derivatives suggests the existence of a pathway for the resolution of these amyloid-containing lesions that may also have therapeutic relevance.[9]

NFTs of fibrous proteins form within nerve cell bodies, axons, and dendrites (Fig. 19.2). They are also occasionally observed in isolation after degeneration of the neurons in which they were formed. NFTs are highly phosphorylated and, as a result, are argentophilic.[10,11] In electron micrographs of negatively stained prepa-

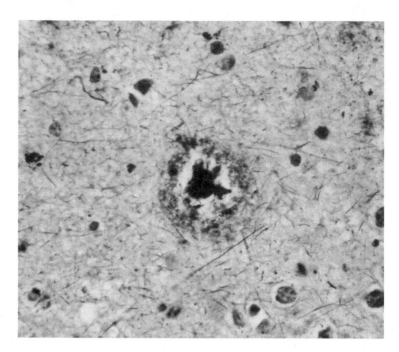

Figure 19.1a. Photomicrographs of senile plaques. **A.** Frontal cortex, Bielschowsky silver stain, 400 × magnification.

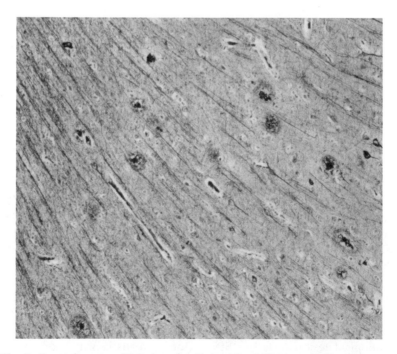

Figure 19.1b. B. Frontal cortex, Bielschowsky silver stain, 100 × magnification.

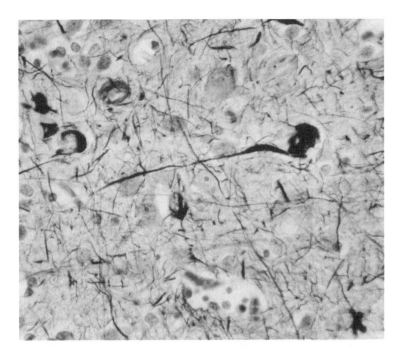

Figure 19.2a. Photomicrographs of neurofibrillary tangles. **A.** Frontal cortex, Bielschowsky silver stain, 400 × magnification.

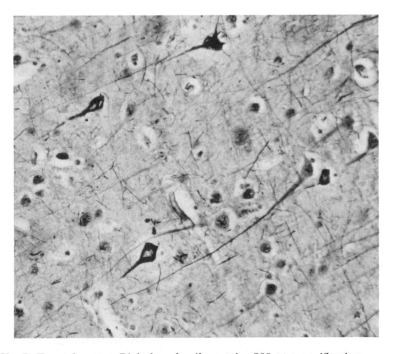

Figure 19.2b. B. Frontal cortex, Bielschowsky silver stain, 200 × magnification.

rations, NFTs consist of paired helical filaments (PHFs) that are ≈20 nm in diameter.[12–16] Cortical densities of NFTs correlate positively with dementia severity among patients with AD and may provide a more proximal reflection of neuronal damage responsible for the clinical phenotype of dementia.[4,6,17]

Postmortem studies have revealed that older individuals who were not demented prior to death have very few mature SPs in their neocortices, which appear to increase only modestly in number with advancing age.[4,18,19] The accumulation of SPs is relatively specific for AD among patients with acquired cognitive impairment, while NFTs accumulate in response to a variety of degenerative, toxic, and traumatic insults to the brain.[20–22] As a result, the neuropathological diagnosis of definite AD relies upon the detection of age-specific densities of SPs.[23]

Substantial densities of NFTs develop with increasing age even among individuals without dementia. However, their proliferation is largely limited to the hippocampus and inferior temporal cortex.[4,18,19] This observation suggests that the age-related accumulation of NFTs in the hippocampus of nondemented elders may reflect neuronal degeneration that corresponds to a more benign age-associated memory impairment rather than AD. Modest age-related decreases in the levels of cholinergic markers in the hippocampus also support this view.[24]

In addition to SPs and NFTs, additional pathological changes are observed in the brains of patients with AD. These include the deposition of amyloid in the microvasculature of the brain and meningeal vessels, leading to cerebral amyloid angiopathy.[25,26] Although amyloid angiopathy is not invariably observed in the brains of patients with AD, it can be severe enough in some patients to produce hemorrhage. Granules located within membrane-limited vacuoles resembling lysosomes occur frequently in the cytoplasm of hippocampal pyramidal cells in AD.[27–29] Although the significance of granulovacuolar de-

generation is uncertain, this characteristic appears to be a harbinger of cell death among this vulnerable population of cells in AD.[28] Ultrastructural studies have also revealed disruptions of the Golgi apparatus in populations of neurons lacking NFTs, which may reflect early events in the pathophysiology of this disorder.[30] Hirano bodies, rod-shaped eosinophilic cytoplasmic inclusions originally described in Guamanian patients with the amyotrophic lateral sclerosis (ALS)-Parkinsonism-dementia complex are also commonly observed in the hippocampal pyramidal cells of patients with AD.[31,32] While their significance is unclear, Hirano bodies appear to contain actin and may be another reflection of cytoskeletal pathology in AD.[33]

Gross examination of the brains of patients with AD reveals atrophy of the cerebral cortex, ventricular dilatation, and a decrease in overall brain weight. These changes result from the combination of a loss of large neurons and dendrites and an apparent shrinkage of the neurons that remain. However, the considerable interindividual differences in these gross characteristics among patients with AD, the lack of specificity of these changes for AD among the other degenerative dementias, and the more modest changes in these parameters that occur with age among nondemented older individuals limits their diagnostic and clinical utility.[18,34] Volumetric determinations of specific structures that undergo atrophy in AD may have greater discriminating power.

Although AD typically leads to diffuse cortical atrophy in the late stages of the disorder, this endpoint is typically reached as the result of progressive multifocal degeneration. The multifocal nature of this degenerative process is reflected in the heterogeneity of the clinical presentations of patients who suffer from AD. For example, patients rarely present with comparable levels of impairment in all areas of cognition, and the specific progression of cognitive deficits can vary considerably from patient to patient.[35–39] Specific neurological symptoms often reflect disproportionate neuronal degeneration in functionally different brain areas.[40–42] Moreover, patients who develop clinically significant depression appear to do so in response to accelerated degeneration of the brainstem aminergic nuclei, especially the locus ceruleus.[34,42–45]

A significant minority of patients with AD suffer from concurrent degenerative brain disorders (especially Parkinson's disease) or cerebrovascular disease that contribute to the severity of the dementia.[23,46–53] In fact, early studies suggest that AD and Parkinson's disease occur together at a rate significantly higher than expected from chance alone.[54] This area of investigation has led to identification of the Lewy body variant of AD (ADLBV). This variant of AD is defined by the presence of cytoplasmic inclusion bodies resembling Lewy bodies in diffuse areas of the neocortex that require immunohistochemical staining with antiubiquitin antibodies for reliable detection.[55–57] Patients with ADLBV have reduced (or absent) numbers of neocortical NFTs, more severe cholinergic deficits, and greater nigrostriatal degeneration.[55,56,58–60] Retrospective clinicopathological studies suggest that patients who suffer from this subtype of AD are more prone to develop delirium, hallucinations, depression, and extrapyramidal symptoms.[55,58–62]

Constituents of Senile Plaques and Neurofibrillary Tangles

Both diffuse plaques and the central cores of mature SPs are complex agglomerations of proteins, the most common of which is amyloid,[3,63] a generic term describing insoluble fibrillar aggregates with a β-pleated sheet structure. As a consequence of this shared conformation, amyloid-containing structures are identifiable by their birefringence when stained with Congo red and illuminated with polarized light. In the brains of patients with AD, the amyloid that accumulates in SPs and

blood vessel walls is composed of the ≈4-kDa amyloid protein (Aβ).[2,3] The Aβ in SPs and vascular amyloid is a mixture of peptides ranging from 39 to 43 amino acids in length.[63,64] Possible sources of the Aβ include neurons, the circulation, and cells in the walls of the cerebrovasculature. However, at least some of the Aβ in parenchymal SPs may be neuronally derived. In addition to amyloid, SPs contain a large number of additional proteins that may provide clues about the pathophysiology of AD. These include synaptic proteins, apolipoproteins, growth factors and receptors, proteases and their inhibitors, heat-shock proteins, proteoglycans, intercellular adhesion and basement membrane proteins, and a variety of proteins related to the immune system (Table 19.1).

Available evidence suggests that, initially, normal neurites in the vicinity of diffuse plaques may be recruited by unaggregated Aβ or other growth factors[65,66] and subsequently rendered dystrophic by toxic effects of amyloid aggregates that are mediated through either direct or indirect mechanisms.[67–75] These neurites have a variety of neurotransmitter phenotypes and probably reflect the predominant neurotransmitters used in the local area of each SP.[76] Dystrophic neurites contain prominent NFTs.

Paired helical filaments are composed primarily of tau, a family of microtubule-associated phosphoproteins whose structural gene is located on chromosome 17.[77–80] NFTs stain heavily with silver as well as Alz-50, a monoclonal antibody that reacts only minimally with normal brain tissue. The antigen to which Alz-50 binds is a 68-kDa protein (A68) that appears to be a hyperphosphorylated tau derivative.[81–84] The participation of tau in the dynamic structure of the cytoskeleton is normally controlled by its state of phosphorylation, which is mediated through protein kinases and phosphatases. In AD, incompletely understood disturbances in this process lead to the hyperphosphorylation of tau protein, which assembles into

Table 19.1. Molecules Associated with Senile Plaque Amyloid

Acute phase reactants	**Proteases/inhibitors**
Heat shock proteins	Trypsin
Amyloid P component	Cathepsin B and D
Coagulation factors	α 1-antichymotrypson
Tissue factor	α 1-antitrypsin
Thrombin	α2-macroglobulin
Hageman factor	Protease nexin I
Complement proteins/	**Other enzymes**
inhibitors	Acetylcholinesterase
Clq	Butyrylcholinesterase
CM, C3c	Dopamine β hydroxylase
C4d	Protein kinase C
Cl Inhibitor	(βII isoform)
C4-binding protein	**Proteoglycans**
Vitronectin	Heparan sulfate
Clusterin	proteoglycan
Protectin	Chondroitin sulfate
Growth factors/receptors	proteoglycan
bFGF	Dermatan sulfate
TGF-β1	proteoglycan
SLIR	**Others**
Midkine	Apolipoproteins
EGFR	Ubiquitin
α-2-macroglobulin R	Synapsin
	Spectrin
	Laminin
	ICAM-1
	Lactoferrin

bFGF, fibroblast growth factor-basic; TGT-bl, transforming growth factor-b1; EGFR, epidermal growth factor receptor; SLIR, somatostatin-like immuno-reactivity; ICAM-1 intercellular adhesion moecule-1. Modified from: McGeer PL, Klegeris A, Walker DG, et al. Pathological proteins in senile plaques. *Tohoku J Exp Med* 1994;174:269–277.

PHFs.[11,85] Disruption of microtubule assembly/disassembly by hyperphosphorylated tau and the formation of PHF may lead to neuronal compromise through interference with normal intracellular trafficking of essential components.

Biology of Amyloid

Aβ is derived from the proteolysis of a larger amyloid precursor protein (APP) (Fig. 19.3). Amyloid precursor protein is encoded by a large gene, including 18 exons and encompassing ≈400 kb of DNA, located in the middle of the long arm of chromosome 21.[86,87] Expression of the APP gene involves the alternate splicing of pre-mRNA species into three transcripts that encode APP molecules of 695, 751, and 770 amino acids in length.[86–91] The largest and intermediate-sized forms (APP$_{770}$, APP$_{751}$) contain a 56-amino-acid domain resembling a Kunitz serine-protease inhibitor that is lacking from the smallest form. The largest form (APP$_{770}$) differs from APP$_{751}$ by the inclusion of an internal 19-amino-acid sequence of unknown function. Its ubiquitous expression in mammalian tissues and evolutionary conservation suggests that APP may have important biological functions.[92–96] APP also appears to be a member of a larger family of APP-like proteins that may share

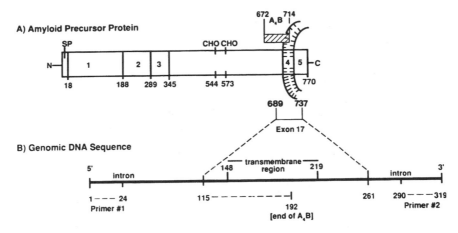

Figure 19.3. Structure of the amyloid precursor protein (**A**) and the respective genomic DNA sequence in proximity to exon 17 (**B**). The structure of APP$_{770}$ is shown with numbers referring to the positions of amino acids that demarcate functional domains. *N*, extracellular amino terminus; *SP*, signal peptide; *1*, cysteine-rich domain; *2*, highly negatively charged domain; *3*, Kunitz-type serine protease inhibitor; *4*, transmembrane domain; *5*, intracellular domain; *C*, carboxyl terminus. The amino and carboxyl terminal residues of the A$_4$β peptide are presented with respect to the APP transmembrane domain. The positions of nucleotides corresponding to the termini of the transmembrane domain and the carboxyl terminus of the A$_4$β are shown. (Reproduced with permission from: Zubenko GS, Stiffler S, Kopp U, et al. Lack of variation in the nucleotide sequence corresponding to the transmembrane domain of the β-amyloid precursor protein in Alzheimer's disease. *Am J Med Genet* 1993;48:131–136.)

some of its biological activities but lack the Aβ sequence.[97,98]

A soluble cleavage product of APP$_{751}$ is identical to protease nexin II/factor XIa inhibitor, a molecule that participates in hemostasis and wound healing.[99,100] However, the role of APP in the central nervous system (CNS) is not well defined. Indirect evidence suggests that APP may participate in mediating cell adhesion and in supporting cell growth.[65,66,101–104]

The APPs are integral membrane glycoproteins that mature through the constitutive secretory pathway and are modified by the addition of *N*- and *O*-linked oligosaccharides, sialic acid, tyrosine sulfate, and phosphate.[105–107] A fraction of synthesized APP is transported to the cell surface.[107–109] Some of these molecules are cleaved by an α-secretase in the midportion of the Aβ sequence (aa687), producing nonamyloidogenic products.[108–113] The larger of these represents almost the entire ectocellular domain of APP, which includes epitopes of Aβ at its

carboxyl terminus and can be detected in cerebrospinal fluid.[114] The remaining ≈10-kDa product remains embedded in the cell membrane.

This observation stimulated the search for an "alternative pathway" of APP processing that could lead to the formation and secretion of Aβ. Some of the full-length APP molecules on the cell surface undergo endocytosis via clathrin-coated vesicles directed by a consensus-targeting sequence in the APP cytoplasmic tail.[115] Internalized APP molecules appear either to be rapidly recycled to the surface or to enter an endosomal/lysosomal pathway that contains the proteases necessary to generate smaller carboxyl-terminal derivatives containing the Aβ sequence.[108,116,117] Whether lysosomal proteolysis leads ultimately to the formation and secretion of Aβ itself is unclear. Additional candidates for the intracellular sites mediating the formation of Aβ include other membrane compartments such as endosomes and the Golgi apparatus.

Regulation of the expression and metabolic fate of APP is complex and incompletely understood. Expression of APP appears to be increased by neuronal injury or ischemia/oxidative stress,[118] exposure to cytokines released by activated microglia including interleukin-1 and basic fibroblast growth factor,[119] and by trisomy 21.[120,121] Neuronal stimulation by cholinergic agonists and other neurotransmitters (e.g., serotonin, vasopressin, bradykinin) that activate the phospholipase C/protein kinase C–dependent signal-transduction pathway stimulates the cleavage of APP by α-secretase and the production of nonamyloidogenic products.[122,123] In contrast, the passage of APP molecules into the amyloidogenic "alternate" pathway is favored by events (often cytotoxic) that lead to increased intracellular free calcium[124] and by certain pathogenic mutations in the presenilin genes that produce early-onset familial AD.[125-128] Pathogenic mutations at or near the amino and carboxyl termini of the Aβ sequence, that produce early-onset familial AD, also alter the proteolytic processing of Aβ in ways that favor amyloidogenesis (see Genetics of AD section).

Aβ is synthesized as a mixture of peptides with a common amino terminus that range from 39 to 43 amino acids in length. This observation suggests that the amino terminus is generated by an endoproteolytic cleavage (β-secretase) whereas the microheterogeneity in the carboxyl terminus may result from progressive digestion by a carboxypeptidase (γ-secretase). The carboxyl terminus of Aβ has an important influence on the tendency of Aβ molecules to aggregate, with the longer peptides Aβ_{1-42} and Aβ_{1-43} favoring fibril formation.[129,130] In fact, Aβ molecules ending in A$\beta_{42(43)}$ may be the predominant species in SP amyloid and may provide the nucleation site for Aβ of shorter lengths.[63,131] The aggregation of Aβ into fibrils may also be enhanced by interactions with apolipoproteins and other potential molecular chaperones.[132-137]

Steady levels of extracellular Aβ deposits appear to reflect a balance between formation and clearance. The low-density lipid (LDL) receptor-related protein-1 (LRP-1) is a multifunctional neuronal receptor for both apolipoprotein E (apoE) and α2-macroglobulin (α2M) that mediates the clearance of both apoE/Aβ and α2M/Aβ complexes.[138,139] This receptor also participates in the clearance of Aβ species from the brain across the blood brain barrier.[140] As a result, the accumulation of cerebral Aβ may result from an imbalance between the formation/secretion of Aβ and the rate of clearance of this material from the brain parenchyma. While the association of the APOE4 allele with AD has been established in many populations worldwide, studies also suggest that variants of the structural genes for LRP-1[141] and α2M may also confer more modest increases in the risk of AD (see Genetics of AD section).

While soluble monomeric Aβ have neuroprotective and trophic properties,[65,66,101-104] aggregates of Aβ appear to be neurotoxic.[67-75] The direct toxic effects of Aβ fibrils on neurons may be mediated through a number of mechanisms including perturbations of intracellular calcium homeostasis, activation of protein kinases, generation of free radicals (oxidative injury), and induced abnormalities in ion channels. Its neurotoxic effects in vivo may also involve indirect effects, including the activation of inflammatory and immune mechanisms that produce cytotoxicity[142] and the sensitization of neurons to excitotoxicity or other physiological stressors.[68]

Neurotransmitters and their Receptors

AD is a complex, multisystem disease involving a variety of neurotransmitters and neuromodulators. Disturbances of these neurotransmitter systems result from presynaptic events that affect the synthesis and release of neurotransmitters at specific locations as well as postsynaptic changes that influence signal transduction and the modulation of cellular responses. Reported presynaptic alterations in AD include decrements in tissue levels of neurotransmitters and their metabolites, reduced levels of respective biosynthetic enzymes, uptake of neurotransmitter precursors, synaptic release of neurotransmitters, and the reuptake of neurotransmitters released at synaptic clefts. Postsynaptic disturbances typically include reductions in receptor binding sites, although disruptions of receptoreffector coupling and signal transduction through second-messenger systems have also been described.

Understanding the complex array of pre- and postsynaptic changes that occur in particular brain neurotransmitter systems in AD is facilitated by placing these findings in an anatomical, cellular, and, when possible, functional context. For example, the loss of presynaptic cholinergic functions that are widely observed throughout the neocortex and hippocampus is largely attributable to the degeneration of cholinergic neurons whose cell bodies reside in the basal forebrain and whose role in memory and learning is well established. This approach has been used to review the more consistently reported disturbances in neurotransmitter systems of the neocortex, hippocampus, and their subcortical afferents (Tables 19.2 and 19.3).

Afferent Neurons

One of the most consistently reported and profound pathological changes in AD is the loss of cholinergic neurons in the basal forebrain (especially the basal nucleus of Meynert) whose projections innervate the neocortex and hippocampus.[143-146] This process is reflected in a loss of the biosynthetic enzyme choline acetyltransferase (ChAT) and decreases in acetylcholinesterase, choline uptake, and the synthesis and release of acetylcholine from cortical tissue slices.[147-153] Several studies have reported significant negative correlations of ChAT activity with the

density of SPs in the neocortex and hippocampus.[18,154-157] Since the cholinergic system plays an important role in memory and learning,[158,159] its degeneration in AD seems likely to contribute to the development of dementia. Reduced cholinergic innervation of the cortex and basal ganglia may also have an attenuating effect on the emergence of depression and parkinsonian features in AD.[34]

The basis for the enhanced vulnerability of cholinergic neurons in patients with AD is unclear. One factor may be related to their need to draw on a limited supply of choline for multiple purposes, including the synthesis of structural components of cell membranes (phosphatidyl choline and sphingomyelin), second-messenger molecules, and the neurotransmitter acetylcholine.[160,161] Despite its key role in neuronal metabolism, brain cells lack the capacity to synthesize choline *de novo*. As a result, they are almost entirely dependent upon the availability of dietary choline for their existence.[162-166] The significant decline in the uptake of circulating choline into brain that develops with age may disproportionately compromise cholinergic neurons whose need for choline is the greatest.[167] This phenomenon may also contribute to the modest and inconsistent effects of increases in dietary choline and its precursor lecithin in ameliorating the memory and cognitive impairments of patients with AD.[168-174]

While muscarinic M_1 receptors probably represent the principal postsynaptic cholinergic receptor subtype in the CNS, at least a subpopulation of muscarinic M_2 receptors appears to function as presynaptic autoreceptors.[175,176] The muscarinic M_3 and M_4 receptors have been defined pharmacologically and by cloning experiments, although their anatomical localizations and functions remain unknown.[177,178] No consistent changes or only modest reductions in total, M_1, and M_2 muscarinic receptor binding have been reported in neocortical, hippocampal, and subcortical brain regions from patients with AD.[179] These inconsistencies

Table 19.2.   Neurotransmitter Disturbances in AD

Afferent Neurotransmitters	Histopathology		Neurochemistry
Ach	Loss of cholinergic neurons in basal forebrain, NFTs	↓	ChAT, AChE, choline uptake, ACh synthesis and release, and receptor changes
5-HT	Loss of serotonergic cells from dorsal and median raphe, NFTs	↓	5-HT, 5-HIAA, 5-HT uptake, 5-HT$_2$ receptor binding
NE	Loss of cells from locus ceruleus, NFTs	↓	NE, DPH, NE uptake
DA	Loss of cells from the substantia nigra and ventral tegmental area, NFTs (ADLBV much greater than pure AD); Lewy bodies in ADLBV	↓ ↓	DA, HVA, and TH, in caudate, hippocampus, and amygdala; D$_1$ and D$_2$ receptors in some regions; (for both, ADLBV much greater than pure AD)

Intrinsic Neurotransmitters	Histopathology		Neurochemistry
Glu	Loss of pyramidal cells from neocortex and hippocampus, GVD, NFTs	↓ ↓ ↓	Glu levels (esp. hippocampus); Receptor binding
GABA	GAD immunoreactivity in SPs	↓ ↓ ↓	GABA (esp. inferior temporal); GABA uptake; Receptor binding
Somatostatin	NFTs in somatostatin-containing neurons	↓	Somatostatin-like immunoreactivity in cortex
CRF	Loss of cortical interneurons?	↓	CRF-like immunoreactivity in cortex

ACh, acetylcholine; ChAT, choline acetyltransferase; AChE, acetylcholine esterase; 5-HT, 5-hydroxytryptamine (serotonin); 5-HIAA, 5-hydroxyindoleacetic acid; NE, norepinephrine; DβH, dopamine β-hydroxylase; Glu, glutamate; GVD, granulovacuolar degeneration; GABA, γ-aminobutyric acid; DA, dopamine; ADLBV, AD-Lewy body variant; HVA, homovanillic acid; TH, tyrosine hydroxylase.

may result in part from a complex sequence of events, including progressive loss of presynaptic cholinergic afferents accompanied by the transient upregulation of cholinergic receptors on postsynaptic neurons. However, the functional status of these receptors remains uncertain. Reduced coupling of the M$_1$ receptor to its corresponding G protein occurs, resulting in decreased high-affinity-ligand binding.[180,181] This phenomenon may limit the effectiveness of cholinergic augmentation strategies, including those that involve the use of cholinomimetic agents or acetylcholinesterase inhibitors,[182] and compound the obstacle to dietary strategies posed by age-associated reduction in choline uptake into the brain.

The density of cholinergic nicotinic receptors in the brain is substantially lower than that of muscarinic receptors, and their function in the CNS is unknown.[183] However, they appear to be located on both pre- and postsynaptic sites, suggesting that a fraction of them may serve as autoreceptors. In contrast to muscarinic receptors, substantial reductions in nicotinic receptor binding in the neocortex and hippocampus have been consistently reported in AD.[184–186] This may at least

Table 19.3.   Neurotransmitter Receptor Disturbances in AD

Afferent Neurotransmitters	Receptor Subtype	G Protein-Linked (GP) or Ligand-Gated (LG)	
		Channel	Receptor Disturbance
Ach	Muscarinic M_1	GP	No consistent change; possible G protein uncoupling
	Muscarinic M_2	GP	No change or modest $\downarrow$ (presynaptic autoreceptor?)
	Muscarinic M_3	GP	?
	Muscarinic M_4	GP	?
	Nicotinic	LG	Substantial $\downarrow$ in neocortex and hippocampus (pre- and postsynaptic)
5-HT	1A	GP	No consistent change, although modest
	1B	GP	$\downarrow$ in 5-HT$_{1A}$ binding has been
	1C	GP	reported
	1D	GP	
	2	GP	Substantial $\downarrow$ in neocortex, hippocampus, and subcortical regions
NE	3	LG	
	$\alpha 1$	GP	No consistent change
	$\alpha 2$	GP	$\downarrow$, when agonist binding is measured (presynaptic autoreceptor?)
DA	$\beta 1$	GP	No consistent change
	$\beta 2$	GP	No consistent change
	$\beta 3$	GP	?
	D_1	GP	No consistent change. Possible U protein uncoupling.
	D_2	GP	$\downarrow$ in basal ganglia
	D_3	GP	?
	D_4	GP	
	D_5	GP	

Intrinsic Neurotransmitters	Receptor Subtype	G Protein-Linked (GP) or Ligand-Gated (LG)	
		Channel	Receptor Disturbance
Ghi	NMDA	LG	$\downarrow$ in cortex, $\downarrow$ in hippocampus, $\downarrow$ ion channels
	AMPA	LG	$\downarrow$ in hippocampus (also in glia)
	Kainate	LG	No consistent changes
	Metabotropic	GP	$\downarrow$ in hippocampus
GABA	GABA$_A$	LG	Inconsistent changes in neocortex. Modest $\downarrow$ in hippocampus
	GABA$_B$	GP	$\downarrow$ neocortex and hippocampus (few studies)

ACh, acetylcholine; 5-HT, 5-hydroxytryptamine; NE, norepinephrine; DA, dopamine; Glu, glutamate; GABA, γ-aminobutyric acid.

partially reflect the loss of presynaptic cholinergic terminals.

Degeneration of the major brainstem aminergic nuclei that occurs in AD is likely to contribute to disturbances in perception, mood, thought, and behavior ("noncognitive" disturbances) that are common and important sources of suffering and excess disability.[34,43,187,188] Projections from the dorsal and median raphe nuclei provide extensive serotonergic innervation of the forebrain. The noradrenergic cells of the locus ceruleus project axons widely to both the neocortex and the hippocampus. AD is associated with the loss of neuronal cells from both of these nuclei, and a substantial fraction of those that remain develop NFTs.[43,189–192] The neurochemical correlates of this process include decrements in levels of these amine neurotransmitters, their metabolites, and their respective biosynthetic enzymes as well as in the presynaptic reuptake of both neurotransmitters in their projection areas.[34,148,193–195] While the bulk of the evidence of disturbances in brain neurotransmitter systems in AD derives from postmortem studies, the cholinergic, serotonergic, and noradrenergic deficits have been confirmed in living patients through examination of brain tissue removed for diagnostic purposes.[196,197]

Three serotonergic receptor classes have been defined by both pharmacologic and molecular biological studies.[198,199] The 5-HT$_{1A}$ receptor produces slow hyperpolarization of neurons through a G protein–mediated mechanism. In contrast, 5-HT$_2$ and 5-HT$_3$ receptors lead to neuronal depolarization.[200] The excitatory effect of 5-HT$_2$ receptors appears to result from their localization on glutamatergic pyramidal neurons in the cortex.[201] Absent or modest reductions in 5-HT$_1$ receptors occur in AD,[202–205] while substantial reductions in 5-HT$_2$ receptors occur and may reflect the loss of pyramidal cells.[204] These events may lead to a change in the net effect of brain serotonergic neurotransmission favoring the inhibition of neuronal firing. The therapeutic effect of 5-HT$_{1A}$ antagonists (SSRIs) on disturbances of mood and behavior in AD[206] may result from a reduction in 5-HT$_{1A}$-mediated hyperpolarization.[207]

The only consistently reported change in noradrenergic receptor binding in AD is a reduction in α_2-receptors and an increase in β_2 receptors that is observed when agonist binding is measured.[208,209] Since the α_2-receptor is likely to function as a presynaptic autoreceptor, this observation is probably a reflection of the loss of noradrenergic afferents in the neocortex and hippocampus.

Most dopaminergic neurons in the brain reside in the pars compacta of the substantia nigra and the ventral tegmental area, although some evidence suggests that a small fraction of intrinsic cortical neurons of primates may use this neurotransmitter as well.[210] Dopaminergic neurons in the substantia nigra project primarily to the basal ganglia through the nigrostriatal system. The neocortical system, which arises from the ventral tegmental area, projects more widely to the prefrontal, cingulate, and entorhinal cortex as well as other limbic structures. Although five dopamine receptor subtypes have been cloned, reliable binding assays exist only for D$_1$ and D$_2$ receptors.[198,211] Both receptor subtypes appear to reside predominantly on postsynaptic neurons, although a subset of D$_2$ receptors are located on presynaptic dopaminergic nerve terminals.[212]

The role of dopaminergic systems in AD is complex and remains the subject of considerable research interest. In AD without Lewy body pathology, only modest cell loss from the substantia nigra and ventral tegmental area occurs,[213,214] with concomitant reductions in dopamine, its metabolite homovanillic acid, and the biosynthetic enzyme tyrosine hydroxylase.[34,197,215–218] The density of D$_1$ receptors appears to be unaffected or modestly reduced in the neocortex and basal ganglia.[219–222] However, somewhat larger reductions have been observed in autoradiographic studies of the hippocampus and nucleus accumbens.[220,221] Interestingly, selective loss of high-affinity D_1 receptors has been reported in the frontal cortex of patients with AD[219] and resembles the apparent decoupling of the M_1 muscarinic receptor from its respective G protein. Both of these phenomena may result from abnormalities of neuronal membranes (see section on Cell Membranes). The loss of D_2 receptors has been more consistently reported and probably reflects the loss of dopaminergic terminals in these regions.[219] Deficits in all of these dopaminergic indices are considerably greater when Lewy bodies are present in the neocortex and substantia nigra.[58,218] The Lewy body variant of AD also appears to be associated with greater cholinergic deficits.[55,223]

Intrinsic Neurons

Glutamate, the principal excitatory neurotransmitter in the brain, is released by intrinsic pyramidal neurons and spiny stellate interneurons in the neocortex and hippocampus.[224] Of relevance to AD, glutamate is the neurotransmitter used by cortico-cortical association pathways, the perforant pathway from entorhinal cortex to dentate gyrus, and both intrinsic and efferent hippocampal pathways.[225–230] Like cholinergic neurons, substantial loss of pyramidal neurons occurs in AD, and those pyramidal neurons that remain often develop NFTs and granulovacuolar degeneration, indicating neuronal dysfunction and harbingers of cell death.[26–29,224,231] Decreases in tissue levels of glutamate in the neocortex have been reported along with even larger reductions in the hippocampus.[232–234]

Glutamate exerts its effects through four classes of receptors, three of which consist of ligand-gated ion channels.[230,235] N-Methyl-D-aspartate (NMDA) receptors are present at high concentrations throughout the brain, especially in the neocortex and hippocampus, where their distribution overlaps considerably with that of N-acetylaspartylglutamate (AMPA) receptors.[236–239] Both of these glutamate receptors contain ion channels that are permeable to calcium ions. As a result, both NMDA and AMPA receptors participate in two phenomena that may be important in the pathophysiology of AD: long-term potentiation (LTP) and excitotoxicity. LTP refers to marked and enduring enhancement in the responsiveness of postsynaptic hippocampal neurons that results from brief tetanic stimulation of presynaptic fibers, a process that appears to occur physiologically.[240–242] As such, LTP is an electrophysiological model for learning and memory that involves the major synaptic pathways of the hippocampus. Overstimulation of NMDA and AMPA receptors can lead to excessive calcium influx into neurons resulting in cell damage or death, a process termed excitotoxicity.[243] Excitotoxicity contributes to neuronal death caused by stroke or trauma, and the administration of NMDA receptor antagonists affords a degree of neuroprotection in these contexts.[244,245] Indirect evidence suggests that excitotoxicity may play a contributing role in the neurodegeneration that occurs in AD.[68,234,246–248]

Although divergent reports have appeared, the preponderance of available evidence suggests that NMDA receptors are reduced in the neocortex and hippocampus in AD.[204,249–255] These changes have been demonstrated by the loss of both NMDA binding sites and ion channels in these regions. AMPA receptor binding is also reduced in the hippocampus.[204,256,257] However, the presence of AMPA receptors on glial cells, which proliferate in AD, may obscure even larger reductions in neuronal AMPA receptors.[258–260]

Less is known about kainate and metabotropic receptors. Like AMPA receptors, kainate and metabotropic regions appear to be present on glial cells as well as neurons.[259,261] Moreover, metabotropic receptors represent the only G-protein–linked glutamate-receptor subtype.[262] Inconsistent changes in kainate receptor binding have been reported in AD.[251,252,254,263] Metabotropic receptor binding in the hippocampus may be reduced in AD,[257] although relatively few studies address this issue.

γ-aminobutyric acid (GABA) is the predominant intrinsic neurotransmitter in the neocortex and hippocampus. According to estimates, GABA-containing neurons account for 30 to 40% of all intrinsic cortical neurons. Most inhibitory interneurons, nonspiny stellate cells, and bipolar cells use GABA or neuropeptides as neurotransmitters.[223] The evidence implicating GABA-ergic neurons in AD includes significant reductions of GABA in widespread cortical areas, reduced uptake of GABA into synaptosomes prepared from the neocortex and hippocampus, and the presence of the biosynthetic enzyme glutamic acid decarboxylase immunoreactivity in SPs.[150,232] Reductions in somatostatin-like immunoreactivity (SLIR) and corticotropin-releasing factor–like immunoreactivity in the cortex have also been consistently reported in AD, with the formation of NFTs in SLIR-positive interneurons.[264–266] The concordant abnormalities of these neurotransmitter systems in AD is not surprising, since GABA and SLIR appear to be colocalized in a subset of cortical neurons.[264]

GABA exerts its effects through two receptor subtypes, $GABA_A$ and $GABA_B$.[268] The former is a ligand-gated ion channel that allows the influx of chloride ions, resulting in neuronal hyperpolarization. It is allosterically controlled by benzodiazepines and barbiturates. The less abundant $GABA_B$ receptor is a G-coupled receptor whose stimulation produces slow postsynaptic inhibitory potentials. AD is associated with normal levels or modest reductions in $GABA_A$ receptors in the neocortex and hippocampus.[238,260–272] Reductions in $GABA_B$ receptor binding have also been described, although only a few studies of $GABA_B$ receptor changes in AD have been reported.[270,273]

Energy Metabolism

Positron emission tomography (PET) using 2-[^{18}F]fluoro-2-deoxy-D-glucose (^{18}FDG PET) provides a method for measuring glucose metabolism in the cortical and subcortical brain regions of living subjects.[274–276] ^{18}FDG PET studies of patients with AD widely report regional reductions in resting glucose metabolism, especially in the parietal and temporal areas.[277–282] These metabolic changes appear to develop early in the course of AD, at or before the onset of symptoms.[283–287] As a consequence, refinements of this technique may contribute to early identification of asymptomatic individuals with this diathesis, when the greatest potential exists for therapeutic intervention. Like most biological abnormalities that have been described in AD, the distributions of ^{18}FDG PET measures of regional cerebral glucose metabolism in patients with AD, individuals at risk for AD, and nondemented controls exhibit substantial overlap.[280,286–288] Furthermore, reductions in cerebral glucose metabolism have also been reported for cognitively intact older patients with late-life depression and Parkinson's disease, although the pattern of affected brain regions may partially differentiate among these disorders.[288–290] As a result, this approach currently has limited usefulness for the diagnosis of AD in individual patients. However, refinements in functional brain imaging promise to provide new insights into the clinical biology of AD as well as other psychiatric disorders.[291]

Reductions in cerebral glucose metabolism among patients with AD are often attributed to neuronal loss and reduced basal synaptic activity.[292] However, abnormalities of glucose transport, glycolysis, or oxidative phosphorylation also have the potential to contribute to these characteristics. Alterations in mitochondrial energy metabolism in AD have been reported from in vitro and in vivo studies of brain tissue and nonneural tissue.[293,294] Biochemical studies have revealed reductions in the specific activities of cytochrome oxidase, a component of the electron transport chain, as well as succinate dehydrogenase and ketoglutarate dehydrogenase, which catalyze steps in the Krebs cycle.[295-298] Of these abnormalities, reduction in ketoglutarate dehydrogenase has been the most consistently replicated in brain tissue and fibroblasts from patients with AD. The variable reductions observed in cytochrome oxidase activity are consistent with the hypothesis that they may arise from secondary damage to the mitochondrial genome, which encodes 3 of the 13 subunits of this complex.[297] Alternatively, alterations in post-translational modification or protein trafficking in AD may compromise the subunits encoded by nuclear genes.

In vivo ^{31}P magnetic resonance spectroscopy (^{31}P MRS) provides an opportunity to evaluate brain energy metabolism not available through autopsy studies. Reductions in the relative amounts of phosphocreatine and ADP, the immediate precursors of ATP, have been reported in the prefrontal cortex of AD patients with mild impairment and appear to normalize as the dementia worsens.[294] This observation (although controversial)[280] suggests an elevation in the oxidative metabolic rate of brain tissue early in the disorder that attenuates with advancing degeneration.

Two additional studies suggest that brain oxidative stress may contribute to the pathophysiology of AD. Coronary artery disease was reported to be associated with an elevation in the density of cortical SPs among patients without AD,[299] and women with a history of myocardial infarction also have a significantly higher cumulative incidence of AD.[300] This phenomenon may also contribute to the common concurrence of AD and cerebrovascular disease among demented patients in autopsy studies.

Cell Membranes

Biophysical studies using ^{31}P magnetic resonance and fluorescence spectroscopy, small-angle x-ray diffraction, and differential scanning calorimetry reveal AD-associated alterations in the structural and dynamic properties of brain cell membranes that are likely to be functionally significant.[294,301,302] Biophysical changes of the magnitude reported are likely to produce alterations in signal transduction and the intercellular transport of small molecules in several ways. The intrinsic activities of integral membrane proteins, including receptors, ion channels, and enzymes, are sensitive to changes to their local environments and often require localization in lipid domains of defined composition for optimal activity. In addition, signal transduction across cell membranes requires coordinated interactions between activated receptors and their local effectors, including G proteins. Alterations in membrane structural and biophysical properties can also have deleterious consequences for the efficiency of receptor-effector coupling and the subsequent modulation of second and third messengers.[303-305] These mechanisms may contribute to reported reductions in high-affinity M_1 muscarinic and D_1 dopaminergic receptor densities in AD.[176,177,219]

Brain Cell Membranes

Alterations of brain membrane lipid composition that occur in AD are summarized in Table 19.4. A series of in vitro and in

Table 19.4. Alterations of Brain Membrane Lipid Composition in AD

	PHOSPHOLIPIDS
↓	Phosphatidylcholine and ethanolamine, phosphatidic acid
↓	PME (early?), PDE (late?), phosphatidylserine, sphingomyelin, cardiolipin (mitochondria)
→	Phosphatidyl inositol
	NEUTRAL LIPIDS
↓	Cholesterol
↑	Ubiquinone (mitochondria)
?	Dolichols, gangliosides

PME, phosphomonesters; PDE, phosphodiesters.

vivo ^{31}P MRS studies suggest an increase in brain phosphomonoesters early in the course of AD followed by increased brain phosphodiesters later in the disorder.[294,306] In these studies, reduced phosphatidylcholine levels, like ChAT-specific activity, correlates with the density of SPs. Increases in the level of brain phosphatidylserine have also been reported in AD, and L-phosphoserine may have toxic effects, including the perturbation of normal cell membrane structure, binding to NMDA receptors, and inhibition of choline acetyltransferase activity.[307–309] Elevations in the levels of both cardiolipin and ubiquinone, lipids that are concentrated in mitochondria and participate in the electron transport chain, have been interpreted as physiological responses to oxidative stress.[294,310] Analyses of the fatty acid composition of brain phospholipids reveal a relative increase in fatty acid unsaturation compatible with abnormalities in 6 desaturase activity in AD.[311–313]

Small-angle x-ray diffraction studies of neural plasma membranes from the temporal cortices of patients who died with AD reveal a 4Å reduction in lipid bilayer width that is associated with a 30% decrease in unesterified membrane cholesterol.[314] Moreover, experimental restoration of the cholesterol content results in normalization of the membrane bilayer width and electron density profile, strongly suggesting that cholesterol deficit plays an important role in the perturbation of neuronal membranes in AD. Reductions in membrane cholesterol and increased fatty acid unsaturation are important determinants favoring increased membrane fluidity.[315]

Inconsistent changes in levels of dolichols and gangliosides have been reported in the brains of patients with AD: While the overall level of dolichols appears to decline, the amount of dolichol phosphate increases.[310,316] This moiety plays a key role in the biosynthesis of glycoproteins containing asparagine-linked oligosaccharides, including APP, and may reflect an accelerated rate of glycoprotein

synthesis.[317] Gangliosides appear to be relatively concentrated at synaptic terminals and to be among the components of NFTs.[318] Although changes in the level of brain gangliosides are inconsistent, the levels of GM_1 and GD_{1a} in CSF appear to rise in patients with AD and may reflect the release of gangliosides during neuritic degeneration.[319]

Peripheral Cells

Abnormalities of cell membrane structure and function have been reported in several nonneural tissues from patients with AD.[320,321] The most thoroughly characterized of these is increased platelet membrane fluidity (PMF), as reflected in decreased fluorescence anisotropy of 1,6-diphenyl-1,3,5-hexatriene (DPH) in labeled membranes at 37°C.[301] This finding was replicated by several independent research groups during the last decade, each of which recruited subjects from clinical populations in their respective locations on three continents.[322–327] In aggregate, these published studies include approximately 500 patients and controls and incorporate strategies to control for the potential effects of age, sex, concurrent medical conditions, and medication exposure. Increased PMF in AD is also seen using an independent technique, electron spin resonance spectroscopy.[328] Only one report failed to find an association between PMF and AD, perhaps because of differences in laboratory methods.[329]

Increased PMF appears to be unrelated or weakly related to sex,[330–332] to remain stable during adulthood,[330–333] and to be associated relatively specifically with AD among the mental disorders that produce cognitive impairment in late life.[301,322,330] In cross-sectional studies, increased PMF identifies among patients with AD a subgroup with distinct clinical features. AD patients with increased PMF suffer from earlier symptomatic onset (approximately 5 years),[330,334] more rapidly progressive decline,[330] and lower prevalence of focal electroencephalographic slowing[335] and risk factors for stroke.[336] In light of these findings, the AD subgroup with increased PMF may represent a more homogeneous group of patients whose dementias are more likely to result from a purely degenerative etiology rather than ischemia or a mixture of etiologies. Evaluations of the cognitive impairments of patients with AD do not reveal any specific cognitive deficits, or spectrum of cognitive deficits, associated with increased PMF.[337]

While increased PMF is not associated exclusively with familial forms of AD, increased PMF itself appears to be a familial trait that aggregates in the asymptomatic, first-degree relatives of patients with AD.[331,334] Moreover, this phenotype is vertically transmitted in families so ascertained through probands with clinically diagnosed or autopsy-confirmed AD.[328] These findings exclude nonspecific concomitants of chronic illness or medication history as the cause of increased PMF in patients with AD and suggest that this molecular phenotype antedates the onset of dementia in these individuals. A complex segregation analysis of continuous DPH anisotropy values found evidence for the existence of a single major locus that could explain 80% of the variance in PMF among the members of these families.[332] Furthermore, the initial results from a prospective study of an AD high-risk cohort suggest that this phenotype is a risk factor for AD.[338]

What is the mechanism by which increased PMF may elevate the risk of developing AD? If cerebral ischemia plays some as yet undefined role in the development of AD, platelets may contribute directly to the biology of this disorder through their participation in atherogenesis and thrombosis. Another possibility derives from the fact that platelets are a rich source of APP and have the potential to contribute to the development of AD by delivering APP or its amyloidogenic derivatives to endothelial cells of the cerebral vasculature.[339–342] Both of these mechanisms involve the direct participation of platelets

in the pathogenesis of AD and suggest that agents modulating platelet function may have a place in the treatment of this disorder. The mechanism by which antiinflammatory agents, such as aspirin and other nonsteroidal antiinflammatory agents (NSAIDs), appear to exert a protective effect against AD may warrant reconsideration in this light. Recent evidence from in vitro, animal, and human studies suggests that inhibitors of the cholesterol biosynthetic enzyme 3-hydroxy 30methylglutaryl CoA reductase (statins) reduce the level of Aβ as well as cholesterol in blood and brain.[343] Although the mechanism by which this effect on Aβ levels is uncertain, may derive from reduced β-secretase activity, which is cholesterol-dependent. Retrospective human studies suggest that treatment with cholesterol-lowering statin drugs may reduce the risk of AD by up to 70%.[344–346] Moreover, treatment with atorvastatin (Lipitor) significantly attenuates the deposition of Aβ in the PSAPP transgenic mouse model of AD.[347] Since atorvastatin does not cross the blood-brain barrier, these findings suggest that the clinical and pharmacologic actions of statins on AD pathology may be peripherally mediated. These findings also raise the possibility that platelets, the largest reservoir of APP in the body, may play a direct role in the pathophysiology of AD. Alternatively, substantive evidence suggests that the increased risk of AD associated with increased PMF is conferred by the expression of the *PMF* locus in the CNS. Regardless of mechanism, continued investigation of the cellular and molecular events that give rise to increased membrane fluidity of platelets may provide insight into the pathophysiology of AD.

The results of ultrastructural,[324,348,349] biochemical,[324,350,351] and biophysical[325,331,348–350] studies suggest that increased PMF in AD results from the accumulation of a functionally abnormal internal membrane compartment resembling smooth endoplasmic reticulum (SER).[351] Because the SER plays an important role in both maturation and localization of cellular proteins,[352,353] especially glycoproteins, a functional defect in this (or a related) organelle, or an alteration in membrane/protein trafficking, may lead to the synthesis of inappropriately modified proteins along with the improper localization of proteins or complex carbohydrates within or outside the cell. This model provides a potential mechanism by which cell viability could be compromised by the loss of important enzymes, structural proteins, or proteins in the plasma membrane required for signal transduction or endo/exocytosis, or could result in formation of toxic molecules. Among the proteins in this final category are those that have the potential to become cytotoxic through a membrane-dependent change from α-helical to β-pleated sheet conformations, including amyloid and prion proteins.[354] The conversion of both of these membrane proteins to their respective pathological forms requires passage through internal membrane compartments resembling ER.[116,354,355]

It seems plausible that the *PMF* locus may control the efficiency of a rate-limiting step in this process. Interestingly, the greatest concentrations of APP and presenilins are localized within the SER or the early Golgi.[128,348] Moreover, mutations in the presenilin structural genes produce increased risk of AD with varying ages of onset, as well as increased production of long Aβ peptides that have an enhanced propensity for aggregation.[127,129] These observations further suggest that the site of the internal membrane abnormality associated with increased PMF may be appropriately positioned to alter the processing of APP in a way that favors the formation and secretion of amyloidogenic products. Since the SER also plays a central role in calcium homeostasis, an abnormality of this compartment could produce a variety of toxic effects mediated by a dysregulation in calcium-sensitive regulatory cascades.[318,321] Elevations in intracellular levels of free calcium have also

been reported to enhance the amyloidogenic processing of APP.[124]

Inflammation and Immune Mechanisms

Considerable evidence implicates inflammatory and immune mechanisms in the neurodegeneration that occurs in AD.[142,357] Microglia are widely distributed in the brain and function as the counterparts of monocytes in blood and macrophages in peripheral tissues. In AD, cells exhibiting the morphological and biochemical features of activated microglia cluster within or near SPs and NFTs. At these locations, activated microglia attach to targets for phagocytosis by modifications in their spectra of surface receptors.[358,359] Once attached, activated microglia release a number of compounds that have direct toxic effects on local cells.[360,361] They also secrete cytokines that attract T lymphocytes, albeit in modest numbers, and express major histocompatible complex proteins that enable them to potentially interact with these T cells.[362,363] Diffuse Aβ deposits do not appear to trigger the activation of microglia and, as previously described, the molecular events that lead to the conversion of diffuse Aβ deposits to SPs remain unknown.

Complement proteins appear to be synthesized in the normal brain by microglia and possibly by astrocytes and certain neurons as well.[364,365] The synthesis of these proteins is greatly enhanced in patients with AD, and proteins derived from the activation of the classical pathway are richly deposited in both diffuse Aβ deposits and SPs (see Table 19.1). In vitro studies suggest that complement activation is initiated by the interaction of component C1q with Aβ (and possibly other molecules), followed by the binding of this complex to local target cells.[366,367] This event both labels the target for eventual phagocytosis and triggers a cascade of proteolytic cleavages of complement proteins that generate peptides with immune-stimulating activity. This pathway terminates in the assembly of the membrane attack complex, which attaches to available cells, disrupts membrane integrity, and leads to cell lysis. Dystrophic neurites in SPs stain intensely for the membrane attack complex, suggesting that this process contributes to their demise.[362]

The actions of the complement system are normally kept in check by a fail-safe mechanism involving a number of protease inhibitors. These include at least three inhibitors of the membrane attack complex: clusterin, vitronectin, and protectin.[368–370] The enhanced expression of these proteins in the brains of patients with AD strongly suggests a physiological response to destructive autolytic events in the brain mediated by complement activation.[368,371,372]

Evidence of the possible beneficial effects of antiinflammatory agents including corticosteroids, ACTH, NSAIDs, and aspirin in delaying the age at onset and slowing the rate of progression of AD have been reported in retrospective studies of twin pairs,[373,374] clinical populations,[375] and population-based epidemiological samples.[376,377] Initial results from a controlled study of indomethacin have been encouraging in this regard,[378] although findings from subsequent prospective studies have been inconsistent.[379]

Infectious Agents and Toxins

Prions cause transmissible and genetic neurodegenerative disorders of humans and other vertebrate animals.[354] These spongiform encephalopathies include kuru, Creutzfeldt-Jacob disease (CJD), and Gerstmann-Sträussler-Schenker disease (GSS) among humans, as well as scrapie and bovine spongiform encephalopathy ("mad cow" disease) among livestock. Prions are composed largely, and perhaps exclusively, of an altered isoform of the normal cellular prion protein.[380] In the inherited prion diseases (forms of CJD

and GSS), the conformational change is induced by mutations in the prion structural gene.[354,381] Sporadic/transmissible cases arise from infection by an altered isoform that interacts with and converts normally occurring prion protein molecules to the altered isoform. This process appears to occur in the ER or Golgi and results from a conformational change in the native prion protein.[382–387] How altered prion isoforms produce neurodegeneration remains unknown. Some prion diseases are associated with the development of AD-like neuropathological lesions in the brain including SPs and NFTs.[388–392] However, the amyloid in these SPs is composed of prion protein rather than $A\beta$. This morphological similarity and a potentially shared intracellular site of abnormal posttranslational modification suggests an overlap in the pathophysiology of the human prion diseases with AD.

The neurotoxic potential of aluminum has been established by experiments performed in vitro as well as in vivo.[393] Animal models demonstrate a variety of biochemical abnormalities, cytotoxic changes, and behavioral disturbances that are dependent on the specific forms of aluminum administered, dose, route of administration, and duration of exposure. Moreover, considerable epidemiological, biochemical, and clinical evidence implicate aluminum toxicity in the dialysis encephalopathy of humans.[394–402] A few acute cases of possible aluminum neurotoxicity have also been reported among individuals with high occupational exposures.[403–406] However, the role of aluminum exposure in the etiology of dementia remains uncertain.

The hypothesis that aluminum might have a causal role in AD was suggested by reports of elevated levels of aluminum in the brains of patients with this disorder and especially by the presence of aluminum in neurons containing NFTs and in the cores of SPs.[407–410] However, these findings have not been consistently reported. Furthermore, their specificity and etiological significance have been questioned; the deposition of aluminum in dying cells and lesions composed of hyperphosphorylated proteins may be epiphenomenological.[411–413] Discrepancies between the profile of neuropathological and neurochemical changes that occur in AD and those reported in dialysis encephalopathy and animal models of aluminum neurotoxicity further weaken this hypothesis.[412,413] Epidemiological studies of occupational exposure to aluminum, levels of aluminum in drinking water, and exposure to aluminum-containing compounds (e.g., antacids, history of peptic ulcer disease, analgesics, antiperspirants) also yield inconsistent results.[393] On the whole, the epidemiological evidence of an association between aluminum exposure and AD has been negative or weakly positive. While initial attempts to slow the progression of AD through the reduction of dietary aluminum or chelation therapy with desferrioxamine mesylate seemed promising,[414] the design and interpretation of this study have been criticized, and reports of subsequent controlled studies confirming these results have not been forthcoming. In summary, exposure to aluminum as critical for the development of most cases of AD seems unlikely.

The compound 1-methyl-4-phenyl-1,2,3,6-tetrahydropyridine (MPTP) is a potent neurotoxin with selective effects on dopaminergic neurons.[415,416] Exposure of primates to MPTP results in a profound depletion of dopamine in the striatum and the emergence of Parkinson's disease.[417] While exposure to MPTP itself is responsible for few cases of this disorder, a greater number of cases may result from exogenous or endogenous MPTP-like compounds.[418] Their toxic effects may be mediated alone or in concert with other degenerative processes and may be accentuated by genetic or age-related decrements in detoxification systems.[419] Monoamine oxidase B inhibitors, including deprenyl, protect against MPTP-induced neurotoxicity in animal models.[420] Deprenyl is also effective in the acute and maintenance treatment of Parkinson's disease and may slow its progression.[421–424] These results are consistent with a role for MPTP-like toxins in the pathogenesis of some cases of PD. Although a fraction of AD patients manifest Lewy body pathology, MPTP-oids are unlikely to account for the range of neuropathological and neurochemical abnormalities that occur in AD.

The potential contributions of excitotoxicity, oxidative stress, and cell membrane abnormalities to the pathogenesis of AD have been described above. Evidence supporting the involvement of these processes in the biology of ALS, Parkinson's disease, and Huntington's disease has also been reported.[425] The involvement of excitotoxicity in development or progression of neurodegenerative disorders with prominent movement disturbances is attractive in light of the strong glutamatergic innervation of the corpus striatum. The deleterious consequences of superoxide free radicals are most clearly illustrated by familial forms of ALS that result from mutations in the structural gene for superoxidase dismutase, which normally detoxifies these radicals.[426,427] The peroxidation of membrane lipids by accumulating superoxide radicals has the potential to alter membrane structure and fluidity with resulting abnormalities in membrane-related functions. Since these radicals are largely impermeable to cell membranes, internal cell membrane compartments including the ER, Golgi, and mitochondria may be primarily affected. It is tempting to speculate that this process may be related to disturbances of posttranslational modification, protein/membrane trafficking, and cellular energy metabolism described in these neurodegenerative disorders, as well as the fragmentation of the Golgi apparatus reported in both AD and ALS.[30,428]

During at least the last two centuries, the inhabitants of Guam and nearby islands have suffered from a common, progressive neurodegenerative disorder that has been characterized as the ALS-Parkinsonism-dementia complex.[31] Although an environmental etiological factor is suspected, none has yet been unambiguously identified. Initial suspects included cycasins and the excitotoxic amino acid L-β-methylaminoalanine (L-βMAA), which are prominent components of flour derived from the seeds of the false sago palm used by these Pacific islanders as a food staple and for medicinal purposes.[429] Cycasins were initially suspected because a metabolite of this compound has DNA-methylating potential and is neuroteratogenic. However, the role of cycasins in causing the ALS-Parkinson-dementia complex remains speculative. L-βMAA has emerged as an unlikely cause of this disease complex because of its relatively weak excitotoxicity in vivo, its low abundance in cycad flour, and its inability to produce effects in animal models that resemble those of the disease complex.[430,431]

Mechanisms of Cell Death

Neuronal death in the brains of patients with AD appears to occur by mechanisms of both necrosis and apoptosis. While these pathways may overlap to some extent, they are typically triggered by different events, are manifested by distinguishable cytologic and biochemical features, and have somewhat different outcomes.[432] Necrosis usually results from physical injury, is not genetically controlled, is typified by the destruction of organelles and the plasma membrane, and results in the release of cellular debris that often stimulates a local inflammatory response. In contrast, apoptosis or programmed cell death represents a genetically controlled response to specific developmental or environmental stimuli. Cells undergoing apoptosis manifest shrinkage, membrane blebbing, chromatin condensation, and DNA fragmentation. The last two characteristics have commonly been used to identify apoptotic cells in formalin-fixed, paraffin-embedded sections of brain tissue. In vivo, apoptotic cells and their fragments undergo phagocytosis by microglia and do not stimulate an inflammatory response.

Several lines of evidence implicate apoptosis in the loss of neurons from vulnerable brain areas in AD. Increased oxidative damage, disturbances of calcium homeostasis, reduction in neurotrophic factors, deposition of β amyloid aggregates, and reduced energy metabolism are all characteristic of the central neurodegeneration that occurs in AD,[433] and all of these conditions induce or stimulate apoptosis in cultured neuronal cell lines.[434] DNA fragmentation-labeling techniques have been used to identify substantial numbers of cells in vulnerable cortical regions (frontal, temporal, hippocampus) that appear to have initiated the apoptosis pathway in AD victims, a process that occurs to a substantially lesser extent in normal aging.[435-439] These observations do not appear to result from DNA damage occurring during the postmortem interval or from agonal factors,[434,440] and is consistent with evolving research on one of the regulatory functions of the presenilin genes.[441,442] These findings have recently been extended to studies of the degeneration of the aminergic nuclei of the brain stem in AD.[443]

Genetics of Alzheimer's Disease

Age at onset of dementia has emerged as an important descriptive variable for classifying genes that influence the development of AD (Table 19.5). Although they are uncommon, most cases of AD that become symptomatic before the age of 60 appear to arise from highly penetrant, autosomal dominant genetic lesions. These include mutations in the structural genes for the APP located on chromosome 21,[128,444-446] presenilin 1 *(PSN1)* located on chromosome 14,[447-451] presenilin 2 *(PSN2)* located on chromosome 1,[452,453] as well as trisomy 21.[453] The association of trisomy 21 with cognitive impairment and

Table 19.5. AD Susceptibility Loci

Locus	Chromosome	Proportion of all AD Cases Affected	Clinical Phenotype	Aβ Phenotype
GENES WITH PATHOGENIC MUTATIONS				
APP mutations	21	<1%	Rare early-onset FAD, autosomal dominant	↑ Production of total Aβ and Aβ$_{42(43)}$ peptides
Presenilin 1 mutations	14	<5%	Majority of early-onset FAD, some with intermediate onset (60–70 yr), autosomal dominant	↑ Production of total Aβ$_{42(43)}$ peptides
Presendin 2 mutations	1	<1%	Early-onset FAD, Volga Germans, autosomal dominant	↑ Production of total Aβ$_{42(43)}$ peptides
GENES WITH POLYMORPHISMS THAT INCREASE RISK				
APOE, ε4 allele	19	~50%	Typical-onset (60s+) FAD and sporadic AD, dose effect on risk	↑ Density of Aβ plaques and vessel wall deposits

the proliferation of cortical SPs among individuals who live into the 4th decade may be the consequence of an *APP* gene dosage effect.[120,121]

Six pathogenic missense mutations in the APP gene have been identified, five of which produce early-onset familial AD (FAD). Three result in single amino acid substitutions at codon 717 (codon numbering based on 770aa form of APP), three amino acids distal to the carboxyl terminus of the Aβ sequence (see Fig. 19.3).[455–457] A fourth mutant APP allele produces early onset FAD as the result of the substitution of two amino acids at codons 670 and 671, which immediately precede the amino terminus of the Aβ sequence.[458] The locations of these pathogenic mutations suggest that they produce AD by affecting the proteolytic cleavage events that generate Aβ from its precursor. The remaining two pathogenic APP mutations are located in the middle of the Aβ coding sequence. A missense

mutation at codon 692 has been shown to cosegregate with a disorder characterized by presenile dementia and cerebral hemorrhage in a Dutch family.[459] An adjacent missense mutation in codon 693 produces hereditary cerebral hemorrhage with amyloidosis, Dutch type (HCHWA-D).[460]

Cells transfected with these mutant APP alleles either overproduce Aβ or synthesize an increased proportion of Aβ$_{1-42(43)}$ peptides. A transgenic mouse model has recently been described that overexpresses the APP$_{695}$ isoform containing the missense substitutions at positions 670 and 671 that result in early-onset FAD.[461] These mice overproduce both Aβ$_{1-40}$ and Aβ$_{1-42(43)}$, develop amyloid-containing SPs in the cortex, and manifest memory and behavioral abnormalities by 9 to 10 months of age. Further studies of this and other transgenic models may provide compelling evidence of the causal role of APP mutations in the pathogenesis of early-onset FAD in humans.[462] This approach is likely to provide an important tool for further dissecting the biology of AD, as well as an efficient means for screening potential therapeutic agents.

Amyloid precursor protein mutations account for only a small fraction (2 to 3%) of all early-onset FAD cases.[463] Genetic linkage analysis used to search the genome for additional *FAD* loci led to identification of a second *FAD* locus on chromosome 14,[447] which has been cloned and identified as the structural gene for presenilin 1.[451] Mutations in *PSN1* appear to account for most cases of early-onset FAD.[448,450–458,464–468] The *PSN2* locus is identified by the high homology of its predicted protein product to that of presenilin 1.[452,453,469] One or two missense mutations in *PSN2* cosegregate with early-onset FAD in families descended from a colony of ethnic Germans who lived in the Volga valley of Russia during the 18th and 19th centuries.[451,453,469] Hydrophobicity analyses of the presenilins suggest that they contain seven transmembrane domains. Sequence homology studies with proteins from *Caenorhabditis elegans* suggest that the presenilins may play a role in the membrane trafficking of specialized Golgi-derived organelles or in signal transduction from the cell surface to the nucleus.[469,470] The presenilins are predominantly located in the ER and early Golgi of transfected cells.[356] Moreover, fibroblasts from individuals bearing pathogenic *PSN* mutations secrete elevated levels of $A\beta_{1-42(43)}$.[125–127] These results suggest that the pathogenicity of these *PSN* mutations may result from an alteration in the metabolic fate of APP leading to the overproduction of long $A\beta$ peptides that have an increased propensity for aggregation.

Mutations in the *APP, PSN1,* and *PSN2* loci appear to account for most cases of early-onset FAD but only about 5% of all AD cases (471). Synergism between genome scanning and candidate gene strategies led to an observed association of the ε4 allele of *APOE*,[134,472,473] the structural gene for an apolipoprotein involved in lipid transport and metabolism, with both

sporadic (no family history) and FAD cases with more typical late-ages at onset.[134,474–476] This association is now well established in many populations throughout the world.[445,471,475,477–484] The *APOE* ε4 frequency among AD patients is typically in the range of 0.30 to 0.40 (higher in familial cases and patients with prominent amyloid angiopathy) compared with 0.10 to 0.15 in most older nondemented control populations. Consistent with these estimates, approximately 10% of AD patients are homozygous for the ε4 allele, about 40% are heterozygous for the ε4 allele, and about 50% lack the ε4 allele. In contrast, the *APOE* ε2 allele appears to confer an independent protective effect against development of late-onset AD.[485,486]

While the *APOE* ε4 allele is a known risk factor for cardiovascular disease,[487–491] the elevation in the ε4 frequency appears to be relatively specific for AD among the causes of dementia.[474,475,492–494] Patients with AD and cortical Lewy bodies also manifest increased ε4 allele frequency.[217,495–498] Moreover, evidence of an association of the ε4 allele with subtypes of late-life depression may represent prodromes or antecedents of AD.[499,500]

Retrospective studies suggest that the *APOE* ε4 allele produces increased age-specific risk of developing late-onset and sporadic early onset AD[480,501–503] and reduced longevity.[504] Whether these manifestations result from an effect of the ε4 allele in lowering the age at onset or are an inevitable consequence of aging remains controversial. Both female gender[484] and head injury[485] appear to increase the risk of developing AD through a synergistic interaction with the *APOE* ε4 allele. Cross-sectional [18]FDG PET studies report reductions of cerebral glucose metabolism in at-risk ε4 carriers and cognitively intact ε4 homozygotes.[286,287] Presence of an ε4 allele also emerges as a risk factor for development of dementia in a longitudinal study of elderly patients with mild cognitive impairment.[507] Prospective, longitudinal studies of the effect of the *APOE* ε4 allele on the age-specific cumulative incidence of AD among cognitively intact individuals are conspicuously absent from the literature.

Experiments performed in vitro suggest that the ε4 isoform of APOE may serve as a molecular chaperone that facilitates the conversion of monomeric Aβ to aggregates with a β-pleated sheet conformation.[134–137,473,508,509] This observation offers a mechanism by which the ε4 allele may promote cerebral amyloidogenesis and the development of AD. It is also consistent with the dose effect manifested by the *APOE* ε4 allele on the density of cortical SPs in the brains of patients who develop this disorder.[475,510,511] While the molecular chaperone hypothesis has the largest body of evidence to support it at the current time, additional mechanisms have been proposed to explain the effect of the *APOE* genotype on the risk of developing AD. It has been suggested that Aβ may be removed from the extracellular space by the resorption of Aβ-APOE complexes, a process that may be mediated by the low-density lipoprotein receptor or low-density lipoprotein receptor-related protein.[510] APOE also binds to the tau protein and may influence the formation of NFTs.[512,513] In addition, APOE appears to be a neural-injury response protein that may facilitate neuronal repair by transporting lipids to the site of injury.[514] In some model systems of neural repair, the E4 isoform outperforms the E3 isoform in promoting neurite outgrowth.[515] Alternatively, the allelic associations between the *APOE* locus and AD may result from linkage disequilibrium with a neighboring bona fide AD susceptibility gene.

These four loci explain about half of the heritability of AD, underscoring the importance of searching for vulnerability genes that remain to be detected.[516] Increased PMF identifies a prominent subgroup of AD patients with distinct clinical features, is relatively specific for this disorder, and appears to be controlled by the inheritance of a single major locus,

PMF (see Cell Membranes section). Initial evidence from a prospective study suggests that increased PMF is associated with a 7-fold increase in the age-specific risk of AD among asymptomatic first-degree relatives.[338] Results of cross-sectional studies of AD patients, family studies, and this prospective study suggest that this locus may be among a new class of genes that affect the risk of developing AD with an intermediate age at onset between 65 and the early 70s.[330,334,338] Antemortem determinations of increased PMF are accompanied by greater hippocampal densities of SPs and a higher rate of cerebral amyloid angiopathy among patients who die with AD. This observation is likely to be related to an altered metabolic fate of platelet APP in these patients, as suggested by immunological studies of platelet APP and its derivatives.

Subsequent efforts to identify susceptibility genes for AD with typical ages at onset have relied on association or linkage approaches that employ genome-wide panels of highly polymorphic, anonymous DNA markers, or studies of single genes whose known functions identify them as potential candidates for susceptibility genes based on pathophysiologic models of AD. A systematic survey of the human genome, conducted at an average resolution of 10cM, for the identification of simple sequence tandem repeat polymorphisms (SSTRPs) that target new risk genes for AD by virtue of linkage disequilibrium showed allelic associations with AD for 6 of the 391 SSTRPs in the CHLC Human Screening Set/Weber Version 6 (Research Genetics, Inc., Huntsville, AL): D1S518, D1S547, D10S1423, D12S1045, D19S178, and DXS1047.[517] These allelic associations were replicated in an independent sample of autopsied AD cases and controls recruited from a geographically disparate site. The association of the large D19S178 alleles with AD appeared to arise from linkage disequilibrium with the *APOE* ε4 allele, while the remaining five markers appeared to identify novel AD risk loci.

An association of the D10S1423 234bp allele with AD has been reported in three independent samples of AD cases and controls in Boston, Pittsburgh, and Bonn.[517,518] In addition, the effects of carrying either or both of the D10S1423 234bp and APOE ε4 alleles on the age-specific risk of developing AD were determined in a prospective, longitudinal, double-blind assessment of an at-risk population of 325 asymptomatic first-degree relatives of AD probands.[519] The age-specific risk of developing AD was greatest for individuals carrying both alleles (Mantel-Cox statistic = 20.12, df = 3, p = 0.0002; Breslow statistic = 13.36, df = 3, p = 0.004). In the resulting best-fitting Cox proportional hazards model, only individuals who carried both risk alleles exhibited a risk ratio that differed significantly from 1 (risk ratio = 16.2, p = 0.008, 95% C.I. = 2.1 to 128.3). After controlling for these genotypes, female gender was also significantly associated with increased risk of developing AD (risk ratio = 5.1, p = 0.02, 95% C.I. = 1.2 to 21.1). Neither age at recruitment nor years of education made significant contributions to the model.

At least four genes reside within approximately 1 Mb of D10S1423: VIM, the structural gene for vimentin, a major component of intermediate filaments; DNMT2, which encodes DNA (cytosine-5-)-methyltransferase 2; CUBN, which encodes cubilin, an intrinsic factor-cobalamin receptor; and BMI1, which encodes a murine leukemia viral oncogene homologue; all of these have been cytogenetically localized within or adjacent to 10p13. All of these genes are plausible candidates for susceptibility genes for AD, illustrating one of the limitations of the candidate gene approach. In addition to facilitating the absorption of the intrinsic factor- vitamin B_{12} complex, cubilin is a high-affinity apolipoprotein A-I receptor that facilitates the endocytosis of high-density lipoprotein (HDL) holoparticles and their subsequent transport to endosomes/lysosomes where they are digested.[520,521] This endocytic process resembles that of low-density lipoproteins (LDL) and appears to involve the participation of the coreceptor megalin, a member of the LDL receptor family.[520,521] Moreover, cubilin-mediated HDL endocytosis is inhibitable by apolipoproteins including A-I, A-II, and E.[520] These features provide a biochemical basis for interactions between apolipoproteins, including apolipoprotein E, and cubilin as part of a physiologic process that is likely to be relevant to the neurodegeneration/repair that occurs in AD.

The clinical, neuropathological, and neurochemical phenotypes of subjects who carry each of these candidate susceptibility alleles were explored in a group of 50 autopsy-confirmed cases of AD followed longitudinally prior to death and who lacked other brain diseases (Table 19.6).[522–524] Consistent with previous reports, *APOE* ε4 carriers exhibited greater densities of SPs and NFTs than noncarriers. Carriers of the D12S1045 91bp allele manifest symptomatic onset and death at earlier ages, increased density of NFTs, and a substantially greater reduction in cortical dopamine levels compared to AD patients who lacked this allele. This exaggerated reduction in cortical dopamine levels is also shared by subjects who carry risk alleles at the D10S1423 and DXS1047 loci. The latter two genotypic groups have similar phenotypes that also include the relative preservation of cortical norepinephrine levels. Carriers of the susceptibility alleles at the D1S518 and D1S547 loci do not differ phenotypically from the corresponding noncarrier genotype, although carriers of the D1S518 195bp allele tended to have lower densities of cortical NFTs than noncarriers. The observations that several of these alleles modulate biological variables that are relevant to the pathophysiology of AD further support their candidacy as AD susceptibility loci.

Three of these six candidate risk alleles for AD appear to modulate cortical levels of the amine neurotransmitters dopamine and norepinephrine in important ways. As a result, their inheritance may in-

Table 19.6. Phenotypic Characterization of Six Susceptibility Alleles in 50 Autopsied AD Cases

Allele	Clinical Features		Histopathologic Features[a]		Neurochemical Features[b]	
	AAO	AAD	SP	NFT	NE	DA
APOE E4	NA	NA	↑	↑	NA	NA
D12S1045 91bp	↓	↓	NA	↑	NA	↓
D10S1423 234bp	NA	NA	NA	NA	↑	↓
DXS1047 202bp	NA	NA	NA	NA	↑	↓tr
D1S518 195bp	NA	NA	NA	↓tr	NA	NA
D1S547 286bp	NA	NA	NA	NA	NA	NA

(↑) Positive association, (↓) negative association, (↓tr) negative trend. (NA) no association. AAO, age at onset; AAD, age at death; SP, senile plaque density; NFT, neurofibrillary tangle density; NE, norepinephrine levels; DA, dopamine levels.
[a]None of the alleles manifested an association with cerebral amyloid angiopathy.
[b]None of the alleles manifested an association with cortical choline acetyltransferase activities or serotonin levels.

fluence the development of behavioral disturbances that are common sources of excess morbidity in AD. For example, the emergence of clinically significant depression in the context of primary dementia is associated with degeneration of the dopaminergic neurons in the substantia nigra and noradrenergic neurons in the locus ceruleus.[42–45,187,188] These genotypes may also contribute to the development of psychosis, apathy, and extrapyramidal symptoms, as well as to interindividual differences in response to the therapeutic or adverse effects of medications that involve these aminergic systems. In addition to their relevance to the behavioral manifestations of AD, emerging evidence suggests that these AD susceptibility loci may be shared with psychiatric disorders whose symptomatic onsets occur earlier in life.[525]

Five genome-wide linkage scans for susceptibility genes for typical onset AD have been completed, all of which provide evidence consistent with the acceptance of APOE as a bona fide risk gene for AD[526,527]; at least four additonal chromosomal regions were identified in at least two studies, including chromosomes 12, 10, 9, and 6. Consistent with the large and burgeoning knowledge base related to the complex pathophysiology of AD, the list of candidate genes at these and other locations is also substantial and growing. Favorite candidate genes currently include the following: those that encode α_2-macroglobulin, the LDL receptor-like protein 1, and the transcription factor CP2 on chromosome 12; insulin-degrading enzyme and urokinase-type plasminogen activator on chromosome 10; tumor necrosis factor-α on chromosome 6; and the interleukins, angiotensin I-converting enzyme, and cathepsin D. Inherited or acquired alterations in the mitochondrial genome may also contribute to the risk of developing AD.[528]

Etiologic Model

As this chapter reflects, recent literature on AD is rich with descriptions of neurobiological perturbations with the potential for contributing to the etiology of this disorder. These observations are integrated into a hypothetical model of the etiopathogenesis of AD presented in Figure 19.4. Although it will undoubtedly require revision and elaboration as our

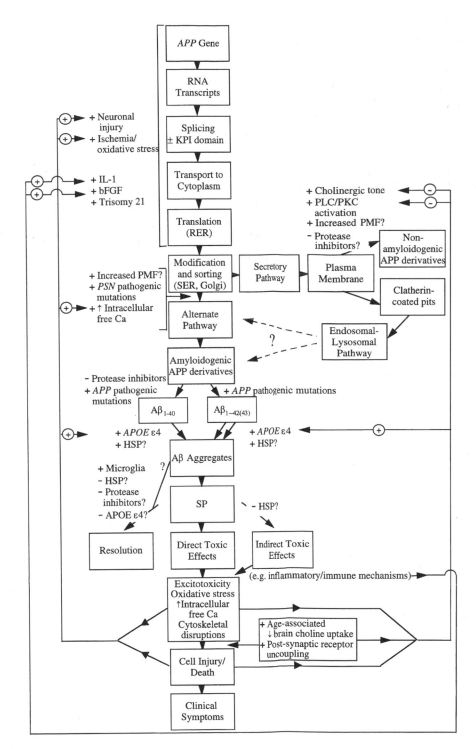

Figure 19.4. Hypothesized etiological model of AD.

knowledge base expands, this model may contribute to our understanding of the natural history and clinical biology of AD and to the design of potential pharmacotherapeutic strategies.

The expression of the structural gene for APP is a convenient place to begin an exploration of the model. This process includes transcription, splicing of mRNA transcripts, and transport of the resulting mRNA species into the cytoplasm where translation occurs. The individual steps in this process, and those that follow, are highly complex, and the interconnecting arrows serve as proxies for numerous intervening reactions. Expression of *APP* is enhanced by neuronal injury, ischemia/oxidative stress, IL-1, and bFGF, and is inhibited by cholinergic stimulation. Expression of *APP* is also enhanced in patients with trisomy 21, possibly as the result of an increased number of *APP* genes. Co- and posttranslational modification of APP occurs in the SER and Golgi apparatus where protein sorting and the subsequent destination of modified proteins is determined.

APP molecules that pass into the secretory pathway appear on the cell surface where they may be cleaved by α-secretase into nonamyloidogenic products, a process facilitated by cholinergic stimulation and other neurotransmitters that activate the phospholipase C/protein kinase C signal transduction pathway (e.g., serotonin, vasopressin, bradykinin). In a fraction of cases, APP molecules on the cell surface undergo endocytosis and entry into the endosomal-lysosomal system. Potentially amyloidogenic carboxyl-terminal derivatives appear to be present in this cellular compartment, but whether this pathway merges with (or is part of) the "alternate" pathway predominantly responsible for the generation of Aβ is uncertain. Pathogenic *PSN* mutations, alleles that confer increased PMF, and events that lead to increased intracellular calcium appear to produce a preferential flow of APP molecules into the alternate pathway. Missense mutations that alter the amino acid com-

position of APP at or near the amino or carboxyl terminus of Aβ can alter the proteolytic processing of APP in a way that favors the formation of excess A$\beta_{1\text{-}40}$, A$\beta_{1\text{-}42(43)}$, or both. Endogenous protease inhibitors (perhaps including the APP KPI sequence) may slow this process.

The E4 isoform of *APOE* may serve as a molecular chaperone, along with certain proteoglycans, that facilitate the conversion of soluble Aβ monomers to aggregates with a β-pleated sheet conformation. These diffuse amyloid aggregates are then converted to SPs by an unknown mechanism. The density of SPs also depends on a poorly understood mechanism for clearance of these morphological lesions that may be mediated by microglia and inhibited by protease inhibitors and the encapsulation of SPs by heparin sulfate proteoglycans. Aβ may also form complexes with APOE and be cleared from the extracellular space by resorption mediated by LDL receptors.

Mature SPs produce cytotoxicity through both direct and indirect mechanisms. The latter includes activation of microglia, complement, and formation of the membrane attack complex. Activated microglia release compounds toxic to neighboring cells and secrete both IL-1 and bFGF, which further stimulate the synthesis of APP. Encapsulation of SPs by proteoglycans may inhibit activation of these inflammatory/immune processes. Both pathways induce cytotoxicity through excitotoxicity, oxidative stress, increased intracellular free calcium, cytoskeletal disruptions, and membrane lysis. Evidence also suggests that inherited or environmentally mediated alterations in these processes may act as risk factors for AD. Cell membrane alterations may contribute to this pathogenic pathway in several ways. In addition to unfavorably affecting the balance between the nonamyloidogenic and amyloidogenic processing of APP, alterations in membrane trafficking may impair the delivery of proteins encoded by nuclear genes to mitochondria and other organelles. Dec-

rements in mitochondrial functions may result, contributing to oxidative stress. In addition, nuclei without a full complement of normal proteins may manifest abnormalities of gene expression and DNA synthesis. Plasma membrane alterations have been suggested as the basis for the uncoupling of M_1 and D_1 receptors at postsynaptic locations. Reduced postsynaptic signal transduction may further inhibit the nonamyloidogenic processing of APP within intrinsic cortical neurons, and contribute to the metabolic burden of presynaptic neurons that release excess neurotransmitters in futile attempts to maintain homeostasis. Cholinergic neurons are likely to be the most vulnerable to the resulting increased metabolic stress because of multiple and competing cellular needs for choline, the inability to synthesize choline, and age-associated decrement in the uptake of this nutrient into the brain. According to the model, this cascade of events leads to neuronal injury and death, with the resulting manifestation of clinical symptoms.

Changes in the levels of proteoglycans and protease inhibitors modulate the pathway in ways that may have opposing effects on neurodegeneration. For example, increased synthesis and deposition of proteoglycans at the sites of evolving SPs may augment accumulation of these lesions by facilitating Aβ aggregation and inhibiting their elimination. However, encapsulation of SPs by proteoglycans may inhibit their stimulatory actions on the inflammation and immune systems. Similarly, elevation in levels of endogenous or exogenously administered protease inhibitors may slow the proteolytic conversion of APP to $A\beta_{1-40}$ and $A\beta_{1-42(43)}$ and the activation of the complement cascade, but also have the potential to enhance the flow of APP into the alternate pathway and to interfere with the elimination of amyloid aggregates and SPs. For these reasons predicting the net effect of elevations or decreases in proteoglycans and endogenous protease inhibitors on the neurodegeneration predicted by the model is diffi-

cult. However, compounds with specificity for one or more of these steps may influence the process in a particular direction and provide an opportunity for therapeutic intervention.

One of the most important features of the hypothesized model is that it predicts the recruitment of additional pathological cascades and an ever-increasing rate of neurodegeneration. The cytotoxic and cytolytic consequences of the model accelerate the synthesis of APP, alter its processing in favor of the alternate pathway, and facilitate the assembly of Aβ and long Aβ fragments into aggregates that are converted to SPs. Moreover, the initiation of additional neurodegenerative cascades, including inflammatory/immune mechanisms, excitotoxicity, oxidative stress, cytoskeletal disruptions, and alterations of intracellular calcium homeostasis is likely to compromise neurons and supporting cells that produce synergistic effects with the potential for these destructive processes to become self-perpetuating. Preexisting cell membrane characteristics may facilitate the pathogenic process along with those produced as casualties of oxidative stress and neurodegeneration. These predictions are consistent with the natural history of AD. Even cases of AD resulting from mutations that profoundly influence the synthesis and fate of APP do not appear to produce clinical manifestations until age 40 or later. Typical patients have an average age in the 70s at onset. Yet progression from symptomatic onset to end-stage dementia and death occurs in only 8 to 10 years.[529]

These features also have important implications for the design of potential pharmacotherapeutic interventions in AD. Because of the recruitment of multiple neurodegenerative cascades and the accelerating nature of the disease process, studies that recruit subjects at the earliest possible stage of the diathesis are the most likely to detect beneficial effects of individual drugs (or other interventions). Unfortunately, clinical diagnosis of AD is least reliable when symptoms are mild or

equivocal and progression is not yet evident. Such efforts could most profitably benefit from the recruitment of at-risk individuals, identified by a battery of risk factors (e.g., positive family history, risk genes, in vivo spectroscopy, other biological "markers"), who are asymptomatic or only mildly affected. Although such approaches require substantive sample sizes and longitudinal designs, the alternative is to risk discounting an agent or approach that has genuine beneficial effects on forestalling AD in vulnerable individuals.

An additional strategy worthy of consideration is coadministration of agents that together might impede multiple neurochemical pathways that contribute to the progression of the disease in symptomatic individuals. This approach is analogous to that often used in chemotherapy for cancer and AIDS.

Conclusions and Future Directions

Concluding with a reconsideration of whether AD, as currently defined, more closely resembles a disease with a unitary etiology or a syndrome with multiple contributing etiologies seems appropriate. Most familial, early-onset cases of AD appear to result from the inheritance of autosomal dominant mutations that produce major perturbations in the biosynthesis and fate of APP. At least in the early stages, these disorders, and perhaps a fraction of cases with more typical ages at onset, can be conceptualized as primary cerebral amyloidoses. However, the progression of the disorder, regardless of age at onset, appears to involve additional neurochemical cascades that make their own contributions to the neurodegeneration that typifies AD. From this perspective, most AD cases more closely resemble a syndrome (e.g., anemia) than a unitary disease entity (e.g., sickle cell disease).

The future of research in this area seems bright. Application of established neurochemical and neuropathological approaches augmented by in vivo methods and genetic strategies, including ongoing development of transgenic models of AD, should support the continued exponential growth of our understanding of the pathophysiology of AD. In the process, new and unexpected insights into the biology of the brain and the function of the nervous system will also undoubtedly occur. The resulting knowledge and experimental tools make the search for successful therapeutic interventions to prevent or arrest the progression of AD among the most hopeful of the complex disorders of aging. Integration, both operationally and conceptually, across these areas of investigation will be key to designing the best experiments and gleaning the greatest understanding from a large and growing information base. Meanwhile, substantive alleviation of suffering and excess disability can be gained by successful management of the psychiatric and other comorbid medical conditions that often afflict patients with AD, along with proper attention to the education and support of their families and other caregivers.

Acknowledgment. This work was supported by research grants MH43261 and MH47346, and Independent Scientist Award MH00540 from the National Institute of Mental Health.

References

1. Alzheimer A. Uber eine eigenartige Erkrankung der Hirnrinde. *Allg Z Pschiatr Psych-Gericht Med* 1907;64:146–148.
2. Glenner GG, Wong CW. Alzheimer's disease: initial report of the purification and characterization of a novel cerebrovascular amyloid protein. *Biochem Biophys Res Commun* 1984;120:885–890.
3. Masters CL, Simms G, Weinman NA, et al. Amyloid plaque core protein in Alzheimer disease and Down syndrome. *Proc Natl Acad Sci USA* 1985;82:4245–4249.
4. Arriagada PV, Marzloff K, Hyman BT. Distribution of Alzheimer-type pathologic changes in nondemented elderly individuals matches the pattern in Alzheimer's disease. *Neurology* 1992;42:1681–1688.
5. Berg L, McKeel DW, Miller JP, et al. Neuro-

pathological indexes of Alzheimer's disease in demented and nondemented persons aged 80 years and older. *Arch Neurol* 1993;50:349–358.

6. Bierer LM, Hof PR, Purohit DP, et al. Neocortical neurofibrillary tangles correlate with dementia severity in Alzheimer's disease. *Arch Neurol* 1995;52:81–88.

7. Yamaguchi H, Hirai S, Mortimatsu M, et al. Diffuse type of senile plaques in brain of Alzheimer-type dementia. *Acta Neuropathol* 1988;7: 113–119.

8. Joachim CL, Morris JH, Selkoe DJ. Diffuse senile plaques occur commonly in the cerebellum in Alzheimer's disease. *Am J Pathol* 1989; 135:309–319.

9. Hyman BT, Marzloff K, Arriagada PV. The lack of accumulation of senile plaques or amyloid burden in Alzheimer's disease suggests a dynamic balance between amyloid deposition and resolution. *J Neuropathol Exp Neurol* 1993; 52:594–600.

10. Iqbal K, Grundke-Iqbal I. Ubiquitination and abnormal phosphorylation of paired helical filaments in Alzheimer's disease. *Mol Neurobiol* 1991;5:399–410.

11. Grundke-Iqbal I, Iqbal K, Quinlan M, et al. Microtubule-associated protein tau. A component of Alzheimer paired helical filaments. *J Biol Chem* 1986;261:6084–6089.

12. Kidd M. Paired helical filaments in electron microscopy of Alzheimer's disease. *Nature* 1963; 197:192–193.

13. Wisniewski WM, Narang HK, Terry RD. Neurofibrillary tangles of paired helical filaments. *J Neurol Sci* 1976;27:173–181.

14. Wisniewski HM, Merz PA, Iqbal K. Ultrastructure of paired helical filaments of Alzheimer's neurofibrillary tangle. *J Neuropathol Exp Neurol* 1984;43:643–656.

15. Wischik CM, Crowther RA, Stewart M, Roth M. Subunit structure of paired helical filaments in Alzheimer's disease. *J Cell Biol* 1985;100: 1905–1912.

16. Goldman JE, Yen S-H. Cytoskeletal protein abnormalities in neurodegenerative diseases. *Ann Neurol* 1986;19:209–223.

17. Tomlinson BE, Blessed G, Roth M. Observations on the brains of non-demented old people. *J Neurol Sci* 1968;7:331–356.

18. Zubenko GS, Moossy J, Martinez AJ, et al. A brain regional analysis of morphologic and cholinergic abnormalities in Alzheimer's disease. *Arch Neurol* 1989;46:634–638.

19. Giannakopoulos P, Hof PR, Mottier S, et al. Neuropathological changes in the cerebral cortex of 1258 cases from a geriatric hospital: retrospective clinicopathological evaluation of a 10-year autopsy population. *Acta Neuropathol* 1994;87:456–468.

20. Wisniewski K, Jervis GA, Moretz RC, Wisniewski H. Alzheimer neurofibrillary tangles in diseases other than senile and presenile dementia. *Ann Neurol* 1979;5:288–294.

21. Ishii T, Nakamura Y. Distributions and ultrastructure of Alzheimer's neurofibrillary tangles in postencephalitis parkinsonism of Economo type. *Acta Neuropathol* (Berlin) 1981;55:59–62.

22. Halper J, Scheithauer BW, Okazaki H, Laws ER. Meningio-angromatosis: a report of six cases with special reference to the occurrence of neurofibrillary tangles. *J Neuropathol Exp Neurol* 1986;45:426–446.

23. Mirra SS, Heyman A, McKeel D, et al. and participating CERAD neuropathologists. The consortium to establish a registry for Alzheimer's disease (CERAD). *Neurology* 1991;41:479–486.

24. Davies P. Neurotransmitter-related enzymes in senile dementia of the Alzheimer type. *Brain Res* 1979;171:319–327.

25. Mountjoy CQ, Tomlinson BE, Gibson RH. Amyloid and senile plaques and cerebral blood vessels. A semiquantitative investigation of a possible relationship. *J Neurol Sci* 1982;57: 89–103.

26. Vinters HV, Secor DL, Read SL, et al. Microvasculature in brain biopsy specimens from patients with Alzheimer's disease: an immunohistochemical and ultrastructural study. *Ultrastruct Pathol* 1994;18:333–348.

27. Tomlinson BE, Kitchener D. Granulovacuolar degeneration of hippocampal pyramidal cells. *J Pathol* 1972;106:165–185.

28. Ball MJ. Neuronal loss, neuro-fibrillary tangles and granulovacuolar degeneration in the hippocampus with ageing and dementia. *Acta Neuropathol* 1977;37:111–118.

29. Xu M, Shibayama H, Kobayashi H, et al. Granulovacuolar degeneration in the hippocampal cortex of aging and demented patients—a quantitative study. *Acta Neuropathol* 1992;85: 1–9.

30. Stieber A, Mourelatos Z, Gonatas NK. In Alzheimer's disease the Golgi apparatus of a population of neurons without neurofibrillary tangles is fragmented and atrophic. *Am J Pathol* 1996; 148:415–426.

31. Hirano A. Pathology of amyotrophic lateral sclerosis. In: Gajdusek DC, Gibbs CJ, Alpers, eds. *Slow, latent and temperate virus infections.* Washington, DC: Natl Inst Neurol Disease and Blindness, monograph no. 2, 1965:23–27.

32. Gibson PH, Tomlinson BE. Numbers of Hirano bodies in the hippocampus of normal and demented people with Alzheimer disease. *J Neurol Sci* 1977;33:199–206.

33. Goldman JE. The association of actin with Hirano bodies. *J Neuropathol Exp Neurol* 1983;42: 146–152.

34. Zubenko GS, Moossy J, Kopp U. Neurochemical correlates of major depression in primary dementia. *Arch Neurol* 1990;47:209–214.

35. Crystal HA, Horoupian DS, Katzman R. Biopsy-proved Alzheimer disease presenting as a right parietal lobe syndrome. *Ann Neurol* 1981;12: 186–188.

36. Martin A, Brouwers P, Lalonde F, et al. Towards a behavioral typology of Alzheimer's disease. *J Clin Exp Neuropsychol* 1986;8:594–610.

37. Huff FJ, Becker JT, Belle SH, et al. Cognitive deficits and clinical diagnosis of Alzheimer's disease. *Neurology* 1987;37:1119–1124.

38. Becker JT, Huff FJ, Nebes RD, et al. Neuropsychological function in Alzheimer's disease. Pattern of impairment and rates of progression. *Arch Neurol* 1988;45:263–268.

39. Jagust WJ, Davies P, Tiller-Borcich JK. Focal Alzheimer's disease. *Neurology* 1990;40:14–19.

40. Leverenz J, Sumi SM. Parkinson's disease in patients with Alzheimer's disease. *Arch Neurol* 1986;43:662–664.

41. Ditter SM, Mirra SS. Neuropathologic and clinical features of Parkinson's disease in Alzheimer's disease patients. *Neurology* 1987;37: 754–760.

42. Förstl H, Burns A, Levy R, et al. Neurologic signs in Alzheimer's disease. Results of a prospective clinical and neuropathologic study. *Arch Neurol* 1992;49:1038–1042.

43. Zubenko GS, Moossy J. Major depression in primary dementia: clinical and neuropathologic correlates. *Arch Neurol* 1988;45:1182–1186.

44. Zweig RM, Ross CA, Hedreen JC, et al. The neuropathology of aminergic nuclei in Alzheimer's disease. *Ann Neurol* 1988;24:233–242.

45. Chan-Palay V. Depression and senile dementia of the Alzheimer type: catecholamine changes in the locus ceruleus—basis for therapy. *Dementia* 1990;1:253–261.

46. Alafuzoff I, Iqbal K, Friden H, et al. Histopathological criteria for progressive dementia disorders: clinical-pathological correlation and classification by multivariate data analysis. *Acta Neuropathol* 1987;74:209–225.

47. Wade JPH, Mirsen TR, Hachinski VC, et al. The clinical diagnosis of Alzheimer's disease. *Arch Neurol* 1987;44:24–29.

48. Joachim CL, Morris JH, Selkoe DJ. Clinically diagnosed Alzheimer's disease: autopsy results in 150 cases. *Ann Neurol* 1988;24:50–56.

49. Morris JC, McKeel DW, Fulling K, et al. Validation of clinical diagnostic criteria for Alzheimer's disease. *Ann Neurol* 1988;24:17–22.

50. Boller F, Lopez OL, Moossy J. Diagnosis of dementia: clinicopathologic correlations. *Neurology* 1989;39:76–79.

51. Mendez MF, Mastru AR, Sung JH, et al. Clinically diagnosed Alzheimer disease: neuropathologic findings in 650 cases. *Alzheimer Dis Assoc Disord* 1992;6:35–43.

52. Kazee AM, Cox C, Richfield EK. Substantia nigra lesions in Alzheimer disease and normal aging. *Alzheimer Dis Assoc Disord* 1995;9:61–67.

53. Victoroff J, Mack WJ, Lyness SA, Chiu HC. Multicenter clinicopathological correlation in dementia. *Am J Psychiatry* 1995;152:1476–1484.

54. Boller F, Mizutani T, Roessmann U, Gambetti P. Parkinson disease, dementia, and Alzheimer's disease: clinicopathological correlations. *Ann Neurol* 1980;7:329–335.

55. Hansen L, Salmon D, Galasko D, et al. The Lewy body variant of Alzheimer's disease: a clinical and pathologic entity. *Neurology* 1990; 40:1–8.

56. Lippa CF, Smith TW, Swearer JM. Alzheimer's disease and Lewy body disease: a comparative clinicopathological study. *Ann Neurol* 1994;35: 81–88.

57. Kazee AM, Han LY. Cortical Lewy bodies in Alzheimer's disease. *Arch Pathol Lab Med* 1995; 119:448–453.

58. Perry EK, Marshall E, Perry RH, et al. Cholinergic and dopaminergic activities in senile dementia of Lewy body type. *Alzheimer Dis Assoc Disord* 1990;4:87–95.

59. Perry EK, McKeith I, Thompson P, et al. Topography, extent, and clinical relevance of neurochemical deficits in dementia of Lewy body type, Parkinson's disease, and Alzheimer's disease. *Ann NY Acad Sci* 1991;640:197–202.

60. Förstl H, Burns A, Luthert P, et al. The Lewy-body variant of Alzheimer's disease. Clinical and pathological findings. *Br J Psychiatry* 1993; 162:385–392.

61. McKeith IG, Perry RH, Fairbairn AF, et al. Operational criteria for senile dementia of Lewy body type (SDLT). *Psychol Med* 1992a;22: 911–922.

62. Weiner MF, Risser RC, Cullum CM, et al. Alzheimer's disease and its Lewy body variant: a clinical analysis of postmortem verified cases. *Am J Psychiatry* 1996;153:1269–1273.

63. Gravina SA, Ho L, Eckman CB, et al. Amyloid β protein (Aβ) in Alzheimer's disease brain. *J Biol Chem* 1995;270:7013–7016.

64. Roher AE, Lowenson JD, Clarke S, et al. β-amyloid-(1–42) is a major component of cerebrovascular amyloid deposits: implications for the pathology of Alzheimer's disease. *Proc Natl Acad Sci USA* 1993;90:10836–10840.

65. Saitoh T, Sunsdmo M, Roch J-M, et al. Secreted form of amyloid β protein precursor is involved in the growth regulation of fibroblasts. *Cell* 1989;58:615–622.

66. Koo EH, Park L Selkoe DJ. Amyloid β-protein as a substrate interacts with extracellular matrix to promote neurite outgrowth. *Proc Natl Acad Sci USA* 1993;90:4748–4752.

67. Yankner BA, Caceles A, Duffy LK. Nerve growth factor potentiates the neurotoxicity of βamyloid. *Proc Natl Acad Sci USA* 1990;87:9020–9023.

68. Koh J-Y, Yang LL, Cotman CW. β-Amyloid protein increases the vulnerability of cultured cortical neurons to excitotoxic damage. *Brain Res* 1990;565:345–348.

69. Cotman CW, Pike CJ, Copani A. β-Amyloid neurotoxicity: a discussion of in vitro findings. *Neurobiol Aging* 1992;13:587–590.

70. Kosik K, Coleman P. Special issue: is β-amyloid neurotoxic? *Neurobiol Aging* 1992;5:535–630.

71. Price DL, Borchelt DR, Walker LC, Sisodia SS. Toxicity of synthetic Aβ peptides and modeling of Alzheimer's disease. *Neurobiol Aging* 1992;13: 623–625.

72. Pike CJ, Burdick D, Walencewicz AJ, et al. Neurodegeneration induced by β-amyloid peptides in vitro: the role of peptide assembly state. *J Neurosci* 1993;13:1676–1687.

73. Hensley K, Carney JM, Mattson MP, et al. A model for β-amyloid aggregation and neurotoxicity based on free radical generation by the peptide: relevance to Alzheimer disease. *Proc Natl Acad Sci USA* 1994;91:3270–3274.

74. Lorenzo A, Yankner B. Beta-amyloid neurotoxicity requires fibril formation and is inhibited by Congo red. *Proc Natl Acad Sci USA* 1994;91: 12243–12247.

75. Harris ME, Hensley K, Butterfield DA, et al. Direct evidence of oxidative injury produced by the Alzheimer's β-amyloid peptide (1–40)

in cultured hippocampal neurons. *Exp Neurol* 1995;131:193–202.

76. Walker LC, Kitt CA, Cork LC, et al. Multiple transmitter systems contribute neurites to individual senile plaques. *J Neuropathol Exp Neurol* 1988;47:138–144.

77. Delacourte A, Defossez A. Alzheimer's disease: tau proteins, the promoting factors of microtubule assembly, are major components of paired helical filaments. *J Neurol Sci* 1986;76:173–186.

78. Goedert M, Wischik CM, Crowther RA, et al. Cloning and sequencing of the cDNA encoding a core protein of the paired helical filament of Alzheimer disease: identification as the microtubules-associated protein tau. *Proc Natl Acad Sci USA* 1988;85:4051.

79. Iqbal K, Grunke-Iqbal I, Smith AJ, et al. Identification and localization of a tau peptide to paired helical filaments of Alzheimer's disease. *Proc Natl Acad Sci USA* 1989;86:5646.

80. Lee VM. Unraveling the mystery of the paired helical filaments of Alzheimer's disease. *J Natl Inst Health Res* 1991;3:52–56.

81. Wolozin BL, Pruchnicki A, Dickson DW, Davies P. A neuronal antigen in the brains of patients with Alzheimer's disease. *Science* 1986;232:648.

82. Wolozin BL, Davies P. Alzheimer related neuronal protein A68: specificity and distribution. *Ann Neurol* 1987;22:521.

83. Ksiezak-Reding H, Binder LI, Yen SH. Alzheimer disease proteins (A68) share epitopes with tau but show distinct biochemical properties. *J Neurosci Res* 1990;25:420–430.

84. Lee VM, Balin BJ, Otvos L, Trojanowski JQ. A68: a major subunit of paired helical filaments and derivatized forms of normal tau. *Science* 1991;251:675–678.

85. Baudier J, Lee SH, Cole RD. Separation of the different microtubule-associated tau protein species from bovine brain and their mode II phosphorylation by Ca^{2+}/phospholipid-dependent protein kinase C. *J Biol Chem* 1987;262:17584–17590.

86. Kang J, Lemaire HG, Unterbeck A, et al. The precursor of Alzheimer's disease amyloid A4 protein resembles a cell-surface receptor. *Nature* 1987;325:733–736.

87. Yoshikai SI, Sasaki H, Doh-ura K, et al. Genomic organization of the human amyloid beta-protein precursor gene. *Gene* 1990;87:257–263.

88. Kitaguchi N, Takahashi Y, Tokushima Y, et al. Novel precursor of Alzheimer's disease amyloid protein shows protease inhibitory activity. *Nature* 1988;331:530–532.

89. Ponte P, Gonzalez-DeWhitt P, Schilling J, et al. A new A4 amyloid mRNA contains a domain homologous to serine proteinase inhibitors. *Nature* 1988;331:525–532.

90. Tanzi RE, McClatchey AI, Lampert ED, et al. Protease inhibitor domain encoded by an amyloid protein precursor mRNA associated with Alzheimer's disease. *Nature* 1988;331:528–530.

91. König G, Mönnign U, Czech C, et al. Identification and differential expression of a novel alternative splice isoform of the β/A4 amyloid precursor protein (APP) mRNA in leukocytes and brain microglial cells. *J Biol Chem* 1992;267:10804–10809.

92. Selkoe DJ, Bell DS, Podlisny MB, et al. Conservation of brain amyloid proteins in aged mammals and humans with Alzheimer's disease. *Science* 1987;235:873–877.

93. Selkoe DJ, Podlinsly MB, Joachim CL, et al. β-Amyloid precursor protein of Alzheimer disease occurs as 110- to 135-kilodalton membrane-associated proteins in neural and nonneural tissues. *Proc Natl Acad Sci USA* 1988;85:7341–7345.

94. Tanzi RE, St George-Hyslop PH, Haines JL, et al. The genetic defect in familial Alzheimer's disease is not tightly linked to the amyloid beta-protein gene. *Nature* 1987;329:156–157.

95. Zimmermann K, Herget T, Salbaum JM. Localization of the putative precursor of Alzheimer's disease—specific amyloid at nuclear envelopes of adult human muscle. *EMBO J* 1988;7:367–372.

96. Yamada T, Sasaki H, Dohura K, et al. Structure and expression of the alternatively-spliced forms of mRNA for the mouse homolog of Alzheimer's disease amyloid beta protein precursor. *Biochem Biophys Res Commun* 1989;158:906–912.

97. Sprecher CA, Grant FJ, Grimm G, et al. Molecular cloning of the cDNA for a human amyloid precursor protein homolog: evidence for a multigene family. *Biochemistry* 1993;32:4481–4486.

98. Wasco W, Gurubhagavatula S, Paradis M, et al. Isolation and characterization of *APLP2* encoding a homologue of the Alzheimer's associated amyloid β protein precursor. *Nat Genet* 1993;5:95–99.

99. Smith RP, Higuchi DA, Broze GJ. Platelet coagulation factor XIa-inhibitor, a form of Alzheimer amyloid precursor protein. *Science* 1990;248:1126–1128.

100. Van Nostrand WE, Schmaier AH, Farrow JS, Cunningham DD. Protease nexin-II (amyloid β-protein precursor): a platelet α-granule protein. *Science* 1990;248:745–748.

101. Schubert D, Jin LW, Saitoh T, Cole G. The regulation of amyloid β protein secretion and its modulatory role in cell adhesion. *Neuron* 1989;3:689–694.

102. Mattson M, Cheng B, Culwell A, et al. Evidence for excitoprotective and intraneuronal calcium-regulating roles for secreted forms of the β-amyloid precursor protein. *Neuron* 1993;10:243–254.

103. Small GW, Okonek A, Mandelkern MA, et al. Age-associated memory loss: initial neuropsychological and cerebral metabolic findings of a longitudinal study. *Int Psychogeriatr* 1994;6:21–43.

104. Qiu WQ, Ferreira A, Miller C, et al. Cell-surface beta-amyloid precursor protein stimulates neurite outgrowth of hippocampal neurons in an isoform-dependent manner. *J Neurosci* 1995;15:2157–2167.

105. Dyrks T, Weidermann A, Multhaup J, et al. Identification, transmembrane orientation and biogenesis of the amyloid A_4 precursor of Alzheimer's disease. *EMBO J* 1988;7:949–957.

106. Oltersdorf T, Fritz LC, Schenk DB, et al. The secreted form of the Alzheimer's amyloid precursor protein with the Kunitz domain is protease nexin-II. *Nature* 1989;341:144–147.

107. Weidemann A, Kauonig G, Bunke D, et al. Identification, biogenesis, and localization of precursors of Alzheimer's disease A4 amyloid protein. *Cell* 1989;57:115–126.

108. Haass C, Koo EH, Mellon A, et al. Targeting of cell-surface β-amyloid precursor protein to lysosomes: alternative processing into amyloid-bearing fragments. *Nature* 1992;357:500–503.

109. Sisodia SS. β-Amyloid precursor protein cleavage by a membrane-bound protease. *Proc Natl Acad Sci USA* 1992;89:6075–6079.

110. Esch FS, Keim PS, Beattie EC, et al. Cleavage of amyloid β peptide during constitutive processing of its precursor. *Science* 1990;248:1122–1124.

111. Sisodia SS, Koo EH, Beyreuther K, et al. Evidence that β-amyloid protein in Alzheimer's disease is not derived by normal processing. *Science* 1990;248:492–495.

112. Anderson JP, Esch FS, Keim PS, et al. Exact cleavage site of Alzheimer amyloid precursor in neuronal PC-12 cells. *Neurosci Lett* 1991;128:126–128.

113. Wang R, Meschia JF, Cotter RJ, Sisodia SS. Secretion of the β/A4 amyloid precursor protein. Identification of a cleavage site in cultured mammalian cells. *J Biol Chem* 1991;266:16960–16964.

114. Pasternack JM, Palmert MR, Usiak M, et al. Alzheimer's disease and control brain contain soluble derivatives of the amyloid protein precursor that end within the β amyloid protein region. *Biochemistry* 1992;31:10936–10940.

115. Lai A, Sisodia SS, Trowbridge IS. Characterization of sorting signals in the β-amyloid precursor protein cytoplasmic domain. *J Biol Chem* 1995;270:3565–3573.

116. Golde TE, Estus S, Younkin LH, et al. Processing of the amyloid protein precursor to potentially amyloidogenic derivatives. *Science* 1992;255:728–730.

117. Yamazaki T, Koo EH, Selkoe DJ. Trafficking of cell-surface amyloid beta-protein precurser. II. Endocytosis, recycling, and lysomal targeting detected by immunolocalization. *J Cell Sci* 1996;109:999–1008.

118. Nukina N, Kanazawa I, Mannen T, Uchida Y. Accumulation of amyloid precursor protein and beta-protein immunoreactivities in axons injured by cerebral infarct. *Gerontology* 1992;38:10–14.

119. Araujo DM, Cotman CW. Beta-amyloid stimulates glial cells in vitro to produce growth factors that accumulate in senile plaques in Alzheimer's disease. *Brain Res* 1992;569:141–145.

120. Bendotti C, Forloni G, Morgan R, et al. Neuroanatomical localization and quantification of amyloid precursor protein mRNA by in situ hybridization in the brains of normal, aneuploid and lesioned mice. *Proc Natl Acad Sci USA* 1988;85:3628–3632.

121. Rumble B, Retallack R, Hilbich C, et al. Amyloid A4 protein and its precursor in Down's syndrome and Alzheimer's disease. *N Engl J Med* 1989;320:1446–1452.

122. Buxbaum JD, Oishi M, Chen HI, et al. Cholinergic agonists and interleukin 1 regulate processing and secretion of the Alzheimer beta/A4 amyloid protein precursor. *Proc Natl Acad Sci USA* 1992;89:10075–10078.

123. Nitsch RM, Blusztajn JK, Pittas AG, et al. Evidence for a membrane defect in Alzheimer disease brain. *Proc Natl Acad Sci USA* 1992;89:1671–1675.

124. Querfurth HW, Selkoe DJ. Calcium ionophore increases amyloid beta peptide production by cultured cells. *Biochemistry* 1994;33:4550–4561.

125. Haltia M, Vitanen M, Sulkava R, et al. Chromosome 14-encoded Alzheimer's disease: genetic and clinicopathological description. *Ann Neurol* 1994;36:362–367.

126. Song XH, Suzuki N, Bird T. et al. Plasma amyloid β protein (Aβ) ending at Aβ42(43) is increased in carriers of familial AD linked to chromosome 14. *Soc Neurosci Abstr* 1995;21:1501.

127. Scheuner D, Eckman C, Jensen M, et al. The amyloid β-protein deposited in the senile plaques of Alzheimer's disease is increased in vivo by the presenilin 1 and 2 and APP mutations linked to familial Alzheimer's disease. *Nat Med* 1996;2:864–870.

128. Selkoe DJ. Amyloid β-protein and the genetics of Alzheimer's disease. *J Biol Chem* 1996;271:18295–18298.

129. Jarrett JT, Berger EP, Lansbury PT. The carboxy terminus of the beta amyloid protein is critical for the seeding of amyloid formation: implications for the pathogenesis of Alzheimer's disease. *Biochemistry* 1993;32:4693–4697.

130. Jarrett JT, Lansbury PT. Seeding "one dimensional crystallization" of amyloid: a pathogenic mechanism in Alzheimer's disease and scrapie? *Cell* 1993;73:1055–1058.

131. Jwatsubo T, Okada S, Suzuki N, et al. Visualization of Aβ$_{42(43)}$-positive and Aβ$_{40}$-positive senile plaques with end-specific Aβ-monoclonal antibodies: evidence that an initially deposited Aβ species is Aβ$_{1-42(43)}$. *Neuron* 1994;13:45–53.

132. Buee L, Ding W, Anderson JP, et al. Binding of vascular heparan sulfate proteoglycan to Alzheimer's amyloid precursor protein is mediated in part by the N-terminal region of A4 peptide. *Brain Res* 1993;627:199–204.

133. Ghiso J, Matsubara E, Koudinov A, et al. The cerebrospinal-fluid soluble form of Alzheimer's amyloid beta is complexed to SP-40, 40 (apolipoprotein J), an inhibitor of the complement membrane-attack complex. *Biochem J* 1993;293:27–30.

134. Strittmatter WJ, Saunders AM, Schmechel D, et al. Apolipoprotein E: high-avidity binding to β-amyloid and increased frequency of type 4 allele in late onset familial Alzheimer disease. *Proc Natl Acad Sci USA* 1993;90:1977–1981.

135. Castaño EM, Prelli F, Wisniewski T, et al. Fibrillogenesis in Alzheimer's disease of amyloid β peptides and apolipoprotein E. *Biochem J* 1995; 306:599–604.

136. Evans KC, Berger EP, Cho CG, et al. Apolipoprotein E is a kinetic but not a thermodynamic inhibitor of amyloid formation: implications for the pathogenesis and treatment of Alzheimer disease. *Proc Natl Acad Sci USA* 1995;92: 763–767.

137. Wisniewski T, Golabek AA, Kida E, et al. Conformational mimicry in Alzheimer's disease. Role of apolipoproteins in amyloidogenesis. *Am J Pathol* 1995;147:238–244. Implications for therapy. *Am J Psychiatry* 1994;151:1105–1113.

138. Hyman BT, Strickland D, Rebeck GW. Role of the low-density lipoprotein receptor-related protein in beta-amyloid metabolism and Alzheimer disease. *Arch Neurol* 2000;57:646–50.

139. Kang DE, Pietrzik CU, Baum L, et al. Modulation of amyloid beta-protein clearance and Alzheimer's disease susceptibility by the LDL receptor-related protein pathway. *J Clin Invest* 2000;106:1159–66

140. Shibata M, Yamada S, Kumar SR, et al. Clearance of Alzheimer's amyloid-ss(1-40) peptide from brain by LDL receptor-related protein-1 at the blood-brain barrier. *J Clin Invest* 2000; 106:1489-9

141. Sanchez L, Alvarez V, Gonzalez P, et al. Variation in the LRP-associated protein gene (LRPAP1) is associated with late-onset Alzheimer disease. *Am J Med Genet* 2001;105:76–8

142. Aisen PS, Davis KL. Inflammatory mechanisms in Alzheimer's disease: implications for therapy. *Am J Psychiatry* 1994;151:1105–1113.

143. Whitehouse PJ, Price DL, Struble RG, et al. Alzheimer's disease and senile dementia: loss of neurons in the basal forebrain. *Science* 1982; 215:1237–1239.

144. Arendt T, Bigl V, Arendt A, Tennstedt A. Loss of neurons in the nucleus basalis of Meynert in Alzheimer's disease, paralysis agitans, and Korsakoff's disease. *Acta Neuropathol* 1983;61: 101–108.

145. McGeer PL, McGeer EG, Suzuki J, et al. Aging, Alzheimer's disease, and the cholinergic system of the basal forebrain. *Neurology* 1984;34: 741–745.

146. Saper CB, German DC, White CL. Neuronal pathology in the nucleus basalis and associated cell groups in senile dementia of the Alzheimer's type: possible role in cell loss. *Neurology* 1985;35:1089–1095.

147. Pope A, Hess HH, Lewin E. Microchemical pathology of the cerebral cortex in pre-senile dementias. *Trans Am Neurol* 1964;89:15–16.

148. Bowen DM, Smith CB, White P, Davison AN. Neurotransmitter-related enzymes and indices of hypoxia in senile dementia and other abiotrophies. *Brain* 1976;99:459–496.

149. Davies P, Maloney AJ. Selective loss of central cholinergic neurons in Alzheimer's disease. *Lancet* 1976;2:1403.

150. Rossor MN, Garrett NJ, Johnson AL, et al. A post-mortem study of the cholinergic and GABA systems in senile dementia. *Brain* 1982; 105:313–330.

151. Bird TD, Stranahan S, Sumi SM, Raskind M. Alzheimer's disease: choline acetyltransferase activity in brain tissue from clinical and pathological subgroups. *Ann Neurol* 1983;14: 284–293.

152. Bowen DM, Allen SJ, Benton JS, et al. Biochemical assessment of serotonergic and cholinergic dysfunction and cerebral atrophy in Alzheimer's disease. *J Neurochem* 1983;41:266–272.

153. Sims NR, Bowen DM, Allen SJ, et al. Presynaptic cholinergic dysfunction in patients with dementia. *J Neurochem* 1983;40:503–509.

154. Perry EK, Tomlinson BE, Blessed G, et al. Correlation of cholinergic abnormalities with senile plaques and mental test scores in senile dementia. *Br Med J* 1978;2:1457–1459.

155. Mountjoy CQ, Rossor MN, Iversen LL, Roth M. Correlation of cortical cholinergic and GABA deficits with quantitative neuropathological findings in senile dementia. *Brain* 1984;107: 507–518.

156. Neary D, Snowden JS, Mann DMA, et al. Alzheimer's disease: a correlative study. *J Neurol Neurosurg Psychiatry* 1986;49:229–237.

157. Dickson DW, Crystal HA, Bevona C, et al. Correlations of synaptic and pathological markers with cognition of the elderly. *Neurobiol Aging* 1995;3:285–304.

158. Drachman DA, Leavitt J. Human memory and the cholinergic system. *Arch Neurol* 1974;30: 113–121.

159. Bartus RT, Dean RL, Beer B, Lippa AS. The cholinergic hypothesis of geriatric memory dysfunction. *Science* 1982;217:408–417.

160. Blusztajn JK, Wurtman RJ. Choline and cholinergic neurons. *Science* 1983;221:614–620.

161. Wurtman RJ, Blusztajn JK, Maire J-C. "Autocannibalism" of choline-containing membrane phospholipids in the pathogenesis of Alzheimer's disease: an hypothesis. *Neurochem Int* 1985;7:369–372.

162. Tucek S. Problems in the organization and control of acetylcholine synthesis in brain neurons. *Prog Biophys Mol Biol* 1984;44:1–46.

163. Wurtman RJ. Choline metabolism as a basis for the selective vulnerability of cholinergic neurons. *Trends Neurosci* 1992;15:117–122.

164. Zeisel SH. Choline: an important nutrient in brain development, liver function and carcinogenesis. *J Am Coll Nutr* 1992;11:473–481.

165. Klein J, Gonzalez R, Köppen A, Löffelholz K. Free choline and choline metabolites in rat brain and body fluids. *Neurochem Int* 1993;22: 293–300.

166. Scremin OU, Jenden DJ. Acetylcholine turnover and release. *Prog Brain Res* 1993;98: 191–195.

167. Cohen BM, Renshaw PF, Stoll AL, et al. Decreased brain choline uptake in older adults. *JAMA* 1995;274:902–907.

168. Brinkman S, Sniff R, Meyer J, et al. Lecithin and memory training in suspected Alzheimer's disease. *J Gerontol* 1982;37:4–9.

169. Kaye W, Sitaram N, Weingartner H, et al. Modest facilitation of memory in dementia with combined lecithin and anticholinesterase treatment. *Biol Psychiatry* 1982;17:275–280.

170. Pomara N, Domino E, Yoon H, et al. Failure of single dose lecithin to alter aspects of central cholinergic activity in Alzheimer's disease. *J Clin Psychiatry* 1983;44:293–295.

171. Wettstein A. No effect from double-blind trial of physostigmine and lecithin in Alzheimer's disease. *Ann Neurol* 1983;13:210–212.

172. Smith R, Vroulis G, Johnson R, Morgan R. Comparison of therapeutic response to long-term treatment with lecithin vs. piracetam plus lecithin in patients with Alzheimer's disease. *Psychopharmacol Bull* 1984;20:542–545.

173. Little A, Levy R, Chuagui-Kidd C, et al. A double-blind, placebo-controlled trial of high dose lecithin in Alzheimer's disease. *J Neurol Neurosurg Psychiatry* 1985;48:736–742.

174. Duffy F, McAnulty G, Albert M, et al. Lecithin: absence of neurophysiologic effect in Alzheimer's disease by EEG topography. *Neurology* 1987;37:1015–1019.

175. Raiteri M, Leardi R, Marchi M. Heterogeneity of presynaptic muscarinic receptors regulating neurotransmitter release in the rat brain. *J Pharmacol Exp Ther* 1984;228:209–214.

176. Mash DC, Flynn DD, Potter LT. Loss of FM2 muscarine receptors in the cerebral cortex in Alzheimer's disease and experimental cholinergic denervation. *Science* 1985;228:1115–1117.

177. Bonner TI. The molecular basis of muscarinic receptor diversity. *Trends Pharmacol Sci* 1989;10: 148–151.

178. McKinney M, Anderson DJ, Vella-Rountree L, et al. Pharmacological profiles for rat cortical M_1 and M_2 muscarinic receptors using selective antagonists: comparison with N1E-15 muscarinic receptors. *J Pharmacol Exp Ther* 1991;257: 1121–1129.

179. Greenamyre JT, Maragos WF. Neurotransmitter receptors in Alzheimer disease. *Cerebrovasc Brain Metab Rev* 1993;5:61–94.

180. Smith CJ, Perry EK, Perry RH, et al. Guanine nucleotide modulation of muscarinic receptor binding in postmortem human brain—a preliminary study in Alzheimer's disease. *Neurosci Lett* 1987;82:227–232.

181. Flynn DD, Weinstein DA, Mash DC. Loss of high-affinity agonist binding to M1 muscarinic receptors in Alzheimer's disease: implications for the failure of cholinergic replacement therapies. *Ann Neurol* 1991;29:256–262.

182. Marin DB, Davis KL. Experimental therapeutics. In: Bloom FE, Kupfer DJ, eds. *Psychopharmacology: the fourth generation of progress.* New York: Raven Press, 1995:1417–1426.

183. Woolf NJ, Butcher LL. Cholinergic systems: synopsis of anatomy and overview of physiology and pathology. In: Scheibel AB, Wechsler AF, eds. *The biological substrates of Alzheimer's disease.* New York: Academic Press, 1989:73–86.

184. Flynn DD, Mash DC. Characterization of L-[^{3}H]nicotine binding in human cerebral cortex: comparison between Alzheimer's disease and normal. *J Neurochem* 1986;47:1948–1954.

185. Whitehouse PJ, Martino AM, Antuono PG, et al. Nicotinic acetylcholine binding sites in Alzheimer's disease. *Brain Res* 1986;371:146–151.

186. Araujo DM, Lapchak PA, Robitaille Y, et al. Differential alteration of various cholinergic markers in cortical and subcortical regions of human brain in Alzheimer's disease. *J Neurochem* 1988;50:1914–1923.

187. Zubenko GS, Moossy J, Martinez AJ, et al. Neuropathological and neurochemical correlates of psychosis in primary dementia. *Arch Neurol* 1991b;48:619–624.

188. Zubenko GS. Clinicopathological and neurochemical correlates of major depression and psychosis in primary dementia. *Int Psychogeriatr,* 1996;8:219–223.

189. Tomlinson BE, Irving D, Blessed G. Cell loss in the locus coeruleus in senile dementia of Alzheimer type. *J Neurol Sci* 1981;49:419–428.

190. Iversen LL, Rossor MN, Reynolds GP, et al. Loss of pigmented dopamine-β-hydroxylase positive cells from locus coeruleus in senile dementia of Alzheimer's type. *Neurosci Lett* 1983;39:95–100.

191. Curcio CA, Kemper T. Nucleus raphe dorsalis in dementia of the Alzheimer type: neurofibrillary changes and neuronal packing density. *J Neuropathol Exp Neurol* 1984;43:359–368.

192. Yamamoto T, Hirano A. Nucleus raphe dorsalis in Alzheimer's disease: neurofibrillary tangles and loss of large neurons. *Ann Neurol* 1985;17: 573–577.

193. Yates CM, Simpson J, Russell D, Gordon A. Cholinergic enzymes in neurofibrillary degeneration produced by aluminum. *Brain Res* 1980; 197:269–274.

194. Cross AJ, Crow TJ, Perry EK, et al. Reduced dopamine-beta-hydroxylase activity in Alzheimer's disease. *Br Med J* 1981;1:93–94.

195. Winblad B, Adolfsson R, Carlsson A, Gottfries CG. Biogenic amines in brains of patients with Alzheimer's disease. In: Corkin S, Davis KL, Growdon JH, et al., eds. *Alzheimer's disease: a report of progress in research (aging).* New York: Raven Press, 1982;19:25–33.

196. Bowen DM, Benton JS, Spillane JA, et al. Choline acetyltransferase activity and histopathology of frontal neocortex from biopsies of demented patients. *J Neurol Sci* 1982;57:191–202.

197. Palmer AM, Francis PT, Bowen DM, et al. Catecholaminergic neurons assessed ante-mortem in Alzheimer's disease. *Brain Res* 1987;414: 365–375.

198. Hyman SE, Nestler EJ. *The molecular foundations of psychiatry.* Washington, DC: American Psychiatric Press, 1993.

199. Peroutka SJ. 5-Hydroxytryptamine receptor subtypes: molecular, biochemical and physiological characterization. *Trends Neurosci* 1988; 11:496–500.

200. Davies MF, Deisz RA, Prince DA, et al. Two distinct effects of 5-hydroxytryptamine on single cortical neurons. *Brain Res* 1987;423:347–352.

201. Leysen JE, Van Gompel P, Verwimp M, et al. Role and localization of serotonin-2 receptor binding sites: effects of neuronal lesions. In: Mandel P, DeFeudis FV, eds. *CNS receptors from molecular pharmacology to behavior.* New York: Raven Press, 1983:373–383.

202. Coyle JT, Price DL, DeLong MR. Alzheimer's disease: a disorder of cortical cholinergic innervation. *Science* 1983;219:1184–1190.

203. Middlemiss DN, Palmer AN, Edel N, et al. Binding of the novel serotonin agonist 8-hydroxy-2-(di-n-propylamino) tetralin in normal and Alzheimer brain. *J Neurochem* 1986;46:993–996.

204. Jansen KLR, Faull RLM, Dragunow M, et al. Alzheimer's disease: changes in hippocampal N-methyl-D-aspartate, quisqualate, neurotensin, adenosine, benzodiazepine, serotonin and opioid receptors—an autoradiographic study. *Neuroscience* 1990;39:613–627.

205. O'Neill C, Fowler CJ, Wiehager B, et al. Coupling of human brain cerebral cortical α₂-adrenoceptors to GTP-binding proteins in Alzheimer's disease. *Brain Res* 1991;563:39–43.

206. Gottfries CG, Karlsson I, Nyth AL. Treatment of depression in elderly patients with and without dementia disorders. *Int Clin Psychopharmacol* 1992;5:55–64.

207. Bowen DM, Francis PT, Pangalos MN, et al. Treatment strategies for Alzheimer's disease. *Lancet* 1992;339:132–133.

208. Kalaria RN, Andorn AC, Tabaton M, et al. Adrenergic receptors in aging and Alzheimer's disease: increased β₂-receptors in prefrontal cortex and hippocampus. *J Neurochem* 1989;53:1772–1781.

209. Meana JJ, Barturen F, Garro MA, et al. Decreased density of presynaptic α₂-adrenoceptors in postmortem brains of patients with Alzheimer's disease. *J Neurochem* 1992;58:1896–1904.

210. Lewis DA, Morrison JH. Noradrenergic innervation of monkey prefrontal cortex: a dopamine-β-hydroxylase immunohistochemical study. *J Comp Neurol* 1989;282:317–330.

211. Civelli O, Bunzow JR, Grandy DK, et al. Molecular biology of the dopamine receptors. *Eur J Pharmacol Mol Pharmacol Sect* 1991;207:277–286.

212. Starke K, Gothert M, Kilbinger H. Modulation of neurotransmitter release by presynaptic autoreceptors. *Physiol Rev* 1989;69:864–989.

213. Mann DMA, Yates PO, Marcyniuk B. Dopaminergic neurotransmitter systems in Alzheimer's disease and in Down's syndrome in middle age. *J Neurol Neurosurg Psychiatry* 1987;50:341–344.

214. Torak RM, Morris JC. The association of ventral tegmental area histopathology with adult dementia. *Arch Neurol* 1988;45:497–501.

215. Adolfsson R, Gottfries CG, Roos BE, Winblad B. Changes in the brain catecholamine in patients with dementia of Alzheimer type. *Br J Psychiatry* 1979;135:216–223.

216. Yates CM, Allison Y, Simpson J, et al. Dopamine in Alzheimer's disease and senile dementia. *Lancet* 1979;ii:851–852.

217. Arai H, Kosaka K, Iizuka T. Changes of biogenic amines and their metabolites in postmortem brains from patients with Alzheimer-type dementia. *J Neurochem* 1984;43:388–393.

218. Langlais PJ, Thal L, Hansen L, et al. Neurotransmitters in basal ganglia and cortex of Alzheimer's disease with and without Lewy bodies. *Neurology* 1993;43:1927–1934.

219. Cross AJ, Crow TJ, Ferrier IN, et al. Striatal dopamine receptors in Alzheimer-type dementia. *Neurosci Lett* 1984c;52:1–6.

220. Rinne JO, Rinne JK, Laasko K, et al. Reduction in muscarinic receptor binding in limbic areas of Alzheimer brain. *J Neurol Neurosurg Psychiatry* 1984;47:651–653.

221. Cortes R, Probst A, Palacios JM. Decreased densities of dopamine D1 receptors in the putamen and hippocampus in senile dementia of the Alzheimer type. *Brain Res* 1988;475:164–167.

222. De Keyser J, Ebinger G, Vauquelin G. D1-dopamine receptor abnormality in frontal cortex points to a functional alteration of cortical cell membranes in Alzheimer's disease. *Arch Neurol* 1990;47:761–763.

223. Perry EK, Irving D, Kerwin JM, et al. Cholinergic transmitter and neurotrophic activities in Lewy body dementia: similarity to Parkinson's and distinction from Alzheimer disease. *Alzheimer Dis Assoc Disord* 1993;7:69–79.

224. Francis PT, Webster MT, Chessel IP, et al. Neurotransmitters and second messengers in aging and Alzheimer's disease. *Ann NY Acad Sci* 1993;695:19–26.

225. Stone TW. Amino acids as neurotransmitters of corticifugal neurones in the rat: a comparison of glutamate and aspartate. *Br J Pharmacol* 1979;67:545–551.

226. Storm-Mathisen J, Iverson LL. Uptake of [³H]glutamic acid in excitatory nerve endings: light and electron microscopic observations in the hippocampal formation of the rat. *Neuroscience* 1979;4:1237–1253.

227. Zaczek R, Hedreen JC, Coyle JT. Evidence for a hippocampal-septal glutamatergic pathway in the rat. *Exp Neurol* 1979;65:145–156.

228. Streit P. Glutamate and aspartate as transmitter candidates for systems of the cerebral cortex. In: Jones EJ, Peters A, eds. *Cerebral cortex, vol. 2.* New York: Plenum Press, 1984:119–143.

229. Manzoni T, Barbarest P, Fabri M. D-[³H]Aspartate retrograde labelling of association neurones in area S1 of the cat. *Neurosci Lett* 1986;67:175–180.

230. Young AB, Fagg GE. Excitatory amino acid receptors in the brain: membrane and receptor autoradiographic approaches. *Trends Pharmacol Sci* 1990;11:126–133.

231. Proctor AW, Palmer AM, Stratmann GC, et al. Glutamate/aspartate-releasing neurons in Alzheimer's disease. *N Engl J Med* 1986;314:1711–1712.

232. Ellison DW, Beal MF, Mazurek MF, et al. A postmortem study of amino acid neurotransmitters in Alzheimer's disease. *Ann Neurol* 1986;20:616–621.

233. Sasaki H, Muramoto O, Kanazawa I, et al. Regional distribution of amino acid transmitters in post-mortem brains of presenile dementia of Alzheimer type. *Ann Neurol* 1986;19:263–269.

234. Greenamyre JT, Young AB. Excitatory amino acids and Alzheimer's disease. *Neurobiol Aging* 1989;10:593–602.

235. Watkins JC, Evans RH. Excitatory amino acid transmitters. *Annu Rev Pharmacol Toxicol* 1981;21:165–204.

236. Monaghan DT, Holets VR, Toy DW, et al. Anatomical distribution of four pharmacologically distinct ^{3}H-L-glutamate binding sites. *Nature* 1983;306:176–179.

237. Monaghan DT, Yao D, Cotman CW. Distribution of [^{3}H]AMPA binding sites in rat brain determined by quantitative autoradiography. *Brain Res* 1984;324:160–164.

238. Greenamyre JT, Penney JB, Young AB, et al. Alterations of L-glutamate binding in Alzheimer's and Huntington's diseases. *Science* 1985; 227:1496–1499.

239. Jansen KLR, Dragunow M, Faull RLM. [^{3}H]Glycine binding sites, NMDA and PCP receptors have similar distributions in the human hippocampus: an autoradiographic study. *Brain Res* 1989;482:174–178.

240. Collingridge GL. Long term potentiation in the hippocampus: mechanisms of initiation and modulation by neurotransmitters. *Trends Pharmacol Sci* 1985;6:407–411.

241. Harris EW, Ganong AH, Cotman CW. Long-term potentiation in the hippocampus involves activation of N-methyl-D-aspartate receptors. *Brain Res* 1984;323:132–137.

242. Morris RGM, Anderson E, Lynch GS, et al. Selective impairment of learning and blockade of long-term potentiation by an N-methyl-D-aspartate receptor antagonist, AP5. *Nature* 1986; 319:774–776.

243. Meldrum B, Garthwaite J. Excitatory amino acid neurotoxicity and neurodegeneration disease. *Trends Pharmacol Sci* 1990;11:379–387.

244. Faden AI, Demediuk P, Panter SS, et al. The role of excitatory amino acids and NMDA receptors in traumatic brain injury. *Science* 1989; 244:798–800.

245. Benveniste H. The excitotoxin hypothesis in relation to cerebral ischemia. *Cerebrovasc Brain Metab Rev* 1991;3:213–245.

246. Maragos WF, Greenamyre JT, Penney JB, Young AB. Glutamate dysfunction in Alzheimer's disease: an hypothesis. *Trends Neurosci* 1987bf:65–68.

247. Greenamyre JT, Maragos WF, Albin RL, et al. Glutamate transmission and toxicity in Alzheimer's disease. *Prog Neuropsychopharmacol Biol Psychiatry* 1988;12:421–430.

248. Dodd PR, Scott HL, Wetphalen RI. Excitotoxic mechanisms in the pathogenesis of dementia. *Neurochem Int* 1994;25:203–219.

249. Maragos WF, Chu DCM, Young AB, et al. Loss of hippocampal [^{3}H]TCP binding in Alzheimer's disease. *Neurosci Lett* 1987a;74:371–376.

250. Monaghan DT, Geddes JW, Yao D, et al. [^{3}H]TCP binding sites in Alzheimer's disease. *Neurosci Lett* 1987;73:197–200.

251. Repressa A, Duyckaets C, Tremblay E, et al. Is senile dementia of the Alzheimer type associated hippocampal plasticity? *Brain Res* 1988; 457:355–359.

252. Chalmers DT, Dewar D, Graham DI, et al. Differential alterations of cortical glutamatergic binding sites in senile dementia of the Alzheimer type. *Proc Natl Acad Sci USA* 1990;87: 1352–1356.

253. Ninomiya H, Fukunaga R, Taniguchi T, et al. [^{3}H]N-[1-(2-thienyl)cyclohexyl]-3,4-piperidine ([^{3}H]TCP) binding in human frontal cortex: decreases in Alzheimer-type dementia. *J Neurochem* 1990;54:526–532.

254. Penney JB, Maragos WF, Greenamyre JT, et al. Excitatory amino acid binding sites in the hippocampal region of Alzheimer's disease and other dementias. *J Neurol Neurosurg Psychiatry* 1990;53:314–320.

255. Ulas J, Brunner LC, Geddes JW, et al. N-Methyl-D-aspartate receptor complex in the hippocampus of elderly, normal individuals and those with Alzheimer's disease. *Neuroscience* 1992;49: 45–61.

256. Dewar D, Chalmers DT, Shand A, et al. Selective reduction of quisqualate (AMPA) receptors in Alzheimer's cerebellum. *Ann Neurol* 1990;28:805–810.

257. Dewar D, Chalmers DT, Graham DI, et al. Glutamate metabotropic and AMPA binding sites are reduced in Alzheimer's disease: an autoradiographic study of the hippocampus. *Brain Res* 1991;553:58–64.

258. Backus KH, Kettenmann H, Schachner M. Pharmacological characterization of the glutamate receptor in cultured astrocytes. *J Neurosci Res* 1989;22:274–282.

259. Usowicz MM, Gallo V, Cull-Candy SG. Multiple conductance channels in type-2 cerebellar astrocytes activated by excitatory amino acids. *Nature* 1989;339:380–383.

260. Glaum SR, Holzwarth JA, Miller RJ. Glutamate receptors activate Ca^{2+} mobilization and Ca^{2+} influx into astrocytes. *Proc Natl Acad Sci USA* 1990;87:3454–3458.

261. Tanabe Y, Masu M, Ishii T, et al. A family of metabotropic glutamate receptors. *Neuron* 1992;8:169–179.

262. Schoepp DD, Johnson BG, Monn JA. Inhibition of cyclic AMP formation by a selective metabotropic glutamate receptor agonist. *J Neurochem* 1992;58:1184–1188.

263. Geddes JW, Monaghan DT, Cotman CW, et al. Plasticity of hippocampal circuitry in Alzheimer disease. *Science* 1985;230:1179–1181.

264. Candy JM, Gascoigne AD, Biggins JA, et al. Somatostatin immunoreactivity in cortical and some subcortical regions in Alzheimer's disease. *J Neurol Sci* 1985;71:315–323.

265. Roberts GW, Crow TJ, Polak JM. Location of neuronal tangles in somatostatin neurones in Alzheimer's disease. *Nature* 1985;314:92–94.

266. Taminga CA, Foster NL, Chase TN. Reduced brain somatostatin levels in Alzheimer's disease. *N Engl J Med* 1985;313:1294–1295.

267. Schmechel DE, Vickrey BG, Fitzpatrick D, et al. GABAergic neurons of mammalian cerebral cortex: widespread subclass defined by somatostatin content. *Neurosci Lett* 1984;47:227–232.

268. Sivilotti L, Nistri A. GABA receptor mechanisms in the central nervous system. *Prog Neurobiol* 1991;36:35–92.

269. Cross AJ, Crow TJ, Ferrier IN, et al. Serotonin receptor changes in dementia of the Alzheimer type. *J Neurochem* 1984b;43:1574–1581.

270. Chu DC, Penney JB, Young AB. Quantitative autoradiography of hippocampal GABA$_B$ re-

ceptor changes in Alzheimer's disease. *Neurosci Lett* 1987b;82:246–252.

271. Greenamyre JT, Penney JB, D'Amato CJ, et al. Dementia of the Alzheimer's type: changes in hippocampal L-[³H] glutamate binding. *J Neurochem* 1987;48:543–551.

272. Vogt BA, Crino PB, Volicer L. Laminar alterations in γ-aminobutyric acid$_A$, muscarinic and β adrenoceptors and neuron degeneration in cingulate cortex in Alzheimer's disease. *J Neurochem* 1991;57:282–290.

273. Chu DC, Penney JB, Young AB. Cortical GABA$_B$ and GABA$_A$ receptors in Alzheimer's disease: a quantitative autoradiographic study. *Neurology* 1987a;37:1454–1459.

274. Phelps ME, Huang SC, Hoffman EJ, et al. Tomographic measurement of local cerebral glucose metabolic rate in humans with (F-18) 2-fluoro-2-deoxyglucose: validation of method. *Ann Neurol* 1979;6:371–388.

275. Rivich M, Kuhl D, Wolf A, et al. The ¹⁸F-fluorodeoxyglucose method for the measurement of local cerebral glucose utilization in man. *Circ Res* 1979;44:127–137.

276. Huang SC, Phelps ME, Hoffman EJ, et al. Noninvasive determination of local cerebral metabolic rate of glucose in man. *Am J Physiol* 1980;238:E69–E82.

277. McGeer EG, Peppard RP, McGeer PL, et al. ¹⁸Fluorodeoxyglucose positron emission tomography studies in presumed Alzheimer cases, including 13 serial scans. *Can J Neurol Sci* 1990;17:1–11.

278. Kumar A, Schapiro MB, Grady CL, et al. High-resolution PET studies in Alzheimer's disease. *Neuropsychopharmacology* 1991;4:35–46.

279. Smith GS, de Leon MJ, George AE, et al. Topography of cross-sectional and longitudinal glucose metabolic deficits in Alzheimer's disease: pathophysiologic implications. *Arch Neurol* 1992;49:1142–1150.

280. Murphy DGM, Bottomley PA, Salerno JA, et al. An in vivo study of phosphorus and glucose metabolism in Alzheimer's disease using magnetic resonance spectroscopy and PET. *Arch Gen Psychiatry* 1993;50:341–349.

281. Mielke R, Herholz K, Grond M, et al. Clinical deterioration in probable Alzheimer's disease correlates with progressive metabolic impairment of association areas. *Dementia* 1994;5:36–41.

282. Minoshima S, Frey KA, Koeppe RA, et al. A diagnostic approach in Alzheimer's disease using three-dimensional stereotactic surface projections of fluorine-18-FDG PET. *J Nucl Med* 1995;36:1238–1248.

283. Kuhl DE, Small GW, Riege WH, et al. Cerebral metabolic patterns before the diagnosis of probable Alzheimer's disease. *J Cereb Blood Flow Metab* 1987;7:S406.

284. Grady CL, Haxby JV, Horwitz B, et al. Longitudinal study of the early neuropsychological and cerebral metabolic changes in dementia of the Alzheimer type. *J Clin Exp Neuropsychol* 1988;10:576–596.

285. Haxby JV, Grady CL, Koss E, et al. Longitudinal study of cerebral metabolic asymmetries and associated neuropsychological patterns in early

286. dementia of the Alzheimer type. *Arch Neurol* 1990;47:753–760.

286. Small GW, Mazziotta JC, Collins MT, et al. Apolipoprotein E type 4 allele and cerebral glucose metabolism in relatives at risk for familial Alzheimer disease. *JAMA* 1995;273:942–947.

287. Reiman EM, Caselli RJ, Yun LS, et al. Preclinical evidence of Alzheimer's disease in persons homozygous for the ε4 allele for apolipoprotein E. *N Engl J Med* 1996;334:752–758.

288. Kumar A, Newberg A, Alavi A, et al. Regional cerebral glucose metabolism in late-life depression and Alzheimer disease. A preliminary positron emission tomography study. *Proc Natl Acad Sci USA* 1993;90:7019–7023.

289. Prohovnik I, Mayeux R, Sackheim HA, et al. Cerebral perfusion as a diagnostic marker of early Alzheimer's disease. *Neurology* 1988;38:931–937.

290. Schapiro MB, Pietrini P, Grady CL, et al. Reductions in parietal and temporal cerebral metabolic rates for glucose are not specific for Alzheimer's disease. *J Neurol Neurosurg Psychiatry* 1993;56:859–864.

291. Rapoport SI. Anatomic and functional brain imaging in Alzheimer's disease. In: Bloom FE, Kupfer DJ, eds. *Psychopharmacology: the fourth generation of progress.* New York: Raven Press. 1995:1401–1415.

292. Mazziotta JC, Phelps ME. Positron emission tomography studies of the brain. In: Phelps M, Mazziotta J, Schelber H, eds. *Positron emission tomography and autoradiography: principles and applications for the brain and heart.* New York: Raven Press, 1986:493–579.

293. Blass JP, Gibson GE. The role of oxidative abnormalities in the pathophysiology of Alzheimer's disease. *Rev Neurol* 1991;147:513–525.

294. Pettegrew JW, McClure RJ, Kanfer JN, et al. The role of membranes and energetics in Alzheimer's disease. In: Terry RD, Katzman R, Bick KL, eds. *Alzheimer disease.* New York: Raven Press, 1994:369–386.

295. Bowen DM, Davison AN. Biochemical studies of nerve cells and energy metabolism in Alzheimer's disease. *Br Med Bull* 1986;1:75–80.

296. Sorbi S, Mortilla M, Piacentini S, et al. Altered hexokinase activity in skin cultured fibroblasts and leukocytes from Alzheimer's disease patients. *Neurosci Lett* 1990;117:165–168.

297. Kish SJ, Bergeron C, Rajput A, et al. Brain cytochrome oxidase in Alzheimer's disease. *J Neurochem* 1992;59:776–779.

298. Simonian NA, Hyman BT. Functional alterations in Alzheimer's disease: diminution of cytochrome oxidase in the hippocampal formation. *J Neuropathol Exp Neurol* 1993;52:580–585.

299. Sparks DL, Hunsaker JC III, Scheff SW, et al. Cortical senile plaques in coronary artery disease, aging and Alzheimer's disease. *Neurobiol Aging* 1990;11:601–607.

300. Aronson MK, Ooi WL, Morgenstern H, et al. Women: myocardial infarction and dementia in the very old. *Neurology* 1990;40:1102–1106.

301. Zubenko GS. Biological correlates of clinical heterogeneity in primary dementia. *Neuropsychopharmacology* 1992;6:77–93.

302. Roth GS, Joseph JA, Mason RP. Membrane alterations as causes of impaired signal transduction in Alzheimer's disease and aging. *Trends Neurosci* 1995;18:203–206.

303. Heron DS, Shinitzky M, Hershkowitz M, et al. Lipid fluidity markedly modulates the binding of serotonin to mouse brain membrane. *Proc Natl Acad Sci USA* 1980;77:7463–7467.

304. Hershkowitz M, Heron D, Samuel D, et al. The modulation of protein phosphorylation and receptor binding in synaptic membranes by changes in lipid fluidity: implications for ageing. *Prog Brain Res* 1982;56:419–434.

305. Yeagle PL, Young J, Rice D. Effects of cholesterol on (Na + , K +)-ATPase ATP hydrolyzing activity in kidney. *Biochemistry* 1988;27: 6449–6452.

306. McClure RJ, Kanfer JN, Panchalingam K, et al. Alzheimer's disease: membrane-associated metabolic changes. *Ann NY Acad Sci* 1994;747: 110–124.

307. Klunk WE, McClure RJ, Pettegrew JW. L-Phosphoserine, a metabolite elevated in Alzheimer's disease, interacts with specific L-glutamate receptor subtypes. *J Neurochem* 1991;56: 1997–2003.

308. Andriamampandry C, Kanfer JN. The inhibition of cytosolic human forebrain choline acetyltransferase activity by phospho-L-serine phosphomonoester that accumulates during early stages of Alzheimer's disease. *Neurobiol Aging* 1993;14:367–372.

309. Mason RP, Trumbore MV, Pettegrew JW. Membrane interactions of phosphomonester elevated early in Alzheimer's disease. *Neurobiol Aging* 1995;16:531–539.

310. Soderberg M, Edlund C, Alafuzoff I, et al. Lipid composition in different regions of the brain in Alzheimer's disease/senile dementia of the Alzheimer's type. *J Neurochem* 1992;59: 1646–1653.

311. Nkada T, Kwee IL, Ellis WG. Membrane fatty acid composition shows delta-6-desaturase abnormalities in Alzheimer's disease. *Neuroreport* 1990;1:153–155.

312. Kwee IL, Nakada T, Ellis WG. Elevation in relative levels of brain membrane unsaturated fatty acids in Alzheimer's disease: high resolution proton spectroscopic studies of membrane lipid extracts. *Magn Reson Med* 1991;21:49–54.

313. Soderberg M, Edlund C, Kristensson K, et al. Fatty acid composition of brain phospholipid in ageing and in Alzheimer's disease. *Lipids* 1991;26:421–425.

314. Mason RP, Shoemaker WJ, Shajenko L, et al. Evidence for changes in the Alzheimer's disease brain cortical membrane structure mediated by cholesterol. *Neurobiol Aging* 1992;13: 413–419.

315. Shinitzky M, Barenholz Y. Fluidity parameters of lipid regions determined by fluorescence polarization. *Biochim Biophys Acta* 1978;515: 367–394.

316. Soderberg M, Edlund K, Kristensson K, et al. Lipid compositions of different regions of the human brain during aging. *J Neurochem* 1990; 54:415–423.

317. Struk DK, Lennarz WJ. The function of saccharide-lipids in synthesis of glycoproteins. In: Lennarz WJ, ed. *The biochemistry of glycoproteins and proteoglycans.* New York: Plenum Press, 1980:35–73.

318. Emory CR, Ala TA, Frey WH. Ganglioside monoclonal antibody (A2B5) labels for Alzheimer's neurofibrillary tangles. *Arch Neurol* 1987; 37:768–772.

319. Blennow K, Davidsson P, Wallin A, et al. Gangliosides in cerebral spinal fluid in "probable" Alzheimer's disease. *Arch Neurol* 1991;48: 1032–1035.

320. Blass JP, Gibson GE. Nonneural markers in Alzheimer disease. *Alzheimer Dis Assoc Disord* 1992; 6:205–224.

321. Sweet RA, Zubenko GS. Peripheral markers in Alzheimer's disease. In: Burns A, Levy R, eds. *Dementia.* London: Chapman and Hall, 1994: 387–403.

322. Hicks N, Brammer MJ, Hymas N, et al. Platelet membrane properties in Alzheimer and multi-infarct dementias. *Alzheimer Dis Assoc Disord* 1987;1:90–97.

323. Eagger S, Hajimohammadreza I, Fletcher K, et al. Platelet membrane fluidity, family history, and severity and age of onset in Alzheimer's disease. *Int J Geriatr Psychiatry* 1990;5:395–400.

324. Hajimohammadreza I, Brammer MJ, Eagger S, et al. Platelet and erythrocyte membrane changes in Alzheimer's disease. *Biochim Biophys Acta* 1990;1025:208–214.

325. Piletz JE, Sarasua M, Whitehouse P, et al. Intracellular membranes are more fluid in platelets of Alzheimer's disease patients. *Neurobiol Aging* 1991;12:401–406.

326. van Rensburg SJ, Carstens ME, Potocnik FCV, et al. Membrane fluidity of platelets and erythrocytes in patients with Alzheimer's disease and the effect of small amounts of aluminum on platelet and erythrocyte membranes. *Neurochem Res* 1992;17:825–829.

327. Kálmán J, Dey I, Ilona SV, et al. Platelet membrane fluidity and plasma malondialdehyde levels in Alzheimer's demented patients with and without family history of dementia. *Biol Psychiatry* 1994;35:190–194.

328. Kaakkola S, Rosenberg PH, Alila A, et al. Platelet membrane fluidity in Alzheimer's disease and multi-infarct dementia: a spin label study. *Acta Neurol Scand J Suppl* 1991;84:18–21.

329. Kukull WA, Hinds TR, Schellenberg GD, et al. Increased platelet membrane fluidity as a diagnostic marker for Alzheimer's disease: a test in population-based cases and controls. *Neurology* 1992;42:607–614.

330. Zubenko GS, Cohen BM, Reynolds CF, et al. Platelet membrane fluidity in Alzheimer's disease and major depression. *Am J Psychiatry* 1987b;144:860–868.

331. Zubenko GS, Wusylko M, Boller F, et al. Family study of platelet membrane fluidity in Alzheimer's disease. *Science* 1987d;238:539–542.

332. Chakravarti A, Slaugenhaupt S, Zubenko GS. Inheritance pattern of platelet membrane fluidity in Alzheimer's disease. *Am J Hum Genet* 1989;44:799–805.

333. Zubenko GS, Teply I. Longitudinal study of platelet membrane fluidity in Alzheimer's disease. *Biol Psychiatry* 1988;24:918–924.

334. Zubenko GS, Huff FJ, Beyer J, et al. Familial risk of dementia associated with a biologic subtype of Alzheimer's disease. *Arch Gen Psychiatry* 1988c;45:889–893.

335. Zubenko GS, Brenner RP, Teply I. Electroencephalographic correlates of increased platelet membrane fluidity in Alzheimer's disease. *Arch Neurol* 1988a-:1009–1013.

336. Zubenko GS, Brenner RP, Teply I. Risk factors for stroke and platelet membrane fluidity in Alzheimer's disease. *Stroke* 1991a;22: 997–1003.

337. Zubenko GS, Huff FJ, Becker J, et al. Cognitive function and platelet membrane fluidity in Alzheimer's disease. *Biol Psychiatry* 1988b;24: 925–936.

338. Zubenko GS, Teply I, Winwood E, et al. Prospective study of increased platelet membrane fluidity as a risk factor for Alzheimer's disease: results at five years. *Am J Psychiatry* 1996b;153: 420–423.

339. Bush AI, Martins RN, Rumble B, et al. The amyloid precursor protein of Alzheimer's disease is released by human platelets. *J Biol Chem* 1990; 265:15977–15983.

340. Cole GM, Galasko D, Shapiro IP, Saitoh T. Stimulated platelets release amyloid beta-protein precursor. *Biochem Biophys Res Commun* 1990;170:288–295.

341. Schlossmacher MG, Ostaszewski BL, Hecker LI, et al. Detection of distinct isoform patterns of the β-amyloid precursor protein in human platelets and lymphocytes. *Neurobiol Aging* 1992;13:421–434.

342. Di Luca M, Pastorino L, Cattabeni F, et al. Abnormal pattern of platelet APP isoforms in Alzheimer's disease and Down syndrome. *Arch Neurol* 1996;53:1162–1166.

343. Wolozin B. Cholesterol and Alzheimer's disease. *Biochem Soc Trans* 2002;30:525–9.

344. Wolozin B, Iwasaki K, Vito P, et al. Participation of presenilin 2 in apoptosis: Enhanced basal activity conferred by an Alzheimer mutation. *Science* 1996;274:1710–1713.

345. Jick H, Zornberg GL, Jick SS, et al. Statins and the risk of dementia. *Lancet* 2000;356:1627–31.

346. Yaffe K, Barrett-Connor E, Lin F, et al. Serum lipoprotein levels, statin use, and cognitive function in older women. *Arch Neurol* 2002; 378–84.

347. Petanceska SS, DeRosa S, Olm V, Diaz N, Sharma A, Thomas-Bryant T, Duff K, Pappolla M, Refolo LM. Statin therapy for Alzheimer's disease: will it work? *J Mol Neurosci* 2002;19: 155–61.

348. Zubenko GS, Cohen BM, Boller F, et al. Platelet membrane abnormality in Alzheimer's disease. *Ann Neurol* 1987a;22:237–244.

349. Zubenko GS, Malinakova I, Chojnacki B. Proliferation of internal membranes in platelets from patients with Alzheimer's disease. *J Neuropathol Exp Neurol*, 1987c;46:407–418.

350. Cohen BM, Zubenko GS, Babb S. Abnormal platelet membrane composition in Alzheimer's disease. *Life Sci* 1987;40:2445–2451.

351. Zubenko GS. Endoplasmic reticulum abnormality in Alzheimer's disease: selective alteration in platelet NADH–cytochrome C reductase activity. *J Geriatr Psychiatry Neurol* 1989; 2:3–10.

352. Palade G. Intracellular aspects of the process of protein secretion. *Science* 1975;189:347–358.

353. Hubbard SC, Ivatt RJ. Synthesis and processing of asparagine-linked oligosaccharides. *Annu Rev Biochem* 1981;5:555–583.

354. Prusiner SB. Molecular biology of prion diseases. *Science* 1991;252:1515–1522.

355. Estus S, Golde E, Kunishita T, et al. Potentially amyloidogenic, carboxyl-terminal derivatives of the amyloid protein precursor. *Science* 1992; 255:726–728.

356. Haass C. Presenile because of presenilin: the presenilin genes and early onset Alzheimer's disease. *Curr Opinion Neurol* 1996;9:254–259.

357. McGeer PL, Rogers J, McGeer EG. Neuroimmune mechanisms in Alzheimer disease pathogenesis. *Alzheimer Dis Assoc Disord* 1994;8: 149–158.

358. Rozemuller JM, Eikelenboom P, Pals ST, et al. Microglial cells around amyloid plaques in Alzheimer's disease express leucocyte adhesion molecules of the LFA-1 family. *Neurosci Lett* 1989;101:288–292.

359. McGeer PL, Kawamata T, Walker DG, et al. Microglia in degenerative neurological disease. *Glia* 1993;7:84–92.

360. Banati RB, Gehrmann J, Schubert P, et al. Cytotoxicity of microglia. *Glia* 1993;7:111–118.

361. Giulian D. Reactive glia as rivals in regulating neuronal survival. *Glia* 1993;7:102–110.

362. McGeer PL, Akiyama H, Iagaki S, McGeer EG. Immune system response in Alzheimer's disease. *Can J Neurol Sci* 1989;16:516–527.

363. Tooyama I, Kimura H, Akiyama H, et al. Reactive microglia express class I and class II major histocompatibility antigens in Alzheimer disease. *Brain Res* 1990;523:273–280.

364. Johnson SA, Lampert-Etchels M, Rozovsky I, et al. Complement mRNA in the mammalian brain: responses to Alzheimer's disease and experimental brain lesioning. *Neurobiol Aging* 1992;13:641–648.

365. Walker DG, McGeer PL. Complement gene expression in human brain: comparison between normal and Alzheimer disease cases. *Mol Brain Res* 1992;14:109–116.

366. Rogers J, Cooper NR, Webster S, et al. Complement activation by β-amyloid in Alzheimer disease. *Proc Natl Acad Sci USA* 1992;89: 10016–10020.

367. Jiang H, Burdick D, Glabe CG, et al. β-Amyloid activates complement by binding to a specific region of the collagen-like domain in the C1q A chain. *J Immunol* 1994;152:5050–5059.

368. Murphy DE, Hutchinson AJ, Hurt SD, et al. Characterization of the binding of [3H]-CGS 19755: a novel N-methyl-D-aspartate antagonist with nanomolar affinity in rat brain. *Br J Pharmacol* 1988;95:932–938.

369. Preisner KT, Podack ER, Müller-Eberhard HJ. SC5b-8 and SC5b-9 complexes of complement: ultrastructure and localization of the S-protein

within the macromolecules. *Eur J Immunol* 1989;19:69–75.

370. Rosse WF. Phosphatidylinositol-linked proteins and paroxysmal nocturnal hemoglobinuria. *Blood* 1990;75:1595–1601.

371. May PC, Lampert-Etchells M, Johnson SA, et al. Dynamics of gene expression for a hippocampal glycoprotein elevated in Alzheimer's disease and in response to experimental lesions in rat. *Neuron* 1990;5:831–839.

372. McGeer PL, Walker DG, Akiyama H, et al. Detection of the membrane inhibitor of reactive lysis (CD59) in disease neurons of Alzheimer brain. *Brain Res* 1991;544:315–319.

373. Breitner JCS, Gau BA, Welsh KA, et al. Inverse association of anti-inflammatory treatments and Alzheimer's disease: initial results of a co-twin control study. *Neurology* 1994;44:227–232.

374. Breitner JCS, Welsh KA, Helms MJ, et al. Delayed onset of Alzheimer's disease with non-steroidal anti-inflammatory and histamine H2 blocking drugs. *Neurobiol Aging* 1995;16:523–530.

375. Rich JB, Rasmusson DX, Folstein MF, et al. Nonsteroidal anti-inflammatory drugs in Alzheimer's disease. *Neurology* 1995;45:51–55.

376. Canadian Study of Health and Aging. Risk factors for Alzheimer's disease in Canada. *Neurology* 1994;44:2073–2080.

377. Anderson K, Launer LJ, Ott A, et al. Do nonsteroidal anti-inflammatory drugs decrease the risk for Alzheimer's disease? The Rotterdam study. *Neurology* 1995;45:1441–1445.

378. Rogers J, Kirby LC, Hempelman SR, et al. Clinical trial of indomethacin in Alzheimer's disease. *Neurology* 1993;43:1609–1611.

379. in t' Veld BA, Ruitenberg A, Hofman A, et al. Nonsteroidal antiinflammatory drugs and the risk of Alzheimer's disease. *N Engl J Med* 2001;345:1515–21.

380. Pruisiner SB. Novel proteinaceous infectious particles cause scrapie. *Science* 1982;216:136–144.

381. DeArmond SJ, Pruisner SB. The neurochemistry of prion diseases. *J Neurochem* 1993;61:1589–1601.

382. Doms RW, Russ G, Yewdell JW. Brefeldin A redistributes resident and itinerant Golgi proteins to the endoplasmic reticulum. *J Cell Biol* 1989;109:61–72.

383. Caughey B, Raymond GJ. The scrapie-associated form of PrP is made from a cell surface precursor that is both protease- and phospholipase-sensitive. *J Biol Chem* 1991;266:18217–18223.

384. Taraboulos A, Raeber A, Borchelt D, et al. Brefeldin A inhibits protease-resistant prion protein synthesis in scrapie-infected cultured cells. *FASEB J* 1991;5:A1177.

385. Taraboulos A, Raeber AJ, Borchelt DR, et al. Synthesis and trafficking of prion proteins in cultured cells. *Mol Biol Cell* 1992;3:851–863.

386. Borchelt DR, Taraboulos A, Prusiner SB. Evidence for synthesis of scrapie prion proteins in the endocytic pathway. *J Biol Chem* 1992;267:6188–6199.

387. Cohen FE, Pan K-M, Huang Z, et al. Structural clues to prion replication. *Science* 1994;264:530–531.

388. Ghetti B, Tagliavini F, Masters CL, et al. Gerstmann-Straussler-Scheinker disease. II. Neurofibrillary tangles and plaques with PrP-amyloid coexist in an affected family. *Neurology* 1989;39:1453–1461.

389. Giaccone G, Tagliavini F, Verga L, et al. Neurofibrillary tangles of the Indiana kindred of Gerstmann-Straussler-Scheinker disease share antigenic determinants with those of Alzheimer's disease. *Brain Res* 1990;530:325–329.

390. Ghagliavini F, Prelli F, Ghisto J, et al. Amyloid protein of Gerstmann-Straussler-Scheinker disease (Indiana kindred) is an 11-kd fragment of prion protein with an N-terminal glycine at codon 58. *EMBO J* 1991;10:513–519.

391. Dlouhy SR, Hsiao K, Farlow MR, et al. Linkage of the Indiana kindred of Gerstmann-Straussler-Scheinker disease to the prion protein gene. *Nat Genet* 1992;1:64–67.

392. Hsiao K, Dloughy S, Ghetti B, et al. Mutant prion proteins in Gerstmann-Straussler-Scheinker disease with neurofibrillary tangles. *Nat Genet* 1992;1:68–71.

393. Rifat SL, Eastwood MR. The role of aluminum in dementia of Alzheimer's type: a review of the hypotheses and summary of the evidence. In: Burns A, Levy R, eds. *Dementia*. London: Chapman and Hall, 1994:268–280.

394. Alfrey AC, LeGendre GR, Kaehny WD. The dialysis encephalopathy syndrome: possible aluminum intoxication. *N Engl J Med* 1976;294:184–188.

395. Platts MM, Goode GC, Hislop JS. Composition of the domestic water supply and the incidence of fractures and encephalopathy in patients on home dialysis. *Br Med J* 1977;2:657–660.

396. McDermott JR, Smith AI, Ward MK, et al. Brain-aluminum concentration in dialysis encephalopathy. *Lancet* 1978;1:901–904.

397. Ackrill PA, Ralston AJ, Day JP, et al. Successful removal of aluminum from patients with dialysis encephalopathy. *Lancet* 1980;2:692–693.

398. Alfrey AC. Aluminum metabolism in uremia. *Neurotoxicology* 1980;1:43–53.

399. Crapper DR, Quittkat S, Krishnan SS, et al. Intranuclear aluminum content in Alzheimer's disease, dialysis encephalopathy and experimental aluminum encephalopathy. *Acta Neuropathol* 1980;50:19–24.

400. Arze RS, Parkinson IS, Cartlidge NEF, et al. Reversal of aluminum dialysis encephalopathy after desferrioxamine treatment. *Lancet* 1981;2:1116.

401. Chang TMS, Barre P. Effect of desferrioxamine on removal of aluminum and iron by coated charcoal haemoperfusion and haemodialysis. *Lancet* 1983;2:1051–1053.

402. Alfrey AC. Systemic toxicity of aluminum in man. *Neurobiol Aging* 1986;7:543–544.

403. Spofforth J. Cases of aluminum poisoning. *Lancet* 1921;1:1301.

404. MacLaughlin AIG, Kazantzis G, King E. Pulmonary fibrosis and encephalopathy associated with the inhalation of aluminum dust. *Br J Ind Med* 1962;19:253–263.

405. Longstreth WT, Rosenstock L, Heyer NJ. Potroom palsy? Neurologic disorder in three aluminum smelter workers. *Arch Intern Med* 1985; 145:1972–1975.

406. Kobayashi S, Hirota N, Saito K, et al. Aluminum accumulation in tangle-bearing neurons of Alzheimer's disease with Balant's syndrome in a long-term aluminum refiner. *Acta Neuropathol* 1987;74:47–52.

407. Crapper DR, Krishnan SS, Dalton AJ. Brain aluminum distribution in Alzheimer's disease and experimental neurofibrillary degeneration. *Science* 1973;180:511–513.

408. Duckett S, Galle P. Electron microscope microprobe studies of aluminum in the brains of cases of Alzheimer's disease and aging patients. *J Neuropathol Exp Neurol* 1980;39:350.

409. Perl DP, Brody AR. Alzheimer's disease: x-ray spectrometric evidence of aluminum accumulation in neurofibrillary tangle-bearing neurons. *Science* 1980;208:297–299.

410. Candy JM, Oakley AE, Klinowski J, et al. Aluminosilicates and senile plaque formation in Alzheimer's disease. *Lancet* 1986;1:354–357.

411. Crapper-McLachlan DR. Review: aluminum and Alzheimer's disease. *Neurobiol Aging* 1986; 7:525–532.

412. Ghetti B, Bugiani O. 'Aluminum's disease' and Alzheimer's disease. *Neurobiol Aging* 1986;7: 536–537.

413. Wisniewski HM. No evidence for aluminum in etiology and pathogenesis of Alzheimer's disease. *Neurobiol Aging* 1986;7:532–535.

414. Crapper-McLachlan DR, Dalton AJ, Kruck TPA, et al. Intramuscular desferrioxamine in patients with Alzheimer's disease. *Lancet* 1991; 337:1304–1308.

415. Elsworth JD, Deutch AY, Redmond DE Jr, et al. Symptomatic and asymptomatic 1-methyl4-phenyl-1,2,3,6-tetrahydropyridine (MPTP) treated primates: biochemical changes in striatal regions. *Neuroscience* 1989a;33:323–331.

416. Elsworth JD, Redmond DE Jr, Sladek JR Jr, et al. Reversal of MPTP-induced parkinsonism in primates by fetal dopamine cell transplants: In: Franks AJ, Ironside JW, Mindham RHS, eds. *Function and dysfunction of the basal ganglia.* Manchester: Manchester University Press, 1989b: 161–180.

417. Langston JW, Ballard PA, Tetrud JW, Irwin I. Chronic parkinsonism in humans due to a product of meperidine-analog synthesis. *Science* 1983;219:979–980.

418. Tanner CM, Langston JW. Do environmental toxins cause Parkinson's disease? A critical review. *Neurology* 1990;40:17–30.

419. Stevenson GB, Heafield MTE, Waring RH, Williams AC. Xenobiotic metabolism in Parkinson's disease. *Neurology* 1989:39:883–887.

420. Heikkila RE, Manzino L, Cabbat FS. Protection against the dopaminergic neurotoxicity of 1-methyl-4-phenyl-1,2,4,6-tetrahydropyridine by monoamine oxidase inhibitors. *Nature* 1984; 311:467–469.

421. Golbe JI. Deprenyl as symptomatic therapy in Parkinson's disease. *Clin Neuropharmacol* 1988; 11:387–400.

422. Parkinson Study Group. Effect of deprenyl on the progression of disability in early Parkinson's disease. *N Engl J Med* 1989;321: 1364–1371.

423. Parkinson Study Group. Effects of tocopherol and deprenyl on the progression of disability in early Parkinson's disease. *N Engl J Med* 1993; 328:176–183.

424. Elizan TS, Moros DA, Yahr MD. Early combination of selegiline and low-dose levodopa as initial symptomatic therapy in Parkinson's disease. *Arch Neurol* 1991;48:31–34.

425. Plaitakis A, Shashidharan P. Amyotrophic lateral sclerosis, glutamate, and oxidative stress. In: Bloom FE, Kupfer DJ, eds. *Psychopharmacology: the fourth generation of progress.* New York: Raven Press, 1995:1531–1543.

426. Zubenko GS: Molecular neurobiology of Alzheimer's disease (syndrome?). *Harvard Review of Psychiatry,* 1997;5:1–37.

427. Rosen DR. Mutations in Cu/Zn superoxidase dismutase gene are associated with familial amyotrophic lateral sclerosis. *Nature* 1993;364: 362.

428. Deng H-X, Hentati A, Tainer JA, et al. Amyotrophic lateral sclerosis and structural defects in Cu,Zn superoxide dismutase. *Science* 1993;261: 1047–1051.

429. Mourelatos Z, Yachnis A, Rorke L, et al. The Golgi apparatus of motor neurons in amyotrophic lateral sclerosis. *Ann Neurol* 1993;33: 608–615.

430. Spencer PS, Nunn PB, Hugon J, et al. Guam amyotrophic lateral sclerosis-parkinsonism-dementia linked to a plant excitant neurotoxin. *Science* 1987;237:517–522.

431. Duncan MW, Steele JC, Kopin IJ. 2-Amino-3-(methylamino)-propanoic acid (BMAA) in cycase flour: an unlikely cause of amyotrophic lateral sclerosis and parkinsonism-dementia of Guam. *Neurology* 1990;40:767–772.

432. Kerr JF, Wylie AH, Currie AR: Apoptosis: a basic biological phenomenon with wide-ranging implications in tissue kinetics. *Br J Cancer* 26:239–257, 1972.

433. Zubenko GS: Molecular neurobiology of Alzheimer's disease (syndrome?). *Harvard Review of Psychiatry,* 1997;5:1–37.

434. Cotman CW, Su JH: Mechanisms of neuronal death in Alzheimer's disease. *Brain Pathology* 1996;6:493–506.

435. Su JH, Anderson AJ, Cummings BJ, et al. Immunohistochemical evidence for apoptosis in Alzheimer's disease. *NeuroReport* 1994;5:2529–2533.

436. Dragunow M, Fauli RLM, Lawlor P, et al. In situ evidence for DNA fragmentation in Huntington's disease striatum and Alzheimer's disease temporal lobes. *NeuroReport* 1995;6: 1053–1057.

437. Lassmann H, Bancher C, Breitschopf H, et al: Cell death in Alzheimer's disease evaluated by DNA fragmentation in situ. *Acta Neuropathol* 1995;89:35–41.

438. Smale G, Nichols NR, Brady DR, et al. Evidence for apoptotic cell death in Alzheimer's disease. *Exp Neurol* 1995;133:225–230.

439. Thomas LB, Gates DJ, Richfield EK, et al. DNA end labeling (TUNEL) in Huntington's dis-

ease and other neuropathological conditions. *Exp Neurol* 1995;133:265–272.

440. Anderson AJ, Su JH, Cotman CW. DNA damage and apoptosis in Alzheimer's disease: colocalization with c-Jun immunoreactivity, relationship to brain area, and effect of postmortem delay. *J Neurosci* 1996;16:1710–1719.

441. Vito P, Ghayur T, D'Adamio L. Generation of anti-apoptotic presenilin-2 polypeptides by alternative transcription, proteolysis, and caspase-3 cleavage. *J Biol Chem* 1997;272: 28315–28320.

442. Wolozin B, Iwasaki K, Vito P, Ganjei JK, Lacana E, Sunderland T, Zhao B, Kusiak JW, Wasco W, D'Adamio L: Participation of presenilin 2 in apoptosis: Enhanced basal activity conferred by an Alzheimer mutation. *Science* 1996;274: 1710–1713.

443. Zubenko GS. Lack of variation in the nucleotide sequence corresponding to the transmembrane domain of the β-amyloid precursor protein in Alzheimer's disease. *Am J Med Genet* (Neuropsychiatr Genet) 1993;48:131–136.

444. Zubenko GS, Stiffler S, Kopp U, et al. Lack of variation in the nucleotide sequence corresponding to the transmembrane domain of the β-amyloid precursor protein in Alzheimer's disease. *Am J Med Genet* (Neuropsychiatr Genet) 1993;48:131–136.

445. Schellenberg GD. Progress in Alzheimer's disease genetics. *Curr Opinion Neurol* 1995;8: 262–267.

446. Sisodia SS, Price DL. Role of the β-amyloid protein in Alzheimer's disease. *FASEB J* 1995;9: 366–370.

447. Schellenberg GD, Bird TD, Wijsman EM, et al. Genetic linkage evidence for a familial Alzheimer's disease locus on chromosome 14. *Science* 1992;258:668–671.

448. Campion D, Flaman JM, Brice A, et al. Mutations of the presenilin 1 gene in families with early-onset Alzheimer's disease. *Hum Mol Genet* 1995;4:2373–2377.

449. Clark RF, Alzheimer's Disease Collaborative Group. The structure of the presenilin 1 (S182) gene and identification of six novel mutations in early onset AD families. *Nat Genet* 1995;11:219–222.

450. Cruts M, Backhovens H, Wang SY, et al. Molecular genetic analysis of familial early-onset Alzheimer's disease linked to chromosome 14q24.3. *Hum Mol Genet* 1995;4:2363–2371.

451. Sherrington R, Govaev EI, Liang Y, et al. Cloning of a gene bearing missense mutations in early-onset familial Alzheimer's disease. *Nature* 1995;375:754–760.

452. Levy-Lahad E, Wijsman EM, Nemens E, et al. A familial Alzheimer's disease locus on chromosome 1. *Science* 1995a;269:970–972.

453. Levy-Lahad E, Wasco W, Poorkaj P, et al. Candidate gene for the chromosome 1 familial Alzheimer's disease locus. *Science* 1995b;269: 973–977.

454. Holland AJ. Down's syndrome and dementia of the Alzheimer type. In: Burns A, Levy R, eds. *Dementia.* London: Chapman and Hall, 1994: 695–708.

455. Chartier-Harlin MC, Crawford F, Houlden H, et al. Early-onset Alzheimer's disease caused by

mutations at codon 717 of the β-amyloid precursor protein gene. *Nature* 1991;353:844–846.

456. Goate AM, Chartier-Harlin CM, Mullan M, et al. Segregation of a missense mutation in the amyloid precursor protein gene with familial Alzheimer's disease. *Nature* 1991;349:704–706.

457. Murrell J, Farlow M, Ghetti B, et al. A mutation in the amyloid precursor protein associated with hereditary Alzheimer's disease. *Science* 1991;254:97–99.

458. Mullan M, Crawford F, Axelman K, et al. A pathogenic mutation for probable Alzheimer's disease in the APP gene at the N-teminus of β-amyloid. *Nat Genet* 1992;1:345–347.

459. Hendricks L, van Diujn CM, Cras P, et al. Presenile dementia and cerebral hemorrhage linked to a mutation at codon 692 of the β-amyloid precursor gene. *Nat Genet* 1992;1: 218–221.

460. Levy E, Carman MD, Fernandez-Madrid JJ, et al. Mutation of the Alzheimer's disease amyloid gene in hereditary cerebral hemorrhage, Dutch type. *Science* 1990;248:1124–1126.

461. Hsiao K, Chapman P, Nilsen S, et al. Correlative memory deficits, Aβ elevation, and amyloid plaques in transgenic mice. *Science* 1996;274: 99–102.

462. Price DL, Sisodia SS. Cellular and molecular biology of Alzheimer's disease and animal models. *Annu Rev Med* 1994;45:435–446.

463. Tanzi RE, Vaula G, Romano DM. Assessment of amyloid β-protein precursor gene mutations in a large set of familial and sporadic Alzheimer disease cases. *Am J Hum Genet* 1992;51:273–282.

464. St George-Hyslop P, Haines J, Rogaev E, et al. Genetic evidence for a novel familial Alzheimer's disease locus on chromosome 14. *Nat Genet* 1992;2:330–334.

465. van Broeckhoven C, Backhovens H, Cruts M, et al. Mapping of a gene predisposing to early-onset Alzheimer's disease to chromosome 14q24.3. *Nat Genet* 1992;2:335–339.

466. Nechiporuk A, Fain P, Kort E, et al. Linkage of familial Alzheimer disease to chromosome-14 in 2 large early-onset pedigrees: effects of marker allele frequencies on LOD scores. *Am J Med Genet* 1993;48:63–66.

467. Alzheimer's Disease Collaborative Group. The structure of the presenilin 1 (S182) gene and identification of six novel mutations in early onset AD families. *Nat Genet* 1995;11:219–222.

468. Sahara N, Yahagi YI, Takagi H. Identification and characterization of presenilin I-467, I-463 and I-374. *FEBS Lett* 1996;381:7–11.

469. Rogaev EI, Sherrington R, Rogaeva EA, et al. Familial Alzheimer's disease in kindreds with missense mutations in a gene on chromosome 1 related to the Alzheimer's disease type 3 gene. *Nature* 1995;376:775–778.

470. Leviatan D, Greenwald I. Facilitation of lin-12-mediated signaling by sel-12, a *Cenorhabditis elegans S182* Alzheimer's disease gene. *Nature* 1995;377:351–354.

471. Pericak-Vance MA, Haines JL. Genetic susceptibility to Alzheimer's disease. *Trends Genet* 1995; 11:504–508.

472. Pericak-Vance MA, Bebout JL, Gaskell PC, et al. Linkage studies in familial Alzheimer disease: evidence for chromosome 19 linkage. *Am J Hum Genet* 1991;48:1034–1050.

473. Wisniewski T, Frangione B. Apolipoprotein E: a pathological chaperone protein in patients with cerebral and systemic amyloid. *Neurosci Lett* 1992;135:235–238.

474. Saunders AM, Strittmatter WJ, Schmechel D, et al. Association of apolipoprotein E allele ε4 with late-onset familial and sporadic Alzheimer's disease. *Neurology* 1993;43:1467–1472.

475. Zubenko GS, Stiffler S, Stabler S, et al. Association of the apolipoprotein E ε4 allele with clinical subtypes of autopsy-confirmed Alzheimer's disease. *Am J Med Genet* (Neuropsychiatr Genet) 1994;54:199–205.

476. Payami H, Kaye J, Heston LL, et al. Apolipoprotein E genotype and Alzheimer's disease. *Lancet* 1993;342:738.

477. Menzel H, Kladetzky R, Assmann G. Apolipoprotein E polymorphism and coronary artery disease. *Arteriosclerosis* 1983;3:310–315.

478. Noguchi S, Murakami K, Yamada N. Apolipoprotein-E genotype and Alzheimer's disease. *Lancet* 1993;342:737.

479. Ueki A, Kawano M, Namba Y, et al. A high frequency of apolipoprotein E4 isoprotein in Japanese patients with late-onset nonfamilial Alzheimer's disease. *Neurosci Lett* 1993;163:166–168.

480. Dai XY, Nanko S, Hattori M, et al. Association of apolipoprotein E4 with sporadic Alzheimer's disease is more pronounced in early onset type. *Neurosci Lett* 1994;175:74–76.

481. Yoshizawa T, Yamakawkobayashi K, Komatsuzaki Y, et al. Dose-dependent association of apolipoprotein E allele epsilon 4 with late-onset, sporadic Alzheimer's disease. *Ann Neurol* 1994;36:656–659.

482. Hendrie HC, Hall KS, Hui S, et al. Apolipoprotein E genotypes and Alzheimer's disease in a community study of elderly African Americans. *Ann Neurol* 1995;37:118–120.

483. Kamboh MI, Sanghera DK, Ferrell RE, DeKosky ST. APOE*4-associated Alzheimer's disease risk is modified by α1-antichymotrypsin polymorphism. *Nat Genet* 1995;10:86–88.

484. Maestre G, Ottman R, Stern Y, et al. Apolipoprotein E and Alzheimer's disease: ethnic variation in genotypic risks. *Ann Neurol* 1995;37:254–259.

485. Chartier-Harlin MC, Parfitt M, Legrain S, et al. Apolipoprotein E, ε4 allele as a major risk factor for sporadic early and late-onset forms of Alzheimer's disease: analysis of the 19q13.2 chromosomal region. *Hum Mol Genet* 1994;3:569–574.

486. Corder EH, Saunders AM, Risch NJ, et al. Protective effect of apolipoprotein E type 2 allele for late onset Alzheimer's disease. *Nat Genet* 1994;7:180–184.

487. Cumming AM, Robertson FW. Polymorphism at the apoprotein-E locus in relation to risk of coronary disease. *Clin Genet* 1984;25:310–313.

488. Lenzen HJ, Assmann G, Buckwalsky R, Schulte H. Association of apolipoprotein E polymorphism, low-density lipoprotein cholesterol, and coronary artery disease. *Clin Chem* 1986;32:778–781.

489. Davignon J, Gregg RE, Sing CF. Apolipoprot-

ein E polymorphism and atherosclerosis. *Arteriosclerosis* 1988;8:1–21.

490. van Bockxmeer FM, Mamotte CDS. Apolipoprotein ε4 homozygosity in young men with coronary heart disease. *Lancet* 1992;340:879–880.

491. Eichner JE, Kuller LH, Orchard TJ, et al. Relation of apolipoprotein E phenotype to myocardial infarction and mortality from coronary artery disease. *Am J Cardiol* 1993;71:160–165.

492. Marder K, Maestre G, Cote L, et al. The apolipoprotein ε4 allele in Parkinson's disease with and without dementia. *Neurology* 1994;44:1330–1331.

493. Pickering-Brown SM, Mann DM, Bourke JP, et al. Apolipoprotein E4 and Alzheimer's disease pathology in Lewy body disease and other beta-amyloid-forming diseases. *Lancet* 1994;343:1155.

494. Koller WC, Glatt SL, Hubble JP, et al. Apolipoprotein E genotypes in Parkinson's disease with and without dementia. *Ann Neurol* 1995;37:242–245.

495. Galasko D, Saitoh T, Xia Y, et al. The apolipoprotein E allele ε4 is over-represented in patients with the Lewy body variant of Alzheimer's disease. *Neurology* 1994;44:1950–1951.

496. Harrington CR, Louwagie J, Rossau R, et al. Influence of apolipoprotein E genotype on senile dementia of the Alzheimer and Lewy body types. Significance for etiological theories of Alzheimer's disease. *Am J Pathol* 1994;145:1472–1484.

497. St Clair D, Norman J, Perry R, et al. Apolipoprotein E epsilon 4 allele frequency in patients with Lewy body dementia, Alzheimer's disease and age-matched controls. *Neurosci Lett* 1994;176:45–46.

498. Lippa CF, Smith TW, Saunders AM, et al. Apolipoprotein E genotype and Lewy body disease. *Neurology* 1995;45:97–103.

499. Krishnan KRR, Ritchie JC, Tupler LA, et al. Letter to the editor. *Neurology* 1994;44:2420–2421.

500. Zubenko GS, Henderson R, Stiffler JS, et al. Association of the *APOE* ε4 allele with clinical subtypes of late life depression. *Biol Psychiatry* 1996a;40:1008–1016.

501. Corder EH, Saunders AM, Strittmatter WJ, et al. Gene dose of apolipoprotein E type-4 allele and the risk of Alzheimer's disease in late onset families. *Science* 1993;261:921–923.

502. Okuizumi K, Onodera O, Tanaka H, et al. ApoE-epsilon 4 and early-onset Alzheimer's. *Nat Genet* 1994;7:10–11.

503. van Duijn CM, de Knijff P, Cruts M, et al. Apolipoprotein E4 allele in a population-based study of early-onset Alzheimer's disease. *Nat Genet* 1994;7:74–78.

504. Schachter F, Faure-Delanef L, Guenot F, et al. Genetic associations with human longevity at the APOE and ACE loci. *Nat Genet* 1994;6:29–32.

505. Payami H, Zareparsi S, Montee KR, et al. Gender difference in apolipoprotein E-associated risk for familial Alzheimer disease: a possible clue to the higher incidence of Alzheimer disease in women. *Am J Hum Genet* 1996;58:803–811.

506. Mayeux R, Ottman R, Maestre G, et al. Synergistic effects of traumatic head injury and apolipoprotein ε4 in patients with Alzheimer's disease. *Neurology* 1995;45:555–557.

507. Petersen RC, Smith GE, Ivnik RJ, et al. Apolipoprotein E status as a predictor of the development of Alzheimer's disease in memory-impaired individuals. *JAMA* 1995;273:1274–1278.

508. Ladu MJ, Falduto MT, Manelli AM, et al. Isoform-specific binding of apolipoprotein E to beta-amyloid. *J Biol Chem* 1994;269: 23403–23406.

509. Ma JY, Yee A, Brewer HB, et al. Amyloid-associated proteins alpha(1)-antichymotrypsin and apolipoprotein E promote assembly of Alzheimer beta-protein into filaments. *Nature* 1994; 372:92–94.

510. Rebeck GW, Reiter JS, Strickland DK, Hyman BT. Apolipoprotein E in sporadic Alzheimer's disease: allelic variation and receptor interactions. *Neuron* 1993;11:575–580.

511. Schmechel D, Saunders A, Strittmatter W, et al. Increased amyloid β-peptide deposition in cerebral cortex as a consequence of apolipoprotein E genotype in late-onset Alzheimer disease. *Proc Natl Acad Sci USA* 1993;90: 9649–9653.

512. Strittmatter WJ, Saunders AM, Goedert M, et al. Isoform-specific interactions of apolipoprotein E with microtubule-associated protein tau: implications for Alzheimer disease. *Proc Natl Acad Sci USA* 1994a;91:11183–11186.

513. Strittmatter WJ, Weisgraber KH, Goedert M, et al. Hypothesis: microtubule instability and paired helical filament formation in the Alzheimer disease brain are related to apolipoprotein E genotype. *Exp Neurol* 1994b;125:163–171.

514. Poirier J. Apolipoprotein E in animal models of DNS injury and in Alzheimer's disease. *Trends Neurosci* 1994;17:525–530.

515. Nathan BP, Bellosta S, Sanan DA, et al. Differential effects of apolipoproteins E3 and 34 on neuronal growth in vitro. *Science* 1994;264: 850–852.

516. Roses AD, Devlin B, Conneally PM, et al. Measuring the genetic contributions of APOE in late-onset Alzheimer's disease. *Am J Hum Genet* 1995;57:A202.

517. Zubenko GS, Hughes HB, Stiffler JS, et al. A genome survey for novel Alzheimer's disease risk loci: Results at 10cM resolution. *Genomics* 1998;50:121–128.

518. Majores M, Bagli M, Papassotiropoulos A, et al. Allelic association between the D10S1423 marker and Alzheimer's disease in a German population. *Neuroscience Letters* 2000;289: 224–226.

519. Zubenko GS, Hughes HB, Stiffler JS. D10S1423 identifies a susceptibility locus for Alzheimer's disease in a prospective, longitudinal, double-blind study of asymptomatic individuals. *Mol Psychiatry* 2001;6:413–419.

520. Hammad SM, Stefansson S, Twal WO, et. al. Cubilin, the endocytic receptor for intrinsic factor-vitamin B_{12} complex, mediates high-density lipoprotein holoparticle endocytosis. *Proc Natl Acad Sci USA* 1999;96:10158–10163

521. Kozyraki R, Fyfe J, Kristiansen M, et. al. The intrinsic factor-vitamin B_{12} receptor, cubilin, is a high-affinity apolipoprotein A-I receptor facilitating endocytosis of high-density lipoprotein. *Nature Medicine* 1999;5:656–661.

522. Zubenko GS, Hughes HB, Stiffler JS. Clinical and neurobiological correlates of D10S1423 genotype in Alzheimer's disease. *Biol Psychiatry* 1999;46:740–749.

523. Zubenko GS, Hughes HB, Stiffler JS. Clinical and neurobiological correlates of DXS1047 genotype in Alzheimer's disease. *Biol Psychiatry* 1999;46:173–181.

524. Zubenko GS, Hughes HB, Stiffler JS. Neurobiological correlates of a putative risk allele for Alzheimer's disease on chromosome 12q. *Neurology* 1999;52:725–732.

525. Zubenko GS. Do susceptibility loci contribute to the expression of more than one mental disorder? A view from the genetics of Alzheimer's disease (Millennium Article). *Mol. Psychiatry,* 2000;5:131–136.

526. Myers AJ, Goate AM. The genetics of late-onset Alzheimer's disease. *Curr Opin Neurol* 2001;14: 433–440.

527. Selkoe DJ, Podlisny MB. Decipering the genetic basis of Alzheimer's disease. *Annu Rev Genomics Hum Genet.* 3:67–99, 2002.

528. Mattson MP. Contributions of mitochondrial alterations, resulting from bad genes and a hostile environment, to the pathogenesis of Alzheimer's disease. *Int Rev Neurobiol* 2002;53: 387–409.

529. Berg L, Miller JP, Storandt M, et al. Mild senile dementia of the Alzheimer type: 2. Longitudinal assessment. *Ann Neurol* 1988;23:477–484.

Supplemental Readings

General

Bachman DL, Wolf PA, Linn R, et al. Prevalence of dementia and probable senile dementia of the Alzheimer type in the Framingham Study. *Neurology* 1992;42:115–119.

Brayne C, Gill C, Huppert FA, et al. Incidence of clinically diagnosed subtypes of dementia in an elderly population. Cambridge Project for Later Life. *Br J Psychiatry* 1995;167:255–262.

Wisniewski KG, Wisniewski M. Age-associated changes and dementia in Down's syndrome. In: Reisenberg B, ed. *Alzheimer's disease: the standard reference.* New York: Free Press, 1983:319–326.

Diagnosis

Brown GG, Levine SR, Gorell JM, et al. In vivo ^{31}P NMR profiles of Alzheimer's disease and multiple subcortical infarct dementia. *Neurology* 1989; 39:1423–1427.

Folstein M, Folstein S, McHugh PR. "Mini-Mental Status": a practical method for grading the cognitive state of patients for the clinician. *J Psychiatr Res* 1975;12:189.

Khachaturian ZS. Diagnosis of Alzheimer's disease. *Arch Neurol* 1985;42:1097–1105.

McKeith I, Fairbairn A, Perry R, et al. Neuroleptic

sensitivity in patients with senile dementia of Lewy body type. *Br Med J* 1992b;305:673–678.

Rosen WG, Mohs RC, Davis KL. A new rating scale for Alzheimer's disease. *Am J Psychiatry* 1984;141: 1356–1364.

Schneider LS, Olin JT. Clinical global impressions in Alzheimer's clinical trials. *Int Psychogeriatr* 1996;8: 277–288.

Tariot PN, Blazina L. The psychopathology of dementia. In: Morris JC, ed. *Handbook of dementing illnesses.* New York: Marcel Dekker, 1993: 461–475.

Neuropathology

Bahmanyar S, Higgins G, Goldgaber D, et al. Localization of amyloid beta protein messenger RNA in brains from patients with Alzheimer's disease. *Science* 1987;237:77–80.

Beal MF. Oxidative damage in Alzheimer's disease pathogenesis. *Neurobiol Aging* 1996;17:S141.

Blessed G, Tomlinson BE, Roth M. The association between quantitative measures of dementia and of senile change in the cerebral grey matter of elderly subjects. *Br J Psychiatry* 1968;114:797–811.

Breitner JCS, Gau BA, Welsh KA, et al. Inverse association of anti-inflammatory treatments and Alzheimer's disease: initial results of a co-twin study. *Neurology* 1994;44:227–232.

Buell SJ, Coleman PD. Dendritic growth in the aged human brain and failure of growth in senile dementia. *Science* 1979;206:854–856.

Davies P. Neurochemical studies: an update on Alzheimer's disease. *J Clin Psychiatry* 1988;49(suppl 5):23–28.

Delabar J, Goldgaber D, Lamour Y, et al. Beta amyloid gene duplication in Alzheimer's disease and karyotypically normal Down syndrome. *Science* 1987;235:1390–1392.

Esch F, Keim P, Beattie E, et al. Cleavage of amyloid beta peptide during constitutive processing of its precursor. *Science* 1990;248:1122–1124.

Fox JH, Penn R, Clasen R, et al. Pathological diagnosis in clinically typical Alzheimer's disease. *N Engl J Med* 1985;313:1419–1420.

Gottfries CG. Alzheimer's disease. A critical review. *Compr Gerontol* 1988;2:47–62.

Hirano A, Malamud N, Elizan TS, et al. Amyotrophic lateral sclerosis and parkinsonism-dementia complex on Guam. Further pathologic studies. *Arch Neurol* 1966;15:35–51.

Hyman B, VanHoesen GW, Demasio AR, et al. Alzheimer's disease: cell-specific pathology isolates the hippocampal formation. *Science* 1984;225: 1168–1170.

Joachim CL, Selkoe DJ. Minireview: amyloid protein in Alzheimer's disease. *J Gerontol* 1989;44: B77–82.

Koskik K. The molecular and cellular pathology of Alzheimer neurofibrillary lesions. *J Gerontol* 1989; 44:B55–58.

Krigman MR, Feldman RG, Bensch K. Alzheimer's presenile dementia. A histochemical and electron microscopic study. *Lab Invest* 1965;14: 381–396.

Lal H, Sohal RS, Forster MJ. Models of age-associated free-radical brain damage. *Neurobiol Aging* 1996; 17:S23.

LeBel CP, Bondy SC. Mini-review: oxygen radicals: common mediators of neurotoxicity. *Neurotoxicol Teratol* 1991;13:341–346.

Martin EM, Wilson RS, Penn RD, et al. Cortical biopsy results in Alzheimer's disease: correlation with cognitive deficits. *Neurology* 1987;37: 1201–1204.

Marx J. Brain protein yields clues to Alzheimer's disease. *Science* 1989;243:1664–1666.

Mazurek M, Beal M, Bird E, et al. Vasopressin in Alzheimer's disease: a study of post-mortem brain concentrations. *Ann Neurol* 1986;20: 665–670.

Mirra SS, Heyman A, McKeel D, et al. The consortium to establish a registry for Alzheimer's disease (CERAD). Part II: Standardization of the neuropathological assessment of Alzheimer's disease. *Neurology* 1991;41:479–486.

Neary D, Snowden JS, Mann DMA, et al. Alzheimer's disease: a correlative study. *J Neurol Neurosurg Psychiatry* 1986;49:229–237.

Palmert M, Gold ET, Cohen M, et al. Amyloid protein precursor messenger RNAs: differential expression in Alzheimer's disease. *Science* 1988; 241:1080–1084.

Rogers J, Kirby LC, Hempelman SR, et al. Clinical trial of indomethacin in Alzheimer's disease. *Neurology* 1993;43:1609–1611.

Roses A, Pericak-Vance M, Haynes C, et al. Genetic linkage studies in Alzheimer's disease (AD). *Neurology* 1988;38(suppl 1):173.

Rossor MN, Garrett NJ, Johnson AL, et al. A post-mortem study of the cholinergic and GABA systems in senile dementia. *Brain* 1982;105: 313–330.

Rumble B, Retallack R, Hilbich C, et al. Amyloid a4 protein and its precursor in Down's syndrome and Alzheimer's disease. *N Engl J Med* 1989;320: 1446–1452.

Sajdel-Sulkowska E, Chou W, Salim M, et al. Genetic expression of amyloid and glial-specific protein in the Alzheimer brain. *J Am Geriatr Soc* 1988;36: 558–564.

Schellenberg G, Bird T, Wijsman E. Absence of linkage of chromosome c1q21 markers to familial Alzheimer's disease. *Science* 1988;241:1507–1510.

Selkoe D. Deciphering Alzheimer's disease: the pace quickens. *Trends Neurosci* 1987;10:181–184.

Selkoe D, Bell D, Podlisny M, et al. Concentration of brain amyloid proteins in aged mammals and humans with Alzheimer's disease. *Science* 1987; 235:873–877.

Selkoe DJ. Deciphering Alzheimer's disease: the amyloid precursor protein yields new clues. *Science* 1990;248:1058–1060.

Selkoe DJ. The molecular pathology of Alzheimer's disease. *Neuron* 1991;1:989–992.

Sisodia S, Koo E, Beyruther K, et al. Evidence that beta amyloid in Alzheimer's disease is not derived by normal processing. *Science* 1990;248: 492–495.

Smith CD, Carney JM, Starke-Reed PE, et al. Excess brain protein oxidation and enzyme dysfunction in normal aging and in Alzheimer's disease. *Proc Natl Acad Sci* 1991;88:10540–10543.

St George-Hyslop P, Tanzi R, Polinski R, et al. Absence of duplication of chromosome 21 genes in familial and sporadic Alzheimer's disease. *Science* 1987;238:664–666.

St George-Hyslop PH, Tanzi RE, Polinski RJ, et al. The genetic defect causing familial Alzheimer's disease maps on chromosome 21. *Science* 1987; 235:885–890.

Tanzi R, Gusella J, Watkins P, et al. Amyloid beta protein gene: CDNA, MRNA distribution, and genetic linkage near the Alzheimer locus. *Science* 1987;235:880–884.

Terry RD. The fine structure of neurofibrillary tangles in Alzheimer's disease. *J Neuropathol Exp Neurol* 1963;22:622–642.

Terry RD, Peck A, DeTeresa R, et al. Some morphometric aspects of the brain in senile dementia of the Alzheimer type. *Ann Neurol* 1981;10:184–192.

Volicer L, Crino PB. Review: involvement of free radicals in dementia of the Alzheimer-type: a hypothesis. *Neurobiol Aging* 1990;11:567–571.

Wolozin B, Pruchnicki A, Dickson D, et al. A neuronal antigen in the brains of Alzheimer's patients. *Science* 1986;232:648–650.

Genetics

Alzheimer's Disease Collaborative Group. Apolipoprotein E genotype and Alzheimer's disease. *Lancet* 1993;342:737–738.

Breitner J, Folstein M. Familial Alzheimer dementia: a prevalent disorder with specific clinical features. *Psychol Med* 1984;14:63–80.

Corder EH, Saunders AM, Risch MJ, et al. Apolipoprotein E type 2 allele and the risk of late onset Alzheimer's disease. *Nat Genet* 1994;7:180–183.

Corder EH, Saunders AM, Strittmatter WJ, et al. Gene dose of apolipoprotein E type 4 allele and the risk of Alzheimer's disease in late onset families. *Science* 1993;261:921–923.

Farrer L, O'Sullivan D, Cuppels A, et al. Assessment of genetic risk for Alzheimer's disease among first degree relatives. *Ann Neurol* 1989;25: 485–493.

Goate A, Chartier-Harlin MC, Mullan M, et al. Segregation of a missense mutation in the amyloid precursor protein gene with familial Alzheimer's disease. *Nature* 1991;349:704–706.

Heston L, Mastri A, Anderson E, et al. Dementia of the Alzheimer-type: clinical genetics, natural history, and associated conditions. *Arch Gen Psychiatry* 1981;38:1085–1090.

Kay D. The genetics of Alzheimer's disease. *Br Med Bull* 1986;42:19–23.

Kay D. Heterogeneity in Alzheimer's disease: epidemiological and family studies. *Trends Neurosci* 1987;10:194–196.

Levy-Lahad E, Wasco W, Poorkaj P, et al. Candidate gene for the chromosome 1 familial Alzheimer's disease locus. *Science* 1995;269:973–977.

Martin R, Gerteis G, Gabrielle W. A family genetic study of dementia of the Alzheimer-type. *Arch Gen Psychiatry* 1988;48:894–900.

Mayeux R, Stern Y, Ottman R, et al. The apolipoprotein epsilon 4 allele in patients with Alzheimer's disease. *Ann Neurol* 1993;34:752–754.

Mohs R, Breitner J, Silverman J, et al. Alzheimer's disease: morbid risk among first degree relatives approximates 50% by 90 years of age. *Arch Gen Psychiatry* 1987;44:405–408.

Nee L, Polinsky R, Eldridge R, et al. A family with histologically confirmed Alzheimer's disease. *Arch Neurol* 1983;40:203–208.

Rocca W. The etiology of Alzheimer's disease: epidemiologic contributions with emphasis on the genetic hypothesis. *J Neural Transm* 1987;24(suppl): 3–12.

Rogaev EI, Sherrington R, Rogaeva EA, et al. Familial Alzheimer's disease in kindreds with missense mutations in a gene on chromosome 1 related to the Alzheimer's disease type 3 gene. *Nature* 1995;376:775–778.

Saunders AM, Strittmatter WJ, Schmechel D, et al. Association of apolipoprotein E allele E4 with late onset familial and sporadic Alzheimer's disease. *Neurology* 1993;43:1467–1472.

Sherrington R, Rogaev EI, Liang Y, et al. Cloning of a gene bearing missense mutations in early-onset familial Alzheimer's disease. *Nature* 1995;375: 754–760.

Zubenko G, Huff K, Beyer J, et al. Familial risk of dementia associated with a biological subtype of Alzheimer's disease. *Arch Gen Psychiatry* 1988;45: 889–893.

Infections

Bruce M. Scrapie and Alzheimer's disease. *Psychol Med* 1984;14:497–500.

Cuara R, Grady C, Haxby J, et al. Positron emission tomography in Alzheimer's disease. *Neurology* 1986;36:879–887.

Friedland R, May C, Dahlberg J. The viral hypothesis of Alzheimer's disease. *Arch Neurol* 1990;47: 177–178.

Goudsmit J, Morrow C, Asher D, et al. Evidence for and against the transmissibility of Alzheimer's disease. *Neurology* 1980;30:945–950.

Mozar H, Bal D, Howard J. Perspectives on the etiology of Alzheimer's disease. *JAMA* 1987;257: 1503–1507.

Prusiner S. Prions and neurodegenerative diseases. *N Engl J Med* 1987;317:1571–1581.

Somerville R. Ultrastructural links between scrapie and Alzheimer's disease. *Lancet* 1985;1:504–506.

Werter PG, Murgas D, Pomerantz S. AIDS as a cause of dementia in the elderly. *J Am Geriatr Soc* 1988; 36:139–141.

Neurochemistry

Adolfsson R, Gottfries C, Roos B, Winblad B. Changes in the brain catecholamines in patients with dementia of Alzheimer's-type. *Br J Psychiatry* 1979;135:216–223.

Arai H, Kosaka K, Iizuka R. Changes of biogenic amines and their metabolites in post-mortem brains from patients with Alzheimer's-type dementia. *J Neurochem* 1984;43:388–393.

Bartus R, Dean R, Beer B, Lippa A. The cholinergic hypothesis of geriatric memory dysfunction. *Science* 1982;217:408–417.

Beal M, Martin J. Neuropeptides in neurological disease. *Ann Neurol* 1986;20:547–565.

Beal M, Mazurek M, Tran V, et al. Reduced numbers of somatostatin receptors in the cerebral cortex in Alzheimer's disease. *Science* 1985;225:289–291.

Bondareff W, Mountjoy C, Roth M. Selective loss of neurones of origin of adrenergic projection to cerebral cortex (nucleus locus coeruleus) in senile dementia. *Lancet* 1981;2:783–784.

Bowen D. Neurotransmitters in Alzheimer's disease. *Age* 1988;11:104–110.

Bowen D, Allen S, Benton J, et al. Biochemical assessment of serotonergic and cholinergic dysfunction and cerebral atrophy in Alzheimer's disease. *J Neurochem* 1983;41:266–272.

Caporaso GL, Takei K, Gandy SE, et al. Morphologic and biochemical analysis of the intracellular trafficking of the Alzheimer β/A4 amyloid precursor protein. *J Neurosci* 1994;14:3122–3138.

Cheng AVT, Ferrier IN, Morris CM, et al. Cortical serotonin-S_2 receptor binding in Lewy body dementia, Alzheimer's and Parkinson's diseases. *J Neurol Sci* 1991;106:50–55.

Coyle J, Price D, DeLong M. Alzheimer's disease: a disorder of cortical innervation. *Science* 1983;219:1184–1190.

Cross A, Crow T, Perry E, et al. Reduced dopamine-beta-hydroxylase activity in Alzheimer's disease. *Br Med J* 1981;282:93–94.

Cross AJ, Crow TJ, Johnson JA, et al. Studies on neurotransmitter receptor systems in the neocortex and hippocampus in senile dementia of the Alzheimer-type. *J Neurol Sci* 1984a;64:109–117.

Crow T, Cross A, Cooper S, et al. Neurotransmitter receptors and monoamine metabolites in the brains of patients with Alzheimer-type dementia and depression, and suicides. *Neuropharmacology* 1984;23(12B):1561–1569.

D'Amato R, Zweig R, Whitehouse P, et al. Aminergic systems in Alzheimer's disease and Parkinson's disease. *Ann Neurol* 1987;22:229–236.

Davies P, Katzman R, Terry RD. Reduced somatostatin-like immunoreactivity in cerebral cortex from cases of Alzheimer disease and Alzheimer senile dementia. *Nature* 1980;288:279–280.

Davies P, Wolozin B. Recent advances in the neurochemistry of Alzheimer's disease. *J Clin Psychiatry* 1987;48(suppl 5):23–30.

DeSouza E, Whitehouse P, Kuhar M, et al. Alzheimer's disease: reciprocal changes in corticotropin releasing factor (CRF)-like immunoreactivity and CRF receptors in cerebral cortex. *Nature* 1986;319:593.

Deutsch S, Morihisa J. Glutamatergic abnormalities in Alzheimer's disease and a rationale for clinical trials with L-glutamate. *Clin Neuropharmacol* 1988;11(1):18–35.

Emson PC, Lindvall O. Neuroanatomical aspects of neurotransmitters affected in Alzheimer's disease. *Br Med Bull* 1986;42:57–62.

Fliers E, Swaab D. Neuropeptide changes in aging and Alzheimer's disease. *Progr Brain Res* 1986;70:141–151.

Forssell LG, Hellstrom A, Ericsson K, et al. Early stages of late onset Alzheimer's disease. Diagnostic criteria, protein metabolism, precursor loading effects, neurochemical and neuropsychological applications. *Acta Neurol Scand Suppl* 1989;121(2):1–95.

Francis P, Bowen D, Lole S, et al. Somatostatin content and release measured in cerebral biopsies from demented patients. *J Neurol Sci* 1987;78:1–16.

Francis P, Palmer A, Sims N, et al. Neurochemical studies of early onset Alzheimer's disease. *N Engl J Med* 1985;313:7–11.

Gottfries C. Alzheimer's disease and senile dementia: biochemical characteristics and aspects of treatment. *Psychopharmacology* 1985;86:245–252.

Gottfries C, Adolfsson R, Aquilonius S, et al. Biochemical changes in dementia disorders of Alzheimer type. *Neurobiol Aging* 1983;4:261–271.

Hardy J, Cowburn R, Barton A, et al. A disorder of cortical GABAergic innervation in Alzheimer's disease. *Neurosci Lett* 1987;73:192–196.

Husain M, Nemeroff C. Neuropeptides and Alzheimer's disease. *J Am Geriatr Soc* 1990;38:918–925.

Mazurek M, Beal M, Bird E, et al. Oxytocin in Alzheimer's disease: post-mortem brain levels. *Neurology* 1987;37:1001–1003.

McGeer E, Singh E, McGeer P. Sodium-dependent glutamate binding in senile dementia. *Neurobiol Aging* 1987;8:219–223.

McGeer P, McGeer E, Suzuki J, et al. Aging, Alzheimer's disease and the cholinergic system of the basal forebrain. *Neurology* 1984;34:741–745.

McGeer PL, McGeer EG. Enzymes associated with the metabolism of catecholamines, acetylcholine and GABA in human controls and patients with Parkinson's disease and Huntington chorea. *Neurochem* 1976;26:65–76.

Morrison J, Rogers J, Schar S, et al. Somatostatin immunoreactivity in neuritic plaques of Alzheimer patients. *Nature* 1985;314:90–92.

Mountjoy C, Rossor M, Iversen L, et al. Correlations of cortical cholinergic and GABA deficits with quantitative neuropathological findings in senile dementia. *Brain* 1984;107:507–518.

Neary D, Snowdon J, Mann D, et al. Alzheimer's disease: a correlative study. *J Neurol Psychiatry* 1986;49:229–237.

Parker WD. Cytochrome oxidase deficiency in Alzheimer's disease. *Ann NY Acad Sci* 1991;640:59–64.

Perry EK, Perry RH, Gibson PH, et al. A cholinergic connection between normal aging and senile dementia in the human hippocampus. *Neurosci Lett* 1977;6:85–89.

Perry RH, Blessed G, Perry EK, et al. Histochemical observations on the cholinesterase activities in the brains of elderly normal and demented (Alzheimer-type) patients. *Age Ageing* 1980;9:9–16.

Perry T, Yong V, Burgeron C, et al. Amino acids, glutathione, and glutathione transferase activity in the brains of patients with Alzheimer's disease. *Ann Neurol* 1987;21:331–336.

Quirion R, Martel JC, Robitaille Y, et al. Neurotransmitter and receptor deficits in senile dementia of the Alzheimer type. *Can J Neurol Sci* 1986;13:503–510.

Reynolds GP, Arnold L, Rossor MN, et al. Reduced binding of [^{3}H]ketanserin to cortical 5-HT$_2$ receptors in senile dementia of the Alzheimer type. *Neurosci Lett* 1984;44:47–51.

Reinikainen K, Paljarvi L, Halonen T, et al. Dopaminergic system and monoamine oxidase B activity in Alzheimer's disease. *Neurobiol Aging* 1988;9:245–252.

Reinikainen K, Reikinen P, Jolkkonen J, et al. Decreased somatostatin-like immunoreactivity in cerebral cortex and cerebral spinal fluid in Alzheimer's disease. *Brain Res* 1987;402:103–108.

Rinne JO, Sako E, Paljarvi L, et al. Brain dopamine D-1 receptors in senile dementia. *J Neurol Sci* 1986;73:219–230.

Roberts E, Chase TN, Tower DB, eds. *GABA in nervous system function*. New York: Raven Press, 1976.

Roberts G, Crow T, Polak J. Location of neuronal tangles and somatostatin neurones in Alzheimer's disease. *Nature* 1985;314:92–94.

Rossor M, Iversen L. Noncholinergic abnormalities in Alzheimer's disease. *Br Med Bull* 1986;42: 70–74.

Rossor M, Iversen L, Reynolds G, et al. Neurochemical characteristics of early and late onset types of Alzheimer's disease. *Br Med J* 1984;288:961–964.

Rossor MN, Emson PC, Mountjoy CQ, et al. Reduced amounts of immunoreactive somatostatin in the temporal cortex in senile dementia of Alzheimer type. *Neurosci Lett* 1980;20:373–377.

Rossor MN, Garret N, Johnson A, et al. A post-mortem study of the cholinergic and GABA systems in senile dementia. *Brain* 1982;105:313–330.

Sasaki H, Muramoto O, Kanazawa I, et al. Regional distribution of amino acid transmitters in postmortem brains of presenile and senile dementia of Alzheimer-type. *Ann Neurol* 1986;19:263–269.

Simpson MDC, Cross AJ, Slater P, et al. Loss of cortical GABA uptake sites in Alzheimer's disease. *J Neural Transm* 1988;71:219–226.

Sims N, Bowen D, Allen S, et al. Presynaptic cholinergic dysfunction in patients with dementia. *J Neurochem* 1983;40:503–509.

Sparks D, DeKosky S, Markesbery W. Alzheimer's disease: aminergic-cholinergic alterations in hypothalamus. *Arch Neurol* 1988;45:994–999.

Sunderland T, Rubinow D, Tariot P, et al. CSF somatostatin in patients with Alzheimer's disease, older depressed patients, and age-matched control subjects. *Am J Psychiatry* 1987;144:1313–1316.

Walker LC, Kitt CA, Struble RG, et al. Glutamic acid decarboxylase-like immunoreactive neurites in senile plaques. *Neurosci Lett* 1985;59:165–169.

White WF, Nadler JV, Hamberger A, et al. Glutamate as a transmitter of hippocampal perforant path. *Nature* 1977;270:356–357.

Whitehouse P, Martino A, Antuono P, et al. Nicotinic acetylcholine binding sites in Alzheimer's disease. *Brain Res* 1986;371:146–151.

Whitehouse P, Price D, Clark A, et al. Alzheimer's disease: evidence for selective loss of cholinergic neurons in the nucleus basalis. *Ann Neurol* 1981; 10:122–126.

Whitehouse P, Vale W, Sweig R, et al. Reductions in corticotropin releasing factor-like immunoreactivity in cerebral cortex in Alzheimer's disease, Parkinson's disease, and progressive supranuclear palsy. *Neurology* 1987;37:905–909.

Whitford G. Alzheimer's disease and serotonin: a review. *Neuropsychobiology* 1986;15:133–142.

Zubenko GS, Huff FJ, Becker J, et al. Cognitive function and platelet membrane fluidity in Alzheimer's disease. *Biol Psychiatry* 1988;24:925–936.

Zubenko GS, Teply I. Longitudinal study of platelet membrane fluidity in Alzheimer's disease. *Biol Psychiatry* 1988;24:918–924.

Neurotoxicity

Barnes D. NMDA receptors trigger excitement. *Science* 1988;239:254–256.

Bharucha B. A case control study of association with medical conditions and surgical procedures. *Neurology* 1983;33(suppl 2):85.

Candy J, Edwardson J, Klinowsky J, et al. Colocalization of aluminum and silicone in senile plaques. In: Traber J, Gisbon W, eds. *Senile dementia of the Alzheimer-type*. Berlin: Springer-Verlag, 1985: 183–197.

Crapper D, Krishnon S, Palton A. Brain aluminum distribution in Alzheimer's disease and experimental neurofibrillary degeneration. *Science* 1973;180:511–513.

French L, Schuman L, Mortimer J, et al. A case control study of dementia of the Alzheimer-type. *Am J Epidemiol* 1985;121:414–421.

Greenamyre J. The role of glutamate in neurotransmission and in neurologic disease. *Arch Neurol* 1986;43:1058–1063.

Heyman A, Wilkinson W, Stafford J, et al. Alzheimer's disease: a study of epidemiological aspects. *Ann Neurol* 1984;15:335–341.

Langston J, Irwin I, Langston E, et al. Pargyline prevents MPTP-induced parkinsonism in primates. *Science* 1984;225:1481–1482.

MacVicar BA, Baker K, Crichton SA. Kainic acid evokes a potassium efflux from astrocytes. *Neuroscience* 1988;25:721–725.

Maragos W, Greenamyre J, Penny J, et al. Glutamate dysfunction in Alzheimer's disease: an hypothesis. *Trends Neurosci* 1987;10:65–68.

Martyn C, Osmond C, Edwardson E. Geographical relation between Alzheimer's disease and aluminum in drinking water. *Lancet* 1989;1:59–62.

McLachlan D, Van Berkum M. Aluminum: a role in degenerative brain disease associated with neurofibrillary degeneration. *Progr Brain Res* 1986;70: 399–408.

Nicoletti F, Meek JL, Iadarola MJ, et al. Coupling of inositol phosphate phospholipid metabolism with excitatory amino acid recognition sites in rat hippocampus. *J Neurochem* 1985;46:40–46.

Poirier J. Pathophysiology and biochemical mechanisms involved in MPTP-induced parkinsonism. *J Am Geriatr Soc* 1987;35:660–668.

Shalat S, Seltzer B, Pidcock C, et al. A case control study of medical and familial history and Alzheimer's disease. *Am J Epidemiol* 1986;124:540.

Shore D, Wyatt R. Aluminum and Alzheimer's disease. *J Nerv Ment Dis* 1983;171:553–558.

Sladeczak F, Pin JP, Recasens M, et al. Glutamate stimulates inositol phosphate formation in striatal neurones. *Nature* 1985;317:717–720.

Perl D, Good P. The association of aluminum, Alzheimer's disease, and neurofibrillary tangles. *J Neural Transm* 1987;24(suppl):205–211.

Tanner C. The toll of environmental toxins in the etiology of Parkinson's disease. *Trends Neurosci* 1989;12:49–53.

Plasticity

Buell S, Coleman P. Dendritic growth in the aged human brain and failure of growth in senile dementia. *Science* 1979;206:854–856.

Buell S, Coleman PD. Quantitative evidence for selective dendritic growth in normal human aging but not in senile dementia. *Brain Res* 1981;214: 23–41.

Fine R, Rubin J. Specific trophic factor-receptor interactions: key selective elements in brain development and "regeneration." *J Am Geriatr Soc* 1988;36:457–466.

Hefti F, Will B. Nerve growth factor is a neurotropic factor for forebrain cholinergic neurons: implications for Alzheimer's disease. *J Neural Transm* 1987;24(suppl 1):309–315.

Perry E. Hypothesis linking plasticity, vulnerability and nerve growth factor to basal forebrain cholinergic neurons. *Int J Geriatr Psychiatry* 1990;5: 223–231.

Chapter 20

Treatment of Dementia

Lon Schneider

Pierre Tariot

Carl Salzman

Alzheimer's disease (AD) affects about 25 million individuals throughout the world[1] and is increasing substantially as populations age.[2] The cost in both human and economic terms for managing this chronic illness with its progressive loss of cognitive and intellectual functions is enormous. Recent research, focused on the underlying pathophysiology of AD and related dementias, holds the possibility for developing treatments that target specific AD symptoms. Current antidementia treatments reviewed in this chapter produce modest, short-term improvement in memory and other cognitive functions.

Before the 1980s, medications were generally proposed for dementia treatment on the basis of clinical experience or prevailing theories of dementia and aging. Drugs included psychostimulants, vasodilators, ergoloids, and various medication "cocktails." Only one medication, Hydergine, was approved in the United States for the ill-defined condition "senile mental decline," based on constructs such as "cerebral insufficiency" or "cerebral deterioration." In addition, recognition of functionally significant but mild cognitive impairment has also been the target of clinical trials of medications previously used for AD.

The Food and Drug Administration has now established guidelines that define "antidementia efficacy."[3] Until recently most clinical trials concentrated on elderly patients with well-defined AD. Studies now have also begun to focus on treatment of age-associated memory impairment, mild cognitive impairment, and depressive pseudodementia. In addition, research has begun to investigate treatment of dementia with Lewy bodies. Clinical characteristics of diffuse Lewy body disease are very similar to those of AD. However, they also include fluctuating cognitive impairment with episodic confusion and lucid intervals as well as variable performance over time, often associated with hallucinations and extrapyramidal findings.[4] Subcortical, limbic, and neocortical ubiquitin-staining inclusion bodies are defining features of the syndrome, and decrease in choline acetyltransferase is more pronounced and predictable than in AD without Lewy bodies.[5]

Treatment Implications of Alzheimer's Disease Pathology

The most common form of cognitive decline among older persons, AD, afflicts 5% of people over age 65 years and accounts for the most striking rise in dementia incidence in the very old. Although the causes of AD are unknown, except for rare early-onset familial cases, basic and clinical research efforts offer the hope of discovering etiologies that can be expected to lead to specific treatments or cures.

An increasing number of genes have been associated with AD. For example, mutations of genes on chromosome 1,[6,7] chromosome 14,[8] or, less commonly, chromosome 21[9] have been found to cause the familial form of AD that begins before age 60. For the more common late-onset AD, numerous studies demonstrate a strong association between the apolipo-protein E (ApoE) locus on chromosome 19 and both familial and sporadic AD.[10-12] The ApoE4 allele confers a major dose-related risk for late-onset familial and sporadic AD[13] whereas ApoE-2 confers relative protection.[14]

As the molecular mechanisms resulting from these various genetic mutations and polymorphisms are clarified, treatments aimed at specific pathogenetic pathways will likely emerge. For example, therapies that block abnormal tau phosphorylation or that prevent amyloid deposition may eventually be developed, and the observation that cholinergic mechanisms partly control amyloid precursor protein (APP) processing (see Chapter 19) suggests that cholinergically based therapeutic strategies may modify disease progression in addition to improving symptoms.[15] Another possible pharmacotherapeutic approach is the development of drugs that interfere with β-amyloid formation (e.g., secretase inhibitors, modulators of APP expression, or inhibitors of Aβ aggregation or deposition). Finally, the use of substances that block oxidative processes may prevent AD.

At present, altering neurotransmitter function in AD with pharmacotherapy is the most accessible therapeutic approach. For example, cholinergic deficits, although not the exclusive neurotransmitter alteration in AD, occur early in the disease process and remain a major target of clinical pharmacologic research. In addition, glutamate dysfunction, as well as noradrenergic and serotonergic deficits in AD, suggests a potential use for antidepressant drugs for AD patients. These neurotransmitter systems work together and interact, and animal studies indicate that an intact noradrenergic system is necessary for a cholinesterase inhibitor to improve cholinergic function.[16]

Cholinergic Restitutive Therapies

The dramatic reduction in cholinergic neurotransmission in AD has led to the hypothesis that its potentiation or restoration should improve the cognitive and behavioral impairment associated with AD. The well-established cholinergic defects in AD include decline of cholinergic basocortical projections and reduced activity of cerebral cortical choline acetyltransferase (ChAT), the acetylcholine (ACh) synthesis enzyme, as well as cholinergic cell-body loss in the nucleus basalis. Additionally, correlations may be seen between cortical ChAT reduction or nucleus basalis cell reduction and cortical plaque density. These cholinergic deficits correlate with cognitive decline. The cholinergic hypothesis proposes that cognitive deficits of AD are related to decreases in central acetylcholinergic activity, and that increasing intrasynaptic ACh will enhance cognitive function and clinical well-being.

The medical analogy used to support this restitutive approach is Parkinson's disease, which is characterized by prominent deficits in central dopaminergic neurotransmission. Dopamine agonist therapy can partially ameliorate some of the symptoms of Parkinson's disease without altering the course of illness. By analogy, restoring disordered cholinergic and other neurotransmitter functions in AD can, hypothetically, reduce symptoms. Historically, much emphasis has been placed on cholinergic restitutive strategies because of the prominence of cholinergic dysfunction and its discovery before that of other neurotransmitter disorders.

Three types of investigation focus on cholinergic neurotransmission: (1) studies of efforts to promote cholinergic neurotransmission via administration of acetylcholine precursors ("precursor loading"); (2) studies of reduced degradation of synaptic acetylcholine by inhibition of the enzyme acetylcholinesterase; and (3) use of agents acting on cholinergic receptors (cholinergic agonists).

Cholinergic Precursors

Although many studies of the possible efficacy of cholinergic precursors in AD, such as lecithin (phosphatidyl choline), have been conducted, their results have not been clinically significant. Only one study of older patients who took low doses of lecithin reports significantly improved self-care, orientation, verbal learning, and memory.[17] Most other lecithin trials used small samples and failed to demonstrate improved cognitive performance in AD, and only 10 of 43 acetylcholine precursor trials report *any* positive effect at all.[18] No evidence indicates that the rate of progression of the illness might be altered with chronic administration of lecithin. Furthermore, although lecithin causes increased plasma and red blood cell choline levels, no associated changes have been found in measures of central nervous system (CNS) cholinergic activity such as spectrally analyzed EEG, cortisol, prolactin, and vital signs. Trials in which lecithin was combined with the cholinesterase inhibitor tacrine did not reveal any added benefit.

Recently, however, cytidine diphosphate choline (CDP-choline), another acetylcholine precursor, has been assessed for its therapeutic potential in dementia. Clinical trials have repeatedly shown positive effects of CDP-choline in demented patients.[19] A recent study of patients with AD found that most benefited from a 3-month course of CDPcholine, 1000 mg/day.[20]

Muscarinic Agonists and Antagonists

The rationale for use of direct cholinergic agonists rests on the presence of relatively intact postsynaptic (M_1) cholinergic receptors in contrast to decreased presynaptic (M_2) cholinergic receptors in AD. Cholinergic agonists that have been studied in the past include bethanechol, oxotremorine, pilocarpine, RS-86, and arecoline. These agents have had little or no efficacy and considerable side effects, sug-

gesting that direct stimulation of postsynaptic muscarinic receptors may not be sufficient to treat AD. Various methods of indirect cholinergic enhancement via increasing presynaptic potassium-mediated release of acetylcholine have also failed to be clinically effective.

Cholinesterase Inhibitors

Cholinesterase inhibition has been the most common approach to treatment of the cognitive symptoms of AD and is the only intervention with consistently positive results in clinical trials. Impetus to develop these compounds arose from early studies of physostigmine, a rapidly acting cholinesterase inhibitor that consistently improved memory although improved cognition was modest.[21-26] Physostigmine's very short duration of action (1–2 hours) limits its clinical usefulness.

The mechanism by which the enzyme acetylcholinesterase (AchE) hydrolizes acetylcholine is well understood and has led to other more clinically useful cholinesterase inhibitors. By inhibiting actions of this enzyme, the amount of acetylcholine available for intrasynaptic cholinergic receptor stimulation increases. An acetylcholinesterase inhibitor can work on either of two sites, an ionic subsite or a catalytic esterase subsite to prevent the interaction between ACh and AChE. Different approaches to blocking acetylcholinesterase correlate with these differences. For example, tacrine and donepezil act at the ionic subsite, whereas physostigmine and rivastigmine act at the catalytic esterase subsite. Butyrylcholinesterase may also be inhibited (by rivastigmine). Some medications compete with acetylcholine for binding to the enzyme. For example, galantamine, a cholinesterase inhibitor, competes with acetylcholine for acetylcholinesterase, and rivastigmine is a cholinesterase inhibitor that is highly selective for the postsynaptic receptor for acetylcholinesterase. Currently available cholinesterase inhibitors appear in Table 20.1; controlled trials

Table 20.1. FDA-Approved Drugs to Improve Cognitive Function in Alzheimer's Disease.

Drug	Pharmacodynamics	Absorption	Bioavailability	Peak Plasma (hr)	Elimination Half-life (hr)	Protein Binding	Metabolism	How Supplied	Initial Dosage	Maintenance Dosage	Clinical Comments
Tacrine (Cognex)	Noncompetitive, reversible cholinesterase inhibitor, both butyrl- and acetyl-cholinesterase inhibitor, also multiple other actions	Delayed by food	17%	1–2	2–4	55%	Via 1A2, nonlinear pharmacokinetics; hepatotoxicity requires regular monitoring of serum ALTs.	10, 20, 30, and 40 mg capsules	10 mg q.i.d.	30 or 40 mg, q.i.d.	120 to 160 mg/d are efficacious doses. Reversible direct hepatotoxicity in about 1/3 patients, requiring initial biweekly transaminase monitoring and dose titration. Not commonly used
Donepezil (Aricept)	Noncompetitive, reversible acetyl-cholinesterase inhibitor	Not affected by food	100%	3–4	70	96%	Via 2D6, 3A4. Non linear pharmacokinetics at 10 mg/d	5 and 10 mg tablets	5 mg q.d.	5–10 mg, q.d.	5 and 10 mg are both effective doses; 10 mg may be somewhat more efficacious in some trials; higher doses not tested.

Drug	Mechanism							Forms			Comments
Rivastigmine (Exelon)	Noncompetitive cholinesterase inhibitor, both butryrl and acetyl-cholinesterase inhibitor, may differentially affect different acetyl-cholinesterase	Delayed by food	40%	1.4–2.6	<5	40%	Hydrolysis by esterases and excreted in urine (non hepatic). Duration of cholinesterase inhibition longer than plasma half-life. Non-linear pharmacokinetics	1.5, 3, 4.5, and 6 mg capsules	1.5 mg b.i.d	3, 4.5, or 6 mg b.i.d.	Available as a liquid concentrate. Effective dosage range 3–6 mg bid. Doses of 4.5 mg bid may be most optimal. May be taken with food.
Galantamine (Reminyl)	Competitive, reversible cholinesterase inhibitor, modulates nicotine receptors	Delayed by food	90%	1	7	18%	Via 2D6, 3A4	4, 8, and 12 mg capsules Solution 4 mg/mL	4 mg b.i.d	8 or 12 mg b.i.d.	Effective dosage range is 8–16 mg bid. 8 mg bid is the modal optimal dose.

Note: pharmacodynamic effects of some cholinesterase inhibitors are longer than their elimination half-lives. Drugs that inhibit of induce the cytochrome enzymes above might be expected to increase or decrease blood levels. For the most part clinically however, drug interactions with donepezil, rivastigmine and galantamine have not been problems.
Initial doses should be maintained for at least 2 and preferably 4 to 6 weeks before increasing. Adverse events may occur with dosage titration.
The FDA approved indication for these drugs is: "indicated for the treatment of mild to moderate dementia of the Alzheimer's type."
Websites for prescribing information on cholinesterase inhibitors: tacrine, *http://www.horizor.pharm.com/downloads/Cognex2.pdf*; donepezil, *www.aricept.com/productinfo.htm* *http://www.pfizer.com*, rivastigmine, *http://www.novartis.com*, *http://www.pharma.us.novartis.com/product/pi/pdf/exelon.pdf*; galantamine, *www.us.reminyl.com/Reminyl/Reminyl.pdf* *http://www.us.reminyl*, *http://www.janssen.com*.

are shown in Table 20.2; and adverse effects of these drugs appear in Table 20.3.

Tacrine was the only cholinesterase inhibitor with FDA approval for treatment of cognitive symptoms in AD from September 1993 to December 1996, at which time donepezil received marketing approval. Studies of tacrine have consistently shown a dose-response effect: Patients who receive 80 mg/day of tacrine over 6 to 12 weeks perform better on cognitive testing than patients who receive 40 mg/ day or patients who receive placebo[27,28]; patients who receive 160 mg/day perform better than those who receive lower doses over 30 weeks.[29]

Plasma level/response relationships from some studies report a mean serum tacrine level of 8.4 ng/mL after 12 weeks (average dose approximately 132 mg/ day), and modest but significant correlations between improvements on the MMSE and plasma tacrine levels as well as plasma levels of tacrine's 1-OH metabolite.[30] Improved MMSE scores occur in

Table 20.2. Placebo-Controlled, Randomized Cholinesterase Inhibitor Clinical Trials.

Citation	Duration (wk)	Number	Age (y)	Dose (mg/d)
Tacrine				
Knapp et al. 1994	26	663	73	120
				160
Donepezil				
Rogers et al. 1998b	24	473	73	5
				10
Burns et al. 1999	24	818	72	5
				10
Tariot et al. 2001	24	208	86	10
Feldman et al. 2001	52	2xx		
Winblad et al. 2001		286	72	10
Rivastigmine				
Corey-Bloom et al. 1998	26	699	75	1–4
				6–12
Rosler et al. 1999		725	72	1–4
				6–12
Galantamine				
Tariot et al. 2000	24	978	77	8
				16
				24
Raskind et al. 2000	24	636	75	24
				32
Wilcock et al. 2000	24			

Rounded to two figures. All trials had 58% to 64% female subjects except for tacrine (Knapp et al 1994, 53%), and donepezil nursing home trial (Tariot et al 2001, 82%). Dropouts are for all reasons to avoid bias, not just those attributed to side effects.

Table 20.3.   Adverse Effects of Cholinesterase Inhibitors in Placebo-Controlled, Randomized Clinical Trials.

Drug	Adverse Events
Tacrine	Nausea, vomiting, diarrhea, dyspepsia, myalgia, anorexia, dizziness, confusion, insomnia, rare agranulocytosis Approximately 50% of patients will develop direct, reversible hepatotoxicity manifested by elevated transaminases Drug interactions may include increased cholinergic effects with bethanacol and increased plasma tacrine levels with cimetidine or fluvoxamine. These may occur by inhibition of P450 1A2. Association of tacrine with haloperidol may increase parkinsonism. Tacrine increases theophylline concentration
Donepezil	Nausea, diarrhea, insomnia, vomiting, muscle cramps, fatigue, anorexia, dizziness, abdominal pain, myasthenia, rhinitis, weight loss, anxiety, syncope (2 vs 1%)
Rivastigmine	Nausea, vomiting, anorexia, dizziness, abdominal pain, diarrhea, malaise, fatigue, asthenia, headache, sweating, weight loss, somnolence, syncope (3 vs 2%). Severe vomiting with esophageal rupture may occur rarely
Galantamine	Nausea, vomiting, diarrhea, anorexia, weight loss, abdominal pain, dizziness, tremor, syncope (2 vs 1%)

Adverse event estimates vary widely among the cholinesterase inhibitors from study to study; relative adverse event rates among drugs are thus difficult to estimate. Cholinergic side effects generally occur early and are related to initiating or increasing medication. They tend to be mild and self-limited. Medications should be restarted at lowest doses after temporarily stopping. See prescribing information referenced in Table 2

General precautions with cholinesterase inhibitors (as indicated in prescribing information)
By increasing central and peripheral cholinergic stimulation cholinesterase inhibitors may:
1. Increase gastric acid secretion, increasing risk of GI bleeding, especially in patients with ulcer disease or those taking antiinflammatories
2. Cause bradycardia from vagal effects on the heart, especially in patients with sick sinus or other supraventricular conduction delay, leading to syncope, falls, and possible injury
3. Exacerbate obstructive pulmonary disease
4. Cause urinary outflow obstruction
5. Increase risk for seizures
6. Prolong effects of succinylcholine-type muscle relaxants

43% of patients with tacrine plasma levels below 10 ng/mL compared with 71% of patients with tacrine levels above 10 ng/mL. In another trial,[28] similar correlations were observed between plasma tacrine levels and cognitive improvements.

Tacrine has also been studied in patients with increased genetic vulnerability to AD as well as in patients with Lewy body dementia. Patients with autopsy-confirmed AD with diffuse Lewy body disease who had been strong responders to tacrine have been reported,[31,32] suggesting that this dementia subtype may respond preferentially to tacrine. In light of observations that AD patients with the ApoE4 allele have an increased risk for the illness and possibly a more rapid course, 83% of patients not carrying the ApoE4 allele show improvement with tacrine treatment whereas nearly 60% of ApoE4 carriers show significant deterioration.[33] Thus cholinergic activity may be selectively compromised in ApoE4 patients, and the ApoE2 and ApoE3 bearers may respond better to acetylcholine-based therapies because they possess sufficient residual acetylcholine activity. Patients with ApoE4 who receive tacrine also tend to do better over the long term than ApoE3 patients with respect to nursing home placement.

Newer cholinesterase inhibitors—donepezil, rivastigmine, galantamine—exert relatively selective acetylcholinesterase inhibition and hold the promise of fewer side effects than tacrine. Data from clinical trials suggest efficacy similar to that of tacrine for many of these newer compounds, with no significant elevation of serum tranaminases and fewer study dropouts but a similar frequency of adverse cholinergic effects.

Donepezil

Donepezil, a piperidine-based cholinesterase inhibitor with dose-dependent activity, shows greater selectivity for acetylcholinesterase than other cholinesterases, and a longer duration of cholinesterase inhibition than tacrine or physostigmine.[34] Characterized by linear pharmacokinetics at therapeutic doses, with a slow clearance (70-hour elimination half-life), it may be given once per day. The drug is extensively bound to plasma protein, including α-1-acid glycoproteins. It is excreted unchanged in the urine and extensively metabolized by the CYP2D6 and 3A3/4 hepatic enzymes to active and inactive metabolites.

Two multicenter, placebo-controlled studies examining donepezil (5 and 10 mg/day vs. placebo) for 12 and 24 weeks respectively, were conducted in the United States in addition to a 24-week trial conducted in Europe. Results of these studies show statistically significant benefit in both cognition and clinician-rated improvement.[34] A trend toward a greater effect with 10 mg/day rather than 5 mg/day was seen during the course of treatment but not at the end of 24 weeks, suggesting possible tolerance to the drug. In both U.S. studies, neuropsychologic scores 3 to 6 weeks after discontinuation of donepezil approach those in the placebo group.

Donepezil is initiated at 5 mg/d and then increased to 10 mg/d after 4 to 6 weeks. Raising the dose earlier increases the risk for cholinergic adverse events. Doses of 5 or 10 mg/d are effective, although 10 mg tends to be somewhat more effective than 5. The most common side effects of donepezil are gastrointestinal, e.g., nausea, vomiting, and diarrhea. Additionally, some patients develop anorexia, muscle cramps, headache, dizziness, syncope, flushing, insomnia, weakness, drowsiness, fatigue, and agitation. Adverse effects are more likely at 10 mg than 5 mg.

Rivastigmine is a selective AChE subtype inhibitor that inhibits butyrylcholinesterase as well. Four placebo-controlled studies suggest the efficacy of this compound. The recommended starting dose of rivastigmine is 1.5 mg twice a day taken with meals. If this dose is well tolerated after a minimum of two weeks of treatment, it may be increased to 3 mg bid. Subsequent increases to 4.5 mg and then 6 mg bid should be based on good tolerability of the current dose and may be considered after a minimum of two weeks of treatment.

Adverse effects are primarily gastrointestinal and occur in the high-dose (6–12 mg/d) group, mainly during dose escalation. Other adverse effects in the higher-dose group include sweating, fatigue, asthenia, weight loss, malaise, dizziness, somnolence, nausea, vomiting, anorexia, and flatulence.

Galantamine is a reversible competitive inhibitor of AChE that also modulates the nicotinic receptor sites, possibly enhancing cholinergic transmission by presynaptic nicotinic stimulation.[35] Large clinical trials indicate that treatment with either 24 or 32 mg/d improves cognition and enhanced activities of daily living. Initial dosing is 4 mg bid, which should be raised to 8 mg bid after 2 to 4 weeks. Principal adverse effects are nausea, vomiting, diarrhea, anorexia, weight loss, abdominal pain, dizziness, and tremor. These events are more frequent earlier in the course of treatment and during dosage titration from 16 to 24 mg/d and higher.

Donepezil, rivastigmine, and galantamine are the cholinesterase inhibitors currently in clinical use. All are mildly to moderately effective for treatment of AD.

Although all three are superior to tacrine, available research studies do not permit determination of whether any one of these three agents is superior to the others. In general, these drugs are best suited for patients with AD of mild to moderate cognitive severity. Optimal duration of treatment with continuing efficacy is unknown, but overall efficacy extends at least to 9 to 12 months. Maintenance treatment can be continued for as long as therapeutic benefit seems apparent. Specific symptoms, dementia subtype, age, gender, and race do not seem to correlate with response to cholinesterase inhibitors.

Anorexia and weight loss may be clinically significant problems over the longer term, especially in older more medically ill individuals as well as nursing home residents. Gastric acid secretion may be increased with cholinesterase inhibitors, thereby increasing a risk for developing ulcers or gastrointestinal bleeding. Patients receiving nonsteroidal antiinflammatory drugs may particularly be at additional risk.

There is emerging evidence that cholinesterase inhibitors may improve behavior.[36,37] Clinical experience suggests that they may be effective for at least mildly disturbed behavior and may delay the onset of more troublesome behaviors. Cholinergic therapies may also have neuroprotective effects by decreasing the production of toxic β amyloid. Cholinergic therapies may also have neuroprotective effects by decreasing the production of toxic β amyoloid and the formation of amyloid plaques.[38-40]

Other Neurotransmitter-Based Approaches

Noncholinergic as well as cholinergic neurotransmitter function may be dysregulated in AD. Strategies for treatment have focused on the catecholamine neurotransmitters, amino acids (excitatory and inhibitory), and peptides.

Catecholamines

Central catecholaminergic disturbances in AD provide a rationale for pharmacologic enhancement of neurotransmitters and therapeutic strategies analogous to those used with cholinergic agents (i.e., precursor loading, degradative enzyme inhibition, and agonist use). Unfortunately, studies of tryptophan, tyrosine, L-dopa and such agonists as clonidine, guancfacine, amantadine, and bromocriptine have failed to demonstrate efficacy.[41-48]

By contrast, monoamine oxidase (MAO) inhibitors demonstrate some acute effects. Selegiline (L-deprenyl), an MAO inhibitor with relatively selective inhibition of MAO_B at the recommended dosage (5 to 10 mg daily), may increase central levels of dopamine and other neurotransmitters without an effect on norepinephrine levels.[49]

Compounds with minimal effects on behavior or cognition include citalopram,[50] zimelidine,[51] tryptophan,[52] alapracolate[53] and *m*-chlorphenylpiperazine,[54] milacemide,[55] and tetraisoazolopyridine.[56] Other attempts to enhance peptide function have failed,[57-63] or have produced only mild effects.[64-66]

Excitatory Amino Acids

The *N*-methyl-D-aspartate (NMDA) receptor, a glutamate receptor subtype, is involved in memory function. When the excitatory amino acid glutamate stimulates the receptor, long-term potentiation of neuronal activity basic to memory formation occurs.[67] AD appears to be accompanied by reduced numbers of cerebral cortical and hippocampal NMDA receptors. Studies aimed at directly enhancing glutaminergic function via the NMDA receptor (milacemide)[55] and γ-aminobutyric acid (GABA) function (tetraisoazolopyridine)[56] have not succeeded. The role of NMDA receptors in AD is still unclear, and studies using NMDA agonists D-cycloserine and milacemide for AD have not been successful.[55,68,69]

Excitatory amino acids such as glutamate and aspartate may either enhance cognitive function or be neurotoxic. On one hand, stimulation of NMDA may improve memory; on the other, excessive stimulation is associated with brain injury.

Another NMDA antagonist, Memantine (1-amino-3,5-dimethyladamantane), has recently been released for clinical use in the United States. Memantine blocks the NMDA receptor channel in the resting state and may provide neuroprotection against the excitotoxic activation of glutamate receptors. Although an initial study showed no effect,[41] recent studies clearly demonstrate that memantine treatment leads to functional improvement and reduced clinical deterioration in moderate to severe AD.[70–72] Two recent studies suggest that the combination of memantine with a cholinesterase inhibitor is safe, and results in statistically improved cognitive function compared with the cholinesterase inhibitor alone.[73,74]

The dose of memantine is 20 mg a day. Most adverse events are mild to moderate; agitation, urinary incontinence, insomnia, diarrhea, and urinary tract infection are the most frequent side effects reported. Agitation is the most common reason for drug discontinuation. Since the memantine data are derived from a research population of patients with moderate to severe impairment, memantine cannot be directly compared with the efficacy of donepezil, rivastigmine, or galantamine, each of which has been tested in mild to moderately impaired individuals. From a clinical perspective, however, memantine study results suggest that this drug may be effectively combined with an effective cholinesterase inhibitor for treatment of a broad spectrum of patients with AD.

Peptides

Several neuropeptide neurotransmitter systems are known to be disturbed in AD, including somatostatin, corticotropin-releasing factor, neuropeptide Y, and substance P. Neuropeptides are also of potential interest because they modulate other neurotransmitter systems (e.g., choliner-

gic and catecholaminergic) that may be dysregulated in AD. A somatostatin analogue administered to a small group of AD patients without cognitive effect may not have been administered in sufficient quantity to enter the CNS; no follow-up was reported.[57]

Arginine vasopressin and several of its analogues have been extensively studied because of their role in cognition. Their use led to modest improvements in behavior, possibly related to improved energy and mood, but no improvement or very mild improvement in memory.[63] The same is true of adrenocorticotrophic hormone agonists, which appear to affect mood and behavior without clear memory or cognitive effects.

Studies of thyrotropin-releasing hormone (TRH) analogues with procholinergic effects have all been negative, although TRH itself has been shown to have possible beneficial cognitive effects in two small pilot studies.[64,65] Endogenous opiates may function as peptide neurotransmitters as well. Although naloxone, an opiate receptor antagonist, was initially reported to improve cognitive function in AD, these findings were not confirmed by more carefully conducted controlled studies. Similar negative effects have been found for the mixed agonist-antagonist, naltrexone. Neither drug is now considered to have any clinical utility in the treatment of dementia.

Nonneurotransmitter Treatment Strategies

Several convergent processes are involved in the neuronal degeneration central to AD. These include oxidative damage, immunological and inflammatory responses, and the release of autodestructive as well as second-messenger enzymes. Some of these may not be specific to AD itself but, rather, may be associated with aging and neuronal death in general. Nevertheless, specific targeted interventions may be effective in modifying the course of the illness.

Antioxidant Agents

Several compounds may function as scavengers of neurotoxic free-oxygen radicals, most notably selegiline, idebonone, and ginkgo. Antioxidant vitamins have also been studied.

Selegiline

The MAO_B inhibitor selegiline, in addition to its role in enhancing catecholamine neurotransmission, also has therapeutic effects[49] that have been linked recently to its antioxidant and neuroprotective properties.[66] Oxidative deamination of endogenous monoamines by MAO results in the formation of hydrogen peroxide and other toxic byproducts such as hydroxyl radicals and superoxide.[67,68] In addition, oxidation of some monoamines by MAO, including dopamine, can produce neurotoxins such as 6-hydroxydopamine and quinine.[69,75,76] Thus, one rationale for beneficial effects of selegiline over the long term is the possible reduction of free radicals and neurotoxins resulting from inhibition of MAO_B activity.[77] Indeed, some in vitro data indicate that selegiline reduces the oxidant stress associated with catabolism of dopamine.[68] If this theoretical rationale is borne out, selegiline may conceivably have a preventive role in the development of neurodegenerative disorders or even the cognitive decline of normal aging. Although "preventive" efficacy data are not available for humans, increased survival has been reported in rodents treated with selegiline.[78,79]

Studies of behavioral effects on patients with dementia indicate that selegiline may improve cooperativeness and reduce anxiety, depression, and agitation.[80-83] Open-label studies show improved cognition in AD,[84-86] but an adequate efficacy trial has never been completed. Selegiline is currently approved for maintaining motor function in Parkinson's disease, and may have efficacy through both its neurotransmitter effects and its chronic antioxidant effects.

Recent longer-term studies with selegiline have yielded mixed results.[87-90] A recently completed multicenter trial demonstrates the value of selegiline combined with vitamin E in prolonging time to nursing home placement.[91]

Idebonone (TAK-147)

In two recently reported trials, idebonone was effective over 6 and 12 months in improving cognitive and global functioning in patients with AD.[92]

Ginkgo

Derived from the bark of the *Ginkgo biloba* tree, ginkgo is associated with activities of EEG alpha waves,[93] and has been studied for the treatment of AD following the strategy discussed for selegiline. Multicenter studies in Europe have reported that ginkgo enhances cognitive function in AD.[94,95] *Ginkgo biloba extract* (GbE) may also exert neuroprotective effects under conditions of hypoxia, inhibit toxic effects of β amyloid,[96,97] and act as a free-radical scavenger.[98-100] In aged animals, oral GbE treatment leads to increased densities of hippocampal muscarinic acetylcholine receptors and cortical 5HT1A receptors[101,102] as well as enhancing high-affinity choline uptake into hippocampal synaptosomes.[103]

Antiinflammatory Medications

Epidemiologic evidence supports the use of nonsteroidal antiinflammatory medications to prevent or delay the onset of AD. A placebo-controlled trial of indomethacin supports a potential role for antiinflammatory drugs.[104] Patients with rheumatoid arthritis who receive chronic antiinflammatory treatment have a lower risk for AD than controls without rheumatoid arthritis.[105] However, a one-year, placebo-controlled trial of low-dose prednisone (10 mg)[106] did not prove effective. Because of gastrointestinal and other potential adverse effects from antiinflammatory agents, newer drugs that may be safer (e.g., cyclo-oxygenase-2 inhibitors) have been tested. Unfortunately the cyclo-oxy-genase-2 inhibitors celecoxib and rofec-oxib, as well as the nonspecific cyclo-oxy-genase inhibitor naprosyn, have not been effective.[107] Overall, it appears that antiin-flammatory medications will not play a role in the treatment or prevention of AD.

Hydergine and Nicergoline

Hydergine (a combination of four dihy-dro derivatives of ergotoxine) is the trade name of a mixture of ergot alkaloids. Dur-ing the era when AD was believed to result from vascular disease, Hydergine was mar-keted as a vasodilator because of its α-ad-renergic antagonistic effects. Minimal evi-dence supports this contention, however. Subsequently, the drug's ability to change cyclic AMP levels led to its classification as a metabolic enhancer. It may also have partial agonist activity at central dopa-mine, serotonin, and noradrenergic re-ceptors.

The longest used putative cognition-enhancing drug, Hydergine, is one of the most commonly prescribed drugs world-wide, although not in the United States. It has mixed and complex actions on cen-tral α-adrenergic, dopaminergic, and se-rotonergic receptors,[108] and is currently used primarily for patients with dementia or age-associated cognitive symptoms. The FDA reviewed and approved Hyder-gine for "idiopathic decline in mental ca-pacity" on several occasions. Data from numerous randomized, double-blind, pla-cebo-controlled clinical trials in a variety of elderly patient populations have gener-ally shown positive effects, although re-sults from some trials were conflicting. Even though many of these trials favored Hydergine over placebo, they are difficult to interpret because of methodologic lim-itations,[108] and the clinical meaning of the results remains unclear. Hydergine is now not commonly prescribed.

Nicergoline, another ergoloid deriva-tive available in Europe, has shown signifi-cant effects on orientation and atten-tion[109] and is currently being tested in clinical trials in the United States.

More than 60 studies have been con-ducted on ergot alkaloids. A review of 22 methodologically adequate studies of Hydergine found that 18 showed positive effects, with best effects at highest doses (up to 4.5 mg/day).[110] Since that time, studies have tended to focus on higher doses and more prolonged therapy. In general, they arrive at the same findings: At doses of up to 7.5 mg/day, patients show slight improvement, particularly later in the course of therapy. The largest and most recent study[111] found no benefi-cial effect, however, whereas mixed results were recently reported with nicergo-line.[108]

Calcium Channel Blockers

Increased intracellular free calcium acti-vates various destructive enzymes (e.g., proteases, endonucleases, phospholi-pases), and may mediate neuronal death from aging and AD.[112] Thus, blocking in-tracellular free calcium could retard neu-ronal death and slow disease progression. One trial of the calcium channel blocker nimodipine found that patients in the low-dose group (30 mg tid) had less mem-ory deterioration after 12 weeks of treat-ment than those receiving placebo or high-dose nimodipine (60 mg thrice daily).[113] A larger study of patients with mixed diagnoses found significant cogni-tive improvement with nimodipine, com-pared with Hydergine and placebo.[114] Ni-modipine continues to be investigated in the United States for its potential clinical efficacy in AD and vascular dementia; it is marketed as a cognition-enhancing agent in Europe.

Neurotrophic Factors

Animal studies suggest that nerve growth factor (NGF) administration counteracts cholinergic atrophy in the nucleus basalis, although no direct evidence supports NGF involvement in AD pathogenesis. Ad-ministering NGF to humans with AD may slow the rate of cholinergic neuronal de-generation, enhance neuronal function, and thus improve behaviors caused by cholinergic deficits.[115,116] NGF does not cross the blood-brain barrier, thus requiring carrier molecules or intraventricular catheter and pump for administration.[115] European trials of intrathecal NGF demonstrated limited success.[116] Other proposed strategies include use of alkaloid-like molecules that cross the blood-brain barrier and may potentiate NGF activity (e.g., K-252b),[117] intraparenchymal administration, tissue transplant, or injection of genetically modified cells.

Estrogens

Estrogens also may improve cognitive function through cholinergic neuroprotective and neurotrophic effects. Estradiol replacement enhances learning in ovariectomized rats and reverses lowered neuronal choline uptake and choline acetyltransferase levels resulting from ovariectomy.[118] The data suggesting that estrogen replacement may be helpful in AD come from several large observational studies and five preliminary controlled and uncontrolled trials.

Observations of an inverse relation between ERT exposure and a diagnosis of dementia as recorded on death certificates suggest estrogen's potential benefit for improving cognitive function in AD.[119] Two recent reports show conflicting results: (1) of 470 women followed for 16 years, those who never took estrogen replacement showed a 54% reduced risk for AD over those who did,[120] and (2) among 1124 elderly women observed over a 5-year period, those who received estrogen replacement for a decade or more showed a 30 to 40% reduced risk of developing AD.[121] These studies, however, were not randomized and require empirical replication. Preliminary trials have found estradiol, estrone, and conjugated estrogens to enhance cognitive function in AD.[66,122–124] Moreover, cognition-enhancing effects on verbal memory have been demonstrated in studies of cognitively intact postmenopausal women.[125] Most postmenopausal women, however,

decide not to take ERT and thus spend much of their later years in an estrogen-deficient state, when their risk for AD is highest.

An analysis of a 30-week tacrine trial indicated that women receiving ERT had a greater response to tacrine than those not receiving ERT.[126] In this clinical trial, approximately 85% of women were taking conjugated estrogens (Premarin) at a median dose of 0.625 mg. Clinical trials assessing whether conjugated estrogens influence cognitive functioning in women with AD, or whether conjugated estrogens delay AD onset have not been successful. Indeed, women treated with Premarin fared somewhat less well, both in cognition and safety, including 5% having deep vein thrombosis.[127,128] On the basis of this information, estrogen replacement cannot be recommended as a treatment for women with AD.

Therapy Affecting the Circulatory System

Investigation of cerebral vasodilators as a treatment strategy is based on the hypothesis that dementia is caused by atherosclerosis of cerebral vessels. Over the years, a significant number of treatment modalities have been proposed to improve cerebrovascular circulation. These include carbon dioxide and carbonic anhydrase inhibitors, anticoagulants, nicotinic acid, tocopherol (vitamin E), hyperbaric oxygen, use of vasodilators such as papaverine, cyclandelate, isoxuprine, and cinnarizine—all aimed at improved oxygen delivery to the brain. None of these strategies proved effective, however, and the hypothesis that faulty circulation is implicated in the dementia process is no longer tenable. Vitamin E 1000 IUBID has been found clinically effective in maintaining patients' activities of daily living and prolonging their time in the community.

Noötropics

The term *noötropic* applies to compounds that enhance memory and learning by direct effects on brain function and metabolism without other physiological effects.[129] Piracetam, a GABA derivative without GABA effects, is considered the prototypic noötropic agent.[130-134] It has a variety of effects on brain neurochemistry, and enhances memory and learning in animals. Most AD-specific studies show no effect, although one report suggests a slightly positive effect when coadministered with lecithin—an unreplicated finding.[135] Other noötropic agents have been tested, such as oxiracetam, and two reports suggest a very slightly positive effect of this drug in patients with organic brain disease.[136,137] Aniracetam and vinpocetine as well as other noötropic compounds show no clear cognitive effect in AD, although they do indicate variable mild effect on mood and overall functional status.

In addition to piracetam, other noötropics include oxiracetam, pramiracetam, aniracetam, CI 933, and BMY 21502—agents that may protect the CNS from potential damage from hypoxia or drug intoxication. Noötropics may also enhance CNS microcirculation through reduced platelet activity and adherence of red blood cells to vessel walls. Despite such effects, an antidementia mechanism has not been established although noötropics are marketed for dementia and cognitive impairment in many countries throughout the world. Controlled and clinical trials of noötropics in AD have produced conflicting results.[55,130-135] At present, this class of drugs is not relevant to the clinician caring for dementia patients.

Combination Treatments

To date, antidementia drugs administered individually have, at best, only modest effects in treating AD. Logic indicates that combinations of drugs with different mechanisms of action could have greater effects than individual medications alone. An unsuccessful example of this approach, however, is the use of choline precursors in attempts to augment cholinesterase inhibitors. A more successful approach suggests the use of cholinergic agonists to augment the effect of cholinesterase inhibitors. Animal studies suggest that an intact noradrenergic system is necessary for a cholinesterase inhibitor to have an effect.[16] Therefore, the addition of a noradrenergic agent may augment a cholinesterase inhibitor.[138,139] Other drug combinations are likely in the future and may include antioxidants, MAO_B inhibitors, antiinflammatories, cholinergics, and others.

Combining the glutamate antagonist memantine with a cholinesterase inhibitor has proven effective for patients in delaying the time they entered a nursing home.[28] A strategy of combining two modestly efficacious treatment approaches is likely to continue in order to improve cognition and quality of life. Therapeutic results, however, are usually modest, and duration of effect beyond one year as well as long-term safety are not known. Nevertheless, at present, use of cholinesterase inhibitors alone or in combination with memantine is the primary therapeutic approach for cognitive defects of AD and associated decrement in quality of life.

Current Clinical Considerations

All patients with complaints of cognitive difficulties or those for whom cognitive impairment is suspected should be evaluated and diagnosed, and illnesses and medications that might exacerbate dementia symptoms should be addressed.

Cholinesterase inhibitors are the best-studied symptomatic treatments for patients with mild to moderate cognitive impairment and should be given as a therapeutic trial of one of three available cholinesterase inhibitors: donepezil, rivastigmine, or galantamine. Choice of drug involves ease of use, dosage regimen, side-effect profile, and reasonable outcome expectations. Many clinicians add memantine to enhance the therapeutic response in patients with more severe cognitive impairment; its efficacy for milder conditions has not yet been studied.

Other treatments still available for prescribing include vitamin E, selegiline, antiinflammatory medications, and estrogens. However, little evidence exists for efficacy of any of these treatments, and antiinflammatory drugs and estrogens may be harmful to some patients with AD.

Treatment issues concerning patients with very mild dementia or subtle cognitive impairment that may be a prodrome to dementia are similar to those for treating mildly to moderately impaired patients. Considerations include whether to start vitamin E and/or deprenyl, or to use a course of antiinflammatory treatment, together with full consideration of risks. In the absence of true prevention studies regarding minimal cognitive impairment, physicians must use their best judgment when consulting with the patient and family.

More research is needed on antidementia drug effects on behavioral symptoms associated with dementia and on patients in severe stages of the disease. Recent genetic discoveries will likely move the field forward but without knowledge of specific pathophysiology, future efforts will emphasize encouraging theoretical leads, sensible empirical trials, and symptomatic treatment research. Despite public excitement from each announced "breakthrough," balanced but conservative interpretations of results from carefully controlled trials should guide clinical practice standards.

CLINICAL VIGNETTES

Case 20.1

Mrs. A, an 87-year-old widow, moved from one city in the northeastern United States to another to be closer to her daughter and grandchildren. Shortly after the move, she began to experience increased forgetfulness. Her daughter confirmed increased cognitive impairment, described as forgetting what she had read in the newspapers or had seen on television, repeating herself, and being confused about the day of the week. Mrs. A was also depressed about having left her lifelong city of residence and felt lonely and isolated. In consultation, it was not clear whether her cognitive impairment was secondary to these emotional symptoms or was an indication of a primary cognitive impairment. The clinician decided, therefore, to offer her treatment with a cholinesterase inhibitor rather than an antidepressant or antianxiety medication in order to avoid side effects of the latter two classes of drugs. Donepezil 10 mg/d was started.

Two months later in follow-up, Mrs. A was still feeling grumpy, isolated, and sad. She was considerably less anhedonic, however, and reported a return of her lifelong great joy in listening to classical music. She was less forgetful and much less disoriented. On Mini-Mental Status examination, she scored 27 out of 30, and perfectly reproduced intersecting pentangles; she also drew a perfect clock face. Mrs. A was considered to have responded to donepezil, and treatment was continued.

Cognitive impairment in very elderly individuals may arise from several sources including emotional dysregulation, worry, a disruption in routine such as relocation, medications, impaired sleep, and, of course, organic dysfunction. A patient like Mrs. A might have responded to another treatment, such as an antidepressant, with improved cognition. In this particular case, the selection of a cholinesterase inhibitor was made on the basis of fewer side effects than an antidepressant or antianxiety agent. Current clinical strategy suggests ongoing maintenance with cholinesterase inhibitors if a therapeutic response has occurred.

Case 20.2

A retired physician, Dr. B, had obvious symptoms of progressive cognitive decline. He had been a leader in his profession, always active, and highly productive, known for his excellent memory. He had written several books, been president of professional organizations, and had a wide group of friends and devoted patients. In his 80s, however, Dr. B became so forgetful that he closed his practice, discontinued professional relationships, and became progressively socially withdrawn. He could no longer remember people's names, recent conversations, or current events. His remote memory, in contrast, was excellent, and he was still able to regale family and friends with stories from past "good old days." He was a dutiful grandfather and enjoyed times with his family but was unable to read, understand the theme of movies, and could not follow conversation among others around him. When alone, he became agitated, restless, and very irritable.

Dr. B's primary care physician decided that Dr. B was clinically depressed and began him on a low dose of an SSRI antidepressant. He became less irritable, and his spirits seemed to lift moderately, but no change in his cognitive abilities appeared; indeed, over the next year they continued to decline even while taking an SSRI. A decision was made to begin galantamine. After 3 months, the family reported that Dr. B's progressive cognitive impairment seemed to have ``plateaued,'' although it certainly did not improve. Because Dr. B experienced no significant side effects, he continued on this medication.

This patient illustrates clearly that cholinesterase inhibitors as a group may slow the progress of late-life dementia but they do not reverse it. In this typical clinical situation, the quality of Dr. B's life was moderately enhanced by the use of the medication, although he never regained his former cognitive abilities.

Case 20.3

Mr. C, a dapper 80-year-old gentleman, came to the clinical consultation cheerful and smiling. He seemed attentive to the discussion of his symptoms between the physician and his wife and always responded positively when asked how he was feeling. It became clear, however, that Mr. C was unable to speak more than a few words (i.e., ``doing just fine,'' ``can't complain,'' ``not bad''). Although these answers were given affably and positively, it was apparent that Mr. C was incapable of thinking rationally or describing his emotional or cognitive experience.

Cognitive decline had been progressive over several years, and a trial of donepezil had no effect. Memantine (10 mg b.i.d.) was started. Over the next 4 months, Mr. C's affable state continued although no significant change in his cognitive status occurred: it neither improved nor worsened. Mr. C's wife reported that he was somewhat easier to live with at home, although he certainly was not thinking more clearly. Because memantine caused no side effects, it was continued.

Memantine, a new antagonist of the neurotransmitter glutamate, has been found to truly slow the progressive deterioration of Alzheimer's disease. However, although this medication may offer a mildly improved quality of life

because it delays cognitive worsening, it does not reverse the essential decline in cognition. When prescribing a cholinesterase inhibitor or memantine, therefore, clinicians must emphasize to the family that no available medication reverses the essential pathology and cognitive decline of late-life dementia. At best, available agents slow progression of the illness; at worst, they have no effect whatsoever. Nevertheless, their use has brought about not infrequent improvement in quality of life for cognitively impaired patients at least for a few months and occasionally a few years.

References

1. Winblad B. *Socio-economic perspectives of dementia and cost-effectiveness of treatments.* 7th International Geneva/Springfield Symposium on Advances in Alzheimer Therapy; 2002 Apr 3–6; Geneva.
2. Henderson AS, Jorm AF. Definition and epidemiology of dementia: a review. In: Maj M, Sartorius N, eds. *Dementia.* 2nd ed. Chichester, England: John Wiley, 2002:1–33.
3. Leber P. Criteria used by Drug Regulatory Authorities. In Qisilbash N, Schneider L, Chui H, et al. eds. *Evidence-based Dementia Practice.* Oxford: Blackwell *Science* Ltd., 2000:376–387.
4. McKeith I, Fairbairn A, Perry R, et al. Neuroleptic sensitivity in patients with senile dementia of Lewy body type. *Br Med J* 1992;305:673–678.
5. Perry RH, Irving D, Blessed G, et al. Senile dementia of Lewy body type, a clinically and neuropathologically distinct form of Lewy body dementia in the elderly. *J Neurol Sci* 1990;95: 119–139.
6. Levy-Lahad E, Wasco W, Poorkaj P, et al. Candidate gene for the chromosome 1 familial Alzheimer's disease locus. *Science* 1995;269: 973–977.
7. Rogaev EI, Sherrington R, Rogaev EA, et al. Familial Alzheimer's disease in kindreds with missense mutations in a gene on chromosome 1 related to the Alzheimer's disease type 3 gene. *Nature* 1995;376:775–778.
8. Sherrington R, Rogaev EI, Liang Y, et al. Cloning of a gene bearing missense mutations in early onset familial Alzheimer's disease. *Nature* 1995;375:754–760.
9. Goate A, Chartier-Harlin MC, Mullan M, et al. Segregation of a missense mutation in the amyloid precursor protein gene with familial Alzheimer's disease. *Nature* 1991;349:704–706.
10. Alzheimer's Disease Collaborative Group. Apolipoprotein E genotype and Alzheimer's disease. *Lancet* 1993;342:737–738.
11. Mayeux R, Stern Y, Ottman R, et al. The apolipoprotein epsilon 4 allele in patients with Alzheimer's disease. *Ann Neurol* 1993; 34:752–754.
12. Saunders AM, Strittmatter WJ, Schmechel D, et al. Association of apolipoprotein E allele E4

with late onset familial and sporadic Alzheimer's disease. *Neurology* 1993;43:1467–1472.

13. Corder EH, Saunders AM, Strittmatter WJ, et al. Gene dose of apolipoprotein E type 4 allele and the risk of Alzheimer's disease in late onset families. *Science* 1993;261:921–923.

14. Corder EH, Saunders AM, Risch MJ, et al. Apolipoprotein E type 2 allele and the risk of late onset Alzheimer's disease. *Nat Genet* 1994;7:180–183.

15. Giacobini F. Cholinomimetic therapy of Alzheimer's disease: does it slow down deterioration? In: Racagni G, Brunello N, Langer SZ, eds. *Recent advances in the treatment of neurodegenerative disorders and cognitive dysfunction.* Acad Biomed Drug Res. Basel: Karger, 1994:51–57.

16. Haroutunian V, Kanof PD, Tsuboyama G, Davis KL. Restoration of cholinomimetic activity by clonidine in cholinergic plus noradrenergic lesioned rats. *Brain Res* 1990;507:261–266.

17. Brinkman S, Sniff R, Meyer J, et al. Lecithin and memory training in suspected Alzheimer's disease. *J Gerontol* 1982;37:4–9.

18. Becker RE, Giacobini E. Mechanisms of cholinesterase inhibition in senile dementia of the Alzheimer type: clinical, pharmacological, and therapeutic aspects. *Drug Dev Res* 1988;12:163–195.

19. de la Morena E. Efficacy of CDP-choline in the treatment of senile alterations in memory. *Ann NY Acad Sci* 1993;640:233–236.

20. Cacabelos R, Alvarez XA, Franco MA, et al. Effect of CDP-choline on cognition and immune function in Alzheimer's disease and multi infarct dementia. *Ann NY Acad Sci* 1993;695:321–323.

21. Christie JE, Shering A, Ferguson J, Glen AIM. Physostigmine and arecoline: effects of intravenous infusions in Alzheimer presenile dementia. *Br J Psychiatry* 1981;138:46–50.

22. Davis KL, Hollander E, Davidson M, et al. Induction of depression with oxotremorine in patients with Alzheimer's disease. *Am J Psychiatry* 1987;144:468–471.

23. Mohs RC, Davis BM, Johns CA, et al. Oral physostigmine treatment of patients with Alzheimer's disease. *Am J Psychiatry* 1985;142:28–33.

24. Stern Y, Sano M, Mayeux R. Effects of oral physostigmine in Alzheimer's disease. *Ann Neurol* 1987;22:306–310.

25. Thal LJ, Masur DM, Sharpless NS, et al. Acute and chronic effects of oral physostigmine and lecithin in Alzheimer's disease. *Prog Neuropsychopharmacol Biol Psychiatry* 1986;10:617–636.

26. Jorm AF. Effects of cholinergic enhancement therapies on memory function in Alzheimer's disease: a meta-analysis of the literature. *Aust NZ J Psychiatry* 1986;20:237–240.

27. Farlow M, Gracon SI, Hershey LA, et al. A 12-week, double-blind, placebo-controlled, parallel-group study of tacrine in patients with probable Alzheimer's disease. *JAMA* 1992;268:2523–2529.

28. Davis KL, Thal LJ, Gamzu E, et al. Tacrine in patients with Alzheimer's disease: a double-blind, placebo-controlled multicenter study. *N Engl J Med* 1992;327:1253–1259.

29. Knapp MJ, Knopman DS, Solomon PR, et al. Controlled trials of high-dose tacrine in patients with Alzheimer's disease. *JAMA* 1994; 271:985–991.

30. Eagger SA, Levy R, Sahakian BJ. Tacrine in Alzheimer's disease. *Lancet* 1991;337:989–992.

31. Levy R, Eagger S, Griffiths M, et al. Lewy bodies and response to tacrine in Alzheimer's disease. *Lancet* 1994;343:176.

32. Wilcock GK, Scott M, Pearsall T. Long-term use of tacrine. *Lancet* 1994;343:294.

33. Poirier J, Dellsle M, Quirion R, et al. Apolipoprotein E4 allele as a predictor of cholinergic deficits and treatment outcome in Alzheimer disease. *Proc Natl Acad Sci USA* 1995;92:12260–12264.

34. Rogers S. Clinical profile of donepezil (E2020). *Neurobiol Aging* 1996;17(4S):S46.

35. Maelicke A, Samochocki M, Jostock R, et al. Allosteric sensitization of nicotinic receptors by galantamine, a new treatment strategy for Alzheimer's disease. *Biological Psychiatry.* 49:279–288.

36. Kaufer DI, Cummings JL, Christine D. Effect of tacrine on behavioral symptoms in Alzheimer's disease: an open-label study. *J Geriatr Psychiatry Neurology* 1996;9:1–6.

37. Raskind MA, Sadowsky CH, Sigmund WR, et al. Effect of tacrine on language, praxis, and noncognitive behavioral problems in Alzheimer's disease. *Arch Neurology* 1997;54:836–840.

38. Inestrosa NC, Alvarez A, Perez CA, et al. Acetylcholinesterase accelerates assembly of amyloid-beta-peptides into Alzheimer's fibrils: possible role of the peripheral site of the enzyme. *Neuron* 1996;16:881–891.

39. Muller D, Mendla K, Farber Sa, et al. Muscarinic M1 receptor agonists increase the secretion of the amyloid precursor protein ectodomain. *Life Sciences* 1997;60:985–991.

40. Nitsch RM, Slack BE, Wurtman RJ, et al. Release of Alzheimer amyloid precursor derivatives stimulated by activation of muscarinic acetylcholine receptors. *Science* 1992;258:304–307.

41. Fleischacker W, Buchgeher A, Schubert H. Memantine in the treatment of senile dementia of the Alzheimer-type. *Prog Neuropsychopharmacol Biol Psychiatry* 1986;10:87–93.

42. Kristensen V, Olsen M, Theilgaard A. Levodopa treatment of presenile dementia. *Acta Psychiatry Scand* 1984;70:470–477.

43. Kushnir SL, Ratner JT, Gregoire PA. Multiple nutrients in the treatment of Alzheimer's disease. *J Am Geriatr Soc* 1987;35:476–477.

44. Mohr E, Schlegal J, Fabbrini G, et al. Clonidine treatment of Alzheimer's disease. *Arch Neurol* 1989;46:376–378.

45. Phuapradit P, Phillips M, Lees AJ, et al. Bromocriptine in presenile dementia. *Br Med J* 1978; 1:1052–1053.

46. Schlegel J, Mohr E, Williams J, et al. Guanfacine treatment of Alzheimer's disease. *Clin Neuropharmacol* 1989;12:124–128.

47. Schubert H, Fleischhacker W. Therapeutische Ansatze ba dementiellen Syndromen. Ergebnisse mit Amantadin Sulfat unter stationaren Bedingungen. *Arztl Praxis* 1979;46:2157–2160.

48. Smith D, Stromgren E, Peterson H, et al. Lack of effect of tryptophan treatment in demented

gerontopsychiatric patients. *Acta Psychiatry Scand* 1984;70:470–477.

49. Tariot PN, Schneider LS, Coleman PD. Treatment of Alzheimer's disease: glimmers of hope? *Chem Ind* 1993;20:801–807.

50. Nyth AL, Gottfries C. The clinical efficacy of citalopram in treatment of emotional disturbances in dementia disorders: a Nordic multicentre study. *Br J Psychiatry* 1990;157:894–901.

51. Cutler NR, Haxby J, Kay AD, et al. Evaluation of zimeldine in Alzheimer's disease. Cognitive and biochemical measures. *Arch Neurol* 1985; 42:744–748.

52. Soininen H, Koskinen C, Helkala E, et al. Treatment of Alzheimer's disease with a synthetic ACTH 4-9 analog. *Neurology* 1985;35:1348–1351.

53. Dehlin O, Hedenrud B, Jansson P, et al. A double-blind comparison of alapracolate and placebo in the treatment of patients with senile dementia. *Acta Psychiatry Scand* 1985;71:190–196.

54. Lawlor BA, Sunderland T, Mellow AM, et al. Hyperresponsivity to the serotonin agonist m-chlorphenylpiperazine in Alzheimer's disease: a controlled study. *Arch Gen Psychiatry* 1989;46:542–549.

55. Dysken MW, Mendels J, LeWitt P, et al. Milacemide: a placebo-controlled study in senile dementia of the Alzheimer type. *J Am Geriatr Soc* 1992;40:503–506.

56. Mohr E, Bruno G, Foster N, et al. GABA-agonist therapy for Alzheimer's disease. *Clin Neuropharmacol* 1986;9:257–263.

57. Cutler NR, Haxby J, Narang PK, et al. Evaluation of an analog of somatostatin (L363, 586) in Alzheimer's disease. *N Engl J Med* 1985;312:725.

58. Henderson VW, Roberts E, Wimer C, et al. Multicenter trial of naloxone in Alzheimer's disease. *Ann Neurol* 1989;25:404–406.

59. Hyman BT, Eslinger PJ, Damasio AR. Effect of naltrexone on senile dementia of the Alzheimer type. *J Neurol Neurosurg Psychiatry* 1985;48:1169–1171.

60. Tariot PN, Sunderland T, Weingartner H, et al. Naloxone and Alzheimer's disease: cognitive and behavioral effects of a range of doses. *Arch Gen Psychiatry* 1986;43:727–732.

61. Weiss BL. Failure of nalmefene and estrogen to improve memory in Alzheimer's disease. *Am J Psychiatry* 1987;144:386–387.

62. Peabody CA, Davies H, Berger PA, et al. Des-amino-D-arginine-vasopressin (dDAVP) in Alzheimer's disease. *Neurobiol Aging* 1986;7:301–303.

63. Wolters EC, Riekkinen P, Lowenthal A, et al. DGAVP (org 5667) in early Alzheimer's disease patients: an international double-blind, placebo-controlled, multicenter trial. *Neurology* 1990;40:1099–1101.

64. Lampe TH, Norris J, Risse SC, et al. Therapeutic potential of thyrotropin-releasing hormone and lecithin co-administration in Alzheimer's disease. In: Iqbal K, McLachlan DRC, Winblad B, Wisniewski HM, eds. *Alzheimer's disease: basic mechanisms, diagnosis and therapeutic strategies.* New York: John Wiley & Sons, 1990:643–648.

65. Mellow AM, Sunderland T, Cohen RM, et al. Acute effects of high-dose thyrotropin releasing hormone infusions in Alzheimer's disease. *Psychopharmacology* 1989;98:403–407.

66. Tatton WG. "Trophic-like" reduction of nerve cell death by deprenyl without monoamine oxidase inhibition. *Neurol Forum* 1993;4:3–10.

67. Cotman C, Monaghan D, Ganong A. Excitatory amino acid neurotransmission: NMDA receptors and Hebb-type synaptic plasticity. *Annu Rev Neurosci* 1988;11:61–80.

68. Chessell IP, Procter AW, Francis PT, et al. D-Cycloserine, a putative cognitive enhancer, facilitates activation of the N-methyl-D-aspartate receptor-ionophore complex in Alzheimer brain. *Brain Res* 1991;565:345–348.

69. Herting RL. Milacemide and other drugs active at glutamate NMDA receptors as potential treatment for dementia. *Ann NY Acad Sci* 1991; 640:237–240.

70. Winblad B, Poritis N. Memantine in severe dementia: results of the [9]M-BEST study (benefit and efficacy in severely demented patients during treatment with memantine). *Int J Geriat Psychiatry* 1999;14:135–146.

71. Reisberg R, Doody R, Stoffler A, et al. Memantine in Moderate-to-Severe Alzheimer's Disease. *N Eng J Med* 2003;348:1333–1341.

72. Wimo A, Winblad B, Stoffler A, et al. Resource utilization and cost analysis of memantine in patients with moderate to severe Alzheimer's Disease. *Pharmacoeconomics* 2003;21:327–340.

73. Hartmann S, Mobius HJ. Tolerability of memantine in combination with cholinesterase inhibitors in dementia therapy. *Int Clin Psychopharmacol* 2003, 18:81–85.

74. Tariot PN, Farlow MR, Grossberg GT, et al. Memantine treatment in patients with moderate to severe Alzheimer disease already receiving donepezil: a randomized controlled trial. *JAMA.* 2004;291:317–324.

75. Graham DG. Catecholamine toxicity: a proposal for the molecular pathogenesis of manganese neurotoxicity and Parkinson's disease. *Neurotoxicol* 1984;5:83–96.

76. Heikkila RF, Manzion L, Cabbat FS, Duvoisin RC. Protection against the dopaminergic neurotoxicity of MPTP by monoamine oxidase inhibitors. *Nature* 1984;311:467–469.

77. Bowen DM, Davison AN. Can the pathophysiology of dementia lead to rational therapy? In: Crook T, Bartus R, Ferris S, Gershon S, eds. *Treatment development strategies for Alzheimer's disease.* Madison, CT: Powley Assoc 1986;35–66.

78. Knoll J. Striatal dopamine dependency of life span in male rats. *Mech Aging Dev* 1988;46:237–262.

79. Tariot PN, Blazina L. The psychopathology of dementia. In: Morris JC, ed. *Handbook of dementing illnesses.* New York: Marcel Dekker 1993:461–475.

80. Schneider LS, Pollock VE, Zemansky MF, et al. A pilot study of low dose L-deprenyl in Alzheimer's disease. *J Geriatr Psychiatry Neurol* 1991;4:143–148.

81. Tariot PN, Cohen RM, Sunderland T, et al. L-Deprenyl in Alzheimer's disease: preliminary

evidence for behavioral change with monoamine oxidase B inhibition. *Arch Gen Psychiatry* 1987;44:427–433.

82. Martini E, Pataky I, Szilagyi K, Venter V. Brief information on an early phase II-study with deprenyl in demented patients. *Pharmacopsychiatry* 1987;20:256–257.

83. Monteverde A, Gnemmi P, Rossi F. Selegiline in the treatment of mild to moderate Alzheimer-type dementia. *Clin Ther* 1990;12:315–322.

84. Falsaperia A, Preti P, Oliani C. Selegiline vs. oxiracetam in patients with Alzheimer-type dementia. *Clin Ther* 1990;12:376–384.

85. Campi N, Todeschini GP, Scarzella L. Selegiline vs. L-acetylcarnitine in the treatment of Alzheimer-type dementia. *Clin Ther* 1990;12:306–314.

86. Milgram NW, Racine RJ, Nellis P, et al. Maintenance on L-deprenyl prolongs life in aged male rats. *Life Sci* 1990;47:415–420.

87. Burke WJ, Roccaforte WH, Wengel SP, et al. L-Deprenyl in the treatment of mild dementia of the Alzheimer type: results of a 15-month trial. *J Am Geriatr Soc* 1993;41:1219–1225.

88. Freedman M, Rewilak D, Xerri T, et al. L-Deprenyl in Alzheimer's disease: cognitive and behavioral effects. The Lancet conference: challenge of the dementias. Edinburgh, UK, April 1996:105.

89. Riekkinen PJ, Koivisto K, Helkala EL, et al. Efficacy and safety of selegiline in the long-term treatment of patients with Alzheimer's disease. *Neurobiol Aging* 1996;17(4S):S144.

90. Sano M, Ernesto C, Klauber MR, et al. Rationale and design of a multicenter study of selegiline and α-tocopherol in the treatment of Alzheimer disease using novel clinical outcomes. *Alzheimer Dis Assoc Disord* 1996;10:132–140.

91. Sano M, Ernesto C, Thomas RG, et al. A controlled trial of seligiline, alpha-tocopherol, or both as treatment for Alzheimer's disease. *N Engl J Med* 1997;333:1216–1222.

92. Gutzmann H, Erzigkeit H, Hadler D. Long-term treatment of Alzheimer's disease with idebenone. *Neurobiol Aging* 1996;17(4S):S141.

93. Salzman C, Lebars P. Effect of ginkgo biloba on the EEG. Unpublished.

94. Itil TM, Eralp E, Tsambis E, et al. Central nervous system effects of ginkgo biloba, a plant extract. *Am J Ther* 1996;3:63–73.

95. Itil T, Martorano D. Natural substances in psychiatry (ginkgo biloba in dementia). *Psychopharmacol Bull* 1995;31:147–158.

96. Bastianetto S, Ramassamy C, Dore S, et al. The Ginkgo biloba extract (Egb 761) protects hippocampal neurons against cell death induced by beta-amyloid. *Eur J Neurosci* 2000;12:1882–1890.

97. Spinnewyn B. Ginkgo biloba extract (ECb 761) protects against delayed neuronal death in gerbil. In: Christen Y, Constentin J, Lacour M, eds. *Effects of Ginkgo biloba extract (Ecb 761) on the Central Nervous Stystem.* Paris: Elsevier, 1992:113–118.

98. Dorman DC, Cote LM, Buck WB. Effects of an extract of Ginkgo biloba on bromethalin-induced cerebral lipid peroxidation and edema in rats. *Am J Vet Res* 1992;53:138–142.

99. Dumont E, Petit E, Tarrade T, et al. UV-C irradiation-induced peroxidative degradation of microsomal fatty acids and proteins: protection by an extract of Ginkgo biloba (EGb 761). *Free Radic Biol Med* 1992;13:197–203.

100. Pietschmann A, Kuklinski B, Otterstein A. [Protection from uv-light-induced oxidative stress by nutritional radical scavengers.] *Zeitschrift fue die Gesamte Innere Medizin und Ihre Grenzgebiete* 1992;47:518–522.

101. Huguet F, Drieu K, Piriou A. Decreased cerebral 5-HT1A receptors during aging: reversal by Ginkgo biloba extract (Egb 761). *J Pharm Pharmacol* 1994;46:316–318.

102. Taylor J. The effects of chronic, oral Ginkgo biloba extract administration on neurotransmitter receptor binding in young and aged Fisher 344 rats. In: Agnoli A, Rapin J, Scapagnini V, Weitbrecht WU, eds. *Effects of Ginkgo biloba extract on organic cerebral impairment.* John Libbey Eurotext Ltd, 1985:31–34.

103. Kristofikova Z, Benesova O, Tejkalova H. Changes of high-affinity choline uptake in the hippocampus of old rats after long term administration of two nootropic drugs (Tacrine and Ginkgo biloba extract). *Dementia* 1992;3:304–307.

104. Rogers J, Kirby LC, Hempelman SR, et al. Clinical trial of indomethacin in Alzheimer's disease. *Neurology* 1993;43:1609–1611.

105. McGeer PL, McGeer E, Rogers J, Sibley J. Anti-inflammatory drugs and Alzheimer's disease. *Lancet* 1987;335:1037.

106. Aisen PS, Davis KL. Inflammatory mechanisms in Alzheimer's disease: implications for therapy. *Am J Psychiatry* 1994;151:1105–1113.

107. Aisen PS, Schafer K, Gundman M, et al. Results of a multicenter trial of rofecoxib and naproxen in Alzheimer's disease. *Neurobiol Aging* 2002;23:S429.

108. Schneider LS, Olin JT. Overview of clinical trials of Hydergine in dementia. *Arch Neurol* 1994;51:787–798.

109. Battaglia A, Bruni G, Ardia A, et al. Nicergoline in mild to moderate dementia: a multicenter, double-blind, placebo-controlled study. *J Am Geriatr Soc* 1989;37:295–302.

110. Hollister L, Yesavage J. Ergoloid mesylates for senile dementias: unanswered questions. *Ann Intern Med* 1990;100:894–898.

111. Thompson T, Filley C, Mitchell D, et al. Lack of efficacy of Hydergine in patients with Alzheimer's disease. *N Engl J Med* 1990;323:445–448.

112. Grobe-Einsler R, Traber J. Clinical results with nimodipine in Alzheimer's disease. *Clin Neuropharm* 1992;15(suppl 1, pt A):416A–417A.

113. Tollefson GD. Short term effects of the calcium channel blocker nimodipine (Bay-e-9736) in the management of primary degenerative dementia. *Biol Psychiatry* 1990;27:1133–1142.

114. Kanowski S, Fischof P, Hiersemenzel R, et al. Wirksamkeitsnachweis von nootropika am beispiel von Nimodipin—ein beitrag zur entwicklung geeigneter klinischer prufmodelle. *Z Gerontopsychol Psychiatr* 1988;1:35–44.

115. Hefti F, Schneider LS. Rationale for the planned clinical trials with nerve growth factor

in Alzheimer's disease. *Psychiatr Dev* 1989;4: 297–315.

116. Olson L. NGF and the treatment of Alzheimer's disease. *Exp Neurol* 1993;124:5–15.

117. Knusel B, Kaplan DR, Winslow JW, et al. K-252b selectively potentiates cellular actions and trk tyrosine phosphorylation mediated by neurotrophin-3. *J Neurochem* 1992;59:715–722.

118. Simpkins JW, Singh M, Bishop J. The potential role for estrogen replacement therapy in the treatment of the cognitive decline and neurodegeneration associated with Alzheimer's disease. *Neurobiol Aging* 1994;15(suppl 2):S195–197.

119. Paganini-Hill A, Henderson VW. Estrogen deficiency and risk of Alzheimer's disease in women. *Am J Epidemiol* 1994;140:256–261.

120. Morrison A, Kawas C, Resnick S, et al. *A prospective study of estrogen replacement therapy and the risk of developing Alzheimer's disease in the Baltimore Longitudinal Study of Aging.* The 8th International Congress on the Menopause, Sydney, Australia, Nov 6, 1996.

121. Tang MX, Jacobs D, Stern Y, et al. Effect of estrogen during menopause on risk and age at onset of Alzheimer's disease. *Lancet* 1996;348: 429–432.

122. Ohkura T, Isse K, Akazawa K, et al. Evaluation of estrogen treatment in female patients with dementia of the Alzheimer type. *Endocr J* 1994; 41:361–371.

123. Honjo H, Ogino Y, Tanaka K, et al. An effect of conjugated estrogen to cognitive impairment in women with senile dementia-Alzheimer's type: a placebo-controlled double blind study. *J Jpn Menopause Soc* 1993;1:167–171.

124. Honjo H, Ogino Y, Naitoh K, et al. In vivo effects by estrone sulfate on the central nervous system-senile dementia (Alzheimer's type). *J Steroid Biochem* 1989;34:521–525.

125. Kampen DL, Sherwin BB. Estrogen use and verbal memory in healthy postmenopausal women. *Obstet Gynecol* 1994;83:979–983.

126. Schneider LS, Farlow MR, Henderson VW, Pogoda JM. Effects of estrogen replacement therapy on response to tacrine in patients with Alzheimer's disease. *Neurology* 1996;46:1580–1584.

127. Henderson VW, Paganini-Hill A, Miller BL, et al. Estrogen for Alzheimer's disease in women: randomized, double-blind, placebo-controlled trial. *Neurology* 2000;54:295–301.

128. Mulnard RA, Cotman CW, Kawas C, et al. Estrogen replacement therapy for treatment of mild to moderate Alzheimer's disease: a randomized controlled trial. Alzheimer's Disease Cooperative Study. *JAMA* 2000;283:1007–1015.

129. Nicholson CD. Pharmacology of nootropic and metabolically active compounds in relation to their use in dementia. *Psychopharmacology* 1990; 101:147–159.

130. Vernon MW, Sorkin EM. Piracetam. An overview of its pharmacological properties and a review of its therapeutic use in senile cognitive disorders. *Drugs Aging* 1991;1:17–35.

131. Chouinard G, Annable L, Ross-Chouinard A, et al. A double-blind, placebo-controlled study

of piracetam in elderly psychiatric patients. *Psychopharmacology* 1981;17:129.

132. Growdon JH, Corkin S, Huff FJ, et al. Piracetam combined with lecithin in the treatment of Alzheimer's disease. *Neurobiol Aging* 1986;7: 269–276.

133. Croisile B, Trillet M, Fondarai J, et al. Long-term and high-dose piracetam treatment of Alzheimer's disease. *Neurology* 1993;43:301–305.

134. Flicker L, Grimley Evans J. Piracetam for dementia or cognitive impairment. *Cochrane Database Syst Rev* 2001;2:CD001011.

135. Smith R, Vroulis G, Johnson R. Comparison of therapeutic response to long-term treatment with lecithin versus piracetam plus lecithin in patients with Alzheimer's disease. *Psychopharmacol Bull* 1984;20:542–545.

136. Moglia A, Sinforiani CE, Zandrini C, et al. Activity of oxiracetam in patients with organic brain syndrome: a neuropsychological study. *Clin Neuropharmacol* 1986;9:S73–S78.

137. Villardita C, Parini J, Grioli S, et al. Clinical and neuropsychological study with oxiracetam versus placebo in patients with mild to moderate dementia. *J Neural Transm* 1987;24(suppl): 293–295.

138. Sunderland T, Molchan S, Lawlor B, et al. A strategy of "combination chemotherapy" in Alzheimer's disease: rationale and preliminary results with physostigmine plus deprenyl. *Int Psychogeriatr* 1992;4(suppl 2):291–309.

139. Schneider LS, Olin J, Pawluczyk S. A double-blind crossover pilot study of L-deprenyl (selegiline) combination with cholinesterase inhibitor in Alzheimer's disease. *Am J Psychiatry* 1993; 150:321–323.

Table 20.2 References

Burns A, Rossor M, Hecker J, et al. The effects of donepezil in Alzheimer's disease—results from a multinational trial. *Dement Geriatr Cogn Disord* 1999;10:237–244.

Corey-Bloom J, Anand R, Veach J, et al. A randomized trial evaluating the efficacy and safety of ENA 713 (rivastigmine tartrate), a new acetylcholinesterase inhibitor, in patients with mild to moderately severe Alzheimer's disease. *International Journal Geriatric Psychopharmacology* 1998;1: 55–65.

Feldman H, Gauthier S, Hecker J, et al. A 24-week, randomized, double-blind study of donepezil in moderate to severe Alzheimer's disease. *Neurology* 2001;57:613–620.

Knapp MJ, Knopman DS, Solomon PR, et al. A 30-week randomized controlled trial of high-dose tacrine in patients with Alzheimer's disease. The Tacrine Study Group. *JAMA* 1994;271:985–991.

Raskind M, Peskind ER, Wessel T, Yuan W. Galantamine in Alzheimer's disease—a 6-month, randomized, placebo-controlled trial with a 6-month extension. *Neurology* 2000;54:2261–2268.

Rogers SL, Farlow MR, Doody RS, et al. A 24-week, double-blind, placebo-controlled trial of donepezil in patients with Alzheimer's disease. Donepezil Study Group. *Neurology* 1998b:136–145.

Rosler M, Anand R, Cicin-Sain A, et al. Efficacy and safety of rivastigmine in patients with Alzheimer's disease: internationl randomized controlled trial. *BMJ* 1999;318:633–638.

Tariot PN, Solomon PR, Morris JC, et al. A 5-month, randomized, placebo-controlled trial of galantamine in AD. The Galantamine USA-10 Study Group. *Neurology* 2000;54:2269–2276.

Tariot PN, Cummings JL, Katz IR, et al. A randomized, double-blind, placebo-controlled study of the efficacy and safety of donepezil in patients with Alzheimer's disease in the nursing home setting. *J Am Geriatr Soc* 2001;49:1590–1599.

Wilcock GK, Lilienfeld S, Gaens E. Efficacy and safety of galantamine in patients with mild to moderate Alzheimer's disease: multicentre randomized controlled trial. Galantamine International-1 Study Group. *BMJ* 2000;321:1445–1449.

Winblad B, Bonura ML, Rossini BM, Battaglia A. Niccrgoline in the treatment of mild-to-moderate Alzheimer's disease: a European multicentre trial. *Clin Drug Invest* 2001;21:621–632.

Supplemental Readings

General Treatment

Abernathy D. Development of memory enhancing agents in the treatment of Alzheimer's disease. *J Am Geriatr Soc* 1987;35:957–958.

Amaducci L. Phosphatidylserine in the treatment of Alzheimer's disease: results of a multicenter study. *Psychopharmacol Bull* 1988;24:130–134.

Amaducci L, Fratiglioni L, Rocca W, et al. Risk factors for clinically diagnosed Alzheimer's disease: a case control study of an Italian population. *Neurology* 1985;36:922–931.

Ambrozi L, Danielczyk W. Treatment of impaired cerebral function in psychogeriatric patients with memantine—results of a phase II double-blind study. *Pharmacopsychiatry* 1988;21:144–146.

Bartus R. Drugs to treat age-related neurodegenerative problems: the final frontier of medical Science? *J Am Geriatr Soc* 1990;38:680–695.

Baskys A, Davis P. *Use of the atypical antipsychotic quetiapine in the treatment of the psychosis associated with Lewy body dementia.* NCDEU Annual Meeting, June 10–13, 2002.

Cholinergic treatment in Alzheimer's disease: encouraging results [Editorial]. *Lancet* 1987;1: 139–142.

Cohen BM, Satlin A, Zubenko GS. S-Adenosyl-L-methionine in the treatment of Alzheimer's disease. *J Clin Psychopharmacol* 1988;8:43–47.

Conti L, Placidi GF, Cassano GB. Ateroid in the treatment of dementia: results of a clinical trial. *Mod Probl Pharmacopsychiatry* 1989;23:76–84.

Cronan-Golomb A. Meeting report: International Study Group on the Pharmacology of Memory Disorders Associated with Aging. *Neurobiol Aging* 1987;8:277–282.

Crook T. Alzheimer's disease: new developments in treatment and symptom management research. *Psychopharmacol Bull* 1988;24:31–38.

Crook T, Bartus R, Ferris S, eds. *Treatment development strategies for Alzheimer's disease.* Madison, CT: Powley, 1986.

Crook TH III. Diagnosis and treatment of normal and pathologic memory impairment in later life. *Semin Neurol* 1989;9:20–30.

Doody RS. Current treatments for Alzheimer's Disease: Cholinesterase inhibitors. *J Clin Psychiatry* 2003;64(suppl 9):11–17.

Dowson J. Drug treatments for cognitive impairment due to ageing and disease: current and future strategies. *Int J Geriatr Psychiatry* 1989;4:345–353.

Dysken M. A review of recent clinical trials in the treatment of Alzheimer's dementia. *Psychiatry Ann* 1987;17:178–191.

Erkinjuntti T, Kurz A, Gauthier S, et al. Efficacy of galantamine in probable vascular dementia and Alzheimer's disease combined with cerebrovascular disease: a randomized trial. *Lancet* 2002; 359:1283–1290.

Gottfries C. Pharmacology of mental aging and dementia disorders. *Clin Neuropharmacol* 1987;10: 313–329.

Grossberg T. Diagnosis and Treatment of Alzheimer's Disease. *J Clin Psychiatry* 2003;64(suppl 9): 3–6.

Kim KY. Quetiapine as treatment of delirium in older adults. NCDEU Annual Meeting, June 10–13, 2002.

Laplane D. Practical management of Alzheimer's disease. *Rev Pract* 1989;39:486–488.

Mintzer JE. The search for better noncholinergic treatment options for Alzheimer's Disease. *J Clin Psychiatry* 2003;64(suppl 9):18–22.

Molloy DW, Cape RD. Acute effects of oral pyridostigmine on memory and cognitive function in SDAT. *Neurobiol Aging* 1989;10:199–204.

New treatment strategies for dementia [Editorial]. *Lancet* 1987;1:114.

Orgogozo J, Spiegel R. Critical review of clinical trials in senile dementia. *Postgrad Med J* 1987;63: 337–343.

Piette F. Inclusion and exclusion clinical criteria to form homogeneous groups of patients in the therapeutic trials of a memory enhancing drug. *Arch Gerontol Geriatr Suppl* 1989;1:195–200.

Pomponi M, Giacobini E, Brufani M. Present state and future development of the therapy of Alzheimer's disease. *Aging* 1990;2:125–153.

Prui SK, Hsu RS, Ho I, Lassman HB. Single dose safety, tolerance, and pharmacokinetics of HP 029 in healthy young men: a potential Alzheimer agent. *J Clin Pharmacol* 1989;29:278–284.

Raskind MA, Peskind ER, Wessel T, et al. Galantamine in AD: A 6-month randomized, placebo-controlled trial with a 6-month extension. *Neurology* 2000;54:2261–2268.

Reifler BV, Teri L, Raskind M, et al. Double-blind trial of imipramine in Alzheimer's disease patients with and without depression. *Am J Psychiatry* 1989;146:45–49.

Sano M. Noncholinergic treatment options for Alzheimer's Disease. *J Clin Psychiatry* 2003;64(suppl 9):23–28.

Schneider LS. New therapeutic approaches to Alzheimer's disease. *J Clin Psychiatry* 1996;57: (suppl)14:30–36.

Spar J. Psychopharmacology of Alzheimer's disease. *Psychiatry Ann* 1984;14:186–189.

Tariot PN, Blazina L. The psychopathology of dementia. In: Morris JC, ed. *Handbook of dementing illnesses.* New York: Marcel Dekker, 1993: 461–475.

Tariot PN, Solomon PR, Morris JC, et al. A 5-month, randomized, placebo-controlled trial of galantamine in AD. *Neurology* 2000;54:2269–2276.

Wenk GL. Neuropathologic changes in Alzheimer's Disease. *J Clin Psychiatry* 2003;64(suppl 9):7–10.

Wurtman R. Strategies in the development of drugs that might be useful in cognitive disorders. *Clin Neuropharmacol* 1986;9(suppl 3):S3–S7.

Neuropathology

Bahmanyar S, Higgins G, Goldgaber D, et al. Localization of amyloid beta protein messenger RNA in brains from patients with Alzheimer's disease. *Science* 1987;237:77–80.

Blass J, Gleason P, Brush D, et al. Thiamine and Alzheimer's disease: a pilot study. *Arch Neurol* 1988; 45:833–835.

Blessed G, Tomlinson BE, Roth M. The association between quantitative measures of dementia and of senile change in the cerebral grey matter of elderly subjects. *Br J Psychiatry* 1968;114:797–811.

Buell SJ, Coleman PD. Dendritic growth in the aged human brain and failure of growth in senile dementia. *Science* 1979;206:854–856.

Caputo C, Salama A. The amyloid proteins of Alzheimer's disease as potential targets for drug therapy. *Neurobiol Aging* 1989;10:451–461.

Cohen G. Oxidative stress in the nervous system. In: Sies H, ed. *Oxidative stress.* London: Academic Press, 1985:383–402.

Cohen G, Spina MB. Deprenyl suppresses the oxidant stress associated with increased dopamine turnover. *Ann Neurol* 1989;26:689–690.

Davies P. Neurochemical studies: an update on Alzheimer's disease. *J Clin Psychiatry* 1988;49(suppl 5):23–28.

Delabar J, Goldgaber D, Lamour Y, et al. Beta amyloid gene duplication in Alzheimer's disease and karyotypically normal Down's syndrome. *Science* 1987;235:1390–1392.

Esch F, Keim P, Beattie E, et al. Cleavage of amyloid beta peptide during constitutive processing of its precursor. *Science* 1990;248:1122–1124.

Fox JH, Penn R, Clasen R, et al. Pathological diagnosis in clinically typical Alzheimer's disease. *N Engl J Med* 1985;313:1419–1420.

Gottfries CG. Alzheimer's disease. A critical review. *Compr Gerontol* 1988;2:47–62.

Hefti F, Hartikka J, Knusel B. Function of neurotrophic factors in the adult and aging brain and their possible roles in the treatment of neurodegenerative diseases. *Neurobiol Aging* 1989;10: 515–533.

Hyman B, VanHoesen GW, Demasio AR, Barnes CL. Alzheimer's disease: cell-specific pathology isolates the hippocampal formation. *Science* 1984; 225:1168–1170.

Joachim CL, Selkoe DJ. Minireview: amyloid protein in Alzheimer's disease. *J Gerontol* 1989;44: B77–82.

Jonsson G. Studies on the mechanisms of 6-hydroxydopamine cytotoxicity. *Med Biol* 1976;54:406–420.

Koskik K. The molecular and cellular pathology of

Alzheimer neurofibrillary lesions. *J Gerontol* 1989; 44:B55–58.

Martin EM, Wilson RS, Penn RD, et al. Cortical biopsy results in Alzheimer's disease: correlation with cognitive deficits. *Neurology* 1987;37:1201–1204.

Marx J. Brain protein yields clues to Alzheimer's disease. *Science* 1989;243:1664–1666.

Mazurek M, Beal M, Bird E, Martin J. Vasopressin in Alzheimer's disease: a study of post-mortem brain concentrations. *Ann Neurol* 1986;20:665–670.

Neary D, Snowden JS, Mann DMA, et al. Alzheimer's disease: a correlative study. *J Neurol Neurosurg Psychiatry* 1986;49:229–237.

Palmert M, Gold ET, Cohen M, et al. Amyloid protein precursor messenger RNAs: differential expression in Alzheimer's disease. *Science* 1988; 241:1080–1084.

Perry EK. Cortical neurotransmitter chemistry in Alzheimer's disease. In: Meltzer HY, ed. *Psychopharmacology: the third generation of progress.* New York: Raven Press, 1987:887–895.

Podlisny M, Lee G, Selkoe D. Gene dosage of the amyloid beta precursor protein in Alzheimer's disease. *Science* 1987;238:669–674.

Roses A, Pericak-Vance M, Haynes C, et al. Genetic linkage studies in Alzheimer's disease (AD). *Neurology* 1988;38(suppl 1):173.

Rumble B, Retallack R, Hilbich C, et al. Amyloid a4 protein and its precursor in Down's syndrome and Alzheimer's disease. *N Engl J Med* 1989;320: 1446–1452.

Sajdel-Sulkowska E, Chou W, Salim M, et al. Genetic expression of amyloid and glial specific protein in the Alzheimer brain. *J Am Geriatr Soc* 1988;36: 558–564.

Schellenberg G, Bird T, Wijsman E. Absence of linkage of chromosome c1q21 markers to familial Alzheimer's disease. *Science* 1988;241:1507–1510.

Selkoe D. Deciphering Alzheimer's disease: the pace quickens. *Trends Neurosci* 1987;10:181–184.

Selkoe D, Bell D, Podlisny M, et al. Concentration of brain amyloid proteins in aged mammals and humans with Alzheimer's disease. *Science* 1987; 235:873–877.

Selkoe DJ. Deciphering Alzheimer's disease: the amyloid precursor protein yields new clues. *Science* 1990;248:1058–1060.

Sisodia S, Koo E, Beyruther K, et al. Evidence that beta amyloid in Alzheimer's disease is not derived by normal processing. *Science* 1990;248: 492–495.

St. George-Hyslop P, Tanzi R, Polinski R, et al. Absence of duplication of chromosome 21 genes in familial and sporadic Alzheimer's disease. *Science* 1987;238:664–666.

St. George-Hyslop PH, Tanzi RE, Polinski RJ, et al. The genetic defect causing familial Alzheimer's disease maps on chromosome 21. *Science* 1987; 235:885–890.

Tanzi R, Bird E, Latt S, Neve R. The amyloid beta protein gene is not duplicated in brains from patients with Alzheimer's disease. *Science* 1987;238: 666–669.

Tanzi R, Gusella J, Watkins P, et al. Amyloid beta protein gene: CDNA, MRNA distribution, and genetic linkage near the Alzheimer locus. *Science* 1987;235:880–884.

Terry RD. The fine structure of neurofibrillary tangles in Alzheimer's disease. *J Neuropathol Exp Neurol* 1963;22:622–642.

Terry RD, Peck A, DeTeresa R, et al. Some morphometric aspects of the brain in senile dementia of the Alzheimer type. *Ann Neurol* 1981;10:184–192.

Whitson J, Selkoe D, Cotman C. Amyloid beta protein enhances the survival of hippocampal neurons in vitro. *Science* 1989;243:1488–1490.

Wolozin B, Davies P. Alzheimer's-related neuronal protein A68: specificity and distribution. *Ann Neurol* 1987;22:521–526.

Wolozin B, Pruchnicki A, Dickson D, Davies P. A neuronal antigen in the brains of Alzheimer's patients. *Science* 1986;232:648–650.

Yankner B, Dawes L, Fisher S, et al. Neurotoxicity of a fragment of amyloid precursor associated with Alzheimer's disease. *Science* 1989;245:417–420.

Genetics

Breitner J, Folstein M. Familial Alzheimer dementia: a prevalent disorder with specific clinical features. *Psychol Med* 1984;14:63–80.

Farrer L, O'Sullivan D, Cuppels A, et al. Assessment of genetic risk for Alzheimer's disease among first degree relatives. *Ann Neurol* 1989;25:485–493.

Heston L, Mastri A, Anderson E, White J. Dementia of the Alzheimer-type: clinical genetics, natural history, and associated conditions. *Arch Gen Psychiatry* 1981;38:1085–1090.

Kay D. The genetics of Alzheimer's disease. *Br Med Bull* 1986;42:19–23.

Kay D. Heterogeneity in Alzheimer's disease: epidemiological and family studies. *Trends Neurosci* 1987;10:194–196.

Martin R, Gerteis G, Gabrielle W. A family genetic study of dementia of the Alzheimer-type. *Arch Gen Psychiatry* 1988;48:894–900.

Mohs R, Breitner J, Silverman J, Davis K. Alzheimer's disease: morbid risk among first degree relatives approximates 50% by 90 years of age. *Arch Gen Psychiatry* 1987;44:405–408.

Nee L, Eldridge R, Sunderland T, et al. Dementia of the Alzheimer-type: clinical and family study of 22 twin pairs. *Neurology* 1987;37:359–363.

Nee L, Polinsky R, Eldridge R, et al. A family with histologically confirmed Alzheimer's disease. *Arch Neurol* 1983;40:203–208.

Rocca W. The etiology of Alzheimer's disease: epidemiologic contributions with emphasis on the genetic hypothesis. *J Neural Transm* 1987;24(suppl):3–12.

Spencer P, Nunn P, Hugon J, et al. Guam amyotrophic lateral sclerosis-Parkinsonism-dementia linked to a plant excitant neurotoxin. *Science* 1987;237:517–522.

Zubenko G, Huff K, Beyer J, et al. Familial risk of dementia associated with a biological subtype of Alzheimer's disease. *Arch Gen Psychiatry* 1988;45:889–893.

Infections

Bruce M. Scrapie and Alzheimer's disease. *Psychol Med* 1984;14:497–500.

Cuara R, Grady C, Haxby J, et al. Positron emission tomography in Alzheimer's disease. *Neurology* 1986;36:879–887.

Friedland R, May C, Dahlberg J. The viral hypothesis of Alzheimer's disease. *Arch Neurol* 1990;47:177–178.

Goudsmit J, Morrow C, Asher D, et al. Evidence for and against the transmissibility of Alzheimer's disease. *Neurology* 1980;30:945–950.

Mozar H, Bal D, Howard J. Perspectives on the etiology of Alzheimer's disease. *JAMA* 1987;257:1503–1507.

Prusiner S. Prions and neurodegenerative diseases. *N Engl J Med* 1987;317:1571–1581.

Somerville R. Ultrastructural links between scrapie and Alzheimer's disease. *Lancet* 1985;1:504–506.

Werter PG, Murgas D, Pomerantz S. AIDS as a cause of dementia in the elderly. *J Am Geriatr Soc* 1988;36:139–141.

Neurochemistry

Adolfsson R, Gottfries C, Roos B, Winblad B. Changes in the brain catecholamines in patients with dementia of Alzheimer's-type. *Br J Psychiatry* 1979;135:216–223.

Allen G, Burns S, Tulipan T, Parker R. Adrenal medullary transplantation to the caudate nucleus in Parkinson's disease: initial clinical results in 18 patients. *Arch Neurol* 1989;46:487–491.

Arai H, Kosaka K, Iizuka R. Changes of biogenic amines and their metabolites in post-mortem brains from patients with Alzheimer's-type dementia. *J Neurochem* 1984;43:388–393.

Bartus R, Dean R, Beer B, Lippa A. The cholinergic hypothesis of geriatric memory dysfunction. *Science* 1982;217:408–417.

Beal M, Martin J. Neuropeptides in neurological disease. *Ann Neurol* 1986;20:547–565.

Beal M, Mazurek M, Tran V, et al. Reduced numbers of somatostatin receptors in the cerebral cortex in Alzheimer's disease. *Science* 1985;225:289–291.

Bondareff W, Mountjoy C, Roth M. Selective loss of neurones of origin of adrenergic projection to cerebral cortex (nucleus locus coeruleus) in senile dementia. *Lancet* 1981;2:783–784.

Bowen D. Neurotransmitters in Alzheimer's disease. *Age* 1988;11:104–110.

Bowen D, Allen S, Benton J, et al. Biochemical assessment of serotonergic and cholinergic dysfunction and cerebral atrophy in Alzheimer's disease. *J Neurochem* 1983;41:266–272.

Chu D, Penney J, Young A. Cortical GABA-B and GABA-A receptors in Alzheimer's disease: a quantitative autoradiographic study. *Neurology* 1987;37:1454–1459.

Coyle J, Price D, DeLong M. Alzheimer's disease: a disorder of cortical innervation. *Science* 1983;219:1184–1190.

Cross A, Crow T, Perry E, et al. Reduced dopamine-beta-hydroxylase activity in Alzheimer's disease. *Br Med J* 1981;282:93–94.

Crow T, Cross A, Cooper S, et al. Neurotransmitter

receptors and monoamine metabolites in the brains of patients with Alzheimer-type dementia and depression, and suicides. *Neuropharmacology* 1984;23:1561–1569.

D'Amato R, Zweig R, Whitehouse P, et al. Aminergic systems in Alzheimer's disease and Parkinson's disease. *Ann Neurol* 1987;22:229–236.

Davies P, Wolozin B. Recent advances in the neurochemistry of Alzheimer's disease. *J Clin Psychiatry* 1987;48(suppl 5):23–30.

DeSouza E, Whitehouse P, Kuhar M, et al. Alzheimer's disease: reciprocal changes in corticotropin releasing factor (CRF)-like immunoreactivity and CRF receptors in cerebral cortex. *Nature* 1986;319:593.

Deutsch S, Morihisa J. Glutamatergic abnormalities in Alzheimer's disease and a rationale for clinical trials with L-glutamate. *Clin Neuropharmacol* 1988; 11:18–35.

Fliers E, Swaab D. Neuropeptide changes in aging and Alzheimer's disease. *Progr Brain Res* 1986;70: 141–151.

Forssell LG, Hellstrom A, Ericsson K, Winblad B. Early stages of late onset Alzheimer's disease. Diagnostic criteria, protein metabolism, precursor loading effects, neurochemical and neuropsychological applications. *Acta Neurol Scand Suppl* 1989;121:1–95.

Francis P, Bowen D, Lole S, et al. Somatostatin content and release measured in cerebral biopsies from demented patients. *J Neurol Sci* 1987;78: 1–16.

Francis P, Palmer A, Sims N, et al. Neurochemical studies of early onset Alzheimer's disease. *N Engl J Med* 1985;313:7–11.

Gottfries C. Alzheimer's disease and senile dementia: biochemical characteristics and aspects of treatment. *Psychopharmacology* 1985;86:245–252.

Gottfries C, Adolfsson R, Aquilonius S, et al. Biochemical changes in dementia disorders of Alzheimer type. *Neurobiol Aging* 1983;4:261–271.

Greenamyre J, Peney J, D'Amato C, Young A. Dementia of the Alzheimer's type, changes in hippocampal L(3H) glutamate binding. *J Neurochem* 1987;48:543–551.

Husain M, Nemeroff C. Neuropeptides and Alzheimer's disease. *J Am Geriatr Soc* 1990;38:918–925.

Lindvall O, Brundin P, Widner H, et al. Grafts of fetal dopamine neurons survive and improve motor function in Parkinson's disease. *Science* 1990;247: 574–577.

Madrazo I, Crucker-Colin R, Diaz V, et al. Open microsurgical autograft of adrenal medulla to the right caudate nucleus in two patients with intractable Parkinson's disease. *N Engl J Med* 1987;316: 831–834.

Madrazo I, Franco-Bourland R, Ostrosky-Solis F, et al. Fetal homotransplants (ventral mesencephalon and adrenal tissue) to the striatum of parkinsonian subjects. *Arch Neurol* 1990;47:1281–1285.

Mazurek M, Beal M, Bird E, Martin J. Oxytocin in Alzheimer's disease: post-mortem brain levels. *Neurology* 1987;37:1001–1003.

McGeer E, Singh E, McGeer P. Sodium-dependent glutamate binding in senile dementia. *Neurobiol Aging* 1987;8:219–223.

McGeer P, McGeer E, Suzuki J, et al. Aging, Alzhei-

mer's disease and the cholinergic system of the basal forebrain. *Neurology* 1984;34:741–745.

Morrison J, Rogers J, Schar S, et al. Somatostatin immunoreactivity in neuritic plaques of Alzheimer patients. *Nature* 1985;314:90–92.

Mountjoy CQ, Rossor M, Iversen L, Roth M. Correlations of cortical cholinergic and GABA deficits with quantitative neuropathological findings in senile dementia. *Brain* 1984;107:507–518.

Neary D, Snowdon J, Mann D, et al. Alzheimer's disease: a correlative study. *J Neurol Psychiatry* 1986; 49:229–237.

Parkinson Study Group. DATATOP: a multi-center controlled clinical trial in early Parkinson's disease. *Arch Neurol* 1989;46:1052–1060.

Perry T, Yong V, Burgeron C, et al. Amino acids, glutathione, and glutathione transferase activity in the brains of patients with Alzheimer's disease. *Ann Neurol* 1987;21:331–336.

Reinikainen K, Paljarvi L, Halonen T, et al. Dopaminergic system and monoamine oxidase B activity in Alzheimer's disease. *Neurobiol Aging* 1988;9: 245–252.

Reinikainen K, Reikinen P, Jolkkonen J, et al. Decreased somatostatin-like immunoreactivity in cerebral cortex and cerebral spinal fluid in Alzheimer's disease. *Brain Res* 1987;402:103–108.

Roberts G, Crow T, Polak J. Location of neuronal tangles and somatostatin neurones in Alzheimer's disease. *Nature* 1985;314:92–94.

Rossor M, Iversen L. Noncholinergic abnormalities in Alzheimer's disease. *Br Med Bull* 1986;42: 70–74.

Rossor M, Iversen L, Reynolds G, et al. Neurochemical characteristics of early and late onset types of Alzheimer's disease. *Br Med J* 1984;288:961–964.

Rossor MN, Garret N, Johnson A, et al. A post-mortem study of the cholinergic and GABA systems in senile dementia. *Brain* 1982;105:313–330.

Sasaki H, Muramoto O, Kanazawa I, et al. Regional distribution of amino acid transmitters in postmortem brains of presenile and senile dementia of Alzheimer-type. *Ann Neurol* 1986;19:263–269.

Schmitt F, Bigley J, McKinnis R, et al. Neuropsychological outcome of zidovudine (AZT) treatment of patients with AIDS and AIDS-related complex. *N Engl J Med* 1988;319:1573–1578.

Shoulson I, Ordoroff C, Oakes D, et al. A controlled clinical trial of baclofen as protective therapy in early Huntington's disease. *Ann Neurol* 1989;25: 252–259.

Sims N, Bowen D, Allen S, et al. Presynaptic cholinergic dysfunction in patients with dementia. *J Neurochem* 1983;40:503–509.

Sparks D, DeKosky S, Markesbery W. Alzheimer's disease: aminergic-cholinergic alterations in hypothalamus. *Arch Neurol* 1988;45:994–999.

Sunderland T, Rubinow D, Tariot P, et al. CSF somatostatin in patients with Alzheimer's disease, older depressed patients, and age-matched control subjects. *Am J Psychiatry* 1987;144:1313–1316.

Tamminga C, Foster N, Fedio P, et al. Alzheimer's disease: low cerebral somatostatin levels correlate with impaired cognitive function and cortical metabolism. *Neurology* 1987;37:161–165.

Whitehouse P, Martino A, Antuono P, et al. Nicotinic acetylcholine binding sites in Alzheimer's disease. *Brain Res* 1986;371:146–151.

Whitehouse P, Price D, Clark A, et al. Alzheimer's disease: evidence for selective loss of cholinergic neurons in the nucleus basalis. *Ann Neurol* 1981; 10:122–126.

Whitehouse P, Vale W, Sweig R, et al. Reductions in corticotropin releasing factor-like immunoreactivity in cerebral cortex in Alzheimer's disease, Parkinson's disease, and progressive supranuclear palsy. *Neurology* 1987;37:905–909.

Whitford G. Alzheimer's disease and serotonin: a review. *Neuropsychobiology* 1986;15:133–142.

Xiang Z, Huguenard JR, Prince DA. Cholinergic switching within neocortical inhibitory networks. *Science* 1998;281:985–988.

Zubenko GS, Huff FJ, Becker J, et al. Cognitive function and platelet membrane fluidity in Alzheimer's disease. *Biol Psychiatry* 1988;24:925–936.

Zubenko GS, Teply I. Longitudinal study of platelet membrane fluidity in Alzheimer's disease. *Biol Psychiatry* 1988;24:918–924.

Neurotoxicity

Barnes D. NMDA receptors trigger excitement. *Science* 1988;239:254–256.

Bharucha B. A case control study of association with medical conditions and surgical procedures. *Neurology* 1983;33(suppl 2):85.

Candy J, Edwardson J, Klinowsky J, et al. Colocalization of aluminum and silicone in senile plaques. In: Traber J, Gisbon W, eds. *Senile dementia of the Alzheimer-type.* Berlin: Springer-Verlag, 1985: 183–197.

Crapper D, Krishnon S, Palton A. Brain aluminum distribution in Alzheimer's disease and experimental neurofibrillary degeneration. *Science* 1973;180:511–513.

French L, Schuman L, Mortimer J, et al. A case control study of dementia of the Alzheimer-type. *Am J Epidemiol* 1985;121:414–421.

Greenamyre J. The role of glutamate in neurotransmission and in neurologic disease. *Arch Neurol* 1986;43:1058–1063.

Heyman A, Wilkinson W, Stafford J, et al. Alzheimer's disease: a study of epidemiological aspects. *Ann Neurol* 1984;15:335–341.

Langston J, Irwin I, Langston E, Forno L. Pargyline prevents MPTP-induced parkinsonism in primates. *Science* 1984;225:1481–1482.

Maragos W, Greenamyre J, Penny J, Young A. Glutamate dysfunction in Alzheimer's disease: an hypothesis. *Trends Neurosci* 1987;10:65–68.

Martyn C, Osmond C, Edwardson E. Geographical relation between Alzheimer's disease and aluminum in drinking water. *Lancet* 1989;1:59–62.

McLachlan D, Van Berkum M. Aluminum: a role in degenerative brain disease associated with neurofibrillary degeneration. *Progr Brain Res* 1986;70: 399–408.

Perl D, Good P. The association of aluminum, Alzheimer's disease, and neurofibrillary tangles. *J Neural Transm* 1987;24(suppl):205–211.

Poirier J. Pathophysiology and biochemical mechanisms involved in MPTP-induced parkinsonism. *J Am Geriatr Soc* 1987;35:660–668.

Shalat S, Seltzer B, Pidcock C, Baker E. A case control study of medical and familial history and Alzheimer's disease. *Am J Epidemiol* 1986;124:540.

Shore D, Wyatt R. Aluminum and Alzheimer's disease. *J Nerv Ment Dis* 1983;171:553–558.

Tanner C. The toll of environmental toxins in the etiology of Parkinson's disease. *Trends Neurosci* 1989;12:49–53.

Plasticity

Buell S, Coleman P. Dendritic growth in the aged human brain and failure of growth in senile dementia. *Science* 1979;206:854–856.

Buell S, Coleman PD. Quantitative evidence for selective dendritic growth in normal human aging but not in senile dementia. *Brain Res* 1981;214: 23–41.

Fine R, Rubin J. Specific trophic factor-receptor interactions: key selective elements in brain development and "regeneration." *J Am Geriatr Soc* 1988;36:457–466.

Hefti F, Will B. Nerve growth factor is a neurotropic factor for forebrain cholinergic neurons: implications for Alzheimer's disease. *J Neural Transm* 1987;24(suppl 1):309–315.

Perry E. Hypothesis linking plasticity, vulnerability and nerve growth factor to basal forebrain cholinergic neurons. *Int J Geriatr Psychiatry* 1990;5: 223–231.

Cholinergic Strategies

Agnoli A, Martucci N, Manna V, et al. The effect of cholinergic and anticholinergic drugs on short-term memory in Alzheimer's disease: a neuropsychologic and computerized electroencephalographic study. *Clin Neuropharmacol* 1983;6: 311–323.

Ahlin A, Nyback H, Junthe T, et al. Tetrahydroaminoacridine in Alzheimer's dementia: clinical and biochemical results of a double-blind crossover trial. *Hum Psychopharmacol Clin Exp* 1991; 6: 109–118.

Ashford JW, Sherman KA, Jumar V. Advances in Alzheimer therapy: cholinesterase inhibitors. *Neurobiol Aging* 1989;10:99–105.

Beller SA, Overall JE, Rhoades HM, Swann AC. Long-term outpatient treatment of senile dementia with oral physostigmine. *J Clin Psychiatry* 1988;49:400–404.

Blackwood D, Christie J. The effects of physostigmine on memory and auditory P300 in Alzheimer-type dementia. *Biol Psychiatry* 1986;21: 557–560.

Brinkman S, Sniff R, Meyer J, et al. Lecithin and memory training in suspected Alzheimer's disease. *J Gerontol* 1982;37:4–9.

Canal N, Imbimbo BP, Lucchelli PE, for the Eptastigmine Study Group. A 25-week, double-blind, randomized, placebo-controlled, trial of eptastigmine in patients with diagnosis of probable Alzheimer's disease. *Eur J Neurol* 1996;3(suppl 5)238.

Christie J, Shering A, Ferguson J, Glenn A. Physostigmine and arecoline: effects of intravenous infusions in Alzheimer presenile dementia. *Br J Psychiatry* 1981;138:46–50.

Corona G, Cucchi M, Frattini P, et al. Clinical and biochemical responses to therapy in Alzheimer's disease and multi-infarct dementia. *Eur Arch Psychiatry Neurol Sci* 1989;239:79–86.

Davies B, Andrewes D, Stargatt R, et al. Tacrine in Alzheimer's disease [Letter]. *Lancet* 1989;2: 163–164.

Davis BM, Mohs RC, Greenwald BS, et al. Clinical studies of the cholinergic deficit in Alzheimer's disease. I: Neurochemical and neuroendocrine studies. *J Am Geriatr Soc* 1985;33:741–748.

Davis K, Mohs R. Enhancement of memory processes in Alzheimer's disease with multiple dose intravenous physostigmine. *Am J Psychiatry* 1982; 139: 1421–1424.

Duffy F, McAnulty G, Albert M, et al. Lecithin: absence of neurophysiologic effect in Alzheimer's disease by EEG topography. *Neurology* 1987;37: 1015–1019.

Fitten J, Perryman K, Gross P, et al. Treatment of Alzheimer's disease with short- and long-term oral THA and lecithin: a double-blind study. *Am J Psychiatry* 1990;147:239–242.

Gauthier S, Bouchard R, Bacher Y, et al. Progress report on the Canadian "Multi-centre Trial" of tetrahydroaminoacridine with lecithin in Alzheimer's disease. *Can J Neurol Sci* 1989;16:543–546.

Gauthier S, Bouchard R, Lamontagne A, et al. Tetrahydroamineoacridine-lecithin combination treatment in patients with intermediate-stage Alzheimer's disease: results of a Canadian double-blind, crossover, multicenter study. *N Engl J Med* 1990;322:1272–1276.

Hammel P, Larrey D, Bernuau J, et al. Acute hepatitis after tetrahydroaminoacridine administration for Alzheimer's disease. *J Clin Gastroenterol* 1990; 12:329–331.

Harbaugh R. Intracerebroventricular cholinergic drug administration in Alzheimer's disease. Preliminary result of a double-blind study. *J Neural Transm* 1987;24(suppl):271–277.

Harbaugh R, Roberts D, Coombs D, et al. Preliminary report: intracranial cholinergic drug infusion in patients with Alzheimer's disease. *Neurosurgery* 1984;15:514–518.

Harrell L, Jope R, Falgout J, et al. Biological and neuropsychological characterization of physostigmine responders and nonresponders in Alzheimer's disease. *J Am Geriatr Soc* 1990;38: 113–122.

Hollander E, Davidson M, Mohs R, et al. RS86 in the treatment of Alzheimer's disease: cognitive and biological effects. *Biol Psychiatry* 1987;22: 1067–1078.

Jenike M, Albert M, Baer L. Oral physostigmine as treatment for dementia of the Alzheimer type: a long-term outpatient trial. *Alzheimer Dis Assoc Disord* 1990;4:226–231.

Jenike M, Albert M, Heller H, et al. Oral physostigmine treatment for patients with presenile and senile dementia of the Alzheimer-type: a double-blind, placebo-controlled trial. *J Clin Psychiatry* 1990;51:3–7.

Kaye W, Sitaram N, Weingartner H, et al. Modest facilitation of memory in dementia with combined lecithin and anticholinesterase treatment. *Biol Psychiatry* 1982;17:275–280.

Levy R. Tacrine in Alzheimer's disease [Letter]. *Lancet* 1989;2:329.

Little A, Levy R, Chuagui-Kidd C, Hand D. A double-blind, placebo-controlled trial of high dose lecithin in Alzheimer's disease. *J Neurol Neurosurg Psychiatry* 1985;48:736–742.

Kumar V, Smith RC, Sherman KA, et al. Cortisol responses to cholinergic drugs in Alzheimer's disease. *Int J Clin Pharmacol Ther Toxicol* 1988;26: 471–476.

Marx J. Alzheimer's drug put on hold: signs of liver damage in test patients brings controversial drug study to temporary halt. *Science* 1987;238: 1041–1042.

Mohs R, Davis B, Johns C, et al. Oral physostigmine treatment of patients with Alzheimer's disease. *Am J Psychiatry* 1985;142:28–33.

Mohs RC, Davis BM, Greenwold BS, et al. Clinical studies of the cholinergic deficit in Alzheimer's disease. II: Psychopharmacologic studies. *J Am Geriatr Soc* 1988;33:749–757.

Molloy D, Cape R. Acute effects of oral pyridostigmine on memory and cognitive function in SDAT. *Neurobiol Aging* 1989;10:199–204.

Muramoto O, Sugishita M, Ando K. Cholinergic system and constructional praxis: a further study of physostigmine in Alzheimer's disease. *J Neurol Neurosurg Psychiatry* 1984;47:485–491.

Nyback H, Nynam H, Ohman G, et al. Preliminary experiences with THA for the amelioration of symptoms of Alzheimer's disease. In: Giacobini E, Becker R, eds. *Current research in Alzheimer's therapy.* New York: Taylor & Francis, 1988:231–236.

Oral tetrohydroaminoacridine in treatment of senile dementia, Alzheimer-type [Editorial]. *N Engl J Med* 1987;316:1603–1606.

Palacios J, Spiegel R. Muscarinic cholinergic agonists: pharmacological and clinical perspectives. *Prog Brain Res* 1986;70:485–497.

Palmer A, Stratmann G, Proctor A, Bowen D. Possible neurotransmitter basis of behavioral changes in Alzheimer's disease. *Ann Neurol* 1988;23: 616–620.

Penn S, Martin E, Wilson R, et al. Intraventricular bethanecol infusion for Alzheimer's disease: result of double-blind and escalating dose trials. *Neurology* 1988;38:219–222.

Perry E. Acetylcholine and Alzheimer's disease. *Br J Psychiatry* 1988;152:737–740.

Perry E, Tomlinson B, Blessed G, et al. Correlation of cholinergic abnormalities with senile plaques and mental test scores in senile dementia. *Br Med J* 1978;2:1457–1459.

Pomara N, Domino E, Yoon H, et al. Failure of single dose lecithin to alter aspects of central cholinergic activity in Alzheimer's disease. *J Clin Psychiatry* 1983;44:293–295.

Roberts F, Lazareno S. Cholinergic treatments for Alzheimer's disease. *Biochem Soc Trans* 1989;17: 76–79.

Rose R, Moulthrop M. Differential responsivity of verbal and visual recognition memory to physostigmine and ACTH. *Biol Psychiatry* 1986;21: 538–542.

Sahakian B, Jones G, Levy R, et al. The effects of nicotine on attention, information processing, and short-term memory in patients with dementia of the Alzheimer type. *Br J Psychiatry* 1989;154: 797–800.

Sattin A, Muhoberac BB, Aprison MH, Schauf CL. Tetrahydroaminoacridine (THA) as a pharmacological probe in Alzheimer's disease (AD) and other neurodegenerative disorders. *Med Hypotheses* 1989;29:155–159.

Shimohama S, Taniguchi T, Fujiwara M, Kameyama M. Changes in nicotinic and muscarinic cholinergic receptors in Alzheimer-type dementia. *J Neurochem* 1986;46:288–293.

Stern Y, Sano M, Mayeux R. Effects of oral physostigmine in Alzheimer's disease. *Ann Neurol* 1987;22: 306–310.

Stern Y, Sano M, Mayeux R. Long-term administration of oral physostigmine in Alzheimer's disease. *Neurology* 1988;38:1837–1841.

Summers W, Majovski V, Marsh G, Candeora K. Oral tetrohydroaminoacridine in long-term treatment of senile dementia, Alzheimer-type. *N Engl J Med* 1986;315:1241–1245.

Summers W, Viesselman J, Marsh G. Use of THA in treatment of Alzheimer-like dementia. *Biol Psychiatry* 1981;16:145–153.

Tariot PN, Cohen RM, Welkowitz JA, et al. Multiple-dose arecoline infusions in Alzheimer's disease. *Arch Gen Psychiatry* 1988;45:901–905.

Thal LJ, Masur DM, Blau AD, et al. Chronic oral physostigmine without lecithin improves memory in Alzheimer's disease. *J Am Geriatr Soc* 1989; 37:42–48.

Vida S, Gauthier L, Gauthier S. Canadian collaborative study of tetrahydroaminoacridine (THA) and lecithin treatment of Alzheimer's disease: effect on mood. *Can J Psychiatry* 1989;34:165–170.

Wettstein A. No effect from double-blind trial of physostigmine and lecithin in Alzheimer's disease. *Ann Neurol* 1983;13:210–212.

Whitehouse P. Neurotransmitter receptor alterations in Alzheimer's disease: a review. *Alzheimer Dis Assoc Disord* 1987;1:9–18.

Whitehouse PJ. Intraventricular bethanechol in Alzheimer's disease: a continuing controversy [Editorial]. *Neurology* 1988;38:307–308.

Indoleaminergic Strategies

Cutler N, Haxby J, Kay A, et al. Evaluation of zimeldine in Alzheimer's disease: cognitive and biochemical measures. *Arch Neurol* 1985;42:744–748.

Dehlin O, Hedenrud B, Jansson P, Norgard J. A double-blind comparison of alaproclate and placebo in the treatment of patients with senile dementia. *Acta Psychiatr Scand* 1985;71:190–196.

Lawlor B, Sunderland T, Mellow A, et al. Hyperresponsivity to the serotonin agonist, *m*-chlorophenyl piperazine, in Alzheimer's disease: a controlled study. *Arch Gen Psychiatry* 1989;46:542–549.

Lawlor BA, Mellow AM, Sunderland T, et al. A pilot study of serotonergic system responsivity in Alzheimer's disease. *Psychopharmacol Bull* 1988;24: 127–129.

Serrby M. Neuroleptic malignant syndrome in Alz-

heimer's disease. *J Am Geriatr Soc* 1986;34: 895–896.

Smith D, Stromgren E, Peterson H, et al. Lack of effect of tryptophan treatment in demented gerontopsychiatric patients. *Acta Psychiatr Scand* 1984;70:470–477.

Neuronal Growth/Plasticity

Ala T, Romero S, Knight F, et al. GM-1 treatment of Alzheimer's disease. *Arch Neurol* 1990;47:1126–1130.

Butcher L, Wolf N. Neurotrophic agents may exacerbate the pathologic cascade of Alzheimer's disease. *Neurobiol Aging* 1989;10:557–570.

Marx J. NGF and Alzheimer's: hopes and fears. *Science* 1990;247:408–410.

Phelps C, Gage F, Growdon J, et al. Potential use of nerve growth factor to treat Alzheimer's disease (ad hoc Working Group on Nerve Growth Factor in Alzheimer's Disease). *Science* 1989;243:11.

Villardita C, Grioli S, Salmeri G, et al. Multi-center clinical trial of brain phosphatidylserine in elderly patients with intellectual deterioration. *Clin Trials J* 1987;24:84–93.

Wesseling H, Agoston S, Vandam G. Effects of 4-aminopyridine in elderly patients with Alzheimer's disease. *N Engl J Med* 1984;310:988–989.

Blood Flow

Prohovanik I, Smith G, Sackeim HA, et al. The early stages of presenile and senile Alzheimer's disease: limited studies of disease severity and cerebral blood flow. In: Fisher A, Hanin I, Lachinon R, eds. *Alzheimer's and Parkinson's diseases*. New York: Plenum, 1986:233–239.

Metabolic Enhancement

Albizzati M, Bassi S, Calloni E, et al. Cyclandelate vs. flunarizone: a double-blind study in a selected group of patients with dementia. *Drugs* 1987; 33(suppl 2):90–96.

Balestreri R, Fontana L, Astengo F. A double-blind, placebo-controlled evaluation of the safety and efficacy of vinpocetine in the treatment of chronic vascular senile cerebral dysfunction. *J Am Geriatr Soc* 1987;35:425–430.

Bergman I, Brane G, Gottfries C, et al. Alaproclate: a pharmacokinetic and biochemical study in patients with dementia of the Alzheimer-type. *Psychopharmacology* 1983;80:279–283.

Davidson M, Zemishlany Z, Mohs R. 4-Aminopyridine in the treatment of Alzheimer's disease. *Biol Psychiatry* 1988;23:485–490.

Gosz K. Oxpentifylline in dementia: a controlled study. *Arch Gerontol Geriatr* 1987;6:19–26.

Growdon J, Corkin S, Huff F, Rosen T. Piracetam combined with lecithin in the treatment of Alzheimer's disease. *Neurobiol Aging* 1986;7: 269–276.

Jenike M, Albert S, Heller H, et al. Combination therapy with lecithin and ergoloid mesylates for

Alzheimer's disease. *J Clin Psychiatry* 1986;47: 249–251.

Lazzari R, Franzese A, Chierichetti S, et al. Multicenter double-blind, placebo-controlled, long-term clinical trial of Hydergine in chronic senile cerebral insufficiency: an interim report. In: Agnoli A, ed. *Aging brain and ergot alkaloids.* Vol. 23. New York: Raven Press, 1983:347–371.

Nicholson C. Pharmacology of nootropics and metabolically active compounds in relation to their use in dementia. *Psychopharmacology* 1990;101: 147–159.

Parnetti L, Ciufetti G, Mercuri M, Senin U. Haemorheological pattern in initial mental deterioration: results of a long-term study using piracetam and pentoxifylline. *Arch Gerontol Geriatr* 1985;4: 141–155.

Passeri M, Cucinotta D, DeMello M, et al. Minaprine for senile dementia. *Lancet* 1985;1:824.

Reynolds C, Perel J, Kupfer D, et al. Open-trial response to antidepressant treatment in elderly patients with mixed depression and cognitive impairment. *Psychiatry Res* 1987;21:111–122.

Saletu B, Linzmayer L, Grunberger J, Pietschmann H. Double-blind, placebo-controlled, clinical, psychometric and neurophysiological investigations with oxiracetam in the organic brain syndrome of late life. *Neuropsychobiology* 1985;13: 44–52.

Sourander L, Portin R, Molsa P, et al. Senile dementia of the Alzheimer-type treated with aniracetam: a new nootropic agent. *Psychopharmacology* 1987;91:90–95.

Sunderland T, Tariot PN, Mueller EA. TRH stimulation test in dementia of the Alzheimer-type, and elder and elderly controls. *Psychiatry Res* 1985;16: 225–269.

Thal L, Salmone D, Lasker B, et al. The safety and lack of efficacy of vinpocetine in Alzheimer's disease. *J Am Geriatr Soc* 1989;37:515–520.

Thienhaus O, Wheeler B, Simon S, et al. A controlled double-blind study of high dose dihydroergotoxine mesylate (Hydergine) in mild dementia. *J Am Geriatr Soc* 1987;35:219–223.

van Loveren-Huiben C, Engelarr H, Hermans M, et al. Double-blind clinical and psychologic study of ergoloid mesylates (Hydergine) in subjects with senile mental deterioration. *J Am Geriatr Soc* 1984; 32:584–588.

Monoaminergic Strategies

Agnoli A, Martucci N, Fabrini G, et al. Monoamine oxidase and dementia: treatment with an inhibitor of MAO-B activity. *Dementia* 1990;1:109–114.

Alber S, Goldberg M, Choi D. N-Methyl-D-aspartate antagonists: ready for clinical trial in brain ischemia? *Ann Neurol* 1989;25:398–403.

Amaducci L, SMID Group. Phosphatidylserine in the treatment of clinically diagnosed Alzheimer's disease. *J Neural Transm* 1987;24(suppl):287–292.

Bonavita E. Study of the efficacy and tolerability of L-acetylcarnitine therapy in the senile brain. *Int J Clin Pharmacol Ther Toxicol* 1986;24:511–516.

Campi N, Todeschini G, Scarzella L. Selegiline (deprenyl) versus L-acetylcarnitine in the treatment

of Alzheimer-type dementia. *Clin Ther* 1990;12: 306–314.

Cohen B, Satlin A, Zubenko G. S-Adenosyl-L-methionine in the treatment of Alzheimer's disease. *J Clin Psychopharmacol* 1988;8:43–47.

Cohen R, Sunerland T, Aulakh C. Antidepressants in states of cognitive dysfunction. *Drug Dev Res* 1984;4:517–532.

Davidson M, Bierer L, Kaminsky R, et al. Combined administration of physostigmine and clonidine to patients with dementia of the Alzheimer type: a pilot safety study. *Alzheimer Dis Assoc Disord* 1989; 3:224–227.

Fleischacker W, Buchgeher A, Schubert H. Memantine in the treatment of senile dementia of the Alzheimer-type. *Prog Neuropsychopharmacol Biol Psychiatry* 1986;10:87–93.

Martini E, Pataky I, Szilagy IK, et al. Brief information on an early phase II study with deprenyl in demented patients. *Pharmacopsychiatry* 1987;20: 256–257.

Meyer J, Rogers R, McClintic K, et al. Randomized clinical trial of daily aspirin therapy in multi-infarct dementia: a pilot study. *J Am Geriatr Soc* 1989; 37:549–555.

Monteverde A, Gnemmi P, Rossi F, et al. Selegeline (deprenyl) in the treatment of mild-to-moderate Alzheimer-type dementia. *Clin Ther* 1990;12: 315–322.

Palmieri G, Palmieri R, Inzoli M, et al. Double-blind controlled trial of phosphatidylserine in patients with senile mental deterioration. *Clin Trial J* 1987;24:73–83.

Piccinin G, Finali G, Piccirilli M. Neuropsychological effects of L-deprenyl in Alzheimer's type dementia. *Clin Neuropharmacol* 1990;13:147–163.

Rai G, Wright G, Scott L, et al. Double-blind, placebo-controlled study of acetyl-L-carnitine in patients with Alzheimer's disease. *Curr Med Res Opin* 1990;11:638–647.

Reding M, Young R, DiPonte P. Amitriptyline in Alzheimer's disease [Letter]. *Neurology* 1983;33: 522–523.

Reinkainen KJ, Palianvi L, Hadonen T, et al. Dopamine system and monoamine oxidase-B activity in Alzheimer's disease. *Neurol Aging* 1988;9: 245–252.

Tariot P, Cohen R, Sunderland T, et al. L-Deprenyl in Alzheimer's disease: preliminary evidence for behavioral change with monoamine oxidase-B inhibition. *Arch Gen Psychiatry* 1987;44:427–433.

Tariot PN, Sunderland T, Cohen RM, et al. Tranylcypromine compared with L-deprenyl in Alzheimer's disease. *J Clin Psychopharmacol* 1988;8: 23–27.

Peptidergic Strategies

Blass J, Reding M, Drachman D, et al. Naloxone in Alzheimer's disease [Letter]. *N Engl J Med* 1983; 309:566.

Henderson V, Roberts E, Wimer C, et al. Naloxone treatment fails in Alzheimer's disease patients. *Ann Neurol* 1989;25:404–406.

Hyman B, Eslinger B, Demasio A. Effect of naltrexone on senile dementia of the Alzheimer-type. *J Neurol Neurosurg Psychiatry* 1985;48:1169–1171.

Jolles J. Neuropeptides in the treatment of cognitive deficits in aging and dementia. *Prog Brain Res* 1986;70:429–440.

Panela J, Blass J. Lack of clinical benefit from naloxone in a dementia day hospital. *Ann Neurol* 1984; 15:308.

Pomara N, Roberts R, Rheiw B, et al. Multiple, single-dose naltrexone administrations fail to affect overall cognitive functioning and plasma cortisol in individuals with probable Alzheimer's disease. *Neurobiol Aging* 1985;6:223–236.

Pomara N, Stanley M, Rhiew HB, et al. Loss of the cortisol response to naltrexone in Alzheimer's disease. *Biol Psychiatry* 1988;23:726–733.

Reisberg B, Ferris S, Anand R, et al. Effects of naloxone in senile dementia. A double-blind trial. *N Engl J Med* 1983;308:721–722.

Steiger W, Mendelson M, Jenkins T, et al. Effects of naloxone in treatment of senile dementia. *J Am Geriatr Soc* 1985;33:155.

Tariot P, Sunderland T, Weingartner H, et al. Naloxone and Alzheimer's disease: cognitive and behavioral effects of a range of doses. *Arch Gen Psychiatry* 1986;43:727–732.

Tariot PN, Goss M, Sunderland T, et al. High dose naloxone in older normal subjects: implications for Alzheimer's disease. *J Am Geriatr Soc* 1988;36: 681–686.

Transplant

Collier T. Neural transplantation in Alzheimer's disease: the evidence from animal models. In: Altman H, Altman B, eds. *Alzheimer's and Parkinson's diseases.* New York: Plenum, 1989:291–324.

Gash D, Collier T, Sladek J. Neural transplantation a review of recent developments and potential applications to aged brain. *Neurobiol Aging* 1985; 6:131–150.

Miscellaneous Therapies

Cardelli M, Russell M, Bagne C, Pomara N. Chelation therapy: unproved modality in the treatment of Alzheimer-type dementia. *J Am Geriatr Soc* 1985;33:548–551.

Fillit H, Weinreb H, Cholst I, et al. Observations in a preliminary open trial of estradiol therapy for senile dementia-Alzheimer's type. *Psychoneuroendocrinology* 1986;11:337–345.

Phelps CH, Gage FH, Growdon JH, et al. Potential use of nerve growth factor to treat Alzheimer's disease. *Neurobiol Aging* 1989;10:205–207.

Serrby M. Neuroleptic malignant syndrome in Alzheimer's disease. *J Am Geriatr Soc* 1986;34: 895–896.

Soininen H, Koskinen C, Helkala E. Treatment of Alzheimer's disease with a synthetic ACTH 4–9 analog. *Neurology* 1985;35:1348–1351.

Van Tiggalen C. Alzheimer's disease/alcohol dementia: association with zinc deficiency and cerebral vitamin B deficiency. *J Orthomol Psychiatry* 1984;13:97–101.

Yamamoto T, Ishihara S, Okada H, et al. In vivo effects by estrone sulfates on the central nervous system—senile dementia (Alzheimer's type). *J Steroid Biochem* 1989;34:511–515.

Other Dementias

Balestreri R, Fontana L, Astengo F. A double-blind controlled evaluation of the safety and efficacy of vinpocetine in the treatment of patients with chronic vascular senile cerebral dysfunction. *J Am Geriatr Soc* 1987;35:425–430.

Blakemore C. Cyclandelate in the treatment of multi-infarct dementia. Interim findings from a multi-center study in general practice. *Drugs* 1987;33(suppl 2):110–113.

Langlais P, Mair R, Whalen P, et al. Memory effect of DL-threo-3-4-dihydrooxiphenylserine (DOPS) in human Korsakoff's disease. *Psychopharmacology* 1988;95:250–254.

Parkinson Study Group. Effect of deprenyl on the progression of disability in early Parkinson's disease. *N Engl J Med* 1989;321:1364–1371.

Pert C, Ruff M, Hill J. AIDS as a neuropeptide disorder: peptide T, VIP and the HIV receptor. *Psychopharmacol Bull* 1988;24:315–319.

Ransmayr G, Plorer S, Gerestenbrand F, Bauer G. Double-blind, placebo-controlled phosphatidylserine in elderly patients with arteriosclerotic encephalopathy. *Clin Trial J* 1987;24:62–72.

Sebul R. Aspirin and MID: notes of caution [Editorial]. *J Am Geriatr Soc* 1989;37:573–575.

Sheardown M, Nielsen E, Hansen A, et al. 2,3-dihydroxy-6-nitro-7-sulfamoyl-benzo(F) quinoxaline: a neuroprotectant for cerebral ischemia. *Science* 1990;247:571–574.

Tetrud J, Langston W. The effect of deprenyl (selegiline) on the natural history of Parkinson's disease. *Science* 1989;245:519–522.

Yarchoan R, Thomas R, Grafman J, et al. Long-term administration of 3-azido-2,3-dideoxythymidine to patients with AIDS-related neurological disease. *Ann Neurol* 1988;23(suppl):S82–S87.

Young A, Greenamyre J, Hollingsworth Z, et al. NMDA receptor losses in putamen from patients with Huntington's disease. *Science* 1988;241: 981–983.

Appendix A

Prescribing Information

Carl Salzman

The drug dosages presented here are meant as recommendations for the ranges appropriate for elderly patients. In many cases, the therapeutic range has not been clearly established. Often, older patients respond to lower doses than those prescribed for younger patients. Some elderly patients, however, may in fact require usual adult dose or higher doses to experience therapeutic effect. Side effects such as sedation, postural hypotension, and anticholinergic toxicity are possible consequences against which dosages must be titrated. Whenever possible, closely following serum levels of medications such as carbamazepine, tricyclic antidepressants, lithium, and valproic acid is critical because older patients have a greater potential for toxicity at lower doses than younger patients.

Drug Names and Geriatric Dosages

Generic Name	Trade Name	Approximate Daily Dose Range (mg)	Brief Comments
FIRST GENERATION ANTIPSYCHOTICS			
Chlorpromazine	Thorazine	10–200	Sedation and orthostatic hypotension limit usefulness for elderly
Fluphenazine	Prolixin	0.25–4	High-potency phenothiazine; EPS common in elderly
Haloperidol	Haldol	0.25–4	High-potency butryrophenone; EPS common in elderly; very low doses may be effective with less EPS
Loxapine	Loxitane	10–100	Midpotency thioxanthine; few studies in elderly
Mesoridazine	Serentil	10–200	Similar to thioridazine
Perphenazine	Trilafon	2–32	Midpotency phenothiazine; EPS common in elderly at higher doses
Pimozide	Orap	0.25–4	No data for use in elderly patients; same action as haloperidol

(continued)

Drug Names and Geriatric Dosages *(continued)*

Generic Name	Trade Name	Approximate Daily Dose Range (mg)	Brief Comments
Thioridazine	Mellaril	10–200	Low-potency phenothiazine; sedation, cardiac arrhythmia, and hypotension may limit high-dose use
Thiothixene	Navane	1–15	High-potency thioxanthine; same action as trifluoperazine
Trifluoperazine	Stelazine	1–15	High-potency phenothiazine; EPS common in elderly in high doses

SECOND GENERATION ANTIPSYCHOTICS

Generic Name	Trade Name	Approximate Daily Dose Range (mg)	Brief Comments
Aripiprazole	Abilify		May be activating and may increase agitation
Clozapine	Clozaril	10–100	May be too sedating and too anticholinergic; agranulocytosis and respiratory problems reported in elderly
Olanzapine	Zyprexa	1.25–10	Dose range not established for elderly; sedating; weight gain; may also be associated with development of diabetes
Quetiapine	Seroquel	25–200	Sedating; useful for sleep and agitation
Risperidone	Risperdal	0.25–2	May be activating; causes EPS; long-acting form available
Ziprasidone	Geodon	20–80	Dose range not established for elderly; may be activating; prolonged QTc interval reported in younger patients

TRICYCLIC ANTIDEPRESSANTS

Generic Name	Trade Name	Approximate Daily Dose Range (mg)	Brief Comments
Amitriptyline	Elavil	10–75	Tertiary amine tricyclic; strong anticholinergic, sedating, and hypotensive side effects
Amoxapine	Asendin	10–300	Secondary amine tricyclic; metabolite may block dopamine and cause EPS
Clomipramine	Anafranil	10–250	See amitriptyline; used to treat OCD but usual therapeutic doses may be toxic to elderly
Desipramine	Norpramin	10–75	Secondary amine recommended for use with elderly; therapeutic plasma levels same as for younger patients
Doxepin	Sinequan	10–75	See amitriptyline
Imipramine	Tofranil	10–75	See amitriptyline
Nortriptyline	Pamelor	10–100	Secondary amine recommended for use with elderly; best studied of all antidepressants for older patients; therapeutic plasma levels same as for younger adults
Protriptyline	Vivactil	5–20	Secondary amine, but strongly anticholinergic; very long elimination half-life; no data on use in elderly
Trimipramine	Surmontil	10–75	See amitriptyline

(continued)

Drug Names and Geriatric Dosages *(continued)*

Generic Name	Trade Name	Approximate Daily Dose Range (mg)	Brief Comments
SELECTIVE SEROTONIN REUPTAKE INHIBITORS			
Citalopram	Celexa	50–20	May be sedating; no significant pharmacokinetic drug interactions
Escitalopram	Lexapro	5–20	See citalopram
Fluoxetine	Prozac	5–40	Upper dose range not established for elderly; may be activating and cause insomnia; long half-life; inhibits CP450 IID6 (see Appendix B)
Fluvoxamine	Luvox	50–150	Dose range for elderly not established; not marketed in U.S. as antidepressant; does not inhibit CP450 11D6; inhibits CP450 IA2 (see Appendix B)
Paroxetine	Paxil	5–20	May be sedating, anticholinergic; strong inhibitor of CP450 11D6
Sertraline	Zoloft	12.5–150	May inhibit CP450 3A/4 at high doses; can cause nausea and gastrointestinal upset; mildly anticholinergic; sedating; inhibits CP450 11D6; does not inhibit CP450 3A/4 (see Appendix B)
NEW AND ATYPICAL ANTIDEPRESSANTS			
Bupropion	Wellbutrin	75–225	Upper dose range not established for elderly; may be activating; extended release form commonly used
Trazodone	Desyrel	25–200	Very sedating; useful addition to other antidepressants for sleep
Mirtazapine	Remeron	7.4–45	Dose range not established for elderly; insufficient research data to guide clinical prescribing; sedating in younger adults
Nefazadone	Serzone	50–200	Upper dose range not established for elderly; sedating
Venlafaxine	Effexor	12.5–225	May cause nausea, headaches, and elevated blood pressure at higher doses; no CP450 isoenzyme interactions; extended release form commonly used
MONOAMINE OXIDASE INHIBITORS			
Phenelzine	Nardil	7.5–30	Caution necessary because of high risk of adverse drug reactions due to increased polypharmacy in elderly; must not be added to mepridine or SSRI antidepressants; hypotension a common side effect
Tranylcypromine	Parnate	5–30	See phenelzine

(continued)

Drug Names and Geriatric Dosages   *(continued)*

Generic Name	Trade Name	Approximate Daily Dose Range (mg)	Brief Comments
ANXIOLYTICS			
Alprazolam	Xanax	0.125–1	Relatively short half-life; may cause rebound and withdrawal if abruptly discontinued; extended release form available; associated with falls, sedation, decreased recall
Chlordiazepoxide	Librium	10–40	Long half-life benzodiazepine; not recommended for routine antianxiety use in elderly; associated with falls, sedation, decreased recall
Clorazepate	Tranxene	3.75–15	See chlordiazepoxide
Clonazepam	Klonopin	0.125–1	Long half-life; very sedating, see alprazolam
Diazepam	Valium	2–20	See chlordiazepoxide
Hydroxyzine	Atarax, Vistaril, Marax	25–100	Strongly antihistaminic; may interfere with cognition; sedating; not routinely used for elderly
Lorazepam	Ativan	10–45	See alprazolam; useful in elderly
Oxazepam	Serax	10–45	Useful in elderly; delayed absorption and onset of action; see alprazolam
Buspirone	Buspar	5–80	Antianxiety effect at low dose unpredictable; modest antiagitation effects at higher doses
HYPNOTICS			
Estazolam	Pro-Som	0.5–2	Moderately long half-life
Flurazepam	Dalmane	7.5–30	Very long half-life; demonstrated toxicity in elderly at high doses; not recommended for routine elderly use
Temazepam	Restoril	7.5–30	Intermediate half-life
Triazolam	Halcion	0.125–0.25	Ultra-short half-life; may be associated with rebound insomnia and need for additional dose during night
Zaleplon	Sonata	5–10	Blood levels and toxicity increased by inhibitors of 3A/4
Zolpidem	Ambien	5–10	Behaves like short half-life benzodiazepine; may have less cognitive impairment than benzodiazepines
MOOD STABILIZERS			
Carbamazepine	Tegretol	50–1200	May cause agranulocytosis; induces its own metabolism and other drugs metabolized by CP450 3A/4 (see Appendix B)
Gabapentin	Neurontin	100-?	Excretion reduced by renal impairment; sedating; useful for sleep and agitation

(continued)

Drug Names and Geriatric Dosages   *(continued)*

Generic Name	Trade Name	Approximate Daily Dose Range (mg)	Brief Comments
Lamotrigine	Lamictal	?	Usefulness in elderly not yet established
Lithium	Eskalith, Lithobid	75–1500	May be effective at very low blood levels (e.g., 0.2–0.4); may cause cognitive side effects resembling dementia
Oxcarbazepine	Trileptal	150-1200	Headache, sedation, and ataxia are side effects; does not inhibit hepatic enzymes but may induce 3A/4 (see Appendix B)
Tiagabine	Gabitril	?	Insufficient data in elderly; dizziness, anxiety, and sedation are common side effects
Topiramate	Topamax	25–100	Usefulness in elderly unclear; cognitive dysfunction at high doses
Valproic acid	Depakene, Depakote	125–1800	May cause weight gain; may impair concentration and recall
Zonisamide	Zonegran	?	Usefulness in the elderly not yet established

STIMULANTS

Generic Name	Trade Name	Approximate Daily Dose Range (mg)	Brief Comments
Amphetamines	Adderall, Dexedrine	? ?	Has not been studied in elderly Has not been studied in elderly All amphetamines cause/increase agitation
Methylphenidate	Ritalin, Concerta	2.5–10 18.5	Frequently used to increase energy in elderly; may increase agitation and interfere with sleep. Extended release form is available
Modafanil	Provigil	50–200	Has not been studied in elderly
Pemoline	Cylert	?	Has not been studied in elderly

COGNITIVE ENHANCERS

Generic Name	Trade Name	Approximate Daily Dose Range (mg)	Brief Comments
Donepezil	Aricept	5–10	Nausea, diarrhea, and insomnia more common at higher dose
Galantamine	Reminyl	16–24	Nausea and vomiting. More common at higher doses
Rivastigmine	Exelon	6–12	Nausea and vomiting are common at higher dose
Tacrine	Cognex	10–80	Frequent GI side effects, ataxia, and elevated LFTs
Memantine	Namenda	5–10	Modesty slows progression of advanced Alzheimer's disease

Enzyme Metabolism and Drug Interactions

Michelle Wiersgalla

Carl Salzman

Virtually all medications taken by the elderly undergo complex hepatic biotransformation (the only exception is lithium, which does not undergo metabolism of any kind prior to excretion). These enzyme systems render medications (the substrates upon which the enzyme exerts its chemical activity) harmless and transform them to water-soluble compounds in preparation for renal excretion. Known collectively as the cytochrome P450 enzyme family (CYP 450), the enzymes most commonly involved in the metabolism of psychotropic drugs are subdivided into subfamilies, or isoenzyme systems: CYP 1A2; CYP 2B6; CYP 2C9/10; CYP 2C19; CYP 2D6; CYP 3A3/4. The names and letters derive from the genetic construction of the isoenzymes and serve to identify the different subfamilies. Considerable overlap occurs in the metabolic function of these isoenzyme families, so medications may be metabolized by more than one isoenzyme.

Many factors, such as age, play an important role in regulating the metabolism of drugs via the CYP 450 enzyme system; Chapter 4 reviews these age-related changes and their clinical consequences. This appendix presents six tables. The first lists psychotropic medications according to the isoenzyme primarily responsible for their metabolism. In Table B.2, the medications are listed alphabetically by therapeutic indication; when more than one isoenzyme is involved in the metabolism, the primary metabolizer is printed in **boldface.** For example, amitriptyline is primarily metabolized by the 2D6 isoenzyme, but 3A3/4, 1A2, 2C9/10, and 2C19 also contribute to its biotransformation.

Isoenzyme activity is a function of physical health of the liver and age, but it is also affected by the presence of drugs or chemicals other than its substrate. Often, other drugs inhibit the activity of an isoenzyme. When this occurs, biotransformation is impaired or delayed, resulting in a rise in the plasma level of the active medication and a delay in its elimination. Since older people are likely to be taking several medications simultaneously (see Chapter 2), this inhibition is of increased concern when treating them. Not all drug inhibition has serious clinical consequences, however. Table B.3 lists inhibitors of CYP 450 isoenzymes; clinically serious or common inhibitions are in **boldface.** Some psychotropic medications significantly inhibit their own metabolism (e.g., paroxetine and fluoxetine). Other medications may inhibit the metabolism of a second medication that is commonly co-prescribed. For example, fluoxetine and paroxetine commonly raise the blood levels of tricyclic antidepressants by inhibiting 2D6; the resultant tricyclic plasma level may increase as much as fourfold.

Some psychotropic drugs may also inhibit enzymes responsible for the bio-transformation of drugs used to treat medical conditions, resulting in potential toxicity. For example, the isoenzyme 3A3/4 metabolizes numerous medications, including calcium channel blockers (e.g., nifedipine, diltiazem, verapamil), antibiotics (e.g., erythromycin, clarithromycin, triacetyloleandomycin), antihistamines (e.g., terfenadine, astemizole), and antiarrythmics (e.g., quinidine, lidocaine). An inhibitor of 3A3/4 such as the antidepressant nefazodone thus might place an elderly person at risk of drug toxicity if prescribed with any of these other medications. The nonpsychotropic medications and their metabolizing enzymes are listed in Table B.4.

Less commonly, some medications or chemical substances may cause an increase in hepatic enzyme activity (i.e., they "induce" the enzyme). When this occurs, plasma levels of the medication may fall below the minimally effective concentration. Well-known inducers of isoenzyme activity include cigarette smoking (1A2) and phenobarbital and phenytoin (3A3/4, 2C9/10, 1A2, 2D6, 2C19). Carbamazepine, a mood stabilizer used to treat mania in the elderly (see Chapter 12), and severe agitation (see Chapter 6) induces its own metabolism so that doses of carbamazepine may require adjustment upward. Common inducers of psychotropic medications are listed in Table B.5.

The main sources for data summarized in Tables B.1–5 are listed at the end of Appendix B.

References

Anderson GD. A mechanistic approach to antiepileptic drug interactions. *Ann Pharmacother* 1998; 32:554–563.

Anderson JR, Nawarskas JJ. Cardiovascular drug-drug interactions. *Cardiol Clin* 2001;19:215–234.

Anonymous. Aripiprazole (Abilify) for schizophrenia. *Med Lett Drugs Ther* 2003;45:15–16.

Arlander E, Ekstrom G, Alm C, et al. Metabolism of ropivacaine in humans is mediated by CYP1A2 and to a minor extent by CYP3A4: an interaction study with fluvoxamine and ketoconazole as in vivo inhibitors. *Clin Pharm Ther* 1998;64:484–491.

Ball SE, Ahern D, Scatina J, Kao J. Venlafaxine: in vitro inhibition of CYP2D6 dependent imipramine and desipramine metabolism; comparative studies with selected SSRIs, and effects on human hepatic CYP3A4, CYP2C9, and CYP1A2. *Br J Clin Pharmacol* 1997;43:619–626.

Brachtendorf L, Jetter A, Beckurts KT, et al. Cytochrome P450 enzymes contributing to the demethylation of maprotiline in man. *Pharmacol Toxicol* 2002;90:144–149.

Brown CS, Markowitz JS, Moore TR, Parker NG. Atypical antipsychotics: Part II: Adverse effects, drug interactions, and costs. *Ann of Pharmacother* 1999;33:210–217.

Caccia S. Metabolism of the newer antidepressants: an overview of the pharmacological and pharmacokinetic implications. *Clin Pharmacokinet* 1998; 34:281–302.

Catterson ML, Preskorn SH, Martin RL. Pharmacodynamic and pharmacokinetic considerations in geriatric psychopharmacology. *Psychiatr Clin North Am* 1997;20:205–218.

Chouinard G, Lefko-Singh K, Teboul E. Metabolism of anxiolytics and hypnotics: benzodiazepines, buspirone, zopiclone, and zolpidem. *Cell Mol Neurobiol* 1999;19:533–552.

Corsini A, Bellosta S, Baetta R, et al. New insights into the pharmacodynamic and pharmacokinetic properties of statins. *Pharmacol Ther* 1999; 84:413–428.

Coutts RT, Urichuk LJ. Polymorphic cytochromes P450 and drugs used in psychiatry. *Cell Mol Neurobiol* 1999;19:325–354.

Curran S, de Pauw K. Selecting an antidepressant for use in a patient with epilepsy: safety considerations. *Drug Safety* 1998;18:125–133.

DeVane CL. Interaction potential of selective serotonin-reuptake inhibitors. *Am J Health-Syst Pharm* 2000;57:1802.

DeVane CL, Markowitz JS. Avoiding psychotropic drug interactions in the cardiovascular patient. *Bull Menninger Clin* 2000;64:49–59.

DeVane CL, Nemeroff CB. An evaluation of risperidone drug interactions. *J Clin Psychopharmacol* 2001;21:408–416.

Dresser GK, Spence JD, Bailey DG. Pharmacokinetic-pharmacodynamic consequences and clinical relevance of cytochrome P450 3A4 inhibition. *Clin Pharmacokinet* 2000;38:41–57.

Ereshefsky L. Pharmacologic and pharmacokinetic considerations in choosing an antipsychotic. *J Clin Psychiatry* 1999;60(suppl 10):20–30.

Ereshefsky L, Dugan D. Review of the pharmacokinetics, pharmacogenetics, and drug interaction potential of antidepressants: focus on venlafaxine. *Depress Anxiety* 2000;12(suppl 1):30–44.

Faucette SR, Hawke RL, Shord SS, et al. Evaluation of the contribution of cytochrome P450 3A4 to human liver microsomal bupropion hydroxylation. *Drug Metab Dispos* 2001;29:1123–1129.

Frye RF, Branch RA. Effect of chronic disulfiram administration on the activities of CYP1A2, CYP2C19, CYP2D6, CYP2E1, and N-acetyltransferase in healthy human subjects. *Br J Clin Pharmacol* 2002;53:155–162.

Ghahramani P, Ellis SW, Lennard MS, et al. Cytochromes P450 mediating the N-demethylation of amitriptyline. *Br J Clin Pharmacol* 1997;43:137–144.

Harvey AT, Preskorn SH. Fluoxetine pharmacokinetics and effect on CYP 2C19 in young and elderly volunteers. *J Clin Psychopharmacol* 2001;21:161–166.

Hemeryck A, De Vriendt C, Belpaire FM. Inhibition of CYP2C9 by selective serotonin reuptake inhibitors: in vitro studies with tolbutamide and (S)-warfarin using human liver microsomes. *Eur J Clin Pharmacol* 1999;54:947–951.

Hesse LM, Vankatakrishnan K, Court MH, et al. CYP 2B6 mediates the in vitro hydroxylation of bupropion: potential drug interactions with other antidepressants. *Drug Metab Dispos* 2000;28:1176–1183.

Hesse LM, von Moltke LL, Shader RI, et al. Ritonavir, efavirenz, and nelfinavir inhibit CYP2B6 activity in vitro; potential drug interactions with bupropion. *Drug Metab Dispos* 2001;29:100–102.

Huang F, Lasseter KC, Janssens L, et al. Pharmacokinetic and safety assessments of galantamine and risperidone after the two drugs are administered alone and together. *J Clin Pharmacol* 2002;42:1341–1351.

Jann MW, Shirley KL, Small GW. Clinical pharmacokinetics and pharmacodynamics of cholinesterase inhibitors. *Clin Pharmacokinet* 2002;41:719–739.

Jeppesen U, Gram LF, Vistisen K, et al. Dose-dependent inhibition of CYP1A2, CYP2C19, and CYP2D6 by citalopram, fluoxetine, fluvoxamine, and paroxetine. *Eur J Clin Pharmacol* 1996;51:73–78.

Kashuba AD, Nafziger AN, Kearns GL, et al. Effect of fluvoxamine therapy on the activities of CYP1A2, CYP2D6, and CYP3A as determined by phenotyping. *Clin Pharm Ther* 1998;64:257–268.

Kobayashi K, Chiba K, Yagi T, et al. Identification of cytochrome P450 isoforms involved in citalopram N-demethylation by human liver microsomes. *J Pharmacol Exp Ther* 1997;280:927–933.

Kobayashi K, Ishizuka T, Shimada N, et al. Sertraline N-demethylation is catalyzed by multiple isoforms of human cytochrome P-450 in vitro. *Drug Metab Dispos* 1999;27:763–766.

Koyama E, Chiba K, Tani M, et al. Reappraisal of human CYP isoforms involved in imipramine N-demethylation and 2-hydroxylation: a study using microsomes obtained from putative extensive and poor metabolizers of S-mephenytoin and eleven recombinant human CYPs. *J Pharmacol Exp Ther* 1997;281:1199–1210.

Lloyd P, Flesch G, Dieterle W. Clinical pharmacology and pharmacokinetics of oxcarbazepine. *Epilepsia* 1994;35(suppl 3):S10–13.

Madsen H, Rasmussen BB, Brosen K. Imipramine demethylation in vivo: impact of CYP1A2, CYP2C19, and CYP3A4. *Clin Pharm Ther* 1997;61:319–324.

Mahmood I, Sahajwalla C Clinical pharmacokinetics and pharmacodynamics of buspirone, an anxiolytic drug. *Clin Pharmacokinet* 1999;36:277–287.

Olesen OV, Linnet K. Fluvoxamine-clozapine drug interaction: inhibition in vitro of five cytochrome P450 isoforms involved in clozapine metabolism. *J Clin Psychopharmacol* 2000;20:35–42.

Olesen OV, Linnet K. Hydroxylation and demethylation of the tricyclic antidepressant nortriptyline by cDNA-expressed human cytochrome P450 isozymes. *Drug Metab Dispos* 1997;25:740–744.

Olesen OV, Linnet K. Metabolism of the tricyclic antidepressant amitriptyline by cDNA-expressed human cytochrome P450 enzymes. *Pharmacology* 1997;55:235–243.

Olesen OV, Linnet K. Studies on the stereoselective metabolism of citalopram by human liver microsomes and cDNA-expressed cytochrome P450 enzymes. *Pharmacology* 1999;59:298–309.

Olver JS, Burrows GD, Norman TR. Third-generation antidepressants: do they offer advantages over the SSRIs? *CNS Drugs* 2001;15:941–954.

Owen JR, Nemeroff CB. New antidepressants and the cytochrome P450 system: focus on venlafaxine, nefazodone, and mirtazepine. *Depress Anxiety* 1998;7(suppl 1):24–32.

Paoletti R, Corsini A, Bellosta S. Pharmacological interactions of statins. *Atheroscler Suppl* 2002;3:35–40.

Pearce RE, Vakkalagadda GR, Leeder JS. Pathways of carbamazepine bioactivation in vitro I: characterization of human cytochromes P450 responsible for the formation of 2- and 3-hydroxylated metabolites. *Drug Metab Dispos* 2002;30:1170–1179.

Poolsup N, Li Wan Po A, Knight TL. Pharmacogenetics and psychopharmacotherapy. *J Clin Pharm Ther* 2000;25:197–220.

Prakash C, Kamel A, Cui D, et al. Identification of the major human liver cytochrome P450 isoform(s) responsible for the formation of the primary metabolites of ziprasidone and prediction of possible drug interactions. *Br J Clin Pharmacol* 2000;49(suppl 1):35S–42S.

Prior TI, Baker GB. Interactions between the cytochrome P450 system and the second-generation antipsychotics. *J Psychiatry Neurosci* 2003;28:99–112.

Prior TI. Chue PS. Tibbo P. Baker GB. Drug metabolism and atypical antipsychotics. *Eur Neuropsychopharmacology* 1999;9:1–9.

Ravindranath V. Metabolism of xenobiotics in the central nervous system: implications and challenges. *Biochem Pharmacol* 1998;56:547–551.

Rasmussen BB, Nielsen TL, Brosen K. Fluvoxamine inhibits the CP2C19-catalysed metabolism of proguanil in vitro. *Eur J Clin Pharmacol* 1998;54:735–740.

Renwick AB, Mistry H, Ball SE, et al. Metabolism of zaleplon by human hepatic microsomal cytochrome P450 isoforms. *Xenobiotica* 1998;28:337–348.

Ring BJ, Eckstein JA, Gillespie JS, et al. Identification of the human cytochromes p450 responsible for in vitro formation of R- and S-norfluoxetine. *J Pharmacol Exp Ther* 2001;297:1044–1050.

Robertson P Jr, Hellriegel ET. Clinical pharmacokinetic profile of modafinil. *Clin Pharmacokinet* 2003;42:123–137.

Rochat B, Amey M, Gillet M, et al. Identification of three cytochrome P450 isozymes involved in N-demethylation of citalopram enantiomers in human liver microsomes. *Pharmacogenetics* 1997; 7:1–10.

Rotzinger S, Baker GB. Human CP 3A4 and the metabolism of nefazodone and hydroxynefazodone by human liver microsomes and heterologously expressed enzymes. *Eur Neuropsychopharmacol* 2002;12:91–100.

Rotzinger S, Fang J, Baker GB. Trazodone is metabolized to m-chlorophenylpiperazine by CYP3A4 from human sources. *Drug Metab Dispos* 1998;26: 572–575.

Shulman RW, Ozdemir V. Psychotropic medications and cytochrome P450 2D6: pharmacokinetic considerations in the elderly. *Can J Psychiatry* 1997;42(suppl 1):4S–9S.

Sternbach H, State R. Antibiotics: neuropsychiatric side effects and psychotropic interactions. *Harv Rev Psychiatry* 1997;5:214–226.

Taavitsainen P, Anttila M, Nyman L, et al. Selegiline metabolism and cytochrome P450 enzymes: in vitro study in human liver microsomes. *Pharmacology & Toxicology* 2000;86:215–221.

Taylor D, Lader M. Cytochromes and psychotropic drug interactions. *Br J Psychiatry* 1996;168:529–532.

Venkatakrishnan K, Greenblatt DJ, von Moltke LL, et al. Five distinct human cytochromes mediate amitriptyline N-demethylation in vitro: dominance of CYP 2C19 and 3A4. *J Clin Pharmacol* 1998;38:112–121.

Venkatakrishnan K, Schmider J, Harmatz JS, et al. Relative contribution of CYP3A to amitriptyline clearance in humans: in vitro and in vivo studies. *J Clin Pharmacol* 2001;41:1043–1054.

Venkatakrishnan K, von Moltke LL, Greenblatt DJ. Nortriptyline E-10-hydroxylation in vitro is mediated by human CYP 2D6 (high affinity) and CYP3A4 (low affinity): implications for interactions with enzyme-inducing drugs. *J Clin Pharmacol* 1999;39:567–577.

von Moltke LL, Greenblatt DJ, Granda BW, et al. Zolpidem metabolism in vitro: responsible cytochromes, chemical inhibitors, and in vivo correlations. *Br J Clin Pharmacol* 1999;48:89–97.

von Moltke LL, Weemhoff JL, Perloff MD, et al. Effect of zolpidem on human cytochrome P450 activity, and on transport mediated by P-glycoprotein. *Biopharm Drug Dispos* 2002;23:361–367.

Wen X, Wang J, Kivisto KT, et al. In vitro evaluation of valproic acid as an inhibitor of human cytochrome 450 isoforms: preferential inhibition of cytochrome P450 2C9 (CYP2C9). *Br J Clin Pharmacol* 2001;52:547.

Wilner KD, Demattos SB, Anziano RJ, et al. Ziprasidone and the activity of cytochrome P450 2D6 in healthy extensive metabolizers. *Br J Clin Pharmacol* 2000;49(suppl 1):43S–47S.

Table B.1   Drugs Metabolized by Cytochrome P-450 Enzymes

CYP 1A2	CYP 2D6	CYP 3A3/4
Acetaminophen	Alprenolol	Acetaminophen
Amitriptyline	Amitriptyline	Adriamycin
Caffeine	Aripiprazole	Alfentanil
Cigarettes	Bisoprolol	Alprazolam
Ciprofloxacin	Bufarolol	Amiodarone
Clomipramine	Carbamazepine	Amitriptyline
Clozapine	Carvedilol	Androstenedione
Fluvoxamine	Chlorpromazine	Aripiprazole
Imipramine	Citalopram	Astemizole
Lidocaine	Clomipramine	Atorvastatin
Maprotiline	Clonidine	Benzphetamine
Mexiletine	Clozapine	Buprenorphine
Modafinil	Codeine	Buspirone
Olanzapine	Debrisoquin	Caffeine
Paracetamol	Deprenyl	Carbamazepine
Phenacetin	Desipramine	Chlordiazepoxide
Propafenone	Dextromethorphan	Cisapride
Propranolol	Donepezil	Citalopram
Ropivacaine	Encainide	Clarithromycin
R-Warfarin	Ethylmorphine	Clomipramine
Selegiline	Flecainide	Clonazepam
Tacrine	Fluoxetine	Clozapine
Theophylline	Fluphenazine	Cocaine
Verapamil	Fluvoxamine	Codeine
Zaleplon	4-Hydroamphetamine	Cortisol
Ziprasidone	Galantamine	Cyclosporine
Zolpidem	Guanoxan	Dapsone
	Haloperidol	Dexamethasone
	Hydrocodone	Dextromethorphan
	Imipramine	Diazepam
	Indoramine	Dihydroepiandrosterone 3-sulfate
	Lidocaine	Diltiazem
	Loxapine	Disopyramide
	Maprotiline	Docetaxel
	mCPP	Donepezil
	Meperidine	Erythromycin
	Methadone	Estradiol
	Methoxyphenamine	Ethinylestradiol
	Metoprolol	Ethosuximide
	Mexiletine	Felbamate
	Mianserin	Felodipine
	Mirtazepine?	Febtanyl
	Morphine	Fluoxetine
	N-Desmethylcitalopram	Fluvastatin
	N–Desmethylclomipramine	Fluvoxamine
	Nefazodone	Galantamine
	Norifluoxetine	Imipramine
	Nortriptyline	Irbesartan
	Olanzapine	Ketoconazole
	Ondansetron	Lidocaine
	Oxycodone	Loratadine
	Paroxetine	Losartan
	Perphenazine	Lovastatin
	Perphexiline	Methadone
	Phenformin	Midazolam

(continued)

Table B.1   *(continued)*

CYP 1A2	CYP 2D6	CYP 3A3/4
	Propafenone	Mirtazepine
	Propranolol	Modafinil
	Risperidone	Nefazodone
	Sertindole	Nicardipine
	Sertraline	Nifedepine
	Simvastatin	Niludipine
	Sparteine	Nimodipine
	Tamoxifen	Nisoldipine
	Tamoxetine	Nitrendipine
	Thioridazine	*O*-Desmethylvenlafaxine
	Timolol	Omeprazole
	Trazodone	Ondansetron
	Trimipramine	Paclitaxel
	Tramadol	Pimozide
	Venlafaxine	Pravastatin
	Zaleplon	Progesterone
	Zolpidem	Propafenone
		Protease inhibitors
		Quetiapine
		Quinidine
		Risperidone
		Selegiline
		Sertindole
		Sertraline
		Sildenafil
		Simvastatin
		Tacrolimus
		Tamoxifen
		Terfenadine
		Testosterone
		Tiagabine
		Trazodone
		Triacetylolenadomycin
		Triazolam
		Valsartan
		Verapamil
		Vinblastine
		Vincristine
		Zaleplon
		Ziprasidone
		Zolpidem
		Zonisamide

CYP 2C9	CYP 2C19	CYP 2B6
Amitriptyline	Amitriptyline	Bupropion
Carbamazepine	Citalopram	Carbamazepine
Clozapine	Clomipramine	Modafinil
Diazepam	Clozapine	Sertraline
Diclofenac	Diazepam	
Fluoxetine	Flecainide	
Fluvastatin	Imipramine	
Glipizide	Indomethacin	
Ibuprofen	Lansoprazole	

(continued)

Table B.1 *(continued)*

CYP 2C9	CYP 2C19	CYP 2B6
Irbesartan	Modafinil	
Losartan	Nelfinavir	
Modafinil	Nortriptyline	
Naproxen	Omeprazole	
Phenobarbital	Phenobarbital	
Phenytoin	Phenytoin	
Rosiglitazone	Primidone	
Sertraline	Propranolol	
S-Warfarin	R-Warfarin	
Tolbutamide	Sertraline	
Torsemide	S-Mephenytoin	
Valproic Acid	Valproic acid	
Valsartan		
Zolpidem		

Table B.2   Metabolizing Enzymes of Psychotropic Drugs

ANTIDEPRESSANTS

Amitriptyline	1A2	Imipramine	1A2
	2C19		2C19
	2D6		**2D6**
	3A3/4		3A3/4
	2C9	Maprotiline	**2D6**
	2C19		1A2
Bupropion	2B6	Mirtazepine	**3A3/4**
Citalopram	**2D6**		2D6
	3A3/4	Nefazodone	3A3/4
	2C19		2D6
Clomipramine	1A2	Nortriptyline	**2D6**
	2019		2C19
	2D6	Paroxetine	2D6
	3A3/4	Sertraline	3A3/4
N-Desmethylclomipramine	2D6		**2D6**
Deprenyl	2D6		2C9
Desipramine	2D6		2B6
Fluoxetine	**2D6**		2C19
	3A3/4	Trazodone	**2D6**
	2C9		3A3/4
Norfluoxetine	2D6	Trimipramine	2D6
Fluvoxamine	**3A3/4**	Venlafaxine	2D6
	1A2	O-Desmethylvenlafaxine	3A3/4
	2D6		

(continued)

Table B.2   *(continued)*

ANTIPSYCHOTICS

Aripiprazole	**3A3/4**		2D6
	2D6	Perphenazine	2D6
Chlorpromazine	2D6	Pimozide	3A3/4
Clozapine	**1A2**	Quetiapine	3A3/4
	3A3/4	Risperidone	**2D6**
	2D6		3A3/4
	2C19	Sertindole	**2D6**
	2C9		3A3/4
Fluphenazine	2D6	Thioridazine	2D6
Haloperidol	2D6	Ziprasidone	1A2
Loxapine	2D6		**3A3/4**
Olanzapine	**1A2**		

ANXIOLYTICS-HYPNOTICS

Alprazolam	3A3/4	Triazolam	3A3/4
Buspirone	3A3/4	Zaleplon	1A2
Chlordiazepoxide	3A3/4		2D6
Clonazepam	3A3/4		**3A3/4**
Diazepam	2C9/10		2C9
	2C19		1A2
	3A3/4	Zolpidem	2D6
Midazolam	3A3/4		**3A3/4**

MOOD STABILIZERS

Carbamazepine	2D6		2B6
	3A3/4	Valproic acid	2C9
	2C9		2C19

COGNITIVE ENHANCERS

Donepezil	2D6		3A3/4
	3A3/4	Tacrine	1A2
Galantamine	2D6		

OTHER PSYCHOTROPICS

Buprenorphine	3A3/4	Modafinil	2B6
Methadone	2D6		1A2
	3A3/4		3A3/4
	2C9		2C19

Table B.3   Inhibitors of Cytochrome P-450 Enzymes

CYP 1A2	CYP 2D6	CYP 3A3/4
Cimetidine	Amitriptyline	**Astemizole**
Ciprofloxacin	Bupropion	**Cimetidine**
Disulfiram	Chlorpromazine	Ciprofloxacin
Erythromycin	**Cimetidine**	Desmethlysertraline
Fluoxetine	Citalopram	**Diltiazem**
Fluvoxamine	Clomipramine	**Erthromycin**
Grapefruit juice	Diphenhydramine	**Fluconazole**
Paroxetine	**Desipramine**	Fluoxetine
Sertraline	**Diltiazem**	**Fluvoxamine**
Theophylline	**Flecainide**	Grapefruit Juice
	Fluoxetine	**Itraconazole**
	Fluphenazine	**Ketoconazole**
	Fluvoxamine	Lovastatin
	Haloperidol	Mapyramine
	Labetalol	Miconazole
	Mirtazepine	Morphine
	N-Desmethylcitalopram	**Nefazodone**
	Norfluoxetine	Norfloxacin
	Paroxetine	**Norfluoxetine**
	Perphenazine	Paroxetine
	Propafenone	Ritonavir
	Quinidine	Saquinavir
	Ritonavir	Sertraline[a]
	Sertraline[a]	**Troleandomycin**
	Thioridazine	**Verapamil**
	Ticlopidine	Zafirlukast
	Venlafaxine	
	Vincristine	
	Yohimbine	

CYP 2C9	CYP 2C19	CYP 2B6
Amiodarone	Cimetidine	Efavirenz
Cimetidine	Clozapine	Nelfinavir
Clozapine	Felbamate	Ritonavir
Fluconazole	Fluoxetine	
Fluoxetine	**Fluvoxamine**	
Fluvastatin	Lansoprazole	
Fluvoxamine	Modafinil	
Isoniazid	Omeprazole	
Itraconazole	Oxcarbazepine	
Ketoconazole	Sertraline	
Lovastatin	Ticlopidine	
Metronidazole	Topiramate	
Modafinil	Tranylcypromine	
Omeprazole	Valproic acid	
Phenytoin		
Propoxyphene		
Ritonavir		
Sertraline		
Trimethoprim		
Valproic acid		
Zafirlukast		

[a] At higher doses, sertraline is a potent inhibitor of 2D6.

Table B.4 Isoenzyme Metabolizers of Nonpsychotropic Medications

Acetaminophen	1A2	Mexiletine	3A3/4
	3A3/4		2D6
Adriamycin	3A3/4		1A2
Alfentanil	3A3/4	Morphine	2D6
Alprenolol	2D6	Naproxen	2C19
	3A3/4		2C9
Androstendione	3A3/4	Nelfinavir	2C19
Astemizole	3A3/4	Nicardipine	2C19
Atorvastatin	3A3/4	Nifedipine	2C9/10
Bisoprolol	2D6	Nicotine	3A3/4
Bufarolol	2D6	Niludipine	3A3/4
Caffeine	1A2	Nimodipine	3A3/4
	3A3/4	Nisoldipine	3A3/4
Captopril	2D6	Nitrendipine	3A3/4
Carvedilol	2D6	Omeprazole	2D6
Ciprofloxacin	1A2		2C19
Cisapride	3A3/4	Ondansetron	2D6
Clarithromycin	3A3/4		3A3/4
Clonidine	2D6	Oxycodone	3A3/4
Cocaine	3A3/4	Paclitaxel	3A3/4
Codeine	2D6	Paracetamol	1A2
	3A3/4	Penicillamine	2D6
Cortisol	3A3/4	Perhexiline	2D6
Cyclosporine	3A3/4	Phenacetin	2D6
Dapsone	3A3/4	Phenformin	3A3/4
Debrisoquin	2D6	Phenobarbital	2C9
Dexamethasone	3A3/4		2C19
Dextromethorphan	2D6	Phenytoin	3A3/4
	3A3/4		1A2
Dextropropoxyphene	2D6		2C9/10
Diclofenac	2C9		2C19
Dihydroepiandrosterone 3-sulfate	3A3/4	Pindolol	2D6
Diltiazem	3A3/4	Pravastatin	3A3/4
Disopyramide	3A3/4	Primidone	2C19
Docetaxel	3A3/4	Progesterone	2C19
Encainide	2D6	Propafenone	1A2
Erythromycin	3A3/4		2D6
Estradiol	3A3/4		3A3/4
Ethinylestradiol	3A3/4	Quinidine	3A3/4
Ethosuximide	3A3/4	Ropivacaine	1A2
Ethylmorphine	2D6	Rosiglitazone	2C9
Felbamate	3A3/4	R-Warfarin	1A2
Felodipine	3A3/4		2C19
Fentanyl	3A3/4	Selegiline	1A2
Flecainide	2D6		3A3/4
	2C19	Sildenafil	3A3/4
Fluvastatin	2C9	Simvastatin	2D6
	3A3/4		3A3/4
Glipizide	2C9	Smoking	1A2
Guanoxan	2D6	Sparteine	2D6
Hexobarbital	2C19	S-Mephenytoin	2D6
Hydrocodone	2D6		2C19
4-Hydroxyamphetamine	2D6	S-Warfarin	2C9/10
Ibuprofen	2C9	Tacrine	1A2
Indomethacin	2C19	Tacrolimus	3A3/4
Indoramine	2D6	Tamoxetine	2D6
Irbesartan	2C9	Tamoxifen	3A3/4
	3A3/4		2D6

(continued)

Table B.4   *(continued)*

Ketoconazole	3A3/4	Terfenadine	3A3/4
Labetolol	2D6	Testosterone	3A3/4
Lansoprazole	2C19	Theophylline	1A2
Lidocaine	2C19	Tiagabine	3A3/4
	2D6	Timolol	2D6
	3A3/4	Tolbutamide	2C9/10
	1A2	Torsemide	2C9
Loratadine	3A3/4	Triacetyloleandomycin	3A3/4
Losartan	2C9	Valsartan	2C9
	3A3/4		3A3/4
Lovastatin	3A3/4	Verapamil	1A2
Meperidine	2D6		3A3/4
S-Mephentoin	2D6	Vinblastine	3A3/4
Mephobarbital	2D6	Vincristine	3A3/4
Methoxyphenamine	2D6	Yohimbine	2D6
Metoprolol	2D6	Zonisamide	3A3/4

Table B.5   Inducers of Cytochrome P-450 Enzymes

CYP 1A2	CYP 2D6	CYP 3A3/4
Carbamazepine	Dexamethasone?	Amiodarone
Charbroiled meat	Phenobarbital?	Carbamazepine
Chlorpromazine	Phenytoin?	Clofibrate?
Clozapine	Rifampin?	Clozapine
Cruciferous vegetables	Ritonavir?	Ethosuxamide
Modafinil		Felbamate
Morphine		Glucocorticoids (high potency)?
Omeprazole		Griseofulvin
Pethidine		Isoniazid
Phenobarbital		Modafinil
Phenytoin		Oxcarbazepine
Primidone		Pethidine
Rifampin		Phenytoin
Smoking		Phenobarbital
		Prednisone
		Primidone
		Rifampin
		Rifabutin
		Ritonavir
		Topiramate

CYP 2C9	CYP 2C19	CYP 2B6
Carbamazepine	Carbamazepine	Clozapine
Phenobarbital	Norethindrone	Modafinil
Phenytoin	Phenobarbital	
Rifampin	Phenytoin	
	Rifampin	

The authors wish to thank Dr. Jayendra Patel, who prepared the drug metabolism tables for Appendix B in *Clinical Geriatric Psychopharmacology,* 3rd ed., upon which these tables are based.

Drug Interactions with Psychotropic Medications

Michelle Wiersgalla

Carl Salzman

Drug interactions are an important feature of treatment of elderly patients who receive psychotropic medications. Nursing home residents, for example, almost always take multiple medications—often 5 to 12 drugs concomitantly. Complicated medication regimens such as these increase the risk of adverse interactions. In addition, the aging process brings about changes in the body's ability to metabolize medications: renal function diminishes, as does the liver's capacity for oxidative metabolism. Consequently, elderly patients are often at higher risk for toxicity. These factors result in a need for caution in prescribing psychotropic medication for the elderly.

The set of tables presented here identify adverse drug interactions involving several classes of psychotropic drugs: antipsychotics, heterocyclic antidepressants, MAO inhibitors, SSRIs, atypical and new antidepressants, mood stabilizers, anxiolytics, and others. For each class, the interacting drugs and clinical effect(s) of the interaction are listed. Also presented are references for each interaction (coded by number) and a scale of clinical significance (coded by letter) to provide a qualitative measure for the various interactions. **Note that new references have been added to this edition which are indicated in bold and are listed in a separate reference list.**

Acknowledgments. The authors wish to thank Dr. Jayendra Patel and Dr. Eric Watsky, who prepared the drug interaction tables for Appendix C in *Clinical Geriatric Psychopharmacology,* 3rd ed. and 2nd ed., respectively, upon which these tables are based.

Table C.1. Adverse Drug Interactions with Antipsychotics

Interacting Drug	Clinical Effect of Interaction
ACE inhibitors	Increased hypotensive effects with chlorpromazine or clozapine (D) **30**, 481
	Increased clozapine levels with lisinopril, leading to drooling, irritability, sleep disturbance* (D) **1**
Activated charcoal	Delayed oral antipsychotic absorption (C) 440
Amphetamines	Decreased appetite suppression by amphetamines (B) 308, 372, 419
	Decreased effectiveness of amphetamines (C) 14, 222
Antacids	Delayed oral antipsychotic absorption (C) 141, 153, 167, 215, 352
Anticholinergics	Increased anticholinergic effects (C) 13, 27, 137, 158
	Delayed onset of effects of acute oral doses of antipsychotics (C) 377, 379, 410,411
	Altered antipsychotic blood levels (C) 26, 275, 377, 379
	Increased risk of hyperthermia (C) 287, 478
Ascorbic acid	Decreased fluphenazine levels (D) 128
β-Blockers	Increased levels of either chlorpromazine or β-blockers* (B) 343, 463
	Additive hypotensive effects and cardiopulmonary arrest (C) 10, **30**
	Increased plasma concentrations of phenothiazines* (C) 342, 343, 406
	Increased risk of neurotoxicity (C) 298
Barbiturates	Reduction of serum levels of antipsychotics* (C) **35**, 102, 153,
	Increased risk of respiratory depression and sedation (B) 124, 270, 469
Benzodiazepines	Reported cases of cardiopulmonary collapse with clozapine (C) **14**, 389,
	Additive CNS depression/increased sedation (B) 18, **14**, 204
	Increased risk of respiratory depression (C) 35, 93
	Increased risk of syncope, orthostatic hypotension (B) **115**
Benztropine	Acute intestinal pseudo-obstruction with haloperidol (D) **10**
Bethanidine	Decreased antihypertensive effects (C) 143, 221
Bromocriptine	Risk of reduced pharmacological effects of bromocriptine and/or antipsychotics (C) 381, 473
Bupropion	Decreased seizure threshold (C) 256
Buspirone	Increased haloperidol levels (C) 163
Carbamazepine	Decreased antipsychotic levels* (B) **8**, 19, **103**, **107**, **108**, 145, 219, 236, 238, 247, 248, 270, 366
	Neurotoxicity with haloperidol (D) 238
	Increased risk of granulocytopenia and possibly agranulocytosis with clozapine (B) 234
Chloroquine	Increased chloroquine levels with phenothiazines (C) 256
Cimetidine	Decreased chlorpromazine absorption (C) 209
	Increased sedation with chlorpromazine (D) 69
	Inhibition of metabolism of antipsychotics* (B) 348
	Increased clozapine levels* (B) 434
Ciprofloxacin	Increased levels of clozapine and olanzapine* (C) **14, 95, 110**
Clarithromycin	Lengthened QTc in combination with pimozide (B) **39**
Clonidine	Delirium with fluphenazine (D) 12
	Potentiated hypotensive effects (C) 182
Coffee/tea	Decreased sedation and risk of exacerbation of psychosis (D) 295
	Delayed clinical effects of antipsychotics (D) 54, 257–259, 468
Debrisoquine	Decreased antihypertensive effects (C) 399
Digoxin	Increased digoxin levels via protein-binding displacement by clozapine (C) 256
Disulfiram	Decreased serum perphenazine levels (C) 188
Enflurane/isoflurane	Profound hypotension with phenothiazines (B) 124, 164, 223
Epinephrine	Hypotension and tachycardia with low-potency antipsychotics (e.g., chlorpromazine and thioridazine) (B) 124, 398
Guanethidine	Reversal of antihypertensive effects with chlorpromazine, haloperidol, thiothixene (C) 143, 221

(continued)

Table C.1.   *(continued)*

Interacting Drug	Clinical Effect of Interaction
Heterocyclic antidepressants	Increased hypotension, sedation, anticholinergic effects (C) 181, 274
	Risk of ventricular arrhythmias with thioridazine (B) 483
	Increase in plasma levels of antipsychotic and/or antidepressant* (C) 133, 173, 174, 237, 274, 316, 414
	Increased risk of seizures (D) 316
	Increased EPS with amoxapine or risperidone (C) **16**, 156,
Imipenem	Hypotension in combination with haloperidol (D) **40**
Indinavir/ritonavir	Increased risperidone levels* (D) **58**
Indomethacin	Drowsiness with haloperidol (D) 45
Kaolin/pectin	Delayed oral antipsychotic absorption (C) 153, 440, 423
L-Dopa	Decreased antiparkinsonian effects of L-Dopa (B) 70, 127, 228, 491
	Risk of exacerbation of psychosis (B) 15
Lithium	Risk of neurotoxicity and delirium-like symptoms (B) 356
	Increased EPS (C) 7, 386, 401
	Decreased chlorpromazine levels, possibly via inhibition of gastric emptying (C) 244, 378
	Increased lithium excretion with chlorpromazine (C) 418
	Ventricular fibrillation associated with chlorpromazine and sudden withdrawal of lithium (D) 432
	Third-degree heart block with mesoridazine (D) 388
	CNS toxicity correlated with antipsychotic dosage (C) 8, 33, 94, 155, 166, 297, 401, 412
Lovastatin	Lengthened QTc interval in combination with quetiapine (C) **41**
MAOIs	Increased effect of antipsychotics by inhibition of metabolism (C) 448
	Increased EPS with phenothiazines (C) 448
	Hepatotoxicity and encephalopathy with iproniazid and prochlorperazine (C) 72
	Increased risk of hypotension (C) 448
	Catatonia with haloperidol and phenelzine (D) 199
Meperidine	Risk of prolonged respiratory depression, hypotension, and CNS toxicity with phenothiazines (B) 240, 263, 427
Methyldopa	Orthostatic hypotension (C) 85
	Reversible dementia with haloperidol (C) 446
	Rare delirium (D) 311
	Paradoxical hypertension (D) 477
Modafinil	Increased clozapine levels* (D) **29**
Narcotics	Increased sedation (C) 223, 427
	Increased hypotension (C) 223, 437
	Increased risk of respiratory depression (C) 223, 240, 263
Nefazodone	Increased haloperidol levels* (C) 132
Olanzapine	Increased EPS in combination with haloperidol (D) **44**
Oral contraceptives	Increased effect of antipsychotic (C) 134
	Increased clozapine levels* (C) **41**
	Tremor and dyskinesia associated with increased chlorpromazine levels* (D) **21**
Oral hypoglycemics	Increased serum glucose; dosage adjustment of antidiabetic medication may be necessary (C) 21, 66, 200, 264, 359
Perphenazine	Increased psychosis, myoclonus, and hypersalivation associated with increased clozapine levels (D) **25**
Phenindione	Decreased bleeding with haloperidol (C) 321
Phenylpropanolamine	Ventricular arrhythmias with thioridazine (B) 84, 161
	Risk of increased psychosis (C) 348
Phenytoin	Increased phenytoin toxicity (C) 207, 260, 465
	Decreased antipsychotic serum levels* (C) **83, 118**, 270

(continued)

Table C.1. *(continued)*

Interacting Drug	Clinical Effect of Interaction
Rifampin	Decreased effect of antipsychotics via induction of metabolism* (C) **57**, 256, 442
Risperidone	Possible neurotoxicity with clozapine (D) **63**
SSRIs	Increased levels of some antipsychotics with fluoxetine (e.g., clozapine, haloperidol, risperidone)* (B) **9, 12**, 76, 162, 439,
	Increased risk of seizure and of CNS depression due to elevated clozapine levels with fluoxetine* (B) **37, 102, 113**
	Increased EPS with fluoxetine (C) **16, 106**, 439
	Increased clozapine levels with paroxetine* (C) 77, **105**
	Parkinsonian symptoms due to elevated risperidone levels with paroxetine (C) **104**
	Increased clozapine levels with fluvoxamine* (B) 113, 229
	Increased levels of haloperidol and thioridazine with fluvoxamine* (C) **9, 20**
	Risk of serotonin syndrome with risperidone and fluvoxamine (C) **96**
	Increased clozapine levels with high doses of citalopram* (D) **13**
Succinylcholine	Prolonged apnea with ECT (D) 370
Tetracycline	Decreased risperidone levels (D) **109**
Thioridazine	Increased quetiapine clearance (C) **93**
Tramadol	Lowered seizure threshold (B) **98**
Trazodone	Additive hypotension with phenothiazines (D) 23
Valproic acid	Prolonged half-life of valproic acid with chlorpromazine (C) 217
	Case of catatonia in combination with risperidone and sertraline (C) **66**
	Altered clozapine levels (D) **24, 83**
Warfarin	Increased levels of warfarin via protein-binding displacement by clozapine (C) 256
	Increased prothrombin time (C) 472
Zolpidem	Increased half-life of chlorpromazine (C) **22, 51**

(A) = Severe interaction; (B) = Significant interaction; (C) = Potentially significant interaction; (D) = Mild interaction or single case; * = Interaction mediated partially or totally through CYP-450 enzyme system.

Table C.2.   Adverse Drug Interactions with Heterocyclic Antidepressants

Interacting Drug	Clinical Effect of Interaction
Alcohol	Increased sedation (C) 121, 265, 471
	Altered TCA levels via effects on TCA metabolism (C) 88, **112**
Amiloride	Hyponatremia with amitriptyline (D) 301
Anticholinergics	Additive anticholinergic effects (B) 22, 220, 223
	Anticholinergic delirium (B) 22
Antipsychotics	Possible ventricular arrhythmias with thioridazine (B) 483
	Increased thioridazine concentration with imipramine, amitriptyline* (B) **28**
	Increased EPS with amoxapine (C) 156
	Increased plasma levels of antipsychotic and/or antidepressant* (C) 133, 173, 174, 237, 274, 316, 414
	Increased maprotiline levels with risperidone* (C) **88**
	Increased sedation, hypotension, anticholinergic effect (C) 181, 274
	Increased risk of seizures (D) 316
β-adrenergic blockers	Increased imipramine levels with labetolol (B)* 198
	Increased hypotensive effect (C) **30**
Barbiturates	Decreased blood levels of TCAs by induction of metabolism* (B) 11, 67, **117**
	Additive respiratory depressive effects (C) 51
Benzodiazepines	Increased sedation, confusion, impaired motor function (C) 42
	Increased TCA levels with alprazolam* (C) 16
	Decreased imipramine levels with diazepam (D) 147
	Decreased desipramine levels with clonazapam (D) 114
Bethanidine	Decreased antihypertensive effects (B) 57, 417
Bupropion	Decreased seizure threshold (C) 256
Buspirone	Hypertension and anxiety with clomipramine (D) 83
Carbamazepine	Decreased TCAs levels and increased heterocyclic metabolites and toxicity* (D) 31, 60, 61
Cholestyramine	Decreased absorption of TCAs (C) **30**
Cimetidine	Increased TCA levels* (B) 5, 194, 300, 302
	Psychosis with cimetidine and imipramine (C) 300
Ciprofloxacin	Increased TCA levels* (C) **110**
Clonidine	Decreased antihypertensive effects (B) 5, 58, 455
	Potential hypertensive crises with imipramine (D) 210
Debrisoquine	Decreased antihypertensive effects (B) 417
Diltiazem	Increased imipramine levels* (C) **30**
Directly acting pressors: epinephrine/ norepinephrine/ phenylephrine/ dopamine	Significant increase in pressor response (B) **34**, 49, 398
Disulfiram	Increased blood levels of antidepressants by inhibition of metabolism (C) 90
	Risk of psychosis and confusional state (C) 284
Estrogen	Decreased therapeutic effect of imipramine (C) 246, 357
	Prolonged half-life of imipramine (C) 4
	Lethargy, headache, tremor, hypotension (C) 246
	Increased incidence of akathisia (C) 255
Grapefruit juice	Increased clomipramine levels* (C) **59**
Guanethidine	Elevated blood pressure (B) 239, 266, 294, 306
Indirectly acting pressors: dobutamine/ephedrine	Decreased pressor effects (B) **34**
L-Dopa	Increased agitation, tremor, rigidity (C) 129, 368
	Decreased plasma levels via impaired gastrointestinal absorption (D) 310

(continued)

Table C.2. *(continued)*

Interacting Drug	Clinical Effect of Interaction
Lithium	Increased lithium tremor (C) 226, 371
	Seizures with amitriptyline (D) 422
	Myoclonus (C) 118
Local anesthetic dissolved in epinephrine	Increased nasal bleeding in nasal surgery (C) 390
MAOIs	Toxic reaction if TCAs added to MAOI; can occur if TCA is abruptly substituted for MAOI; fatalities possible (A) 216, 320, 325, 391, 409, 438
	Disseminated intravascular coagulation with clomipramine (D) 37, 438
	Inhibition of TCA metabolism; TCA blood levels and rsk of toxicity increased (B) 181, 398
	Increased incidence of mania (C) 112
Methadone/morphine	Additive analgesic effects (C) 241, 334
	Increased morphine levels (C) 461
	Increased TCA levels (C) 283
Methyldopa	Agitation, tremor, and tachycardia with amitriptyline (C) 126, 480
Methylphenidate	Increased TCA levels (B) 152, 479
Modafinil	Increased clomipramine levels* (D) **48**
Oral anticoagulants	Increased bioavailability of dicumarol (B) 354
	Increased bleeding/increased warfarin effect (D) **30**, 252, 462
Oxybutynin	Decreased clompramine levels* (D) **49**
Phenylbutazone	Delayed absorption with desipramine (C) 96
Phenytoin	Decreased TCA blood levels* (B) 207, 313, 314, 350
Propafenone	Increased desipramine concentration* (D) **30**
Quinidine	Increased TCA levels* (B) 429
	Additive type la antiarrhythmic effects with serious consequences (B) 44
Rifampin	Decreased nortriptyline levels* (D) **38**
SSRIs	Significantly increased TCA levels* (B) 20, 39, 235, 392, 457
Sulfonylureas	Increased incidence of hypoglycemia (C) 449
Testosterone	Paranoid psychosis with aggression (C) 485
Valproic acid	Increased valproate levels (C) 256
	Inhibition of TCA metabolism* (C) 83
Verapamil	Increased TCA levels (C) 256

(A) = Severe interaction; (B) = Significant interaction; (C) = Potentially significant interaction; (D) = Mild interaction or single case; * = Interaction mediated partially or totally through CYP-450 enzyme system.

Table C.3.   Adverse Drug Interactions with Monoamine Oxidase Inhibitors

Interacting Drug	Clinical Effect of Interaction
Alcohol	Risk of hypertensive crises (A) 355, 433, 435
	Increased CNS depression (C) 47, 476
	Malignant hyperthermia (D) 304
Amantadine	Elevated blood pressure (D) 218
Amine-containing foods	Hypertensive crises, strokes, and death (A) 46, 292, 365, 393, 433
Amphetamines	Increased blood pressure (B) 63, 105, 165, 273, 299, 320
Anticholinergics	Enhanced CNS depression (C) 89, 109
Antipsychotics	Increased risk of hypotension (C) 448
	Increased EPS with phenothiazines (C) 448
	Increased effect of antipsychotics via decreased metabolism (C) 448
	Catatonia with haloperidol and phenelzine (D) 199
	Hepatotoxicity and encephalopathy with iproniazid and prochlorperazine (C) 72
Aspartame	Headache and diaphoresis with phenelzine (D) 150
Barbiturates	Enhanced CNS depression (C) 120
Benzodiazepines	Disinhibition and generalized edema with chlordiazepoxide (C) 169,338
Buspirone	Increased blood pressure (B) 89
Codeine	Enhanced CNS depression (C) 73
Dextromethorphan	Fatalities and toxic reactions (B)
	Increased blood pressure (A) 380, 425
Dopamine	Increased blood pressure (B) 416
Ephedrine	Increased blood pressure (B) 110, 165, 416
Fenfluramine	Confusion (C) 256
General anesthetics	Enhanced CNS depression (C) 404
	Labile blood pressure with atracurium (D) 404
Guanethidine	Decreased antihypertensive effect (C) 183
Heterocyclic antidepressants	Toxic reaction if TCAs added to or abruptly substituted for MAOI; fatalities possible (A) 216, 320, 325, 391, 409, 438
	Inhibition of TCA metabolism; TCA blood levels and toxicity increased (B) 181, 398
	Increased incidence of mania (C) 112
	Disseminated intravascular coagulation with clomipramine (D) 37, 438
Insulin/sulfonylureas	Enhanced or prolonged hypoglycemic reaction (B) 9, 97–99, 339, 454, 475
	Increased hypotension (C) 99
Levarterenol	Increased blood pressure (B) 49, 135, 165, 416
L-Dopa	Acute hypertension (B) 212
Lithium	Tardive dyskinesia with tranylcypromine (C) 428
L-Tryptophan	Serotonin syndrome (A) 256
Meperidine	Known fatalities; toxic reaction and coma; report of agitation and delirium with selegiline (A) 63, 73, 139, 165, 223, 416, 464, 499
Mephentermine	Increased blood pressure (B) 223
Metaraminol	Increased blood pressure (B) 206, 416
Methyldopa	Excitation and hallucinations with pargyline (D) 340
Methylphenidate	Increased blood pressure (B) 223, 416
Morphine	Hypotension (C) 256
Nefazodone	Toxicity (B) 256
Phenylephrine	Increased blood pressure (B) 49, 135, 110
Phenylpropanolamine	Increased blood pressure (B) 103, 211, 289
Procaine hydrochloride (dissolved in epinephrine)	Increased blood pressure (B) 49, 165, 416
Propoxyphene	Enhanced CNS depression (C) 73, 157
Pseudoephedrine	Increased blood pressure (B) 489

(continued)

Table C.3.   *(continued)*

Interacting Drug	Clinical Effect of Interaction
Reserpine	Frank mania with nialamide (D) 172 Hypomania (C) 256 Increased hypotension (C) 111
SSRIs/serotonin agonists	Sudden death secondary to hyperserotonergic states; 5-week interval required between discontinuation of fluoxetine and start of MAOI (A) 148, 171, 256, 431
Succinylcholine	Prolonged apnea with phenelzine(B) 50
Sulfisoxazole	Ataxia and paresthesias (D) 55
Sympathomimetics	Fatalities, cardiac arrhythmias, hyperpyrexia, and cerebral vascular hemorrhage (A) 355
Thiazide diuretics	Increased hypotension (C) 416
Tranylcypromine	Hypertensive reaction with other MAOIs, particularly if switched abruptly (A) 36, 81, 318
Venlafaxine	Toxicity (B) 256

(A) = Severe interaction; (B) = Significant interaction; (C) = Potentially significant interaction; (D) = Mild interaction or single case; * = Interaction mediated partially or totally through CYP-450 enzyme system.

Table C.4.   Adverse Drug Interactions with Selective Serotonin Reuptake Inhibitors (SSRIs)

Interacting Drug	Clinical Effect of Interaction
Adderall/methylphenidate	Tachyarrhythmias in combination with sertraline (D) **46**
Antiarrhythmics—Type 1C	Increased levels of antiarrhythmics (e.g., propafenone)* (B) **5**, 256
Antipsychotics	Increased levels of some antipsychotics with fluoxetine (e.g., haloperidol, clozapine)* (B) 76, 162, 439
	Significantly increased clozapine levels with fluvoxamine* (B) 113, 229
	Increased clozapine levels with paroxetine* (C) 77
	Increased EPS with fluoxetine (C) 439
	Increased agitation/increased symtpoms of serotonin syndrome with combination of paroxetine and risperidone (C) **60**
	Worsened OCD symptoms with combination of fluoxetine and risperidone (D) **6**
Atorvastatin/lovastatin/ simvastatin	Risk of myositis and rhabdomyolysis with fluoxetine* (B) **5**
β-Blockers	Increased frequency of bradycardia with metoprolol/propranolol/ carvedilol and fluoxetine (B) **5**, 375
	Increased levels of propranolol with fluvoxamine* (C) 375
Benzodiazepines	Increased alprazolam levels with fluvoxamine and paroxetine (C) **9**
Buprenorphine/methadone	Inhibition of metabolism by fluoxetine and fluvoxamine* (D) **54**
Caffeine	Increased adverse effects of caffeine in combination with fluvoxamine* (C) **34**, **113**
Carbamazepine	Increased levels of carbamazepine with fluoxetine and fluvoxamine (B) **9**, 341
Cimetidine	Increased paroxetine levels* (B) 32
Codeine	Increased codeine levels* (C) 256
Cyclobenzaprine	Lengthened QTc with fluoxetine (C) **82**
Cyclosporine	Increased cyclosporine levels with fluoxetine and fluvoxamine* (C) **113**, **116**
Cyproheptadine	Loss of antidepressant activity (B) 87, 146
Diazepam	Increased half-life of diazepam (C) 267
Diuretics	SIADH with sertraline and fluoxetine (C) 92
Grapefruit juice	Decreased sertraline metabolism* (C) **67**
Heterocyclic antidepressants	Significantly increased TCA levels* (B) 20, 39, 235, 392, 457
Hypoglycemic agents	Increased hypoglycemia, mostly with fluoxetine (C) 256
	Increased glimepiride concentrations with fluvoxamine (D) **87**
Lamotrigine	Increased lamotrigine levels with sertraline (C) **107**
Lithium	Lithium neurotoxicity possibly due to SSRI-induced SIADH (C) 138, 348
	Fever, increased bilirubin, leucocytosis (C) 319
	Increased lithium levels with fluoxetine (C) 184, 387
L-Tryptophan	Mild serotonin syndrome (C) 430
	Worsened OCD symptoms (C) 430
MAOIs	Serotonin syndrome and fatality; 5-week interval required between discontinuing fluoxetine and starting MAOI (A) 148, 171, 256, 431
Oral anticoagulant	Increased risk of bleeding (C) **30**, 32, 91, 484
	Increased warfarin concentration with fluvoxamine* (B) 375
Phenytoin	Increased phenytoin levels* (C) **76**, **86**, 256
Quinidine	Decreased clearance with fluvoxamine* (C) **26a**
Rifampin	Risk of sertraline discontinuation symptoms due to decreased sertraline level* (D) **38**, **77**
Ropivacaine	Increased concentration with fluvoxamine* (D) **7**, **56**
Terfenadine/astemizole/ cisapride	Theoretical risk of ventricular arrhythmia (?A) 256

(continued)

Table C.4. *(continued)*

Interacting Drug	Clinical Effect of Interaction
Theophylline	Increased theophylline levels with fluvoxamine, which may result in coma, seizures, and supraventricular tachycardia* (B) 56, 136
Tolbutamide	Increased tolbutamide levels with sertraline* (C) **9**
Tramadol	Decreased seizure threshold (B) **98**
Trazodone	Increased levels of trazodone with fluoxetine (D) 20
Valproic acid	Increased valproic acid levels with fluoxetine (C) **73**
Zolpidem	Faster onset of action and incresed effect of zolpidem with sertraline (D) **3**
	Reports of visual hallucinations with SSRIs (D) **33**

(A) = Severe interaction; (B) = Significant interaction; (C) = Potentially significant interaction; (D) = Mild interaction or single case; * = Interaction mediated partially or totally through CYP-450 enzyme system.

Table C.5.   Adverse Drug Interactions with Atypical and New Antidepressants

Interacting Drug	Clinical Effect of Interaction
	NEFAZODONE
Atovastatin/lovastatin/ simvastatin	Risk of myositis and rhabdomyolysis* (B) **5, 26, 30, 90**
Benzodiazepines	Increased levels of triazolobenzodiazepines* (B) 34, 132
Cyclosporine/tacrolimus	Increased cyclosporine/tacrolimus concentrations* (C) **42, 116, 119**
Digoxin	Elevation of digoxin levels* (B) **30**, 132
Haloperidol	Increased haloperidol levels* (C) 132
MAOIs	Toxicity (B) 256
Nonsedating antihistamines	Increased levels of astemizole and terfenadine, such that *torsades de pointes* may occur and may be fatal* (A) 348
Oral contraceptives	Increased estrogen concentration (C) **2**
Sildenafil	May increase sildenafil levels* (D) **92**
	VENLAFAXINE
Benzodiazepines	Increased levels of diazepam and alprazolam* (D) **89**
Cimetidine	Increased levels in at-risk populations (C) **89**, 256
Diphenhydramine	Decreased venlafaxine metabolism (C) 68
Haloperidol	Decreased haloperidol clearance (C) **89**
Indinavir	Decreased indinavir levels (C) **69**
MAOIs	Toxicity (B) 256
TCAs	Increased levels of imipramine and desipramine* (C) **89**
	BUPROPION
Antipsychotics	Decreased seizure threshold (C) 256
Carbamazepine	Induction of bupropion metabolism* (D) **107**
Cyclosporine	Decreased cyclosporine levels (C) **70**
TCAs	Decreased seizure threshold (C) 256
	TRAZODONE
Antipsychotics	Additive hypotension with phenothiazines (D) 23
β-Blockers	Increased hypotensive effect (C) **30**
Coumadin	Decreased prothrombin and prothromboplastin times (D) 189
Fluoxetine	Increased levels (D) 20
Isopropamide	Increased urinary retention (D) 80
Ketoconazole	Decreased metabolism of trazodone* (C) **120**
Phenytoin	Increased serum levels (D) 122
Ritonavir	Altered trazodone clearance (C) **120**

(A) = Severe interaction; (B) = Significant interaction; (C) = Potentially significant interaction; (D) = Mild interaction or single case; * = Interaction mediated partially or totally through CYP-450 enzyme system.

Table C.6.   Adverse Drug Interactions with Mood Stabilizers

Interacting Drug	Clinical Effect of Interaction

LITHIUM

ACE inhibitors	Decreased lithium clearance and increased lithium levels, with risk of neurotoxicity (B) **5**, **32**, 123, 286, 312, 360, 407
Acetazolamide	Increased lithium clearance (C) **30**, **32**
Aminophylline	Decreased lithium levels via increased renal clearance (C) **32**, 445
Amphetamine	Decreased activating and euphoric effects of amphetamine (D) 151, 453
Angiotensin receptor blockers: candesartan/ losartan/valsartan	Increased lithium concentration with risk of lithium toxicity (C) **5**, **30**, **38**, **121**
Antipsychotics	Neurotoxicity and delirium-like symptoms (B) 356
	CNS toxicity correlated with antipsychotic dosage (C) 8, 33, 94, 155, 166, 297, 401, 412
	Increased EPS (C) 7, 386, 401
	Increased lithium excretion with chlorpromazine (C) 418
	Third-degree heart block with mesoridazine (D) 388
	Ventricular fibrillation associated with chlorpromazine and sudden withdrawal of lithium (D) 432
	Decreased chlorpromazine levels, possibly by inhibition of gastric emptying (C) 244, 378
Benzodiazepines	Increased serum lithium levels with clonazepam (C) 253
	Hypothermia associated with diazepam (D) 315
Caffeine	Decreased lithium levels via increased renal clearance (C) **32**, 225
Calcitonin	Decreased lithium levels (D) **91**
Carbamazepine	Carbamazepine-induced water intoxication and hyponatremia, with risk of lithium toxicity (C) 82, 160
	Increased risk of neurotoxicity (C) 82, 159, 349, 403
	Carbamazpeine-induced renal failure may lead to lithium intoxication (D) **80**
Clonidine	Decreased antihypertensive effect (C) 168
Decamethonium/ pancuronium/ succinylcholine	Prolonged apnea during ECT (B) 52, 190, 201, 220, 226, 288, 374
Digitalis	Cardiac arrhythmias via depletion of intracellular potassium (D) 486
	Decreased response to lithium (D) 79
Diltiazem	Increased lithium levels (D) 451
	Risk of neurotoxicity (C) **30**
Heterocyclic antidepressants	Increased lithium tremor (C) 226, 371
	Seizures with amitriptyline (D) 422
	Myoclonus (C) 118
Insulin	Adjustment in insulin dosage may be required early in lithium treatment due to altered glucose tolerance (C) 402, 458–460
Iodide salts	Synergistic action in precipitation of hypothyroidism (C) 233, 400
Levofloxacin	Risk of lithium toxicity (C) **111**
Loop diuretics	Increased lithium effect and toxicity due to decreased renal lithium clearance with furosemide (C) **30**, **32**, 326
MAOIs	Tardive dyskinesia with tranylcypromine (C) 428
Mazindol	Increased lithium toxicity (D) 195
Methyldopa	Neurotoxicity associated with increased lithium levels (C) 68, 331, 333, 467, 492
Metronidazole 24 Spectinomycin 25, 95 Tetracycline **110**, 185, 281 }	Increased lithium effect and toxicity via decreased renal clearance (B)
Norepinephrine	Decreased pressor response to norepinephrine (C) 142, 151
Osmotic diuretics	Decreased lithium levels (B) **32**, 445

(continued)

Table C.6.   *(continued)*

Interacting Drug	Clinical Effect of Interaction

LITHIUM (*Con't*)

Phenytoin	Increased risk of neurotoxicity for both drugs (C) 277, 369, 426
Potassium-sparing diuretics	Increased lithium concentration (C) **30**
Propranolol	Increased bradycardia (C) 38
Prostaglandin inhibitors **32**	
Aspirin 41	
Celecoxib **74**	
Diclofenac **72, 84**, 373	
Ibuprofen 361, 364	
Indomethacin 154, 364	
Ketorolac 441	Significantly decreased lithium clearance and increased lithium levels (C)
Naproxen 363	
Phenylbutazone 408	
Piroxicam 243, 466	
Rofecoxib **74**	
Sulindac 299, 362, 363	
Psyllium hydrophilic mucilloid	Decreased lithium absorption (D) 346
Sodium bicarbonate 445	
Sodium chloride 29, 115, 214	Decreased lithium levels via increased renal clearance (C)
Urea 445	
SSRIs	Increased lithium levels with fluoxetine (C) 184, 387
	Fever, increased bilirubin, leucocytosis with fluoxetine (C) 319
	Lithium-induced neurotoxicity possibly due to SSRI-induced SIADH (C) 138, 348
Sulfamethoxazole/ trimethoprim	Altered lithium levels (C) **110**, 117,
Theophylline	Decreased lithium levels due to increased renal clearance (C) **32**, 347, 405
Thiazide diuretics	Increased lithium levels; 50% dose reduction may be necessary (B) 43, 202, 203, 214, 227, 269, 278, 421
Topiramate	Decreased lithium levels (D) **107**
Verapamil	Altered lithium levels (C) **30**, 474
	Sinus bradycardia (C) 125
	Choreoathetosis (D) 192
	Neurotoxicity (D) 358

CARBAMAZEPINE

Antipsychotics	Decreased antipsychotic levels* (C) 19, **28, 32**, 145, 219, 236, 238, 247, 248, 270
	Decreased clozapine levels* (B) **32**, 366
	Increased risk of granulocytopenia and possibly of agranulocytosis with clozapine (B) 234
	Neurotoxicity with haloperidol (D) 238
	Decreased carbamazepine level with risperidone (C) **85**
Benzodiazepines	Decreased clonazepam and alprazolam levels (D) 17, **32**, 261, 436
Bupropion	Decreased bupropion concentration* (B) **32**, 245
Calcium channel blockers	Increased carbamazepine levels and risk of neurotoxicity with diltiazem and verapamil (B) **5, 30**, 30, **32**, 59, 131, 279
	Decreased bioavailability of felodipine; decreased calcium channel blockade with felodipine (B) **5**, 71
Cimetidine	Transient inhibition of carbamazepine metabolism during first week* (B) **32**, 106, 107, 443
Corticosteroids	Increased clearance of corticosteroids* (C) 328
Cyclosporine	Increased clearance of cyclosporine* (B) 493
Danazol	Significantly increased carbamazepine levels and risk of neurotoxicity (B) 254, 497

(continued)

Table C.6.   *(continued)*

Interacting Drug	Clinical Effect of Interaction
	CARBAMAZEPINE (*Con't*)
Doxycycline	Increased doxycycline metabolism (C) 230, 317, 345
Felbamate	Increased felbamate clearance* (D) **43**
Grapefruit juice	Increased carbamazepine levels* (C) **59**
Heterocyclic antidepressants	Decreased TCA levels and increased heterocyclic metabolites and toxicity* (B) 31, 60, 61
Indinavir	Decreased indinavir concentration and risk of failure of antiretroviral therapy* (C) **53**
Isoniazid	Toxicity secondary to increased carbamazepine levels (B) **32**, 48, 452, 488
Ketoconazole	Increased carbamazepine levels* (C) **32**
Lithium	Increased polyuria, ataxia, and dizziness (C) 82, 160
	Increased risk of neurotoxicity (C) 82, **83**, 159, 349, 403
Macrolide antibiotics	Significant increase in carbamazepine levels and toxicity, including risk of heart block, with erythromycin and troleandomycin* (A) **32**, 74, 191, 293, 296, 487, 490, 498
Mebendazole	Decreased mebendazole levels (C) 276
Methadone	Decreased methadone levels (C) 40
Nefazodone	Increased carbamazepine concentration* (D) **89**
Neuromuscular blocking agents	Significantly shortened postoperative recovery times (B) 385
Oral anticoagulant	Decreased warfarin concentrations* (B) 187, 242, 290, 344, 384
Oral contraceptives	Decreased contraceptive drug levels and increased risk of pregnancy* (A) **32**, 100, 101, 193
Phenobarbital/ phenytoin/primidone	Decreased carbamazepine serum levels* (C) 78, 86, 205, 231
	Increased serum phenytoin levels* (D) 496
Propoxyphene	Increased carbamazepine levels and risk of toxicity* (C) 108, 186, 327, 495
Ritonavir/efavirenz	Carbamazepine toxicity* (D) **11, 15**
SSRIs	Increased levels of carbamazepine with fluoxetine (B) **4, 32**, 341
Theophylline	Decreased theophylline and/or carbamazepine levels* (B) 305, 383
Thyroid hormones	Induction of metabolism of thyroid replacement hormones* (C) 1, 232
Valproic acid	Altered valproic acid and/or carbamazepine levels; close monitoring is required* (C) **4, 32**, 53, 268, 280, 282, 291, 309, 336, 367, 424
Vincristine	Increased vincristine clearance with combination of carbamazepine and phenytoin (C) **116a**
	VALPROIC ACID
Antipsychotics	Prolonged half-life of valproic acid with chlorpromazine (C) 217
	Altered levels of risperidone and/or valproic acid (C) **31**
	Case of acute generalized edema with risperidone (D) **100**
Barbiturates	Barbiturate intoxication via inhibition of metabolism (C) 65, 337, 482
Benzodiazepines	Increased sedation and absence seizure activity with clonazepam (D) 62, 224, 261, 436
	Increased half-life of diazepam (C) 119
Carbamazepine	Altered valproic acid and/or carbamazepine levels; close monitoring is required* (C) 53, 268, 280, 282, 291, 309, 336, 367, 424
Cholestyramine	Decreased valproic acid concentration (C) **30**
Ethosuximide	Prolonged half-life (C) 353
Felbamate	Decreased valproic acid clearance (D) **43**
Heterocyclic antidepressants	Increased valproate levels (C) 256
Lamotrigine	Increased lamotrigine levels (C) **4**, 256
	Risk of Stevens-Johnson syndrome (B) 256
	Decreased valproic acid levels (C) **4**
Magnesium/aluminum hydroxide	Increased valproate levels (C) 256

(continued)

Table C.6.   *(continued)*

Interacting Drug	Clinical Effect of Interaction
	VALPROIC ACID (*Con't*)
Phenytoin	Altered phenytoin and/or valproic acid levels* (C) 64, 104, 196, 291, 309, 335, 376
Salicylates	Increased hepatotoxic metabolites of valproate (C) 2
	Valproic acid toxicity via increased free levels and decreased clearance (C) 2, 144, 170, 332
Tiagabine	Slightly decreased valproic acid levels (D) 4
Topiramate	Decreased valproic acid levels (C) 4
Zidovudine	Increased zidovudine levels (C) 71
	LAMOTRIGINE
Acetaminophen	Increased lamotrigine clearance (C) 4
Carbamazepine	Decreased lamotrigine levels (C) 4
Phenobarbital	Decreased lamotrigine levels (C) 4
Phenytoin	Decreased lamotrigine levels (C) 4
Valproic acid	Increased lamotrigine levels (C) 4, 256
	Risk of Stevens-Johnson syndrome (B) 256
	Decreased valproic acid levels (C) 4
	OXCARBAZEPINE
Oral contraceptives	Decreased estrogen/progesterone levels* (C) 36
	TOPIRAMATE
Digoxin	Slight increase in digoxin clearance (D) 4
Oral contraceptives	Decreased hormone levels* (C) 4
Phenobarbital	Decreased topiramate concentration (D) 4
	GABAPENTIN
Maalox	10–20% decreased gabapentin bioavailability (D) 4

(A) = Severe interaction; (B) = Significant interaction; (C) = Potentially significant interaction; (D) = Mild interaction or single case; * = Interaction mediated partially or totally through CYP-450 enzyme system.

Table C.7. Adverse Drug Interactions of Anxiolytics-Hypnotics

Interacting Drug	Clinical Effect of Interaction
	BENZODIAZEPINES
Alcohol	Increased sedation (B) 262, 271
	Additive CNS depressant effects; increased BZ absorption and impaired elimination (B) 272
	Behavioral dyscontrol and adverse psychomotor effects with alcohol and BZs (B) 444
Antacids	Delayed oral absorption of BZs (D) 180, 215, 397
Anticholinergics	Delayed oral absorption of BZs (D) 420
Antipsychotics	Increased risk of respiratory depression (C) 35, 93
	Increased sedation (B) 18, 204
	Two cases of cardiopulmonary collapse with clozapine (C) 389
Barbiturates/narcotics	Increased sedation (B) 179, 435
Buprenorphine	Case reports of fatalities with combination of buprenorphine and BZs (B) 97
Caffeine	Diminished BZ effects (C) **51**
Calcium channel blockers	Increased half-life of BZs metabolized by CYP 3A3/4 enzymes* (B) 28, **30**
Carbamazepine	Decreased clonazepam and alprazolam levels (D) 17, 261, 436
Cholestyramine	Increased half-life of lorazepam (C) **30**
Cimetidine	Increased cognitive impairment with midazolam (C) **22**
Digoxin	Increased digoxin levels with diazepam (D) 75, 324, 447
Disulfiram	Inhibition of metabolism of some BZs (C) 285, 395
Erythromycin/ troleandomycin	Inhibition of midazolam and triazolam metabolism* (C) 330, 351, 470
Fluoxetine	Increased half-life of diazepam* (C) 267
	Increased plasma levels of alprazolam* (C) **9**
Fluvoxamine	Increased plasma levels of alprazolam; risk of impaired motor performance and memory* (C) **9**
Grapefruit juice	Increased bioavailability of diazepam, midazolam, triazolam* (C) **59**
H$_2$ blockers	Decreased oral diazepam levels with ranitidine (C) 249
	Significantly increased benzodiazepine levels and risk of CNS toxicity with cimetidine* (C) 116, 176–178, 250, 251
Heterocyclic antidepressants	Increased sedation, confusion, impaired motor function (C) 42
	Increased TCA levels with alprazolam* (C) 16
	Decreased imipramine levels with diazepam (D) 147
	Decreased desipramine level with clonazepam (D) 114
Intraconazole/ketoconazole	Significantly increased midazolam and triazolam blood levels* (B) 175, 329, 456
Isoniazid	Increased toxicity of some BZs via inhibition of metabolism* (D) 322, 323
L-Dopa	Decreased effect of L-Dopa with chlordiazepoxide (D), 213, 494
Lithium	Increased serum lithium levels with clonazepam (C) 253
	Hypothermia associated with diazepam (D) 315
MAOIs	Disinhibition and generalized edema with chlordiazepoxide (C) 169, 338
Metoprolol	Decreased negative chronotropic effect with chlordiazepoxide (C) 307
Nefazodone	Increased levels of triazolobenzodiazepines* (C) 34, 132
Oral contraceptives	Inhibition of metabolism of long-acting BZs and increased toxicity (D) 6, 382
Phenytoin	Decreased clinical effect of BZs by hepatic enzymes induction* (C) 197, 413, 415
	Alteration of clinical effects of phenytoin (D) 130, 208, 435
Probenecid	Significantly increased lorazepam levels (C) 3
Protease inhibitors	Increased levels of BZs metabolized by CYP3A3/4* (C) **47**, 348
Rifampin	Increased clearance of BZs* (D) 322
Succinylcholine	Decreased neuromuscular blockage (D) 140, 149

(continued)

Table C.7.   *(continued)*

Interacting Drug	Clinical Effect of Interaction
	BENZODIAZEPINES (*Con't*)
Valproic acid	Increased sedation and absence seizure activity with clonazepam (D) 62, 224, 261, 436
	Increased half-life of diazepam (C) 119
	Increased lorazepam concentration (C) **71**
	BUSPIRONE
Carbamazepine	Decreased buspirone levels* (D) **75**
Diltiazem/verapamil	Decreased metabolism of buspirone (D) **30, 75**
Erythromycin	Increased buspirone levels* (D) **62, 75**
Fluvoxamine	Increased buspirone levels* (D) **64**
Grapefruit juice	Increased buspirone levels* (D) **59, 75**
Haloperidol	Increased haloperidol levels (C) 163
Heterocyclic antidepressant	Hypertension and anxiety with clomipramine (D) 83
Itraconazole	Increased buspirone levels* (D) **62, 75**
MAOIs	Increased blood pressure (B) 89
Phenytoin	Decreased buspirone levels* (D) **75**
Rifampin	Increased clearance of buspirone* (C) **38, 75**
Ritonavir	Parkinsonian symptoms with combination of ritonavir and buspirone (D) **23**
Warfarin	Increased anticoagulant effects (C) **30**
	OTHER ANXIOLYTICS-HYPNOTICS
Chlorpromazine	Increased sedative effects with zolpidem (C) **51**
Cimetidine	Decreased clearance of zaleplon (C) **51**
	Increased sleep duration and decreased alertness with zolpidem (C) **51**
Ethanol	Increased CNS depression with chloral hydrate (B) 396
	Unexpected reactions such as flushing, tachycardia, and headache with chloral hydrate (C) 396
	Increased sedative effects with zolpidem (C) **51**
Flumazenil	Reversal of sedative effect of zolpidem (C) **51**
Fluoxetine	Shortened duration of action of zolpidem (D) **22**
Imipramine	Increased sedative effect of zolpidem (C) **51**
	Additive motor effects with zaleplon (C) **51**
Ketoconazole	Increased zolpidem effects* (C) **51**
Oral anticoagulants	Transient potentiation of warfarin hypoprothrombinemic effect with chloral hydrate (B) 303, 450
Rifampin	Decreased levels of zolpidem and zaleplon* (D) **51**
Ritonavir	Decreased metabolism of zolpidem* (D) **22**
Sertraline	Shortened onset of action and/or increased effect of zolpidem (D) **51**
Thioridazine	Increased reaction time with zaleplon (D) **51, 52**

(A) = Severe interaction; (B) = Significant interaction; (C) = Potentially significant interaction; (D) = Mild interaction or single case; * = Interaction mediated partially or totally through CYP-450 enzyme system.

Table C.8.   Adverse Drug Interactions with Other Psychotropics

Interacting Drug	Clinical Effect of Interaction
	STIMULANTS
Acetazolamide	Decreased clearance of dextroamphetamine (D) **30**
Anticonvulsants	Increased levels of phenytoin and phenobarbital with methylphenidate (C) 256
	Decreased methylphenidate levels with carbamazepine* (D) **10**
Citalopram	Risk of serotonin syndrome with dextroamphetamine (D) **94**
Clonidine	Adverse cardiovascular effects with methylphenidate (C) **30**
	Four cases of sudden death with combination of clonidine and methylphenidate (A) **78**
Cyclosporine	Increased cyclosporine levels with methylphenidate (C) **70**
Ethinyl estradiol	Induction of hormone metabolism by modafinil* (D) **99**
Guanethidine	Decreased pressor effect with methylphenidate (C) 256
Heterocyclic antidepressants	Increased TCA levels with methylphenidate (B) **78**, 152, 479
	Cases of hypertension, agitation, and blood dyscrasia with combination of imipramine and methylphenidate (C) **78**
L-Dopa	Increased motor effects of L-Dopa with methylphenidate (D) **17**
MAOIs	Hypertension (B) **78**, 223, 416
Phenytoin	Phenytoin toxicity with methylphenidate (C) **78**
Pressor agents	Increased pressor effect with methylphenidate (C) 256
Sertraline	Case reports of confusion, visual hallucinations, seizures in combination with methylphenidate (C) **78**
Triazolam	Induction of triazolam metabolism by modafinil (D) **99**
Venlafaxine	Risk of serotonin syndrome with dextroamphetamine (D) **94**
	SUBSTANCE ABUSE/DEPENDENCE TREATMENT AGENTS
Antiretroviral agents	Increased levels of AZT, ddI with methadone* (C) **45**
Benzodiazepines	Additive respiratory depression with methadone (C) **18**
Clarithromycin	Case report of toxic epidermal necrolysis with disulfiram (D) **79**
Grapefruit juice	Increased methadone levels* (D) **59**
Nevirapine	Decreased methadone levels; risk of opiate withdrawal symtpoms* (C) **45, 50**
NSAIDs	Increased rate of hepatic transaminase elevation with naltrexone (C) **61**
Zidovudine	Increased methadone levels* (C) **81**
	COGNITIVE ENHANCERS
Amantadine	Potentiation of anticholinergic effects resulting in nocturnal confusion and hallucinations (C) 394
Antipsychotics	Altered antipsychotic blood levels (C) 26, 275, 377, 379
	Delayed onset of effects of acute oral doses of antipsychotics (C) 377, 379, 410, 411
	Increased anticholinergic effects (C) 13, 27, 137, 158
	Increased risk of hyperthermia (C) 287, 478
Cimetidine	Increased tacrine levels* (D) **55**
Erythromycin	Increased bioavailability of galantamine* (D) **55**
Fluvoxamine	Inhibition of tacrine metabolism* (D) **55, 65**
Heterocyclic antidepressants	Additive anticholinergic effects (C) 22, 220, 223
	Anticholinergic delirium (B) 22
Hormone replacement therapy	Increased tacrine levels* (D) **55**
Ketoconazole	Increased donepezil levels* (D) **55, 114**
	Increased bioavailability of galantamine* (D) **55**
MAOIs	Risk of enhanced CNS depression (C) 89, 109
Paroxetine	Adverse GI effects and agitation in combination with donepezil (D) **19, 55**
	Increased bioavailability of galantamine* (D) **55**
Sertraline	Case of fulminant hepatitis with donepezil (D) **55**
Theophylline	Decreased theophylline clearance with tacrine (D) **55**

(A) = Severe interaction; (B) = Significant interaction; (C) = Potentially significant interaction; (D) = Mild interaction or single case; * = Interaction mediated partially or totally through CYP-450 enzyme system.

References

1. Aanderud S, Myking OL, Strandjord RE. The influence of carbamazepine on thyroid hormones and thyroxine binding globulin in hyperthyroid patients substituted with thyroxine. *Clin Endocrinol* 1981;15:247–252.

2. Abbott FS, Kassam J, Orr JM, Farrell K. The effects of aspirin on valproic acid metabolism. *Clin Pharmacol Ther* 1986;40:94–100.

3. Abernethy DR, Greenblatt DJ, Ameer B, et al. Probenecid impairment of acetaminophen formation. *J Pharmacol Exp Ther* 1985;234: 345–349.

4. Abernethy DR, Greenblatt DJ, Shader RI. Imipramine disposition in users of oral contraceptive steroids. *Clin Pharmacol Ther* 1984;35: 792–797.

5. Abernethy DR, Greenblatt DJ, Shader RI. Imipramine-cimetidine interaction: impairment of clearance and enhanced bioavailability. *J Pharmacol Exp Ther* 1984;229:702–705.

6. Abernethy DR, Greenblatt DJ, Divoll M, et al. Impairment of diazepam metabolism by low-dose estrogen-containing oral contraceptive steroids. *N Engl J Med* 1982;306:791–792.

7. Addonizio G, Roth SD, Stokes PE, Stoll PM. Increased extrapyramidal symptoms with addition of lithium to neuroleptics. *J Nerv Ment Dis* 1988;176:682–685.

8. Addy RO, Foliart RH, Suran AS, et al. EEG observations during combined haloperidol lithium treatment. *Biol Psychiatry* 1986;21:2: 170–176.

9. Adnitt PI. Hypoglycemic action of monoamine oxidase inhibitors (MAOI). *Diabetes* 1968;17: 628–633.

10. Alexander HE, McCarty K, Giffen MB. Hypotension and cardiopulmonary arrest associated with concurrent haloperidol and propranolol therapy. *JAMA* 1984;252:87–88.

11. Alexanderson B, Evans DAP, Sjoqvist F. Steadystate plasma levels of nortriptyline in twins: influence of genetic factors and drug therapy. *Br Med J* 1969;5:764–768.

12. Allen RM, Klemenbaum A. Delirium associated with combined fluphenazine-clonidine therapy. *J Clin Psychiatry* 1979;40:236–237.

13. Alpert M, Diamond F, Laski EM. Anticholinergic exacerbation of phenothiazine-induced extrapyramidal syndrome. *Am J Psychiatry* 1976; 133:1073–1075.

14. Angrist B, Lee HK, Gershon S. The antagonism of amphetamine-induced symptomatology by a neuroleptic. *Am J Psychiatry* 1974;131:817–819.

15. Angrist B, Sathanathan G, Gershon S. Behavioral effects of L-dopa in schizophrenic patients. *Psychopharmacologia* 1973;31:1–12.

16. Antal EJ, et al. Multicenter evaluation of the kinetic and clinical interaction of alprazolam and imipramine. *Clin Pharmacol Ther* 1986;39: 178.

17. Arana GW, Epstein S, Molloy M, Greenblatt DJ. Carbamazepine-induced reduction of plasma alprazolam concentrations: a clinical case report. *J Clin Psychiatry* 1988;49:11:448–449.

18. Arana GW, Orusteen ML, Kaufer F, et al. The use of benzodiazepines for psychotic disorders: a literature review and preliminary clinical findings. *Psychopharmacol Bull* 1986;22:77–87.

19. Arana GW, Goff DC, Friedman H, et al. Does carbamazepine-induced reduction of plasma haloperidol levels worsen psychotic symptoms? *Am J Psychiatry* 1986;143:5:650–651.

20. Aranow RB, Aranow AB, Hudsson II, Pope HG, et al. Elevated antidepressant plasma levels after addition of fluoxetine. *Am J Psychiatry* 1989;146:911–913.

21. Arneson G. Phenothiazine derivatives and glucose metabolism. *J Neuropsychiatry* 1964;5: 181–185.

22. Arnold SE, Kahn RJ, Faldetta LL, et al. Tricyclic antidepressants and peripheral anticholinergic activity. *Psychopharmacology* 1981;74:325–328.

23. Asayesh K. Combination of trazodone and phenothiazines: a possible additive hypotensive effect. *Can J Psychiatry* 1986;31:857–858.

24. Ayd FJ Jr. Metronidazole-induced lithium intoxication. *Int Drug Ther Newslett* 1982;17:15.

25. Ayd FJ Jr. Possible adverse drug-drug interaction report: lithium intoxication in a spectinomycin-treated patient. *Int Drug Ther Newslett* 1978;13:15.

26. Ayd FJ Jr. Do antiparkinson drugs interfere with the therapeutic effects of neuroleptics? *Int Drug Ther Newslett* 1974;9:8.

27. Babayan EA, Rudenko GM, Lepakhin VK. Neuroleptics and antipsychotic drugs. In: Dukes MNG, ed. *Side effects of drugs annual 5.* Amsterdam: Excerpta Medica, 1981:41.

28. Backman JT, Olkkola JT, Aranko K, et al. Dose of midazolam should be reduced during diltiazem and verapamil treatments. *Br J Clin Pharmacol* 1994;37:221–225.

29. Baer L, Glassman AH, Kassir S. Negative sodium balance in lithium carbonate toxicity. Evidence of mineralocorticoid blockade. *Arch Gen Psychiatry* 1973;29:823–827.

30. Bahls F, Ozuna K, Ritchie DE. Interactions between calcium channel blockers and the anticonvulsants, carbamazepine and phenytoin. *Neurology* 1991;41:740–742.

31. Baldessarini RJ, Teicher MH, Cassidy JW, Stein MH. Anticonvulsant cotreatment may increase toxic metabolites of antidepressants and other psychotropic drugs. *J Clin Psychopharmacol* 1988;8:5:381–382.

32. Bannister BJ, Houser VP, Hulse JD, et al. Evaluation of the potential for interactions of paroxetine with diazepam, cimetidine, warfarin, and digoxin. *Acta Psychiatr Scand* 1989;80(suppl 350):102–106.

33. Baptista T. Lithium-neuroleptic combination and irreversible brain damage. *Acta Psychiatr Scand* 1986;73:1:111.

34. Barbhaiya RH, Shukla UA, Kroboth PD, et al. Coadministration of nefazodone and benzodiazepines, II: a pharmacokinetic interaction study with triazolam. *J Clin Psychopharmacol* 1995;15:320–326.

35. Battaglia J, Thornton L, Young C. Loxapine-lorazepam-induced hypotension and stupor. *J Clin Psychopharmacol* 1989;9:3:227–228.

36. Bazire SR. Sudden death associated with switching monoamine oxidase inhibitors. *Drug Intell Clin Pharm* 1986;20:954–956.

37. Beaumont G. Drug interactions with clomipramine (Anafranil). *J Int Med Res* 1973;1:480.

38. Becker D. Lithium and propranolol: possible synergism? *J Clin Psychiatry* 1989;50:12:473.

39. Bell IR, Cole JO. Fluoxetine induces elevation of desipramine level and exacerbation of geriatric nonpsychotic depression. *J Clin Psychopharmacol* 1988;8:6:447–448.

40. Bell J, Seres V, Bowron P, et al. The use of serum methadone levels in patients receiving methadone maintenance. *Clin Pharmacol Ther* 1988;43:623–629.

41. Bendz H, Feinberg M. Aspirin increases serum lithium ion levels. *Arch Gen Psychiatry* 1984;41:310–311.

42. Beresford TP, Feinsilver DL, Hall RC. Adverse reactions to a benzodiazepine-tricyclic antidepressant compound. *J Clin Psychopharmacol* 1981;1:392–394.

43. Berkowitz HL. Drug interactions [Letter]. *Hosp Community Psychiatry* 1987;38:886.

44. Bigger JT, Giardina EG, Perel JM, et al. Cardiac antiarrhythmic effect of imipramine hydrochloride. *N Engl J Med* 1977;296:206–208.

45. Bird HA, le Gallez P, Wright V. Drowsiness due to haloperidol/indomethacin in combination. *Lancet* 1983;1:830–831.

46. Blackwell B, Marley E, Price J, et al. Hypertensive interaction associated with monoamine oxidase inhibitors and food stuffs. *Br J Psychiatry* 1967;113:349–365.

47. Blackwell B, Schmidt GL. Drug interactions in psychopharmacology. *Psychiatr Clin North Am* 1984;7:625–637.

48. Block SH. Carbamazepine-isoniazid interaction. *Pediatrics* 1982;69:494–495.

49. Boakes AJ, Laurence DR, Teon PC, et al. Interactions between sympathomimetic amines and antidepressant agents in man. *Br Med J* 1973;1:311–315.

50. Bodley PO, Halwax K, Potts L. Low serum-pseudocholinesterase levels complicating treatment with phenelzine. *Br Med J* 1969;3:510–512.

51. Borden EC, Rostrand SG. Recovery from massive amitriptyline overdosage [Letter]. *Lancet* 1968;1:1256.

52. Borden H. The use of pancuronium bromide in patients receiving lithium carbonate. *Can Soc J* 1974;21:79–82.

53. Bowdle TA, Levy RH, Cutler RE. Effects of carbamazepine on valproic acid kinetics in normal subjects. *Clin Pharmacol Ther* 1979;26:629–634.

54. Bowen S. Effect of coffee and tea on blood levels and efficacy of antipsychotic drugs [Letter]. *Lancet* 1981;1:1217.

55. Boyer WF, Lake CR. Interaction of phenelzine and sulfisoxazole. *Am J Psychiatry* 1983;140:264–265.

56. Van den Brekel, Harrington L. Toxic effects of theophylline caused by fluvoxamine. *Can Med Assoc J* 1994;151:1289–1290.

57. Briant RH, George CF. The assessment of potential drug interactions with a new tricyclic antidepressant drug. *Br J Clin Pharmacol* 1974;1:113.

58. Briant RH, Reid JL, Dollery CT. Interaction between clonidine and desipramine in man. *Br Med J* 1973;1:522–523.

59. Brodie MJ, Macphee GJ. Carbamazepine neurotoxicity precipitated by diltiazem. *Br Med J* 1986;292:1170–1171.

60. Brosen K, Kragh-Sorensen P. Concomitant intake of nortriptyline and carbamazepine. *Ther Drug Monit* 1993;15:258–260.

61. Brown CS, Wells BG, Cold JA, et al. Possible influence of carbamazepine on plasma imipramine concentration in children with attention-deficit hyperactivity disorder. *J Clin Psychopharmcol* 1990;10:359–362.

62. Browne TR, Watson WA. Interaction between clonazepam and sodium valproate. *N Engl J Med* 1979;300:678–679.

63. Brownlee G, Williams GW. Potentiation of amphetamine and pethidine by monoamine oxidase inhibitors. *Lancet* 1963;1:669.

64. Bruni J, Gallo JM, Lee CS, et al. Interactions of valproic acid with phenytoin. *Neurology* 1980;30:1233–1236.

65. Bruni J, Wilder BJ, Perchalski RJ, et al. Valproic acid and plasma levels of phenobarbital. *Neurology* 1980;30:94–97.

66. Buckle RM, Guillebaud J. Hypoglycemic coma occurring during treatment with chlorpromazine and orphenadrine. *Br Med J* 1967;4:599–600.

67. Burrows GD, Davies B. Antidepressants and barbiturates [Letter]. *Br Med J* 1971;4:113.

68. Byrd GJ. Methyldopa and lithium carbonate: suspected interaction [Letter]. *JAMA* 1975;233:320.

69. Byrne A, O'Shea B. Adverse interaction between cimetidine and chlorpromazine in two cases of chronic schizophrenia. *Br J Psychiatry* 1989;155:413–415.

70. Campbell JB. Long-term treatment of Parkinson's disease with levodopa. *Neurology* 1970;20:12:18–22.

71. Capewell S, Freestone S, Critchley JA, et al. Reduced felodipine bioavailability in patients taking anticonvulsants. *Lancet* 1988;2:480–482.

72. Capron J, Gineston JL, Opolon P, et al. Fulminating lethal hepatitis due to the interaction of iproniazid and prochlorperazine. *Gastroenterol Clin Biol* 1980;4:123–127.

73. Caranasos GJ. Drug reactions and interactions in the patient undergoing surgery. *Med Clin North Am* 1979;63:1245–1255.

74. Carranco E, Kareus J, Co S, et al. Carbamazepine toxicity induced by concurrent erythromycin therapy. *Arch Neurol* 1985;42:187–188.

75. Castillo-Ferrando JR, Garcia M, Carmona J. Digoxin levels and diazepam [Letter]. *Lancet* 1980;2:368.

76. Centorrino F, Baldessarini RJ, Kando J, et al. Serum concentrations of clozapine and its major metabolites: effects of cotreatment with fluoxetine or valproate. *Am J Psychiatry* 1994;151:123–125.

77. Centorrino F, Baldessarini RJ, Frankenberg FR, et al. Serum levels of clozapine and norclozapine in patients treated with selective serotonin reuptake inhibitors. *Am J Psychiatry* 1996;153:820–822.

78. Cereghino JJ, Brock JT, Van Meter JC, et al.

The efficacy of carbamazepine combinations in epilepsy. *Clin Pharmacol Ther* 1975;18: 733–741.

79. Chambers CA, Smith AH, Naylor GJ. The effect of digoxin on the response to lithium therapy in mania. *Psychol Med* 1982;12:57–60.

80. Chan C, Ruskiewicz R. Anticholinergic side effects of trazodone combined with another pharmacologic agent. *Am J Psychiatry* 1990;147: 4:533.

81. Chandler JD. Switching MAOIs. *J Clin Psychopharmacol* 1987;7:438.

82. Chaudhry RP, Waters BG. Lithium and carbamazepine interaction: possible neurotoxicity. *J Clin Psychiatry* 1983;44:30–31.

83. Chignon JM, Lepine JP. Panic and hypertension associated with single dose of buspirone. *Lancet* 1989;2:46.

84. Chouinard G, Ghadirian AM, Jones BD. Death attributed to ventricular arrhythmias induced by thioridazine in combination with a single Contac-C capsule. *Can Med Assoc J* 1978;119: 729–730.

85. Chouinard G, Dinard G, Prenoveau Y, Tetreault L. Alpha-methyldopa-chlorpromazine interaction in schizophrenic patients. *Curr Ther Res Clin Exp* 1973;15:60–72.

86. Christiansen J, Dam M. Influence of phenobarbital and diphenylhydantoin on plasma carbamazepine levels in patients with epilepsy. *Acta Neurol Scand* 1973;49:543–546.

87. Christensen RC. Adverse interaction of paroxetine and cyproheptadine [Letter]. *J Clin Psychiatry* 1995;56:433–434.

88. Ciraulo DA, Barnhill JG, Jaffe JH. Clinical pharmacokinetics of imipramine and desipramine in alcoholics and normal volunteers. *Clin Pharmacol Ther* 1988;43:509–518.

89. Ciraulo DA, Shader RI, Greenblatt DJ, Creelman WL. *Drug interactions in psychiatry.* Baltimore: Williams & Wilkins, 1989.

90. Ciraulo DA, Barnhill J, Boxenbaum H. Pharmacokinetic interaction between disulfiram and antidepressants. *Am J Psychiatry* 1985;142: 1373–1374.

91. Claire RJ, Servis ME, Cram DL Jr. Potential interaction between warfarin sodium and fluoxetine [Letter]. *Am J Psychiatry* 1991;148:1604.

92. Cohen BJ, Mahelsky M, Adler L. More cases of SIADH with fluoxetine [Letter]. *Am J Psychiatry* 1990;147:948–949.

93. Cohen S, Khan A. Respiratory distress with use of lorazepam in mania. *J Clin Psychopharmacol* 1987;7:3:199–200.

94. Cohen W, Cohen N. Lithium carbonate, haloperidol, and irreversible brain damage. *JAMA* 1974;230:1283–1287.

95. Conroy RW. Possible adverse drug-drug interaction report: lithium intoxication in a spectinomycin-treated patient. *Int Drug Ther Newslett* 1978;13:15.

96. Consolo S, Morselli PL, Zaccala M, Garattini S. Delayed absorption of phenylbutazone caused by desmethylimipramine in humans. *Eur J Pharmacol* 1970;10:239–242.

97. Cooper AJ. Action of mebanazine, a monoamine oxidase inhibitor antidepressant drug in diabetes. II. *Int J Neuropsychiatry* 1966;2: 342–345.

98. Cooper AJ, Ashcroft G. Potentiation of insulin hypoglycaemia by MAOI antidepressant drugs. *Lancet* 1966;1:407–409.

99. Cooper AJ, Keddie KM. Hypotensive collapse and hypoglycaemia after mebanazine, a monoamine oxidase inhibitor. *Lancet* 1964;1: 1133–1134.

100. Coulam CB, Annegers JF. Do anticonvulsants reduce the efficacy of oral contraceptives? *Epilepsia* 1979;20:519–525.

101. Crawford P, Chadwick DJ, Martin C, et al. The interaction of phenytoin and carbamazepine with combined oral contraceptive steroids. *Br J Clin Pharmacol* 1990;30:892–896.

102. Curry SH, Davis JM, Janowsky DS, Marshall JH. Factors affecting chlorpromazine plasma levels in psychiatric patients. *Arch Gen Psychiatry* 1970; 22:209–215.

103. Cuthbert MF, Greenberg MP, Morley SW. Cough and cold remedies: potential danger to patients on monoamine oxidase inhibitors. *Br Med J* 1969;1:404–406.

104. Dahlqvist R, Borga O, Rane A, et al. Decreased plasma protein binding of phenytoin in patients on valproic acid. *Br J Clin Pharmacol* 1979; 8:547–552.

105. Dally PJ. Fatal reaction associated with tranylcypromine and methylamphetamine [Letter]. *Lancet* 1962;1:1235.

106. Dalton MJ, Powell JR, Messenheimer JA Jr, Clark J. Cimetidine and carbamazepine: a complex drug interaction. *Epilepsia* 1986;27: 553–558.

107. Dalton MJ, Powell JR, Messenheimer JA Jr. The influence of cimetidine on a single dose carbamazepine pharmacokinetics. *Epilepsia* 1985;26: 127–130.

108. Dam M, Kristensen CB, Zaitansen BS, Christiansen J. Interaction between carbamazepine and propoxyphene in man. *Acta Neurol Scand* 1977;566:603–607.

109. Davidson J, Zung WW, Walker JI. Practical aspects of MAO inhibitor therapy. *J Clin Psychiatry* 1984;45:81–84.

110. Davies B, Bannister R, Sever P. Pressor amines and monoamine-oxidase inhibitors for treatment of postural hypotension in autonomic failure. Limitations and hazards. *Lancet* 1978; 1:172–175.

111. Davies TS. Monoamine oxidase inhibitors and rauwolfia compounds [Letter]. *Br Med J* 1960; 739.

112. de la Fuente JR, Berlanga C, Leon-Andrade C. Mania induced by tricyclic-MAOI combination therapy in bipolar treatment resistant depression: case reports. *J Clin Psychiatry* 1986;47:1: 40–41.

113. Dequardo JR, Roberts M. Elevated clozapine levels after fluvoxamine initiation. *Am J Psychiatry* 1996;153:840–841.

114. Deicken RF. Clonazepam-induced reduction in serum desipramine concentration. *J Clin Psychopharmacol* 1988;8:1:71–73.

115. Demers RG, Heninger GR. Sodium intake and lithium treatment in mania. *Am J Psychiatry* 1971;128:100–104.

116. Desmond PV, Patwardhan RV, Schenker S, Speeq KV Jr. Cimetidine impairs elimination of chlordiazepoxide (Librium) in man. *Ann Intern Med* 1980;93:266–268.

117. Desvilles M, Sevestre P. Effect paradoxal de l'association lithium et sulfamethoxazol-trimetroprime. *Nouv Presse Med* 1982;11:3267–3268.

118. Devanand DP, Sackeim HA, Brown RP. Myoclonus during combined tricyclic antidepressant and lithium treatment. *J Clin Psychopharmacol* 1988;8:6:446–447.

119. Dhillon SA, Richens A. Valproic acid and diazepam interactions in vivo. *Br J Clin Pharmacol* 1982;13:553–560.

120. Domino EF, Sullivan TS, Luby ED. Barbiturate intoxication in a patient treated with a MAO inhibitor. *Am J Psychiatry* 1962;118:941–943.

121. Dorian P, Sellers EM, Reed KL, et al. Amitriptyline and ethanol: pharmacokinetic and pharmacodynamic interaction. *Eur J Clin Pharmacol* 1983;25:325–331.

122. Dorn JM. A case of phenytoin toxicity possibly precipitated by trazodone. *J Clin Psychiatry* 1986;47:89–90.

123. Douste-Blazy PH, Rostin M, Livarek B, et al. Angiotensin converting enzyme inhibitors and lithium treatment [Letter]. *Lancet* 1986;1:1448.

124. Dripps RD, Vandam LD, Pierce EC, et al. The use of chlorpromazine in anesthesia and surgery. *Ann Surg* 1955;142:774–785.

125. Dubovsky SL, Franks RD, Allen S. Verapamil: a new antimanic drug with potential interactions with lithium. *J Clin Psychiatry* 1987;48:371–372.

126. Dunphy TW. The pharmacist's role in the prevention of adverse drug interactions. *Am J Hosp Pharm* 1969;26:366–377.

127. Duvoisin RC. Diphenidol for levodopa induced nausea and vomiting. *JAMA* 1972;221:1408.

128. Dysken MW, Cumming RJ, Channon RA, Davis JM. Drug interaction between ascorbic acid and fluphenazine. *JAMA* 1979;24:2008.

129. Edwards M. Adverse interaction of levodopa with tricyclic antidepressants. *Practitioner* 1982;226:1447–1449.

130. Edwards VE, Eadie MJ. Clonazepam—a clinical study of its effectiveness as an anticonvulsant. *Proc Aust Assoc Neurol* 1973;10:61–66.

131. Eimer M, Carter BL. Elevated serum carbamazepine concentrations following diltiazem initiation. *Drug Intell Clin Pharm* 1987;21:340–342.

132. Ellingrod VJ, Perry PJ. Nefazodone: a new antidepressant or another "me too" drug? *Am J Health-system Pharm* 1995;52:2799–2812.

133. El-Yousef MK, Manier DH. Tricyclic antidepressants and phenothiazines [Letter]. *JAMA* 1974;229:1419.

134. El-Yousef MK, Manier DH. Estrogen effects on phenothiazine derivative blood levels [Letter]. *JAMA* 1974;226:827–828.

135. Ellis J, Laurence DR, Mattie H, Prichard BN. Modification by monoamine oxidase inhibitors of the effect of some sympathomimetics on blood pressure. *Br Med J* 1967; 2:75–78.

136. Ereshefsky L, Riesenman C, Lam YF. Serotonin selective reuptake inhibitor drug interactions and the cytochrome P450 system. *J Clin Psychiatry* 1996;57:17–25.

137. Evans DL, Rogers JF, Peiper SC. Intestinal dilatation associated with phenothiazine therapy: a case report and literature review. *Am J Psychiatry* 1979;136:970–972.

138. Evans M, Marwick P. Fluvoxamine and lithium: an unusual interaction [Letter]. *Br J Psychiatry* 1990;156:286.

139. Evans-Prosser CGD. The use of pethidine and morphine in the presence of MAO inhibitors. *Br J Anaesth* 1968;40:279–282.

140. Fahmy NR, Malek NS, Lappas DG. Diazepam prevents some adverse effects of succinylcholine. *Clin Pharmacol Ther* 1979;26:395–398.

141. Fann WE, Davis JM, Janowsky DS, et al. Chlorpromazine: effects of antacids on its gastrointestinal absorption. *J Clin Pharmacol* 1973;13:388–390.

142. Fann WE, Davis JM, Janowsky DS, et al. Effects of lithium on adrenergic function in man. *Clin Pharmacol Ther* 1972;13:71–77.

143. Fann WE, Janowsky DS, Davis JM, Dates JA. Chlorpromazine reversal of the anti-hypertensive action of guanethidine [Letter]. *Lancet* 1971;2:436–437.

144. Farrell K, Orr JM, Abbott FS, et al. The effect of acetylsalicylic acid on serum free valproate concentrations and valproate clearance in children. *J Pediatr* 1982;101:142–144.

145. Fast DK, Jones BD, Kusalic M, Erickson M. Effect of carbamazepine on neuroleptic plasma levels and efficacy. *Am J Psychiatry* 1986;143:1:117–118.

146. Feder R. Reversal of antidepressant activity of fluoxetine by cyproheptadine in three patients. *J Clin Psychiatry* 1991;52:163–164.

147. Feet PO, Larsen S, Robak OH. A double-blind study in outpatients with primary non-agitated depression treated with imipramine in combination with placebo, diazepam or dixyrazine. *Acta Psychiatr Scand* 1986;72:4:334.

148. Feighner JP, Boyer WF, Tyler DL, Neborsky RJ. Adverse consequences of fluoxetine-MAO inhibitor combination therapy. *J Clin Psychiatry* 1990;51:6:222–225.

149. Feldman SA, Crawley BE. Interaction of diazepam with the muscle relaxant drugs. *Br Med J* 1970;2:336–338.

150. Ferguson JM. Interaction of aspartame and carbohydrates in an eating-disordered patient. *Am J Psychiatry* 1985;142:271.

151. Flemenbaum A. Does lithium block the effects of amphetamine? A report of three cases. *Am J Psychiatry* 1974;131:820–821.

152. Flemenbaum A. Hypertensive episodes after adding methylphenidate (Ritalin) to tricyclic antidepressants. *Psychosomatics* 1972;8:265–268.

153. Forrest FM, Forrest IS, Sorr MT. Modification of chlorpromazine metabolism by some other drugs frequently administered to psychiatric patients. *Biol Psychiatry* 1970;2:53–58.

154. Frölich JC, Leftwich R, Ragheb M, et al. Indomethacin increases plasma lithium. *Br Med J* 1979;1:1115–1116.

155. Fruncillo RJ, Gibbons WJ, Vlasses DH, Fergusson RK. Severe hypotension associated with concurrent clonidine and antipsychotic medication. *Am J Psychiatry* 1985;142:274.

156. Fuller MA, Sajatovic M. Neurotoxicity resulting

from a combination of lithium and loxapine. *J Clin Psychiatry* 1989;50:5:187.

157. Gaffney GR, Tune LE. Serum neuroleptic levels and extrapyramidal side effects in patients treated with amoxapine. *J Clin Psychiatry* 1985; 46:10:428–429.

158. Garbutt JC. Potentiation of propoxyphene by phenelzine. *Am J Psychiatry* 1987;144:251–252.

159. Gershon S, Neubaver H, Sundland DM. Interaction between some anticholinergic agents and phenothiazines. *Clin Pharmacol Ther* 1965; 6:749–756.

160. Ghose K. Interaction between lithium and carbamazepine. *Br Med J* 1980;280:1122.

161. Ghose K. Effect of carbamazepine in polyuria associated with lithium therapy. *Pharmakopsychiatr Neuro-Psychopharmakol* 1978;11:241–245.

162. Giles TD, Modlin RK. Death associated with ventricular arrhythmia and thioridazine. *JAMA* 1968;205:108–110.

163. Goff DC, Midha KK, Brotman AW, et al. Elevation of plasma concentrations of haloperidol after the addition of fluoxetine. *Am J Psychiatry* 1991;148:790–792.

164. Goff DC, Midha KK, Brotman AW, et al. An open trial of buspirone added to neuroleptics in schizophrenic patients. *J Clin Psychopharmacol* 1991;11:193–197.

165. Gold MI. Profound hypotension associated with preoperative use of phenothiazines. *Anesth Analg Cleveland* 1974;53:844–848.

166. Goldberg LI. Monoamine oxidase inhibitors. Adverse reactions and possible mechanisms. *JAMA* 1964;190:456–462.

167. Goldney RD, Spence ND. Safety of the combination of lithium and neuroleptic drugs. *Am J Psychiatry* 1986;143:7:882–884.

168. Goldstein BJ. Interaction of antacids with psychotropics. *Hosp Community Psychiatry* 1982;33: 96.

169. Goodnick PJ, Meltzer HY. Neurochemical changes during discontinuation of lithium prophylaxis. I. Increases in clonidine-induced hypotension. *Biol Psychiatry* 1984;19:883–889.

170. Goonewardene A. Gross oedema occurring during treatment for depression. *Br Med J* 1977; 1:879–880.

171. Goulden KJ, Dooley JM, Camfield PR, et al. Clinical valproate toxicity induced by acetylsalicylic acid. *Neurology* 1987;37:1392–1394.

172. Graber MA, Hoehns TB, Perry PJ. Sertraline-phenelzine drug interaction: a serotonin syndrome reaction. *Ann Pharmacother* 1994;28: 732–735.

173. Gradwell BG. Psychotic reactions and phenelzine. *Br Med J* 1960;2:1018.

174. Gram LF, Overo KF. Drug interaction: inhibiting effect of neuroleptics on metabolism of tricyclic antidepressants in man. *Br Med J* 1972;1: 463–465.

175. Gram LF, Overo K, Kirk L. Influence of neuroleptics and benzodiazepines on metabolism of tricyclic antidepressants in man. *Am J Psychiatry* 1974;131:863–866.

176. Greenblatt DJ, von Moltke LL, Harmatz JS, et al. Interaction of triazolam and ketoconazole [Letter]. *Lancet* 1995;345:191.

177. Greenblatt DJ, Abernethy DR, Koepke HH, Shader RI. Interaction of cimetidine with oxazepam, lorazepam, and flurazepam. *J Clin Pharmacol* 1984;24:187–193.

178. Greenblatt DJ, Abernethy DR, Morse DS, et al. Clinical importance of the interaction of diazepam and cimetidine. *N Engl J Med* 1984;310: 1639–1643.

179. Greenblatt DJ, Abernethy DR, Divoll M, et al. Old age, cimetidine, and disposition of alprazolam and triazolam [Abstract]. *Clin Pharmacol Ther* 1983;33:253.

180. Greenblatt DJ, Allen MD, Noel BJ, Shader RI. Acute overdosage with benzodiazepine derivatives. *Clin Pharmacol Ther* 1977;21:497–514.

181. Greenblatt DJ, Shader RI, Harmatz JS, et al. Influence of magnesium and aluminum hydroxide mixture on chlordiazepoxide absorption. *Clin Pharmacol Ther* 1976;19:234–239.

182. Griffen JP, D'Arcy PF. *A manual of adverse drug interactions*. Bristol, Conn.: Wright, 1984.

183. Gulati OD, Dave BT, Gokhale SD, Shah KM. Antagonism of adrenergic neuron blockade in hypertensive subjects. *Clin Pharmacol Ther* 1966; 7:510–514.

184. Hadley A, Cason MP. Mania resulting from lithium-fluoxetine combination. *Am J Psychiatry* 1989;146:12:1637–1638.

185. Halaris AE. The use of lithium in psychiatric practice. *Psychiatr Ann* 1983;13:53.

186. Hansen BS, Dam M, Brandt J, et al. Influence of dextropropoxyphene on steady-state serum level and protein binding of three anti-epileptic drugs in man. *Acta Neurol Scand* 1980;61: 357–367.

187. Hansen JM, Siersboek-Nielsen K, Skovsted L. Carbamazepine induced acceleration of diphenylhydantoin and warfarin metabolism in man. *Clin Pharmacol Ther* 1971;12:539–543.

188. Hansen LB, Larsen N. Metabolic interaction between perphenazine and disulfiram. *Lancet* 1982;2:1472.

189. Hardy JL, Sirois A. Reduction of prothrombin and partial thromboplastin times with trazodone. *Can Med Assoc J* 1986;135:1372.

190. Havdala HS, Borison RL, Diamond BI. Potential hazards and applications of lithium in anesthesiology. *Anesthesiology* 1979;50:534–537.

191. Hedrick R, Williams F, Morin R, et al. Carbamazepine-erythromycin interaction leading to carbamazepine toxicity in four epileptic children. *Ther Drug Monit* 1983;5:405–407.

192. Helmuth D, Ljaljevic Z, Ramirez L. Choreoathetosis induced by verapamil and lithium treatment. *J Clin Psychopharmacol* 1989;9:454–455.

193. Hempel E, Klinger W. Drug stimulated biotransformation of hormonal steroid contraceptives: clinical implications. *Drugs* 1976;12: 442–448.

194. Henauer SA, Holister LE. Cimetidine interaction with imipramine and nortriptyline. *Clin Pharmacol Ther* 1984;35:183–187.

195. Hendy MS, Dove AF, Arblaster PL. Mazindol-induced lithium toxicity. *Br Med J* 1980;280: 684–685.

196. Henriksen O, Johanessen SI. Clinical and pharmacokinetic observations on sodium valproate: 5-year follow-up study in 100 children with epilepsy. *Acta Neurol Scand* 1982;65:504–523.

197. Hepner GW, Jesell ES, Lipton A, et al. Disposition of aminopyrine, antipyrine, diazepam and indocyanine green in patients with liver disease or on anticonvulsant drug therapy: diazepam breath test and correlations in drug elimination. *J Lab Clin Med* 1977;90:440–456.

198. Hermann DJ, Krol TF, Dukes GE, et al. Comparison of verapamil, diltiazem, and labetalol on the bioavailability and metabolism of imipramine. *J Clin Pharmacol* 1992;32:176–183.

199. Herrmann N, Lieff SJ. Drug-induced catatonia. *Can J Psychiatry* 1988;33:7:633–634.

200. Hiles BH. Hyperglycaemia and glycosuria following chlorpromazine therapy. *JAMA* 1956; 162:1651.

201. Hill GE, Wong KC, Hodges MR. Potentiation of succinylcholine neuromuscular blockade by lithium carbonate. *Anesthesiology* 1976;44:439–442.

202. Himmelhoch JM, Poust RI, Mallinger J, et al. Adjustment of lithium dose during lithium-chlorothiazide therapy. *Clin Pharmacol Ther* 1977;22:225–227.

203. Himmelhoch JM, Forrest J, Neil JF, Detre TP. Thiazide-lithium synergy in refractory mood swings. *Am J Psychiatry* 1977;134:149–152.

204. Holden J. Thioridazine and chlordiazepoxide, alone and combined in the treatment of acute schizophrenia. *Compr Psychiatry* 1968;9:633–643.

205. Hooper WD, Dubetz DK, Eadie MJ, Tyrer JH. Preliminary observations on the clinical pharmacology of carbamazepine. *Proc Aust Assoc Neurol* 1974;11:189–198.

206. Horler AR, Wynne NA. Hypertensive crisis due to pargyline and metaraminol. *Br J Med* 1965; 3:460–461.

207. Houghton GW, Richens A. Inhibition of phenytoin metabolism by other drugs used in epilepsy. *Int J Clin Pharmacol Biopharm* 1975;12:210–216.

208. Houghton GW, et al. The effect of benzodiazepines and pheneturide on phenytoin metabolism in man. *Br J Clin Pharmacol* 1974;1:344P.

209. Howes CA, Pullar T, Sourindhrin I, et al. Reduced steady-state plasma concentrations of chlorpromazine and indomethacin in patients receiving cimetidine. *Eur J Clin Pharmacol* 1983; 24:99–102.

210. Hui KK. Hypertensive crisis induced by interaction of clonidine with imipramine. *J Am Geriatr Soc* 1983;31:164–165.

211. Humberstone PM. Hypertension from cold remedies [Letter]. *Br Med J* 1969;1:846.

212. Hunter KR, Boakes AJ, Laurence DR, Stern GM. Monoamine oxidase inhibitors and L-dopa. *Br Med J* 1970;3:388.

213. Hunter KR, Stern GM, Laurence DR. Use of levodopa with other drugs. *Lancet* 1970;2:1283–1285.

214. Hurtig HI, Dyson WL. Lithium toxicity enhanced by diuresis [Letter]. *N Engl J Med* 1974; 290:748.

215. Hurwitz A. Antacid therapy and drug kinetics. *Clin Pharmacokinet* 1977;2:269–280.

216. Insel TR, Roy BF, Cohen RM, Murphy DL, et al. Possible development of the serotonin syndrome in man. *Am J Psychiatry* 1982;139:954–955.

217. Ishizaki T, Chiba K, Saito M, et al. The effects of neuroleptics (haloperidol and chlorpromazine) on the pharmacokinetics of valproic acid in schizophrenic patients. *J Clin Psychopharmacol* 1984;4:254–261.

218. Jack RA, Daniel DG. Possible interaction between phenelzine and amantadine. *Arch Gen Psychiatry* 1984;41:726.

219. Jann MW, Ereshefsky L, Saklad SR, et al. Effects of carbamazepine on plasma haloperidol levels. *J Clin Psychopharmacol* 1985;5:106–109.

220. Janowsky D, David JM, el-Yousef MK, Serkerke HJ. Combined anticholinergic agents and atropine-like delirium. *Am J Psychiatry* 1972;129:360–361.

221. Janowsky DS, el-Yousef MK, Davis JM, Fann WE. Antagonism of guanethidine by chlorpromazine. *Am J Psychiatry* 1973;130:808–812.

222. Janowsky DS, Davis JM. Methylphenidate, dextroamphetamine, levamphetamine effects on schizophrenic patients. *Arch Gen Psychiatry* 1976;33:304–308.

223. Janowsky EC, Risch C, Janowsky DS. Effects of anesthesia on patients taking psychotropic drugs. *J Clin Psychopharmacol* 1981;1:14–20.

224. Jeavons PM, Clark JE, Maheshwari MC. Treatment of generalized epilepsies of childhood and adolescence with sodium valproate (Epilim). *Dev Med Child Neurol* 1977;19:9–25.

225. Jefferson JW. Lithium tremor and caffeine intake: two cases of drinking less and shaking more. *J Clin Psychiatry* 1988;49:72–73.

226. Jefferson JW, Greist JH, Bandhuin M. Lithium: interactions with other drugs. *J Clin Psychopharmacol* 1981;1:124–134.

227. Jefferson JW, Kalin NH. Serum lithium levels and long-term diuretic use. *JAMA* 1979;241:1134–1136.

228. Jenkins RB, Groh RH. Psychic effects in patients treated with levodopa [Letter]. *JAMA* 1970;212:2265.

229. Jerling M, Lindstrom L, Bondesson U, et al. Fluvoxamine inhibition and carbamazepine induction of the metabolism of clozapine: evidence from a therapeutic drug monitoring service. *Ther Drug Monit* 1994;16:368–374.

230. Johannessen SI. Antiepileptic drugs: pharmacokinetic and clinical aspects. *Ther Drug Monit* 1981;3:17–37.

231. Johannessen SI, Strandjord RE. The influence of phenobarbital and phenytoin on carbamazepine serum levels. In: Schneider H, Janz D, Garoner-Thorpe C, et al., eds. *Clinical pharmacology of antiepileptic drugs*. New York: Springer-Verlag, 1975:201–205.

232. Joffe RT, Gold PW, Uhde TW, et al. The effects of carbamazepine on the thyrotropin response to thyrotropin-releasing hormone. *Psychiatry Res* 1984;12:161–166.

233. Jorgensen JV, Brandup F, Schroll M. Possible synergism between iodine and lithium carbonate [Letter]. *JAMA* 1973;223:192–193.

234. Junghan U, Albers M, Moggon B. Increased risk of hematological side effects in psychiatric patients treated with clozapine and carbamazepine? *Pharmacopsychiatry* 1993;26:262.

235. Kahn DG. Increased plasma nortriptyline concentration in a patient cotreated with fluoxetine. *J Clin Psychiatry* 1990;51:1:36.

236. Kahn EM, Schulz Sc, Perel JM, Alexander JE. Change in haloperidol level due to carbamazepine—a complicating factor in combined medication for schizophrenia. *J Clin Psychopharmacol* 1990;10:1:54–57.

237. Kane F, Taylor T. An unusual reaction to combined imipramine-thorazine therapy. *Am J Psychiatry* 1963;120:187–188.

238. Kanter GL, Yerevanian BI, Ciccone S. Case report of a possible interaction between neuroleptics and carbamazepine. *Am J Psychiatry* 1984;141:1101–1102.

239. Kaumann A, Basso N, Aramendia P. Cardiovascular effects of desmethylimipramine and guanethidine. *Pharmacol Exp Ther* 1965;147:54–64.

240. Keeri-Szanto M. The mode of action of promethazine in potentiating narcotic drugs. *Br J Anaesth* 1974;46:918–924.

241. Kellstein DE, Malseed RJ, Goldstein FJ. Contrasting effects of acute vs. chronic tricyclic antidepressant treatment on central morphine analgesia. *Pain* 1984;20:323–324.

242. Kendall AG, Boivin M. Warfarin-carbamazepine interaction [Letter]. *Ann Intern Med* 1981;94:280.

243. Kerry R, Owen G, Michaelson S. Possible toxic interaction between lithium and piroxicam. *Lancet* 1983;1:418–419.

244. Kerzner B, Rivera-Calimlim L. Lithium and chlorpromazine interaction. *Clin Pharmacol Ther* 1979;19:109.

245. Ketter TA, Jenkins JB, Schroeder DH, et al. Carbamazepine but not valproate induces bupropion metabolism. *J Clin Psychopharmacol* 1993;15:327–333.

246. Khurana RC. Estrogen-imipramine interaction [Letter]. *JAMA* 1972;222:702.

247. Kidron R, Averbuch I, Klein E, Belmaker R. Carbamazepine-induced reduction of blood levels of haloperidol in chronic schizophrenia. *Biol Psychiatry* 1985;20:219–222.

248. Klein E, Bental E, Lerer B, Belmaker R. Combination of carbamazepine and haloperidol v. placebo and haloperidol in excited psychoses: a controlled study. *Arch Gen Psychiatry* 1984;41:165–170.

249. Klotz U, Reimann IW, Ohnhaus EE. Effect of rantidine on the steady state pharmacokinetics of diazepam. *Eur J Clin Pharmacol* 1983;24;357–360.

250. Klotz U, Reimann I. Elevation of steady-state diazepam levels by cimetidine. *Clin Pharmacol Ther* 1981;30:513–517.

251. Klotz V, Reimann I. Delayed clearance of diazepam due to cimetidine. *N Engl J Med* 1980;302:1012.

252. Koch-Weser J. Hemorrhagic reactions and drug interactions in 500 warfarin-treated patients [Abstract]. *Clin Pharmacol Ther* 1973;14:139.

253. Koczerginski D, Kennedy SH, Swinson RP. Clonazepam and lithium—a toxic combination in the treatment of mania? *Int* Clin Psychopharmacol 1989;4:195–99.

254. Kramer G, Neisohn M, von Unruh GE, Eichelbaum M. Carbamazepine-danazol drug interaction: its mechanism examined by a stable isotope technique. *Ther Drug Monit* 1986;8:387–392.

255. Krishnan KRR, France RD, Ellinwood EH Jr. Tricyclic induced akathisia in patients taking conjugated estrogens. *Am J Psychiatry* 1984;141:696–697.

256. Krishnan KRR. Psychotropic drug interactions. *Prim Psychiatry* 1996;3:21–45.

257. Kulhanek F, Linde OK. Coffee and tea influence pharmacokinetics of antipsychotic drugs [Letter]. *Lancet* 1981;2:359.

258. Kulhanek F, et al. Interaction of coffee and tea with neuroleptics. *Dtsch Apoth Ztg* 1980;120:1771.

259. Kulhanek F, Linde OK, Meisenberg G. Precipitation of antipsychotic drugs in interaction with coffee or tea [Letter]. *Lancet* 1979;2:1130.

260. Kutt H, McDowell F. Management of epilepsy with diphenylhydantoin. *JAMA* 1968;203:969–972.

261. Lai AA, Levy RH, Cutler RE. Time-course of interaction between carbamazepine and clonazepam in normal man. *Clin Pharmacol Ther* 1978,24:316–323.

262. Laisi U, et al. Pharmacokinetic and pharmacodynamic interactions of diazepam with different alcoholic beverages. *Eur J Clin Pharmacol* 1979;16:263.

263. Lambertsen CJ, Wendel H, Longenhagen JB. The separate and combined respiratory effects of chlorpromazine and meperidine in normal men controlled at 46 mm Hg alveolar PCO_2. *J Pharmacol Exp Ther* 1961;131:381–393.

264. Lancaster NP, Jones DH. Chlorpromazine and insulin in psychiatry. *Br Med J* 1954;2:565–567.

265. Landauer AA, Milner G, Patman J. Alcohol and amitriptyline effects on skills related to driving behavior. *Science* 1969;163;1467–1468.

266. Leishman AWD, Matthews HL, Smith AJ. Antagonism of guanethidine by imipramine. *Lancet* 1963;1:112.

267. Lemberger L, Rowe H, Bosomworth JC, et al. The effect of fluoxetine on the pharmacokinetics and psychomotor responses of diazepam. *Clin Pharmacol Ther* 1988;43:412–419.

268. Levy RH, Moreland TA, Morselli PL, et al. Carbamazepine-valproic acid interaction in man and rhesus monkey. *Epilepsia* 1984;25:338–345.

269. Levy ST, Forrest JN Jr, Heninger GR. Lithium-induced diabetes insipidus: manic symptoms, brain and electrolyte correlates, and chlorothiazide treatment. *Am J Psychiatry* 1973;130:1014–1018.

270. Linnoila M, Viukari M, Vaisanen K, Auvinen J. Effect of anticonvulsants on plasma haloperidol and thioridazine levels. *Am J Psychiatry* 1980;137:819–821.

271. Linnoila M, Saario I, Olkoniemi J, et al. Effect of two weeks' treatment with chlordiazepoxide or flupenthixole, alone or in combination with alcohol on psychomotor skills related to driving. *Arzneimittelforschung* 1975;25:1088–1092.

272. Linnoila M, Hakkinen S. Effects of diazepam and codeine, alone and in combination with alcohol on simulated driving. *Clin Pharmacol Ther* 1974;15:368–373.

273. Lloyd JTA, Walker DR. Death after combined dexamphetamine and phenelzine [Letter]. *Br Med J* 1965;2:168–169.

274. Loga S, Curry S, Lader M. Interaction of chlorpromazine and nortriptyline in patients with schizophrenia. *Clin Pharmacokinet* 1981;6:454–462.

275. Loga S, Curry S, Lader M. Interactions of orphenadrine and phenobarbitone with chlorpromazine: plasma concentrations and effects in man. *Br J Clin Pharmacol* 1975;2:197–208.

276. Luder PJ, Siffert B, Witassek F, et al. Treatment of hydatid disease with high oral doses of mebendazole: long-term follow-up of plasma mebendazole levels and drug interactions. *Eur J Clin Pharmacol* 1986;31:443–448.

277. MacCallum WAG. Interaction of lithium and phenytoin. *Br Med J* 1980;280:610–611.

278. Macfie AC. Lithium poisoning precipitated by diuretics. *Br Med J* 1975;1:516.

279. Macphee GJ, McInnes GT, Thompson GG, Brodie MJ. Verapamil potentiates carbamazepine neurotoxicity: a clinically important interaction. *Lancet* 1986;1:700–703.

280. MacPhee GJ, Mitchell JR, Wisemen L, et al. Effect of sodium valproate on carbamazepine disposition and psychomotor profile in man. *Br J Clin Pharmacol* 1988;25:59–66.

281. McGennis AJ. Lithium carbonate and tetracycline interaction. *Br Med J* 1978;1:1183.

282. McKauge L, Tyrer JH, Eadie MJ. Factors influencing simultaneous concentrations of carbamazepine and its epoxide in plasma. *Ther Drug Monit* 1981;3:63–70.

283. Maany I, Dhopesh V, Arndt IO, et al. Increase in desipramine serum levels associated with methadone treatment. *Am J Psychiatry* 1989;146:12:1611–1613.

284. Maany I, Hayashida M, Pfeffer SL, Kron RE. Possible toxic interaction between disulfiram and amitriptyline. *Arch Gen Psychiatry* 1982;39:743–744.

285. MacLeod SM, Sellers EM, Giles HG, et al. Interaction of disulfiram with benzodiazepines. *Clin Pharmacol Ther* 1978;24:583–589.

286. Mahieu M, Houvenagel E, Leduc JJ, Choteau P. Lithium-inhibiteurs de l'enzyme de conversion: une association a eviter? [Letter]. *Presse Med* 1988;17:281.

287. Mann SC, Boger WP. Psychotropic drugs, summer heat and humidity, and hyperpyrexia: a danger restated. *Am J Psychiatry* 1978;135:1097–1100.

288. Martin BA, Kramer PM. Clinical significance of the interaction between lithium and a neuromuscular blocker. *Am J Psychiatry* 1982;139:1326–1328.

289. Mason AMS, Buckle RM. "Cold" cures and monoamine-oxidase inhibitors [Letter]. *Br Med J* 1969;1:845–846.

290. Massey EW. Effect of carbamazepine on coumadin metabolism. *Ann Neurol* 1983;13:691–692.

291. Mattson RH, Cramer JA, Williamson PD, Novelly RA. Valproic acid in epilepsy: clinical and pharmacological effects. *Ann Neurol* 1978;3:20–25.

292. McGrath PJ, Stuart JW, Quitkin FU. A possible

293. Mesdjian E, Dravet C, Cenraud B, Roger J. Carbamazepine intoxication due to triacetyloleandomycin administration in epileptic patients. *Epilepsia* 1980;21:489–496.

294. Meyer JF, McAllister CK, Goldberg LI. Insidious and prolonged antagonism of guanethidine by amitriptyline. *JAMA* 1970;213:1487–1488.

295. Mikkelsen EJ. Caffeine and schizophrenia. *J Clin Psychiatry* 1978;39:732–736.

296. Miles MV, Tennison MB. Erythromycin effects on multiple-dose carbamazepine kinetics. *Ther Drug Monit* 1989;11:1:47–52.

297. Miller F, Menninger J. Lithium-neuroleptic neurotoxicity is dose dependent. *J Clin Psychopharmacol* 1987;7:89–91.

298. Miller FA, Rampling D. Adverse effects of combined propranolol and chlorpromazine therapy. *Am J Psychiatry* 1982;139:1198–1199.

299. Miller LG, Bowman RC, Bakht F. Sparing effect of sulindac on lithium levels. *J Fam Pract* 1989;28:5:592–593.

300. Miller ME, Perry CJ, Siris SG. Psychosis in association with combined cimetidine and imipramine treatment. *Psychosomatics* 1987;28:4:217–219.

301. Miller MG. Tricyclics as a possible cause of hyponatremia in psychiatric patients. *Am J Psychiatry* 1989;146:6:807.

302. Miller DD, Macklin M. Cimetidine-imipramine interaction: a case report. *Am J Psychiatry* 1983;140:351–352.

303. Miller RR, Greenblatt DJ. Hypnotics. In: Miller RR, Greenblatt DJ, eds. *Drug effects in hospitalized patients.* New York: Wiley, 1976:171–191.

304. Mirchandani H, Reich LE. Fatal malignant hyperthermia as a result of ingestion of tranylcypromine combined with white wine and cheese. *J Forensic Sci* 1985;30:217–220.

305. Mitchell EA, Dower JC, Green RJ. Interaction between carbamazepine and theophylline [Letter]. *NZ Med J* 1986;1:69–70.

306. Mitchell JR, Arias L, Oates JA. Antagonism of the antihypertensive action of guanethidine sulfate by desipramine hydrochloride. *JAMA* 1967;202:973–976.

307. Mittal SR, Mathur AK. Drug interaction between metoprolol and chlordiazepoxide. *Int J Cardiol* 1986;13:372–374.

308. Modell W, Hussar AE. Failure of dextroamphetamine sulfate to influence eating and sleeping patterns in obese schizophrenic patients: clinical and pharmacological significance. *JAMA* 1965;193:275–278.

309. Monks A, Richens A. Effect of single doses of sodium valproate on serum levels and protein binding in epileptic patients. *Clin Pharmacol Ther* 1980;27:89–95.

310. Morgan JP, Rivera-Calimlim L, Messina F, et al. Imipramine-mediated interference with levodopa absorption for the gastrointestinal tract in man. *Neurology* 1975;25:1029–1034.

311. Nadel I, Wallach M. Drug interaction between haloperidol and methyldopa. *Br J Psychiatry* 1979;135:484.

312. Navis GJ, de Jong PE, de Zeeuw D. Volume ho-

L-deprenyl-induced hypertensive reaction [Letter]. *J Clin Psychopharm* 1989;9:310–311.

meostasis, angiotensin converting enzyme inhibition, and lithium therapy. *Am J Med* 1989;86: 621.

313. Nawishy S, et al. Kinetic interaction of mianserin in epileptic patients on anticonvulsant drugs. *Br J Clin Pharmacol* 1982;13:612P.

314. Naylor GJ, McHarg A. Profound hypothermia on combined lithium carbonate and diazepam treatment. *Br Med J* 1977;2:22.

315. Nelson JC, Jatlow PI. Neuroleptic effect on desipramine steady-state plasma concentrations. *Am J Psychiatry* 1980;137:1232–1234.

316. Neuvonen PJ, Penttila O. Interaction between doxycycline and barbiturates. *Br Med J* 1974;1: 535–536.

317. Nies A. Monoamine oxidase inhibitors. In: Paykel ES, ed. *Handbook of affective disorders.* New York: Guilford, 1982:245.

318. Noveske FG, Hahn KR, Flynn RJ. Possible toxicity of combined fluoxetine and lithium [Letter]. *Am J Psychiatry* 1989;146:1515.

319. Nymark M, Nielsen IM. Reactions due to the combination of monoamine oxidase inhibitors with thymoleptics, pethidine, or methylamphetamine. *Lancet* 1963;2:524–525.

320. Oakley DP, Lautch LL. Haloperidol and anticoagulant treatment [Letter]. *Lancet* 1963;2: 1231.

321. Ochs HR, Greenblatt DJ, Roberts GM, Dengler HJ. Diazepam interaction with antituberculosis drugs. *Clin Pharmacol Ther* 1981;29:671–678.

322. Ochs HR, Greenblatt DJ, Knuchel M. Differential effect of isoniazid on triazolam oxidation and oxazepam conjugation. *Br J Clin Pharmacol* 1983;16:743–746.

323. Ochs HR, Greenblatt DJ, Verburg-Ochs B. Effect of alprazolam in digoxin kinetics and creatinine clearance. *Clin Pharmacol Ther* 1985;38: 595–598.

324. Oefele Kv, Grohmann R, Ruther E. Adverse drug reactions in combined tricyclic and MAOI therapy. *Pharmacopsychiatry* 1986;19:243.

325. Oh TE. Furosemide and lithium toxicity. *Anesth Intensive Care* 1977;5:60–62.

326. Oles KS, Mirza W, Penry JK. Catastrophic neurologic signs due to drug interaction: Tegretol and Darvon. *Surg Neurol* 1989;32:144–151.

327. Olivesi A. Modified elimination of prednisolone in epileptic patients on carbamazepine monotherapy, and in women using low-dose oral contraceptives. *Biomed Pharmacother* 1986; 40:301–308.

328. Olkkola KT, Backman JT, Neuvonen PJ. Midazolam should be avoided in patients receiving the systemic antimycotics ketoconazole or itraconazole. *Clin Pharmacol Therap* 1994;55: 481–485.

329. Olkkola KT, Aranko K, Luurila H, et al. A potentially hazardous interaction between erythromycin and midazolam. *Clin Pharmacol Ther* 1993;53:298–305.

330. O'Regan JB. Adverse interaction of lithium carbonate and methyldopa [Letter]. *Can Med Assoc J* 1976;115:385.

331. Orr J, Abott FS, Farrell K, et al. Interaction between valproic acid and aspirin in epileptic children: serum protein binding and meta-

332. Osanloo E, Deglin JH. Interaction of lithium and methyldopa. *Ann Intern Med* 1980;92: 433–434.

333. Ossipov MH, Malseed RJ, Goldstein F. Augmentation of central and peripheral morphine analgesia by desipramine. *Arch Int Pharmacodyn Ther* 1982;259:222–229.

334. Palm R, Silseth C, Alvan G. Phenytoin intoxication as the first symptom of fatal liver damage induced by sodium valproate. *Br J Clin Pharmacol* 1984;17:597–599.

335. Panesar SK, Orr JM, Farrell K, et al. The effect of carbamazepine on valproic acid disposition in adult volunteers. *Br J Clin Pharmacol* 1989; 27:3:323–328.

336. Patel IH, Levy RH, Cutler RE. Phenobarbital-valproic acid interaction. *Clin Pharmacol Ther* 1980;27:515–521.

337. Pathak SK. Gross oedema during treatment for depression [Letter]. *Br Med J* 1977;2:1220.

338. Patrignani A, Miele V. The influence of MAOI on the glycemic balance: the potentiation of insulin hypoglycemia by beta-phenylethylhydrazine (Nardil). *J Psychiatr Neuropathol* 1968; 96:29–43.

339. Paykel ES. Hallucinosis on combined methyldopa and pargyline. *Br Med J* 1966;5490:803.

340. Pearson HJ. Interaction of fluoxetine with carbamazepine. *J Clin Psychiatry* 1990;51:3:126.

341. Peet M, Middlemiss DN, Yates RA. Pharmacokinetic interaction between propranolol and chlorpromazine in schizophrenic patients. *Lancet* 1980;2:978.

342. Peet M, Middlemiss DN, Yates RA. Propranolol in schizophrenia. II. Clinical and biochemical aspects of combining propranolol with chlorpromazine. *Br J Psychiatry* 1981;138:112–117.

343. Penry JK, Newmark ME. The use of antiepileptic drugs. *Ann Intern Med* 1979;90:207.

344. Penttila O, Neuvonen PJ, Aho K, Lehtovaara R. Interaction between doxycycline and some antiepileptic drugs. *Br Med J* 1974;2:470–472.

345. Perlman BB. Interaction between lithium salts and isphagula husk. *Lancet* 1990;335:416.

346. Perry PJ, Calloway RA, Cook BL, Smith RE. Theophylline precipitated alterations of lithium clearance. *Acta Psychiatr Scand* 1984;69: 528–537.

347. Perry PJ, Alexander B, Liskow BI. *Psychotropic drug handbook.* Washington, DC: American Psychiatric Press, 1997.

348. Perucca E, Richens A. Interaction between lithium and carbamazepine. *Br Med J* 1980;280: 863.

349. Perucca E, Richens A. Interaction between phenytoin and imipramine. *Br J Clin Pharmacol* 1977; 4:485–486.

350. Phillips JP, Antal EJ, Smith RB. A pharmacokinetic drug interaction between erythromycin and triazolam. *J Clin Psychopharmacol* 1986;6: 297–299.

351. Pinell OC. Drug-drug interactions of chlorpromazine and antacid. *Clin Pharmacol Ther* 1978; 23:125.

352. Pisani F, Narbone MC, Trunfio C, et al. Val-

proic acid-ethosuximide interaction: a pharmacokinetic study. *Epilepsia* 1984;25:229–233.

353. Pond SM, Graham GG, Birkett DJ, et al. Effects of tricyclic antidepressants on drug metabolism. *Clin Pharmacol Ther* 1975;18:191–199.

354. Ponto LB, Perry PJ, Liskow BI, et al. Tricyclic antidepressant and monoamine oxidase inhibitor combination therapy. *Am J Hosp Pharm* 1977;34:954–961.

355. Prakash R, Reed RM, Bass AD. Neurotoxicity with combined administration of lithium and a neuroleptic. *Compr Psychiatry* 1982;23:567–571.

356. Prange AJ Jr, et al. Estrogen may well affect response to antidepressant (Medical News). *JAMA* 1972;219:143.

357. Price WA, Giannini AJ. Neurotoxicity caused by lithium-verapamil synergism. *J Clin Psychopharmacol* 1986;26:8:717–719.

358. Proakis AG, Browitz JL. Blockage of insulin release by certain phenothiazines. *Biochem Pharmacol* 1974;23:1693–1700.

359. Pulik M, Lida H. Interaction lithium-inhibiteurs de l'enzyme de conversion [Letter]. *Presse Med* 1988;17:755.

360. Ragheb MA. Ibuprofen can increase serum lithium level in lithium-treated patients. *J Clin Psychiatry* 1987;48:161–163.

361. Ragheb MA, Powell AL. Failure of sulindac to increase serum lithium levels. *J Clin Psychiatry* 1986;47:33–34.

362. Ragheb MA, Powell AL. Lithium interaction with sulindac and naproxen. *J Clin Psychopharmacol* 1986;6:3:150–154.

363. Ragheb MA, Ban TA, Buchanan D, Frolich JC. Interaction of indomethacin and ibuprofen with lithium in manic patients under a steady-state lithium level. *J Clin Psychiatry* 1980;41:397–398.

364. Raisfeld IH. Cardiovascular complications of antidepressant therapy. *Am Heart J* 1972;82:129–133.

365. Raitasuo V, Lehtovaara R, Huttunen MO. Carbamazepine and plasma levels of clozapine [Letter]. *Am J Psychiatry* 1993;150:169.

366. Rambeck B, Salke-Treumann A, May T, et al. Valproic acid induced carbamazepine-10-11-epoxide toxicity in children and adolescents. *Eur Neurol* 1990;30:79–83.

367. Rampton DS. Hypertensive crisis in a patient given Sinemet, metoclopramide, and amitriptyline. *Br Med J* 1977;2:607–608.

368. Raskin DE. Lithium and phenytoin interaction [Letter]. *J Clin Psychopharmacol* 1984;4:120.

369. Regan AG, Aldrete JA. Prolonged apnea after administration of promazine hydrochloride following succinylcholine infusion. *Anesth Analg* 1967;46:315–318.

370. Reginaldi D, Tondo L, Floris G, et al. Poor prophylactic lithium response due to antidepressants. *Int Pharmacopsychiatry* 1981;16:124–128.

371. Reid AA. Pharmacological antagonism between chlorpromazine and phenmetrazine in mental hospital patients. *Med J Aust* 1964;1:187–188.

372. Reimann IW, Frölich JC. Effect of diclofenac on lithium kinetics. *Clin Pharmacol Ther* 1981;30:348–352.

373. Reimherr FW, Hodges MR, Hill GE, Wong KC. Prolongation of muscle relaxant effects by lith-ium carbonate. *Am J Psychiatry* 1977;134:205–206.

374. Riesenman C. Antidepressant drug interactions and the cytochrome P450 system: a critical appraisal. *Pharmacotherapy* 1995;15:84S–99S.

375. Reunanen MI, et al. Low serum valproic acid concentrations in epileptic patients on combination therapy. *Curr Ther Res* 1980;28:456.

376. Richens A, Nawishy S, Trimble M. Antidepressant drugs, convulsions and epilepsy. *Br J Clin Pharmacol* 1983;15:2955–2985.

377. Rivera-Calimlim L, Nasrallah H, Strauss J, Lasagna L. Clinical response and plasma levels: effect of dose, dosage schedules, and drug interactions on plasma chlorpromazine levels. *Am J Psychiatry* 1976;133:646–652.

378. Rivera-Calimlim L, Kerzner B, Karch FE. Effect of lithium on plasma chlorpromazine levels. *Clin Pharmacol Ther* 1978;23:451–455.

379. Rivera-Calimlim L, Castaneda L, Lasagna L. Effects of mode of management on plasma chlorpromazine in psychiatric patients. *Clin Pharmacol Ther* 1973;14:978–986.

380. Rivers N, et al. Possible lethal reaction between Nardil and dextromethorphan [Letter]. *Can Med Assoc J* 1970;103:85.

381. Robbins RJ, Kern PA, Thompson TL 2nd. Interactions between thioridazine and bromocriptine in a patient with a prolactin-secreting pituitary adenoma. *Am J Med* 1984;76:5:921–923.

382. Roberts RK, Desmond PV, Wilkinson GR, Schenkers. Disposition of chlordiazepoxide: sex differences and effects of oral contraceptives. *Clin Pharmacol Ther* 1979;25:826–831.

383. Rosenberry KR, Defusco CJ, Mansmann HC Jr, McGeady SJ. Reduced theophylline half-life induced by carbamazepine therapy. *J Pediatr* 1983;102:472–474.

384. Ross JR, Beeley L. Interaction between carbamazepine and warfarin. *Br Med J* 1980;2:1415–1416.

385. Roth S, Ebrahim ZY. Resistance to pancuronium in patients receiving carbamazepine. *Anesthesiology* 1987;66:691–693.

386. Sachdev PS. Lithium potentiation of neuroleptic-related extrapyramidal side effects. *Am J Psychiatry* 1986;143:7:942.

387. Salama AA, Shafey M. A case of severe lithium toxicity induced by combined fluoxetine and lithium carbonate [Letter]. *Am J Psychiatry* 1989;146:278.

388. Salama AA. Complete heart block associated with mesoridazine and lithium carbonate. *J Clin Psychiatry* 1987;48:3:123.

389. Sassim N, Grohmann R. Adverse drug reactions with clozapine and simultaneous application of benzodiazepines. *Pharmacopsychiatry* 1988;21:306–307.

390. Schecter GL, Brease DA, Powell J. Adverse effects of tricyclic antidepressants during nasal surgery. *Otolaryngol Head Neck Surg* 1982;90:223.

391. Schmauss M, Kapfhammer HP, Meyr P, Hoff P. Combined MAO-inhibitor and tri-(tetra) cyclic antidepressant in therapy resistant depression: a retrospective study. *Prog Nueropsychopharmacol Biol Psychiatry* 1988;12:523–532.

392. Schraml F, Benedetti G, Hoyle K, Clayton A. Fluoxetine and nortriptyline combination therapy. *Am J Psychiatry* 1989;146:12: 1636–1637.

393. Shulman KI, Walker SE, MacKenzie S, et al. Dietary restriction, tyramine, and the use of monoamine oxidase inhibitors. *J Clin Psychopharmacol* 1989;9:397–402.

394. Schwab RS, England AC, Poskanzer DC, et al. Amantadine in the treatment of Parkinson's disease. *JAMA* 1969;208:1168–1170.

395. Sellers EM. Inhibition of chlordiazepoxide biotransformation by disulfiram. *Clin Res* 1976;24: 652A.

396. Sellers EM, Carr G, Bernstein JG, et al. Interaction of chloral hydrate and ethanol in man, II: hemodynamics and performance. *Clin Pharmacol Ther* 1972;13:50–58.

397. Shader RI, Ciraulo DA, Greenblatt DJ, Harmatz JS. Steady-state plasma desmethyldiazepam during long-term clorazepate use: effect of antacids. *Clin Pharmacol Ther* 1982;31:180–183.

398. Shader RI, DiMascio A. *Psychotropic drug side effects: clinical and theoretical perspectives.* Baltimore: Williams & Wilkins, 1970.

399. Shinn AF, Shrewsbury RP. *Evaluations of drug interactions.* 3rd ed. St. Louis: CV Mosby, 1985.

400. Shopsin B, Shenkman L, Blum M, Hollander CS. Iodine and lithium-induced hypothyroidism: documentation of synergism. *Am J Med* 1973;55:695–699.

401. Shopsin B, Gershon S. Cogwheel rigidity related to lithium maintenance. *Am J Psychiatry* 1975;132:536–538.

402. Shopsin B, Stern S, Gershon S. Altered carbohydrate metabolism during treatment with lithium carbonate. *Arch Gen Psychiatry* 1972;26: 566–571.

403. Shukla S, Godwin CD, Long LE, Miller MG. Lithium-carbamazepine neurotoxicity and risk factors. *Am J Psychiatry* 1984;141:1604–1606.

404. Sides CA. Hypertension during anaesthesia with monoamine oxidase inhibitors. *Anaesthesia* 1987;42:633–635.

405. Sierles FS, Ossowski MG. Concurrent use of theophylline and lithium in a patient with chronic obstructive lung disease and bipolar disorder. *Am J Psychiatry* 1982;139:117–118.

406. Silver JM, Yudofsky SC, Kogan M, Katz BL. Elevation of thioridazine plasma levels by propranolol. *Am J Psychiatry* 1986;143:1290.

407. Simon G. Combination angiotensin converting enzyme inhibitor/lithium therapy contraindicated in renal disease. *Am J Med* 1988;85: 893–894.

408. Singer L, Imbs JL, Schmidt M, et al. Baise de la clearance renale du lithium sous l'effet de la phenylbutazone. *Encephale* 1978;4:33–40.

409. Singh H. Atropine-like poisoning due to tranquilizing agents. *Am J Psychiatry* 1960;117:360.

410. Singh MM, Kay SR. Therapeutic reversal with benztropine in schizophrenics. *J Nerv Ment Dis* 1975;160:258–266.

411. Singh MM, Smith JM. Reversal of some therapeutic effects of an antipsychotic agent by an antiparkinsonian drug. *J Nerv Ment Dis* 1973; 157:50–58.

412. Singh SV. Lithium carbonate-fluphenazine

413. Siris JH, Pippenger CE, Werner WL, Masland RL. Anticonvulsant drug-serum levels in psychiatric patients with seizure disorders. Effects of certain psychotropic drugs. *NY State J Med* 1974; 74:1554–1556.

414. Siris SG, Adan F, Lee A, et al. Patterns of plasma imipramine-desipramine concentration in patients receiving concomitant fluphenazine decanoate. *J Clin Psychiatry* 1988;49: 64–65.

415. Sjö O, Hvidberg B, Naestoff J, Lund M. Pharmacokinetics and side-effects of clonazepam and its 7-amino metabolite in man. *Eur J Clin Pharmacol* 1975;8:249–254.

416. Sjoqvist F. Psychotropic drugs (2). Interaction between monoamine oxidase (MAO) inhibitors and other substances. *Proc R Soc Med* 1965; 58:967–978.

417. Skinner C, Coull DC, Johnston AW. Antagonism of the hypotensive action of bethanidine and debrisoquine by tricyclic antidepressants. *Lancet* 1969;2:564–566.

418. Sletten I, Pichardo J, Korol B, Greshon S. The effect of chlorpromazine on lithium excretion in psychiatric subjects. *Curr Ther Res* 1966;8: 441–446.

419. Sletten IW, Ognjanou V, Menendez S, et al. Weight reduction with chlorphentermine and phenmetrazine in obese psychiatric patients during chlorpromazine therapy. *Curr Ther Res Clin Exp* 1967;9:570–575.

420. Snyder SH, Greenberg D, Yamumura HJ. Antischizophrenic drugs and brain cholinergic receptors: affinity for muscarinic sites predicts extrapyramidal effects. *J Psychiatr Res* 1974;11: 91–95.

421. Solomon JG. Lithium toxicity precipitated by a diuretic. *Psychosomatics* 1980;21:425.

422. Solomon JG. Seizures during lithium-amitriptyline therapy. *Postgrad Med* 1979;66:145–146.

423. Sorby DL, Liu G. Effects of adsorbents on drug absorption. II. Effect of an antidiarrheal mixture on promazine absorption. *J Pharm Sci* 1966;55:504.

424. Sovner R. A clinically significant interaction between carbamazepine and valproic acid [Letter]. *J Clin Psychopharmacol* 1988;8:448–449.

425. Sovner R, Wolfe J. Interaction between dextromethorphan and monoamine oxidase inhibitor therapy with isocarboxazid [Letter]. *N Engl J Med* 1988;319:1671.

426. Speirs J, Hirsch SR. Severe lithium toxicity with "normal" serum concentrations. *Br Med J* 1978;1:815–816.

427. Stambaugh JE, Wainer IW. Drug interaction: meperidine and chlorpromazine, a toxic combination. *J Clin Pharmacol* 1981;21:140–146.

428. Stancer HC. Tardive dyskinesia not associated with neuroleptics. *Am J Psychiatry* 1979;136:727.

429. Steiner E, Dumont E, Spina E, Dahlquist R. Inhibition of desipramine 2-hydroxylation by quinidine and quinine. *Clin Pharmacol Ther* 1988;43:577–581.

430. Steiner W, Fontaine R. Toxic reaction following the combined administration of fluoxetine

and L-tryptophan: five case reports. *Biol Psychiatry* 1986;21:1067–1071.

431. Sternbach H. Danger of MAOI therapy after fluoxetine withdrawal [Letter]. *Lancet* 1988;2:850.

432. Stevenson RN, Blanchard C, Patterson DL. Ventricular fibrillation due to lithium withdrawal—an interaction with chlorpromazine? *Postgrad Med J* 1989;65:936–938.

433. Stewart MM. MAOI and food: fact and fiction. *Adverse Drug React Bull* 1976;58:200–203.

434. Szymanski S, Lieberman JA, Picou D, et al. A case report of cimetidine-induced clozapine toxicity. *J Clin Psychiatry* 1991;52:21–22.

435. Stockley I. *Drug interactions: a source book of adverse interactions, their clinical importance, mechanisms and management.* Oxford, England: Blackwell Scientific, 1981.

436. Sunaoshi W, Miura H, Shirai H. Influence of concurrent administration of carbamazepine on the plasma concentrations of clonazepam. *Jpn J Psychiatry Neurol* 1988;42:589–591.

437. Swett C, Cole JO, Hartz SC, et al. Hypotension due to chlorpromazine. *Arch Gen Psychiatry* 1977;34:661–663.

438. Tackley RM, Tregaskis B. Fatal disseminated intravascular coagulation following a monoamine oxidase inhibitor/tricyclic interaction. *Anaesthesia* 1987;42:760–763.

439. Takeda M, Nishinuma K, Yamashita S, et al. Serum haloperidol levels of schizophrenics receiving treatment for tuberculosis. *Clin Neuropharmacol* 1986;9:386–397.

440. Tate JL. Extrapyramidal symptoms in a patient taking haloperidol and fluoxetine [Letter]. *Am J Psychiatry* 1989;146:399.

441. Tatro DS, ed. *Drug interaction facts.* St. Louis: JB Lippincott, 1988.

442. Tatro DS. *Drug interaction facts on disk.* St. Louis, MO: Facts and Comparisons, 1996.

443. Telerman-Toppet N, Duret ME, Coers C. Cimetidine interaction with carbamazepine. *Ann Intern Med* 1981;94:544.

444. Terrell HB. Behavioral dyscontrol associated with combined use of alprazolam and ethanol. *Am J Psychiatry* 1988;145:1313.

445. Thomsen K, Schou M. Renal lithium excretion in man. *Am J Physiology* 1968;215:823–827.

446. Thornton WE. Dementia induced by methyldopa and haloperidol. *N Engl J Med* 1976;294:1222.

447. Tollefson G, Lesar T, Grothe D, Garvey M. Alprazolam-related digoxin toxicity. *Am J Psychiatry* 1984;141:1612–1613.

448. Tollefson G. Monoamine oxidase inhibitors: a review. *J Clin Psychiatry* 1983;44:280–288.

449. True B, Perry J, Burns EA. Profound hypoglycemia with the addition of a tricyclic antidepressant to maintenance sulfonylurea therapy. *Am J Psychiatry* 1987;144:1220–1221.

450. Udall JA. Clinical implications of warfarin interaction with five sedatives. *Am J Cardiol* 1975;35:67–71.

451. Valdiserri EV. A possible interaction between lithium and diltiazem: case report. *J Clin Psychiatry* 1985;46:540–541.

452. Valsalan VC, Cooper GL. Carbamazepine intoxication caused by interaction with isoniazid. *Br Med J* 1982;285:261–262.

453. Van Kammen DP, Murphy DL. Attenuation of the euphoriant and activating effects of D- and L-amphetamine by lithium carbonate treatment. *Psychopharmacologia* 1975;44:215–224.

454. van Praag HM, Leijnse B. The influence of some antidepressives of the hydrazine type on the glucose metabolism in depressed patients. *Clin Chim Acta* 1963;8:466–475.

455. van Spanning HW, van Zwieten PA. The interference of tricyclic antidepressants with the central hypotensive effect of clonidine. *Eur J Pharmacol* 1973;24:402–404.

456. Varhe A, Olkkola KT, Neuvonen PJ. Oral triazolam is potentially hazardous to patients receiving systemic antimycotics ketoconazole or itraconazole. *Clin Pharmacol Therap* 1994;56(6 part 1):601–607.

457. Vaughan DA. Interaction of fluoxetine with tricyclic antidepressants. *Am J Psychiatry* 1988;145:1478.

458. Vendsborg PB. Lithium treatment and glucose tolerance in manic-melancholic patients. *Acta Psychiatr Scand* 1979;59:306–316.

459. Vendsborg PB, Prytz S. Glucose tolerance and serum lipids in man after long-term lithium administration. *Acta Psychiatr Scand* 1976;53:64–69.

460. Vendsborg PB, Rafaelson OJ. Lithium in man. Effect of glucose tolerance and serum electrolytes. *Acta Psychiatr Scand* 1973;49:601–610.

461. Ventafridda V, Ripamontl C, De Conno F, et al. Antidepressants increase bioavailability of morphine in cancer patients. *Lancet* 1987;1:8543:1204.

462. Vesell ES, Passananti GT, Greene FE. Impairment of drug metabolism in man by allopurinol and nortriptyline. *N Engl J Med* 1970;283:1484–1488.

463. Vestal RE, Kornhauser DM, Hollifield JW, Shand DG. Inhibition of propranolol metabolism by chlorpromazine. *Clin Pharmacol Ther* 1979;25:19–24.

464. Vigran IM. Dangerous potentiation of meperidine hydrochloride by pargyline hydrochloride. *JAMA* 1964;187:953–954.

465. Vincent FM. Phenothiazine-induced phenytoin interaction. *Ann Intern Med* 1980;93:56–57.

466. Walbridge DG, Bazire SR. An interaction between lithium carbonate and piroxicam presenting as lithium toxicity. *Br J Psychiatry* 1985;147:206–207.

467. Walker N, et al. Lithium-methyldopa interactions in normal subjects. *Drug Intel Clin Pharmacol* 1980;14:638.

468. Wallace SM, Suveges LG, Blackburn JL, et al. Oral fluphenazine and tea and coffee drinking. *Lancet* 1981;2:691.

469. Wallis R. Potentiation of hypnotics and analgesia. *NY State J Med* 1955;55:243–245.

470. Warot D, Bergougnan L, Lamiable D, et al. Troleoandomycin-triazolam interaction in healthy volunteers: pharmacokinetic and psychometric evaluation. *Eur J Clin Pharmacol Ther* 1979;25:19–24.

471. Warrington SJ, Ankier SL, Turner P. Evalua-

472. Weiner M. Effect of centrally active drugs on the action of coumarin anticoagulants. *Nature* 1966;212:1599.

473. Weingarten JC, Thompson TL II. The effect of thioridazine on prolactinoma growth in a schizophrenic man: case report. *Gen Hosp Psychiatry* 1985;7:364–366.

474. Weinrauch LA, Belok S, D'Elia JA. Decreased serum lithium during verapamil therapy. *Am Heart J* 1984;108:1378–1380.

475. Weiss J, Weiss S, Weiss B. Effects of iproniazid and similar compounds on the gastrointestinal tract. *Ann NY Acad Sci* 1959;80:854–859.

476. Weller RA, Preskorn SH. Psychotropic drugs and alcohol: pharmacokinetics and pharmacodynamic interactions. *Psychosomatics* 1984;25:301–303.

477. Westervelt FB, Atuk NO. Methyldopa-induced hypertension. *JAMA* 1974;227:557.

478. Westlake RJ, Rastegar A. Hyperpyrexia from drug combinations. *JAMA* 1973;225:1250.

479. Wharton RN, Perel JM, Dayton PG, Malitz S. A potential clinical use for methylphenidate (Ritalin) with tricyclic antidepressants. *Am J Psychiatry* 1971;127:1619–1695.

480. White AG. Methyldopa and amitriptyline. *Lancet* 1965;2:441.

481. White WB. Hypotension with postural syncope secondary to the combination of chlorpromazine and captopril. *Arch Intern Med* 1986;146:1833–1834.

482. Wilder BJ, Willmore LJ, Bruni J, Villarreal HJ. Valproic acid: interaction with other anticonvulsant drugs. *Neurology* 1978;28:892–896.

483. Wilens TE, Stern TA. Ventricular tachycardia associated with desipramine and thioridazine. *Psychosomatics* 1990;31:100–103.

484. Wilner KD. The effects of sertraline on the pharmacodynamics of warfarin in healthy volunteers [Abstract]. *Biol Psychiatry* 1991;29:345S.

485. Wilson IC, Prange AJ Jr, Lara PP. Methyltestosterone with imipramine in man: conversion of depression to paranoid reaction. *Am J Psychiatry* 1974;131:21–24.

486. Winters WD, Ralph DD. Digoxin-lithium drug interaction. *Clin Toxicol* 1977;10:487.

487. Wong YY, Ludden TM, Bell RD. Effect of erythromycin on carbamazepine pharmacokinetics. *Clin Pharmacol Ther* 1983;33:460–464.

488. Wright JM, Stokes EF, Sweeney VP. Isoniazid-induced carbamazepine toxicity and vice versa. *Med Intel* 1982;307:1325–1327.

489. Wright SP. Hazards with monoamine-oxide inhibitors: a persistent problem [Letter]. *Lancet* 1978;1:284–285.

490. Wroblewski BA, Singer WD, Whyte J. Carbamazepine-erythromycin interaction: case studies and clinical significance. *JAMA* 1986;255:1165–1167.

491. Yaryura-Tobias JA, Wolpert A, Dana L, Merlis S. Action of L-dopa in drug induced extrapyramidalism. *Dis Nerv Syst* 1970;31:60–63.

492. Yassa R. Lithium-methyldopa interaction. *Can Med Assoc J* 1986;134:141–142.

493. Yee GC, McGuire TR. Pharmacokinetic drug interactions with cyclosporin, part I. *Clin Pharmacokinet* 1990;19:319–332.

494. Yosselson-Superstine S, Lipman AG. Chlordiazepoxide interaction with levodopa. *Ann Intern Med* 1982;96:259–260.

495. Yu Y, Huang CY, Chin D, et al. Interaction between carbamazepine and dextropropoxyphene. *Postgrad Med J* 1986;62:231–233.

496. Zielinski JJ, Haidukewych D, Leheta BJ. Carbamazepine-phenytoin interactions: elevation of plasma phenytoin concentrations due to carbamazepine co-medication. *Ther Drug Monit* 1985;7:51–53.

497. Zielinski JJ, Lichten EM, Haidukewych D. Clinically significant danazol-carbamazepine interaction. *Ther Drug Monit* 1987;9:24–27.

498. Zitelli BJ, Howrie DL, Altman H, Maroon TJ. Erythromycin induced drug interactions. *Clin Pediatr* 1987;26:117–119.

499. Zornberg GL, Bodkin JA, Cohen BM. Severe adverse interaction between pethidine and selegiline [Letter]. *Lancet* 1991;337:246.

New Table References (Bold in Table)

Abraham G, Grunberg B, Gratz S. Possible interaction of clozapine and lisinopril. *Am J Psychiatry* 2001;158:969.

Adson DE, Kotlyar M. A probable interaction between a very low-dose oral contraceptive and the antidepressant nefazodone: a case report. *J Clin Psychopharmacol* 2001;21:618–619.

Allard S, Sainati SM, Roth-Schechter BF. Coadministration of short-term zolpidem with sertraline in healthy women. *J Clin Pharmacol* 1999;39:184–191.

Anderson GD. A mechanistic approach to antiepileptic drug interactions. *Ann Pharmacother* 1998;32:554–563.

Anderson JR, Nawarskas JJ. Cardiovascular drug-drug interactions. *Card Clin* 2001;19:215–234.

Andrade C. Risperidone may worsen fluoxetine-treated OCD. *J Clin Psychiatry* 1998;59:255–256.

Arlander E, Ekstrom G, Alm C, et al. Metabolism of ropivacaine in humans is mediated by CYP1A2 and to a minor extent by CYP3A4: an interaction study with fluvoxamine and ketoconazole as in vivo inhibitors. *Clin Pharmacol Ther* 1998;64:484–491.

Armstrong SC, Cozza KL. Consultation-liaison psychiatry drug—drug interactions update. *Psychosomatics* 2000;41:541–543.

Baker GB, Fang J, Sinha S, et al. Metabolic drug interactions with selective serotonin reuptake inhibitor (SSRI) antidepressants. *Neuro & Behav Rev* 1998;22:325–333.

Behar D, Schaller J, Spreat S. Extreme reduction of methylphenidate levels by carbamazepine. *J Amer Acad Child Adol Psych* 1998;37:1128–1129.

Berbel GA, Latorre IA, Porta EJ, et al. Protease inhibitor-induced carbamazepine toxicity. *Clin Neuropharmacol* 2000;23:216–218.

Bondolfi G, Eap CB, Bertschy G, et al. The effect of fluoxetine on the pharmacokinetics and safety of risperidone in psychiatric patients. *Pharmacopsychiatry* 2002;35:50–56.

Borba CP, Henderson DC. Citalopram and clozapine: potential drug interaction. *J Clin Psychiatry* 2000;61:301–302.

Brown CS, Markowitz JS, Moore TR, et al. Atypical antipsychotics: Part II: Adverse effects, drug interactions, and costs. *Ann Pharmacotherapy* 1999; 33:210–217.

Burman W, Orr L. Carbamazepine toxicity after starting combination antiretroviral therapy including ritonavir and efavirenz. *AIDS* 2000;14: 2793–2794.

Caley CF. Extrapyramidal reactions from concurrent SSRI and atypical antipsychotic use. *Can J Psych—Revue Canadienne de Psychiatrie* 1998;43: 307–308.

Camicioli R, Lea E, Nutt JG, et al. Methylphenidate increases the motor effects of L-Dopa in Parkinson's disease: a pilot study. *Clin Neuropharm* 2001; 24:208–213.

Caplehorn JR, Drummer OH. Fatal methadone toxicity: signs and circumstances, and the role of benzodiazepines. *Austr & NZ J Pub Health* 2002; 26:358–362; discussion 362–363.

Carrier L. Donepezil and paroxetine: possible drug interaction. *J Am Ger Soc* 1999;47:1037.

Carrillo JA, Ramos SI, Herraiz AG, et al. Pharmacokinetic interaction of fluvoxamine and thioridazine in schizophrenic patients. *J Clin Psychopharmacol* 1999;19:494–499.

Chetty M, Miller R. Oral contraceptives increase the plasma concentrations of chlorpromazine. *Ther Drug Monit* 2001;23:556–558.

Chouinard G, Lefko-Singh K, Teboul E. Metabolism of anxiolytics and hypnotics: benzodiazepines, buspirone, zopiclone, and zolpidem. *Cell Mol Neurobiol* 1999;19:533–552.

Clay PG, Adams MM. Pseudo-Parkinson disease secondary to ritonavir-buspirone interaction. *Ann Pharmacotherapy* 2003;37:20–25.

Conca A, Beraus W, Konig P, et al. A case of pharmacokinetic interference in comedication of clozapine and valproic acid. *Pharmacopsychiatry* 2000; 33:234–235.

Cooke C, de Leon J. Adding other antipsychotics to clozapine. *J Clin Psychiatry* 1999;60:710.

Corsini A, Bellosta S, Baetta R, et al. New insights into the pharmacodynamic and pharmacokinetic properties of statins. *Pharmacol Ther* 1999; 84:413–428.

Daniel WA, Syrek M, Haduch A, et al. Pharmacokinetics and metabolism of thioridazine during coadministration of tricyclic antidepressants. *Br J Pharmacol* 2000;131:287–295.

Daniel WA, Syrek M, Haduch A, et al. Pharmacokinetics of phenothiazine neuroleptics after chronic coadministration of carbamazepine. *Polish J Pharmacology* 1998;50:431–442.

Dequardo JR. Modafinil-associated clozapine toxicity. *Am J Psychiatry* 2002;159:1243–1244.

DeVane CL, Markowitz JS. Avoiding psychotropic drug interactions in the cardiovascular patient. *Bull Menninger Clin* 2000;64.

DeVane CL, Nemeroff CB. An evaluation of risperidone drug interactions. *J Clin Psychopharmacol* 2001;21:408–416.

Dunner DL. Drug interactions of lithium and other antimanic/mood-stabilizing medications. *J Clin Psychiatry* 2003;64(Suppl 5):38–43.

Elko CJ, Burgess JL, Robertson WO. Zolpidem-associated hallucinations and serotonin reuptake inhibition: a possible interaction. *J Toxicol Clin Toxicol* 1998;36:195–203.

Ereshefsky L, Dugan D. Review of the pharmacokinetics, pharmacogenetics, and drug interaction potential of antidepressants: focus on venlafaxine. *Depress Anxiety* 2000;12(Suppl 1):30–44.

Facciola G, Avenoso A, Spina E, et al. Inducing effect of phenobarbital on clozapine metabolism in patients with chronic schizophrenia. *Ther Drug Monit* 1998;20:628–630.

Fattore C, Cipolla G, Gatti G, et al. Induction of ethinylestradiol and levonorgestrel metabolism by oxcarbazepine in healthy women. *Epilepsia* 1999; 40:783–787.

Ferslew KE, Hagardorn AN, Harlan GC, et al. A fatal drug interaction between clozapine and fluoxetine. *J Forensic Sci* 1998;43:1082–1085.

Finch CK, Chrisman CR, Baciewicz AM, et al. Rifampin and rifabutin drug interactions: an update. *Arch Int Med* 2002;162:985–992.

Flockhart DA, Drici MD, Kerbusch T, et al. Studies on the mechanism of a fatal clarithromycin-pimozide interaction in a patient with Tourette syndrome. *J Clin Psychopharmacol* 2000;20:317–324.

Franco-Bronson K, Gajwani P. Hypotension associated with intravenous haloperidol and imipenem. *J Clin Psychopharmacol* 1999;19:480–481.

Furst BA, Champion KM, Pierre JM, et al. Possible association of QTc interval prolongation with coadministration of quetiapine and lovastatin. *Biol Psychiatry* 2002;51:264–265.

Garton T. Nefazodone and cyp450 3a4 interactions with cyclosporine and tacrolimus1. *Transplantation* 2002;74:745.

Glue P, Banfield CR, Perhach JL, et al. Pharmacokinetic interactions with felbamate: in vitro-in vivo correlation. *Clin Pharmacokinet* 1997;33:214–224.

Gomberg RF. Interaction between olanzapine and haloperidol. *J Clin Psychopharmacol* 1999;19:272–273.

Gourevitch MN, Friedland GHJ. Methadone and antiretroviral mediations, part II. *AIDS Clin Care* 1999;11:30–31.

Gracious BL. Atrioventricular nodal re-entrant tachycardia associated with stimulant treatment. *J Child Adoles Psychopharmacol* 1999;9:125–128.

Greenblatt DJ, von Moltke LL, Harmatz JS, et al. Differential impairment of triazolam and zolpidem clearance by ritonavir. *JAIDS* 2000;24:129–136.

Grozinger M, Hartter S, Hiemke C, et al. Interaction of modafinil and clomipramine as comedication in a narcoleptic patient. *Clin Neuropharmacol* 1998;21:127–129.

Grozinger M, Hartter S, Hiemke C, et al. Oxybutynin enhances the metabolism of clomipramine and dextrorphan possibly by induction of a cytochrome P450 isoenzyme. *J Clin Psychopharmacol* 1999;19:287–289.

Heelon MW, Meade LB. Methadone withdrawal when starting an antiretroviral regimen including nevirapine. *Pharmacotherapy* 1999;19: 471–472.

Hesse LM, Von Moltke LL, Greenblatt DJ. Clinically important drug interactions with zopiclone, zolpidem, and zaleplon. *CNS Drugs* 2003;17: 513–532.

Hetta J, Broman JE, Darwish M, et al. Psychomotor effects of zaleplon and thioridazine coadministration. *Eur J Clin Pharmacol* 2000;56:211–217.

Hugen PW, Burger DM, Brinkman K, et al. Carbamazepine–indinavir interaction causes antiretroviral therapy failure. *Ann Pharmacotherapy* 2000; 34:465–470.

Iribarne C, Picart D, Dreano Y, et al. In vivo interactions between fluoxetine or fluvoxamine and methadone or buprenorphine. *Fundam Clin Pharmacol* 1998;12:194–199.

Jann MW, Shirley KL, Small GW. Clinical pharmacokinetics and pharmacodynamics of cholinesterase inhibitors. *Clin Pharmacokinet* 2002;41:719–739.

Jokinen MJ, Ahonen J, Neuvonen PJ, et al. The effect of erythromycin, fluvoxamine, and their combination on the pharmacokinetics of ropivacaine. *Anesthesia Analgesia* 2000;91:1207–1212.

Joos AAB, Frank UG, Kaschka WP. Pharmacokinetic interaction of clozapine and rifampicin in a forensic patient with atypical mycobacterial infection. *J Clin Psychopharmacol* 1998;18(1):83–85.

Jover F, Cuadrado JM, Andreu L, et al. Reversible coma caused by risperidone-ritonavir interaction. *Clin Neuropharmacol* 2002;25:251–253.

Kane GC, Lipsky JJ. Drug-grapefruit juice interactions. *Mayo Clin Proc* 2000;75(9):933–942.

Karki SD, Masood GR. Combination risperidone and SSRI-induced serotonin syndrome. *Ann Pharmacotherapy* 2003;37:388–391.

Kim SW, Grant JE, Adson DE, et al. A preliminary report on possible naltrexone and nonsteroidal analgesic interactions. *J Clin Psychopharmacol* 2001;21:632–634.

Kivisto KT, Lamberg TS, Neuvonen PJ. Interactions of buspirone with Itraconazole and rifampicin: effects on the pharmacokinetics of the active 1-(2-pyrimidinyl)-piperazine metabolite of buspirone. *Pharmacol Toxicol* 1999;84:94–97.

Kontaxakis VP, Havaki-Kontaxaki BJ, Stamouli SS, et al. Toxic interaction between risperidone and clozapine: a case report. *Prog Neuropsychopharmacol Biol Psychiatry* 2002;26:407–409.

Lamberg TS, Kivisto KT, Laitila J, et al. The effect of fluvoxamine on the pharmacokinetics and pharmacodynamics of buspirone. *Eur J Clin Pharmacol* 1998;54:761–766.

Larsen JT, Hansen LL, Spigset O, et al. Fluvoxamine is a potent inhibitor of tacrine metabolism in vivo. *Eur J Clin Pharmacol* 1999;55:375–382.

Lauterbach EC. Catatonia-like events after valproic acid with risperidone and sertraline. *Neuropsychiatry, Neuropsychol Behav Neurol* 1998;11:157–163.

Lee AJ, Chan WK, Harralson AF, et al. The effects of grapefruit juice on sertraline metabolism: an in vitro and in vivo study. *Clin Ther* 1999;21: 1890–1899.

Lessard E, Yessine MA, Hamelin BA, et al. Diphenhydramine alters the disposition of venlafaxine through inhibition of CYP2D6 activity in humans. *J Clin Psychopharmacol* 2001;21:175–184.

Levin GM, Nelson LA, DeVane CL, et al. A pharmacokinetic drug-drug interaction study of venla

faxine and indinavir. *Psychopharmacol Bull* 2001; 35:62–71.

Lewis BR, Aoun SL, Bernstein GA, et al. Pharmacokinetic interactions between cyclosporine and bupropion or methylphenidate. *J Child Adolesc Psychopharmacol* 2001;11:193–198.

Liston HL. Markowitz JS. DeVane CL. Drug glucuronidation in clinical pharmacology. *J Clin Psychopharmacol* 21:500–15, 2001 Oct.

Lucas RA, Gilfillan DJ, Bergstrom RF. A pharmacokinetic interaction between carbamazepine and olanzapine: observations on a possible mechanism. *Eur J Clin Pharmacol* 1998;54:639–643.

Lucena MI, Blanco E, Corrales MA, et al. Interaction of fluoxetine and valproic acid. *J Psychiatry* 1998; 155:575.

Lundmark J, Gunnarsson T, Bengtsson F. A possible interaction between lithium and rofecoxib. *Br J Clin Pharmacol* 2002;53,3.

Mahmood I, Sahajwalla C. Clinical pharmacokinetics and pharmacodynamics of buspirone, an anxiolytic drug. *Clin Pharmacokinet* 1999;36:277–287.

Mamiya K, Kojima K Yakawa E, et al. Phenytoin intoxication induced by fluvoxamine. *Ther Drug Monit* 2001;23:75–77.

Markowitz JS, DeVane CL. Rifampin-induced selective serotonin reuptake inhibitor withdrawal syndrome in a patient treated with sertraline. *J Clin Psychopharmacol* 2000;20:109–110.

Markowitz JS, Morrison SD, DeVane CL. Drug interactions with psychostimulants. *Int Clin Psychopharmacol* 1999;14:1–18.

Masia M, Gutierrez F, Jimeno A, et al. Fulminant hepatitis and fatal toxic epidermal necrolysis (Lyell disease) coincident with clarithromycin administration in an alcoholic patient receiving disulfiram therapy. *Arch Int Med* 2002;162: 474–476.

Mayan H, Golubev N, Dinour D, et al. Lithium intoxication due to carbamazepine-induced renal failure. *Ann Pharmacotherapy* 2001;35:560–562.

McCance-Katz EF, Rainey PM, Friedland G, et al. Effect of opioid dependence pharmacotherapies on zidovudine disposition. *Am J Addict* 2001;10: 296–307.

Michalets EL, Smith LK, Van Tassel ED. Torsade de pointes resulting from the addition of droperidol to an existing cytochrome P450 drug interaction. *Ann Pharmacotherapy* 1998;32:761–765.

Monaco F, Cicolin A. Interactions between anticonvulsant and psychoactive drugs. *Epilepsia* 40 Suppl 10:S71–S76.

Monji A, Maekawa T, Miura T, et al. Interactions between lithium and non-steroidal anti-inflammatory drugs. *Clin Neuropharmacol* 2002;25: 241–242.

Mula M, Monaco F. Carbamazepine-risperidone interactions in patients with epilepsy. *Clin Neuropharmacol* 2002;25:97–100.

Nelson MH, Birnbaum AK, Remmel RP. Inhibition of phenytoin hydroxylation in human liver microsomes by several selective serotonin re-uptake inhibitors. *Epilepsy Res* 2001;44:71–82.

Niemi M, Backman JT, Neuvonen M, et al. Effects of fluconazole and fluvoxamine on the pharmacokinetics and pharmacodynamics of glimepiride. *Clin Pharmacol Ther* 2001;69:194–200.

Normann C, Lieb K, Walden J. Increased plasma concentration of maprotiline by coadministration of risperidone. *J Clin Psychopharmacol* 2002; 22:92–94.

Owen JR, Nemeroff CB. New antidepressants and the cytochrome P450 system: focus on venlafaxine, nefazodone, and mirtazepine. *Depress Anxiety* 1998;7(Suppl 1):24–32.

Paoletti R, Corsini A, Bellosta S. Pharmacological interactions of statins. *Atheroscler Suppl* 2002;3: 35–40.

Passiu G, Bocchetta A, Martinelli V, et al. Calcitonin decreases lithium plasma levels in man: preliminary report. *Int J Clin Pharmacol Res* 1998;18: 179–181.

Pies R. Safety of sildenafil for antidepressant-related sexual dysfunction. *J Clin Psych* 1999;60:792.

Potkin SG, Thyrum PT, Alva G, et al. The safety and pharmacokinetics of quetiapine when coadministered with haloperidol, risperidone, or thioridazine. *J Clin Psychopharmacol* 2002;22:121–130.

Prior FH, Isbister GK, Dawson AH, et al. Serotonin toxicity with therapeutic doses of dexamphetamine and venlafaxine. *Med J Aust* 2002;176: 240–241.

Raaska K, Neuvonen PJ. Ciprofloxacin increases serum clozapine and N-desmethylclozapine: a study in patients with schizophrenia. *Eur J Clin Pharmacol* 2000;56:585–589.

Reeves RR, Mack JE, Beddingfield JJ. Neurotoxic syndrome associated with risperidone and fluvoxamine. *Ann Pharmacotherapy* 2002;36:440–443.

Reynaud M, Petit G. Six deaths linked to concomitant use of buprenorphine and benzodiazepines. *Addiction* 1998;93.

Ripple MG, Pestaner JP, Levine BS, et al. Lethal combination of tramadol and multiple drugs affecting serotonin. *Am J Forensic Med Pathol* 2000;21: 370–374.

Robertson P Jr, Hellriegel ET, Arora S, et al. Effect of modafinil on the pharmacokinetics of ethinyl estradiol and triazolam in healthy volunteers. *Clin Pharmacol Ther* 2002;71:46–56.

Sanders RD, Lehrer DS. Edema associated with addition of risperidone to valproate treatment. *J Clin Psychiatry* 1998;59:689–690.

Sheikh RA, Prindiville T, Yasmeen S. Haloperidol and benztropine interaction presenting as acute intestinal pseudo-obstruction. *Am J Gastroenterol* 2001;96:934–935.

Spina E, Avenoso A, Facciola G, et al. Effect of fluoxetine on the plasma concentrations of clozapine and its major metabolites in patients with schizophrenia. *Int Clin Psychopharmacol* 1998;13: 141–145.

Spina E, Avenoso A, Facciola G, et al. Plasma concentrations of risperidone and 9-hydroxyrisperidone: effect of comedication with carbamazepine or valproate. *Ther Drug Monit* 2000;22: 481–485.

Spina E, Avenoso A, Facciola G, et al. Plasma concentrations of risperidone and 9-hydroxyrisperidone during combined treatment with paroxetine. *Ther Drug Monit* 2001;23:223–227.

Spina E, Avenoso A, Salemi M, et al. Plasma concen-

trations of clozapine and its major metabolites during combined treatment with paroxetine or sertraline. *Pharmacopsychiatry* 2000;33:213–217.

Spina E, Avenoso A, Scordo MG, et al. Inhibition of risperidone metabolism by fluoxetine in patients with schizophrenia: a clinically relevant pharmacokinetic drug interaction. *J Clin Psychopharmacol* 2002;22:419–423.

Spina E, Perucca E. Clinical significance of pharmacokinetic interactions between antiepileptic and psychotropic drugs. *Epilepsia* 2002;43(Suppl 2): 37–44.

Spina E, Scordo MG, Avenoso A, et al. Adverse drug interaction between risperidone and carbamazepine in a patient with chronic schizophrenia and deficient CYP2D6 activity. *J Clin Psychopharmacol* 2001;21:108–109.

Steele M, Couturier J. A possible tetracycline-risperidone-sertraline interaction in an adolescent. *Can J Clin Pharmacol* 1999;6:15–17.

Sternbach H, State R. Antibiotics: neuropsychiatric side effects and psychotropic interactions. *Harv Rev Psychiatry* 1997;5:214–226.

Takahashi H, Higuchi H, Shimizu T. Severe lithium toxicity induced by combined levofloxacin administration. *J Clin Psychiatry* 2000;61:949–950.

Tanaka E, Misawa S. Pharmacokinetic interactions between acute alcohol ingestion and single doses of benzodiazepines, and tricyclic and tetracyclic antidepressants—an update. *J Clin Pharm Ther* 1998;23:331–336.

Taylor D, Lader M. Cytochromes and psychotropic drug interactions. *Br J Psychiatry* 1996;168: 529–532.

Tiseo PJ, Perdomo CA, Friedhoff LT. Concurrent administration of donepezil HCl and ketoconazole: assessment of pharmacokinetic changes following single and multiple doses. *Br J Clin Pharmacol* 1998;46 Suppl 1:30–34.

Tupala E, Niskanen L, Tiihonen J. Transient syncope and ECG changes associated with the concurrent administration of clozapine and diazepam. *J Clin Psychiatry* 1999;60:619–620.

Vella JP, Sayegh MH. Interactions between cyclosporine and newer antidepressant medications. *Am J Kidney Dis* 1998;31:320–323.

von Bahr C, Steiner E, Koike Y, et al. Time course of enzyme induction in humans: effect of pentobarbital on nortriptyline metabolism. *Clin Pharmacol Ther* 1998;64:18–26.

Wong YW, Yeh C, Thyrum PT. The effects of concomitant phenytoin administration on the steady-state pharmacokinetics of quetiapine. *J Clin Psychopharmacol* 2001;21:89–93.

Wright DH, Lake KD, Bruhn PS, et al. Nefazodone and cyclosporine drug-drug interaction. *J Heart Lung Transplant* 1999;18:913–915.

Zalma A, von Moltke LL, Granda BW, et al. In vitro metabolism of trazodone by CYP3A: inhibition by ketoconazole and human immunodeficiency viral protease inhibitors. *Biol Psychiatry* 2000;47: 655–661.

Zwanzger P, Marcuse A, Boerner RJ, et al. Lithium intoxication after administration of AT1 blockers. *J Clin Psychiatry* 2001;62:208–209.

Index